Textbook of

PEDIATRIC
RHEUMATOLOGY

SEVENTH EDITION

Textbook of
PEDIATRIC
RHEUMATOLOGY

Ross E. Petty

Ronald M. Laxer

Carol B. Lindsley

Lucy R. Wedderburn

ELSEVIER

ELSEVIER

1600 John F. Kennedy Blvd.
Ste 1800
Philadelphia, PA 19103-2899

TEXTBOOK OF PEDIATRIC RHEUMATOLOGY,
SEVENTH EDITION

ISBN: 978-0-323-24145-8

Previous editions copyrighted 2011, 2005, 2001, 1995, 1990, 1982.

Library of Congress Cataloging-in-Publication Data
Textbook of pediatric rheumatology.
    Textbook of pediatric rheumatology / [edited by] Ross E. Petty, Ronald M. Laxer, Carol B. Lindsley,
Lucy Wedderburn. – 7th edition.
        p. ; cm.
    Textbook of pediatric rheumatology
    Pediatric rheumatology
    Preceded by Textbook of pediatric rheumatology / [edited by] James T. Cassidy ... [et al.]. 6th ed. c2011.
    Includes bibliographical references and index.
    ISBN 978-0-323-24145-8 (hardcover : alk. paper)
    I. Petty, Ross E., editor.   II. Lindsley, Carol B., editor.   III. Laxer, Ronald M., editor.   IV. Wedderburn,
Lucy, editor.   V. Title.   VI. Title: Textbook of pediatric rheumatology.   VII. Title: Pediatric rheumatology.
    [DNLM: 1. Rheumatic Diseases.   2. Arthritis.   3. Child.   4. Connective Tissue Diseases.   5. Vasculitis.
WE 544]
    RJ482.R48
    618.92′723–dc23
                                                                                                2015004728

Content Strategist: Michael Houston
Content Development Specialist: Laura Schmidt
Publishing Services Manager: Patricia Tannian
Project Manager: Kate Mannix
Design Direction: Paula Catalano

Printed in China

Last digit is the print number: 9   8   7   6   5   4   3   2   1

To the memory of James Thomas Cassidy: scholar, mentor, colleague, and friend.

To
Beryl, Edda, Bart, and Jerry.

And to
our patients, who continue to inspire us.

PREFACE

The publication of the seventh edition of the *Textbook of Pediatric Rheumatology* marks 33 years since the publication of the first edition. The changes in the discipline of pediatric rheumatology during that time have been profound, and the *Textbook* has attempted to keep up with important developments in our understanding of rheumatic diseases in childhood and their diagnosis and management. The *Textbook* will provide an up-to-date synthesis of the state of knowledge of rheumatic diseases of childhood for students, physicians, and health care professionals involved in the management of these children and adolescents.

To that end, this edition incorporates new chapters and contributions from new authors. The challenge of maintaining a book of reasonable size while incorporating new information has necessitated deleting some old information. Some chapters have been shortened, and all chapters have been thoroughly revised, updated, and, in some instances, rewritten. The globalization of the specialty of pediatric rheumatology is recognized by the inclusion of information about diagnosis and management of childhood rheumatic diseases in the southern hemisphere. We wish to acknowledge senior authors whose contributions to previous editions of the book have been so important: Dr. Balu Athreya, Dr. Michael Dillon, Dr. Allison Eddy, Dr. Fernanda Falcini, Dr. Edward Giannini, Dr. Wietse Kuis, Dr. Deborah Wenkert, and the late Dr. David Glass. The editors are indebted to the current authors for their willingness to share their expertise and for the time and effort put into their contributions.

The death of Jim Cassidy, the founding editor, is noted with sadness and a sense of loss, and the editors have endeavored to maintain and enhance the intellectual standard and clarity of writing he espoused in the first six editions.

The editors and authors are grateful to the thousands of readers of the *Textbook* who have made it the standard reference in the field of pediatric rheumatology.

Ross E. Petty
Ronald M. Laxer
Carol B. Lindsley
Lucy R. Wedderburn

Jonathan Akikusa, MBBS
Paediatric Rheumatologist
Rheumatology Service, Department of General Medicine
Paediatrician
Department of General Medicine
Royal Children's Hospital
Melbourne, Victoria, Australia

Salvatore Albani, MD, PhD
Director
Translational Research for Infectious and Inflammatory Disease
    Center
Adjunct Professor
Sanford Burnham Medical Research Institute
La Jolla, California

Roger Allen, MBBS, FRACP
Department of Rheumatology
Royal Children's Hospital
Melbourne, Victoria, Australia

Khaled Alsaeid, MD
Professor of Pediatrics
Department of Pediatrics
Kuwait University
Jabryah, Kuwait

Tadej Avčin, MD, PhD
Professor of Pediatrics
Department of Pediatrics
University of Ljubljana;
Head
Department of Allergology, Rheumatology, and Clinical Immunology
Children's Hospital, University Medical Center
Ljubljana, Slovenia

Paul S. Babyn, MDCM, FRCPC
Professor and Head of Medical Imaging
Saskatoon Health Region
University of Saskatchewan
Saskatoon, Saskatchewan, Canada

Arvind Bagga, MD
Professor
Department of Pediatrics
All India Insitute of Medical Sciences
New Delhi, India

Karyl S. Barron, MD
Deputy Director, Division of Intramural Research
National Institute of Allergy and Infectious Diseases
National Institutes of Health
Bethesda, Maryland

Mara L. Becker, MD, MSCE
Director, Division of Rheumatology
Department of Pediatrics
Children's Mercy Kansas City
Kansas City, Missouri

Susanne M. Benseler, MD, PhD
Section Chief, Rheumatology
Department of Pediatrics
Alberta Children's Hospital;
Associate Professor
Department of Pediatrics
University of Calgary
Calgary, Alberta, Canada

Timothy Beukelman, MD, MSCE
Associate Professor
Department of Pediatrics
Division of Rheumatology
University of Alabama at Birmingham
Birmingham, Alabama

Paul Brogan, PhD, FRCPCH
Reader in Vasculitis
Honorary Consultant Paediatric Rheumatologist
Infection Immunity and Rheumatology Section
University College London Institute of Child Health
London, Great Britain

Hermine I. Brunner, MD, MSc, MBA
Professor of Pediatrics
Division of Rheumatology
Cincinnati Children's Hospital Medical Center
University of Cincinnati
Cincinnati, Ohio

Rubèn Burgos-Vargas, MD
Investigator in Medical Sciences
Department of Rheumatology
General Hospital of Mexico;
Professor of Medicine
National Autonomous University of Mexico
Mexico City, Mexico

Jill Buyon, MD
Director
Division of Rheumatology
Director
Lupus Center
Departments of Joint Disease and Medicine
Center for Musculoskeletal Care
New York University Langone Medical Center
New York, New York

David A. Cabral, MBBS

Ross Petty Chair and Clinical Professor
Department of Pediatrics
Division of Rheumatology
British Columbia Children's Hospital
University of British Columbia
Vancouver, British Columbia, Canada

Sharon Choo, MBBS, FRACP, FRCPA

Departments of Allergy and Immunology and Laboratory Services
Royal Children's Hospital
Parkville, Australia

Rolando Cimaz, MD

Associate Professor
Department of Pediatrics
University of Florence
Florence, Italy

Robert Allen Colbert, MD, PhD

Senior Investigator
National Institute of Arthritis, Musculoskeletal, and Skin Diseases
National Institutes of Health
Bethesda, Maryland

William G. Cole, MBBS, MSc, PhD, FRCSC

Director
Pediatric Surgery
University of Alberta
Edmonton, Alberta, Canada

Iris Davidson, BSR

Children's Program
Mary Pack Arthritis Center
Pediatric Rheumatology Division
British Columbia Children's Hospital
Vancouver, British Columbia, Canada

Fabrizio De Benedetti, MD, PhD

Division of Rheumatology
Bambino Gesù Children's Hospital
Rome, Italy

Andrea S. Doria, MD, PhD, MSc

Radiologist
Clinician-Scientist
Research Director
Diagnostic Imaging
The Hospital for Sick Children;
Associate Professor
Medical Imaging
University of Toronto
Toronto, Ontario, Canada

Frank Dressler, Dr. Med

Pediatric Rheumatologist
Pediatric Pneumology, Allergology, and Neonatology
The Children's Hospital of MHH
Hannover, Germany

Ciarán M. Duffy, MBBCh, MSc, FRCPC, FRCPI

Professor and Chairman
Department of Paediatrics
University of Ottawa;
Chief of Paediatrics
Department of Paediatrics
Children's Hospital of Eastern Ontario
Ottawa, Ontario, Canada

Despina Eleftheriou, MBBS,PhD

Senior Lecturer
Paediatric and Adolescent Rheumatology Department
Institute of Child Health and Great Ormond Street Hospital
London, United Kingdom

Brian M. Feldman, MD, MSc, FRCPC

Division Head, Rheumatology
Department of Rheumatology
The Hospital for Sick Children;
Professor
Departments of Pediatrics & Medicine and Health Policy
    Management & Evaluation
Dalia Lana School of Public Health
University of Toronto
Toronto, Ontario, Canada

Polly J. Ferguson, BS, MD

Director
Pediatric Rheumatology
Associate Professor of Pediatrics—Rheumatology
University of Iowa Carver College of Medicine
Iowa City, Iowa

Robert Fuhlbrigge, MD, PhD

Associate Professor of Pediatrics and Dermatology
Harvard Medical School;
Attending in Rheumatology
Division of Immunology
Boston Children's Hospital
Boston, Massachusetts

Marco Gattorno, MD

Pediatria II
G. Gaslini Institute
University of Genoa
Genoa, Italy

Alexei A. Grom, MD

Professor
Department of Pediatrics
University of Cincinnati College of Medicine;
Attending Physician
Department of Rheumatology
Cincinnati Children's Hospital Medical Center
Cincinnati, Ohio

Philip J. Hashkes, MD, MSc
Head, Pediatric Rheumatology Unit
Department of Pediatrics
Shaare Zedek Medical Center;
Associate Professor of Pediatrics
Hebrew University Medical School
Jerusalem, Israel;
Associate Professor of Medicine and Pediatrics
Cleveland Clinic Lerner School of Medicine
Case Western Reserve University
Cleveland, Ohio

Kristin Houghton, MD, MSc, FRCPC, Dip Sports Med, FAAP
Clinical Associate Professor
Department of Paediatrics
British Columbia Children's Hospital
University of British Columbia,
Vancouver, British Columbia, Canada

Hans-Iko Huppertz, MD
Professor of Pediatrics
Head and Director
Children's Hospital (Prof.-Hess-Kinderklinik)
Bremen, Germany;
Children's Hospital
Georg-August-University
Göttingen, Germany

Norman T. Ilowite, MD
Professor
Department of Pediatrics
Albert Einstein College of Medicine;
Division Chief
Pediatric Rheumatology
Children's Hospital at Montefiore
New York, New York

Edgar Jaeggi, MD
Staff Cardiologist
Department of Cardiology
Head
Fetal Cardiac Program
The Hospital for Sick Children;
Professor
Department of Paediatrics
University of Toronto
Toronto, Ontario, Canada

Daniel L. Kastner, MD, PhD
Scientific Director
Division of Intramural Research
National Human Genome Research Institute
Bethesda, Maryland

Adam Kirton, MD, MSc, FRCPC
Associate Professor
Pediatrics & Clinical Neurosciences
University of Calgary
Calgary, Alberta, Canada

Marisa Klein-Gitelman, MD, MPH
Professor of Pediatrics
Northwestern University Feinberg School of Medicine;
Head, Division of Rheumatology
Ann & Robert H. Lurie Children's Hospital of Chicago
Chicago, Illinois

Gay Kuchta, OT
Children's Program
Mary Pack Arthritis Center
Pediatric Rheumatology Division
British Columbia Children's Hospital
Vancouver, British Columbia, Canada

Jerome Charles Lane, MD
Associate Professor of Pediatrics
Northwestern University Feinberg School of Medicine
Division of Kidney Diseases
Ann & Robert H. Lurie Children's Hospital of Chicago
Chicago, Illinois

Ronald M. Laxer, MDCM, FRCPC
Professor
Departments of Pediatrics and Medicine
University of Toronto;
Division of Rheumatology
The Hospital for Sick Children
Toronto, Ontario, Canada

Claire LeBlanc, MD, Dip Sports Med, FRCPC
Associate Professor
Department of Pediatrics
McGill University
Montreal, Quebec, Canada

Steven J. Leeder, PharmD, PhD
Marion Merrell Dow Endowed Chair in Pediatric Clinical
  Pharmacology
Director, Division of Clinical Pharmacology, Toxicology,
  & Therapeutic Innovation
Department of Pediatrics
Children's Mercy Kansas City
Kansas City, Missouri

G. Elizabeth Legger, MD
Consultant Pediatric Rheumatologist
Department of Pediatric Rheumatology
University Medical Center Groningen
Beatrix Children's Hospital
University of Groningen
Groningen, The Netherlands

Suzanne C. Li, MD, PhD
Senior Attending
Department of Pediatrics
Joseph M. Sanzari Children's Hospital
Hackensack University Medical Center
Hackensack, New Jersey;
Associate Professor
Department of Pediatrics
Rutgers-University of Medicine and Dentistry of New Jersey,
Newark, New Jersey

Carol B. Lindsley, MD, FAAP, MACR

Professor
Department of Pediatrics
University of Kansas School of Medicine;
Chief of Pediatric Rheumatology
Department of Pediatrics
University of Kansas Medical Center
Kansas City, Kansas

Dan Lovell, MD, MPH

Joseph E. Levinson Chair and Professor of Pediatrics
Division of Rheumatology
Chairman, Pediatric Rheumatology
Collaborative Study Group
Cincinnati Children's Hospital Medical Center
Cincinnati, Ohio

Outi Makitie, MD, PhD

Professor
Children's Hospital
University of Helsinki
Helsinki, Finland

Alberto Martini, MD

Professor, Pediatria II
G. Gaslini Institute
University of Genoa
Genoa, Italy

Frederick W. Miller, MD, PhD

Chief
Environmental Autoimmunity Group, Clinical Research Branch
Program of Clinical Research
National Institute of Environmental Health Sciences
National Institutes of Health
Bethesda, Maryland

Kimberly Morishita, MD, MHSc, FRCPC

Clinical Assistant Professor
Department of Pediatrics
Division of Rheumatology
British Columbia Children's Hospital and University of British
    Columbia
Vancouver, British Columbia, Canada

Peter A. Nigrovic, MD

Assistant Professor of Medicine
Harvard Medical School;
Staff Pediatric Rheumatologist
Division of Immunology
Boston Children's Hospital
Boston, Massachusetts

Kiem G. Oen, MD

Professor
Department of Pediatrics and Child Health
University of Manitoba
Winnipeg, Manitoba, Canada

Kathleen M. O'Neil, MD

Professor of Pediatrics
Indiana University School of Medicine;
Chief
Section of Rheumatology
Riley Hospital for Children at Indiana University Health,
Indianapolis, Indiana

Seza Ozen, MD

Professor
Pediatric Rheumatology
Hacettepe University Faculty of Medicine
Ankara, Turkey

Peri H. Pepmueller, MD

Associate Professor
Depatements of Pediatrics and Internal Medicine
Saint Louis University
St. Louis, Missouri

Ross E. Petty, MD, PhD, FRCPC

Professor Emeritus, Pediatric Rheumatology
Department of Pediatrics
University of British Columbia
Vancouver, British Columbia, Canada

Elena Pope, MD, MSc

Section Head
Fellowship Director
Pediatric Dermatology
The Hospital for Sick Children;
Associate Professor
University of Toronto
Toronto, Ontario, Canada

Sampath Prahalad, MD, MSc

Marcus Professor of Pediatric Rheumatology
Department of Pediatrics
Emory University School of Medicine;
Associate Professor
Department of Human Genetics
Emory University School of Medicine
Atlanta, Georgia

Berent Prakken, MD, PhD

Professor of Pediatric Immunology
Department of Pediatric Immunology
University Medical Center Utrecht,
Utrecht, The Netherlands

Michael Rapoff, PhD

Ralph L. Smith Professor of Pediatrics
Department of Pediatrics
University of Kansas Medical Center
Kansas City, Kansas

Lisa G. Rider, MD

Deputy Chief
Environmental Autoimmunity Group, Clinical Research Branch
National Institute of Environmental Health Sciences
National Institutes of Health,
Bethesda, Maryland

Carlos Daniel Rosé, MD, CIP, FAAP
Division Chief
Professor of Pediatrics
Department of Pediatrics
Division of Rheumatology
duPont Children's Hospital
Thomas Jefferson University,
Wilmington, Delaware

James T. Rosenbaum, AB, MD
Professor
Ophthalmology, Medicine, and Cell Biology
Oregon Health and Science University
Portland, Oregon

Alan M. Rosenberg, MD
Professor
Department of Pediatrics
University of Saskatchewan College of Medicine
Saskatoon, Saskatchewan, Canada

Johannes Roth, MD, FRCP, RhMSUS
Associate Professor of Pediatrics
University of Ottawa;
Chief, Division of Pediatric Rheumatology
Children's Hospital of Eastern Ontario
Ottawa, Ontario, Canada

Ricardo Alberto Guillermo Russo, MD
Head
Department of Immunology & Rheumatology
Garrahan Hospital
Buenos Aires, Argentina

Rayfel Schneider, MBBCh, FRCPC
Professor
Department of Paediatrics
University of Toronto;
Associate Chair (Education)
Department of Paediatrics
The Hospital for Sick Children
Toronto, Ontario, Canada

**Christiaan Scott, MBChB, FCPaed(SA),
Grad Cert Paed Rheum (UWA)**
Associate Professor and Head
Department of Paediatric Rheumatology
University of Cape Town
Red Cross War Memorial Children's Hospital
Cape Town, Western Cape, South Africa

David D. Sherry, MD
Director, Pain Amplification Program, Rheumatology
Department of Pediatrics
The Children's Hospital of Philadelphia;
Professor of Pediatrics
Department of Pediatrics
Perelman School of Medicine at the University of Pennsylvania
Philadelphia, Pennsylvania

Earl Silverman, MD, FRCPC
Professor
Department of Pediatrics
The Hospital for Sick Children
University of Toronto;
Senior Associate Scientist
Program in Experimental Medicine
The Hospital for Sick Children Research Institute
Toronto, Ontario, Canada

Mary Beth Son, MD
Division of Immunology
Boston Children's Hospital
Boston, Massachusetts

Robert P. Sundel, MD
Director of Rheumatology
Department of Medicine
Boston Children's Hospital;
Associate Professor of Pediatrics
Harvard Medical School
Boston, Massachusetts

Susan D. Thompson, PhD
Professor
Center for Autoimmune Genomics and Etiology
Division of Rheumatology
Cincinnati Children's Hospital Medical Center;
Department of Pediatrics
University of Cincinnati College of Medicine
Cincinnati, Ohio

Karin Tiedemann, MBBS
Professor
Children's Cancer Centre
Royal Children's Hospital
Melbourne, Victoria, Australia

Shirley M.L. Tse, MD, FRCPC
Associate Professor of Paediatrics
University of Toronto;
Staff Rheumatologist
Program Director
Division of Rheumatology
Department of Paediatrics
The Hospital for Sick Children
Toronto, Ontario, Canada

Lori Tucker, MD
Clinical Associate Professor in Pediatrics
Department of Pediatric Rheumatology
British Columbia Children's Hospital
University of British Columbia
Vancouver, British Columbia, Canada

Yosef Uziel, MD, MSc

Head, Pediatric Rheumatology unit
Department of Pediatrics
Meir Medical Center
Kfra-Saba, Israel;
Department of Pediatrics
Sackler School of Medicine
Tel Aviv University
Tek Aviv, Israel

Joris van Montfrans, MD, PhD

Department of Pediatric Immunology and Infectious Diseases
Division of Pediatrics
University Medical Center Utrecht
Utrecht, The Netherlands

Janitzia Vazques-Mellado, MD, PhD

Investigator in Medical Sciences
Department of Rheumatology
General Hospital of Mexico;
Professor of Medicine
Faculty of Medicine
National Autonomous University of Mexico
Mexico City, Mexico

Leanne Ward, MD, FRCPC, FAAP

Senior Scientist
CHEO Research Institute;
Research Chair
Pediatric Bone Health
Associate Professor
University of Ottawa;
Director, Pediatric Bone Health Clinical and Research Programs
Children's Hospital of Eastern Ontario
Ottawa, Ontario, Canada

Lucy R. Wedderburn, MD, MA, PhD, FRCP

Professor in Paediatric Rheumatology
Institute of Child Health
University College London;
Consultant in Paediatric Rheumatology
Department of Rheumatology
Great Ormond Street Hospital National Health Service Trust
London, Great Britain

Carine Wouters, MD, PhD

Professor of Pediatrics
University of Leuven;
Consultant Pediatric Rheumatologist
Leuven University Hospital
Leuven, Belgium

James Wright, MD, MPH, FRCSC

Professor of Surgery, Public Health Sciences, Health Policy,
    Management, and Evaluation
University of Toronto;
Senior Scientist
Child Health Evaluative Sciences Research Institute
The Hospital for Sick Children
Toronto, Ontario, Canada

Nico M. Wulffraat, MD, PhD

Professor
Pediatric Rheumatology
Department of Pediatric Rheumatology
Wilhelmina Children's Hospital
University Medical Center Utrecht
Utrecht, The Netherlands

Lawrence Zemel, MD

Professor
Department of Pediatrics
University of Connecticut School of Medicine
Farmington, Connecticut
Division Head, Pediatric Rheumatology
Connecticut Childrens Medical Center
Hartford, Connecticut

Francesco Zulian, MD

Professor
Department of Pediatrics
University of Padua,
Padua, Italy

CONTENTS

CHAPTER 1

Pediatric Rheumatology: The Study of Rheumatic Diseases in Childhood and Adolescence

Ross E. Petty

WHAT ARE RHEUMATIC DISEASES?

Rheumatic diseases are a diverse group of chronic diseases united by the presence of chronic inflammation, usually of unknown cause, affecting structures of the musculoskeletal system, blood vessels, and other tissues. Pediatric rheumatology, the study of rheumatic diseases in children and adolescents, had its origins in the first half of the 20th century, principally as a study of chronic inflammatory arthritis, the most common of the childhood rheumatic diseases.

HISTORICAL ASPECTS

Archeological evidence supports the existence of chronic arthritis in children as long ago as 900 AD.[1,2] The first English-language reference to "rheumatism" in children is in the 1545 text by Thomas Phaire.[3] In this work, the author refers to the "stifnes or starckenes of the limmes" resulting from exposure of a child to cold, a complaint that may not represent any specific rheumatic disease. Three hundred years later (1864) Cornil described a woman in whom polyarthritis had developed when she was 12 years old.[4] Autopsy at 28 years of age documented ankylosis of some joints and synovial proliferation with marked destruction of cartilage in others. Several small case series were published in the last half of the 19th century,[5,6] but the disease was thought to be very rare.[7] The diversity of chronic arthritis was recognized in the latter part of the 19th century. In 1883, Barlow chaired a discussion on rheumatism in childhood at a meeting of the British Medical Association, Section of Diseases of Children.[8] In the report of this meeting, the term *rheumatism* was used to describe poststreptococcal disease, including acute rheumatic fever. Barlow recognized the extent and complexity of these disorders in childhood: "For there are in children many affections of joints, and of structures around joints, which do not suppurate, and yet are not rheumatic; and there is much rheumatism in children which does not affect joints." Disorders known today as toxic synovitis of the hip, acute pyogenic arthritis, syphilitic arthritis, hemophiliac arthropathy, Henoch–Schönlein purpura, poststreptococcal arthritis, and acute rheumatic fever, including carditis,

arthritis, nodules, erythema marginatum, and chorea, are all identifiable in this paper.

In 1891, Diamant-Berger published the first detailed account of chronic arthritis in 38 children whom he had seen or whose cases had been documented in the literature.[9] In 1896, George Frederic Still described 22 cases of acute and chronic arthritis in children, almost all of whom were observed at the Hospital for Sick Children, London.[10] This treatise, written under the mentorship of Barlow,[11] documented the clinical characteristics and the differing modes of onset of disease in these children. Still was the first English physician to confine his practice to diseases of children and the first professor of pediatrics at King's College Hospital Medical School, London. After his classic study, however, he rarely returned to the field of pediatric rheumatology. In the same year, Koplick[12] described the first American child with chronic arthritis.

Although these publications that described arthritis in childhood marked important milestones in the early development of pediatric rheumatology, other rheumatic diseases were identified in children in the 19th century. The clinical characteristics of leukocytoclastic vasculitis were described by Schönlein[13] and Henoch[14] in the early to mid-1800s. Juvenile dermatomyositis was first identified by Unverricht[15] and others in 1887, although it was not until the mid-1960s that significant experience with this disease in childhood was reported. Systemic lupus erythematosus (SLE) has been recognized in children since at least 1904.[16] The original description of scleroderma was in a 17-year-old girl,[17] but the disease was rarely diagnosed in children until the early 1960s. Ankylosing spondylitis was perhaps first identified in a child[18]—it was certainly known to occur in childhood in the 1950s[19]—but specific studies of the disorder in children did not emerge until the late 1960s.[20,21]

As awareness of the broader spectrum of rheumatic diseases in children and adolescents emerged, it slowly became apparent that there was a body of knowledge and expertise—pediatric rheumatology—that was related to, but quite separate from, adult rheumatology, pediatrics, and orthopedics. Professor Eric Bywaters and Dr. Barbara Ansell at the Canadian Red Cross Memorial Hospital in Taplow, England, were among the earliest (1940s and 1950s) clinician-investigators to be identified with the new discipline. Dr. Elizabeth Stoeber at Garmisch-Partenkirchen, Germany, also pioneered the field in the mid-twentieth century. The second generation of pediatric rheumatologists emerged in the 1950s and 1960s in the United States, Canada, and many countries in Europe, and in 1976, the first North American pediatric rheumatology meeting, Park City I,[22] and the European League Against Rheumatism/World Health Organization (EULAR/WHO) Workshop on the Care of Rheumatic Children in Oslo in 1977[23] laid the groundwork for the development of the discipline. Reminiscences of some of the pioneers of pediatric rheumatology are recommended to the interested reader.[24-31] A summary of the history of arthritis in children has been published by Hayem.[32]

Pediatric rheumatology continues to grow and evolve. More recent additions to the family of rheumatic diseases in children include Kawasaki disease, which was described in detail in 1967,[33] although its clinical characteristics in infants dying of "polyarteritis nodosa" were described by Munro-Faure in 1959.[34] Other rheumatic diseases, such as neonatal lupus, and an ever-growing array of autoinflammatory disorders have more recently been identified. The discovery of *Borrelia burgdorferi* as the etiologic agent responsible for Lyme arthritis is but one example of the role that infection plays in rheumatic diseases. Noninflammatory musculoskeletal pain syndromes are more recent additions to the expanding list of disorders that cause musculoskeletal pain and dysfunction in children and adolescents. Many of the diseases or their complications are confined to the childhood and adolescent population but have lasting effects on health, quality of life, and socioeconomic well-being throughout life.

PEDIATRIC RHEUMATOLOGY TODAY

Today the specialty of pediatric rheumatology is concerned with the diverse group of disorders described in this book, most of which are systemic disorders that require great expertise for prompt diagnosis and optimal management. There are few definitive diagnostic tests, sparse pathognomonic clinical signs, and therapy too often lacks specificity. This specialty requires a diagnostic and therapeutic approach to the "whole" child and family unit, and careful observation over long periods. Sometimes only the passage of time makes a diagnosis possible.

The spectrum of disease in children seen in specialized pediatric rheumatology clinics varies considerably, reflecting referral biases as well as geographically differing frequencies of specific diseases (Table 1-1). In addition to the diagnoses listed in Table 1-1, there are children with related disorders such as chronic anterior uveitis, Raynaud

phenomenon, and autoinflammatory diseases that may be unaccounted for in these registries.

THE BURDEN OF DISEASE

Fundamental to estimating the burden of pediatric rheumatic diseases in a society is the question: "How many children and adolescents have each of the identifiable rheumatic diseases?" It has been difficult to accurately establish the extent of childhood rheumatic disease.[38,39] In many of the most densely populated areas of the world, incidence and prevalence data for such diseases do not exist. In the developed world, inconsistencies of definition and classification, the rarity of occurrence for many of these disorders, and the brevity of follow-up have hindered the accumulation of a substantial body of epidemiological data.

It is apparent that some diseases are much more prevalent in children of certain ethnicities (e.g., SLE is more common in children of Asian origin than in those of European origin; Kawasaki disease is much more common in children of Japanese ancestry than in others). Using prevalence data derived from one ethnic group cannot, therefore, be used to accurately determine the prevalence in another ethnic group. Community-based studies provide insight into disease prevalence that is more representative than those originating from tertiary care centers. One such study by Manners and Diepeveen[40] in Western Australia reported the prevalence of chronic arthritis in 12-year-old school children at 4 per 1,000, and documented that many cases of chronic arthritis in children were undiagnosed and untreated. In Finland, Kunnamo and colleagues[41] surveyed all children under 16 years of age who had swelling or limitation of joint motion, walked with a limp, or had hip pain, as determined by a primary care physician, pediatrician, or orthopedic surgeon. All of these patients were subsequently examined by a single group of pediatric rheumatologists. Overall, the incidence of arthritis was estimated at 109 per 100,000 children per year. Transient synovitis of the hip accounted for 48%, other acute transient arthritis for 24% (Henoch–Schönlein purpura, serum sickness), chronic arthritis for 17%, septic arthritis for 6%, and reactive arthritis for 5%. Connective tissue diseases such as SLE were not identified in this survey.

The effect of childhood rheumatic diseases on life expectancy, their contribution to morbidity and costs of medical care, and the effect on quality of life are all important outcome parameters for which little information exists, even in North America and Europe; there is no information whatsoever on the global scene. There can be little doubt, however, that many children with, for example, arthritis beginning at 2 or 3 years of age will carry a lifelong burden in one or more of these

TABLE 1-1   Relative Frequencies (%) of Diagnoses of Children Seen in Pediatric Rheumatology Clinics in North America, the United Kingdom, and South Africa

	USA[35]	CANADA[36]	UK[37]	SOUTH AFRICA*
	1996	1996	1996	2013
JRA/JCA/JIA	33.1	50.0	61.7	65.6
Noninflammatory disorders	34.9	40.6	32.6	5.8
Vasculitis	10.2	3.0	1.9	5.8
SLE	7.1	3.9	1.3	11.6
Juvenile dermatomyositis	5.2	1.6	2.3	4.8
Systemic scleroderma	0.9	0.2	0.2	2.1
Acute rheumatic fever	8.6	0.7	0	4.2

*Data generously provided by Dr. Lawrence Okongo'o and Dr. Christiaan Scott; Red Cross War Memorial Children's Hospital, and Groote Schuur Hospital, Cape Town, South Africa.

TABLE 1-2 Mortality in Children with Rheumatic Diseases

	OBSERVED DEATHS	EXPECTED DEATHS	SMR (CI)
SLE	17	5.6	3.06 (1.78-4.90)
Juvenile dermatomyositis	5	1.9	2.64 (0.86-6.17)
All JRA	19	33.5	0.57 (0.34-0.89)
Systemic JRA	6	3.3	1.80 (0.66-3.92)
Primary vasculitis*	4	0.8	4.71 (1.28-12.07)

*Excluding Henoch–Schönlein purpura and Kawasaki disease.
SMR: standardized mortality rate.
Data from P.J. Hashkes, B.M. Wright, M.S. Lauer, et al., Mortality outcomes in pediatric rheumatology in the US, Arthritis Rheum. 62 (2010) 599–608.

areas. Indications of increased cardiovascular morbidity[42] and malignancy[43] have been studied. The expense and inconvenience for other members of the family are also significant.

A number of studies have estimated the cost of caring for a child with juvenile idiopathic arthritis.[44-47] Although newer therapies, such as biological response modifiers, are expensive, the added cost of the therapy is at least partially offset by the reduced morbidity and improved quality of life.[48]

MORTALITY

A number of reports have described increased mortality in most rheumatic diseases in childhood. Hashkes and colleagues[39] have reported a detailed analysis of mortality in a large number of patients cared for by pediatric rheumatologists in the United States between 1992 and 2001 (Table 1-2). Not unexpectedly, the highest mortality rates are seen in children with SLE, juvenile dermatomyositis, systemic juvenile idiopathic arthritis (JIA), and primary vasculitis. Patients with other types of JIA did not have an increased mortality rate. Limitations of this study include the relatively short period of follow-up.

ADVANCES AND CHALLENGES IN PEDIATRIC RHEUMATOLOGY

Dramatic advances in understanding the nature of inflammation and the possibility of specifically regulating the aberrant immune inflammatory response are revolutionizing the treatment of rheumatic diseases of childhood. Better understanding of the genetics of rheumatic diseases are pointing the way to therapeutic targeting at an even more fundamental level: the gene. Recognition of the autoinflammatory diseases and their genetic basis illuminates a heretofore obscure and confusing group of childhood disorders.

Mortality from diseases such as chronic arthritis complicated by amyloidosis, dermatomyositis, and SLE has been dramatically reduced since the 1970s, although morbidity and mortality remain serious threats to the child with SLE, vasculitis, scleroderma, and other diseases. Disability associated with many rheumatic diseases has been minimized, and the quality of life has been enhanced. Two decades ago, a significant number of children with JIA or dermatomyositis required long-term ambulation aids; today, this is unusual. Nonetheless, major challenges remain. Major improvements in the short- and medium-term outcomes of these and other rheumatic diseases have not always been matched by improvement in long-term outcome. For example,

half of children with chronic arthritis have active disease 10 years after onset,[49] and children with SLE accumulate visceral damage with the passage of time, which affects the quality of life, in spite of much better control of acute, life-threatening events.

The reasons for these improvements in outcomes are multiple; chief among them are the establishment of a body of knowledge and expertise and involvement of a multidisciplinary team of health professionals in diagnosis and care. Therapeutic landmarks of importance to the child with a rheumatic disease include the introduction of cortisone for treatment of rheumatoid arthritis; its influence on pediatric rheumatology has been profound. Intraarticular corticosteroid therapy has improved disease management in children with oligoarthritis, and methotrexate has radically improved the course and outcome of disease in children with polyarthritis. More judicious use of glucocorticoids and cytotoxic drugs has minimized toxicity and maximized effectiveness in diseases such as SLE and dermatomyositis. The biologics have been therapeutic game changers. Pharmacogenetics promises the possibility of fine-tuning therapy, both with respect to dose of drug used and with the selection of a drug that is likely to be most effective and least likely to produce side effects.

Family support organizations, such as the American Juvenile Arthritis Organization in the United States, and similar groups in many other countries, help promote education and research and provide psychosocial support for patients and families.

For the child to receive the best available medical care, early recognition and diagnosis are critical. Limited exposure of medical students and trainees in pediatrics to learning clinical examination skills and the fundamentals of pediatric rheumatology must therefore be addressed.[50] The challenge and reward of a career in pediatric rheumatology must be conveyed to pediatric trainees in order to close the gap between need and supply of pediatric rheumatologists.[51]

Increasing communication and collaboration in research worldwide is leading to a better understanding of the childhood rheumatic diseases. The enhanced effectiveness of collaborative research is increasingly recognized through participation in clinical trials led by the Pediatric Rheumatology Collaborative Study Group (PRCSG), the Pediatric Rheumatology International Trials Organization (PRINTO), the Childhood Arthritis and Rheumatology Research Alliance (CAARA), and the Canadian Association of Pediatric Rheumatology Investigators (CAPRI). Such organizations enable the study of therapeutic interventions in chronic arthritis and rarer connective tissue diseases. The establishment of collaborative disease and therapeutics registries in North America and Europe will add substantially to our knowledge of vasculitis, JIA, SLE, and other rheumatic diseases.

The globalization of pediatric rheumatology and the establishment of expertise in the less industrialized areas of the world, where most of the global population reside, promises to extend the benefits of advanced diagnostic methodology and therapeutics to millions of children with rheumatic diseases. Documentation and characterization of rheumatic diseases in these populations will undoubtedly illuminate the understanding of pediatric rheumatic diseases in general.

REFERENCES

9. M.S. Diamant-Berger, Du Rhumatisme Noueux (Polyarthrite Déformante), Lecrosnier et Babe, Chez Les Enfants, Paris, 1891. (Reprinted by Editions Louis Parente, Paris, 1988).
10. G.F. Still, On a form of chronic joint disease in children, Med. Chir. Trans. 80 (1897) 47, Reprinted in Am. J. Dis. Child. 132 (12) (1978) 195–200.
11. J.H. Keen, George Frederic Still—Registrar, Great Ormond Street Children's Hospital, Br. J. Rheumatol. 37 (1998) 1247.
16. W. Osler, On the visceral manifestations of the erythema group of skin diseases, Am. J. Med. Sci. 127 (1904) 1.

19. F.D. Hart, N.F. Maclagan, Ankylosing spondylitis: a review of 184 cases, Ann. Rheum. Dis. 14 (1955) 77–83.

20. J. Schaller, S. Bitnum, R.J. Wedgwood, Ankylosing spondylitis with childhood onset, J. Pediatr. 74 (1969) 505–516.

21. J.R. Ladd, J.T. Cassidy, W. Martel, Juvenile ankylosing spondylitis, Arthritis Rheum. 14 (1971) 579–590.

22. J.G. Schaller, V. Hanson (Eds.), Proceedings of the first ARA Conference on the Rheumatic Diseases of Childhood, Arthritis Rheum. 20 (Suppl. 2) (1977) 145–638.

23. E. Munthe (Ed.), The care of rheumatic children, EULAR Monograph No. 3, EULAR Publishers, Basle, 1978.

24. E.G. Bywaters, The history of pediatric rheumatology, Arthritis Rheum. 20 (Suppl.) (1977) 145–152.

32. F. Hayem, The history of chronic joint diseases in children, Rev. Rhum. Engl. Ed. 66 (1999) 499–504.

33. T. Kawasaki, Acute febrile mucocutaneous syndrome with lymphoid involvement with specific desquamation of the fingers and toes in children, Arerugi 16 (1967) 178–222.

34. H. Munro-Faure, Necrotizing arteritis of the coronary vessels in infancy: case report and review of the literature, Pediatrics 23 (1959) 914–926.

39. P.J. Hashkes, B.M. Wright, M.S. Lauer, et al., Mortality outcomes in pediatric rheumatology in the US, Arthritis Rheum. 62 (2010) 599–608.

40. P.J. Manners, D.A. Diepeveen, Prevalence of juvenile chronic arthritis in a population of 12-year old children in urban Australia, Pediatrics 98 (1996) 84–90.

41. I. Kunnamo, P. Kallio, P. Pelkonen, Incidence of arthritis in urban Finnish children. A prospective study, Arthritis Rheum. 29 (1986) 1232–1238.

42. J. Barsalou, T.J. Bradley, E.D. Silverman, Cardiovascular risk in pediatric-onset rheumatic diseases, Arthritis Res. Therapy 15 (2013) 212–224.

43. B.L. Nordstrom, D. Mines, Y. Gu, et al., Risk of malignancy in children with juvenile idiopathic arthritis not treated with biologics, Arthritis Care Res. 64 (2012) 1352–1364.

44. J. Thornton, M. Lunt, D.M. Ashcroft, et al., Costing juvenile idiopathic arthritis: examining patient-based costs during the first year after diagnosis, Rheumatology (Oxford) 47 (2008) 985–990.

45. K. Minden, M. Niewerth, J. Listing, et al., Burden and cost of illness in patients with juvenile idiopathic arthritis, Ann. Rheum. Dis. 63 (2004) 836–842.

46. K. Minden, What are the costs of childhood-onset rheumatic disease?, Best Prac. Res. Clin. Rheumatol. 20 (2006) 223–240.

47. S. Bernatsky, C. Duffy, P. Malleson, et al., Economic impact of juvenile idiopathic arthritis, Arthritis Rheum. 57 (2007) 44–48.

48. J. Haapasarri, H.J. Kautiainen, H.A. Isomäki, M. Hakala, Etanercept does not essentially increase the total costs of the treatment of refractory juvenile idiopathic arthritis, J. Rheumatol. 33 (2004) 2286–2289.

49. K. Oen, P. Malleson, D. Cabral, et al., Disease course and outcome of juvenile rheumatoid arthritis in a multicenter cohort, J. Rheumatol. 299 (2002) 1989–1999.

50. S. Jandial, A. Myers, E. Wise, et al., Doctors likely to encounter children with musculoskeletal complaints have low confidence in their clinical skills, J. Pediatr. 154 (2009) 267–271.

51. N. Pineda, L.J. Chamberlain, J. Chan, et al., Access to pediatric subspecialty care: a population study of pediatric rheumatology inpatients in California, Arthritis Care Res. 63 (2011) 998–1005.

Entire reference list is available online at www.expertconsult.com.

CHAPTER 2

Structure and Function

Ross E. Petty

Inflammation, the fundamental pathologic process in rheumatic diseases, may disrupt the anatomy and function of any structure or tissue. Those structures primarily affected in rheumatic diseases are the connective tissues, muscles, and blood vessels. Abnormalities that occur secondary to damage to these structures may be widespread. This chapter is intended as a brief overview of selected aspects of the anatomy and biology of tissues relevant to the basic understanding of rheumatic diseases of childhood and as a stimulus for further study.

THE SKELETON

The adult skeleton consists of 206 individual bones. It is the scaffold on which muscles, connective tissue structures, blood vessels, and skin are supported; it protects the vital organs; permits movement through articulations and attachment of muscles and tendons; it is a repository of minerals such as calcium, and other ions and hormones; and is the location of hematopoiesis. Many of these functions may be disturbed in the rheumatic diseases.

BONES

Classification of Bones

Bones can be classified as *membranous* or *endochondral*, depending on the manner of their ossification. Bones of the skull, face, and the clavicle are membranous bones, and ossification takes place within mesenchymal tissue condensations. The cortex of tubular bones is also influenced by membranous (subperiosteal) bone formation. Bones of the remainder of the skeleton ossify within a cartilaginous matrix (endochondral ossification).

Structure of Bones

Bones consist of cortical bone, which forms the external surface, and trabecular bone, which lies beneath the cortex. Trabecular bone predominates in the vertebral bodies and the flat bones of the pelvis and skull, whereas tubular bones of the appendicular skeleton have prominent cortical bone, which provides strength.

Long bones of the appendicular skeleton have four parts: the epiphysis, which is separated from the metaphysis by the physis, and the diaphysis, which joins the two metaphyses and provides length. Apophyses, such as the tibial tuberosity, are like epiphyses in that they are the site of new bone formation, but they do not contribute to bone length; instead, they lay down new bone in response to traction.

Cortical bone comprises tightly packed osteons (Haversian systems) that consist of osteocytes in lacunae and bone matrix arranged in a lamellar pattern, surrounding a central Haversian canal containing blood vessels and nerves. The osteons communicate with each other via canaliculi. Trabecular bone is much less organized and consists of interconnecting trabeculae, larger blood vessels, and bone marrow.

With the exception of articular surfaces, bones are covered by periosteum. The fibrous outer layer is the site of attachment of muscles, whereas the inner layer contains osteoblasts that generate new bone.

Growth of Bones

Linear growth of bone occurs at the physis, or growth plate. Circumferential growth is accounted for by periosteal deposition of new bone. Hyaline cartilage cells are arranged in columns in the metaphysis subjacent to the physis. Proliferation of these cells results in elongation of the long bone. The relative contributions to growth at the major physes of the limbs are shown in Table 2-1. Growth of the appendicular skeleton ceases at the time of completion of ossification of the iliac apophyses, although the height of the vertebral bodies may continue to increase and contribute to overall height until the third decade of life. Skeletal bone age can be determined by radiographic identification of the onset of secondary ossification in the long bones and by physeal closure. In general, ossification centers appear earlier, and physes fuse earlier in girls than in boys. Joint inflammation accelerates the development of bone. Factors that influence growth at the physis include thyroxine, growth hormone, and testosterone. Growth hormone and insulin-like growth factor 1 (IGF-1) act together to facilitate the achievement of peak bone mass during puberty. Testosterone stimulates the physis to undergo rapid cell division, with resultant physeal widening during the growth spurt (the anabolic effect). Estrogens suppress the growth rate by increasing calcification of the matrix, a prerequisite to epiphyseal closure. A vast array of genetic abnormalities result in abnormalities of the structure of bones, some of which, such as pseudorheumatoid dysplasia, may mimic inflammatory joint disease.

Vascular Supply

The arterial supply to the diaphysis and metaphysis of a long bone arises from a nutrient artery that penetrates the diaphysis and terminates in the child in end arteries at the epiphyseal plate.[1,2] Epiphyses are supplied by juxtaarticular arteries, which also supply the synovium via a complex network of arterial and arteriovenous anastomoses and capillary beds. Not until growth has ceased and the epiphyseal plate has ossified does arterial communication begin between the metaphyseal and epiphyseal-synovial circulations.

JOINTS

Classification of Joints

Joints may be classified as *fibrous, cartilaginous,* or *synovial* (Table 2-2). Fibrous joints (synarthroses) are those in which little or no motion

TABLE 2-1   Relative Contributions of Individual Physes to the Length of the Bone and Limb

GROWTH AREA		CONTRIBUTION TO TOTAL GROWTH (%)	
		OF BONE	OF LIMB
Humerus	Proximal	80	40
	Distal	20	10
Radius/Ulna	Proximal	20	10
	Distal	80	40
Femur	Proximal	30	15
	Distal	70	40
Tibia/Fibula	Proximal	55	27
	Distal	45	18

Data from J.A. Ogden, Skeletal Injury in the Child, Lea & Febiger, Philadelphia, 1982.

TABLE 2-2   Joints Classified by Structure

Fibrous	Bones separated by fibrous connection
Suture	Bones of the skull
Syndesmosis	Bones united by interosseous ligament
	Sacroiliac interosseous ligament
	Distal tibiofibular and radioulnar interosseous membranes
Cartilaginous	Bones separated by cartilage and allowing minimal movement
Symphysis	Bones separated by cartilaginous disk
	Symphysis pubis
	Sternomanubrial joint
	Intervertebral disk
Synchondrosis	Temporary joints in fetal life; bones separated by hyaline cartilage
	Growth plate (physis)
Synovial	Bones covered by hyaline cartilage are separated by joint "space" lined with synovial membrane producing synovial fluid (SF), surrounded by a joint capsule, allowing free movement

TABLE 2-3   Synovial (Diarthrodial) Joints Classified by Shape

Plane joints	Intercarpal, intertarsal
Spheroidal	Hip, shoulder
Cotylic	Metacarpophalangeal
Hinge	Interphalangeal
Condylar	Knee, temporomandibular joint
Trochoid or pivot	Radioulnar, atlanto-odontoid
Sellar	Carpometacarpal joint

underlying cartilage and, together with a high concentration of hyaluronan at the site, the attraction of water into the newly forming joint space.[4] The most important signals for joint morphogenesis are provided by the cartilage-derived morphogenetic protein 1 (CDMP1) and the bone morphogenetic proteins (BMPs).[5-7] The joint "cavity" is occupied at first by hyaluronic acid–rich joint fluid secreted by fibroblast-like cells lining the synovial membrane. Continued development of the diarthrodial joint depends on fetal movement,[8] which induces formation of cartilage and synovial membrane and without which the "cavity" regresses and becomes filled with fibrous tissue,[9] as occurs in arthrogryposis. The synovial lining forms from the interzone subsequent to cavitation, and the development of other structures, such as bursae, intraarticular fat, tendons, muscle, and capsule, quickly ensues. The whole process takes place between the fourth and seventh weeks of gestation, except for the temporomandibular joint[10] and the sacroiliac joint,[11] which develop several weeks later.

Anatomy of Synovial Joints

The bones of the articular surfaces of diarthrodial (synovial) joints are usually covered by hyaline cartilage. The synovial membrane attaches at the cartilage–bone junction so that the entire joint "space" is surrounded by either hyaline cartilage or synovium. The temporomandibular joint is unusual in that the surface of the condyle is covered by fibrocartilage (fibroblasts and type I collagen).[10] In the sacroiliac joint, the sacral side is covered by thicker hyaline cartilage, whereas the iliac side of the joint is covered by fibrocartilage.[11] In some synovial joints, intraarticular fibrocartilaginous structures are present. A disk (or meniscus) separates the temporomandibular joint into two spaces; the knee joint contains two menisci that separate the articular surfaces of the tibia and femur; and the triangular fibrocartilage of the wrist joins the distal radioulnar surfaces. Other intraarticular structures include the anterior and posterior cruciate ligaments of the knee, the interosseous ligaments of the talocalcaneal joint, and the triangular ligament of the femoral head. These structures are actually extrasynovial, although they cross through the joint space.

ARTICULAR CARTILAGE

The hyaline cartilage (principally type II collagen) covers subchondral bone, facilitates relatively frictionless motion and absorbs the compressive forces generated by weight-bearing.[12-14] In children, hyaline cartilage is somewhat compressible. The cartilage is firmly fixed to subchondral bone in adults by collagen fibrils, although there is little collagen at the osteochondral interface in the growing child.[15] The cartilage's margins blend with the synovial membrane and the periosteum of the metaphysis of the bone. It is composed of chondrocytes within an extracellular matrix (ECM) and becomes progressively less cellular throughout the period of growth; the cell volume in adult articular cartilage is less than 2%.[12] The matrix consists of collagen

occurs, and the bones are separated by fibrous connective tissue. Cartilaginous joints (amphiarthroses) are those in which little or no motion occurs, but the bones are separated by cartilage. Synovial (diarthrodial) joints are those in which considerable motion occurs, and a joint space lined with a synovial membrane is present between the bones. The synovial joint is the site of inflammation in most of the chronic arthritides of childhood. Diarthrodial joints may be further classified according to their shape (Table 2-3).

Development of Synovial Joints

Within the mesenchyme of the limb buds, cells destined to become chondrocytes are surrounded by the perichondrium (the source of new chondrocytes). Between the developing bones, the perichondrium is called the *interzone*. Cavitation occurs in this location, resulting in the formation of a joint "space."[3] Whether this results from enzymatic action or apoptosis is not certain. It is thought that differential growth rates result in slight negative pressure in the more slowly growing interzone, thereby facilitating separation of the interzone from the

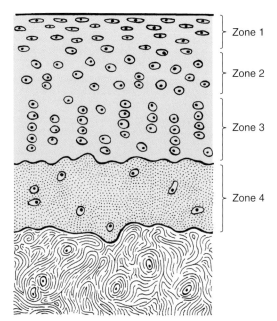

FIGURE 2-1 Organization of articular cartilage. In zone 1, adjacent to the joint space, the chondrocytes are flattened. In zone 2, the chondrocytes are more rounded, and in zone 3 they are arranged in perpendicular columns. The tide mark separates zone 3 from zone 4, which is impregnated with calcium salts. Bone is beneath zone 4. (Courtesy J.R. Petty.)

Zone 1

Zone 2

Zone 3

Zone 4

fibers, which contribute to tensile strength, and ground substance composed of water and proteoglycan, which contributes resistance to compression.[16,17]

Cartilage Zones

Articular hyaline cartilage is organized into four zones (Fig. 2-1). Zones 1, 2, and 3 represent a continuum from the most superficial area of zone 1, in which the long axes of the chondrocytes and collagen fibers are parallel to the surface; through zone 2, in which the chondrocytes become rounder and the collagen fibers are oblique; to zone 3, in which the chondrocytes tend to be arranged in columns perpendicular to the surface. This organization is markedly disturbed in the chronic infantile neurocutaneous and articular syndrome (CINCA) (also called *neonatal onset multisystem inflammatory disorder* [NOMID]).[18] The *tidemark*, a line that stains blue with hematoxylin-eosin, separates zone 3 from zone 4 and represents the level at which calcification of the matrix begins. Chondrocytes in each of the cartilage zones differ not only in appearance but also in metabolic activity, gene expression, and response to stimuli.[19] In the child, end capillaries proliferate in zone 4, eventually leading to replacement of this area by bone. This is probably the manner in which the chondrocytes are nourished. In the adult, however, constituent replacement through the exchange of synovial fluid with cartilage matrix may play the predominant role.

Chondrocytes

Chondrocytes are primarily mesodermal in origin and are the sole cellular constituents of normal cartilage. Their terminal differentiation determines the character of the cartilage (hyaline, fibrous, or elastic).[19] Chondrocytes in articular cartilage persist and ordinarily do not divide after skeletal maturity is attained. Those in the epiphyseal growth plate differentiate to facilitate endochondral ossification, after which they may undergo apoptosis or become osteoblasts.[20] Chondrocytes

are responsible for the synthesis of the two major constituents of the matrix—collagen and proteoglycan—and enzymes that degrade matrix components (collagenase, neutral proteinases, and cathepsins).[20] This dual function places the chondrocyte in the role of regulating cartilage synthesis and degradation. The pericellular region immediately surrounding the chondrocyte contains type VI collagen and the proteoglycans contain decorin and aggrecan.[12] Chondrocytes in zone 1 produce superficial zone protein (lubricin), which is important in maintaining relatively frictionless joint motion. Synthesis of this protein is defective in the camptodactyly-arthropathy-coxa vara-pericarditis syndrome.[21]

Extracellular Matrix

The ECM of hyaline cartilage consists of collagen fibers (which contribute tensile strength), water, diverse structural and regulatory proteins, and proteoglycans. The ECM is heterogeneous and can be subdivided into three compartments. A thin inner rim of aggrecan-rich matrix surrounds the chondrocytes and lacks cross-linked collagen. An outer rim contains fine collagen fibrils. The remainder of the ECM consists primarily of aggrecan, which binds via the link protein to hyaluronan (Fig. 2-2).[19] The endoskeleton of hyaline cartilage consists of a network of collagen fibrils, 90% of which are type II collagen, with minor components of collagen types IX and X.[20]

Proteoglycans

Proteoglycans are macromolecules consisting of a protein core to which 50 to 100 unbranched *glycosaminoglycans* (chondroitin sulfate [CS] and O-linked keratan sulfate [KS]) are attached.[22-24] At least five different protein cores have been defined. The principal proteoglycan of hyaline cartilage is called *aggrecan*. Its attachment to hyaluronan is stabilized by a link protein to form large proteoglycan aggregates with molecular weights of several million (Fig. 2-2).[12,16,17] With increasing age, the size of the proteoglycan aggregate increases, the protein and KS content increase, and the CS content decreases.[24,25] CS chains also become shorter with increasing age, and the position of the sulfated moiety changes, from a combination of 4-sulfated and 6-sulfated *N*-acetylgalactosamine at birth to mainly 6-sulfated *N*-acetylgalactosamine in the adult.[25-27] The significance to inflammatory joint disease, if any, of these and other age-related changes, is unknown.

Collagens

Collagens, the most abundant structural proteins of connective tissues, are trimeric ECM proteins containing a characteristic glycine-X-Y repeating triple helical structure, with a high proline and hydroxyproline content.[28-30] There are at least 28 different collagen α chain trimers grouped into three major classes: fibril forming, fibril-associated collagens with interrupted triple helices (FACIT), and non-fibril-forming collagens that include network-forming and transmembrane collagens (Table 2-4). Fibrillar collagen triple helices are arranged in a quarter-stagger pattern to form fibrils.[30] Many are tough, fibrous proteins that provide structural strength to the tissues of the body.[31] FACIT collagens are non-fibrillar collagens attached to the surface of fibrillar collagens. Type XIV is a FACIT collagen attached to type II collagen and regulates fiber diameter.[30] Network-forming collagens (types IV, VI, VIII, and X) form networks that are often three-dimensional. Transmembrane collagens (types XIII, XVII, XXIII, and XXV) have both an intracellular and an extracellular domain. Types I, II, and III are among the most common proteins in humans. Type II collagen, the principal constituent that accounts for more than half the dry weight of cartilage, is a trimer of three identical α-helical chains. Collagen types III, VI, IX, X, XI, XII, and XIV are all present in minute quantities in the mature

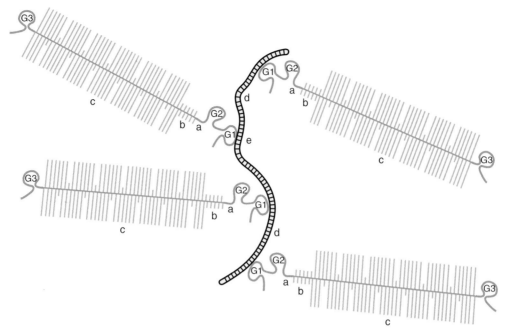

FIGURE 2-2 The structure of the proteoglycan aggregate of cartilage. The proteoglycan monomer consists of a core protein (a) of variable length that contains three globular domains: *G1* (located at the aminoterminus and containing the hyaluronate binding region), *G2*, and *G3*. Link protein (e) stabilizes the aggregate by binding simultaneously to the hyaluronate chain (d) and G1. Glycosaminoglycan molecules are attached to the core protein in specific regions: keratan sulfate (b) and chondroitin sulfate (c).

cartilage matrix.[32] The content of types IX and XI collagen is greater in young animals (20%) than in mature animals (3%).[28]

Collagen synthesis is minimal in the mature animal. The degree of stable cross-linking of collagen fibers increases with advancing age.[33] This may contribute to the increased rigidity and decreased tensile strength of old cartilage.

Collagen undergoes extensive changes in primary and tertiary structure after it is secreted from the fibroblast into the extracellular space as a triple-helical procollagen.[34] Specific peptidases cleave the amino and carboxyl extension peptides, yielding collagen molecules that form cross-links and fibrils via lysyl and hydroxylysyl residues in some types. Glycosylation also occurs at this posttranslational stage.

Collagen genes are named for the type of collagen (e.g., COLI) and the fibril (e.g., A1), and they encode the large triple-helical domain common to human collagens. Mutations in the collagen genes account for human diseases such as Ehlers-Danlos syndrome and osteogenesis imperfecta.[35,36]

Proteinases for Collagen and Cartilage

The proteinases (endopeptidases) are proteolytic enzymes active in homeostatic remodeling of the ECM during health and in its degradation during inflammation. These enzymes occur both intracellularly and extracellularly in tissue fluids and plasma and have been classified into five categories based on functional catalytic groups[37]: the *metalloproteinases* and *serine proteinases*, which are active at neutral to slightly alkaline pH, and the *cysteine, aspartic,* and *threonine proteinases*, which are most active at acid pH (Table 2-5).

The metalloproteinases, which are activated by calcium and stabilized by zinc ions, consist of more than 10 well-characterized enzymes.[37] They are active in the degradation or remodeling of collagens and are known to be synthesized by rheumatoid synovium. Collagenases are inhibited naturally by α_2-macroglobulin and by the *tissue inhibitor of*

metalloproteinase (TIMP). *Stromelysin* is a neutral proteinase synthesized by cultured fibroblasts and synovium. Other members of this family, the *gelatinases*, are active in the remodeling of collagen-containing tissues.

The serine proteinases are a family of endopeptidases that participate in matrix degradation either directly or by activating precursors of the metalloproteinases. They include many of the enzymes of pathways involving coagulation, fibrinolysis, complement activation, and kinin generation: plasmin, plasminogen activator, kallikrein, and elastase. Serine proteinase inhibitors constitute 10% of the plasma proteins. The cysteine proteinases that degrade ECM include cathepsins B and L, which are lysosomal enzymes associated with inflammatory reactions. The aspartic proteinases are primarily lysosomal proteinases active at acid pH. Cathepsin D is the major representative of this family that degrades proteoglycans and is present in the lysosomes of most cells. Threonine proteinases are associated with the proteasome.[37]

SYNOVIUM

Synovial Membrane

The synovial membrane is a vascular connective tissue structure of ectodermal origin that lines the capsules of all diarthrodial joints and has important intraarticular regulatory functions.[38] The synovium consists of the intima—specialized fibroblasts, one to three cells in depth, overlying a loose meshwork of type I collagen fibers—and the subintima—containing blood vessels, lymphatics, fat pads, unmyelinated nerves, and isolated cells such as mast cells (Fig. 2-3). There is no basement membrane separating the joint space from the subsynovial tissues. Increased vascular permeability in inflammation contributes to the increase in joint fluid (effusion) seen in inflamed joints. The synovial membrane is discontinuous, and within the joint space there are so-called *bare areas* between the edge of the cartilage and the

TABLE 2-4 Some Types of Collagen

SUBCLASS AND TYPE	COMPOSITION	TISSUE DISTRIBUTION
Fibril-Forming Collagens		
Type I	α1(I), α2(I)	Most connective tissues; abundant in bone, skin, and tendons
Type II	α1(II)	Cartilage, intervertebral disk, vitreous humor
Type III	α1(III)	Most connective tissues, particularly skin, lung, and blood vessels
Type V	α1(V), α2(V), α3(V)	Tissues containing type I collagen, quantitatively minor component
Type XI	α1(XI), α2(XI), α3(XI)	Cartilage, intervertebral disk, vitreous humor
Type XXIV	α1(XXIV)	Fetal skeleton
Type XXVII	α1(XXVII)	Fetal skeleton
Type XXVIII	α1(XXVIII)	Surrounds peripheral glial cells
FACIT Collagens		
Type IX	α1(IX), α2(IX), α3(IX)	Cartilage, intervertebral disk, vitreous humor
Type XII	α1(XII)	Tissues containing type I collagen
Type XIV	α1(XIV)	Tissues containing type I collagen
Type XVI	α1(XVI)	Several tissues
Type XIX	α1(XIX)	Rhabdomyosarcoma cells
Type XX	α1(XX)	Corneal epithelium
Type XXI	α1(XXI)	Fetal blood vessel walls
Type XXII	α1(XXII)	Basement membrane myotendinous junction
Non-Fibril-Forming Collagens		
Type IV*	α1(IV), α2(IV), α3(IV), α4(IV), α5(IV), α6(IV)	Basement membranes
Type VIII*	α1(VIII), α2(VIII)	Several tissues, especially endothelium
Type X*	α1(X)	Hypertrophic cartilage
Type VI*	α1(VI), α2(VI), α3(VI)	Most connective tissues
Type VII	α1(VII)	Skin, oral mucosa, cervix, cornea
Type XIII†	α1(XIII)	Endomysium, perichondrium, placenta, mucosa of the intestine, meninges
Type XVII†	α1(XVII)	Skin, cornea
Type XXIII†	α1(XXIII)	Prostate
Type XXV		Neurons
Type XV†	α1(XV)	Skeletal and heart muscle, placenta
Type XVIII	α1(XVIII)	Many tissues, especially kidney, liver, and lung
Type XXVI	Not a FACIT collagen	Neonatal testes and ovaries

*Network-forming collagens.
†Transmembrane collagens.

TABLE 2-5 Some Proteinases for Collagen and Cartilage Substrates and Their Inhibitors

ENZYME	SUBSTRATE	INHIBITOR
Metalloproteinases		
Collagenases	Types I, II, and III collagens, and GAGs	Tissue inhibitor of metalloproteinases (TIMP)
Gelatinase	Types IV and V and denatured collagens and elastin	TIMP
Stromelysin	Fibronectin, GAGs, elastin, collagens	TIMP
Serine Proteinases		
Plasmin	Metalloproteinases	α2-Antiplasmin
Elastase	Various collagens and GAGs	α1-Plasminogen inactivator
Cathepsin G	GAGs, type II collagen, elastin, TIMP	α1-Plasminogen inactivator
Plasminogen activators	Proplasminogen	
Cysteine Proteinases		
Cathepsin B	Type II collagen, GAGs, link protein	Cystatins
Cathepsin L	Type I collagen, GAGs, link protein, elastin	Cystatins
Aspartic Proteinases		
Cathepsin D	GAGs, type II collagen	α2-Macroglobulin
Threonine Proteinases	Misfolded and denatured proteins	

GAGs, Glycosaminoglycans.

attachment of the synovial membrane to the periosteum of the metaphysis. These bare areas are especially vulnerable to damage (erosion) by inflamed synovium (pannus) in inflammatory joint diseases. Folds, or villi, of synovium provide for unrestricted motion of the joint and for augmented absorptive area.

The synoviocytes are of two predominant types, a subdivision that may reflect different functional states rather than different origins. Synovial A cells are thought to be of macrophage origin,[38] capable of phagocytosis and pinocytosis, have numerous microfilopodia, have a prominent Golgi apparatus, and synthesize hyaluronic acid, which is essential to maintain the non-adherent properties of the synovium. Synovial B cells are more fibroblast-like, have a prominent rough endoplasmic reticulum, and synthesize fibronectin, laminin, types I and III collagen, enzymes (collagenase, neutral proteinases), catabolin, and lubricin, which is also synthesized by chondrocytes at the surface of hyaline cartilage, and which contributes significantly to lubrication of the cartilage surfaces.

Synovial Fluid

Synovial fluid (SF), present in very small quantities in normal synovial joints, has two functions: lubrication and nutrition.[39,40] Normal fluid is clear and pale yellow; SF is a combination of a filtrate of plasma, which enters the joint space from the subsynovial capillaries, and hyaluronic acid, which is secreted by the synoviocytes. Hyaluronic acid provides the high viscosity of normal SF and, with water, its lubricating properties.[41] Concentrations of small molecules (electrolytes, glucose)

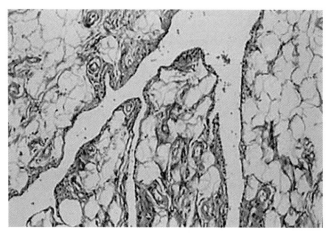

FIGURE 2-3 Photomicrograph of normal synovial membrane histology.

TABLE 2-6	Normal Synovial Fluid	
CHARACTERISTIC	MEAN OR REPRESENTATIVE VALUE	REFERENCE NO.
Volume	0.13-3.5 mL (adult knee)	43
pH	7.3-7.4	44
Relative viscosity	235	43
Cl, HCO_3^-	Slightly higher than serum	43
Na, K, Ca, Mg	Slightly lower than serum	43
Glucose	Serum value ± 10%	45
Total protein	1.7-2.1 g/dL	46
Albumin	1.2 g/dL	47
α1 globulin	0.17 g/dL	
α2 globulin	0.15 g/dL	
β globulin	0.23 g/dL	
γ globulin	0.38 g/dL	
Immunoglobulin G	13% of serum value	48
Immunoglobulin M	5% of serum value	
Immunoglobulin E	22% of serum value	49
$α_2$-Macroglobulin	3% of serum value	48
Transferrin	24% of serum value	
Ceruloplasmin	16% of serum value	
CH_{50}	30-50% of plasma value	50
Hyaluronic acid	300 mg/dL	51
Cholesterol	7.1 mg/dL	47
Phospholipid	13.8 mg/dL	47

are similar to those in plasma, but larger molecules (e.g., complement components) are present in low concentrations relative to plasma unless an inflammatory state alters vasopermeability. Notably absent from SF are elements of the coagulation pathway (fibrinogen, prothrombin, factors V and VII, tissue thromboplastin, and antithrombin).[42] As a result, normal SF is resistant to clotting. There appears to be free exchange of small molecules between SF of the joint space and water bound to collagen and proteoglycan of cartilage. Characteristics of normal SF are listed in Table 2-6.

Synovial Structures

Synovium lines bursae, tendon sheaths, and joints.[15] Bursae facilitate frictionless movement between surfaces, such as subcutaneous tissue and bone, or between two tendons. Bursae located near synovial joints frequently communicate with the joint space. This is particularly evident at the shoulder, where the subscapular bursa or recess communicates with the glenohumeral joint, and around the knee, where the suprapatellar pouch, the posterior femoral recess, and occasionally other bursae communicate with the knee joint. Tendon sheaths lined with synovial cells are prominent around tendons as they pass under the extensor retinaculum at the wrist and at the ankle. Although they are closely associated with joints, tendon sheaths do not communicate with the synovial space.

JOINT CAPSULE

The joint capsule is composed of dense connective tissue, reinforced by ligaments and sometimes tendons, and is lined by the synovial membrane. It is attached to bone via fibrocartilaginous entheses. It encloses the joint, contains the synovial fluid, limits joint mobility, and provides stability.[52] In patients with hypermobility syndromes associated with mutations in collagen genes, the joint capsule is particularly lax.

CONNECTIVE TISSUE STRUCTURES

Other Connective Tissue Constituents

In addition to collagens, a number of specialized tissues derived from embryonic mesoderm contribute to connective tissue structures other than cartilage. *Elastin* occurs in association with collagen in many tissues, especially in the walls of blood vessels and in certain ligaments.[53] Fibers of elastin lack the tensile strength of collagens but can stretch and then return to their original length. Elastin is produced by fibroblasts and by smooth muscle cells. *Fibronectin* is a dimeric glycoprotein with a molecular weight of 450,000 that acts as an attachment protein in the ECM.[54] It is produced by many different cell types, including macrophages, dedifferentiated chondrocytes, and fibroblasts, and has the ability to bind to collagens, proteoglycans, fibrinogen, actin, and to cell surfaces and bacteria. Fibronectin is present in plasma and as an insoluble matrix throughout loose connective tissues, especially between basement membranes and cells. *Laminin* is a major constituent of the basement membrane, together with type IV collagen.[55] *Reticulin* may be an embryonic form of type III collagen. It is present as a fine branching network of fibers widespread in the spleen, liver, bone marrow, and lymph nodes.

Tendons

Tendons are specialized connective tissue structures that, via the enthesis, attach muscle to bone.[56] In addition to water, they contain type I collagen and small amounts of elastin and type III collagen, the latter forming the *epitenon* and *endotenon*. The type III collagen fibers are densely packed in a parallel configuration in a proteoglycan matrix containing elongated fibroblasts.

Ligaments and Fasciae

Ligaments and fasciae join bone to bone and, like tendons, are composed of type I collagen. So-called elastic ligaments, such as the ligamenta flava and ligamentum nuchae, predominantly contain elastin.

Entheses

An enthesis is the site of attachment of tendon, ligament, fascia, or capsule to bone. There are two types of entheses: fibrous and fibrocartilaginous. Fibrous entheses are found at the attachment of tendon to the metaphysis or diaphysis, and are composed of dense fibrous tissue. They are thought to be of little importance in rheumatic diseases.[57] Fibrocartilaginous entheses are present on epiphyses of long bones and on small bones of the hands and feet. They appear to be more important in inflammatory disease. It includes the peritenon, which is continuous with the periosteum; collagen fibers of the tendon or ligament, which insert into the bone *(Sharpey's fibers)*; the adjoining fibrocartilage; and bone not covered by periosteum. Benjamin and colleagues have proposed the concept of the enthesis organ complex that includes adjacent bursae, fat pads, and connective tissues. Entheses have been the subject of extensive reviews.[57,58]

SKELETAL MUSCLE

Anatomy

Skeletal muscle makes up approximately 40% of the adult body mass and consists of about 640 separate muscles that support the skeleton and permit movement and locomotion. Skeletal muscle forms during embryogenesis from mesodermal stem cells. A skeletal muscle is surrounded by the connective tissue *epimysium*. Within the muscle, *fascicles* are covered by connective tissue *perimysium*. Each fascicle contains many individual muscle fibers, which are the basic structural units of skeletal muscle (Fig. 2-4). Muscle fibers are elongated, multinucleated cells surrounded by connective tissue *endomysium* (reticulin, collagen), which is richly supplied with capillaries. Within each fiber is a large number of *myofibrils*, consisting of highly organized interdigitated *myofilaments* of actin and myosin.[59] Each myofilament has approximately 180 myosin molecules with a molecular weight of 500,000, a long tail, and a double head. The myofilament is composed of the myosin tails; the myosin heads project in a spiral arrangement. Lying parallel to the myosin molecules are *actin filaments* (F-actin) composed of globular subunits of G-actin with a molecular weight of 42,000. Two actin filaments are coiled around each other as a helix, with a second protein, *tropomyosin B*, lying in the groove. A regulatory protein, *troponin*, is located at intervals along this structure. This complex structure is demonstrable by light or electron microscopy as striations. *Creatine kinase,* bound to the myosin filaments at regular intervals, is essential for the generation of energy for muscle contraction

Muscle Contraction

The functional ability of muscle to produce coordinated movements is governed by the conversion of chemical to mechanical energy by actomyosin.[60] Calcium diffusion in the myoplasm and binding to thin-filament regulatory proteins are stimulated by the action potential of the α-motor neuron. Variation in the properties of the types of motor fibers and motor units and recruitment of motor units result in the specific patterns of movement. The properties of the motor unit are influenced by the genetic makeup of the individual, muscular conditioning, and the presence of any disease that results in joint pain or immobilization, or metabolic, hormonal, or nutritional disturbances.[61,62]

Types of Muscle Fibers

Muscle fibers constitute 85% of muscle tissue. Muscle fibers are heterogeneous in function and biochemical markers (Table 2-7).[63] Older classifications identified two major fiber types. Most muscles contain both types. Type I (slow) fibers are narrower, have poorly defined myofibrils, are irregular in size, have thick Z bands (electron-dense noncontractile protein that anchors the actin molecules and demarcates sarcomeres), and are rich in mitochondria and oxidative enzymes but poor in phosphorylases. They are associated with sustained contraction. Type II (fast) fibers have fewer mitochondria and are poor in oxidative enzymes but rich in phosphorylases and glycogen. Types I and II muscle fibers can be differentiated histochemically (Fig. 2-5).[64] Muscles differ in the proportions of each fiber type. The diaphragm

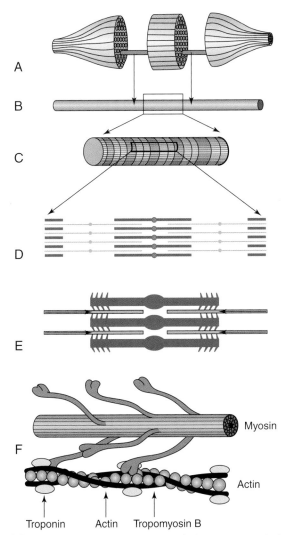

FIGURE 2-4 Schematic representation of the anatomy of skeletal muscle: **A,** fascicle; **B,** fiber; **C,** myofibrils; **D,** actin and myosin; **E** and **F,** enlargement of actin and myosin filaments showing the actin filaments coiled around each other and associated with tropomyosin B lying in the groove. (Courtesy J.R. Petty.)

Labels in figure: Myosin; Actin; Troponin; Actin; Tropomyosin B

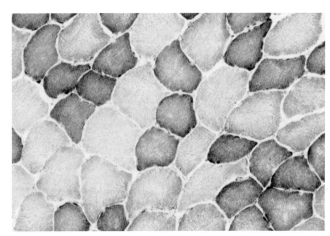

FIGURE 2-5 In this photomicrograph of normal skeletal muscle, type 1 fibers are pale and type 2 fibers are dark.

TABLE 2-7   Characteristics of Muscle Fiber Types

CHARACTERISTIC	TYPE I	TYPE IIA	TYPE IIB	TYPE IIC
Size	Moderate	Small	Large	Small
Color	Red	White	White	White
Myoglobin content	High	Medium	Low	High
Mitochondria	Many	Intermediate	Few	Intermediate
Blood supply	+++	+	+	+
ATPase (pH 4.4)	High	Low	Low	–
ATPase (pH 10.6)	Low	High	High	–
Lipid	High	Low	Low	–
Glycogen	Low	High	High	Variable
Metabolic characteristics				
Oxidative (aerobic)	High	Intermediate	Low	High
Glycolytic (anaerobic)	Moderate	High	High	High
Function				
Contraction time	Slow and sustained	Fast twitch	Fast twitch	Moderate twitch
Resistance to fatigue	High	Moderate	Low	Moderate

contains predominantly slow fibers, and small muscles contain predominantly fast fibers. Classifications of fiber types on the basis of the myosin heavy-chain isoform they contain identify four major types in muscles of the axial skeleton and limbs (types I, IIA, IIB, and IIC) (Table 2-7). In addition, there are minor fiber types in muscles of the head and neck.[63] Muscle conditioning leads to adaptations in the contractile and structural proteins and fiber species within the genetic potential of the individual. Strength training results in hypertrophy of type IIB, and endurance training leads to metabolic alterations in type I and type IIA fibers.[65-67]

VASCULATURE

Inflammation of blood vessels—vasculitis—is one of the major categories of the rheumatic diseases. Blood vessel size, type, and location are often characteristic of specific vasculitides. The innermost layer of all blood vessels (tunica intima) is formed by the mesoderm-derived endothelial cells. Characteristics of endothelial cells vary from location to location in their anatomical characteristics and expression of ligands and receptors, accounting, at least in part, for the disease-restricted distribution of affected vessels.[68] The cells produce a variety of vaso-regulatory substances (nitric oxide, prostacyclin, platelet activating factor, endothelin-1) that influence inflammatory processes through vasodilatation or vasoconstriction. The internal elastic lamina separates the intima from the media. The middle layer (tunica media) consists of smooth muscle and elastin fibers, and is responsible for the ability of vessels to dilate and constrict under the control of the autonomic nervous system via the nervi vasorum. It is particularly prominent in arteries, compared with veins. The external elastic lamina separates the media from the tunica adventia, which consists principally of collagen fibers and nutrient blood vessels (vasa vasorum). Enzymatic degradation of the elastin leads to aneurysm formation in Kawasaki disease.

REFERENCES

1. M. Liew, W.C. Dick, The anatomy and physiology of blood flow in a diarthrodial joint, Clin. Rheum. Dis. 7 (1981) 131–148.
2. J.C. Edwards, V. Morris, Joint physiology relevant to the rheumatologist? Br. J. Rheumatol. 37 (1998) 121–125.
3. C.W. Archer, G.P. Dowthwaite, P. Francis-West, Development of synovial joints, Birth Defects Res. C Embryo Today 69 (2003) 144–155.
5. C.J. Edwards, P.H. Francis-West, Bone morphogenetic proteins in the development and healing of synovial joints, Semin. Arthritis Rheum. 31 (2001) 33–42.
6. A.H. Reddi, Cartilage morphogenetic proteins: role in joint development, homoeostasis, and regeneration, Ann. Rheum. Dis. 62 (Suppl. II) (2003) ii73–ii78.
7. R.J.U. Lories, F.P. Luyten, Bone morphogenetic proteins signalling in joint homeostasis and disease, Cytokine Growth Factor Rev. 16 (2005) 287–298.
9. A.A. Pitsillides, Identifying and characterizing the joint cavity-forming cell, Cell Biochem. Funct. 21 (2003) 235–240.
10. L. Wang, N.S. Detamore, Tissue engineering the mandibular condyule, Tissue Eng. 13 (2007) 1955–1971.
11. V. Bowen, J.D. Cassidy, Macroscopic and microscopic anatomy of the sacroiliac joint from embryonic life until the eighth decade, Spine 6 (1981) 620–628.
12. A.R. Poole, T. Kohima, T. Yasuda, et al., Composition and structure of articular cartilage, Clin. Orthop. 391S (2001) S26–S33.
13. L.C. Dijkgraaf, L.G. de Bont, G. Boering, et al., Normal cartilage structure, biochemistry, and metabolism: a review of the literature, J. Oral Maxillofac. Surg. 53 (1995) 924–929.
14. H.E. Jasin, Structure and function of the articular cartilage surface, Scand. J. Rheumatol. 10 (Suppl.) (1995) 51–55.
17. N.P. Cohen, R.J. Foster, V.C. Mow, Composition and dynamics of articular cartilage: structure, function, and maintaining healthy state, J. Orthop. Sports Phys. Ther. 28 (1998) 203–215.
18. J. Feldman, A.-M. Prieur, P. Quartier, et al., Chronic infantile neurocutaneous and articular syndrome is caused by mutations in CIAS1, a gene highly expressed in polymorphonuclear cells and chondrocytes, Am. J. Hum. Genet. 71 (2002) 198–203.
19. S. Chubinskaya, K.E. Kuettner, Regulation of osteogenic proteins by chondrocytes, Int. J. Biochem. Cell Biol. 35 (2003) 1323–1340.
20. C.W. Archer, P. Francis-West, The chondrocyte, Int. J. Biochem. Cell Biol. 35 (2003) 401–404.
21. M.L. Warman, Human genetic insights into skeletal development, growth, and homeostasis, Clin. Orthop. 379 (2000) 540–554.
22. A.D. Lander, Proteoglycans: master regulators of molecular encounter? Matrix Biol. 17 (1998) 465–472.
23. P.J. Roughley, The structure and function of cartilage proteoglycans, Eur. Cell. Mater. 12 (2006) 92–101.
24. J.T. Gallagher, The extended family of proteoglycans: social residents of the pericellular zone, Curr. Opin. Cell Biol. 1 (1989) 1201–1218.

25. R.V. Iozzo, Matrix proteoglycans: from molecular design to cellular function, Annu. Rev. Biochem. 67 (1998) 609–652.
26. M.T. Bayliss, S.Y. Ali, Age-related changes in the composition and structure of human articular-cartilage proteoglycans, Biochem. J. 176 (1978) 683–693.
27. P.J. Roughley, Age-associated changes in cartilage matrix, Clin. Orthop. 391S (2001) S153–S160.
28. D. Eyre, Articular cartilage and changes in arthritis: collagen of articular cartilage, Arthritis Res. 4 (2002) 30–35.
29. M. van der Rest, R. Garrone, Collagen family of proteins, FASEB J. 5 (1991) 2814–2823.
30. M.K. Gordon, R.A. Hahn, Collagens, Cell Tissue Res. 339 (2010) 247–257.
31. J. Uitto, L.W. Murray, B. Blumberg, et al., Biochemistry of collagen in diseases, Ann. Int. Med. 106 (1986) 740–756.
32. M.T. Bayiliss, S.Y. Ali, Age-related changes in the composition of human articular-cartilage proteoglycans, Biochem. J. 176 (1978) 683–693.
33. N.C. Avery, A.J. Bailey, Enzymic and non-enzymic cross-linking mechanisms in relation to turnover of collagen: relevance to aging and exercise, Scand, J. Med. Sci. Sport 15 (2005) 231–240.
34. K. Piez, Molecular and aggregate structures in the collagens, in: K.A. Piez, A.H. Reddi (Eds.), Extracellular Matrix Biochemistry, Elsevier, New York, 1984.
35. E.M. Carter, C.L. Raggio, Genetic and orthopedic aspects of collagen disorders, Curr. Opin. Pediatr. 21 (2009) 46–54.
36. R. Jobling, R. D'Souza, N. Baker, et al., The collagenopathies: review of clinical phenotypes and molecular correlations, Curr. Rheumatol. Rep. 16 (2014) 394–407.
37. T.E. Cawston, D.A. Young, Proteinases involved in matrix turnover during cartilage and bone breakdown, Cell Tissue Res. 339 (2010) 221–235.
38. M.D. Smith, The normal synovium, Open Rheumatol. J. 5 (Suppl. 1:M2) (2011) 100–106.
39. C.W. McCutchen, Lubrication of joints, in: L. Sokoloff (Ed.), The Joints and Synovial Fluid, Academic Press, New York, 1978.
40. P.A. Simkin, Synovial perfusion and synovial fluid solutes, Ann. Rheum. Dis. 54 (1995) 424–428.
41. J.R. Levick, J.N. McDonald, Fluid movement across synovium in healthy joints: role of synovial fluid macromolecules, Ann. Rheum. Dis. 54 (1995) 417–423.
46. N.R. Rose, E.C. de Marcario, J.L. Fahey (Eds.), Manual of Clinical Laboratory Immunology, 4th ed., American Society for Microbiology, Washington, DC, 1992.

47. R.A. Gatter, H.R. Schumacher, A Practical Handbook of Joint Fluid Analysis, 2nd ed., Lea & Febiger, Philadelphia, 1992.
52. J.R. Ralphs, M. Benjamin, The joint capsule: structure, function, ageing and disease, J. Anat. 184 Part III (1994) 503–509.
53. A.K. Baldwin, A. Simpson, R. Steer, et al., Elastic fibers in health and disease, Expert Rev. Mol. Med. 15 (2013) e8.
54. J.E. Schwarzbauer, D.W. DeSimone, Fibronectins, their fibrillogenesis and in vivo functions, Cold Spring Harb. Perspect Biol. 3 (2011) pii: a005041.
55. M. Aumailley, The laminin family, Cell Adh Migr. 7 (2013) 48–55.
56. J.J. Canoso, Bursae, tendons and ligaments, Clin. Rheum. Dis. 7 (1961) 189–221.
57. P. Claudepierre, M.-C. Voisin, The entheses: histology, pathology and pathophysiology, Joint Bone Spine 72 (2005) 32–37.
58. M. Benjamin, T. Kumai, S. Milz, et al., The skeletal attachment of tendons: tendon "entheses", Comp. Biochem. Physiol. A 133 (2002) 931–945.
59. B.A. Gowitzke, M. Milner, Scientific Basis of Human Movement, Williams & Wilkins, Baltimore, 1988.
60. J. Squire, The Structural Basis of Muscular Contraction, Plenum Press, New York, 1981.
61. J.A. Faulkner, T.P. White, Adaptations of skeletal muscle to physical activity, in: C. Bouchard, R.J. Shephard, T. Stephens (Eds.), Exercise, Fitness, and Health, Human Kinetics, Champaign, IL, 1990.
62. R.R. Heffner Jr. (Ed.), Muscle Pathology, Churchill Livingstone, New York, 1984.
63. S. Schiaffino, C. Reggiani, Fiber types in mammalian skeletal muscle, Physiol. Rev. 91 (2011) 1447–1531.
64. R.S. Staron, Human skeletal muscle fiber types: delineation, development, and distribution, Can. J. Appl. Physiol. 22 (1997) 307–327.
65. M. Zhang, K. Koishi, I.S. McLennan, Skeletal muscle fiber types. Detection methods and embryonic determinants, Histol. Histopathol. 13 (1998) 201–207.
66. F.W. Booth, B.S. Tseng, M. Flück, et al., Molecular and cellular adaptation of muscle in response to physical training, Acta Physiol. Scand. 162 (1998) 343–350.
67. A.W. Taylor, L. Bachman, The effects of endurance training on muscle fibre types and enzyme activities, Can. J. Appl. Physiol. 24 (1999) 41–53.
68. D.B. Cines, E.S. Pollak, C.A. Buck, et al., Endothelial cells in physiology and in the pathophysiology of vascular disorders, Blood 91 (1998) 3527–3561.

Entire reference list is available online at www.expertconsult.com.

3 | CHAPTER

Inflammation and Its Mediators

Marco Gattorno, Alberto Martini

The immune system, the function of which is to protect against infections, comprises two branches: a more primitive one called *innate* (natural, native) *immunity* and the more recently evolved one called *adaptive* (specific) *immunity*. Innate and adaptive immunity are not two separate compartments but an integrated system of host defense, sharing bidirectional interactions fundamental to both the inductive phase and the effector phase of the immune response. The innate immune system constitutes the first line of host defense during infection and therefore plays a crucial role in the early recognition and subsequent triggering of the proinflammatory response to invading pathogens. The adaptive immune system, on the other hand, is responsible for elimination of pathogens in the late phase of infection, the maintenance of immunological tolerance, and the generation of immunological memory.

The cells of the immune system originate from pluripotent hematopoietic stem cells that give rise to stem cells of more limited potential (lymphoid and myeloid precursors). The immune system functions by means of a complex network of cellular interactions that involve cell surface proteins and soluble mediators such as cytokines.

CELLS OF INNATE IMMUNITY

The innate immune system is the first line of defense against microorganisms and is conserved in plants and animals. It is phylogenetically ancient compared with the more evolved form of immunity, which exists only in vertebrates. The principal components of innate immunity are (1) physical and chemical barriers such as epithelia and antimicrobial substances produced at epithelial surfaces, (2) circulating effector proteins such as the complement components and cytokines, and (3) cells with innate phagocytic activity: neutrophils, macrophages, and natural killer (NK) cells.

Phagocyte surface receptors recognize highly conserved structures characteristic of microbial pathogens that are not present in mammalian cells. The binding of microbial structures to these receptors triggers cells to engulf the bacterium and induces cytokines, chemokines, and costimulators that recruit and activate antigen-specific lymphocytes and initiate adaptive immune responses. Thus, innate immunity not only represents an early effective defense mechanism against infection but also provides the "warning" of the presence of an infection against which a subsequent adaptive immune response has to be mounted.[1] The pivotal role of this compartment in the effector phase of the immune response is discussed later.

Phagocytes

Cells of the phagocyte system originate from a common lineage in the bone marrow, circulate in the blood in inactive form and are recruited and activated in the peripheral tissues in case of infection, tissue injury

or other proinflammatory stimuli. *Monocytes* are the classical example of immature circulating phagocytes, characterized by a granular cytoplasm with many phagocytic vacuoles and lysosomes. Once they enter in the tissues, monocytes mature into *macrophages*. Macrophages are strategically placed in all organs and tissues where they act as "sentinels" together with dendritic cells. In fact, one of their major roles is to recognize and respond to microbes and to amplify the response against a potentially harmful stimulus. Depending on the tissues in which they are found, macrophages are known with a number of different names: Kupffer cells in the liver, microglial cells in the central nervous system, alveolar macrophages in the airways. These cells are the prototype of the effector cells of innate immunity. Once activated, macrophages initiate a number of crucial events which include phagocytosis and destruction of ingested microbes, and production of proinflammatory cytokines and other mediators of inflammation that lead to further recruitment of cells of innate immunity (monocytes, neutrophils) and provide signals to cells (T and B cells) of adaptive immunity.[2]

Neutrophils, the other major group of phagocytes, are the most abundant type of circulating leukocytes. Their nucleus is segmented into three to five lobules, hence the term *polymorphonuclear leukocytes*. The cytoplasm is characterized by the presence of two types of granules. *Specific granules* contain enzymes, including lysozyme, elastase, and collagenase. The *azurophilic granules* are lysosomes containing enzymes and microbicidal substances. Neutrophils are the first cells that enter the site of infection and represent the prevalent cell type in the early phases of the inflammatory response. Within 1 or 2 days neutrophils are almost completely replaced by newly recruited monocytes–macrophages that represent the dominant effector cells in the later stages of inflammation.[2]

The Pattern Recognition Receptors

The innate immune response relies on recognition of evolutionarily conserved structures on pathogens called *pathogen-associated molecular patterns* (PAMPs), through a limited number of germ line–encoded *pattern recognition receptors* (PRRs) (Table 3-1, Fig. 3-1).[3,4] Among them the family of Toll-like receptors (TLRs) has been studied most extensively.[4,5] PAMPs are characterized by being invariant among entire classes of pathogens and distinguishable from "self." This characteristic allows a limited number of germ line–encoded PRRs to detect the presence of many microbial infections. Finally, since PAMPs are essential for microbial survival, mutations or deletions of PAMPs are lethal, reducing the possibility that microbes undergo PAMP mutations in order to escape recognition by the innate system.[6]

Many classes of PPRs are present on the surface of cells of the innate immune system where they act as "tissue sentinels" through the continuous monitoring of peripheral tissues for the possible invasion of

TABLE 3-1   Examples of Pathogen-Associated Molecular Patterns (PAMPs) and Respective Pattern Recognition Receptors (PRRs)

MOLECULAR PATTERN	ORIGIN	RECEPTOR	MAIN EFFECTOR FUNCTION
LPS	Gram-negative bacteria	TLR4, CD14	Macrophage activation
Unmethylated CpG nucleotides	Bacterial DNA	TLR9	Macrophage, B-cell, and plasmacytoid cell activation
Terminal mannose residues	Microbial glycoprotein and glycolipids Phagocytosis	(1) Macrophage mannose receptor (2) Plasma mannose-binding lectin	
Complement activation Opsonization			
LPS, dsRNA	Bacteria, viruses	Macrophage scavenger receptor	Phagocytosis
Zymosan	Fungi	TLR2, Dectin-1	Macrophage activation
dsRNA	Viral	TLR3, RIG-I*	IFN type I production
ssRNA	Viral	TLR7/8, MDA5*	IFN type I production
N-formylmethionine residues	Bacteria	Chemokine receptors	Neutrophil and macrophage activation and migration
MDP	Gram-positive and Gram-negative bacteria	NOD2,* NALP1*	Macrophage activation

dsRNA, Double-stranded RNA; *IFN*, interferon; *LPS*, lipopolysaccharide; *MDP*, muramyl dipeptide; *ssRNA*, single-stranded RNA; *TLR*, Toll-like receptor.
*Cytoplasmic.

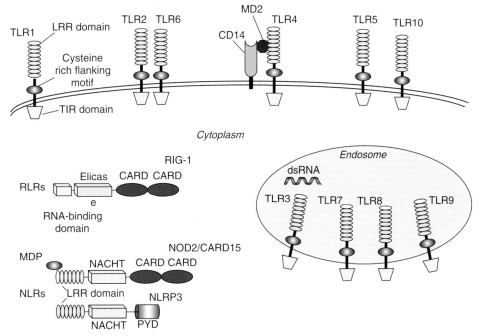

FIGURE 3-1 Localization and structure of cellular pattern recognition receptors. Toll-like receptors (TLRs) are membrane-bound receptors localized at the cellular or endosomal membranes. In addition, there are intracellular (cytosolic) receptors that function in the pattern recognition of bacterial and viral pathogens. NOD2/CARD15 and NALP3 belong to the NLR (nucleotide-binding oligomerization domain [NOD]-like receptors) family. Most NLRs contain a leucine-rich repeat (LRR) domain for PAMPs recognition, such as muramyl dipeptide (MDP) for NOD2/CARD15. RIG-I (retinoic-acid-inducible gene I) represents an example of a class of intracellular sensors of viral nucleic acids grouped under the term of RIG-I-like receptors (RLRs). Thanks to its C-terminal helicase domain, RIG-I binds viral RNA and becomes activated to transduce CARD-dependent signaling ultimately resulting in an antiviral response mediated by type I interferon production.

microbial pathogens. TLRs are a large class of PPR characterized by an extracellular leucine-rich repeat (LRR) domain and an intracellular Toll/IL-1 receptor (TIR) domain (Fig. 3-2). To date, 13 TLRs have been identified in humans, and they each recognize distinct PAMPs derived from various microbial pathogens, including viruses, bacteria, fungi, and protozoa (Table 3-2).[3,7]

Certain TLRs (TLR1, -2, -4, -5, -6, -10) are expressed at the cell surface and mainly recognize bacterial products unique to bacteria, whereas others (TLR3, -7, -8, -9, -11, -12, -13) are located almost exclusively in intracellular compartments, including endosomes and lysosomes (Fig. 3-2) and are specialized in recognition of nucleic acids, with self- versus nonself-discrimination provided by the exclusive

TABLE 3-2   Toll-Like Receptors Identified in Humans

TLR	CELLULAR LOCALIZATION	LIGAND (S)	MICROBIAL SOURCE
TLR1	Cell surface	Lipopeptides	Bacteria, mycobacteria
TLR2	Cell surface	Zymosan	Fungi
		Peptidoglycans	Gram-positive bacteria
		Lipoteichoic acids	Gram-positive bacteria
		Lipoarabinomannan	Mycobacteria
		Porins	*Neisseria*
		Envelope glycoproteins	Viruses (e.g., measles, HSV, CMV)
TLR3	Endolysosomal compartment	dsRNA	Viruses
TLR4	Cell surface and endolysosomal compartment	LPS	Gram-negative bacteria
		Lipoprotein	Many pathogens
		HSP60	*Chlamydia pneumoniae*
		Fusion protein	RSV
TLR5	Cell surface	Flagellin	Bacteria
TLR6	Cell surface	Diacyl lipopeptides	Mycoplasma
		Lipoteichoic acid	Gram-positive bacteria
TLR7	Endolysosomal compartment	ssRNA and short dsRNA	Viruses and bacteria
TLR8	Endolysosomal compartment	ssRNA and short dsRNA	Viruses and bacteria
TLR9	Endolysosomal compartment	Unmethylated CpG DNA	Bacteria, protozoa, viruses
TLR10	Cell surface	Unknown	—
TLR11	Endolysosomal compartment	Profilin and flagellin	Apicomplexan parasites
TLR12	Endolysosomal compartment	Profilin	Apicomplexan parasites
TLR13	Endolysosomal compartment	Bacterial 23S rRNA	Gram-negative bacteria

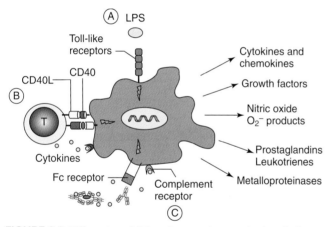

FIGURE 3-2 Different modalities of macrophage activation. **A**, Recognition of conserved molecular constituents of microbes (in the figure, LPS: lipopolysaccharide) by specific receptors (i.e., Toll-like receptors, mannose-receptor, scavenger-receptors). **B**, T-cell-mediated activation via IFN-γ and CD40-CD40-ligand (L) interaction. **C**, Recognition of antibodies, immune complexes, and complement by the membrane receptors for the Fc fragment of immunoglobulins and complement receptors. The main effector soluble mediators produced after macrophage activation are also shown.

localization of the ligands rather than solely based on a unique molecular structure different from that of the host.[4,5,8]

The key cell types expressing TLRs are antigen-presenting cells (APCs), including macrophages, dendritic cells (DCs), and B lymphocytes. Ligand binding to TLRs through PAMP–TLR interaction induces receptor oligomerization, which triggers intracellular signal transduction, resulting in the generation of an antimicrobial proinflammatory response that is also able to involve and orient the adaptive immune system.

In addition to transmembrane receptors on the cell surface and in endosomal compartments, there are intracellular (cytosolic) receptors that function in the pattern recognition of bacterial and viral pathogens. These include nucleotide-binding oligomerization domain (NOD)-like receptors (NLRs)[9,10,11] and the intracellular sensors of viral nucleic acids, such as RIG-I (retinoic-acid-inducible gene I) or melanoma differentiation-associated gene 5 (MDA5), grouped under the term *RIG-I-like receptors* (RLRs)[4] (Fig. 3-1).

NLRs are a family of about 23 intracellular proteins with a common protein-domain organization but diverse functions[12] (Table 3-3). NLRs are composed of a variable N-terminal effector region consisting of caspase recruitment domain (CARD), pyrin domain (PYD), acidic domain, or baculovirus inhibitor repeats (BIRs), a centrally located NOD (or NACTH) domain that is critical for activation, and C-terminal leucine-rich repeats (LRRs) that sense PAMPs (Fig. 3-1). NOD and NLRP subfamilies are the most characterized among NLRs.[11]

The proteins of the NOD subfamily—NOD1 and NOD2—are involved in sensing bacterial molecules derived from synthesis and degradation of peptidoglycan.[13] Whereas NOD1 recognizes diaminopimelic acid produced primarily by Gram-negative bacteria,[14] NOD2 is activated by muramyl dipeptide (MDP), a component of both Gram-positive and Gram-negative bacteria.[15] The NLRP subfamily of NLRs has 14 members, and at least some of these are involved in the induction of the inflammatory response mediated by the IL-1 family of cytokines, which includes interleukin (IL)-1β and IL-18.[16] These cytokines are synthesized as inactive precursors that are cleaved by the proinflammatory caspases, such as caspases 1, 4, 5. These caspases are activated in a multisubunit complex called the inflammasome.

Most PRRs sense not only pathogens but also misfolded/glycated proteins or exposed hydrophobic portions of molecules released at high levels by injured cells; this has therefore been termed *damage-associated molecular pattern* (DAMP).[17,18] DAMP molecules, including high-mobility group box 1 protein (HMGB-1), heat-shock proteins

TABLE 3-3 The Human NOD-Like Receptor (NLR) Family Classification

NAME*	OTHER NAMES	MICROBIAL MOTIFS RECOGNIZED	NLR FAMILY
CIITA	NLRA, C2TA		NLRA
NAIP	NLRB1, BIRC1		NLRB
NOD1	NLRC1, CARD4,	GM-tripeptide	NLRC
NOD2	NLRC2, CARD15, BLAU	MDP	
NLRC3	NOD3	Flagellin from	
NLRC4	CARD12, IPAF	Salmonella, Shigella,	
NLRC5	NOD27	Listeria, Pseudomonas	
NLRP1	NALP1, CARD7	MDP	NLRP
NLRP2	NALP2, PYPAF2	Bacterial RNA, viral	
NLRP3	NALP3, CIAS1, Cryopyrin, PYPAF3	RNA, uric acid crystals, LPS, MDP	
NLRP4	NALP4, PYPAF4		
NLRP5	NALP5, PYPAF8		
NLRP6	NALP6, PYPAF5		
NLRP7	NALP7, PYPAF3		
NLRP8	NALP8, NOD16		
NLRP9	NALP9, NOD6		
NLRP10	NALP10, NOD8		
NLRP11	NALP11, PYPAF6, NOD17		
NLRP12	NALP12, PYPAF2, Monarch1		
NLRP13	NALP13, NOD14		
NLRP14	NALP14, NOD5		
NLRXI	NOD9		NLRX

*According to the Human Genome Organization Gene Nomenclature Committee (HGNC).

(HSPs), uric acid, altered matrix proteins, and S100 proteins, represent important *danger signals* that mediate inflammatory responses through TLRs or NLRPs, or other specific receptor like RAGE (receptor for advanced glycation end products) after release from activated or necrotic cells. The term *alarmins* has also been proposed for DAMP molecules.[17] A prototypic DAMP molecule—the nuclear protein HMGB-1—is either passively released by necrotic cells or actively secreted with delay by activated cells.[19] S100A8, S100A9, and S100A12 (also called *calgranulins*) are calcium-binding proteins expressed in the cytoplasm of phagocytes and secreted by activated monocytes or neutrophils.[20] Once released from cells, calgranulins exert numerous extracellular functions. Secreted S100A8/A9 complexes bind specifically to endothelial cells and directly activate the microvascular endothelium, leading to loss of barrier function, apoptosis of endothelial cells, upregulation of thrombogenic factors, and an increase of junctional permeability. S100A8/A9 and S100A12 upregulate expression and affinity of the integrin receptor on neutrophils and facilitate their adhesion to fibrinogen and to fibronectin and the adhesion of monocytes to the endothelium *in vitro*. In addition, the S100A8/A9 complex, as well as S100A8 itself, bind to and signal directly through the lipopolysaccharide receptor complex including TLR4, MD2, and CD14. The binding to both receptors is able to induce the activation of a number of intracellular proinflammatory pathways (see below).[21] The phagocyte-specific calgranulins S100A8, A9, and A12 are secreted by activated phagocytes and bind to PRRs, which mediates downstream signaling and promotes both inflammation and autoimmunity in a number of immune-mediated conditions.[21]

Downstream Effects of the Stimulation of PRRs

Phagocytosis. The binding of microbes to phagocytes through PRRs initiates the process of phagocytosis of microorganisms and their subsequent destruction in phagolysosomes.[22] The activation of phagocytes through PPRs also induces effector molecules such as inducible nitric oxide synthase and other antimicrobial peptides that can directly destroy microbial pathogens. This is particularly true for polymorphonuclear neutrophils, which are the major contributors on the immediate innate immune response. Their capacity of phagocytosis exceeds that of macrophages, but their capacity to synthesize RNA and proteins is low.[2] Neutrophils are the major source of oxidants, including reactive oxygen species (ROS) and reactive nitrogen species (RNS), which participates in regulation of the immune response and intracellular killing of bacterial pathogens. The main source of ROS in neutrophils is the membrane-bound enzyme complex nicotinamide adenine dinucleotide phosphate (NADPH) oxidase.

Peptides are generated from microbial proteins and presented by professional APCs, such as DCs to T cells to initiate adaptive immune response. Following antigen uptake DCs become activated and migrate to regional lymph nodes to present antigenic peptides in the context of relevant major histocompatibility complex (MHC) molecules. During this process, phagocytosis, upregulation of costimulatory molecules (including CD80, CD86, and CD40, and antigen-presenting MHC molecules), switches in chemokine receptor expression, and cytokine secretion are all events that are regulated through the recognition of pathogens by PRRs expressed on DCs.[22]

The intracellular signaling after stimulation of PPRs. Upon engagement of TLRs by individual PAMPs, a number of different signaling pathways are triggered. Signal transduction is mediated initially by a family of adapter molecules, which at least in part determines the specificity of the response.[4,23] Recruitment of one or several adapter molecules to a given TLR is followed by activation of downstream signal transduction pathways via phosphorylation, ubiquitination, or protein–protein interactions, ultimately culminating in activation of transcription factors that regulate the expression of genes involved in inflammation and antimicrobial host defense[6] (Fig. 3-2). TLR-induced signaling pathways can be broadly classified on the basis of their utilization of different adapter molecules, i.e., dependent on or independent of the adapter MyD88 or TIR domain-containing adapter inducing interferon (IFN)-γ (TRIF), and, additionally, their respective activation of individual kinases and transcription factors.[4,23] Three major signaling pathways responsible for mediating TLR-induced responses include (1) nuclear factor kB (NF-κB), (2) mitogen-activated protein kinases (MAPKs), and (3) IFN regulatory factors (IRFs).[24] Whereas NF-κB and MAPKs play central roles in induction of a proinflammatory response, IRFs are essential for stimulation of IFN production[4,6] (Fig. 3-3).

Following ligand binding, TLRs dimerize and undergo conformational changes required for the subsequent recruitment of cytosolic TIR domain-containing adapter molecules.[23]

MyD88,[25] is involved in signaling triggered by all TLRs, with the exception of TLR3, and plays a major role in TLR-induced signal transduction.[26] In response to TLR4 stimulation by an appropriate PAMP, MyD88 associates with the cytoplasmic part of the receptor and recruits members of the IL-1 receptor (IL-1R)-associated kinase (IRAK) family. IRAK1 or IRAK2 associate with TRAF6, which catalyzes the synthesis of transforming growth factor-activated protein kinase1 (TAK1) and the IκB kinase (IKK) subunit NF-κB essential modifier

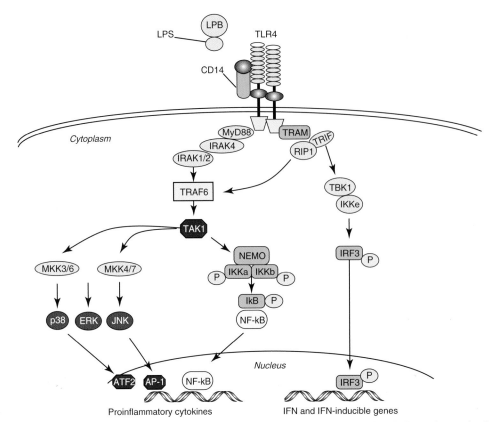

FIGURE 3-3 Toll-Like receptors signaling pathways: MyD88-dependent and MyD88-independent activation of TLR4. Lipopolysaccharide (LPS) binds to the CD14 molecule present on phagocyte surface. Then, the LPS-CD14 complex associates to TLR4 for the subsequent intracellular signaling. The lipopolysaccharide binding protein (LPB) is a circulating protein that binds to LPS in the blood or extracellular fluid, forming a complex that facilitate LPS binding to CD14. The MyD88-dependent signaling pathway is responsible for the early-phase NF-κB and mitogen-activated protein kinases (MAPKs) activation that control the induction of proinflammatory cytokines (see text). The MyD88-independent pathway ultimately activates IFN regulatory factor 3 (IRF-3), which is required for the induction of interferon (IFN)-β and IFN-inducible genes. This latter pathway also mediates the late-phase NF-κB and MAPK activation through the activation of TRAF-6 and TAK1.

(NEMO). TAK1 then stimulates two distinct pathways involving the IKK complex and the MAPK pathway, respectively[4,27] (Fig. 3-3).

NF-κB exists in an inactive form in the cytoplasm physically associated with its inhibitory protein inhibitor of NF-κB (IκB). Upon inflammatory stimuli, IκB is phosphorylated and degraded releasing NF-κB dimers, which translocate to the nucleus. Phosphorylation of IκB is performed by IκB kinase (IKK). NF-κB binds to promoters or enhancers of target genes in the nucleus leading to increased transcription and expression.[4,7,27]

MAPKs are an important kinase family involved in rapid downstream inflammatory signal transduction resulting in activation of several nuclear proteins and transcription factors.[28] MAPK pathways are activated through sequential phosphorylations, beginning with activation of MAPK kinase kinase (MAPKKK), which phosphorylates and activates MAPK kinase (MAPKK), which in turn activates MAPK by phosphorylation. MAPK pathways include p38, JNK, and ERK. The pathways p38 and JNK phosphorylate and activate transcription factors such as ATF-2 and AP-1, which are necessary for the upregulation of several proinflammatory molecules.[28] Cytosolic pattern recognition receptors like NLRs and intracellular sensors of viral nucleic acids (RIG and DAI) exert the same function played by the membrane-bound PRRs. For example, the stimulation of NOD1 or NOD2 by bacterial-derived peptidoglycan fragments results in the activation of NF-kB and MAPKs, which drive the transcription of numerous genes involved in both innate and adaptive immune responses.[4,7,29]

Innate immune cells can be activated through interaction with a number of other cells and soluble factors of the immune system as a response of pathogen recognition. Thus macrophage and neutrophils are activated by immune complexes and complement fragments through the binding with immunoglobulin and complement receptors expressed on their surface (Fig. 3-2). The functional activity of macrophages upon stimulation of PPRs is highly influenced by the environmental conditions and by the interaction with other cells. In response to signals derived from microbes, damaged tissues, or activated lymphocytes, it has been suggested that macrophages may develop into one of two different states: the classically activated M1 phenotype and the alternatively activated M2 phenotype[30] (Fig. 3-4). T helper (Th)1-related cytokines such as IFN-γ, as well as microbicidal stimuli, polarize macrophages to an M1 phenotype. M1 macrophages produce high levels of IL-12 and IL-23 and other molecules engaged in inflammatory, microbicidal, and tumoricidal activities (Fig. 3-4). In contrast, Th2 cytokines such as IL-4 and IL-13 polarize macrophages to an alternatively activated (or M2) phenotype, characterized by immunomodulatory mediators such as IL-10, IL-1 decoy receptor,

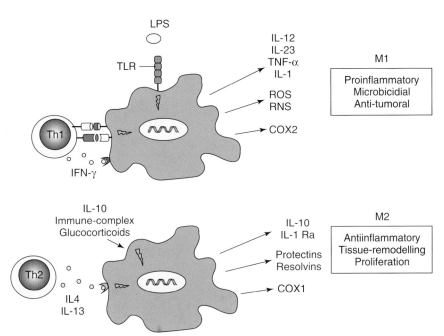

FIGURE 3-4 Schematic representation of the M1- and M2-polarization of macrophages. *COX,* Cyclo-oxygenases; *IL,* interleukin; *IL1Ra,* IL-1 receptor antagonist; *IFN,* interferon; *LPS,* lipopolysaccharide; *ROS,* reactive oxygen species; *RNS,* reactive nitrogen specis; *Th,* T helper; *TNF,* tumor necrosis factor.

and IL-1 receptor antagonist (IL1Ra). M2 macrophages dampen inflammation, promote tissue remodeling and repair, help in parasite clearance and tumor progression, and possess immunoregulatory functions[31] (Fig. 3-4).

The Inflammasome and Its Role in the Secretion of IL-1β

The role of some cytosolic PRRs is complementary to that of membrane-bound TLRs for the activation of the inflammatory response: an example is the role of some NLRP proteins in the activation and secretion of the active form of IL-1β (Fig. 3-4). Unlike most cytokines, IL-1β (together with IL-18 and IL-33) lacks a secretory signal peptide and is externalized by through a nonclassical pathway, arranged in two steps.[32,33] TLR ligands such as LPS induce gene expression and synthesis of the inactive IL-1β precursor (pro-IL-1β). The activation of caspase-1 then catalyzes cleavage of pro-IL-1β to the 17kd active form.[16,34] The protein complex responsible for this catalytic activity is termed the *inflammasome.*[35] The inflammasome is composed of the adapter ASC (apoptosis-associated speck-like protein containing a CARD), pro-caspase-1, and an NLR family member (such as NLRP1, NLRP3 or Ipaf [Ice protease-activating factor]).[35] Oligomerization of these proteins through CARD/CARD interactions results in activation of caspase-1, which cleaves the accumulated IL-1 precursor, resulting in secretion of biologically active IL-1.[16] A growing number of NLR proteins have been shown to have the capacity to activate caspase-1, each recognizing different danger signals or PAMPs through their respective receptors[36,37] (Fig. 3-5).

NLRP3 has been ascribed a role in recognition of adenosine triphosphate (ATP),[34] uric acid crystals,[36] viral RNA,[38] and bacterial DNA.[39] These stimuli play a crucial second hit for the secretion of IL-1β (Fig. 3-6). Indeed, monocytes stimulated with LPS alone release approximately only 20% of IL-1β.[40] A second stimulus, such as exogenous ATP, strongly enhances proteolytic maturation and secretion of IL-1β.[41] ATP-triggered IL-1β secretion is mediated by P2X7 receptors expressed on the surface of monocytes.[42] Notably, knockout mice deficient in cryopyrin cannot activate caspase-1 upon LPS and ATP stimulation, resulting in lack of IL-1β secretion.[34] Mutations in the cryopyrin gene in humans are associated with diseases characterized by excessive

production of IL-1β, called *cryopyrinpathies,*[16,43,44] which belong to the group of the autoinflammatory diseases (see also Chapter 47).

Recent evidence suggests a role for oxidative stress in the activation of the NLRP3-inflammasome.[45,46] The exposure of human monocyte to PAMPs and DAMPs induces oxidative stress in the cells through the production of ROS. The extent to which ROS accumulate in the cells is determined by the antioxidant systems that enable cells to maintain redox homeostasis.[47] Under normal conditions, these systems balance the constitutive generation of ROS. Both events—oxidant and antioxidant—are required for the secretion of IL-1β after DAMP or PAMP triggering[48,49] (Fig. 3-6).

An additional pathway of activation of NLR3 inflammasome has been recently identified.[50] Increased intracellular Ca2+ and decreased cellular cyclic AMP (cAMP) are able to induce NLRP3 activation through calcium-sensing receptor (CASR). Ca2+ or other CASR agonists (gadolinium or R-568) activate the NLRP3 inflammasome in the absence of exogenous ATP, whereas knockdown of CASR reduces inflammasome activation in response to known NLRP3 activators.[50]

Dendritic Cells

DCs are specialized APCs that originate from the bone marrow and play a critical role in the processing and presentation of antigen to T cells during the adaptive immune response[51,52]; they can be considered as a bridge between innate and adaptive immunity. At the immature stage of development, DCs act as sentinels in the epithelia of peripheral tissues (skin, gastrointestinal, and respiratory systems) continuously sampling the antigenic environment. These cells are morphologically identified by their extensive membrane projections. Recognition of microbial or viral products through PRR on the surface of phagocytes initiates the migration of DCs to lymph nodes where they mature (express costimulatory molecules) to present antigen to T cells.[51,53]

DCs control or influence many aspects of T-cell responses; this is further elaborated in Chapter 4. For example, under the control of DCs, helper T cells acquire the capacity to produce powerful cytokines such as IFN-γ to activate macrophages to resist infection by facultative and obligate intracellular microbes (Th1 cells); or IL-4, -5, and -13 to mobilize white cells that resist helminths (Th2 cells); or IL-17 to

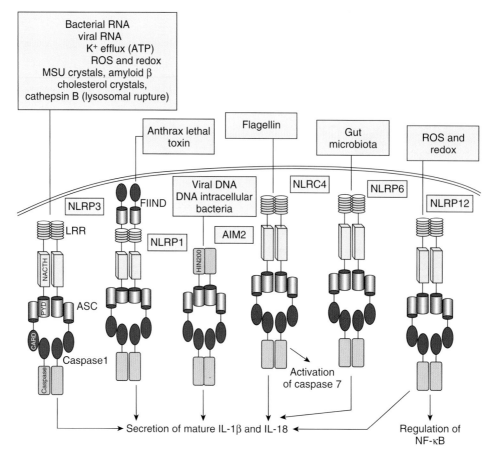

FIGURE 3-5 The inflammasomes. Different exogenous and endogenous stimuli are able to activate the NLRP3 and other inflammasomes belonging to the NLR (Nod-like receptor) family. A second class of inflammasomes has also been described that do not contain NLRs but instead contain members of the PYHIN family. The PYHIN proteins are characterized by the presence of a PYD and one or two HIN-200 DNA-binding domains.

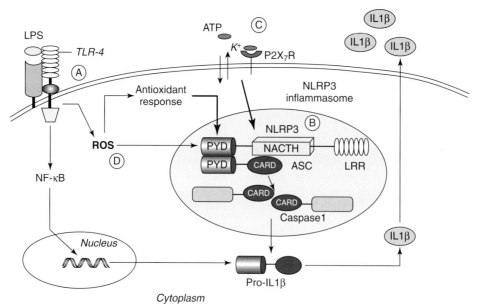

FIGURE 3-6 Role of cryopyrin (NALP3) in the activation of inflammasome and induction of IL-1β secretion. **A**, Toll-like receptor (TLR) ligands, such as LPS, are the first signal for gene expression and synthesis of the inactive IL 1β precursor (pro-IL-1β). **B**, After stimulation, NLRP3 oligomerizes and becomes available for the binding of the adapter protein ASC (apoptosis-associated speck-like protein containing a CARD). This association activates directly two molecules of caspase-1, which, in turn converts pro-IL-1 β to the mature, active 17 kDa form. A second stimulus, such as exogenous ATP (**C**) or ROS (reactive oxygen species) and antiredox response (**D**), strongly enhances proteolytic maturation and secretion of IL-1β.

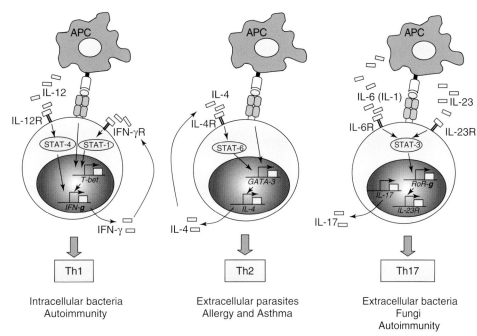

FIGURE 3-7 The role of dendritic cells in the differentiation of Th1, Th2, and Th17 effector T cells. Cytokines produced in the innate immune response to microbes or early in adaptive immune response influence the differentiation of naïve CD4+ T cells into Th1, Th2, and Th17 cells. IL-12 produced by antigen-presenting cells induces the transcription of interferon (IFN)-γ (Th1 development) through a STAT-4 dependent pathway. The transcription factor T-beta, produced in response to IFN-γ, amplifies the Th1 response. The stimulation of naïve T cells in presence of IL-4 favors the differentiation of Th2 cells through a STAT-6 dependent pathway. The transcription factor GATA-3 is critical for Th2 differentiation. In humans, IL-1, IL-6, and IL-23 induce the transcription of IL-17 (Th17 development) through a STAT-3 dependent pathway. The transcription factor RoR-γt is critical for IL-17 and expression of IL-23 receptor that is essential for the stabilization and amplification of Th17 response. For sake of simplicity, other cytokines produced by Th1 (IL-2, TNF-α, lymphotoxin), Th2 (IL-5, IL-10, IL-13), and Th17 (IL-21, IL-22) are not reported in the present figure.

mobilize phagocytes at body surfaces to resist extracellular bacilli (Th17 cells) (Fig. 3-7).[54] Alternatively, DCs can guide T cells to become suppressive by making IL-10 (T regulatory cells) or by differentiating into FOXP positive regulatory T cells (see also Chapter 4).

Plasmocytoid DCs (pDCs) are a distinct subtype of DCs that display the unique capacity to secrete large amounts of type I IFN (α/β) in response to certain viruses and other microbial stimuli (they are also called *plasmacytoid interferon producing cells*). Viral nucleic acids, as well as self-nucleoproteins internalized in the form of immune complexes, trigger TLR7 and TLR9 expressed by pDCs, leading to type I IFN production.[55] Plasmocytoid DCs have been implicated in several autoimmune conditions including systemic lupus erythematous (see Chapter 23) and juvenile dermatomyositis (see Chapter 26).

Natural Killer Cells

Natural killer (NK) cells are large lymphocytes characterized by the presence of cytoplasmic granules containing proteins with proteolytic activities (perforin, granzymes) that lack antigen-specific receptors but are able to kill abnormal cells such as some tumor cells and virus-infected cells.[56] Activation of NK cells is regulated through activating and inhibitory cell surface receptors.[57] The inhibitory receptors bind to self-class I MHC molecules, which are normally expressed on the surface of the majority of cell types (Fig. 3-6). The ligands for activating receptors are only partially known. The engagement of both inhibitory and activating receptors results in a dominant effect of the inhibitory receptors. The infection of host cells, for example, by some viruses, leads to the loss of class I MHC from their surface and exposes

these cells to the exclusive activity of activating receptors (Fig. 3-8).[56] Once activated, NK cells release the contents of their granules. Perforin creates pores in target cell membranes, and granzymes enter into the cells through the perforin pores, inducing the death of target cells by apoptosis, with the same mechanism of cytolysis used by CD8 cytotoxic T cells.

Other important activities of NK cells include their ability to recognize (via Fc receptors) and destroy antibody-coated cells (a process called *antibody-dependent cell-mediated cytotoxicity* [ADCC]), and to produce high amounts of IFN-γ, a potent stimulator of macrophage activity, as well as tumor necrosis factor (TNF)-α, granulocyte macrophage colony-stimulating factor (GMCSF), and other cytokines and chemokines. Production of these soluble factors by NK cells in early innate responses influences the recruitment and function of other hematopoietic cells. In turn, activated macrophages produce IL-12, a potent inducer of NK cell IFN-γ production and cytolytic activity (Fig. 3-8).

Two major subsets of NK cells are found in human subjects according to their level of expression of CD56, namely CD56dim and CD56bright. CD56dim NK cells represent the 90% of NK cells in peripheral blood. They are fully mature and mediated cytotoxicity response. In contrast, CD56bright cells are more immature and play a major role in the cytokine production. Moreover, this immature subpopulation is better able to leave the circulation and constitute the majority of NK cells found in lymphoid organs.[58] Familial hemophagocytic lymphohistiocytosis (FHL) is a genetically heterogeneous disorder caused by mutations in genes involved in the secretory lysosome-dependent exocytosis

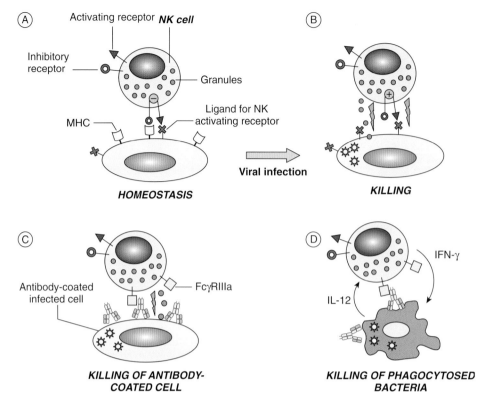

FIGURE 3-8 Functional properties of NK cells. **A**, The inhibitory receptors bind to self-class I MHC molecules that are normally expressed on the surface of the majority of cell types. **B**, The infection of the host cells by virus leads to the loss of class I MHC from their surface and exposes the infected cells to the exclusive activity of activating receptors and subsequent killing. **C**, NK cells recognize antibody-coated cells trough the Fc receptors expressed on their surface and subsequently kill the infected cell. **D**, NK cells respond to IL-12 produced by macrophages during phagocytosis and secrete IFN-γ, which, in turn, further on activate macrophage to kill phagocytosed microbes.

pathway, and it is clinically characterized by a hyperinflammatory syndrome usually triggered by viral infections. Children with autoimmune diseases, especially systemic juvenile idiopathic arthritis (sJIA), may develop a clinical syndrome closely resembling FLH called *macrophage activation syndrome* (MAS). Even if patients with MAS have normal or reduced NK function, reduced expression of perforin and heterozygous mutations in one FHL-related genes have been observed (see also Chapter 16).

Fibroblasts

Fibroblasts, together with cartilage cells, bone cells, and fat cells, belong to the family of connective-tissue cells. All of these cells are specialized in the secretion of collagenous extracellular matrix (ECM) and provide mechanical strength to tissue by providing a supporting framework to the ECM itself. Connective-tissue cells play a central part in repair mechanisms. Tissue fibroblasts may play an active role in the effector arm of the inflammatory response and in immune mediated diseases. During inflammation, proinflammatory cytokines produced by tissue macrophages activate tissue fibroblasts to produce cytokines, chemokines, prostaglandins (PGE_2), and proteolytic enzymes such as metalloproteinases. The failure to switch off activated tissue fibroblasts has been proposed as a possible mechanism leading to chronic inflammation, through the persistent overexpression of chemokine and proinflammatory cytokines, and consequent continuous recruitment of leukocytes within tissues.[59] The late mechanisms play a crucial role in the pathogenesis of scleroderma (see Chapter 27).

Connective tissue contains a mixture of distinct fibroblast lineages including "mature" fibroblasts with a lesser capacity of transformation, and immature fibroblasts (called also *mesenchimal* fibroblasts) that are capable of differentiating into several different cell lineages. Moreover, fibroblast precursors with a multipotent character also circulate in blood and, due to their similarity with stromal cells of bone marrow, are called *mesenchymal stem cells*.

Molecules of Innate Immunity
The Complement System

The complement system consists of several normally inactive plasma proteins, which, after activation under particular conditions, interact to generate products that mediate important effector functions, including promotion of phagocytosis lysis of microbes and stimulation of inflammation. Activation of complement involves sequential proteolytic steps that generate an enzymatic cascade similar to that of the coagulation system.[60]

There are three major pathways of complement activation (Fig. 3-9). The *alternative* pathway is related to the direct binding of one of the complement proteins, C3b to microbial cells. The *classical* pathway involves a more sophisticated mode of activation, in which a plasma protein, C1 binds to the C_H2 domains of immunoglobulin (Ig) G or to C_H3 domains of IgM that have bound antigen. The same proteins involved in the classical pathway can be activated in absence of antibodies by plasma proteins (mannose-binding lectin [MBL] or ficolins) (*lectin* pathway). Activation of the lectin pathway occurs through direct

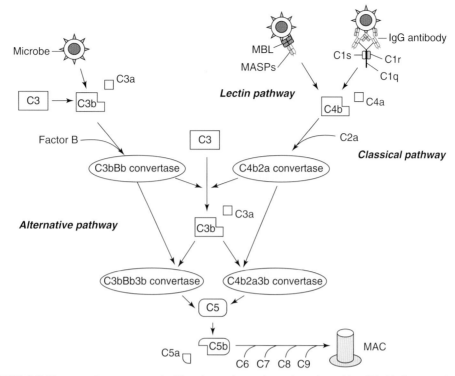

FIGURE 3-9 The complement cascade. The alternative pathway is activated by C3b binding to microbial cell wall, after spontaneous cleavage of free circulating C3. Thereafter, C3b binds to factor B forming a C3bBb convertase. The classical pathway is initiated by the binding of the trimolecular complex C1 (C1q, C1r, C1s) to antigen–antibody complexes. The same proteins involved in the classical pathway can be activated in absence of antibodies by a plasma protein called mannose-binding lectin (MBL), which binds to mannose residues on microbial glycoproteins and glycolipids (lectin pathway). The following binding with the C4b and C2a subunits leads to the formation of the C4b2a convertase. The three pathways of complement activation converge into a central protein, C3, which is cleaved into two fragments. The larger fragment (C3b) activates C5 with subsequent generation of C5b, which is the initiator of the formation of a complex of the complement proteins C6, C7, C8, and C9, which is assembled on the membrane of microbes (membrane attack complex, MAC). *MASP*, MBL-associated serine proteases.

recognition of carbohydrate or acetylated PAMPs by MBL and ficolins, respectively, in association with MBL-associated serine proteases (MASPs).[61]

The three pathways of complement activation converge upon a central protein (C3), which is cleaved into two fragments. The larger fragment (C3b) becomes covalently attached to microbes where it acts as an opsonin to stimulate phagocytosis and activates C5 with subsequent generation of C5b. C5b initiates the formation of a complex of the complement proteins C6, C7, C8, and C9 (membrane attack complex [MAC]); the MAC then forms a pore that causes lysis of the target cell (Fig. 3-9). During complement activation smaller complement fragments (C3a, C4a, C5a) are generated and released into the circulation. These exert several proinflammatory effects including activation of mast cells and neutrophils, and an increase in vascular permeability.[60,62] Another function of complement is to bind to antigen–antibody complexes, promoting their solubilization and their clearance by phagocytes. Complement has a pivotal role in the clearance of apoptotic blebs by the phagocytic system.[63] The implications of this mechanism in the pathogenesis of SLE have been recently pointed out[60,64] (see also Chapter 23).

The biological activities of complement are mediated by the binding of complement fragments to membrane receptors. Receptors for the fragments of C3 are best characterized (Table 3-4). Type 1 complement receptor (CR1, CD35) is expressed by almost all blood cells and

promote phagocytosis of C3b-coated microbes. CR1 expressed on erythrocytes binds to circulating immune complexes with attached C3b. In this way circulating erythrocytes are able to transport immune complexes to the liver and spleen, where they are removed from erythrocyte surface and cleared. Type 2 complement receptor (CR2, CD21) is present on B lymphocytes and follicular dendritic cells of lymph node germinal centers. Its main function is to act as coreceptor for B-cell activation by antigen (discussed below) and to stimulate the trapping of antigen–antibody complexes in germinal centers. Type 3 and type 4 complement receptors are members of the integrin family and are expressed by the cells of innate immunity (neutrophils, NK cells, mononuclear phagocytes). The binding of CR3 or CR4 promotes the activation of these cells and the phagocytosis of microbes opsonized with C3b.

Genetic deficiencies of classical pathway components (C1q, C1r, C2, and C4) causing diseases that resemble SLE are dealt with in Chapter 46.[65] This may be related to the role of the early complement components in the clearance of apoptotic cells and circulating immune complexes. Deficiency of C3 is associated with serious pyogenic infections while defects of the terminal complement components (C5-C9) are associated with an increased risk of disseminated *Neisseria* infections (see also Chapter 46).

Activation of the complement cascade is regulated by a number of circulating and cell membrane proteins that prevent activation on

TABLE 3-4 Complement Receptors

RECEPTOR	CELL TYPES	LIGANDS	FUNCTION

CR1 (CD35)	B and T cells
	Erythrocytes
	Monocytes,
	  macrophages
	Eosinophils
	FDC, neutrophils
		C3b, C4b,
		iC3b
			C3b and C4b decay
			Clearance of
			  immune
			  complexes
			Phagocytosis

CR2 (CD21)	B cell
	FDC
	Upper airways
	  epithelium
		C3d, C3dg,
		iC3b
			Activation of B cell
			  (coreceptor)
			Antigen presentation
			  in germinal
			  centers
			Receptor for EBV

CR3 (CD11b/
CD18)
	Macrophages
	Neutrophils, NK
	  cells
	Dendritic cells,
	  FDCs
		iC3b, ICAM	Phagocytosis
			Adhesion to
			  endothelium (via
			  ICAM)

CR4 (CD11c/ CD18)	Macrophages Neutrophils, NK cells Dendritic cells	iC3b	Phagocytosis

EBV, Epstein–Barr virus; *FDC*, follicular dendritic cells; *ICAM*, intracellular adhesion molecule; *NK*, natural killer.

normal host cells and limit the duration of complement activation on microbial cells and antigen–antibody complexes. The C1 inhibitor (C1 INH) regulates the proteolytic activity of C1, the initiator of the classical pathway of complement activation. Deficiency of this protein causes hereditary angioneurotic edema (see Chapter 46). A number of membrane proteins (membrane cofactor protein [MCP], type 1 complement receptor [CR1], decay-accelerating factor [DAF]) and the plasma protein factor H prevent the activation of C3b if it is deposited on the surfaces of normal mammalian cells. Acquired somatic mutations in the phosphatidylinositol glycan class A (PIGA) gene in the hematopoietic stem cells (HSCs) of patients affected by paroxysmal nocturnal hemoglobinuria. The presence of these mutations leads to production of blood cells with decreased glycosyl phosphatidylinositol-anchored cell surface proteins, making red blood cells derived from the clone more sensitive to complement-mediated hemolysis. Similarly, the rare deficiency of factor H is characterized by an excess alternative pathway activation leading to C3 consumption and glomerulonephritis.

Other Circulating Proteins

A number of circulating proteins behave as secreted PPRs by their ability to specifically recognize microbial PAMPs and promote innate immunity. MBL belonging to the collectin family of proteins has a collagen-like domain separated by a neck region from a calcium-dependent (C-type) lectin.[61,66] MBL binds carbohydrates with terminal mannose and fucose, typically found on surface glycoproteins of bacterial, but not mammalian, cells. MBL is structurally similar to the C1q, binds the C1q receptor present on phagocytes, and may activate complement. Thus MBL is able to opsonize microbes and induce phagocyte activation via the C1q receptor.[61]

C-reactive protein (CRP) and serum amyloid protein (SAP) are plasma proteins belonging to the family of pentraxins.[67] They are abundantly produced during the acute phase of inflammation by

the liver and bind to phosphorylcholine present on the microbial membranes. Moreover they are also able to activate the classical complement pathway and to act as opsonins for neutrophils. The lipopolysaccharide binding protein (LPB) is a circulating protein that binds to LPS in the blood or extracellular fluid, forming a complex that facilitates LPS binding to CD14. Other circulating proteins that participate in innate immunity include defensins, which are diverse members of a large family of antimicrobial peptides, contributing to the antimicrobial action of granulocytes, mucosal host defense in the small intestine, and epithelial host defense in the skin and elsewhere.[68,69]

THE INFLAMMATORY RESPONSE

The acute inflammatory response triggered by infection or tissue injury involves the coordinated delivery of blood components (plasma and leukocytes) to the site of infection or injury. During bacterial infections this response is triggered by PPRs of the innate immune system, such as TLRs and membrane or intracellular sensors. This initial recognition of infection is mediated by tissue-resident macrophages and mast cells, leading to the production of a variety of inflammatory mediators (vasoactive amines, cytokines, chemokines, eicosanoids, and products of proteolytic cascades).[70] This response leads to a local inflammatory exudate: plasma proteins and leukocytes (mainly neutrophils) migrate from blood vessels to the extravascular tissues at the site of infection (or injury) through the postcapillary venules. The activated endothelium of the blood vessels allows selective extravasation of neutrophils and, later, other leukocytes. After their recruitment to the site of infection, neutrophils become activated, either by direct contact with pathogens or through the actions of cytokines secreted by tissue-resident cells. The neutrophils attempt to kill the invading agents by releasing the toxic contents of their granules, which include ROS and RNS, and proteolytic enzymes (proteinase 3, cathepsin G, and elastase 5). The lack of specificity of these highly potent effectors do not prevent the possible damage to host tissue, as collateral effect.[70]

A successful acute inflammatory response results in the elimination of the infectious agents followed by a resolution and repair phase. Conversely, if the acute inflammatory response fails to eliminate the pathogen, the inflammatory process persists and acquires new characteristics. In this case, the neutrophil infiltration is gradually replaced by recently immigrated monocytes differentiating into macrophages, and T cells (see also type IV delayed type hypersensitivity below). The characteristics of this inflammatory state can differ depending on the effector class of the T cells (Th1, Th2, Th17) (see Chapter 4). If the combined effect of these cells is insufficient, a chronic inflammatory state may ensue, involving the formation of tertiary lymphoid tissues and granulomas.[71] Unsuccessful attempts by macrophages to engulf and destroy pathogens or foreign bodies can lead to the formation of granulomata, in which the intruders are walled off by layers of macrophages, in a final attempt to protect the host. Chronic inflammation can result not only from the persistence of pathogens, but also from other causes of tissue damage such as autoimmune or autoinflammatory responses, owing to the persistence of self-antigens or DAMPs.

The Recruitment of Leukocytes Into Inflamed Tissue

One of the pivotal mechanisms leading to the initiation and maintenance of tissue inflammation is the migration of leukocytes from the circulation to the site of inflammation.

This is a multistep process involving many different soluble and surface molecules leading to the attachment of circulating cells to endothelial cells and migration through the endothelium (Fig. 3-10).[72,73]

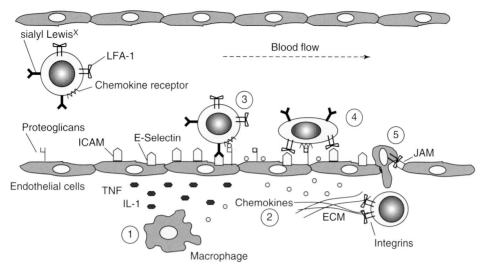

FIGURE 3-10 Recruitment of leukocytes into the inflammatory site. **1,** Proinflammatory cytokines produced by macrophages stimulate the expression of adhesion molecules (selectins and integrin ligands) on the endothelial cells. **2,** Chemokines produced by stromal cells, inflammatory cells and endothelial cells specifically attracts leukocytes bearing specific chemokine receptors. **3,** Leukocytes bearing selectin ligands (i.e., sialyl Lewis^X) weakly adhere to endothelium (rolling). **4,** Leukocytes display a process of integrin affinity maturation stimulated by chemokines. In this way a firm adhesion between leukocytes and endothelium occurs (adhesion). **5,** Transmigration of cells across the endothelial lining into the site of inflammation. The progression of cells through the endothelial cells is allowed by the interaction between other integrins expressed on leukocytes and their specific ligands present at the level of the adherence junction between the endothelial cells (i.e., junctional adhesion molecule [JAM] family) or in the subendothelial extracellular matrix. *ECM,* extracellular matrix; *ICAM,* intracellular adhesion molecule; *IL,* interleukin; *LFA-1,* leukocyte function-associated antigen-1; *TNF,* tumor necrosis factor.

The capture and rolling of circulating cells by activated endothelium is followed by the activation of cells and their firm adhesion to the endothelium, and finally, the migration of cells across the endothelium (diapedesis).[72]

A proinflammatory stimulus (trauma, or infectious or other exogenous agent) leads to the production of proinflammatory cytokines (TNF-α, IL-1) that induce the expression of a series of membrane glycoproteins (selectins) that act as adhesion molecules for circulating leukocytes[74] (Table 3-5). In particular, endothelial (E)-selectin and platelet (P)-derived selectin are selectively expressed on the surface of cytokine-activated endothelial cells. Circulating leukocytes flowing in the bloodstream first loosely adhere to the endothelium through some other constitutively expressed surface glycoproteins (sialyl Lewis^X for E-selectin; P-selectin glycoprotein ligand 1 [PSGL-1] for P-selectin) that allow the sampling of the local environment for signs of inflammation. The second step of leukocyte migration needs their firm adherence to endothelial cells. This is ensured by other surface molecules constitutively expressed on circulating leukocytes, called *integrins*,[75,76] heterodimeric proteins composed of two noncovalently linked polypeptide chains, α and β (Table 3-5). After rolling, leukocytes undergo integrin affinity maturation stimulated by a series of specific cytokines (chemokines, see below). The proinflammatory cytokines (IL-1, TNF-α) mediate overexpression of ligands that are specific for high-affinity integrins; thus firm adhesion between leukocytes and endothelium occurs. During inflammation the very late antigen (VLA)-4 (or α₄β₁) is selectively expressed on leukocytes and mediates their adhesion to activated endothelial cells expressing its ligand, vascular adhesion molecule (VCAM)-1.[76] Similarly, the leukocyte function-associated antigen-1 (LFA-1 or CD11aCD18) binds to its specific ligand, the intracellular adhesion molecule (ICAM). The

specific inhibition of integrins involved in leukocyte recruitment is a therapeutic target pathway in autoimmune diseases.[73,76]

The final step in leukocyte recruitment is the transmigration of cells across the endothelial lining into the site of inflammation. This process is facilitated by the interaction between integrins expressed on leukocytes and their specific ligands present at the level of the adherence junction between the endothelial cells (platelet/endothelial cell adhesion molecule [PECAM-1], junctional adhesion molecule [JAM] family), or in the subendothelial extracellular matrix (fibronectin, osteopontin, collagen) (Table 3-5).[73]

During acute inflammation, mast cells and platelets are stimulated to degranulate and secrete a number of vasoactive amines (histamine and serotonin) that cause increased vascular permeability and vasodilation. Other vasoactive peptides that are stored in sensory neurons (such as substance P) can be released after their activation or generated by proteolytic processing of inactive precursors in the extracellular fluid (for example, kinins, fibrinopeptide A, fibrinopeptide B, and fibrin degradation products). Finally, the complement fragments C3a, C4a, and C5a (the anaphylatoxins) are produced by several pathways of complement activation. C5a (and to a lesser extent C3a and C4a) promote granulocyte and monocyte recruitment and induce mast-cell degranulation.[70]

The Soluble Mediators of Inflammation and the Immune Response

A large number of soluble mediators are involved in the initiation and maintenance of the inflammatory and immune response. These mediators play a pivotal role for proper function of the immune response acting as mediators of cell-to-cell cross-talk, effector factors for the

TABLE 3-5 Adhesion Molecules

FAMILY	NAME	CELL DISTRIBUTION	LIGANDS	MAIN FUNCTIONS
(1) Selectins	P-selectin (CD62P)	Endothelium,* PLT	Sialyl Lewis[X]	Initiate leukocyte-endothelium interactions
	E-selectin (CD62E)	Endothelium*	PSGL-1	
	L-selectin (CD62L)	Leukocytes	GlyCAM-1, CD34, MadCAM-1	
(2) Integrins				
β_1 α_{1-2-3}	VLA-1/3	Leukocytes	Laminin, collagens	Cell matrix-adhesion
α_{4-5}	VLA-4-5		JAM-B	Homing to inflamed tissues
α_6	VLA-6		Fibronectin, Laminin	
α_v	CD51CD29		Vitronectin, fibronectin	
β_2 α_L	LFA-1	Leukocytes	ICAM-1/3, JAM-A	Leukocyte adhesion to endothelium
α_M	MAC-1			Interaction T cell–APC
β_3 α_V	Vitronectin receptor	Leukocytes, endothelium, osteoclasts	Fibronectin, fibrinogen, osteopontin, vitronectin, thrombospondin	Cell matrix-adhesion Leukocyte activation Osteoclast activation Angiogenesis
β_4 α_6	CD49CD104	Leukocytes	Laminin	Cell matrix-adhesion
β_5 α_V		Leukocytes Endothelium	Vitronectin	Cell matrix-adhesion Angiogenesis
β_6 α_V		Leukocytes	Fibronectin	Cell matrix-adhesion
β_7 α_4	LPAM-1	Leukocytes	VCAM-1, fibronectin	Homing to lymphoid tissues
(3) Immunoglobulin superfamily	ICAM-1 (CD54)	Endothelium*	LFA-1, MAC-1	Cell adhesion
	ICAM-2 (CD102)	Dendritic cells	LFA-1	Ligands for integrins
	VCAM-1 (CD106)	Endothelium†	VLA-4	
	PECAM (CD31)	Leukocytes, endothelium	PECAM, $\alpha_V\beta_3$	
(4) Cadherins	VE-cadherin	Endothelium lateral junctions	VE-cadherin	Cell to cell adhesion

*Activated endothelial cells.
†Resting endothelial cells.
ICAM, intracellular adhesion molecule; *JAM*, junctional adhesion molecule; *LFA-1*, leukocyte function-associated antigen-1; *MAC-1*, macrophage 1 antigen; *MadCAM1*, mucosal addressin cell adhesion molecule-1; *PECAM*, platelet/endothelial cell adhesion molecule; *PLT*, platelets; *PSGL-1*, P-selectin glycoprotein ligand 1; *VE-cadherin*, vascular endothelial cadherin; *VLA*, very late antigen.

tissue reaction, and in the later phase, inducers of immune homeostasis and tissue repair.

Cytokines, Chemokines, and Growth Factors

Cytokines and chemokines are proteins secreted by the cells of the innate and adaptive immune systems (microbes, antigens, and other signals) that mediate and regulate the immune and inflammatory responses. Although some cytokines are produced in sufficient quantity to circulate and exert exocrine actions, they typically act locally in autocrine or paracrine fashion. Their functions are mediated by cellular receptors. Cytokine receptors consist of one or more transmembrane proteins whose extracellular portions are responsible for cytokine binding, whereas the cytoplasmic portions mediate the triggering of the intracellular signaling pathway. According to their functional properties, cytokines may be classified into five main categories: (1) interleukins; (2) interferons; (3) proinflammatory and antiinflammatory cytokines (Table 3-6); (4) chemokines, a large family of cytokines produced by various cell types that stimulate and regulate leukocyte migration (see also Table 3-7); and (5) growth factors produced by bone marrow stromal cells and leukocytes that stimulate the differentiation and proliferation of immature leukocytes and sustain the phenomena of angiogenesis.

TNF-α represents a prototype proinflammatory cytokine,[77] originally identified as a soluble molecule present in sera of animals treated with LPS that displayed the ability to cause tumor necrosis *in vivo*.[78] After cell activation, TNF-α is synthesized as a membrane protein that is expressed as a homodimer. It is cleaved by membrane-associated metalloproteinases and released as a 17-kD polypeptide, three of which polymerize to form a 51-kD TNF protein. The various biological actions of TNF-α are mediated by two distinct receptors: 55 kD TNF I (TNFRI or p55 receptor) and 75 kD TNFRII (or p75 receptor).[79] The binding of circulating TNF-α to TNFRs leads to recruitment of cytoplasmic proteins, and TNF receptor-associated factors (TRAFs) that initiate intracellular signaling leading to the activation of transcription factors such as NF-kB and activation protein 1 (AP-1) that cause the production of inflammatory mediators and antiapoptotic proteins[79] (Fig. 3-8). In the case of TNFRI, the binding with TNF-α may lead to either inflammation or apoptosis. In the latter case, different signaling proteins (TNF receptor-associated death domain [TRADD]) are involved and leads to the activation of caspases, which eventually results in cell apoptosis (Fig. 3-8). This latter mechanism represents an important strategy for self-limitation of cell activation.

A key function of TNF-α during inflammation is to stimulate the recruitment of phagocytes into the site of inflammation and promote the killing of microbes. TNF-α also induces the expression of adhesion molecules and chemokines by endothelial cells and enhances the affinity of leukocyte integrins for their ligands. It can activate recently recruited monocytes and stimulate the proinflammatory activity of resident fibroblasts. When produced in large amounts, TNF-α may enter the bloodstream and act at distant sites as an endocrine hormone. In this way TNF-α is able to stimulate the hypothalamus to induce fever, to act on hepatocytes for the production of acute phase reactants, and promote metabolic changes leading to wasting of muscle and fat cells (cachexia). Very high levels of circulating TNF-α ($>10^{-7}$ M) play

TABLE 3-6　Functional Classification of Cytokines

CYTOKINE	SIZE AND FORM	RECEPTORS	MAIN CELL SOURCE	MAIN BIOLOGICAL EFFECTS
Interleukins				
IL-2	14-17 kD, monomer	CD25 (α chain)	T cells	Proliferation and activation of T cells, NK cells
		CD122 (β chain)		Proliferation of B cells and antibody synthesis
		CD132 (γ chain)		Fas-mediated apoptosis
IL-4	18 kD, monomer	CD124	T cells (Th2)	Isotype switching to IgE
				Th2 differentiation
				Inhibition of IFN-γ–mediated macrophage activation
				Th1 suppression
IL-5	45 kD homodimer	CD125	T cells (Th2)	Activation and proliferation of eosinophils
				B cell proliferation and IgA production
IL-7	monomer	CD127, CD132	Non T cells	Growth of pre-B cells and pre-T cells
IL-12	Heterodimer of 35 and 40 kD*	IL-12 Rβ1	DCs, B cells	Differentiation of Th1 cells
		IL-12 Rβ2	Macrophages	Synthesis of IFN-γ by T cells and NK cells
IL-13	15 kD, monomer	IL-13 R	T cells (Th2)	B cell proliferation
				Isotype switching to IgE
				Inhibition of macrophage activation
IL-15	13 kD monomer	IL-15 R (CD122)	Macrophages and other non T cells	NK cells and T-cell proliferation
IL-18	17 kD, monomer	IL-1Rrp (α chain)	Macrophage	Synthesis of IFN-γ by T cells and NK cells
		AcPL (β chain)		
IL-23	Heterodimer of 19 and 40 kD*	IL-12 Rβ1	DCs	Differentiation Th17 cells
		IL-23R		
Proinflammatory Cytokines				
IL-1α	17 kD, monomer	CD121a, b	Macrophages, endothelial	Fever
IL-1β	33 kD (precursors)	(IL-1RI and II)	cells, epithelial cells	Activation of endothelial cells and macrophage
				Acute phase reactants
TNF-α	17 kD homotrimer	p55, p75	Macrophages, T cells, NK	Fever
		(TNFRI, TNFRII)	cells	Activation of endothelial cells, macrophage, and neutrophils
				Acute phase reactants
				Apoptosis
				Cachexia
IL-6	19-26 kD, monomer	IL-6R, gp130	T cells, macrophages, endothelial cells	Fever
				Activation of endothelial cells
				Acute phase reactants
				B-cell proliferation
IL-17	150 kD monomer	IL-17AR	Th17 T cells, NK cells, CD8 T cells	Neutrophil migration
				Activation of endothelial cells, macrophage, and neutrophils
IL-22	146 homodimer	IL-22Rαc	Th17 T cells, NK	Acute phase proteins
		IL10Rβc		Proinflammatory
Antiinflammatory Cytokines				
IL-10	34-40 kD homodimer	IL-10 Rα	Macrophages, T cells (Th2, Treg)	Suppression of macrophage function
		CRF2-4		
TGF-β	25 kD homodimer	TGF-βR	T cells (Treg), macrophages	Inhibition of proliferation and effector function of T cells
				Inhibition of B-cell proliferation
Interferons				
Type I IFNs	IFNα: 15-21 kD	CD118 (IFNAR2)	Leukocytes	Antiviral response
	IFNβ: 20-25 kD monomers		Plasmocytoid DC	Activation of NK cells
			Fibroblasts	
IFN-γ	50 kD homodimer	CD119 (IFNGR2)	T cells, NK cells	Macrophage and NK activation
				Induction of MHC-I on somatic cells and MHC-II on APCs
				Th1 differentiation
				Th2 suppression

*IL-12 and IL-23 share the same p40 subunit.

APCs, Antigen-presenting cells; *DC*, dendritic cells; *IL*, interleukin; *IFN*, interferon; *LT*, lymphotoxin; *MIF*, macrophage inhibitory factor; *NK*, natural killer; *R*, receptor; *TNF*, tumor necrosis factor; *Treg*, regulatory T cell.

TABLE 3-7   Chemokines and Chemokines Receptors

CLASS	NAME (PREVIOUS)	MAJOR SOURCES	RECEPTOR	CELLS ATTRACTED	MAIN FUNCTIONS
(1) CXC	CXCL1 (Gro-α)	M, F, Ec	CXCR2	N, M, Tc, NK	Leukocyte recruitment
	CXCL2 (Gro-β)	M, F, Ec	CXCR2	N, M, Tc, NK	Leukocyte recruitment
	CXCL3 (Gro-γ)	M, F, Ec	CXCR2	N, M, Tc, NK	Leukocyte recruitment
	CXCL5 (ENA78)	M, F, Ec	CXCR2	N	Leukocyte recruitment
	CXCL6 (GCP-2)	M, F, Ec	CXCR1	N, M, Tc, NK	Leukocyte recruitment
	CXCL7 (NAP-2)	M, F, Ec	CXCR2	N	Neutrophils activation, angiogenesis
	CXCL8 (IL-8)	M, Mo, F, Ec	CXCR1/2	N, M, Tc, NK	Neutrophils recruitment and activation
	CXCL9 (MIG)	M, Tc, F, Ec	CXCR3	Tc, NK, M	Leukocyte recruitment
	CXCL10 (IP-10)	M, Tc, F, Ec	CXCR3	Tc, NK, M	Leukocyte recruitment, Th1 response
	CXCL11 (I-TAC)	M, Tc, F, Ec	CXCR3	Tc, NK, M	Leukocyte recruitment
	CXCL12 (SDF-1)	Sc	CXCR4	Naïve Tc, Bc	Lymphocyte recruitment
	CXCL13 (BCA-1)	Sc	CXCR5	B cells	Lymphocyte homing to lymphoid organs
(2) CC	CCL1 (I-309)	M, Tc, Ec	CCR8	M, Tc	Leukocyte recruitment
	CCL2 (MCP-1)	M, F	CCR2	M, NK, Tc, F	Activate macrophage and basophils, Th2 response
	CCL3 (MIP1α)	M, Tc, Mc, F	CCR1/5	M, NK, B, DC	Leukocyte recruitment, Th1 response
	CCL4 (MIP1β)	M, Mo, N, Ec	CCR5	M, NK, Tc, DC	Leukocyte recruitment, HIV co-receptor
	CCL5 (RANTES)	Tc, Ec, P	CCR1/5/3	M, NK, Tc, B, E, DC	Activation of basophils and Tc Chronic inflammation
	CCL7 (MCP-3)	M, F, P, Ec	CCR1/2	E, B, NK	Leukocyte recruitment
	CCL8 (MCP-2)	M, F, Ec	CCR2	E, B	Leukocyte recruitment
	CCL11 (Eotaxin)	Ec, M, Ep, Tc	CCR3	E, M, Tc (Th2)	Allergy, Th2 response
	CCL13 (MCP-4)	Ec, M, Ep	CCR2/4	E, B, Tc	Leukocyte recruitment
	CCL17 (TARC)	Ec, M, Ep	CCR4/8	E, B, Tc	T-cell and basophil recruitment
	CCL19 (ELC)	Sc, Ec	CCR7	Tc, DC	Lymphocyte and DC recruitment in lymphoid organs
	CCL20 (MIP-3α)	M, Tc, DC, E, Mc	CCR6	Tc, DC	Lymphocyte and DC recruitment
	CCL21 (SLC)	Sc, Ec	CCR7	Tc, DC	Lymphocyte and DC recruitment in lymphoid organs
	CCL22 (MDC)	Ec, M, Ep	CCR4	E, B	T-cell and basophil recruitment
	CCL25 (TECK)	Ep	CCR9/11	Tc	T-cell migration
	CCL27 (CTACK)	K, Ec	CCR10	Tc	T-cell migration to skin
	CCL28 (MEC)	Ep	CCR3/10	Tc	T-cell migration to skin
(3) C	XCL1 (lymphotactin)	Tc	XCR1	DC, NK, Tm	Lymphocyte trafficking and development
(4) CX₃C	CX₃CL1 (fractalkine)	M, Ec, Mig	CX₃CR1	M, Tc	Leukocyte-endothelium adhesion Brain inflammation

B, Basophils; Bc, B cells; DC, dendritic cells; E, eosinophils; Ec, endothelial cells, Ep, epithelial cells; F, fibroblasts; K, keratinocytes; M, monocytes/macrophages; Mc, mast cells; Mig, microglial cells; Mo, macrophages; NK, natural killer cells; P, platelets; Sc, stromal cells; Tc, T cells; Tm, thymocytes.

a major role in the pathogenesis of septic shock (severe systemic hypotension, disseminated intravascular coagulation, etc.), which is induced by massive LPS-induced production of proinflammatory cytokines. These potentially lethal effects of TNF-α are balanced by mechanisms for the downregulation of TNF activity, related to the shedding of TNF receptors from the surface of activated cells, thus generating circulating soluble receptors that prevent the binding of free TNF-α to cell-bound receptors (Fig. 3-11). This strategy has been successfully adopted for the therapeutic blockade of TNF activities.[77]

IL-1 shares many biological function with TNF.[80,195] Like TNF, its major source is activated macrophages, although neutrophils, epithelial cells, and endothelial cells can also produce IL-1. Two different isoforms of circulating IL-1 (IL-1α and IL-1β), both 33-kD peptides,

are known. Biologically active IL-1α is a 17-kD protein released after cleavage by the intracellular cysteine protease *caspase-1* (previously known as *IL-1α converting enzyme*) after activation of the NLRP3 inflammasome (Fig. 3-6).[81]

There are two membrane receptors for IL-1. The type I receptor is constitutively expressed on many cell types and mediates intracellular transmission of the signal through activation of the IRAK, leading to activation of NF-kB and AP-1 transcription factors (Fig. 3-11).[81,82] The type II receptor, which is expressed only after cell activation, lacks a cytoplasmic tail, and consequently binding with IL-1 does not result in intracellular signal transmission. This is released in a soluble form as a consequence of proteolytic processing or alternative splicing. Thus, its major function is to downmodulate the biological action of IL-1

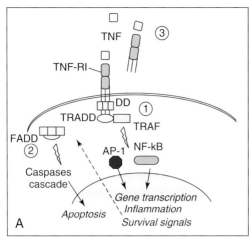
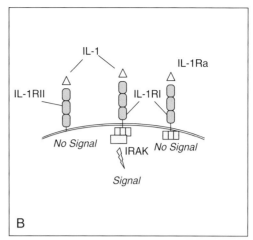

FIGURE 3-11 Mechanisms of cell activation induced by proinflammatory cytokines and strategies for their downregulation. **A,** The binding of circulating TNF-α to TNF receptors (TNFR) leads to the recruitment of cytoplasmic proteins called *TNF receptor associated factors* (TRAFs), which initiate the intracellular signaling; DD: death domain (*1*). In the case of TNFRI, the binding with TNF-α may lead to either inflammation or apoptosis (*2*). In the latter case, different signaling proteins (Fas-associated death domain [FADD]) are involved. The activation of this particular intracellular pathway, due to the loss of survival signals, leads to the activation of caspases cascade that eventually results in cell apoptosis, representing an important strategy for self-limitation of cell activation. Shedding of TNF receptors from the surface of activated cells and prevention of free TNF-α binding to cellular receptors (*3*). **B,** Type I receptor is constitutively expressed on many cell types and mediates the intracellular transmission of the signal after binding with soluble IL-1, through the activation of the IL-1 receptor-associated kinase (IRAK) that eventually leads to cell activation. Type II receptor (decoy receptor), is expressed only after cell activation and lacks a cytoplasmic tail. Thus the binding with IL-1 does not result in intracellular signal transmission. Activated macrophages also secrete a protein with a close structural homology to IL-1, which bind to the same surface receptors but is biologically inactive (IL-1 receptor antagonist, IL-1Ra).

acting as a "decoy" receptor in competition with a type I receptor (Fig. 3-11).[81] A second strategy, which downmodulates IL-1 activities, is the secretion of a protein with a close structural homology to IL-1, which binds to the same surface receptors but is biologically inactive (IL-1 receptor antagonist [IL-1Ra]) (Fig. 3-11).[83,84] This natural pathway of regulation of IL-1 biological activity has been adopted with the use of recombinant IL-1Ra in the treatment of many inflammatory conditions.[85,86] Notably, a genetically determinant defect in the expression of IL-1Ra has been recently associated to a severe neonatal autoinflammatory disease called *DIRA* (deficiency of IL-1 receptor antagonist)[87] (see Chapter 47).

IL-6 is another important cytokine produced by macrophages, some T and B cells, endothelial cells, and tissue fibroblasts during acute and chronic inflammation. Its biological actions are mediated by the specific binding with IL-6 receptor, present on cell membranes or in soluble form; this complex then binds to a signal transducing subunit, called gp130, which is also involved in signal transduction for other cytokines.[88] IL-6 has many proinflammatory functions. It stimulates the synthesis of acute phase reactants by the liver and production of neutrophils from bone marrow. It induces endothelial cells activation, fibroblast proliferation, and osteoclast activation. A large body of evidence has stressed the pivotal role of this cytokine in sJIA. In fact, many of the clinical features peculiar to this disease (chronic anemia, severe growth retardation, osteoporosis, thrombocytosis, amyloidosis) have been related to the biological actions of IL-6.[89] The role of IL-6 in sJIA and its therapeutic implications[90] is further discussed in Chapter 16).

Cells of innate immunity (including DCs) also produce other cytokines that have a pivotal role in the cross-talk between the cells of innate and adaptive immune responses. IL-12, IL-18, and IL-23 (together with IL-1 and IL-6), are key inducers of cell-mediated immunity that may contribute to the differentiation of recently recruited CD4+ helper T cells into IFN-γ–producing Th1 cells or IL-17–producing Th17 cells (Fig. 3-7).

Chemokines. Chemokines are a large family of structurally homologous small cytokines (8-15 kDa) that control the trafficking of leukocytes.[91] According to the motif displayed by the first two cysteine residues near the amino terminus, chemokines are classified in four families: CC, CXC, C, and CX$_3$C (Table 3-7). Chemokines are produced by leukocytes and by many tissue cells (endothelial cells, fibroblast cells, and epithelial cells) in both physiological and pathological conditions. From a functional point of view, chemokines can be broadly classified in two main classes: inflammatory and lymphoid (or homing).[182] The inflammatory chemokines are produced by leukocytes and resident tissues in response to proinflammatory stimuli. Homing chemokines are constitutively expressed in the microenvironment of lymphoid tissues, skin, and mucosa, and are involved in the continuous leukocyte trafficking between circulation and lymphoid structures. Examples include CCL19, CCL21, and CXC13, which play pivotal roles, together with their specific cellular receptors CCR7 and CXCR5, in lymphoid organization in secondary lymphoid organs.[92]

The interaction between chemokines and their cellular receptors induces the activation of intracellular signaling pathways that provoke cytoskeletal rearrangements by stimulating alternating polymerization and depolymerization of actin filaments leading to cell mobilization. The expression of different chemokine receptors on the surface of circulating leukocytes is closely related to their specific function, state of differentiation, and degree of activation (Table 3-7). This complex network of chemokines and cellular receptors allows the selective recruitment of circulating leukocytes to the periphery or to lymphoid organs on the basis of their discrete microenvironment and functional needs.

Many inflammatory chemokines and leukocytes displaying their specific surface receptors have been identified in inflamed tissues. In particular, receptors for inflammatory chemokines, CCR1, CCR2, CCR5, and CXCR3, are regularly detected in tissues where inflammation is characterized by chronic infiltration of macrophages and predominantly T lymphocytes.[93] The selective blockade of inflammatory chemokines and their cellular receptors is a promising possible strategy for the treatment of many autoimmune disorders.[94]

Growth factors. During chronic inflammation a large number of growth factors are secreted by inflammatory cells. Platelet-derived growth factor (PDGF), basic fibroblast growth factor (bFGF), transforming growth factor β (TGF-β), epidermal growth factor (EGF), and vascular endothelial growth factor (VEGF) have been shown to play a role in the induction of *angiogenesis,* the formation of new blood vessels from the preexisting microvascular bed. During chronic inflammation this process provides oxygen and nutrients necessary to the high metabolic requirement of resident cells, and permits the migration and progressive infiltration of newly recruited inflammatory cells.[95]

Prostaglandins and Leukotrienes

Prostaglandins and leukotrienes are acid lipids derived from enzymatic cleavage of arachidonic acid, and are produced by most mammalian cells in response to mechanical, chemical, and immunological stimuli. Arachidonic acid is a member of the ω-6 series of essential fatty acids contained in membrane phospholipids. The activation of the enzyme phospholipase A2 releases arachidonic acid that is further metabolized by two main enzymatic pathways leading to the final production of a class of mediators belonging to the family of bioactive *eicosanoids.*

Cyclooxygenases (COX) are responsible for the production of *prostaglandins* (PGs) both in physiological and pathological conditions. Two different isoforms of COX exist. COX-1 is constitutively expressed in most tissues and at a constant level throughout the cell cycle; PGs are physiologically produced in many tissues and regulate diverse functions, including platelet-dependent homeostasis, renal blood flow, and gastric mucosal integrity. Conversely, COX-2 is normally undetectable in normal tissues but can be rapidly induced in particular cell types (fibroblasts, monocytes, and endothelial cells) upon proinflammatory stimulation. The activation of COX-2 is thought to play a major role in inflammatory reactions.[96] Together with mast cell–derived PGD_2, the most abundant COX-2 product is PGE_2. This can sensitize nerve endings to painful chemical and mechanical stimuli, and acts also as a potent vasodilator. Furthermore, PGE_2 has a crucial role in the induction of fever after stimulation of specialized endothelial cells in hypothalamic tissue by endogenous pyrogens (such as TNF and IL-6).

Leukotrienes (LTs) are derived from the combined actions of 5-lipoxygenases (5-LOX) and 5-LOX-activating protein (FLAP) with initial formation of 5-hydroperoxyeicosatetraenoic acid (5-HPETE), followed by LTA_4. LTB_4 (the hydrolytic product of LTA_4) is the more stable molecule among the LTs. LTB_4 is rapidly synthesized by neutrophils and macrophages upon challenge with stimuli such as microbial pathogens, toxins, aggregated immunoglobulins, and proinflammatory cytokines. It is a powerful chemoattractant, and induces neutrophil aggregation and degranulation, and macrophage production of proinflammatory cytokines, O_2^- and PGE_2.[97]

The study of the metabolism of arachidonic acid in inflammatory responses led to the discovery of lipid molecules called *lipoxins* (LXs)

derived from different enzymatic cascades that are efficient endogenous mediators of inflammation resolution.[98] The interaction between leukocytes and platelets at sites of tissue inflammation leads to the activation in platelets of 5-LOX that generate LTA_4. However, the activation of adherent platelets leads also to the activation of 12-LOX, which results in the production of LXA_4 and LXB_4.[98] A second pathway of LX production occurs in monocytes and macrophages exposed to antiinflammatory cytokines such as IL-4 and IL-13. In this case, LX production is initiated by a 5-LOX, which leads to the generation and release of 15(S)-hydroxyeicosatetraenoic acid (HETE), which in turn is rapidly taken up and converted by polymorphonucleates to LXs.[98] Therefore, in peripheral blood neutrophils, a switch in ecoisanoid biosynthesis from predominantly proinflammatory molecules (PGE_2 and LTB_4) to antiinflammatory LX production occurs. Notably, PGE_5 itself promotes both 5-LOX and 12-LOX gene expression, thus initiating a mechanism of self-limitation of inflammation. LXs display a number of antiinflammatory activities in many animal models of inflammatory diseases, mainly related to inhibition of recruitment of inflammatory cells into the site of inflammation.[70]

Proteolytic Enzymes

Myeloperoxidase and a number of other proteolytic enzymes are abundantly present in the granules of professional phagocytes, such as neutrophils.[99] Among them are serine proteinases (elastases, cathepsin G), acid hydrolases (β-glucuronidase, α-mannosidosis), and peptides with bactericidal activity (lysozyme, defensins, lactoferrin, azurocidin). Matrix metalloproteinases (MMPs) comprise a large family of proteolytic enzymes produced by fibroblasts, macrophages, neutrophils, and chondrocytes upon stimulation with proinflammatory cytokines and growth factors.[100] Their main function is the remodeling of extracellular matrix during tissue resorption. Thus the proteolytic activity of MMPs is thought to represent a crucial component of both physiological (embryonic development, organ morphogenesis, angiogenesis) and pathological (chronic inflammatory diseases, tumors) conditions. MMPs are one of the most important classes of final mediators of tissue damage in many chronic inflammatory conditions, including rheumatoid arthritis.[101]

WHEN DEFECTIVE REGULATION OF INNATE IMMUNITY LEADS TO RHEUMATIC DISEASE

In autoimmune diseases, the cells of innate immunity (DCs, monocytes, and macrophages) play key roles in the orientation of immune response at the moment of antigen presentation or during the effector phase of the immune response, when tissue macrophages exert their proinflammatory functions under stimulation of autoreactive T cells and autoantibodies (this interplay between innate and adaptive immunity is further discussed in Chapter 4). In addition, some paradigms concerning the origin and maintenance of many chronic inflammatory diseases have been modified thanks to lessons learned from a number of inherited inflammatory diseases that are caused by mutations of genes that play a pivotal role in the regulation of the innate immune response (the so-called autoinflammatory diseases). The autoinflammatory diseases are characterized by seemingly unprovoked, recurrent episodes of fever, serositis, arthritis, and cutaneous inflammatory manifestations or by bona fide chronic inflammatory diseases. In these conditions, the usual hallmarks of autoimmunity (high-titer autoantibodies, antigen-specific T cells, human leukocyte antigen [HLA] association, gender disproportion) are absent.[37] A new schema for the classification of the spectrum of immune-mediated and autoinflammatory diseases has been proposed.[102] The autoinflammatory conditions, and the genetic mutations that have been discovered which underlie them, are discussed in detail in Chapter 47, while many autoimmune and immune-mediated conditions, as they occur in children, are discussed in detail in other chapters.

CONCLUSIONS

In the past 16 years a growing number of monogenic chronic inflammatory diseases have been identified that are secondary to mutations in genes involved in the regulatory pathways of innate immunity. The identification of the involved gene has frequently provided important information on a variety of mechanisms involved in the regulation of innate immune response and has opened new perspectives in the understanding of mechanisms leading to chronic inflammation. Thanks to the extraordinary technological advances in the field of genetics (next-generation sequencing), in the next few years we expect to assist to an exponential increase in the identification of new genes, diseases, and intracellular pathways associated with the so-called horror autoinflammaticus[37]; this will probably also radically change our current views on the pathogenesis and treatment of many chronic common inflammatory diseases.

REFERENCES

1. R. Medzhitov, C. Janeway Jr., Innate immunity, N. Engl. J. Med. 343 (5) (2000) 338–344.
2. C. Nathan, Neutrophils and immunity: challenges and opportunities, Nat. Rev. Immunol. 6 (3) (2006) 173–182.
3. R. Medzhitov, Recognition of microorganisms and activation of the immune response, Nature 449 (7164) (2007) 819–826.
4. P. Broz, D.M. Monack, Newly described pattern recognition receptors team up against intracellular pathogens, Nat. Rev. Immunol. 13 (8) (2013) 551–565.
5. R. Medzhitov, Toll-like receptors and innate immunity, Nat. Rev. Immunol. 1 (2) (2001) 135–145.
6. S. Akira, S. Uematsu, O. Takeuchi, Pathogen recognition and innate immunity, Cell 124 (4) (2006) 783–801.
7. T.H. Mogensen, Pathogen recognition and inflammatory signaling in innate immune defenses, Clin. Microbiol. Rev. 22 (2) (2009) 240–273, Table of Contents.
8. K. Takeda, S. Akira, Toll-like receptors in innate immunity, Int. Immunol. 17 (1) (2005) 1–14.
9. J.M. Wilmanski, T. Petnicki-Ocwieja, K.S. Kobayashi, NLR proteins: integral members of innate immunity and mediators of inflammatory diseases, J. Leukoc. Biol. 83 (1) (2008) 13–30.
10. L. Franchi, N. Warner, K. Viani, G. Nunez, Function of Nod-like receptors in microbial recognition and host defense, Immunol. Rev. 227 (1) (2009) 106–128.
11. R.A. Ratsimandresy, A. Dorfleutner, C. Stehlik, An update on PYRIN domain-containing pattern recognition receptors: from immunity to pathology, Front Immunol. 4 (2013) 440.
12. M. Yoneyama, M. Kikuchi, T. Natsukawa, et al., The RNA helicase RIG-I has an essential function in double-stranded RNA-induced innate antiviral responses, Nat. Immunol. 5 (7) (2004) 730–737.
13. T.D. Kanneganti, M. Lamkanfi, G. Nuñez, Intracellular NOD-like receptors in host defense and disease, Immunity 27 (4) (2007) 549–559.
14. M. Chamaillard, M. Hashimoto, Y. Horie, et al., An essential role for NOD1 in host recognition of bacterial peptidoglycan containing diaminopimelic acid, Nat. Immunol. 4 (7) (2003) 702–707.
15. S.E. Girardin, I.G. Boneca, J. Viala, et al., Nod2 is a general sensor of peptidoglycan through muramyl dipeptide (MDP) detection, J. Biol. Chem. 278 (11) (2003) 8869–8872.
16. L. Agostini, F. Martinon, K. Burns, et al., NALP3 forms an IL-1beta-processing inflammasome with increased activity in Muckle-Wells autoinflammatory disorder, Immunity 20 (3) (2004) 319–325.
17. M.E. Bianchi, DAMPs, PAMPs and alarmins: all we need to know about danger, J. Leukoc. Biol. 81 (1) (2007) 1–5.
18. F.G. Goh, K.S. Midwood, Intrinsic danger: activation of Toll-like receptors in rheumatoid arthritis, Rheumatology (Oxford) 51 (1) (2012) 7–23.
19. M.T. Lotze, K.J. Tracey, High-mobility group box 1 protein (HMGB1): nuclear weapon in the immune arsenal, Nat. Rev. Immunol. 5 (4) (2005) 331–342.
20. D. Foell, H. Wittkowski, T. Vogl, J. Roth, S100 proteins expressed in phagocytes: a novel group of damage-associated molecular pattern molecules, J. Leukoc. Biol. 81 (1) (2007) 28–37.
21. C. Kessel, D. Holzinger, D. Foell, Phagocyte-derived S100 proteins in autoinflammation: putative role in pathogenesis and usefulness as biomarkers, Clin. Immunol. 147 (3) (2013) 229–241.
22. D.M. Underhill, H.S. Goodridge, Information processing during phagocytosis, Nat. Rev. Immunol. 12 (7) (2012) 492–502.
23. L.A. O'Neill, A.G. Bowie, The family of five: TIR-domain-containing adaptors in Toll-like receptor signalling, Nat. Rev. Immunol. 7 (5) (2007) 353–364.
24. T. Kawai, O. Takeuchi, T. Fujita, et al., Lipopolysaccharide stimulates the MyD88-independent pathway and results in activation of IFN-regulatory factor 3 and the expression of a subset of lipopolysaccharide-inducible genes, J. Immunol. 167 (10) (2001) 5887–5894.
25. K. Burns, F. Martinon, C. Esslinger, et al., MyD88, an adapter protein involved in interleukin-1 signaling, J. Biol. Chem. 273 (20) (1998) 12203–12209.
26. T. Kawai, O. Adachi, T. Ogawa, et al., Unresponsiveness of MyD88-deficient mice to endotoxin, Immunity 11 (1) (1999) 115–122.
27. C. Wang, L. Deng, M. Hong, et al., TAK1 is a ubiquitin-dependent kinase of MKK and IKK, Nature 412 (6844) (2001) 346–351.
28. L. Chang, M. Karin, Mammalian MAP kinase signalling cascades, Nature 410 (6824) (2001) 37–40.
29. F. Martinon, J. Tschopp, NLRs join TLRs as innate sensors of pathogens, Trends Immunol. 26 (8) (2005) 447–454.
30. A. Mantovani, M. Locati, Orchestration of macrophage polarization, Blood 114 (15) (2009) 3135–3136.
31. A. Mantovani, S.K. Biswas, M.R. Galdiero, et al., Macrophage plasticity and polarization in tissue repair and remodelling, J. Pathol. 229 (2) (2013) 176–185.
32. A. Rubartelli, F. Cozzolino, M. Talio, R. Sitia, A novel secretory pathway for interleukin-1 beta, a protein lacking a signal sequence, EMBO J. 9 (5) (1990) 1503–1510.
33. C. Andrei, C. Dazzi, L. Lotti, et al., The secretory route of the leaderless protein interleukin 1beta involves exocytosis of endolysosome-related vesicles, Mol. Biol. Cell 10 (5) (1999) 1463–1475.
34. S. Mariathasan, D.S. Weiss, K. Newton, et al., Cryopyrin activates the inflammasome in response to toxins and ATP, Nature 440 (7081) (2006) 228–232.
35. F. Martinon, K. Burns, J. Tschopp, The inflammasome: a molecular platform triggering activation of inflammatory caspases and processing of proIL-beta, Mol. Cell 10 (2) (2002) 417–426.
36. F. Martinon, V. Petrilli, A. Mayor, et al., Gout-associated uric acid crystals activate the NALP3 inflammasome, Nature 440 (7081) (2006) 237–241.
37. S.L. Masters, A. Simon, I. Aksentijevich, D.L. Kastner, Horror autoinflammaticus: the molecular pathophysiology of autoinflammatory disease (*), Annu. Rev. Immunol. 27 (2009) 621–668.
38. T.D. Kanneganti, N. Ozoren, M. Body-Malapel, et al., Bacterial RNA and small antiviral compounds activate caspase-1 through cryopyrin/Nalp3, Nature 440 (7081) (2006) 233–236.
39. D.A. Muruve, V. Petrilli, A.K. Zaiss, et al., The inflammasome recognizes cytosolic microbial and host DNA and triggers an innate immune response, Nature 452 (7183) (2008) 103–107.
40. C.A. Dinarello, T. Ikejima, S.J. Warner, et al., Interleukin 1 induces interleukin 1. I. Induction of circulating interleukin 1 in rabbits in vivo and in human mononuclear cells in vitro, J. Immunol. 139 (6) (1987) 1902–1910.
41. D. Perregaux, C.A. Gabel, Interleukin-1 beta maturation and release in response to ATP and nigericin. Evidence that potassium depletion

mediated by these agents is a necessary and common feature of their activity, J. Biol. Chem. 269 (21) (1994) 15195–15203.

42. D. Ferrari, C. Pizzirani, E. Adinolfi, et al., The P2X7 receptor: a key player in IL-1 processing and release, J. Immunol. 176 (7) (2006) 3877–3883.

43. H.M. Hoffman, S. Rosengren, D.L. Boyle, et al., Prevention of cold-associated acute inflammation in familial cold autoinflammatory syndrome by interleukin-1 receptor antagonist, Lancet 364 (9447) (2004) 1779–1785.

44. M. Gattorno, S. Tassi, S. Carta, et al., Pattern of interleukin-1beta secretion in response to lipopolysaccharide and ATP before and after interleukin-1 blockade in patients with CIAS1 mutations, Arthritis Rheum. 56 (9) (2007) 3138–3148.

45. J. Tschopp, K. Schroder, NLRP3 inflammasome activation: the convergence of multiple signalling pathways on ROS production?, Nat. Rev. Immunol. 10 (3) (2010) 210–215.

46. A. Rubartelli, M. Gattorno, M.G. Netea, C.A. Dinarello, Interplay between redox status and inflammasome activation, Trends Immunol. 32 (12) (2011) 559–566.

The entire reference list is available online at www.expertconsult.com.

CHAPTER 4

Adaptive Immunity and Autoimmunity: Translation from Bench to Bedside

Salvatore Albani, Lucy R. Wedderburn, Berent Prakken

THE ADAPTIVE IMMUNE RESPONSE

Most childhood autoimmune diseases are complex, multifactorial diseases. Through interactions with a defined genetic susceptibility, other, mostly unknown, environmental factors play a role in the pathogenesis. This interaction of genetic susceptibility and environment not only determines the onset of a disease but probably also its outcome. The adaptive immune system mediates key interactions at the interface between genetic background and the environment. Understanding adaptive immunity in autoimmune diseases is therefore crucial for our understanding of the immune pathogenesis of autoimmunity, and the generation of new therapeutic targets for drug development. In this chapter the key players in the adaptive immune system and their possible roles in pediatric autoimmune rheumatological diseases such as juvenile idiopathic arthritis (JIA), juvenile dermatomyositis (JDM), and juvenile systemic lupus erythematosus (JSLE) will be reviewed.[1,2] Although much is now known about the interconnections between key players of the adaptive immune system, most data are from adult human subjects or mice; neither sets of data can be fully extrapolated to children or adolescents in whom the developing immune system and mechanisms are known to be distinct.[3]

A group of closely interconnected immune cells including T cells, B cells, and antigen-presenting cells (APCs), together orchestrate the adaptive immune response. A primary function of the adaptive immune system is to offer protection against invading pathogens. The adaptive immune response is traditionally distinguished from the innate immune response by two distinctive properties: specificity and memory. After the initial innate immune response against an invading pathogen, T and B cells are generated that are specific for this antigen. Although the mechanisms of action differ between these different cell types, several fundamental features of adaptive immunity are shared by B and T cells. These include the ability to recognize pathogen components via clonal expression of unique cell surface antigen specific receptors; the ability to rapidly proliferate upon recognition of antigen, along with acquisition of cell lineage-specific immune functions; and the ability to persist after the infection is cleared, combined with the capacity to "remember" the pathogen or antigen, and respond more rapidly and vigorously upon reinfection (immunological memory). Thus, specificity is not lost after an immune response has waned, because so-called memory B cells and T cells are generated and maintained in the immune repertoire long term. This immunological memory ensures that a second encounter with the same antigen can be dealt with more rapidly and effectively. Immunological memory is the basis of one of the earliest and still one of the most effective immune-based interventions, namely vaccination.[4-6]

The adaptive immune system is not an entity that stands or operates alone. Instead, it acts in a close association with the innate immune system (which is discussed in detail in Chapter 3). Innate immunity helps to initiate, drive, and steer the adaptive immune response. Several cell types including dendritic cells (DCs) and the recently recognized innate lymphoid cells (ILCs), exist as a bridge between innate and adaptive immunity.[7,8] Thus the division between adaptive and innate immune cells is not black and white. Adaptive immune cells such as T cells may also carry out innate functions, whereas innate immune cells can act in a more specific way than previously was assumed. For example, while the triggering of a Toll-like receptor (TLR) most likely will lead to a proinflammatory response, it can also lead to temporary immune nonresponsiveness, depending on the timing, the location of the immune response, and local cofactors.

The close interaction between innate and adaptive immune cells is of special importance in chronic inflammatory diseases, such as JIA and other childhood autoimmune diseases.[1,2] In these diseases it may be difficult, if not impossible, to separate entirely the effects of innate and adaptive immune activation. This is particularly the case when analyzing the immune response at the site of inflammation. Instead, in such "real-life" inflammatory environments, a continuous and dynamic interplay takes place, which can involve virtually all immune cells. Innate immune activation is extensively reviewed in Chapter 3; this chapter will focus on adaptive immunity, discuss the most important players of the adaptive immune response, and consider their importance and relevance for chronic inflammation as well as the cross-talk between adaptive and innate immunity.

PLAYERS IN THE ADAPTIVE IMMUNE RESPONSE AND THEIR ROLES IN AUTOIMMUNITY

T Cells

T cells play a central part in the inflammatory response; both helper T cells and cytotoxic T cells are involved in most responses. T-cell immune responses typically involve an interplay of various effector mechanisms: the production of proinflammatory cytokines (including interferon [IFN]-γ tumor necrosis factor-alpha [TNF-α], and interleukin [IL]-17) and the expression of cytolytic effector molecules (including perforin and the granzymes A, B, and K), in addition to interactions with B cells, DCs, and other immune cells.[5,6]

A significant feature of T-cell immunity is the ability of naïve T cells to undergo a program of proliferation and functional differentiation upon activation that results in a large pool of cells.[9-12] All of these cells are capable of recognizing a particular antigen and have acquired the immune functions necessary to control and eventually clear infection. When infection is cleared, the majority of the expanded effector T-cell population dies; this leaves behind a small pool of long-lived memory T cells that can recognize the same antigen that triggered their initial activation. These memory T cells produce a broader array of immune molecules than naïve cells and in larger quantities, and are triggered at lower thresholds. Moreover, unlike naïve cells, they can respond to antigen without the need for further differentiation. These features, combined with persistence at a higher frequency, enable memory T cells to respond more rapidly when there is a secondary infection.

Evidence for the Role of T Cells in Autoimmunity

T cells are thought to play a central role in the immune pathogenesis of many human autoimmune diseases. The three key mechanistic areas that are thought to influence the T-cell arm of the adaptive immune system and its role in autoimmunity[5,10,12] are as follows:

1. **Early development** (commonly called *central tolerance*). Antigens are presented to T-cell clones expressing specific T-cell receptors (TCRs) in the thymus. If there is a strong immune response, T-cell clones are autoreactive and undergo negative selection. Genetic predisposition to a high threshold of T-cell activation (i.e., less TCR signaling) may lead to a reduced selection against autoreactive clones. This, in turn, results in a predisposition to clinical autoimmunity.
2. **Activation/apoptosis** (*peripheral tolerance*). Later in life, when naïve T cells are exposed to antigens, they respond by a similar mechanism of antigen–major histocompatibility complex–TCR signaling events. In this scenario, genetic predisposition to a low threshold of T-cell activation (i.e., stronger TCR signaling) may lead to an overexuberant immune response. Alternatively, high thresholds for T-cell activation might also lead to a predisposition of autoimmunity via a reduction of regulatory T-cell responses or a relative deficiency of apoptosis in responding effector cells.
3. **Polarization.** After antigen exposure, naïve T cells differentiate into memory T cells of a specific subset (e.g., Th1, Th2, Th17), discussed in the following. Polarization into one or another subset is dependent on the balance of cytokines and transcription factors, as well as epigenetic modifications that regulate the distinct functional and phenotypic characteristics of T-cell subsets. Genetic factors also play a role in T-cell differentiation and may influence the threshold to develop into one subset or another. Consequently, there is an influence on the relative proportion of memory T-cell subsets and predisposition to clinical autoimmune disease.

The importance of T cells in autoimmune inflammation has been deduced from diverse sources, including experimental models, the study of human chronically inflamed tissues, and genetic studies. In JIA, various studies have underscored a potential role for T cells in the pathogenesis for most subtypes, with the exception perhaps of the systemic form of JIA, sJIA.[1,13] The case for a role for T cells in JIA is based on multiple lines of evidence. At the onset of the disease, memory T cells with a proinflammatory phenotype are present at the site of inflammation.[14,15] Among these T cells are cells with specificity for autoantigens, such as Hsp60 (heat shock protein 60 kD) and DnaJ.[16,17] Secondly, the skewing of the TCR repertoire at the site of inflammation argues for a specific role of T cells instead of just being "spill over" from systemic inflammation.[18] The fact that these skewed, highly oligoclonal T cells include cells specific for autoantigens has fueled the hypothesis that a pathogenic T-cell response against self-antigens lies at the heart of JIA. However, the picture is not entirely straightforward. For example, in many animal models of arthritis, T cells orchestrate the disease-related immune responses in such a way that they can either protect from arthritis or induce it. In other models, however, arthritis can be induced in the absence of T cells, underscoring that it is not T cells alone that determine arthritis. More "circumstantial" evidence on the importance of T cells in JIA comes from genetic studies.

Genetics That Implicate T-Cell Pathways

A prominent genetic region that is involved in determining risk for human autoimmune diseases is the human leukocyte antigen (HLA) region located on chromosome 6, also known as the human major histocompatibility complex (MHC). MHC molecules can be divided into MHC class I and MHC class II. HLAs A, B, and C code for MHC class I molecules. MHC class I molecules present peptides such as viral peptides from inside the cell to CD8[+] T cells. On the other hand HLA DP, DM, DO, DO, DQ, and DR code for MHC class II molecules, which can present processed antigenic peptides to CD4[+] T cells.

In most complex autoimmune diseases a strong genetic association exists with the HLA region.[19] This link with HLA is further strong evidence for an essential role for T cells in the etiology of autoimmunity. It still remains mostly undefined how this relationship translates into a mechanism, with a few notable exceptions. One possibility is that negative selection in the thymus (see below) in the presence of certain MHC alleles is affected in such a way that it increases the chance of T cells specific for certain MHC–self-peptide combinations to escape negative selection in the thymus.

In both rheumatoid arthritis (RA) and JIA, the strongest genetic associations lie in HLA regions. The HLA associations in some subtypes of JIA (such as oligoarticular JIA), are with different alleles than those in RA[19,20]; in contrast, juvenile-onset polyarticular JIA shares MHC class II allele risk associations closely with RA. Although HLA is the most prominent susceptibility factor in JIA, it only explains around 10% of the total variation of JIA susceptibility. In addition, a large number of non-HLA candidate genes have been found to be associated with JIA, such as genes coding for PTPN22, PTPN2, IL-2RA, MIF, SLC11A6, WISP3, and TNF-α. A genetic study of almost 3000 cases of JIA using the Immunochip platform confirmed associations of a total of 16 non-HLA loci at genome-wide significance, including IL-2/21, STAT4, IL-2RA, IL-2RB, RUNX1, ERAP2, and others.[21] These and other genetic associations point to a central role for the immune system, and more specifically the adaptive immune system in the pathogenesis of JIA. For example, multiple studies have revealed associations with genes related to the IL-2 and IL-2R pathways, which are a crucial for T-cell differentiation and function, again underscoring the importance of T cells to JIA immune pathogenesis.

T-Cell Subsets and Effector Mechanisms

T cells can be grouped into different subsets, based on their phenotype and effector functions. CD8[+] T cells, also called *cytotoxic* or *killer T cells,* express the surface molecule CD8 and are classically important for defense against intracellular pathogens and viruses. They recognize proteins derived from foreign antigens or self-antigens that are expressed on the cell surface of APCs in the context of MHC class I molecules. A main effector mechanism is to kill target cells through the release of various cytotoxic proteins such as granzymes and perforins. CD4[+] T cells, also called *T-helper (Th) cells,* are characterized by surface expression of CD4, and recognize exogenous and self-antigens presented in the context of MHC class II molecules on professional APCs.

A significant feature of T-cell biology is the enormous functional plasticity of naïve T cells.[5,10,22] An example of T-cell functional plasticity is found when naïve helper T cells are activated and may differentiate into distinct functional types, mainly defined by the soluble effector molecules they secrete. Initially three Th cell subsets were recognized:

TABLE 4-1   The Most Important T-Helper Subsets Identified in Humans and Their Possible Relevance in Health and Disease

TH SUBSET	GATE KEEPER TRANSCRIPTION FACTOR	CYTOKINES INVOLVED	RELEVANCE IN HUMANS	PUTATIVE-RELATED DISEASES
Th1	Tbet, STAT4	IFN-γ, IL-12	Protection against microorganism DTH	Autoimmune diseases
Th2	GATA-3	IL-4, IL-5, IL-13	Protection against parasites, allergy, B-cell help, class switching	Allergy
Th3	Unidentified	Transforming growth factor-β (TGF-β)	Mucosal tolerance	Unidentified
Th17	RORC	IL-17 (IL-6, TGF-β)		Autoimmune diseases
Treg	FOXP3	(consumption of) IL-2	Regulation of inflammation	Autoimmune diseases, JIA
Tr1	Unidentified	IL-10	Regulation of inflammation	Diabetes
Tfh	Bcl6	IL-21	Isotype switching and B-cell memory	Variety of inflammatory diseases
Th9	Unidentified	IL-9, TNF-α, and granzyme B	Protection extracellular pathogens	Psoriasis
Th22	Unidentified	IL-22	Protection and damage control	Variety of inflammatory diseases

Th0 cells, Th1 cells, and Th2 cells.[23] Th0 cells are undifferentiated naïve cells, whereas Th1 cells are characterized by the production of IFN-γ and IL-12. Th1 cells are responsible for the delayed type hypersensitivity (DTH) reaction and play a role in the normal adaptive immune response against various (intracellular) microorganisms. Th2 cells provide crucial help for B cells and antibody production. They play a vital role in the defense against parasitic infections and are related to allergic disease. Whereas Th1 cells produce proinflammatory cytokines such as IFN-γ, Th2 cells may have a more antiinflammatory phenotype, and produce predominantly IL-4, IL-5, and IL-10.[22,23]

Because of their apparently opposing cytokine profiles, Th1 and Th2 cells were long thought to be in dynamic balance. However, with increasing understanding of T-cell biology it is clear that this model was oversimplified. Many other T-cell subsets have now been defined, both in mice and in humans, which are unique and significant in their own way, including Th17, regulatory T (Treg) cells, TFh (follicular Th cells), Th22, and Th9 cells (Table 4-1). To date, at least nine distinct Th subsets can be distinguished that are either mostly proinflammatory (such as Th1 and Th17 cells) or mostly antiinflammatory (such Treg and Treg type 1 [Tr1] cells).[5,22] Many of these distinct subsets have been shown to be driven by specific transcription factors (Table 4-1).

The tailoring of helper T-cell responses into distinct functional lineages is a consequence of integration of multiple signals that are present during initial T-cell activation, including local cytokines, other ligand interactions, and metabolic signals.[5,24,25] Indeed, there is heterogeneity of effector function within a responding T-cell population, and no one immune response is uniquely represented by a single Th subset. In fact, there is tailoring of the total T-cell population such that a particular subset may be overrepresented, but many immune responses will involve several types of effector T cell.

T-Cell Subsets in Autoimmunity

In the context of autoimmunity much recent attention has focused on Th1 and Th17 cells.[26,27] Both are considered to be important mediators of a detrimental immune response in autoimmunity. A pathogenic role for Th17 cells has been implicated in JIA as well as several other autoimmune diseases, such as psoriasis and multiple sclerosis. Of special interest is the fact that there is a connection between these proinflammatory Th17 cells and regulatory FOXP3+ Treg cells.[26-29] This interrelationship and its role in childhood autoimmunity is further

discussed below. Deciphering this complex relationship is a prime objective of future research, as it will be indispensable for the development of cell-based therapy in autoimmune diseases.

Regulatory T Cells

On the other end of the spectrum from inflammatory Th cells, are the so-called regulatory T cells, which have gained significant interest over the past decade.[28] Various types of Treg cells are now recognized, of which FOXP3 expressing Treg, and IL-10–producing Treg type 1 cells (Tr1) are among the most studied in humans. FOXP3+ Treg cells are characterized by the expression of the transcription factor FOXP3 and can either be directly derived from the thymus (natural Treg) or induced in the periphery (adaptive Treg).[28,30-32] In experimental models, the presence or absence of FOXP3-expressing Treg cells can determine the presence or absence of disease. In humans, gene mutations in FOXP3 lead to immunodysregulation polyendocrinopathy enteropathy X-linked syndrome (IPEX), a fatal multisystem inflammatory disease with onset early in life, underscoring that in humans Treg cells are also crucial for maintaining immune tolerance.[33,34] On the other hand, in most human autoimmune diseases there seems no quantitative deficiency of Treg cells. Instead, an increased number of Treg cells is often found at sites of inflammation, such as the synovial fluid in JIA.[35,36] However, clearly these are insufficient or unable to suppress inflammation. Whether the Treg cells at the site of inflammation are deficient in function is still a matter of debate.

Also crucial for maintaining peripheral tolerance are Tr1 cells. They are characterized by the production of IL-10 next to other cytokines such as IL-4 and IL-7, and the expression of CD49b and LAG-3. They were first found in studies related to stem-cell transplantation and are now being developed for cell therapy in transplantation setting.[37] However, little is known about their role in JIA. To further complicate our understanding of Treg cells, different functional states can exist within the various subtypes of regulatory cells. For example, FOXP3+ T cells can have a phenotype that resembles Th1, Th2, or Th17 cells and in some circumstances have been shown to produce inflammatory cytokines.[38,39]

T-Cell Plasticity

It is now clear that there is considerable plasticity in the T-cell system such that both Th effector and regulatory cells of one type may change into another functional type.[22,27,40] For example, evidence from both mouse and human autoimmunity has been demonstrated that Th17 cells, when exposed to an inflammatory environment containing IL-12, may convert to double-producing Th1/Th17 or even Th1 cells.[41,42] These "ex-Th17" cells have been shown to produce high levels of the proinflammatory granulocyte-macrophage colony-stimulating factor (GM-CSF) in JIA at the inflamed site.[43]

Similarly, considerable evidence suggests that Th17 and Treg cells may interconvert depending on local cytokines.[27,40] Th17 cell and adaptive Treg cell differentiation are both dependent on transforming growth factor (TGF)-β. In mice the combination of TGF-β with proinflammatory cytokines IL-1β and IL-6 allows the differentiation toward a Th17 phenotype, whereas TGF-β alone induces adaptive Treg cells. Several other factors may influence the balance between Th17 and Treg cells, including IL-2 and retinoic acid (a derivative of vitamin A).[25,26,40] In both human and murine studies, data suggest that Treg cells may convert to Th17 cells under inflammatory conditions.[44,45]

Thus, keeping a healthy immune balance and how this balance is altered in inflammation involves a highly interactive system of communicating T cells that have the ability to adapt easily to a changing environment.[46] This adaptability may be crucial in allowing normal immune responses, because a proinflammatory immune response mounted as a defense against an invading microorganism would lead to serious tissue damage if not controlled properly. However, it will be vital to fully understand what regulates such T-cell plasticity if T cells are to be used in novel cell therapy approaches (for example, infusion of Treg cells).

B Cells and Antibody Production

B cells are crucial players in the adaptive immune response. They are an important part of the defense against pathogens through their capacity to produce antigen-specific, protective antibodies. Moreover, in the constant interaction between cells of the adaptive immune system, B cells are also potent APCs and as such are pivotal for T-cell activation and creating the right immunological environment for the optimal specific immune response. There is much evidence for a role of B cells, and the autoantibody-producing plasma cells they mature into, in the pathogenesis of autoimmunity.[1,2,47,48] In various human autoimmune diseases, hypergammaglobulinemia is a prominent laboratory feature of active disease. In diseases such as systemic lupus erythematosus (SLE) and JDM, the presence of specific autoantibodies is directly related to disease activity or disease subtype.[48] These antibodies are increasingly used as biomarkers to drive clinical care decisions (see Chapters 23 and 26). In both adult and childhood inflammatory arthritis, the presence of autoantibodies, such as antinuclear antibodies (ANAs) in JIA, or rheumatoid factor and anti-cyclic citrullinated peptide (anti-CCP) in RA, are important biomarkers that help both to classify distinct groups of patients, and also serve as prognostic and diagnostic markers (see Chapter 17). Furthermore, these autoantibodies may be present before disease onset. Thus, the fact that anti-CCP antibodies increase the risk for subsequent development of RA, and anti-double stranded DNA (anti-dsDNA) antibodies increase the risk for SLE, indicates there is a direct association between B cells and plasma cells and the development of autoimmune diseases.[49] However, the exact mechanisms through which most autoantibodies contribute to the pathological inflammatory responses or tissue damage in these diseases are still unclear.

In addition to being a source of autoantibodies, it is increasingly clear that B cells and plasma cells also have functional effector diversity and therefore may play important proinflammatory roles in disease through the production of cytokines.[50,51] The robust clinical efficacy of B-cell depletion by anti-CD20 therapy in many systemic autoimmune diseases (RA, SLE, and myositis) underscores the important role of B cells in autoimmunity (see also Chapter 13).

Regulatory B Cells

Recently, the recognition of B cells with an antiinflammatory phenotype has gained attention.[50,51,52,53] Studies in both mice and humans have demonstrated that B cells can have immunosuppressive functions. These so-called regulatory B (Breg) cells have the potential to actively regulate an ongoing immune response, for example, through the production of IL-10 and, more recently demonstrated, IL-35.[53] IL-10–secreting B cells have been shown to promote disease remission in mouse models of autoimmune disorders. Human B cells may also produce IL-10, and there is increasing evidence to support the idea that human IL-1–producing B cells can also inhibit immunity. Human Breg cells have been shown to be within a population of transitional B cells, defined by the phenotype CD19+CD24hiCD38hi and have been shown to be defective in human autoimmune diseases such as lupus.[54,55]

Dendritic Cells

DCs are key regulators of adaptive immunity as part of the first-line defense against microorganisms. They are potent initiators of immune responses as well as mediating immune tolerance (see the next section).[7,56,57] First recognized by Steinman (for which he received the Nobel Prize in 2011) and others more than 40 years ago, DCs form a bridge between innate and adaptive immunity. They are part of lineage of cells that include Langerhans cells, plasmacytoid dendritic cells (pDCs) and monocyte-derived dendritic cells (mDCs); the latter are also referred to as classical dendritic cells or cDCs. DCs can identify and kill potential harmful microorganisms while also processing self-antigens. In doing so they can attract and direct other immune cells and create the proper microenvironment for an effective immune response.

Dendritic Cells in Autoimmunity

DCs may drive both highly inflammatory as well as regulatory responses. The resulting effector response generated will depend in part in levels of costimulatory molecules, cytokines produced by DCs and the strength of APC/T-cell interaction. The mechanisms of action of tolerogenic DCs is still not known, but the production of cytokines (such as IL-10 and TGF-β) and the increased prevalence of tolerogenic versus stimulatory membrane-bound coreceptors appears to have a role.[56] Simultaneously, Treg cells can downregulate the expression of costimulatory molecules (CD80/86) on DCs, through the action of CTLA4, which serves to inhibit antigen presentation to effector T cells.[58]

Much evidence from experimental models indicates that DCs play a key role in autoimmunity. Thus the deficiency of TGF-β signaling specifically in DCs leads to experimental autoimmune colitis, whereas DC-specific knockout of genes associated with human autoimmunity on genome-wide association studies (GWAS), such as Blimp1 and TNFAIP3, leads to autoimmune phenotypes in experimental animals.[59] TNFAIP3, also known as A20, is a ubiquitin-modifier that has a profound antiinflammatory effect, by restricting DC-mediated immune activation, in part through modulating nuclear factor κB (NF-κB) signaling. Interestingly, in the TNFAIP3-deficient mouse model, the disease mimics inflammatory bowel disease, enthesitis, and ankylosing spondylitis (AS),[60] conditions that frequently also occur in humans. On the other hand, DC-l specific knockout of Blimp1 leads to the presence of humoral autoimmunity with a lupuslike serology.[61]

In humans, pDCs can induce T cells to differentiate into suppressor or Treg cells, but they may also be the source of type 1 interferons thought to play a role in SLE and JDM.[7,62,63] Perhaps their most important role in steering the adaptive immune response, whether toward effector or regulatory functions, is their capacity to process antigens and present them to T cells.[64] Because of their central role in immune response initiation and regulation, DCs are important targets for innovative forms of immune therapy.

MAINTAINING IMMUNE TOLERANCE AND BALANCE IN THE ADAPTIVE IMMUNE SYSTEM

Central Tolerance

Maintaining the balance of the adaptive immune system requires an extensive system to keep potential autoreactive T and B cells under control. Prevention of the emergence of autoreactive cells takes place both centrally (at the selection of the repertoire) and in the periphery. In the thymus, T cells are generated that need to have a diverse range of TCRs so that the final repertoire has the potential to cope with an enormous range of different foreign antigens. Similarly, it is crucial that T cells with a TCR with a high affinity for self-antigens are eliminated from the repertoire. This negative selection is dependent on the local expression of tissue-specific antigens in the thymus. This process is controlled by the autoimmune regulator protein (AIRE). Absence of AIRE leads to severe autoimmunity both in animal models and in humans (autoimmune polyendocrinopathy-candidiasis-ectodermal dystrophy syndrome [APECED])[65] (see Chapter 46).

Peripheral Tolerance

Central selection processes are not absolute and not sufficient to prevent harmful autoreactivity. Therefore the immune system harbors other control mechanisms in the periphery. These include the presence of numerous regulatory mechanisms that can be tissue specific and/or cell specific. Of the cellular mechanisms, Treg cells are the best studied, but an increasing body of evidence supports a role for Breg cells, as discussed previously.[31,52] It is clear that DCs also play a key role in maintaining tolerance in part by the generation of Treg cells.[7] In addition, immune control mechanisms are not mediated only by adaptive immunity. Innate immune cells, such as neutrophils, can also have a regulatory, suppressive effect on a potential damaging immune response.

THE INFLAMMATORY RESPONSE OUT OF CONTROL IN AUTOIMMUNITY

Identification of "Self" Versus "Nonself"

The conventional vision of the tolerance process is somewhat dichotomous. It is based on the concept that there is a clear partition between self and nonself, and that the immune system has evolved to ignore self and react against environmental challenges. However, in reality the process of the ontogeny of the most sophisticated part of the immune system, T-cell adaptive immunity, is entirely shaped on recognition of self-antigens, presented in the thymus in the context of self-MHC to immature T cells. T cells whose TCR binds self-antigens with high affinity are deleted, as they would be highly self-reactive, whereas T cells whose TCR binds self-antigens at medium affinity survive and will comprise the mature T-cell repertoire. In the periphery, self-peptides are constantly recognized by the same T cells, and such interactions contribute to maintenance of T-cell clones throughout life. Hence, recognition of self is a necessary and ever-occurring phenomenon for the immune system. Autoimmune disease occurs when the delicate balance between recognition and tolerance tilts toward reactivity. This is most likely to occur in the microenvironment where an autoimmune reaction originates, perhaps in combination with inflammatory triggers such as local infection or tissue damage. Loss of

tolerance is the outcome of environmental, stochastic, and epigenetic elements shaping the cross talk between adaptive and innate immunity.[66-70]

Cross-Talk Between Adaptive and Innate Immunity in Disease

A frequent misconception of the immune system is that it is compartmentalized, with its various components dissected and isolated in "waterproof" compartments. This approach may simplify the sharing of knowledge about individual components of the immune system, and the identifying of potential targets for therapeutic intervention. However, it is important to underscore that the immune system is dynamic and its individual elements profoundly intertwined. In particular, interference in any one individual pathway has effects far beyond the intended target, and eventually involves many components of the immune response. For example, it is evident that JIA, like other autoimmune arthritides, is multifactorial, and several immune pathways contribute etiologically and pathogenetically.

Th17 cells and their relationship to Treg cells in disease

Th17 cells express the transcription factor retinoic acid receptor-related orphan nuclear receptor C (RORC) and secrete the proinflammatory cytokine IL-17.[71] Th17 cells from inflammatory sites such as the joints of children with JIA also frequently produce other cytokines including TNF, GM-CSF, and others.[29,43] As Th17 cells and Treg cells share a close relationship, understanding how these cells interact and what consequence this may have on JIA will help to further understand this complex disease. Patients with active JIA have increased numbers of Th17 cells and reduced numbers of Treg cells compared with healthy controls in peripheral blood. However, at the inflamed site, both these subsets are highly enriched, and there is a reciprocal relationship between Th17 and Treg cells.[29,35] Interestingly, the subset of Treg cells that can also produce IL-17 (identified by the surface marker CD161) is highly enriched in the synovial compartment in JIA and correlates with disease activity.[39] In addition to a potential imbalance between Th17 cells and Treg cells, it appears that the effector T cells within the synovial compartment may be resistant to Treg-mediated suppression.[72] Therefore, Th17/Treg imbalance, Treg cells that have switched to become proinflammatory, and the resistance of Th17 cells to Treg-mediated suppression may all contribute to the pathogenic process in JIA. Key drivers of these switches, and how they may be programmed in terms of epigenetic and transcriptional modulation, remain unknown. Data from mouse models and adult RA suggest that anti-TNF therapies (in particular antibodies to TNF, but not etanercept) may reset an imbalance between Th17 and Treg cells, and induce Treg cells capable of suppressing Th17 responses.[73,74]

Treg cells at the inflamed site colocalize with DCs in the lymphoid aggregate areas of inflamed synovium, but it is thought that this colocalization cannot fully suppress DC activation and function. Interactions between Treg cells and DCs at sites of inflammation may lead to Treg cell proliferation. Murine studies have identified a feedback loop between Treg cells and DCs, regulated by Fms-like tyrosine kinase 3 ligand (Flt3L). Flt3L increased the number of DCs, which induced Treg cell division via MHC class II expression on DCs. This increase in DCs and Treg cells prevented the onset of autoimmune disease in mice.[75] It has been reported that Flt3L levels are elevated in the synovial fluid (SF) of arthritis patients, and administration of Flt3L can alleviate arthritis in the methylated bovine serum albumin (mBSA) model.[76] These findings indicate that Flt3L may act as one important regulator of the immune system via the expansion of DCs and Treg cells.

Monocytes are important players in the synovial microenvironment of autoimmune arthritis. Large numbers of activated monocytes are present in the inflamed joints and contribute to inflammation via secretion of a number of proinflammatory cytokines (e.g., IL-1β, IL-6, IL-7, and TNF-α). These cytokines can potentially affect the differentiation and function of Treg cells. For instance, IL-1β plays a role in the conversion of human Treg cells into IL-17–producing cells and IL-7, whereas TNF-α may abrogate Treg cell function. Also, IL-6, along with an unknown TLR-induced factor, renders effector T cells resistant to Treg-mediated suppression.[77] In JIA the effector resistance demonstrated in synovial T-effector (Teff) cells could be partly replicated by pretreatment of Teff cells with IL-6/TNF.[72] In RA, it has been reported that IL-6, TNF-α, and IL-1-β secreted by synovial monocytes induce expression of both proinflammatory (IL-17, IFN-γ, and TNF-α) and antiinflammatory (IL-10) cytokines by Treg cells. These Treg cells maintain their regulatory phenotype and have an enhanced suppressive ability; they are capable of suppressing IL-17 production.[78] Thus it is possible that despite high levels of proinflammatory cytokines at sites of inflammation, Treg cells may still function effectively.

Fibroblast-like synoviocytes (FLS) are present within the synovial membrane. These cells display an altered phenotype in RA and produce a number of inflammatory mediators including matrix metalloproteases, chemokines, and cytokines. FLS play a major role in RA pathogenesis through the destruction of cartilage and bone and perpetuation of the inflammatory immune response. FLS express the T-cell growth factor IL-15 on their surface, which further stimulates effector T cells to produce proinflammatory cytokines. However, a recent study reported that FLS also induced the proliferation of Treg cells and enhanced their suppressive activity. IL-15 produced by FLS appears to have a dual effect on the balance between Treg cells and effector T cells. It has been reported that FLS from mice with zymosan-induced arthritis express the ligand for glucocorticoid-induced TNF receptor (GITR) and reduce the expression of GITR and FOXP3 in Treg cells via cell-to-cell contact. Furthermore, this interaction increased IL-6 production from FLS, which may cause Treg cells to convert to IL-17–producing cells or inhibit Treg cell suppression. Therefore, the interaction between FLS and Treg cells diminishes the suppressive activity of Treg cells and enhances the proinflammatory activity of FLS, thereby leading to exacerbation of arthritis. To date there are few data about FLS in JIA.[79-82]

Osteoclasts, cartilage, and bone destruction are key features of arthritis. Cytokines such as TNF-α, receptor activator of nuclear factor kappa-B ligand (RANKL), and IL-17 induce an imbalance between bone formation (*osteoblast dependent*) and bone resorption (*osteoclast dependent*) resulting in enhanced bone loss. It has been reported that Treg cells can suppress osteoclast formation and may therefore regulate bone homeostasis. Treg cells have been shown to inhibit the development of collagen-induced arthritis (CIA) in mice and reduce the differentiation of osteoclasts, possibly due to induction of cytokines that inhibit osteoclastogenesis. Moreover, Treg cells have also been shown to suppress inflammation and bone destruction in TNF-mediated arthritis in transgenic mice. However, the bone-protective effects of Treg cells did not reflect improved inflammation but rather had a direct effect on the osteoclasts and osteoclast-mediated bone resorption. Furthermore, adaptive Treg cells may be superior to naturally occurring Treg cells in their ability to suppress osteoclastogenesis, possibly because adaptive Treg cells are more resistant to IL-6–mediated Th17 conversion. Thus, Treg cells both suppress inflammation and autoreactivity, and also directly suppress bone destruction.[83-85]

Condrocytes. Most studies focus on synovial inflammation and hyperplasia with inflammatory pannus, but there are not many studies on the loss of human chondrocytes itself. It is known that the loss of cartilage resulting in cartilage degradation and erosion is an important

pathogenetic mechanism in rheumatic joint diseases. Thus far, chondrocytes have been interpreted as passive participators in inflammatory joint diseases that become damaged during inflammation. However, it is also known that IL-1α and IL-1β are able to induce various cytokines in chondrocytes.[86] Hence, the possible involvement of chondrocytes in the inflammatory process and in the progression of inflammatory joint diseases, which results in disruption of cartilage repair mechanisms and consequently cartilage degradation, has to be considered.

Linking Immune Phenotypes to Clinical Phenotypes

Systemic JIA (sJIA) is characterized by features such as fever, rash, and serositis. Due to the pronounced activation of a patient's innate immune system and the absence of any consistent association with autoantibodies or HLA, it is increasingly believed that sJIA may be a polygenic autoinflammatory syndrome (see Chapter 16). Recent understanding of the roles for IL-1 and IL-6 in pathogenesis of sJIA has translated directly into new and effective treatment pathways for sJIA, by the use of IL-6 and IL-1 blockade.[87-89] Tocilizumab, an anti-IL-6 receptor antibody, has been highly effective in the treatment of sJIA. Anti-IL-1 treatment, either by use of the IL-1R antagonist (anakinra), or anti-IL-1 antibodies such as canakinumab, can also be effective. Some data have suggested the delineation of two subpopulations of this form of disease—one with a pronounced, complete response to IL-1 blockade and another that is resistant to treatment or has an intermediate response. The observation that peripheral blood of sJIA patients has a higher frequency of Th17 cells than controls is interesting given the role of IL-6 in generation of the Th17 cell.[90]

Although the category oligoarticular JIA is clinically heterogeneous, the early onset, ANA-positive form is a well-defined disease that occurs almost exclusively in children[91] and has consistent HLA associations.[20] Patients may have high concentrations of positive ANAs and a high risk of developing chronic iridocyclitis. Based on the current JIA classification criteria from the International League of Associations for Rheumatology (ILAR), oligoarthritis can be distinguished into two categories: persistent oligoarthritis, in which the disease affects four joints or fewer, and extended oligoarthritis, in which more than four joints are affected after the first 6 months of disease. The immunological phenotype has been shown to differ between these two types of oligoarticular JIA, in that the enrichment of Treg cells in the synovial compartment is more marked in persistent than extended oligoarthritis, whereas the synovial enrichment of Th17 cells is more marked in in extended oligoarthritis than persistent oligoarthritis.[29,35] Immunological differences between these two are detectable, in the synovial cells, prior to clinical extension, which may in the future translate to clinical tests that could assist in the prediction of extension.[92]

Rheumatoid factor (RF)-positive polyarthritis, a relatively rare subtype of JIA, is the only form of JIA with positive antibodies to cyclic citrullinated peptides (CCPs), and shares HLA associations with adult-onset RA (see Chapter 17). Enthesitis-related arthritis (ERA) JIA shares features with spondyloarthropathy; many patients are HLA-B27 positive, and the disease can progress to affect sacroiliac joints in about 30% to 40% of patients. Interestingly, ERAP-1 and IL23-R, genes associated with adult AS, are also associated with ERA[93] (see Chapter 19).

RF-negative polyarthritis is a heterogeneous category of JIA. At least two subsets can be identified in this category: one that is similar to adult-onset RF-negative RA (characterized by a symmetric synovitis of large and small joints, onset at school age, and the absence of ANA expression), and another that resembles oligoarthritis. Similarities between this second subset and early-onset oligoarthritis has led some to suggest that pathological mechanisms may be similar in all children with early-onset, ANA-positive arthritis, irrespective of joint count. A major effort is underway to understand the molecular mechanisms a leading to resistance to therapy, for example, in severe JIA.[94]

Translation Into Clinical Practice
Application of Modern Methods to Immune Modulation
The rapid evolution of multiplex, high-throughput technologies (HTT) (genomics, transcriptomics, proteomics, and metabolomics, among others) has provided the opportunity to probe large panels of candidate biomarkers. There are some cases of HTT research yielding a candidate, which can then be combined with traditional clinical laboratory markers to provide a composite score for use in the management of autoimmune disease. However, clinical application of various HTT is limited due to technology. At present, use of single nucleotide polymorphisms (SNPs) and other genetic markers as prognostic biomarkers are constrained by the multifactorial etiology of arthritis. Also, environmental triggers, stochastic events, and epigenetic marks are not captured by genetics. The intrinsic instability of candidate markers that exhibit high biological turnover rates, such as mRNA, and the operator- and procedure-dependent variability of plasma-derived candidates jeopardizes their translation to clinical settings. Proposed synovial candidates require invasive procedures and are therefore less practical, other than where joint aspiration is routine, as in oligoarticular JIA, which supports the case for reliable blood-based assays. In the future a combination of biomarkers, including protein, metabolome, and genetic tests may be used to reclassify diseases and provide prognostic algorithms, as is already the reality in oncology.

The recent advent of biologics, including TNF and other cytokine inhibitors, costimulation blockade and cell-depletion therapies has raised therapeutic expectations for treatment of childhood arthritis from the control of signs and symptoms to a goal of complete remission. However, these objectives are met in only one out of three patients. As of now, patients who will respond to the treatment are phenotypically indistinguishable from those who will not, leaving "trial and error" as the only feasible approach to determining the most effective treatment regimen. Thus, many patients remain exposed to the damage of continued active disease and to the costs and potential side effects of these drugs, with no substantial benefit. Across all autoimmune diseases, the identification of biomarkers that predict responsiveness to therapy is a major unmet medical need.[95] All told, new developments in genetics, immunology, and imaging are instrumental to better define, classify, and treat children with autoimmune rheumatological diseases.

IMMUNE MECHANISMS OF ACTION OF ANTIRHEUMATIC DRUGS
Conventional Therapies for Autoimmune Arthritis
Despite significant progress over the past 20 years, low-dose methotrexate (MTX) therapy, a traditional folate antagonist, and disease-modifying antirheumatic drugs (DMARDs), administered weekly either alone or as part of combination therapy, remains the gold standard treatment of JIA. MTX has been proven safe and convenient, as well as effective. Several potential mechanisms for MTX activity have been proposed; these include antiproliferative, antiinflammatory, and immunosuppressive effects. MTX can affect these mechanisms by inhibiting purine/pyrimidine synthesis or proinflammatory cytokine production; promoting adenosine release or activated T-cell apoptosis; suppressing lymphocyte proliferation, neutrophil chemotaxis, or neutrophil adherence; and reducing serum immunoglobulin (Ig) levels. The mechanism underlying the therapeutic efficacy may be partially attributed to increased production of CD4+CD25+ Treg cells. These

cells specifically downmodulated the T-lymphocyte proliferative response to chicken type II collagen (CCII) but not phytohemagglutinin (PHA), induced a Th1-to-Th2 shift, downregulated Th1 cytokines, and upregulated both Th2 and Th3 cytokines.[96,97]

Although the data are contradictory, it has been reported that established therapies can influence Treg cell populations.[98] In a CIA mouse model, MTX modulated arthritis severity by immune-tolerant effects beyond its known antiproliferative mechanisms. This was attributed to an increased Treg cell population. However, in a study on RA, MTX and infliximab had no effect on Treg cell function, whereas sulfasalazine and leflunomide inhibited the antiproliferative function of Treg cells.[99,100]

Cytokine Blockade
TNF blocking agents infliximab, adalimumab, and etanercept bind soluble and membrane-bound TNF. However, they have different biological effects as demonstrated in complement-dependent and antibody-dependent cell-mediated cytotoxicity assays with a stable cell line expressing TNF. There are differences between etanercept, which is a soluble TNF receptor that also binds lymphotoxin, and the other TNF blockers, which are monoclonal antibodies. These differences in target molecules and signaling may account for the variability in mechanistic effects. An example of how anti-TNF therapy primarily intended to suppress a specific cytokine might affect immune tolerance at large lies in the observation that treatment with infliximab (but not etanercept) resulted in an increase in the percentage of CD4+CD25+ Treg cells in patients with RA who responded to therapy.[73] This increase in the number of Treg cells correlated with clinical improvement. This effect has not yet been reported in JIA.

IL-6 is a proinflammatory cytokine and one of the most important mediators of fever and the acute phase response via stimulation of the JAK–STAT pathway. IL-6 also has a critical role in the proliferation and differentiation of T cells, the terminal differentiation of B cells, and the regulation of Th17 cells. TGF-β induces Th17 cell differentiation in conjunction with IL-6; however, in the absence of IL6, TGF-β induces the differentiation of naturally occurring Treg cells. Hence, it seems likely that blockade of the IL-6 pathway might lead to effects on Treg or Th17 cells and on other proinflammatory cytokines, specifically IL-17 and TNF. To date the data to demonstrate this have been inconclusive in RA, and there have been no published reports in JIA.

Therapies Targeting Costimulatory Molecules
T cells need to receive not only an antigen-specific signal through their T-cell receptors, but also nonspecific costimulatory signals to achieve optimal activation. A particularly important costimulatory signal is that generated by the interaction between CD28 on T cells and CD80 (also known as B71 antigen) or CD86 (also known as B72 antigen) on APCs. T-cell activation is downregulated by CTLA-4, which is expressed on the surface of activated T cells and prevents CD28 from binding to CD80 or CD86. Abatacept (CTLA-4-Ig) inhibits T-cell activation and T cell–dependent B-cell differentiation by acting on recently stimulated T cells, and it has efficacy in JIA.[100,101] In animal models, abatacept converts naïve CD4+CD25- T cells into FOXP3 + Treg cells. It is known that abatacept also expands the numbers of Treg cells, although these findings have not been confirmed in studies of transplant rejection in humans. It may also serve to "strip" costimulatory molecules from APCs, in a similar mechanism to CTLA-4 on Treg cells.[58] Evidence from a mouse model of arthritis suggests that abatacept can also affect Th17 cells by reducing their numbers or inhibiting their function. Notably, CTLA4 expression is reduced in Treg cells from RA patients with active disease, thus providing a rationale for the use of abatacept in therapy.[102]

Therapies Targeting B Cells

B cells secrete proinflammatory cytokines, act as APCs, enhance T-cell activation through B7 costimulatory molecules (CD80 and CD86) and other members of the B7 and CD28 families (such as inducible T-cell costimulator (ICOS) ligand, programmed death-ligand 1 (PD L1), programmed death-ligand 2 (PD L2), CD276, and V-set domain-containing T-cell activation inhibitor 1 (VTCN1)), as well as being precursors to autoantibody-producing plasma cells. TNF and IFN-γ can induce high levels of the B-cell activating factor (BAFF) (also known as B lymphocyte stimulator [BLyS]) and TNF ligand superfamily member [TNFSF]-13B protein in coculture with synovial fibroblasts.[103] BAFF regulates B-cell development as well as survival, activation, and antigen presentation, and is related to APRIL (a proliferation-inducing ligand). Levels of BAFF and APRIL are higher in the synovial fluid of patients with RA, and in blood of both adult and pediatric SLE.[103] In one study of 74 JIA patients, both BAFF and APRIL levels in serum were raised, and correlated with disease activity; within oligoarticular JIA, BAFF levels were higher in those with uveitis than those without.[104] Belimumab, which targets BAFF, has shown modest efficacy in phase II studies in adult RA and efficacy in adult SLE: trials of belimumab in JSLE are ongoing. Atacicept is a recombinant fusion protein that binds to and neutralizes the activity of both BAFF and APRIL. Results of phase IIb trials suggest that this drug is well tolerated and has no obvious safety concerns.

The most developed B cell–based therapy relies on depletion of CD20$^+$ B cells with rituximab, an anti-CD20 monoclonal antibody, which has demonstrated considerable clinical benefit in patients with RA. Early reports of use of rituximab in JIA-associated uveitis are promising, as are some data for B-cell depletion in both adult and childhood onset myositis.[105,106] Whether the ablation of a subset of B cells has direct effects on the mechanisms of immune tolerance or whether the observed clinical effects rely merely on the disruption of some of the pathways mentioned is not yet proved.[102]

Therapies Targeting Kinases

The members of the Janus kinase (JAK) family of nonreceptor tyrosine kinases transduce signals from several cytokines (including IL-6, IL-12, IL-15, IL23, GM-CSF and IFN-γ) that potentially mediate inflammatory pathogenesis. The p38 mitogen-activated protein kinase (MAPK) signaling cascade is involved in a number of cellular processes that are implicated in the pathogenesis, such as the upregulation of inflammatory mediators, including TNF and IL-6. Interestingly, a recent *in vitro* study suggested that MTX may act in part through kinase pathway alteration that was distinct in T cells as compared with FLS.[107,108]

Overall, the development of novel kinase inhibitors for the treatment of arthritis seems to be promising, with several of the agents demonstrating a favorable efficacy profile.[109] In a trial in adult RA of tofacitinib versus MTX, each as monotherapy, tofacitinib was reported to be superior to MTX.[110] However, the side-effect profiles may prove to be an issue for many of these new agents and are yet unknown for children. The induction of immune tolerance by these compounds could be the outcome of direct inhibition of inflammatory pathways together with an indirect restoration of inhibitory mechanisms. Trials of these agents in children with inflammatory disorders are currently being planned.

New Antirheumatic Therapies

Although the exact origin and pathogenesis of JIA remain unknown, research into JIA's pathophysiology has revealed various targets for the development of new antirheumatic therapies. These new therapies may include biological modifier therapies (including recombinant regulatory cytokines, engineered molecules, and monoclonal antibodies [mAbs] targeting proinflammatory cytokines or lymphocyte cell-surface proteins), oral tolerance, gene therapy, and therapeutic vaccination.[102,111] Antigen-specific Treg cells could reinstate immune tolerance, and protocols that expand or induce *de novo* generation of Treg cells are currently under investigation. Recent work has demonstrated both the efficient expansion and induction of Treg cells. However, other cell subsets are also important at inducing Treg cells and may also represent potential cell therapies. For example, Breg cells (CD19$^+$CD24^{hi}CD38^{hi} B cells) have an emerging role in immune tolerance. Interestingly, Breg cells from healthy controls induce Treg cells; however, RA Breg cells fail to induce Treg cell differentiation.[55] Therapies to reinstate Breg cell function are a novel therapeutic avenue currently under investigation.

The next challenge will be to combine genetic and immunological mechanistic studies with new imaging modalities to define the subgroups of patients, individual risk profiles, and response to treatment. Hopefully, these will pave the way for the next generation of clinical trials that aim to restore the immune balance in patients and restrict potential long-term side effects.

FUTURE THERAPEUTICS AND MANIPULATING ADAPTIVE AUTOIMMUNITY

The mechanism of action of biological agents and other drugs described above may reduce or block inflammation but do not restore immunological tolerance.[111] In addition to novel and improved biological agents, it is clear that approaches that are themselves tolerogenic also need to be developed. The ultimate goal of such therapies is to complement the current strategies and maintain disease control using a minimum-treatment regimen.

Antigen-Specific Tolerance

Inducing tolerance against a specific inciting agent could result in the desired downregulation of the autoimmune process while leaving the physiological ability of the immune system to respond effectively to danger intact. Various types of immune cells can contribute to tolerance and are therefore a target of therapeutic attempts to induce antigen-specific tolerance.[102]

Manipulating Dendritic Cell Phenotypes

Some subtypes of DCs, such as immature DCs, can directly induce T cells to differentiate into T cells that have suppressive or regulatory functions. Specifically targeting DCs might prove a successful route to the restoration of immune tolerance in human autoimmune diseases. Tolerogenic DCs can be generated pharmacologically *in vitro,* for example, by exposure to vitamin D and dexamethasone or by manipulation of culture conditions to provide an appropriate microenvironment for their development.[112,113] These insights may lead to avenues by which to "switch" DC to a more tolerogenic phenotype *in vivo* in the future.

Manipulating T-Cell Responses

When contacted with an antigen, T-cell responses range from ignorance to reactivity to tolerance or anergy. The route and frequency of administration as well as the concentration of antigen used can affect the type and intensity of antigen-specific T-cell responses. In this context, the induction of antigen-specific tolerance has been attempted by employing antigenic peptides whose primary sequence has been altered to affect either the affinity or the promiscuity of recognition by the TCR. A promising avenue consists in the induction of tolerance to antigenic peptides that contribute to maintaining inflammation regardless of its original trigger. This concept has been developed and validated in various autoimmune diseases. A peptide derived from the DnaJ heat shock protein is in phase IIb clinical development and appears promising.[114-118] Analog peptides for tolerization have been proposed for JIA.[16] One of the few antigen-specific approaches that have been successful in the clinic is based on the concept of promiscuous engagement of multiple pathogenic T-cell clones. This strategy employed a repetitive, random sequence of a few amino acids as the antigen. The mechanisms of action are not fully understood. However, it seems to involve not only competition for the pathogenic antigens, but also active induction of tolerance via induction of tolerogenic cytokines.[102]

Tolerance Induction and the Microenvironment

The microenvironment is as crucial to the induction of antigen-specific tolerance as is the presence of tolerogenic or proinflammatory mediators. In the mucosal microenvironment, antigen presentation occurs in the presence of tolerogenic stimuli, such as TGF-β and IL-10, and tolerogenic DCs. In mucosal tolerization, the ability of T cells to recognize specific antigens remains unchanged, but the nature of the response is altered, often deviating from an inflammatory to a tolerogenic immune response. The pathways leading to this outcome are not fully understood and probably involve both effector T cells and various types of Treg cells.[102]

TOWARD STRATIFIED MEDICINE: OUTCOMES AND BIOMARKERS

The wide array of technologies and knowledge available based on molecular immunology have not been fully exploited yet in their application to pediatric rheumatic diseases. In addition, information related to the mechanisms of action of immune-therapeutic drugs has not been matched with clinical outcomes. This is partly the consequence of the lack of appropriately powered and controlled studies designed to address mechanistic questions related to the effects of immunotherapy on the pathogenesis of autoimmunity, or clinical trials that are performed without add on mechanistic studies. An important aspect driving immunotherapy is the shift from conservative treatment, often seen as management of disease symptoms in the middle or advanced stages of the disease course, to the concept of early aggressive intervention that seeks to induce remission and, in large part, prevent debilitating damage before onset.

The next generation of immune therapy drugs will face the challenge of matching the efficacy of currently available biologics while also reducing costs and side effects. This challenge can probably be met only by evolving the target focus from nonspecific to disease-related pathogenic mechanisms. One possible avenue will be related to targeting the mechanisms of innate immunity more at the cellular level in an effective way. Inhibition or modulation of innate immunity has, however, inherent risks linked to the possibility that crucial functions of the first line of immune defense might be impaired. Hence it is probable that the field will evolve into integrating approaches targeted to adaptive immunity with the current therapeutic strategies.[111]

Finally, the application of modern treatments and new therapies will be best applied if and when it becomes possible to predict with some accuracy the likelihood of response to any particular treatment, and then to choose drugs using an individualized algorithm, based on reliable biomarkers that are simple to measure. Such prediction algorithms could greatly reduce costs and improve quality of life by selecting only those children likely to respond to first-line agents while

allowing others to progress rapidly to biological or newer therapies. Several recent studies have provided hope that such biomarkers that could predict response or nonresponse to MTX in JIA do exist, and which could be made available at relatively low cost with modern high throughput genomic methods.[119-123] This vision of so-called stratified or personalized medicine in childhood autoimmune disease can become a reality if an increasing number of children are given the opportunity to take part in large, well-structured research cohort studies and clinical trials in order to provide adequate power to test and validate such biomarkers in the future.[124]

REFERENCES

1. B. Prakken, S. Albani, A. Martini, Juvenile idiopathic arthritis, Lancet 377 (9783) (2011) 2138–2149.
2. K. Nistala, L.R. Wedderburn, Update in Juvenile myositis, Curr. Opin. Rheumatol. 25 (6) (2013) 742–746.
5. B.E. Russ, J.E. Prier, S. Rao, et al., T cell immunity as a tool for studying epigenetic regulation of cellular differentiation, Frontiers in Genetics 4 (2013) 218.
7. K.L. Lewis, B. Reizis, Dendritic cells: arbiters of immunity and immunological tolerance, Cold Spring Harbour Perspectives Biol. 4 (8) (2012) 007401.
10. J. Zhu, H. Yamane, W.E. Paul, Differentiation of effector CD4 T cell populations, Annu. Rev. Immunol. 28 (2010) 445–489.
13. L.R. Wedderburn, K. Nistala, Aetiology and pathogenesis of Juvenile idiopathic arthritis, in: G.S. Firestein, et al. (Eds.), Kelley's Textbook of Rheumatology, 9th ed., Elsevier, Philadelphia, 2013.
16. S. Kamphuis, W. Kuis, W. de Jager, et al., Tolerogenic immune responses to novel T-cell epitopes from heat-shock protein 60 in juvenile idiopathic arthritis, Lancet 366 (9479) (2005) 50–56.
19. S. Prahalad, D.N. Glass, A comprehensive review of the genetics of juvenile idiopathic arthritis, Pediatr. Rheumatol. Online J. 6 (2008) 11.
20. J.E. Cobb, A. Hinks, W. Thomson, The genetics of juvenile idiopathic arthritis: current understanding and future prospects, Rheumatology (Oxford) 53 (4) (2014) 592–599.
21. A. Hinks, J. Cobb, M.C. Marion, et al., Dense genotyping of immune-related disease regions identifies 14 new susceptibility loci for juvenile idiopathic arthritis, Nat. Genet. 45 (6) (2013) 664–669.
23. T.R. Mosmann, R.L. Coffman, TH1 and TH2 cells: different patterns of lymphokine secretion lead to different functional properties, Annu. Rev. Immunol. 7 (1989) 145–173.
24. K.C. Verbist, R. Wang, D.R. Green, T cell metabolism and the immune response, Semin. Immunol. 24 (6) (2012) 399–404.
25. J. Barbi, D. Pardoll, F. Pan, Metabolic control of the Treg/Th17 axis, Immunol. Rev. 252 (1) (2013) 52–77.
27. M.T. Palmer, C.T. Weaver, Autoimmunity: increasing suspects in the CD4+ T cell lineup, Nat. Immunol. 11 (1) (2010) 36–40.
31. K. Wing, S. Sakaguchi, Regulatory T cells exert checks and balances on self tolerance and autoimmunity, Nat. Immunol. 11 (1) (2010) 7–13.
35. I.M. de Kleer, L.R. Wedderburn, L.S. Taams, et al., CD4+CD25(bright) regulatory T cells actively regulate inflammation in the joints of patients with the remitting form of juvenile idiopathic arthritis, J. Immunol. 172 (10) (2004) 6435–6443.
38. D.J. Campbell, M.A. Koch, Phenotypical and functional specialization of FOXP3+ regulatory T cells, Nat. Rev. Immunol. 11 (2) (2011) 119–130.
40. R. Basu, R.D. Hatton, C.T. Weaver, The Th17 family: flexibility follows function, Immunol. Rev. 252 (1) (2013) 89–103.
42. K. Nistala, S. Adams, H. Cambrook, et al., Th17 plasticity in human autoimmune arthritis is driven by the inflammatory environment, Proc. Natl. Acad. Sci. U.S.A. 107 (33) (2010) 14751–14756.
52. C. Mauri, Regulation of immunity and autoimmunity by B cells, Curr. Opin. Immunol. 22 (6) (2010) 761–767.
53. C. Mauri, K. Nistala, Interleukin-35 takes the 'B' line, Nat. Med. 20 (6) (2014) 580–581.

56. R.M. Steinman, D. Hawiger, M.C. Nussenzweig, Tolerogenic dendritic cells, Annu. Rev. Immunol. 21 (2003) 685–711.

87. E.D. Mellins, C. Macaubas, A.A. Grom, Pathogenesis of systemic juvenile idiopathic arthritis: some answers, more questions, Nat. Rev. Rheumatol. 7 (7) (2011) 416–426.

88. V. Pascual, F. Allantaz, E. Arce, et al., Role of interleukin-1 (IL-1) in the pathogenesis of systemic onset juvenile idiopathic arthritis and clinical response to IL-1 blockade, J. Exp. Med. 201 (9) (2005) 1479–1486.

98. G. Mijnheer, B.J. Prakken, F. van Wijk, The effect of autoimmune arthritis treatment strategies on regulatory T-cell dynamics, Curr. Opin. Rheumatol. 25 (2) (2013) 260–267.

99. F.A. Cooles, J.D. Isaacs, A.E. Anderson, Treg cells in rheumatoid arthritis: an update, Curr. Rheumatol. Rep. 15 (9) (2013) 352.

102. S. Albani, E.C. Koffeman, B. Prakken, Induction of immune tolerance in the treatment of rheumatoid arthritis, Nat. Rev. Rheumatol. 7 (5) (2011) 272–281.

108. K. Ghoreschi, A. Laurence, J.J. O'Shea, Janus kinases in immune cell signaling, Immunol. Rev. 228 (1) (2009) 273–287.

122. J. Cobb, E. Cule, H. Moncrieffe, et al., Genome-wide data reveal novel genes for methotrexate response in a large cohort of juvenile idiopathic arthritis cases, Pharmacogenomics J. 14 (4) (2014) 356–364.

123. M.B. Calasan, N.M. Wulffraat, Methotrexate in juvenile idiopathic arthritis: towards tailor-made treatment, Expert Rev. Clin. Immunol. 10 (7) (2014) 843–854.

Entire reference list is available online at www.expertconsult.com.

CHAPTER 5

Integrative Genomics

Susan D. Thompson, Sampath Prahalad, Robert Allen Colbert

When viewed from a clinical perspective, few of the common pediatric rheumatic diseases appear to be genetically determined. Family histories are rarely positive for diseases such as juvenile idiopathic arthritis (JIA), and a Mendelian pattern of inheritance would suggest an alternative diagnosis. Pediatric rheumatic diseases share this scenario with autoimmune diseases in general, where the absence of a family history of the specific disease is common, yet a family history of autoimmunity in its various forms is frequent. An exception is spondyloarthritis, which in some families can follow inheritance of human leukocyte antigen (HLA)-B27, although overall penetrance is less than 20%. There is also an expanding list of rare disorders that are often autoinflammatory in nature, caused by single gene defects and inherited in a Mendelian fashion or as a consequence of a new mutation.

The past decade has witnessed remarkable advances in our understanding of the human genome, its variability, and the effects of variants on health and disease. Genetic variability contributes not only to a primary predisposition but also to phenotypic differences, including age of onset and extent and severity of disease, and applies to various forms of JIA and other complex genetic conditions in rheumatology. The well-recognized HLA associations for most of these diseases provide an indication of their genetic nature and involvement of the immune system in pathogenesis. However, although HLA genes may be a necessary part of genetic predisposition, it is now clear that multiple genes outside the major histocompatibility complex (MHC) contribute to risk in a given individual, and there are environmental contributions.

High-throughput technology, including next-generation sequencing, allows for rapid screening of known DNA polymorphisms, routine sequencing of the entire expressed genome (whole exome sequencing), and monitoring the expression of virtually every RNA molecule. The technology is enabling unprecedented discovery of the genetic basis of disease. Understanding how DNA polymorphisms alter gene expression and function (functional genomics) with these basic tools, together with comprehensive and integrative systems biology approaches, will foster a better understanding of human diseases and how to treat them optimally. Here we provide an introduction to the genome with respect to genes, noncoding DNA, and genomic variability, before discussing genetic components of pediatric rheumatic diseases and functional genomic approaches to their understanding.

THE HUMAN GENOME

Organization and Content

The *genome* can be defined as an individual's (or cell's) total genetic information, and *genomics* as the science of mapping, sequencing, and analyzing this information. The sequence of the human genome provides the genetic instructions for human physiology. The first draft of the human genome sequence was reported in 2001,[1,2] followed by a full assembly in 2004.[3] A complete description of The Human Genome Project and its remarkable achievements can be found at the National Human Genome Research Institute (www.nhgri.nih.gov/HGP/).

Protein Coding and Nonprotein Coding DNA

Human genetic information consists of approximately 3.1 billion base pairs of nuclear DNA organized into three components: 22 paired autosomal chromosomes and 2 sex chromosomes. It is striking that less than 2% of our DNA encodes protein (exons), ribosomal RNA (rRNA), or transfer RNA (tRNA). Another 37% contains sequences around or related to genes, such as introns, untranslated regions (UTRs), and pseudogenes.[4] A significant proportion of genetic material is aggregated into repetitive sequences that contribute to the familiar banding pattern that characterizes the morphology of chromosomes. For many years it was thought that much of the noncoding genome was composed of "junk" DNA with little functional significance. However, there has been a transformation in our understanding due in part to the ENCODE Project (http://www.genome.gov/Encode/) intended to produce an *Encyclopedia of Functional DNA Elements*. It is now estimated that 80% of our genome has some function, including transcription factor binding sites and structural elements for histone binding and chromatin formation, with a great deal of noncoding DNA controlling the complexities of gene regulation.[5]

Protein coding DNA encompasses about 21,500 genes that provide the essential information for all proteins in the human body. However, because a single mRNA can be alternately spliced and proteins can be modified posttranslationally (e.g., proteolytic processing, glycosylation, phosphorylation, acetylation), more than one molecular species of a protein from a single gene can exist. This contributes to the inherent complexity of proteome analysis (discussed later in this chapter). There is both qualitative and quantitative variation between different cell types in the genes expressed. For example, a metabolically complex organ such as the liver may express 15,000 genes, many of which are important for hepatic function; the synovium may well express fewer proteins, varying with stage of development and appropriateness for the function of the tissue. The encyclopedia remains to be completed because many cell types and physiological states of these cell types have yet to be investigated.

Noncoding RNA

Regions of nonprotein coding DNA can be transcribed into noncoding RNAs (ncRNAs) that execute a number of important biological

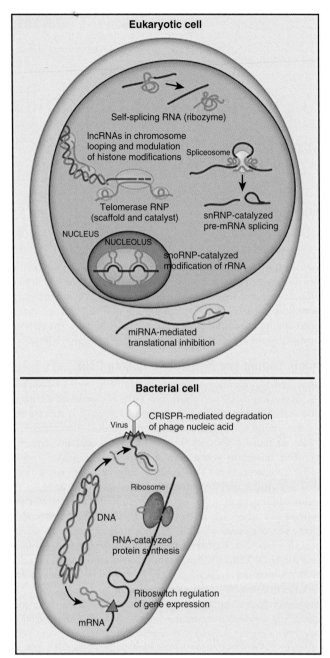

FIGURE 5-1 Examples of the diverse functions of noncoding RNAs in eukaryotic cells. Noncoding RNAs regulate gene expression, including transcription (e.g., lncRNAs), splicing (e.g., snRNP), and mRNA stability and translation (e.g., miRNAs), as well as genome organization and stability (e.g., telomerase RNA). The blue lines indicate DNA, and the red and orange lines, RNA. Ovals are protein components of RNP complexes. (Reprinted from T.R. Cech, J.A. Steitz, The noncoding RNA revolution-trashing old rules to forge new ones, Cell 157 (2014) 77 94, with permission.)

functions. A comprehensive view of this rapidly expanding area of biology is beyond our scope, but a few examples of how ncRNAs function can be instructive (Fig. 5-1). Major classes of regulatory ncRNAs include long noncoding RNA (lncRNA), microRNA (miRNA), small nuclear RNA (snRNA), small nucleolar RNA (snoRNA), self-splicing RNA (ribozymes), and telomerase RNA. Long noncoding RNAs are generally less than 200 nucleotides (nt) in length and are autonomously

transcribed from diverse areas of the genome, including intergenic, intronic, and regulatory regions. They hybridize with other species of RNA or DNA and can bind proteins to form scaffolds in chromatin structure,[6-8] bringing into proximity genes that may be coordinately transcribed despite being distant from one another in the genome. Noncoding RNAs can act in *cis* or in *trans* and are crucial regulators of cell differentiation, organ development, and disease processes. MicroRNAs are generated from primary miRNA (pri-miRNA) transcripts of 80 or more nt in length, after enzymatic processing by Drosha and Dicer. Many pri-miRNAs are generated from introns of protein coding genes and can contain more than one miRNA. MicroRNAs bind to mRNA via complementary sequences at their 5′ end and reduce protein expression, either by facilitating rapid mRNA decay, or through translational inhibition.[9] Small noncoding RNAs complex with proteins to form snRNPs (many of which can be targets of autoantibodies such as anti-Sm in lupus) and the spliceosome complex that removes introns from pre-mRNAs in the nucleus, whereas snoRNAs modify rRNA in the nucleolus. Telomerase RNA complexed with protein provides a scaffold and template for telomeric DNA synthesis, thus contributing to genomic stability. This list of ncRNA species, although incomplete, emphasizes the varied and important functions of the noncoding genome. A greater understanding of the role of ncRNA in normal function will lead to a better appreciation of its role in disease.

Sequence Variation

The Human Genome Project provided a reference genome. However, to characterize genetic influences on disease susceptibility, severity, and response to medications, it was necessary to map sequence variation. The 1000 Genomes Project used DNA sequences obtained from geographically distinct populations around the world[10] to catalog 38 million single nucleotide polymorphisms (SNPs), including 1.4 million short insertions and deletions (indels), and 14,000 large deletions.[11] SNPs are often characterized by the frequency of the variant in a population, with common alleles being present in more than 5% of individuals, uncommon in 0.5-5%, and rare in less than 0.5%. About 10 million of the 38 million human SNPs identified (26%) are classified as *common*. Although the genome and genome structures are broadly the same for all persons (99.9% identity), it is fundamental to the understanding of human diversity and disease susceptibility to recognize that variability is substantial among individuals and can influence health and disease.

The 1000 Genome dataset has been used to provide an estimate of likely pathogenic candidate genes by focusing on rare variants in evolutionarily conserved positions. It is predicted that on average, each person carries between 130 and 400 DNA variants that change a protein's sequence (non-synonymous coding variants), with 2 to 5 of these variants likely to damage protein function, as well as between 10 and 20 complete loss-of-function variants due to premature stop codons (stop-gains), frameshifts or indels in coding sequence, or disruptions in critical mRNA splice sites.[11] These predicted pathological variants, although they may only alter a single expressed gene product, can have effects ranging from deleterious (including fatal) to neutral, or sometimes even result in a gain of function. Clearly, the nature and site of the change (e.g., coding regions, regulatory regions) is important in this regard and can be reflected in changed phenotypes and disease. Although variability is local, the impact may be devastating for the patient. The complement deficiencies are examples of individual gene variability of relevance to autoimmunity; the chromosome 22 deletion associated with JIA[12] is another such example, which, like trisomy 21 (Down syndrome), may also have considerable effects on the expression of a large number of genes.[13]

Throughout the human genome there is a correlation structure linking genetic variation of different loci. Consequently, knowing the genotype at one locus can provide information about the genotype at a second locus. This correlation between variants at different loci is termed linkage disequilibrium (LD). Preceding the 1000 Genomes Project, an international collaborative effort known as the HapMap Project was undertaken to map LD in the human genome (http://hapmap.ncbi.nlm.nih.gov/index.html.en). The HapMap defines regions of LD throughout the genome and identifies SNPs that "tag" these haplotype blocks. The MHC where HLA proteins are encoded is the most comprehensively documented area of LD, with very large haplotype blocks. Specific tag SNPs serve as markers in genome-wide association studies representing large stretches of DNA with highly correlated structure. This facilitates genome-wide testing by limiting the number of SNP genotypes necessary to obtain maximum coverage. The HapMap data has accelerated the search for genes involved in common human diseases, including autoimmune disorders such as JIA and lupus.

The ENCODE project has revealed remarkable insights into gene regulation controlled by nonprotein coding regions of the genome, with implications for human disease. Many regulatory elements at great distance from each other in the linear DNA sequence are physically associated with one another and with expressed genes in live cells. These regulatory regions are statistically associated with sequence variants linked to human disease and will therefore inform our understanding of the consequences of this variation. Together, knowledge of human genome structure and the continued development of functional annotations will potentially improve the power to detect pathological noncoding variants and our understanding of disease mechanisms.[5]

The Epigenome

Epigenetics refers to stably heritable phenotypes resulting from changes in chromosome structure not due to alterations in DNA sequence.[14] Epigenetic changes generally result in structural adaptations of chromosomal regions so as to register, signal, or perpetuate altered activity states.[15] Epigenetic regulation of gene expression occurs through multiple mechanisms, including DNA methylation, histone modifications, and noncoding RNAs (Fig. 5-2).

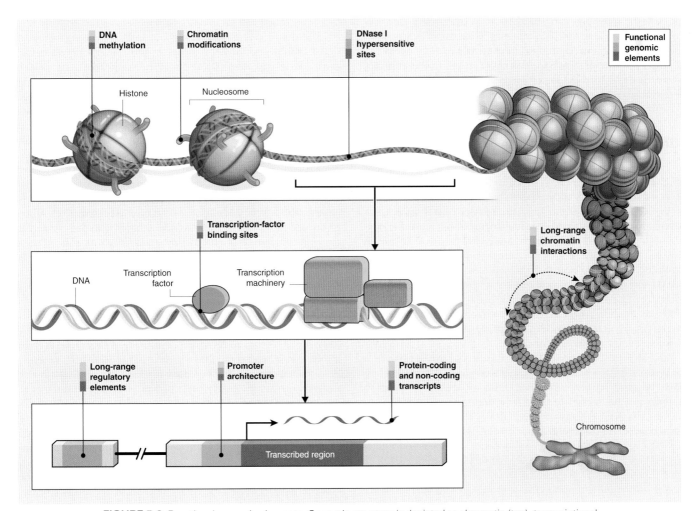

FIGURE 5-2 Functional genomic elements. Genomic structure is depicted as chromatin (top), transcriptional machinery (middle), and gene structure (bottom). Linear regions of DNA wrapped around core histone proteins form nucleosomes that are the elements of chromatin structure. Access to regions of DNA (hypersensitive to DNase I digestion) is regulated by histone and DNA modifications (epigenetic). Open chromatin enables the binding of regulatory machinery including transcription factors and cofactors to gene promoters and enhancers (long-range regulatory elements). The latter may be far removed from transcribed DNA. (Reprinted from J.R. Ecker, ENCODE explained, Nature 489 (2012) 52, with permission.)

DNA methylation is the most commonly studied epigenetic mark in the mammalian genome, and involves enzymatic addition of a methyl group by DNA methyltransferases to cytosine residues adjacent to guanosine (CpG). This typically occurs in long stretches of cytosine-guanine repeats referred to as *CpG islands*, and is often found at or near transcription start sites. These modifications can suppress the binding of transcription factors to gene promoters, alter chromatin structure, or modify methylation-specific regulatory factors, and together play a role in controlling gene expression.[16] The mammalian genome is packaged into nucleosomes, which consist of genomic DNA wrapped around histone octamer scaffolds forming the basic units of chromatin. Chromatin structure is dynamic and serves to regulate access to DNA in response to a variety of signals. The higher order structure of chromatin is dictated not only by enzymatic DNA methylation, but also through posttranslational biochemical modification of histone proteins. Histone modifications are often near the amino terminal end of the protein, which protrudes from the nucleosome structure, as well as within its globular body, where they can directly affect interaction with DNA. In addition to DNA and histone modifications, noncoding RNAs can also regulate the dynamics of the mammalian gene expression and various physiological functions including cell division, differentiation, and apoptosis. Together the features that comprise the epigenome can be thought of as layers controlling gene expression and cellular function, without altering the underlying DNA sequences. Mechanisms controlling their heritability from one cell to its progeny, and in some cases from an entire organism to its offspring, are poorly understood but important areas of investigation. Efforts to comprehensively map epigenetic modifications across the genome are currently under way.[17]

FUNCTIONAL GENOMICS

In its broadest sense, functional genomics refers to the study of how information encoded in the DNA sequence results in the phenotype of the organism. Understanding the mechanisms that enable genotypes to be translated into phenotypes encompasses what Francis Crick referred to in the 1950s as the "central dogma of molecular biology." Although the flow of information from DNA to RNA to protein remains a central tenet, it is not entirely unidirectional, and it is becoming increasingly clear that RNA has many biological functions that do not require its information to be translated into protein. In the context of disease, the concept of functional genomics extends to understanding how genetic differences, both common and uncommon variants as well as mutations, lead to altered phenotypes that manifest as autoimmunity or autoinflammation.

The importance of noncoding or regulatory DNA in disease is underscored by the observation that approximately 93% of SNPs identified by genome-wide association studies (GWAS) of common complex genetic diseases or traits lie within in these DNA regions, whereas less than 5% are in coding DNA.[18] This distribution is not disproportionate because only about 2% of the genome encodes exons. Nevertheless, it emphasizes the need to better understand the effects of common SNPs on gene regulatory networks, sometimes acting at great distances across the genome. This is a challenge for modern biology that requires innovative systems biology and bioinformatics approaches.

Transcriptomics

Transcriptome refers to the set of all RNA molecules from protein coding (mRNA) to noncoding RNA, including rRNA, tRNA, lncRNA, pri-miRNA, and others. Transcriptome may apply to an entire organism or a specific cell type. Methods to comprehensively and systematically

interrogate the expression of virtually all RNA species have been developed and complement global approaches to studying genome sequence, structure, and its variability, which was described previously in the chapter. Microarray (or "chip") technology, and more recently high throughput next generation (NextGen) DNA sequencing, has made assessing the transcriptome a routine laboratory practice.

Methods to Assess the Transcriptome

Microarray-based platforms are frequently used to assess comprehensively the relative or absolute abundance of individual RNA transcripts. DNA oligonucleotide arrays use short oligomers with perfect and single-base pair mismatched oligonucleotides to provide a measure of specificity. For analyzing mRNA, samples are reverse transcribed, and then complementary RNA (cRNA) or complementary DNA (cDNA) containing fluorescent-labeled nucleotides is synthesized. The product is hybridized to the chip, and the fluorescent signal intensity, which is proportional to the abundance of the particular mRNA species in the original sample, is measured at each location on the chip using a high-resolution scanner. Multiple vendors sell microarrays that are designed to provide virtually genome-wide interrogation of known genes or exons. Microarrays for measuring the abundance of noncoding RNAs (lncRNA, miRNA, etc.) are also available.

Sequencing-based approaches to gene expression analysis (e.g., RNA-Seq) utilize ultra-high-throughput DNA sequencing methodology. Basically, purified RNA is broken into conveniently sized fragments, converted into cDNA, and then sequenced using random primers. The transcriptome is assembled using a reference genome, and then various bioinformatics tools for further analysis. The number of reads of a given sequence is directly proportional to the expression level and provides an absolute measure of expression. The initial steps of RNA isolation and selection can be modified to preferentially measure protein coding mRNA or small RNA species (miRNA), or remain unbiased if comprehensive transcriptome analysis is desired. RNA sequencing (RNA-Seq) provides certain advantages over DNA oligonucleotide microarrays, including broader transcriptome coverage with the detection of rare or novel transcripts, alternatively spliced forms, and allele-specific expression. In addition, RNA-Seq can provide better quantitation over a broader dynamic range with reduced noise, enabling more subtle changes to be quantitated reliably.[19,20] A detailed comparison of the strengths and limitations of these approaches to transcriptome analysis is worthwhile before committing significant time and resources to these projects.

Data Analysis

Many aspects of data analysis are specific to the methods used to evaluate the transcriptome, and thus will not be considered here. Nevertheless, a few important points should be considered. Issues of experimental design and quantity, quality, and efficient processing of samples are paramount to obtaining sufficient power to detect statistically significant and biologically meaningful differences. Delayed processing or exposure of cells to heat or cold stress before RNA stabilization can dramatically change gene expression patterns. Estimates of sample sizes depend on the questions being asked, the complexity of the sample (i.e., number of cell or tissue types represented), and variability between samples. Given the issues inherent in the analysis of data generated from tens of thousands of features, conservative P value interpretation and/or multiple testing corrections are often necessary. Several software packages are available for identifying differentially expressed RNAs across multiple samples, recognizing clusters with similar expression, identifying pathways with functional significance, and estimating overall similarity and differences between patterns in complex samples. It is important to recognize that the relative abundance of individual mRNA species does not always correlate with the abundance of the encoded protein. The turnover of many proteins is tightly and specifically regulated. In addition, in complex samples such as tissue, whole blood, or peripheral blood mononuclear cells (PBMCs), where several cell types are represented, increases or decreases in the expression of individual genes may represent differences in the abundance of cell populations.

Validation

Depending on the nature of the study and the conclusions being drawn from the data, there may be a need for validation of RNA expression differences using a second approach. The quantitative real-time polymerase chain reaction (qPCR or real-time PCR) is most commonly used to measure individual complementary DNA that has been produced from the RNA sample. Either a DNA binding dye or fluorescent-labeled oligonucleotides are used to detect an increase in DNA product that accumulates in proportion to the amount of RNA in the original sample. Normalization to RNA species that do not change under the experimental conditions used (often referred to as *housekeeping RNAs*) is critical to properly interpret the results.

Functional Genomics in Rheumatic Diseases

Functional genomics approaches have been used successfully to better understand the complexity and pathogenesis of complex rheumatologic diseases. Oligonucleotide microarrays revealed prominent granulopoiesis and type I interferon (IFN) response "signatures" in PBMCs from patients with juvenile and adult-onset systemic lupus erythematosus (SLE),[21,22] highlighting a role for IFN-α in pathogenesis.[23] The granulopoiesis signature led to the identification of granulocyte precursors that purified with PBMC in new-onset untreated patients. These studies highlighted the type I IFN signature as a potential biomarker for disease activity in SLE, and supported the development of therapeutic agents targeting the IFN axis. Antibodies against IFN-α are currently in clinical development.[24,25]

In juvenile arthritis, PBMC gene expression differences distinguished patients with polyarticular juvenile rheumatoid arthritis (JRA, American College of Rheumatology [ACR] criteria) from healthy controls, and revealed possible differences between the polyarticular and pauciarticular subtypes and juvenile-onset ankylosing spondylitis (AS).[26] Interestingly, differentially expressed genes in polyarticular JIA patients tended to normalize with response to treatment.[27] Subsequent larger studies of untreated patients at disease onset have further distinguished the major subtypes of JIA, including oligoarticular, polyarticular, systemic, and enthesitis-related arthritis based on PBMC gene expression differences.[28] Gene expression differences in active systemic JIA are quite profound and include evidence for interleukin (IL)-1 and IL-6 signaling, an erythropoiesis signature with overexpression of fetal hemoglobins, innate immune signaling, and downregulation of natural killer cell and T-cell networks.[28-31]

Gene expression analyses have also revealed substantial heterogeneity in new-onset polyarticular JIA, with three subgroups reflecting varying strengths of three gene expression signatures.[32] One signature (I), most likely from monocytes, correlated with the presence of autoantibodies (RF and anti-CCP) and was present in two groups of polyarticular JIA subjects but not the third. Another signature (III) with low CD8 expression was associated with reduced numbers of CD8 T cells and increased plasmacytoid dendritic cells. Signature III was almost exclusively found in one group of polyarticular JIA subjects, and many of the gene expression differences were consistent with biological effects of transforming growth factor-β (TGF-β). Using approaches like this together with genetic data, it may be possible to improve classification with a genomics and biomarker-based approach.

These studies emphasize that peripheral blood can be a rich source of information, both in terms of biomarkers and pathogenic mechanisms. In JIA this supports the concept that joint inflammation may be an end result of immune dysregulation, rather than simply a site where joint antigens drive a cross-reactive local inflammatory process. In addition, analysis of complex cell mixtures, such as those present in peripheral blood and synovial fluid, can provide useful information despite the complexity of the sample. It has been striking in these and other studies how small changes in RNA abundance can be powerful means of detecting differences in cell populations rather than simply upregulation or downregulation of genes. Development of bioinformatics methods for computational "deconvolution" of transcriptomic data has greatly facilitated interpretation of such studies.[33,34] The comprehensive nature of transcriptomic approaches affords several advantages, including the ability to measure simultaneously multiple gene products in a pathway, which can be more sensitive and more specific than analyzing individual candidate genes or even cytokines presumed to be driving the signatures. Finally, regardless of the actual identities of the differentially represented transcripts, consistent differences between the groups being compared can serve as gene expression biomarkers that help distinguish disease subtypes, and equally importantly, disease states.[35,36] Further development of biological correlates of active and inactive disease will enrich our clinical definitions and eventually provide a biological definition of remission. It may be possible with genetic and transcriptomic data to use an integrative approach to predict disease severity and outcome.

The remarkable progress in identifying genetic variants associated with susceptibility to common rheumatic diseases has outpaced our understanding of how these variants impact gene function and disease pathogenesis. Nevertheless, certain principles are beginning to emerge. Using an integrative approach, analyzing genetic data with gene expression as a quantitative trait locus (eQTL), common variants in interferon regulatory factor 7 (*IRF7*) were shown to influence IFN-α production,[37] with implications for SLE pathogenesis. Using a similar approach, eQTLs that control monocyte gene expression in response to lipopolysaccharide (LPS) were identified for networks involving IFN-β, *IRF2*, and others. The eQTLs were significantly more often identified for genes identified by GWAS to be involved in susceptibility to autoimmune disease.[38] Together these studies also highlighted the importance of cell-type–specific and condition-specific responses in establishing links between the genetic variants and immune disorders.

Proteomics

Proteome refers to the entire complement of proteins in a cell type or organism. Although methods to detect and measure the proteome of a cell or tissue have advanced significantly, difficulties remain.[39] Current estimates suggest 21,500 proteins are encoded in the human genome, with the number expressed in any individual cell type being significantly smaller. However, the complexity of the proteome is increased substantially by posttranslational modifications such as glycosylation, phosphorylation, and proteolytic processing, and multiple translation products can derive from one differentially spliced mRNA. Comprehensive proteomic studies may need to consider subcellular localization and interacting partners. Proteins are also inherently more complex than DNA/RNA, with 20 amino acid building blocks rather than 4 primary nucleotides, and they cannot be copied or amplified *in vitro*. As a result, methods to assess the proteome are less comprehensive and considerably lower throughput than genomic techniques. In addition, because resolution of proteins on two-dimensional (2D) gels depends primarily on two parameters—relative molecular mass (M_r) and isoelectric point (pI)—there may be considerable overlap in a complex mixture containing thousands of cellular proteins. Methods such as mass spectroscopy (MS), which provides precise mass measurements, are highly sensitive and provide greater resolution than 2D gel separations but are expensive and difficult to automate.

Protein Identification by Mass Spectroscopy Peptide Fingerprinting

The identification of individual proteins separated from complex mixtures has become relatively routine. Single protein "spots" from 2D gel separations can be removed from the gel, proteolytically digested into peptide fragments, and subjected to MS analysis. In matrix-assisted laser desorption ionization, the time of flight provides highly precise fragment masses (fingerprints), which are matched against a database of calculated peptide fragment masses from *in silico* digested proteins based on the specificity of the protease.

It is also possible to obtain peptide sequence information using tandem MS (MS/MS or MS^2), where peptide ion fragments in a complex mixture are isolated in the machine due to their mass (*m/z*), and then fragmented in the gas phase. Because peptides will fragment in a sequence-dependent fashion, in most cases an unambiguous ordering of the amino acids can be obtained from the MS/MS spectrum. This technology has been instrumental in determining the sequences of complex mixtures of peptides derived from HLA class I and class II molecules.[40]

Microarray-Based Methods

Protein or antigen microarrays are being used extensively to assess autoantibody profiles from patients with various autoimmune diseases.[41,42] They offer much higher throughput with smaller sample sizes than traditional enzyme-linked immunosorbent assays (ELISAs) or fluorescence immunoassays. Typically, antigens are immobilized to planar surfaces and reacted with antibody-containing sera or plasma. Antibody-antigen complexes are then visualized with antihuman secondary antibodies conjugated to fluorophores or enzymes, followed by imaging and quantitation. Protein microarrays are more sensitive than conventional ELISAs and offer parallel screening for multiple autoantibodies. The utility of antigen microarrays for screening and discovery is limited by selection bias, because some *a priori* knowledge of relevant antigens is necessary. More recently, high-density arrays with thousands of non-preselected recombinant proteins have been developed and used to identify novel autoantigens in RA[43] and other diseases.

Protein-protein interactions can be mapped using genetic methods known as "yeast two-hybrid screens." Using molecular biological tools, a known or "bait" protein can be expressed as a fusion product with the DNA-binding domain of a transcriptional activator. A different protein ("prey") is expressed as a fusion product with the activation domain of the transcription factor. If the bait and prey interact when expressed in the yeast, the result is activation of transcription of a reporter gene that can easily be detected. This method can be used to study protein-protein interactions of known gene products or to screen entire libraries to discover interaction partners. Variations on this theme have been developed to detect RNA-protein and RNA-RNA interactions.[44,45]

METHODS TO STUDY GENE FUNCTION USING ANIMAL MODELS

To gain a clearer understanding of how a particular gene or its variants function, it is often desirable to turn to animal models. In this section we briefly describe commonly used strategies that have had an important impact on our understanding of disease mechanisms.

Transgenics

DNA introduced into the nuclei of fertilized embryos can incorporate into the host genome and be passed on to subsequent generations. When that DNA encodes a protein, the result is a transgenic animal. Use of foreign genomic DNA with intact regulatory regions can result in tissue- and cell-specific expression and regulation mimicking the pattern seen in the donor organism. Alternatively, cDNA under the control of a nonspecific housekeeping promoter that results in widespread overexpression can be used. Transgenesis is a powerful technique that has been used extensively since the late 1970s, but it has limitations. It usually results in overexpression of the gene of interest; consequently, additional controls need to be considered when interpreting the function of the newly expressed protein.

Targeted Gene Deletion (Knockout) and Knockin Approaches

The discovery and application of homologous recombination led to the production of targeted gene *knockouts* (KOs) in mice in the late 1980s. Briefly, a DNA construct containing a homologous portion of the gene of interest, but with a key region removed and a selection marker added, is introduced into stem cells derived from blastocysts. With homologous recombination, the gene with the key region removed and the selection marker added replaces the wild-type gene. Cells that have the marker are selected usually based on resistance to a drug, and then reintroduced into blastocysts that are then implanted into pseudopregnant female mice. The offspring contain some cells with the targeted (KO) gene and some with the wild-type gene (mosaics). Subsequent rounds of breeding usually result in germ-line transmission of the KO allele, and then generation of homozygous KOs. Depending on what portion of the gene has been targeted, there may be complete loss of expression or, alternatively, expression of a nonfunctional gene product.

It is often desirable to determine the effects of a gene deletion in selected cell types or tissues. This approach can be helpful to dissect complex phenotypes where the impact of the gene is different in different cell types. Cell- or tissue-specific gene deletion can be achieved using Cre-lox technology to create a conditional KO. In this case the targeted gene recombined into the genome contains the region of interest flanked by newly created loxP recognition sites ("floxed"). The floxed gene can be expressed and function normally. However, co-expression of Cre recombinase, a restriction enzyme that recognizes and cleaves loxP sites, will result in removal of the floxed region and creation of a gene KO, but only in the tissue where Cre is expressed. By driving Cre expression from a tissue-specific promoter, the conditional KO can be generated.

Knockins (KIs) are created in a similar fashion to KOs, except that instead of eliminating a key portion of the gene of interest, that region is replaced with a different coding sequence to generate a variant gene product. Conditional KIs can also be produced. These methods have been used to create disease models in which the effects of human gene mutations can be studied in rodents.

GENOME EDITING

Genome editing is the introduction of changes at precise chromosomal DNA sequences. This technology exploits DNA sequence specificity and double-stranded DNA (dsDNA) nuclease activity provided by zinc finger nucleases (ZFNs), transcription activator-like effector nucleases (TALENs), or clustered regularly interspaced short palindromic repeat guide RNA associated with a Cas nuclease (CRISPR/Cas).[46] Cellular repair of dsDNA breaks by nonhomologous end-joining often results in the deletion or insertion of DNA and frameshift mutations. When introduced into the coding sequence of a gene, the result is often a functional KO due to new in-frame stop codons (stop-gains) and/or a nonsense gene product. Homology-directed repair with an added DNA donor template can result in the introduction of precise nucleotide substitutions or larger DNA insertions. This technology is more efficient and less expensive than creating KOs and KIs, and it has been applied to a number of different organisms to create new animal models of human disease without the need to accomplish homologous recombination in embryonic stem cells. Genome editing has also been used in human-induced pluripotent stem cells to correct mutations; it is a promising approach to gene and cell-based therapies for the future.

GENETICS OF PEDIATRIC RHEUMATIC DISEASES

Monogenic Versus Complex Genetic Diseases

Monogenic diseases are controlled primarily by a single gene and thus are typically inherited in a Mendelian fashion, either as autosomal dominant, recessive, or sex-linked traits. Although more than 10,000 Mendelian diseases are now recognized, only a fraction present to a pediatric rheumatology clinic; the ones that do will usually be due to musculoskeletal features including arthritis or joint deformity, periodic fevers, or vasculopathy. Monogenic diseases affecting the musculoskeletal system have been categorized as three groups based on clinical phenotypes of arthritis (e.g., Lesch-Nyhan), contractures or stiff joints (e.g., Gaucher disease), and hypermobility (e.g., Ehlers-Danlos syndrome).[47] The discovery of genes responsible for certain inherited periodic fever syndromes (e.g., familial Mediterranean fever [FMF], TNF receptor-associated periodic syndrome [TRAPS], and cryopyrin-associated periodic syndromes [CAPS]) led to the concept of "autoinflammatory" disease[48] (see Chapter 47). With the increasing capacity to identify causative genes and their functional consequences, molecular analysis becomes more practical and necessary.[49]

Complex genetic traits or diseases are dependent on multiple genes as well as environmental factors and thus exhibit non-Mendelian inheritance patterns. Examples of complex genetic diseases include rheumatoid arthritis (RA), AS, multiple sclerosis, psoriasis and psoriatic arthritis, scleroderma, SLE, and type 1 diabetes mellitus (T1D). Some complex traits also demonstrate an intermediate or endophenotype, which can be measured as biological markers. For instance, antibodies to citrullinated peptide antigens and antinuclear antibodies can be detected years before clinical manifestations in subjects with RA and SLE, respectively.[50,50a] JIA and its various categories display features that suggest a complex genetic trait,[51,52] including a definite but limited family history and few affected members of the extended family, an increased presence of other autoimmune diseases in the family,[53] and HLA associations.

Although some genetic associations in complex genetic rheumatic diseases are strong (e.g., HLA-B27 and its variants provide 23% of heritability in AS; in RA other HLA variants contribute approximately 13% of genetic risk, with 4% or less of risk alleles outside the MHC), these remain the minority.[54] The emerging picture is that the risk alleles identified in genomic screens are common in the general population, have a modest effect on risk, and together explain only a small part of the variance in disease risk. For instance, it has been estimated that the 163 known risk loci for inflammatory bowel disease explain only 13.6% of the variance for Crohn's disease and 7.5% for ulcerative colitis.[55] Although the actual causal variants

for most risk loci identified to date remain to be determined, several themes have emerged; many risk loci are associated with more than one autoimmune disease, and many genes are associated with discrete biological pathways.[56] However, because the number of subjects needed to identify common low-risk alleles is large, performing such studies for pediatric rheumatic diseases often requires international collaboration.

Establishing the Genetic Basis of Rheumatic Diseases

Genomic studies are time-consuming and expensive, and thus quantitation of familial risk to determine the probability that a given disease is a complex genetic trait can be a critical first step. A higher concordance rate for SLE is observed in monozygotic compared with dizygotic twins or siblings (24%-56% versus 2%-5%, respectively),[57] and siblings are estimated to have between 8-fold and 29-fold higher risk of SLE compared with the general population.[58] The concordance rate for JIA in monozygotic twins is 25% to 40%, which is 250 to 400 times the population risk of JIA.[59,60] Sibling recurrence risk ratio (λs) compares the risk in siblings of probands with a disease to the prevalence of disease in the population. Siblings and first cousins of probands with JIA have 12-fold and 6-fold greater risk of JIA, respectively, compared with the general population.[61] These observations establish the genetic basis of these rheumatic diseases, and support ongoing efforts to find the responsible risk genes.

Autoimmunity Is a Shared Trait

Children and relatives of children with JIA have an increased prevalence of other autoimmune disorders.[62-65] Similarly, adults with RA and idiopathic myopathies demonstrate familial clustering of other autoimmune disorders.[66,67] These observations suggested that clinically distinct autoimmune disorders might share common genetic susceptibility factors, many of which have now been identified.[68-70] The concept emerging from these and other observations is the notion that master genes may predispose to autoimmunity in general, with other disease-specific genes and environmental factors influencing the precise phenotype. For example, whereas variants in PTPN22 and STAT4 appear to influence susceptibility to multiple autoimmune phenotypes, the influence of NOD2 and ATG16L1 is so far restricted to inflammatory bowel disease (IBD). Similarly, SNPs in PADI4 appear to be specific to RA, whereas integrin alpha M (ITGAM) variants are more specific to SLE.[71] Meta-analyses of genetic variants associated with clinically distinct autoimmune phenotypes will likely enhance our understanding of common pathways that will be targets for treatment across several diseases.

Principles of Association and Linkage

Association and linkage studies are used to dissect the genetic basis of common diseases.[72,73] Both approaches rely on the co-inheritance of polymorphisms linked to a disease allele. Association studies test whether a phenotype and a marker allele show correlated occurrence in a population. When an association between a marker and a disease is detected, it often implies either that the marker is the disease allele, or that the marker is in LD with the disease allele. LD is a nonrandom association of alleles at two or more loci and is a measure of co-segregation of alleles in a population. Linkage studies provide a complementary approach, and test whether a phenotype and a marker allele show correlated transmission within a pedigree. In genome-wide association and linkage studies the genome is searched for susceptibility loci, and no assumptions are made about the candidacy of particular genes or genomic regions. One limitation of linkage analysis is that it requires the identification of multiplex families, in which many family members have the phenotype of interest.

Principles of Candidate Gene and Genome Wide Studies (Prespecified Gene of Interest)

Two strategies are commonly used in evaluating a disease as a complex trait. One is a candidate gene approach, including selected specific genes or chromosome regions that are tested for disease susceptibility; the other is a comprehensive and unbiased whole genome screen. Although candidate gene studies have the potential to reduce the overall workload by focusing on regions/variants of interest, they have limitations, including the sheer number of potential candidates, possibility for population stratification, and limited knowledge about the function of many genes. Many candidate gene studies that produced initially promising results have proved to be uninformative, in many cases due to lack of reproducibility when larger sample sizes were evaluated. Advances in genome technologies, and the availability of haplotype and LD information from the HapMap Project, now facilitate a comprehensive search for genetic influences, through the performance of GWAS. GWAS offer an unbiased approach to discovering common variants predisposing to a phenotype by systematically examining every genetic region for association. Although GWAS have successfully identified variants associated with susceptibility to complex traits including AS,[74] RA,[75-77] IBD,[76,77] T1D,[78,79] and SLE,[80] they require a large number of well-phenotyped subjects and replication in large independent cohorts that previously have been limiting factors in the search for genes underlying JIA and other pediatric rheumatic diseases. In the era of GWAS, candidate gene association studies are being increasingly used for replication of GWAS findings in independent cohorts and related phenotypes. Selecting "candidate" genes in this manner, rather than based on a preconceived notion of pathogenesis, reduces the likelihood of failure.

GWAS also have limitations. They focus mostly on common variants (frequency greater than 5%), and most loci discovered to date have only modest effects on risk (odds ratio [OR] approximately 1.1-1.2).[75,81-83] Although many SNPs identified to date reside near genes involved in biologically relevant pathways, the causative variants remain to be established. There is a substantial "heritability gap" in RA and other complex traits that is not explained by the genes identified so far by GWAS. Several reasons have been proposed to account for this gap, including the existence of common but as yet undiscovered alleles, rare variants with larger effects, structural variants such as copy number variants, and gene-gene or gene-environment interactions.[84]

Importance of Phenotype, Power, Replication, and Meta-Analysis

Initial findings suggestive of linkage or association require replication in an independent cohort to establish a gene or region for further evaluation. Once a genetic region has been established as linked to or associated with a phenotype of interest, different strategies could be used to identify the causal variant. Sequencing of the entire region or exons can help to identify variants that are in coding regions, or those that alter gene expression. To be successful, GWAS need to be adequately powered to maximize discoveries, and the phenotypes of subjects must be carefully documented. Although population stratification can be a major issue, the current generations of genome-wide genotyping arrays contain thousands of SNP markers that help discern population stratification. It is important to eliminate false positives that result from multiple testing by requiring genome-wide thresholds of significance.

Candidate Gene Studies in Pediatric Rheumatology
Human Leukocyte Antigens

Polymorphisms in HLA class I and class II genes are associated with several rheumatic disorders, with notable examples including HLA-B27 and spondyloarthritis, and the HLA-DRB1 shared epitope alleles and RA. The strongest HLA associations in pediatric rheumatic disease are with various forms of JIA,[85-88] including shared epitope alleles and rheumatoid-factor positive polyarthritis.[89] Various HLA associations exhibit age-specific windows of susceptibility,[86] as well as additive effects. For example, whereas 80% children with one HLA risk allele developed JIA by 9.6 years of age, when four risk alleles were present, 80% of children were affected by 4.7 years. The age-specific effects of HLA alleles on JIA onset were recently confirmed and extended to show that children with early-onset polyarticular JIA clustered with oligoarticular JIA with respect to HLA variation.[88] In some cases using large, well-characterized cohorts, it has been possible to further refine the nature of the HLA associations in RA. Five amino acids in three HLA proteins (three amino acids in HLA-DRβ1, one in HLA-B, and one in HLA-DPβ1), all of which affect peptide binding, were shown to explain the vast majority of HLA-associated risk.[54] Similar efforts in JIA subgroups should be informative, although larger cohorts are needed.

Non-HLA Loci

Many candidate gene studies in JIA have been of limited utility because they were underpowered.[90] Using larger cohorts, the association between *PTPN22* and JIA has now been established, and is more pronounced in certain categories of JIA than others.[91,92] Case control studies have also demonstrated associations between JIA and *STAT4*, *TNFAIP3*, *IL2/IL21* and *IL2RA*, and *TRAF1-C5* loci.[69,93-96] An investigation of 251 trios of childhood-onset SLE families confirmed associations with variants in *SELP* (encodes selectin P) and *IRAK1* (interleukin-1 receptor associated kinase 1).[97] Another association study of 221 children with juvenile dermatomyositis and 203 controls found genetic variants encoding the TNF-α and IL-1α cytokines were associated with disease risk as well as disease severity.[98]

Genome Wide Studies in Pediatric Rheumatology
Linkage Analysis

Linkage studies require ascertainment of families with multiple affected individuals. In pediatric rheumatology, the best examples of linkage studies have been for hereditary periodic fevers. Positional cloning techniques led to the identification of *MEFV* (known initially as *pyrin* or *marenostrin*) as the causative gene for FMF.[99,100] The discovery of this previously unknown gene revealed an important pathway that modulates the innate immune response. Similarly, analysis of several affected families led to the identification of *TNFR1* as the gene responsible for TRAPS,[101] and *MVK* (mevalonate kinase) as causative for hyperimmunoglobulin D with periodic fever syndrome (HIDS).[102] This discovery uncovered the role of an established biochemical pathway in regulating inflammation.

When large collections of families with multiple affected members are unavailable for traditional genome-wide linkage studies, sibling pairs (sib pairs) can be used for nonparametric linkage analysis. A genome-wide linkage study involving 121 affected sib-pair families suggested that genes in the HLA and other regions influence risk of JIA.[103] However, other results were not statistically significant, suggesting that this approach lacked sufficient power to identify most of the causal variants. Analyses stratified by subphenotypes of JIA improved the power to detect linkage.

Genome-Wide Association Studies

GWAS and meta-analyses of GWAS incorporating many thousands of cases and controls have greatly enhanced the identification of common variants predisposing to RA, SLE, AS, IBD, and psoriasis. More than 30 associations have been confirmed in SLE,[104] with many gene products participating in pathways implicated in pathogenesis. Similarly, 98 candidates at 101 risk loci have been reported to be associated with RA, with many of the genes coinciding with targets of approved therapies for RA, suggesting that newly discovered disease-associated loci may provide additional clues to molecular mechanisms of pathogenesis or progression of the phenotype.[105]

The first GWAS in JIA replicated a strong association in the HLA region, with the second strongest signal in the *VTCN1* gene, which encodes B7-H4, a co-stimulatory molecule on antigen-presenting cells, and mediates T-cell interactions.[106] *VTCN1* variants also appear to influence the course of disease in JIA,[107] and were recently found to be associated with RA in a Dutch cohort.[108] A genome-wide association study of 814 cases with JIA followed by a large replication cohort, and gene expression analysis provided evidence of association at 3q13, suggesting a role for a novel gene or genes in pathogenesis.[109]

Immunochip

The Immunochip Consortium was established to investigate shared loci identified in GWAS across multiple autoimmune disorders.[110] The Immunochip interrogates almost 200,000 SNPs, with dense coverage of the MHC, including approximately 180 non-HLA loci that have shown genome-wide evidence of association with one or more of 12 autoimmune diseases. Studies utilizing the Immunochip have been successful in celiac disease,[111] IBD,[55] RA,[112] and AS.[113] Combined analysis of Immunochip data with previously published GWAS results enabled the identification of 163 loci associated with IBD,[55] and overlaps between IBD, AS, and psoriasis. Additionally, there was overlap between susceptibility loci for IBD and mycobacterial infection, suggesting host-microbe interactions have shaped the genetic architecture of inflammatory bowel disease.

The JIA Immunochip Consortium analyzed 2816 cases with oligoarticular and rheumatoid factor (RF)-negative polyarticular JIA and 13,056 controls.[114] In addition to confirming the 3 previously identified loci, 14 new genetic associations were discovered (Fig. 5-3), and 11

potential loci achieved suggestive levels of significance. Many of the loci were shared with RA, T1D, and celiac disease. This study also implicated the IL-2 pathway in JIA pathogenesis. This effort underscores the need for international collaboration to identify predisposing variants for uncommon diseases like JIA.[114]

Whole Exome Sequencing

Despite the success in identifying common variants that predispose an individual to common rheumatic diseases, a substantial proportion of heritability remains unexplained. To address the possibility that there may be rare variants or mutations in causative genes that have escaped detection on current genotyping arrays, many individuals have turned to whole exome sequencing (WES).[84] This approach has been successful in early-onset inflammatory bowel disease,[115,116] and juvenile SLE in a consanguineous kindred.[117] These examples suggest that rare variants with large effects may contribute to complex trait phenotypes and that their discovery with WES is feasible.

CONCLUSION

The immune-mediated inflammatory diseases encountered by pediatric rheumatologists range from rare and sometimes profound autoinflammatory phenotypes, to the more common forms of childhood arthritis, lupus, and spondyloarthritis. From a genetic standpoint, the more common diseases represent complex traits that result from the interaction of multiple gene products with our environment, whereas single genes are being discovered at a rapid pace to be causative for many rare disorders. Eventually, it will be possible to use genetics and biomarkers to better diagnose, classify, and predict treatment response for these complex diseases. Although many of the current treatments used in pediatric rheumatology have been developed without knowledge of how predisposing genes contribute to pathogenesis, new discoveries may lead to the identification of upstream targets that will enable us to envision cures.

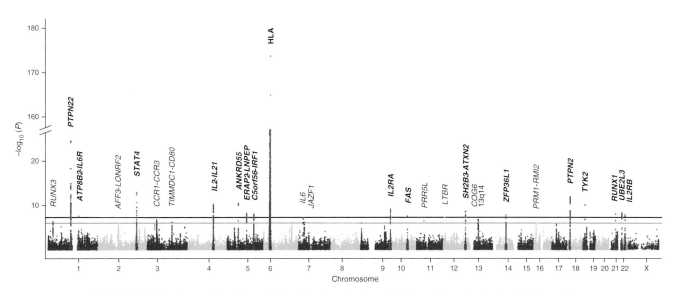

FIGURE 5-3 Manhattan plot of associations in oligoarticular and RF-negative polyarticular JIA. Association statistics (*y* axis) for risk loci (*x* axis) are shown. The upper black line indicates the threshold for genome-wide significance ($P < 5 \times 10^{-8}$). Loci reaching this threshold are highlighted in bold, and individual SNPs mapping to these loci are shown in red. The lower gray line indicates the threshold for suggestive association ($5 \times 10^{-8} < P < 1 \times 10^{-6}$). (Reprinted from A. Hinks, J. Cobb, M.C. Marion, et al., Dense genotyping of immune-related disease regions identifies 14 new susceptibility loci for juvenile idiopathic arthritis, Nat. Genet. 45 (2013) 664–671, with permission.)

REFERENCES

5. ENCODE Project Consortium, An integrated encyclopedia of DNA elements in the human genome, Nature 489 (2012) 57–74.

7. T. Hung, H.Y. Chang, Long noncoding RNA in genome regulation: prospects and mechanisms, RNA Biol. 7 (2010) 582–585.

8. M.C. Tsai, O. Manor, Y. Wan, et al., Long noncoding RNA as modular scaffold of histone modification complexes, Science 329 (2010) 689–693.

9. D.P. Bartel, MicroRNAs: target recognition and regulatory functions, Cell 136 (2009) 215–233.

10. 1000 Genomes Project Consortium, G.R. Abecasis, D. Altshuler, et al., A map of human genome variation from population-scale sequencing, Nature 467 (2010) 1061–1073.

11. 1000 Genomes Project Consortium, G.R. Abecasis, A. Auton, et al., An integrated map of genetic variation from 1,092 human genomes, Nature 491 (2012) 56–65.

14. S.L. Berger, T. Kouzarides, R. Shiekhattar, A. Shilatifard, An operational definition of epigenetics, Genes Dev. 23 (2009) 781–783.

15. A. Bird, Perceptions of epigenetics, Nature 447 (2007) 396–398.

17. L.H. Chadwick, The NIH roadmap epigenomics program data resource, Epigenomics 4 (2012) 317–324.

18. M.T. Maurano, R. Humbert, E. Rynes, et al., Systematic localization of common disease-associated variation in regulatory DNA, Science 337 (2012) 1190–1195.

20. Z. Wang, M. Gerstein, M. Snyder, RNA-Seq: a revolutionary tool for transcriptomics, Nat. Rev. Genet. 10 (2009) 57–63.

25. M. Petri, D.J. Wallace, A. Spindler, et al., Sifalimumab, a human anti-interferon-alpha monoclonal antibody, in systemic lupus erythematosus: a phase I randomized, controlled, dose-escalation study, Arthritis Rheum. 65 (2013) 1011–1021.

28. M.G. Barnes, A.A. Grom, S.D. Thompson, et al., Subtype-specific peripheral blood gene expression profiles in recent-onset juvenile idiopathic arthritis, Arthritis Rheum. 60 (2009) 2102–2112.

29. F. Allantaz, D. Chaussabel, D. Stichweh, et al., Blood leukocyte microarrays to diagnose systemic onset juvenile idiopathic arthritis and follow the response to IL-1 blockade, J. Exp. Med. 204 (2007) 2131–2144.

30. N. Fall, M. Barnes, S. Thornton, et al., Gene expression profiling of peripheral blood from patients with untreated new-onset systemic juvenile idiopathic arthritis reveals molecular heterogeneity that may predict macrophage activation syndrome, Arthritis Rheum. 56 (2007) 3793–3804.

32. T.A. Griffin, M.G. Barnes, N.T. Ilowite, et al., Gene expression signatures in polyarticular juvenile idiopathic arthritis demonstrate disease heterogeneity and offer a molecular classification of disease subsets, Arthritis Rheum. 60 (2009) 2113–2123.

34. S.S. Shen-Orr, R. Gaujoux, Computational deconvolution: extracting cell type-specific information from heterogeneous samples, Curr. Opin. Immunol. 25 (2013) 571–578.

36. K. Jiang, M.B. Frank, Y. Chen, et al., Genomic characterization of remission in juvenile idiopathic arthritis, Arthritis Res. Ther. 15 (2013) R100.

37. M.N. Lee, C. Ye, A.C. Villani, et al., Common genetic variants modulate pathogen-sensing responses in human dendritic cells, Science 343 (2014) 1246980.

38. B.P. Fairfax, P. Humburg, S. Makino, et al., Innate immune activity conditions the effect of regulatory variants upon monocyte gene expression, Science 343 (2014) 1246949.

41. H.T. Maecker, T.M. Lindstrom, W.H. Robinson, et al., New tools for classification and monitoring of autoimmune diseases, Nat. Rev. Rheumatol. 8 (2012) 317–328.

42. J. Sokolove, T.M. Lindstrom, W.H. Robinson, Development and deployment of antigen arrays for investigation of B-cell fine specificity in autoimmune disease, Front Biosci. (Elite Ed.) 4 (2012) 320–330.

43. I. Auger, N. Balandraud, J. Rak, et al., New autoantigens in rheumatoid arthritis (RA): screening 8268 protein arrays with sera from patients with RA, Ann. Rheum. Dis. 68 (2009) 591–594.

46. H. Wang, H. Yang, C.S. Shivalila, et al., One-step generation of mice carrying mutations in multiple genes by CRISPR/Cas-mediated genome engineering, Cell 153 (2013) 910–918.

48. S.L. Masters, A. Simon, I. Aksentijevich, D.L. Kastner, Horror autoinflammaticus: the molecular pathophysiology of autoinflammatory disease (*), Annu. Rev. Immunol. 27 (2009) 621–668.

49. M. Ombrello, K.A. Sikora, D.L. Kastner, Genetics, genomics and their relevance to pathology and therapy, Best Pract. Res. Clin. Rheumatol. 28 (2) (2014) 175–189.

54. S. Raychaudhuri, C. Sandor, E.A. Stahl, et al., Five amino acids in three HLA proteins explain most of the association between MHC and seropositive rheumatoid arthritis, Nat. Genet. 44 (2012) 291–296.

55. L. Jostins, S. Ripke, R.K. Weersma, et al., Host-microbe interactions have shaped the genetic architecture of inflammatory bowel disease, Nature 491 (2012) 119–124.

56. P.K. Gregersen, L.M. Olsson, Recent advances in the genetics of autoimmune disease, Annu. Rev. Immunol. 27 (2009) 363–391.

64. S. Prahalad, E. O'Brien, A.M. Fraser, et al., Familial aggregation of juvenile idiopathic arthritis, Arthritis Rheum. 50 (2004) 4022–4027.

69. S. Prahalad, S. Hansen, A. Whiting, et al., Variants in TNFAIP3, STAT4, and C12orf30 loci associated with multiple autoimmune diseases are also associated with juvenile idiopathic arthritis, Arthritis Rheum. 60 (2009) 2124–2130.

70. E.F. Remmers, R.M. Plenge, A.T. Lee, et al., STAT4 and the risk of rheumatoid arthritis and systemic lupus erythematosus, N. Engl. J. Med. 357 (2007) 977–986.

72. L.R. Cardon, J.I. Bell, Association study designs for complex diseases, Nat. Rev. Genet. 2 (2001) 91–99.

74. Australo-Anglo-American Spondyloarthritis Consortium (TASC), J.D. Reveille, A.M. Sims, et al., Genome-wide association study of ankylosing spondylitis identifies non-MHC susceptibility loci, Nat. Genet. 42 (2010) 123–127.

75. E.A. Stahl, S. Raychaudhuri, E.F. Remmers, et al., Genome-wide association study meta-analysis identifies seven new rheumatoid arthritis risk loci, Nat. Genet. 42 (2010) 508–514.

76. R.H. Duerr, K.D. Taylor, S.R. Brant, et al., A genome-wide association study identifies IL23R as an inflammatory bowel disease gene, Science 314 (2006) 1461–1463.

77. M. Imielinski, R.N. Baldassano, A. Griffiths, et al., Common variants at five new loci associated with early-onset inflammatory bowel disease, Nat. Genet. 41 (2009) 1335–1340.

79. Wellcome Trust Case Control Consortium, Genome-wide association study of 14,000 cases of seven common diseases and 3,000 shared controls, Nature 447 (2007) 661–678.

80. International Consortium for Systemic Lupus Erythematosus Genetics (SLEGEN), J.B. Harley, M.E. Alarcón-Riquelme, et al., Genome-wide association scan in women with systemic lupus erythematosus identifies susceptibility variants in ITGAM, PXK, KIAA1542 and other loci, Nat. Genet. 40 (2008) 204–210.

84. T.A. Manolio, F.S. Collins, N.J. Cox, et al., Finding the missing heritability of complex diseases, Nature 461 (2009) 747–753.

88. J. Hollenbach, S.D. Thompson, T.L. Bugawan, et al., Juvenile idiopathic arthritis and HLA class I and class II interaction and age of onset effects, Arthritis Rheum. 62 (2010) 1781–1791.

89. S. Prahalad, S.D. Thompson, K.N. Conneely, et al., Hierarchy of risk of childhood-onset rheumatoid arthritis conferred by HLA-DRB1 alleles encoding the shared epitope, Arthritis Rheum. 64 (2012) 925–930.

90. S. Prahalad, D.N. Glass, A comprehensive review of the genetics of juvenile idiopathic arthritis, Pediatr. Rheumatol. Online J. 6 (2008) 11.

94. A. Hinks, S. Eyre, X. Ke, et al., Association of the AFF3 gene and IL2/IL21 gene region with juvenile idiopathic arthritis, Genes Immun. 11 (2010) 194–198.

95. A. Hinks, S. Eyre, X. Ke, et al., Overlap of disease susceptibility loci for rheumatoid arthritis and juvenile idiopathic arthritis, Ann. Rheum. Dis. 69 (2010) 1049–1053.

96. A. Hinks, X. Ke, A. Barton, et al., Association of the IL2RA/CD25 gene with juvenile idiopathic arthritis, Arthritis Rheum 60 (2009) 251–257.

100. The International FMF Consortium, Ancient missense mutations in a new member of the RoRet gene family are likely to cause familial Mediterranean fever, Cell 90 (1997) 797–807.

104. Y. Deng, B.P. Tsao, Genetic susceptibility to systemic lupus erythematosus in the genomic era, Nat. Rev. Rheumatol. 6 (2010) 683–692.

105. Y. Okada, D. Wu, G. Trynka, et al., Genetics of rheumatoid arthritis contributes to biology and drug discovery, Nature 506 (2014) 376–381.

106. A. Hinks, A. Barton, N. Shephard, et al., Identification of a novel susceptibility locus for juvenile idiopathic arthritis by genome-wide association analysis, Arthritis Rheum. 60 (2009) 258–263.

107. H.M. Albers, T.H. Reinards, D.M. Brinkman, et al., Genetic variation in VTCN1 (B7-H4) is associated with course of disease in juvenile idiopathic arthritis, Ann. Rheum. Dis. 73 (2014) 1198–1201.

108. N.A. Daha, B.A. Lie, L.A. Trouw, et al., Novel genetic association of the VTCN1 region with rheumatoid arthritis, Ann. Rheum. Dis. 71 (2012) 567–571.

109. S.D. Thompson, M.C. Marion, M. Sudman, et al., Genome-wide association analysis of juvenile idiopathic arthritis identifies a new susceptibility locus at chromosomal region 3q13, Arthritis Rheum. 64 (2012) 2781–2791.

110. A. Cortes, M.A. Brown, Promise and pitfalls of the Immunochip, Arthritis Res. Ther. 13 (2011) 101.

111. G. Trynka, K.A. Hunt, N.A. Bockett, et al., Dense genotyping identifies and localizes multiple common and rare variant association signals in celiac disease, Nat. Genet. 43 (2011) 1193–1201.

112. S. Eyre, J. Bowes, D. Diogo, et al., High-density genetic mapping identifies new susceptibility loci for rheumatoid arthritis, Nat. Genet. 44 (2012) 1336–1340.

113. International Genetics of Ankylosing Spondylitis Consortium (IGAS), A. Cortes, J. Hadler, et al., Identification of multiple risk variants for ankylosing spondylitis through high-density genotyping of immune-related loci, Nat. Genet. 45 (2013) 730–738.

114. A. Hinks, J. Cobb, M.C. Marion, et al., Dense genotyping of immune-related disease regions identifies 14 new susceptibility loci for juvenile idiopathic arthritis, Nat. Genet. 45 (2013) 664–669.

115. E.A. Worthey, A.N. Mayer, G.D. Syverson, et al., Making a definitive diagnosis: successful clinical application of whole exome sequencing in a child with intractable inflammatory bowel disease, Genet. Med. 13 (2011) 255–262.

116. H. Mao, W. Yang, P.P. Lee, et al., Exome sequencing identifies novel compound heterozygous mutations of IL-10 receptor 1 in neonatal-onset Crohn's disease, Genes Immun. 13 (2012) 437–442.

117. A. Belot, P.R. Kasher, E.W. Trotter, et al., Protein kinase cdelta deficiency causes mendelian systemic lupus erythematosus with B cell-defective apoptosis and hyperproliferation, Arthritis Rheum. 65 (2013) 2161–2171.

The entire reference list is available online at www.expertconsult.com.

Trial Design, Measurement, and Analysis of Clinical Investigations

Timothy Beukelman, Hermine I. Brunner

EVIDENCE-BASED MEDICINE AND CLINICAL INVESTIGATION

Today more than ever, clinicians are encouraged to practice *evidence-based medicine* (i.e., the conscientious, explicit, and judicious use of current best evidence in making decisions about the care of individual patients). Inherent to this is the need to appraise the usefulness and quality of clinically relevant research.[1] The strength of evidence depends on many factors, including the rigor of the study design; the selection of patients and appropriate controls; and the meticulousness and appropriateness with which the data were gathered, analyzed, interpreted, and reported.

Clinical research is viewed as a continuum, beginning from basic biomedical research, progressing to clinical science and knowledge, and resulting in improved health of the public. Two major "transitional blocks" are identified that impede efforts to apply science to better human health in an expeditious fashion. The first translational block occurs between basic biomedical research and clinical science and knowledge, and the second block occurs between clinical science and knowledge and improved health. Contributing factors to the first block include lack of study participants willing to participate in research, regulatory burden, fragmented infrastructure, incompatible databases, and a lack of qualified investigators. Contributing to the second block are career disincentives, practice limitations, high research costs, and lack of funding. These obstacles should remain foremost in the reader's mind, with the realization that the design and analysis of studies must be grounded in what is reasonable from logistical, practical, ethical, and economic points of view. This chapter provides readers with enough clinical, epidemiological, and biostatistical skills to assess the literature critically and to determine independently the "strength of the evidence." It also promotes basic skills that facilitate the design, undertaking, and reporting of clinical research. Although this chapter emphasizes clinical research, many of the concepts discussed here are easily translated to the realm of basic science. Whether working in the laboratory or in the clinic, an investigator must understand basic concepts, such as frequency distributions and statistical inferences.

DEFINITION OF CLINICAL RESEARCH

The Nathan Report defines clinical research as "studies of living human subjects, including the laboratory-based development of new forms of technology; studies of the mechanisms of human disease and evaluations of therapeutic interventions (which are known collectively as *translational research*); clinical trials, outcome studies, and health care

research; and epidemiological and behavioral studies."[2] This area of research includes mechanisms of human disease, therapeutic interventions, clinical trials, and the development of new technologies. Human research, per this definition, excludes *in vitro* studies that use human tissues but do not deal directly with patients. Conversely, laboratory or translational research ("bench to bedside"), provided that the identity of the patients from whom the cells or tissues under study are derived is known, constitutes clinical research.

The National Institutes of Health (NIH) considers genomic and behavioral studies as categories of clinical research. In this chapter, clinical trials are considered separately from other types of clinical studies.

PATIENT-ORIENTED RESEARCH

The NIH definition of clinical research groups four categories of investigation under the major heading of patient-oriented research: (1) mechanisms of human disease, (2) therapeutic interventions, (3) clinical trials, and (4) development of new technologies. This chapter emphasizes clinical trial classification and methods. Many of the concepts and much of the terminology presented herein can be generalized to the conduct of clinical studies in any of these four areas of clinical research.

GENERAL TERMINOLOGY AND BASIC CONCEPTS OF CLINICAL STUDIES

All clinical investigations may be divided broadly into observational or experimental studies. In **observational studies,** there is no artificial manipulation of any factor that is to be assessed in the study, and there is no active manipulation of the patient. In observational studies, the subjects have received the "etiological" agent by mechanisms other than active assignment or randomization. Examples may be medication exposure, atmospheric pollutants, and occupational toxins. Observational studies may be either retrospective or prospective. *Retrospective* implies that the data already exist and are retrieved using a systematic approach, but missing data are not retrievable or cannot be verified. In *prospective* observational studies, a cohort is observed prospectively through time, and data are gathered on an ongoing basis. In this case, missing data may possibly be retrieved for purposes of the study, and standardized methods of data verification can be employed. **Experimental studies** are studies in which the investigator artificially manipulates study factors or subjects, such as therapeutic regimen, or some other parameter. In experimental studies, the subjects are observed prospectively, some active maneuver is conducted, and the results of this maneuver are then observed.

OBJECTIVES AND HYPOTHESES

The first step for conducting a clinical study is a research question or hypothesis. A **research question** is a clear, focused, concise, complex, and arguable query around which a particular research is centered. **Hypotheses** are derived from the research question. They are declarative statements about the predicted relationship between two or more variables. Hypotheses are testable, meaning that the variables that are part of a hypothesis must be observable, measurable, and analyzable. However, when formally testing for statistical significance, the hypothesis should be stated as a *null hypothesis.*

The **null hypothesis, H_0,** represents a theory that has been put forward, either because it is believed to be true or because it is to be used as a basis for argument but has not been proved. For example, in a clinical trial of a new drug, the null hypothesis might be that, on average, the new drug is no better than the current drug. Hence the statement for H_0 would be: "There is no difference between the two drugs on average." Special consideration is given to the null hypothesis because it relates to the statement being tested, whereas the **alternative hypothesis** relates to the statement to be accepted if/when the null hypothesis is rejected. The final conclusion, once the test has been carried out, is always given in terms of the null hypothesis. We either "reject H_0 in favor of H_1" or "do not reject H_0"; we never conclude "reject H_1," or even "accept H_1." If we conclude "do not reject H_0," this does not necessarily mean that the null hypothesis is true; it only suggests that there is not sufficient evidence against H_0 in favor of H_1. Rejecting the null hypothesis, then, suggests that the alternative hypothesis may be true.

The **primary objective** of a research study should be coupled with the hypothesis of the study. Study objectives define the specific aims of a study and should be clearly stated in the introduction of the research protocol. The study objective is an active statement about how the study is going to answer the specific research question.

The relation between the research question, hypothesis, and study objectives is exemplified by a study by de Benedetti and colleagues on a randomized trial of tocilizumab in systemic juvenile idiopathic arthritis (SIJA).[3]

- Research question: How does tocilizumab compare with a placebo in managing the signs and symptoms of SJIA?
- Research hypothesis: SJIA signs and symptoms are significantly more improved in patients who receive biweekly intravenous tocilizumab for 12 weeks compared with individuals who receive placebo.
- Objective: To investigate the clinical efficacy and safety of tocilizumab in children with systemic juvenile idiopathic arthritis.

Hypothesis-Generating Versus Hypothesis-Testing Studies

The design of a clinical investigation depends on whether the study intends to generate hypotheses to be tested in future studies or to test specific hypotheses for which the investigator has some existing evidence to support the belief that they are true or not true. *Hypothesis-generating studies* are considered *exploratory.* Studies that are designed as tests of hypotheses, for which there are preliminary data, are often called *pivotal* or *confirmatory* studies. A given study may have confirmatory and exploratory aspects. Each type of study has distinct advantages and disadvantages. The design chosen is always deeply influenced by reality: what is economically, logistically, ethically, and scientifically possible.

A common exercise used by methodologists is to design the best theoretical experiment to answer the research question posed, without regard to time, money, ethics, patient availability, or anything else that could cause a lessening in the quality of the study; a related approach is known as the *infinite data set.*[4] Realizing that there is no such thing as the perfect clinical study, the designer eliminates the most unrealistic "requirement." For example, it is not likely that one can enroll 300 children with active granulomatous angiitis who would agree to the possibility of being randomly assigned to a placebo for 1 year. The study is compromised further and further by reality until one arrives at what can be done in consideration of all the issues. If the resulting study design and its protocol are unacceptable scientifically, perhaps the question cannot (and should not) be answered. The decision to pursue or not to pursue the "compromised" study, based in reality, is one of the most difficult in the entire research process.

EPIDEMIOLOGICAL STUDIES

Clinical epidemiology is a medical science that studies the frequency and determinants of disease development, as well as the diagnostic and therapeutic approaches to disease management in clinical practice. Epidemiology and biostatistics comprise the basic tools of the clinical investigator. Epidemiological methods can be used to answer questions in the following categories.

Studies in *descriptive epidemiology* typically concern themselves with patterns of disease occurrence with respect to person, place, or time. Descriptive epidemiological studies serve as hypothesis-generating studies for studies of causation, much the same way as small exploratory clinical trials serve as preliminary studies for therapeutic confirmatory trials. The *person variable* is concerned with who experiences the disease. A basic tenet is that the disease does not occur at random, but is more likely to develop in some people than in others. Personal factors of potential importance include age, sex, race, ethnicity, socioeconomic status, existing morbidity, health habits, genetics, and epigenetics (i.e., heritable alterations in gene expression caused by mechanisms other than changes in DNA sequence). The *place variable* is concerned with where the disease develops. Variation in place of occurrence can be evaluated at the local, regional, or national level. The *time variable* is concerned with variation in the occurrence of disease in time and its seasonality or periodicity.

A hypothetical example of a descriptive epidemiological study is the investigation of a group of workers in a factory who are suspected of having environmentally acquired lupus. The epidemiologist would investigate the detailed characteristics of the workers to determine whether there are patterns among the workers who do and do not have lupus. Do all types of workers (management through hourly manufacturing employees) show the same rate of disease development? Are people living close to the factory or its effluent affected? Systematic investigation of the patterns of disease allows a more precise hypothesis of causation, particularly if some exposure or dose level is found to be more strongly associated with the illness.

Frequency of Disease Occurrence and Prognosis

The frequency of disease occurrence is an important aspect of understanding a disease process. It can be measured in numerous ways. Epidemiological theory states that incidence is best estimated from prospective studies; prevalence may be calculated by prospective or retrospective approaches.

Incidence is the rate at which newly diagnosed cases develop over time in a population. Mathematically, incidence is equal to the number of new cases (numerator) divided by the number of persons at risk in the population multiplied by the time (duration) of observation (denominator). This rate is expressed in units of cases/person-time. Incidence is related to the concept of risk, defined as the proportion of unaffected individuals who, on average, contract the disease over a specific period. ***Risk of a disease*** is equal to the number of new cases divided by the number of persons at risk. Risk has no units and can have values between 0 (no new occurrences) and 1 (the entire population becomes affected during the risk period). ***Prevalence*** is the total number of existing cases in a defined population at risk of developing a disease, either at a point in time or during some time period. Mathematically, prevalence is equal to the number of existing cases divided by the number of persons in the population at risk of developing the disease. Persons with the disease are subtracted from the denominator because they are no longer at risk of developing it. Prevalence is expressed in different ways: as a proportion (0 to 1), as a percentage (0 to 100), or by actual numbers using a convenient denominator (e.g., cases per 1,000 children). *Point prevalence* is the number of new and old cases in a defined population at a given "instant" in time. *Period prevalence* is the number of new and old cases that exist in a defined population during a given time period (e.g., 1 year).

Prognosis refers to the possible outcomes of a disease and the frequency with which they can be expected to occur. Prognostic factors need not cause the outcome, but must merely be associated with an outcome strongly enough to predict it. Prognosis is narrower in focus and more short-term in aspect than the consequences of disease and treatment that are considered in the field of outcomes research. The six most frequently measured outcomes in outcomes research are known as the ***six D's:*** (1) death, (2) disease, (3) disability, (4) discomfort, (5) dissatisfaction, and (6) dollars. Prognostic studies often use a prospective cohort design. Studies of prognosis in JIA have included the sex of the patient, the age at onset, and a variety of clinical and laboratory variables to estimate outcome.[5-7] Prognostic studies may also evaluate DNA and RNA,[8-15] including pharmacogenetics.[16]

Etiology and Risk of a Disease

In his presidential address to the Royal Society of Medicine in January 1965, Sir Austin Bradford Hill gave his now famous speech titled "The Environment and Disease: Association or Causation."[17] Hill described what have become known as ***Koch's postulates for epidemiologists.*** These postulates describe what evidence should be considered when assessing causation of disease. Satisfaction of all of these criteria is not necessary or sufficient to establish causation, but they serve as a useful guide and include the following:

1. *Strength of the association:* How strong is the association between the factor and the outcome? For example, how significant is the

probability (*P*) value of the association between dietary intake of calcium and bone mineral density among children with juvenile idiopathic arthritis (JIA)?

2. *Consistency of the association:* Does the association between factor and disease persist from one study to the next, even if variations in study design and samples of patients vary substantially?

3. *Specificity of the association:* Is the association limited to specific alleles and types of disease, with little association between the alleles and other diseases? As the study of causation has advanced, including genetic risk, the issue of specificity is considered less important than it previously was.

4. *Temporal correctness:* Did the exposure to the factor occur before the disease? Temporal correctness becomes more difficult to establish in diseases with extended time intervals between exposure and the onset of clinical manifestations of the disease.

5. *Biological gradient:* Is there a dose-response relationship between the factor and the disease? Does increasing the dose or time of exposure to cyclophosphamide result in a subsequent increase in frequency of malignancy?

6. *Biological plausibility:* Does the association make sense with what is currently understood about the disease and its pathogenesis?

7. *Coherence:* Is the association consistent with laboratory science investigations of the disease?

8. *Experiment:* Does the association hold up under experimental conditions? If one reduces the dose or time of exposure to cyclophosphamide, is there a corresponding decrease in the frequency of malignancy?

9. *Analogy:* Are there similar factors that are accepted to be the cause of similar diseases?

No single study can prove indisputably that a potential etiological factor causes a disease, complication, or adverse event. The accumulating body of knowledge concerning factor and disease, or treatment and outcome, finally allows the conclusion that evidence is sufficient to prove a causal link between the two.

Risk of a disease is the likelihood, usually quantified as an incidence rate or cumulative incidence proportion, that an individual will develop a given disease in a given time period. There are several risk measures, among them the ***absolute risk*** of a disease, which is the chance of developing the disease over a time period (see Table 6-1). The same absolute risk can be expressed in different ways. For example, say you have a 1 in 10 risk of developing a certain disease in your life. This can also be said to be a 10% risk, or a 0.1 risk. The absolute risks from different exposures can be compared with each other by calculating the ***absolute risk reduction*** through simple subtraction. For example, if the absolute risk of developing an unwanted outcome with

TABLE 6-1 Terms Associated with Risk Factors and Disease

RISK FACTOR	DISEASE PRESENT	DISEASE ABSENT
Positive	A	B
Negative	C	D

The 2 × 2 table may be used to calculate associations between the risk factor and the disease

TERM	CALCULATION	MEANING
Incidence	$(a + c) / (a + b + c + d)$	Number of new cases among those at risk
Absolute risk	—	Synonymous with incidence
Attributable risk	$[a / (a + b)] - [c / (c + d)]$	Incidence among those with the risk factor *minus* incidence among those without the risk factor (sometimes expressed as a percentage of the incidence rate among those with the risk factor)
Relative risk	$(a / [a + b]) \div (c / [c + d])$	Incidence among those exposed *divided by* incidence among those not exposed
Odds ratio	$(a \times d) / (b \times c)$	Approximation to the relative risk used in case-control studies
Case exposure rate	$a / (a + c)$	Among those *with* the disease, the proportion who had the risk factor
Control exposure rate	$b / (b + d)$	Among those *without* the disease, the proportion who had the risk factor

drug A is 5% and with drug B is 15%, then the absolute risk reduction associated with drug A would be 10%. A related measure is the **number needed to treat,** which is the inverse of the absolute risk reduction. In this example, the number needed to treat is 10 (1 / 0.10 = 10), meaning that for every 10 patients treated with drug A instead of drug B, 1 occurrence of the unwanted outcome is avoided.

An important concept in the study of disease etiology is *relative risk* or *risk ratio (RR)*. RR is used to compare the risk in two different groups of people. For example, research suggests that smokers have a higher risk of developing heart disease compared with (relative to) nonsmokers. An RR ranges from 0 to infinity. The RR indicates the strength of the association between the risk factor and the disease outcome and is calculated by dividing the absolute risk in the group exposed to a risk factor by the absolute risk in the unexposed group. An RR value statistically significantly larger than 1 indicates the exposure is associated with increased risk of disease; an RR value not statistically significantly different from 1 indicates there is no association between the exposure and the risk of disease; and an RR value statistically significantly less than 1 indicates the exposure is associated with decreased risk of disease; that is, the exposure is protective.

An RR used frequently in genetic studies is lambda, indicating familial aggregation of cases. An example is $\lambda_{sibling}$ (λ_s), calculated as the prevalence of a disorder in biological siblings of individuals with the disease divided by the prevalence of the disease in the general population. The λ_s for systemic lupus erythematosus (SLE) has been estimated to be 30, meaning that a sibling of an individual with SLE is 30 times more likely to develop SLE than a member of the general population.[18] *LOD scores (logarithm of odds)* are distinct from λ_s and are commonly used to estimate genetic linkage in families between generic traits or biomarkers, and genetic traits or more than one biomarker.

Table 6-1 presents related terms that are relevant to risk and shows how each may be calculated using a 2 × 2 contingency table. Disease state (present or absent) is considered the dependent variable and is usually placed in the columns (x axis). The risk factor (positive or negative) is considered the independent variable and is usually placed in the rows (y axis).

The RR is calculated differently from the odds ratio and these two terms are not interchangeable. *Odds ratios (ORs)* are used in case-control studies because the retrospective selection of controls does not generally allow for the determination of true incidence rates. Instead, the OR is calculated by dividing the odds of exposure among the cases by the odds of exposure among the controls. The OR is frequently reported in sophisticated epidemiologic studies because it is the effect measure derived from regression models that have binary (yes/no) outcomes (i.e., logistic regression).

Diagnosis of Disease and Classification, and Response Criteria

The diagnosis of disease, as it applies to epidemiology, refers to the performance of screening and diagnostic tests used in populations, rather than the process of differential diagnosis of individual patients. Classification criteria are typically used to identify homogeneous population for studies with the intent to facilitate hypothesis testing. Classification criteria typically employ a set of core variables fashioned into an algorithm. Examples are the classification criteria for juvenile dermatomyositis or scleroderma.[19,20] Although the criteria are often used in clinical practice to support the diagnosis of a rheumatic disease, patients can be diagnosed with a rheumatic disease even if they do not fulfill classification criteria for this disease. Conversely, response criteria provide measures of change to therapy. Examples are the criteria of flare or those of improvement in of JIA.[21,22]

Validity of a Diagnostic or Screening Test or Set of Criteria

The validity of a diagnostic or screening test or set of criteria involves various parameters, as shown in Table 6-2. The table typically is constructed with the presence or absence of disease as the column labels (i.e., x axis) and the test results as the row labels (i.e., y axis). The patients in row 1, column 1, are called *true positives*; patients in row 1, column 2, are *false positives*; patients in row 2, column 1, are *false negatives*; and patients in row 2, column 2, are *true negatives*. **Sensitivity, specificity, positive** and **negative predictive values, false-positive rate** and **false-negative rate,** and **reliability** are terms used to describe the validity of a screening test. Of note, the positive and negative predictive values of a diagnostic test are dependent upon the prevalence of the condition in the population. By contrast, sensitivity and specificity are generally considered to be inherent properties of diagnostic tests.

The utility of diagnostic tests can be evaluated with the use of **likelihood ratios.** The likelihood ratio positive (LR+) and likelihood ratio negative (LR−) are defined in Table 6-2. If one estimates the pretest odds of a patient having a disease, performs the diagnostic test, and then multiplies by the appropriate corresponding likelihood

TABLE 6-2 Estimating the Validity of a Diagnostic Test

TEST RESULT	DISEASE PRESENT	DISEASE ABSENT
Positive	True positive (TP)	False positive (FP)
Negative	False negative (FN)	True negative (TN)

The 2 × 2 table may be used calculate measures of the test's validity

TERM	CALCULATION	MEANING
Sensitivity	TP / (TP + FN)	Proportion (or percentage) of persons *with* the disease who test *positive*
Specificity	TN / (TN + FP)	Proportion (or percentage) of persons *without* the disease who test *negative*
Positive predictive value	TP / (TP + FP)	Proportion (or percentage) of persons who test positive who *have* the disease
Negative predictive value	TN/ (TN + FN)	Proportion (or percentage) of persons who test negative who *do not have* the disease
False-positive rate	FP / (TP + FP)	Proportion (or percentage) of persons who test positive who *do not have* the disease
False-negative rate	FN / (TN + FN)	Proportion (or percentage) of persons who test negative who *have* the disease
Reliability (also called reproducibility)	—	The ability of a test to yield the same result on retesting
Likelihood ratio positive (LR+)	Sensitivity / 1 − specificity	The magnitude of the increase in the odds of disease given a positive test result
Likelihood ratio negative (LR−)	1 − sensitivity / specificity	The magnitude of the decrease in the odds of disease given a negative test result

ratio (LR+ for a positive test result and LR– for a negative result), the result is the posttest odds of the patient having the disease. Odds and probabilities can be interconverted easily [odds = probability / (1 – probability)]. Posttest probabilities of disease generated from likelihood ratios are more refined estimates than the positive predictive value of the test, because they rely on an individual patient's probability of disease rather than the prevalence of disease among the population.

A widely used tool that allows visual comparison of the performance of a set of different criteria, or different cut points for a diagnostic or screening test, is known as the ***receiver operating characteristic (ROC) curve.*** An ROC curve is a plot of the true-positive rate against the false-positive rate–sensitivity on the *y* axis and (1 – specificity) on the *x* axis. An ROC curve informs about the trade-off between sensitivity and specificity for different criteria or cut points; the nearer the curve follows the left upper corner of the ROC space, the more accurate the test is. Conversely, the closer the curve approaches to the 45° diagonal of the ROC space, the less accurate the test is. Tests with an area under the ROC curve of 0.5 or lower are no better than chance to predict whether the disease is present or not. ROC analysis is commonly used to assess the quality of new criteria, diagnostic tests, or predictive tests.[17,23,24] The overall quality of a test can be summarized by the *area under the ROC curve (AUC),* which ranges between 0 and 1. The larger the AUC of a test is, the more accurately the test predicts the disease, in terms of sensitivity and specificity. Figure 6-1 provides a sample of an ROC curve of a new laboratory test for the anticipation of a flare of lupus nephritis with a guide for the interpretation of the area under the ROC curve.[25]

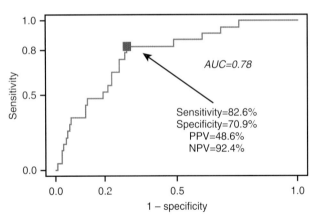

FIGURE 6-1 The receiver operating characteristic (ROC) curve, a plot of the true-positive rate versus false-positive rate (i.e., sensitivity on the *y* axis, and 1 – specificity on the *x* axis). Sensitivity and specificity range between 0 and 1 (or 0% and 100%). ROCs allow one to observe the trade-off between sensitivity and specificity at various cut points of a diagnostic test. Tests of a certain outcome (disease) with ROC curves that are 45° diagonals have an area under the ROC curve of 0.5. These tests are not useful for predicting the outcome (diagnosing the disease). The left most upper point of the ROC curve provides the statistically best trade-off of sensitivity and specificity. Depending on the cutoff point along the ROC curve chosen, the laboratory test yields a certain NPV and PPV. The AUC (0-1) serves as an overall measure of the quality of the test for the diagnosis (here: risk of impending lupus nephritis flare). *NPV,* Negative predictive value; *PPV,* positive predictive value; *AUC,* area under the ROC curve. (Modified from C.H. Hinze, M. Suzuki, M. Klein-Gitelman, et al., Neutrophil gelatinase-associated lipocalin is a predictor of the course of global and renal childhood-onset systemic lupus erythematosus disease activity, *Arthritis Rheum.* 60 [2009] 2772–2781.)

Epidemiological Study Designs Aimed at Establishment of Associations and Cause-Effect Relationships
Case-Controlled Retrospective Study

One of the most common types of study designs used to establish an association, or a cause-effect relationship, is an observational case-controlled retrospective study. In this setting, patients who have the disease are compared with patients who do not have the disease, and data documenting prior exposure to some agent are ascertained retrospectively.

The most frequent statistic to come from this type of study is the OR (see Table 6-1). Provided the disease is rare, the OR estimate is numerically similar to the RR. The choice of an appropriate control group is crucial for the correct inferences to be made about a prior exposure. Controls are chosen with the intent to adjust for personal, socioeconomic, or environmental factors that may influence the development of a disease.

There is no "gold standard" for selecting control subjects, but guidelines exist.[26] One basic principle is that the control patients should be representative of the underlying population from which the cases were derived (i.e., if the controls had developed disease, then they would have been identified as cases for the study). Advantages of case-controlled studies include efficiency, low cost, quick results, and low risk to study subjects. They are particularly advantageous when studying rare outcomes because the persons with the outcome or disease of interest are identified from the beginning of the study. There are several disadvantages of case-controlled studies, however. The temporal relationship of exposure and disease may be obscured. Historical information may be incomplete, inaccurate, or not verifiable; a detailed study of mechanisms of disease is often impossible; and if the study is not well done, results may be biased. For example, persons who develop a disease may remember prior exposures differently than those who do not develop a disease because they suspect a possible causal association in their own minds (i.e., recall bias).

Prospective Cohort Study

The observational approach that most closely resembles an experiment is the prospective cohort study. In this study, a population is defined from which the sample is drawn. Exposure to some factor is established, and subjects are categorized as having been either "exposed" or "not exposed" to a factor thought to contribute risk of some outcome. Each of the two cohorts is monitored prospectively to observe whether the outcome develops. Relative risk is the statistic most commonly used in describing this study. The identification of exposed persons presents several problems. The first is to identify the exposed persons correctly and measure the degree of exposure. This may be done by selecting subjects with some type of unusual occupational or environmental exposure.

The advantages of a prospective observational cohort study are that a clear temporal relationship between exposure and disease is established, and the study may yield information about the length of induction (incubation) of the disease. The design facilitates the study of rare exposures and allows direct calculation of disease incidence rates and thus relative rates or risks.

The disadvantages of cohort studies include the potential for loss to follow-up or alteration of behavior because of the long follow-up time that may be necessary. Cohort studies are not particularly suited for rare diseases when the outcome is onset of the disease. Detailed studies of the mechanisms of the disease typically are impossible in cohort studies. An example of a cohort study designed to detect disease causation is the study by Inman and associates,[28] who prospectively observed a cohort of persons exposed to *Salmonella typhimurium* infection to determine whether reactive arthritis developed. Prospective cohorts or registries also are useful in pediatric rheumatology when the aim is to identify risk factors for development of certain complications or outcomes in a group of children who, typically, have the same disease but vary in predictor or risk variables.[29,30]

Prospective Observational Registries

A patient registry has been defined as the organized collection of uniform observational data to evaluate specific outcomes for a defined population of persons.[31] Registries may be developed to examine the natural history of disease, to analyze the effectiveness and safety of treatments, to measure quality of care, and other purposes. The primary data in registries may be generated by medical encounters (e.g., physician assessments and the results of investigative studies), and these data may be additionally linked to secondary data sources that are collected for other purposes (e.g., outpatient pharmacy billing data). Advantages of prospective observational patient registries include the study of "real-world" patients and conditions with resultant excellent generalizability and the ability to examine clinical questions for which a randomized clinical trial is impractical or unethical. The main disadvantage of registries is common to all observational studies: the potential for bias, especially confounding by indication.

HEALTH SERVICES RESEARCH

Health services research (HSR) can be defined as the multidisciplinary field of scientific investigation that studies how social factors, financing systems, organizational structures and processes, health technologies, and personal behaviors affect access to health care, the quality and cost of health care, and ultimately individual health and well-being. Research domains are individuals, families, organizations, institutions, communities, and populations.[32]

HSR uses a multitude of methods and techniques, and in the following section the ones commonly or increasingly used in pediatric rheumatology are summarized. A comprehensive list can be found at http://www.hsrmethods.org/glossary.aspx.

Among the key methods of HSR are *systematic reviews* that use explicit methods to perform a thorough literature search and critical appraisal of individual studies to identify valid and applicable evidence. Systematic reviews summarize the existing evidence and identify gaps in current knowledge. They are often considered the prerequisite for *meta-analyses*, a statistical procedure for synthesizing quantitative results from different studies. These types of analyses can be used to overcome problems of reduced statistical power of smaller studies, making it a powerful analytical technique. The standard estimates derived by meta-analytic methods are combined probability and average effect size for a set of studies, the stability of these results, and the factors associated with differential treatment outcomes. The evaluation of meta-analyses should include assessment of whether there is a biased selection of studies and judgment about the quality of the data included, as well as the conceptual, methodological, and statistical soundness of the studies. Common challenges in meta-analyses include differences in the outcomes reported by the individual studies or significant heterogeneity in the results of the individual studies such that an aggregate estimate may not be easily interpreted. Despite these potential shortcomings, meta-analysis is a valid approach for overcoming the issues of reduced power because of a small study population or a rare outcome. Important meta-analyses that have influenced medical decisions in rheumatology include those of the

cyclooxygenase-2 inhibitor rofecoxib, which ultimately led to the withdrawal of the product from the market.[33]

The **Cochrane Collaboration** (http://www.cochrane.org) is an international not-for-profit and independent organization that produces and disseminates systematic reviews and meta-analyses of health care interventions and promotes the search for evidence in the form of clinical trials and other studies of interventions.[34]

Decision analysis is another HSR method that is aimed at supporting evidence-based medical decision making. Decision analysis is a means of making complicated medical decisions by including all of the factors that could possibly affect the outcome. Decision analysis uses the form of a decision tree as a diagrammatic representation of the possible outcomes and events that are considered in the decision analytical model. This includes outlining the problem, laying out the options and possible outcomes in explicit detail, assessing the probabilities and values of each outcome, and selecting the "best choice." Few decision analyses have been published in pediatric rheumatology owing to the large amount of evidence generally required to construct an informative decision model, but an example is a decision analysis about the treatment of monoarthritis of the knee in JIA.[35]

Cost-effectiveness analyses are special types of decision analyses that address questions of the cost of health interventions compared with health outcomes. Cost-effectiveness analyses are often done to assess whether the additional costs of new medications are worth paying for by society. Cost-effectiveness analyses often use *quality-adjusted life years (QALYs)* to represent the value of different health outcomes. Using this metric, one year of "perfect health" is assigned a value of 1.0, and death is assigned a value of zero. Individual health states (e.g., moderately active polyarthritis) can be assigned values on this scale using various methodologies to elicit patient preferences. The amount of time spent in a particular health state is then multiplied by its assigned value to determine the number of QALYs for that health outcome. A value often mentioned is the *incremental cost-effectiveness ratio (ICER),* which compares the differences between the costs and health outcomes of the medication being evaluated and the most cost-effective current treatment. One of the challenges of cost-effectiveness studies is selecting the appropriate perspective for the determination of costs. For example, the results of cost-effectiveness analyses are often sensitive to whether or not the indirect costs of disease (e.g., lost time away from employment) are included.

Outcomes research is part of HSR and designed to evaluate the impact of health care on health or economic outcomes. Large population-level data sets are often used to conduct outcomes research, although primary data collection is sometimes conducted. Where large data sets are used, these are often gleaned from administrative or financial data, which may not be ideal for research purposes.

Outcomes research includes *pharmacovigilance* (i.e., the process of detecting, assessing, understanding, and preventing adverse effects of approved drugs), and data from postmarketing reports, including adverse drug event reports, are used. *Pharmacoepidemiology* is the study of the use of and effects of drugs in large groups of people.[36] To complement the information obtained from phase IV studies, pharmacoepidemiology studies frequently make use of data that were collected for other purposes, such as administrative claims billing data. These data sources generally provide detailed patient-level information about physician diagnoses, hospitalizations and other resource utilization, and outpatient medication prescription fills, but they do not contain clinical information, such as physician assessments and results of investigative studies. An example of a pharmacoepidemiology study in pediatric rheumatology is the use of administrative data from the United States Medicaid program to examine the rates of hospitalized infection associated with different treatments in JIA.[37]

HSR also includes *treatment guidelines* and *benchmark development* to standardize therapies and obtain quality parameters for treatment effectiveness.

Other key areas of HSR research are the development and validation of classification and response of disease outcome measures. As the science of clinical research advances, we must update our standards for considering classification and response criteria. Disease outcome measures allow the comparison of patients in a standardized fashion. Details of how to develop and validate classification and response criteria and outcome measures in terms of their reliability, validity, and diagnostic accuracy can be found elsewhere.[38-40]

Regulatory Affairs and Clinical Trials: Useful Guidelines

For simplicity, the generic term *drug* is used in the following discussions. It should be considered synonymous with any medicinal product, vaccine, or biologic agent. The principles discussed can also apply to interventional procedures such as surgery and radiotherapy. Clinical epidemiologists are frequently concerned with evaluating the effectiveness and safety of new therapies.

The **Code of Federal Regulations** of the U.S. Food and Drug Administration (FDA), and in particular Title 21 (Food and Drug), is the most relevant to clinical researchers in the United States. Regulatory activities for clinical research are described in the Good Clinical Practice (GCP) guidance developed by the International Conference on Harmonisation (ICH) of Technical Requirements for Registration of Pharmaceuticals for Human Use. The ICH GCPs represent an international quality standard that various regulatory agencies around the world can transpose into regulations for conducting clinical research. The GCPs include guidelines for human rights protection and how clinical trials should be conducted, and define the responsibilities and roles of clinical investigators and sponsors.

Links to relevant guidance documents for clinical researchers can be found most quickly at the website of the FDA (http://www.fda.gov) and the website of the ICH (http://www.ich.org). Of particular relevance to pediatric rheumatologists is the FDA document titled "Guidance for Industry: Clinical Development Programs for Drugs, Devices and Biological Products for the Treatment of Rheumatoid Arthritis."[41] This document summarizes the position of the FDA on what clinical development programs should consist of, and it provides a framework for conducting studies used to obtain regulatory agency approval of therapies for rheumatoid arthritis or JIA. More recently the FDA issued a draft guidance document specifying pediatric study plans.[42]

Classification of Clinical Trials by Initiator, INDs, NDAs, and BLAs

Before general and specific considerations for individual trials can be discussed, an understanding of the various systems of classification of clinical trials is essential. Clinical trials may be initiated either by industry or by an individual investigator. Trials that are part of a clinical development program and conducted under a sponsor's (pharmaceutical company's) **Investigational New Drug (IND)** submission are usually initiated by industry. Trials undertaken under a sponsor's IND are used frequently by the sponsor in its submission to obtain approval for a new drug, known in the United States and elsewhere as a **New Drug Application (NDA)**. If the NDA is approved by the regulatory agency, the drug may be marketed and labeled for the specific indication (i.e., disease or conditions) stated in the NDA. If the new agent is a biotechnology-derived pharmaceutical, such as a monoclonal antibody, the company files a **Biologic License Application (BLA)**, which is analogous to an NDA for conventional drugs.

Investigator-initiated protocols are typically, but not always, conducted after the drug has been approved for market. The main objective of investigator-initiated protocols may be new dosage regimens or use in diseases other than that for which the drug has obtained an indication. Many such trials are exploratory rather than confirmatory. Funding for investigator-initiated protocols in pediatric rheumatology has come from government agencies, manufacturers, and foundations. Details of the rules and regulations for medication approval in Europe are available at http://www.ema.europa.eu/.

Classification of Clinical Trials by Phase

Phase 0 trial is a term sometimes used to refer to the preclinical or theoretical phase of agent development during which the uses of the drug based on animal models and cellular assays are explored. Clinical drug development programs are often described as consisting of four temporal phases, numbered I through IV by the pharmaceutical industry and by regulatory agencies (Fig. 6-2).[43]

Phase I

Phase I studies are human pharmacology trials with a focus on pharmacokinetics and pharmacodynamics. Both are important in determining a drug's effect. In recent years, the study of *pharmacogenomics* has increasingly occurred (i.e., investigations of how genes affect a person's response to drugs). The goal is to develop medications and drug regimens tailored to the genetic makeup of a person.

Pharmacokinetics can be defined as the study of the time course of drug absorption, distribution, metabolism, and excretion. Study of a drug's pharmacokinetics may progress throughout a clinical development program. This can occur in separate studies or as part of larger trials to determine efficacy and safety. These studies are necessary to assess the clearance of the drug and to anticipate possible accumulation of the drug or its metabolites and the potential for drug-drug interactions. Assessing pharmacokinetics in subpopulations, such as those with impaired renal function or hepatic failure, or in very young children is another important aspect of this phase of studies. Pharmacokinetics data are usually expressed using the following terms[44]:

- *Area under the time-concentration curve* (AUC, or AUC_{0-24} if done over a 24-hour period) is a measure of the total amount of drug absorbed; it is frequently estimated after the drug has reached steady-state levels.
- *Peak concentration* (C_{max}) is the maximum concentration reached at a particular dosage.
- *Time to peak concentration* (T_{max}) is used together with C_{max} to measure the rate of absorption.
- *Cumulative percentage of drug recovered* ($A_c\%$) usually relates to urine data and is the cumulative amount of drug recovered over a specific period (e.g., 24 hours) divided by the initial dose.
- *Elimination (or terminal) half-life* ($t_{1/2}$) is a measure of how long it takes to clear a drug from the system.

Pharmacodynamics is the study of the physiological effects of drugs on the body and the mechanisms of drug action. These studies also typically observe the relationship of drug blood levels to clinical response or to adverse drug events. They may provide early estimates of drug activity and potential efficacy, and they help to establish the dosage regimen used in later phases of drug development.

Phase I studies also provide estimation of initial drug safety and tolerability. **Drug safety** refers to the frequency of adverse drug effects (i.e., physical or laboratory toxicity that could possibly be related to

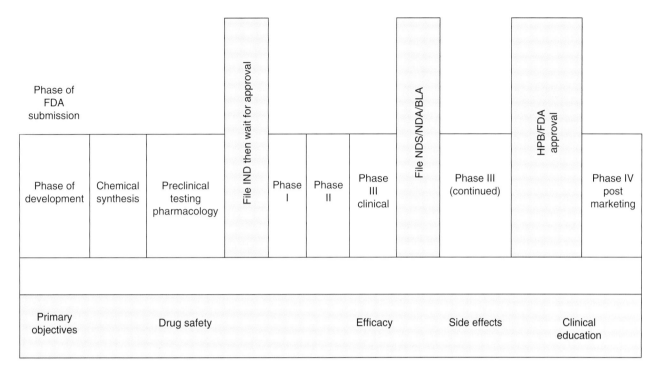

FIGURE 6-2 Study types and the phases of development in which they are performed. This graph shows that study types are not synonymous with phases of development. *BLA,* Biologic license application; *HPB,* health protection branch; *IND,* investigational new drug; *NDA,* new drug application; *NDS,* new drug submission.

the drug) that are treatment emergent (i.e., they develop during treatment and were not present before treatment), or they become worse during treatment compared with the pretreatment state.

Drug tolerability refers to how well subjects are able to tolerate overt adverse drug effects. An *adverse drug effect* is distinguished from an *adverse event* (or experience), which refers to any untoward experience that occurs while a patient is receiving the medication, whether or not it is attributable to the drug. The seriousness of an adverse event dictates how quickly it must be reported to regulatory agencies and to others who may have ongoing experimental protocols. A **serious adverse event** is defined as one that results in death, is life-threatening, requires inpatient hospitalization or prolongation of existing hospitalization, results in persistent or significant disability or incapacity, or is a congenital anomaly or birth defect. Investigators conducting pharmaceutical industry–sponsored studies should be aware that companies may have their own, more strict definition of serious adverse events. The term *severity* is distinguished from *serious* in that *severity* refers to the intensity of a specific event, whereas *serious* refers to the outcome or consequences of the event.

Phase II

Phase II studies are the earliest attempt to establish efficacy in the intended patient population. Many are called *therapeutic exploratory studies* and form the basis for later trials. The hypotheses may be less

well defined than in later studies. These studies may use a variety of different types of study design, including comparisons with baseline status or concurrent controls. In these studies, the eligibility criteria are typically very narrow, leading to a homogeneous population that is carefully monitored for safety. Further studies may establish the drug's safety and efficacy in a broader population after it is determined that a drug does have activity.

In phase II, another aim is to determine more exactly the doses and regimens for later studies. Another important goal is to determine potential study end points, therapeutic regimens (including the use of concurrent medications), and subsets of the disease population (mild versus severe).

Phase III

The primary objective of phase III studies is to confirm a therapeutic benefit. The most typical kind of study is the *therapeutic confirmatory study,* which provides firm evidence of an agent's efficacy and safety. This type of trial always has a predefined hypothesis that is tested. These studies also estimate (with substantial precision) the size of the treatment effect attributable to the drug. Typical for phase III studies are blinding and randomization of treatment allocation. Also incorporated in phase III development are further exploration of the dose-response relationship, study of the drug in a wider population and in different stages of the disease, and the effects of adding other drugs to the agent being investigated. These studies continue to add information to the accumulating safety database.

Phase IV

Phase IV postmarketing surveillance and pharmacovigilance studies aim to accumulate longer-term safety data from large numbers of subjects followed for extended periods, even after the drug has been discontinued in the patient. These types of studies begin after the drug reaches the market and extend the prior demonstration of the drug's safety, efficacy, and dose. The most frequent phase IV study is one of therapeutic use, where it is shown how the drug performs when used in the everyday setting, by patients who may have comorbid conditions or are taking a host of concurrent medications or both. An example of the importance of postmarketing surveillance studies is the discovery of the association between rofecoxib use and increased risk of cardiac events. The FDA has published a guidance document for designers of surveillance and vigilance studies.[46]

Heterogeneity and Investigation in Children

The specific population to be studied is delineated by the inclusion/exclusion criteria. Developers of trials must attempt to reach a compromise between limiting the heterogeneity of the sample and not making the criteria so strict that recruitment of eligible subjects becomes untenable or threatens to restrict the generalizability of results.

The heterogeneity of the patient population that would be allowed to enroll in the trial is influenced by the phase of development. Early exploratory studies are often concerned with whether a drug has any effect whatsoever. In these trials, one may use a very narrow subgroup of the total patient population for which the agent may eventually be labeled. Later phase confirmatory trials typically relax the eligibility criteria to allow for a broader, more heterogeneous sample of the target population. Still, if the criteria for enrollment are too broad, interpretation of treatment effects becomes difficult.

Investigations in children typically are conducted after considerable data have been gathered in an adult population with a similar disease. If clinical development includes children, it is usually appropriate to start with older children before extending the studies to younger children. The exception to the "adults first" rule is when a medication is developed to treat a condition that occurs only in childhood.

The procedures for the development and testing of drugs for children are far from satisfactory; many drugs used to treat children are licensed for use only in adults, drugs are often unavailable in formats suitable for children, and clinical trials involving children raise complex ethical issues. The use of adult products at lower doses or on a less-frequent basis may pose risks to children, as may the use of unlicensed and off-label medicines.[47]

Two U.S. federal acts now mandate that drugs initially developed for use in adults be studied and labeled for children. The *Pediatric Research Equity Act (PREA)* (formerly referred to as the *Pediatric Rule*) requires manufacturers to assess the safety and effectiveness of a drug or biologic product in children if the disease for which the drug was developed in adults also occurs in children. The *Best Pharmaceuticals for Children Act (BPCA)* provides manufacturers with pediatric exclusivity incentives, provides a process for "off-patent" drug development, and requires pediatric study results be incorporated into labeling. For special issues relevant to trials in children, the reader is referred to the FDA guidance document on pediatric research.[48] In 2012, both the BPCA and PREA were made permanent and no longer require renewal by Congress.

Similar legislation was introduced by the European Medicines Agency (EMA) in 2007.[49] To obtain the right to market their medications for use in adults within the European Union, companies are now required to study medicines in pediatric subjects and develop age-appropriate formulations. A Pediatric Drug Committee (PDCO), based at the EMA, is responsible for agreement of the Pediatric Investigation Plan (PIP) with the companies. The PIP contains a full proposal of all the studies and their timings necessary to support the pediatric use of an individual product. More recently, the FDA also provided additional guidance for the industry about pediatric study plans development in line with what has been proposed by EMA,[42] reflecting the updates as were provided in the *FDA Safety and Innovation Act (FDASIA)* of 2011. As a reward or incentive for conducting these studies, companies are entitled to extensions of patent protection and market exclusivity.

Design

The study's phase, objectives, ethics, and feasibility influence the specific design of a trial. New designs have appeared in recent years that reduce the time during which children receive placebo or a known inferior medication.[50,51] More than one type of design may be used to answer the same question. If the same results and conclusions are reached regardless of the design and analysis used, the results are said to show *robustness.* Although a study may be designed as being "pivotal," it is rare that any single trial establishes incontrovertible evidence of an agent's clinical worth.

Comparative and Noncomparative Studies

A *comparative study* implies that some type of comparison is made between the drug under investigation at a particular dosage level and a placebo, another dosage level of the investigational drug, or an active comparator (an existing drug known to be effective for the specific condition). *Noncomparative trials* involve no such comparisons with the investigational agent. Studies that compare the agent with placebo or an active comparator are called *controlled studies.* For a discussion and guidance on the proper selection of a control group, the reader is referred to a guidance document by the FDA. Studies that involve dose escalation or that compare the pharmacokinetics and pharmacodynamics for differing dosage levels of the same drug are not considered controlled in the usual sense.

Open Label Versus Blinded Studies

The phase I and IV studies are usually *open label,* meaning that everyone involved with the study, including the patient and the physician, knows what the patient is receiving. The chief purpose is to gather longer-term safety and efficacy data. Investigator-initiated protocols may also be open if the intent is simply to gather additional information about an agent in another disease or at a dosage level other than that indicated in the label. As one would expect, the possibility of bias in interpretation of safety and efficacy information with open studies is much greater than with blinded studies. Note that phase II and phase III studies may have an open-label extension phase, during which patients who took part in the comparative phase openly receive the investigational drug for an extended period.

Beginning either in late phase I or early phase II, blinded, controlled (comparative) studies are performed. *Blinding* refers to the masking of individuals involved in the assessment of the patient and, in some situations, of the data analyst. The purpose of blinding is to prevent identification of the treatment until any opportunity for bias has passed. These biases include (but are not limited to) decisions about whether to enroll a patient, allocation of patients, clinical assessment of end points, and approaches to data analysis and interpretation. Designs in which the assessor and the patient are blinded are called *double-blind designs.* Designs in which only the patient or only the assessor is blinded to the treatment are called *single-blind designs*. Studies should attempt to maintain blinding until the final patient has completed the study, although this has proved difficult in certain pediatric studies of severe diseases. Clinical studies in humans typically have a steering committee to provide oversight of the trial and a data safety and monitoring plan to provide ongoing monitoring. In large trials and in trials that carry more than minimal risk, the data safety and monitoring plan often includes the formation of a data safety and monitoring board, which meets regularly to assess trial safety, progress, and quality.

Certain studies present challenges to the maintenance of blinding because blinding is either unethical or impractical. Surgical versus nonsurgical interventions prevent the patient and the surgeon from being blinded because they know whether surgery was performed. In this situation, a **blind assessor** may be used to evaluate the patient's condition. The blind assessor may be a physician, nurse, or other health professional who evaluates the patient's response to treatment but is unaware of the treatment being given.

Double-dummy design to maintain blinding. Another situation in which blinding of the patient is difficult is when the dosage administration regimen is different for two drugs being compared. An example in rheumatology is the comparison of methotrexate (administered once weekly) versus hydroxychloroquine (administered once daily). In this case, the *double-dummy design* can be a useful way to maintain the blind. In the example mentioned, patients who are to receive methotrexate take active methotrexate once per week and dummy hydroxychloroquine each day, whereas patients who are to receive hydroxychloroquine receive active hydroxychloroquine each day and dummy methotrexate once per week. Double-dummy designs are limited by ethical issues involving repeated infusions or other aggressive means of delivering the "dummy" agent.

Randomization

The purpose of randomization is to introduce a deliberate element of chance into patient assignment to the treatment groups. Randomization reduces (but does not eliminate) the chance of an unequal distribution of known or unknown prognostic factors among the treatment groups. It also reduces possible bias in the selection and allocation of subjects. Many randomization schemes are currently employed. The simplest form of randomization is *unrestricted randomization*. Patients are assigned to one of two or more treatment groups by a sequential list of treatments. The list of treatments is known as the *randomization schedule*.

Blocked randomization is commonly used to ensure that equal numbers of patients are placed in each treatment group (Table 6-3). Note that in Table 6-3 the assignment to groups is not sequential, but when the block is full, an equal number of patients will have been enrolled into each group. If the blocks are too small, there is a risk of unblinding. If the blocks are too large, they may not be completely filled, increasing the likelihood of unequal assignment to the groups. In more recent pediatric rheumatology studies involving two groups, block sizes of six to eight have been used. Clinical investigators are never made aware of block size during the trial.

Blocks may also be *stratified* by some prognostic factor to ensure equal distribution of the factor among the treatment groups. In multicenter trials, randomization may be stratified by center, such that each center has its own set of blocks. This tends to produce equal numbers of patients in each group at individual centers. In pediatric rheumatology, stratification by center is frequently impossible because only small numbers of patients are enrolled at each center.

If a multicenter trial uses only one randomization schedule for all centers, whether it is unrestricted or stratified, the study is said to be

TABLE 6-3   Example of a Randomization Schedule (Nonstratified, Blocks of 8)*

	PATIENT NUMBER			
Randomization Block 1				
Treatment A	1	2	6	8
Treatment B	3	4	5	7
Randomization Block 2				
Treatment A	12	13	14	15
Treatment B	9	10	11	16

*The first patient entering the study receives treatment A, the second receives treatment A, the third receives treatment B, and so on. The sequence of assignments is random. When the block is full, equal numbers of patients have been enrolled into each treatment group. After block 1 is full, the assignment moves to block 2.

randomized across all centers. Typically, an **interactive voice response system (IVRS)** is used to randomize patients on specific stratification and block size rules using a computer algorithm. If imbalance of one (or at the most two) prognostic factors is found during the enrollment period of a clinical trial, then the randomization scheme may be altered to achieve more balanced groups. This is known as *adaptive randomization*.

Comparative Studies

Randomized controlled trials (RCTs) use comparative designs in which subjects are randomly allocated to two or more specific treatment groups. The comparator may be placebo or an existing therapy that is to be compared with a newly developed active agent. Phase II and early phase III designs often employ a placebo, whereas late phase III and phase IV studies may employ an active comparator. RCTs may be open, single blind, or double blind. In open studies, it is crucial that random allocation to a treatment group be done before knowledge of which treatment the subject is to receive. Various design configurations may employ the basic RCT approach, including parallel, crossover, blinded withdrawal, factorial, and group-sequential studies.

If patients remain in the same group to which they are initially assigned, the study is known as a **parallel group design.**

In **crossover designs,** patients switch from one treatment to the next, often in a randomized manner, and each patient acts as his or her own control for purposes of analysis.

Factorial designs allow for study of the interaction of two treatments that are likely to be used in combination. The simplest factorial design is a 2×2 design in which patients are assigned to receive drug A only, drug B only, both drug A and drug B, or neither drug A nor drug B. Factorial designs are also used to study dose response when two agents are used together. Group sequential designs are particularly well suited to interim analyses. This design implies that the various treatment groups are evaluated for safety and efficacy at periodic intervals during the trial to determine whether the trial should continue or be stopped because of safety or efficacy concerns. Other comparative designs, whose basic approaches are evident from their names, include dose-escalation and fixed-dose, dose-response trials.

A design used to study, among others, etanercept in the treatment of polyarticular JIA is the **blinded withdrawal design.**[50] In this approach, all patients receive active medication long enough to establish whether patients respond (according to a standard definition). Patients who are not classified as "responders" after the prescribed time period are discontinued from the study and considered therapeutic failures. Patients who respond are randomly assigned either (1) to be

TABLE 6-4	Hypotheses Associated with the Different Types of Studies of Assessing Efficacy	
TYPE OF STUDY	**NULL HYPOTHESIS (TO BE REJECTED BASED ON THE CLINICAL TRIAL DATA)**	**RESEARCH HYPOTHESIS**
Traditional comparative (superiority)	There is no difference between the therapies	There is a difference between the therapies
Equivalence	The therapies are not equivalent	The new therapy is equivalent to current therapy
Noninferiority	The new therapy is inferior to the current therapy	The new therapy is not inferior to the current therapy

withdrawn blindly from active medication and given placebo or (2) to continue to receive active medication but in a blind manner. A common phenomenon in blinded withdrawal studies is a mild flare of disease among patients who continue to receive (blinded) active medication after randomization. This is called the *reverse placebo effect* because it is the reverse of the beneficial effect that often is observed in patients who are blindly randomly assigned to placebo. The primary outcome after randomization can be time to flare or percentage who flare (according to a standard definition).

For trials using an ***adaptive design,*** patients are randomized to multiple different active treatments. Patient outcomes are carefully monitored and analyzed during the conduct of the trial, and the randomization scheme is adjusted during the trial to increase the proportion of subjects who receive the treatment that appears to be most favorable. This reduces the number of patients randomized to the less effective treatment, while preserving the statistical power of the study to draw conclusions about the most effective therapy.

Another approach uses an ***end point–driven*** protocol. The outcomes are tallied during the conduct of the trial and when sufficient confidence that the treatment is effective (or not effective) is attained, subject enrollment can be halted and the placebo phase of the study can be terminated. The study of canakinumab in SJIA used an end point–driven design in which the blinded study period was discontinued after a predetermined number of disease flares had occurred.[48]

The ***N-of-1 approach*** repeatedly and randomly crosses over individual patients from one therapy to the next. For example, the randomization scheme may be *A, B, B, A, A, B.* A current pediatric rheumatology example is the N-of-1 study of Hashkes et al.[49] Data from numerous N-of-1 trials in individuals may be combined to increase the sample size, but this is fraught with difficulties and sources of potential bias. Careful consideration of the *"carryover effect"* of the treatment and natural fluctuations of the disease state unrelated to therapy need to occur when planning an N-of-1 trial. The N-of-1 method is most useful in situations where the drug under study has a relatively rapid onset and offset of effect (i.e., has a limited drug carryover effect), and the disease is relatively chronic and stable. Such trials may be poised to emerge as an important part of the methodological armamentarium for comparative effectiveness research and patient-centered outcomes research. By permitting direct estimation of individual treatment effects, N-of-1 trials can facilitate finely graded individualized care, enhance therapeutic precision, improve patient outcomes, and reduce costs.[52]

A trial design that is generating widespread interest is the ***pragmatic trial.*** These studies use randomization of treatment assignment to control for group differences but differ from traditional explanatory trials in several ways. Often, all of the treatment arms in the study are forms of active therapy. Depending on the interventions and the study questions, the randomization may take place at the individual patient level or at the physician or clinical site level, known as *cluster randomization.* Following randomization, the study procedures are generally minimal and are consistent with typical clinical practice. In some cases, the ascertainment of outcome may not require direct interaction with the patients (e.g., death). The results of pragmatic trials are intended to more closely represent real-world outcomes and usually attempt to answer questions about the relative effectiveness of existing accepted treatment approaches.

Intent of Comparative Studies

The type of comparison that one intends to carry out must be decided on before the protocol can be developed. All comparative trials must possess *assay sensitivity,* defined as the ability of a study to distinguish between active and inactive treatments.[53]

Trials that show ***superiority*** are perhaps the most frequent type of comparative studies. They are designed to show superiority of the investigative agent compared with either placebo or an active comparator, or to show a dose-response relationship. In pediatric rheumatology, placebo-controlled studies have become more difficult, because some existing agents are clearly better than placebo. In such situations, the use of a placebo design is considered unethical, and an active comparator is substituted.

In contrast, ***equivalence studies*** aim to demonstrate equivalency (Table 6-4). If the evidence in favor of equivalence is not strong enough, nonequivalence cannot be ruled out. In essence, the null and research hypotheses in testing equivalence are simply those of a traditional comparative study reversed. For ***noninferiority studies,*** the research hypothesis is that the new therapy is either equivalent or superior to the current therapy (Table 6-4). In this setting the term *equivalent* means that the efficacies of the two therapies are close enough so that one cannot be considered superior or inferior to the other. This requires the definition of a constant called the *equivalence margin.* The *equivalence margin* defines a range of values for which the efficacies are "close enough" to be considered equivalent. Therefore, the equivalence margin constitutes the maximum difference between the two treatments that one is willing to accept. Equivalence and noninferiority studies can be difficult to design because of sample size requirements that are often much higher than for superiority trials.[53] Active comparators should be chosen based on convincing, confirmatory trials that are shown to be efficacious in the particular condition. At present for JIA trials, background therapy with methotrexate is often used as an active comparator.

Ethical Requirement for Clinical Equipoise in Comparative Studies

Central to the concept and ethical implications of RCTs is ***clinical equipoise.*** This is defined as honest professional disagreement among expert clinicians about the preferred treatment. Clinical equipoise is widely regarded as an ethical requirement for the design and conduct of RCTs. Underlying clinical equipoise is the norm that no patient should be randomized to treatment known (or thought by the expert clinical community) to be inferior to the established standard of care. Excellent arguments for when placebo trials are appropriate have been presented by Freedman and colleagues.[54-56] According to these authors, the five conditions in which a placebo control may be used are as follows:

- There is no standard treatment
- Standard treatment is no better than placebo

- Standard treatment is placebo
- The net therapeutic advantage of standard treatment has been called into question by new evidence
- Effective treatment exists but is unavailable because of cost or short supply

There are increasing arguments about abandoning the requirement of clinical equipoise for randomized clinical trials.[57] The final arbiter about the ethical acceptability of a trial is always the human subjects or ethics committee.

Conducting a Clinical Trial

With the advent and widespread use of independent for-profit *clinical research organizations* and site management organizations, the quality of clinical trial conduct has increased substantially.

A *coordinating center* is responsible for coordinating almost all trial activities. The role of the study coordinating center is determined in part by whether a clinical research organization is used, and whether the trial is part of a clinical development program or an investigator-initiated protocol.

Site monitoring may be a function of the coordinating center or the clinical research organization. During visits to clinical sites, site monitors—known throughout industry as *clinical research associates*—verify the data on the case report forms against source documentation (i.e., original reports from the laboratory and clinical records).

The study coordinating center may or may not be distinct from the *data coordinating center,* which takes on the overall development of electronic case report forms, data quality assurance procedures, data collation, and data storage. The data coordinating center typically prepares the data for ongoing monitoring and final analysis. *Data collation* refers to the reorganization of the raw data from the case report forms to summary tables and spreadsheets.

The *data safety and monitoring board (DSMB)* of a study is an independent group of experts, and its primary responsibilities are (1) to periodically review and evaluate the accumulated study data for participant safety, study conduct and progress, and, when appropriate, efficacy, and (2) to make recommendations concerning the continuation, modification, or termination of the trial. The DSMB is also responsible for defining its deliberative processes, including event triggers that would call for an unscheduled review, stopping guidelines, and unmasking (unblinding).

The work of the biostatistician of a trial begins with planning of the study and power estimations. At a minimum, the *data analysis plan* considers the following items:

- Identification of the primary and secondary response (outcome) variables
- Calculation of sample size, including assumptions that will be used to justify the sample size, which include the α and β error levels, the difference that one wishes to detect as statistically significant, and how the variance estimate will be obtained

Response Variables

Response variables are defined as outcomes that will be used as the main evidence of the treatment effect of the investigational drug. *Treatment effect* is defined as an effect that is expected to result from a therapy. In comparative trials, the treatment effect of interest is a comparison of two or more agents. In studies designed primarily to observe safety and tolerability of an agent, the "response" variable relates to adverse events or treatment-emergent adverse drug effects, rather than to efficacy.

The choice of *primary response variables* largely depends on the objectives of the trial and should reflect clinically relevant effects. *Secondary response variables* are usually (but not always) associated with the exploratory nature of the study. *Surrogate end points* are outcomes that are intended to relate to a clinically important end point but do not in themselves measure a clinical benefit. In rheumatology, surrogate measures are often so-called composite measures; these integrate or combine multiple relevant variables into a single variable, using a predefined algorithm. Three examples of composite variables are the American College of Rheumatology (ACR) 20 (ACR-20)[58] and the Disease Activity Score[53] for use in trials of adults with rheumatoid arthritis, and the ACR Pediatric-30 for use in trials of children with JIA.[21]

Claims Allowed by the FDA

The claims that the FDA allows for antirheumatic and antiinflammatory therapies for rheumatoid arthritis and JIA heavily rest on the performance of a new medications as measured by standard response variables of structural damage.[41]

The *reduction in signs and symptoms claim* is usually the first to be granted for marketing approval. This claim is typically established in trials of at least 6 months' duration, unless the product belongs to an already well-characterized pharmacological class, in which case trials of 3 months' duration are sufficient to establish efficacy for signs and symptoms. For trials in adults, the FDA recommends that the ACR-20 criteria be used. In studies of JIA, the FDA suggests the ACR JIA-30 be used.

The *major clinical response claim* is awarded to agents that are able to show a response at the ACR-70 level, rather than the 20% improvement needed for a signs and symptoms claim. This claim is based on statistically significant improvement response rates by the ACR-70 definition compared with background therapy in a randomized controlled group. Trial duration should be a minimum of 7 months for an agent that is expected to have a rapid onset of action and longer for agents with less rapid effects.

The *complete clinical response* claim is granted to a drug that produces a remission for at least 6 continuous months by the ACR-20 criteria and by radiographic arrest. Complete clinical response indicates that the patient is in remission, but is still taking antirheumatic drugs. Typically, trials for a complete clinical response last a minimum of 1 year.

The *remission claim* is granted if remission by the ACR definition and radiographic arrest (no radiographic progression by the method of Larsen and colleagues[59] or by the modified method of Sharp and associates[60] are maintained over a continuous 6-month period while the patient is off all antirheumatic therapy. A drug need not be a cure to be awarded a remission claim. A remission claim can be granted even if the patient relapses after 6 months or more of remission. Trials aimed at a remission claim should be at least 1 year in duration. Wallace and colleagues developed a preliminary definition of clinical remission for use in JIA.[61]

The *prevention of disability claim* is granted to drugs for which the primary outcome is a functional ability measure, such as the Childhood Health Assessment Questionnaire or the Arthritis Impact Measurements Scale. In addition, the full effect of JIA on a patient is not captured without the use of a more general health-related measure of quality of life. For this reason, data from a validated measure such as the Medical Outcome Study Short-Form Health Survey (SF-36),[62] the Childhood Health Questionnaire, or the Pediatric Quality of Life Inventory Scales (PedsQL)[63] should also be gathered, and the patient's condition should not worsen on these measures over the duration of the trial.

The *prevention of structural damage* claim is granted to drugs that exhibit either a slowing of radiographic progression or the prevention of new erosions shown by radiography or other measurement tools such as magnetic resonance imaging (MRI). These trials should be at least 1 year in duration.

Other clinical efficacy response variables are possible but such outcome measures must possess a host of validity characteristics, including responsiveness (sensitivity to change within the trial's duration), face (clinical sensibility), content (comprehensiveness), construct (biological sensibility, or how the variable is hypothesized to behave compared with how it does behave), and criterion (does it agree with the gold standard, if one exists) validity.[64] In addition, variables should be reproducible (reliability) and, if more than one variable is chosen, nonredundant with one another.

Analysis Sets (Patients)

Not all patients who enter a trial complete the protocol as it is written. The analysis plan must state the procedures for handling subjects who drop out, are noncompliant, or in some other manner do not follow the protocol specifications. The formation of analysis sets should be aimed at minimizing bias and avoiding an increase in the possibility of an erroneous conclusion that a difference is present between groups when it is not (type I error, described later). The *per-protocol set* (also called *valid cases set, efficacy sample,* or *evaluable subjects sample*) comprises subjects who closely follow and complete the protocol. In practice, consideration of only the per-protocol set results in the loss of valuable information from patients who perhaps completed most of the study or had only one or two minor protocol deviations related to concurrent medication. The *full-analysis set* is also used for the primary analysis. The full-analysis set refers to the intent-to-treat approach and is derived from all randomized patients, including patients who dropped out early or had protocol deviations.

Historically, the *intent-to-treat* analysis meant that all patients, whether they dropped out, were noncompliant, or otherwise deviated from the written protocol, were evaluated for outcome at the time that they would have had their last visit (because one intended to treat them until then). The concept is embodied in the brief saying "Once randomized, analyzed." This approach results in the introduction of substantial bias, however, and is problematic in rheumatology and other specialties in which patients, once off trial, are lost to follow-up and receive various other medications and procedures. It is now common to use a modified intent-to-treat analysis, the *last-observation-carried-forward* approach. This technique involves using the last value obtained for a response variable (no matter when in the trial it was measured) as if it were measured at the scheduled final visit. In this way, the data from individuals who did not complete the trial but who were exposed to the drug long enough to experience treatment effects (if any) can be combined with the data from the per-protocol set.

UNDERSTANDING AND DESCRIBING DATA

Categorical, Ordinal, and Continuous Data

The scale or level of data has important implications for how information is displayed and summarized. All data may be classified into one of the following measurement scales: nominal or categorical, ordinal, or continuous (numerical).

For **categorical variables**, sometimes called *nominal variables* (i.e., "in name only"), each subject can be placed into one of the categories. Variables with two possible outcomes, such as "yes/no" or "male/female," are called *dichotomous*. Categorical variables are expressed as proportions or percentages (i.e., the study population was 75% female and 25% male). The best ways to display categorical data include contingency tables and bar charts.

Ordinal variables have an inherent order. Subjects can be placed in "ranked" or "ordered" categories. Examples of ordinal variables

include the severity scores of swelling (0 to 3+), and tumor staging. Order exists among the categories, but the difference between adjacent categories is not uniform throughout the scale. Ordinal variables are best summarized using percentages and proportions. The entire set of data measured as an ordinal scale may be summarized by a median value.

Continuous variables are observations in which the differences between numbers have meaning on a numerical scale in terms of difference in quantities. Examples are age, height, weight, blood pressure, survival time, and laboratory values such as serum creatinine. Although interval variables all have meaning on a numerical scale, differing degrees of precision are required for different types of studies. Age in a study of adults may be estimated to the closest year; in children, age may have to be estimated to the closest month, and in neonates, to the closest day or hour. Means and medians (discussed later) are used to summarize continuous variables.

When to Convert Higher Levels of Data to Lower Levels

As a rule and in order to increase the accuracy of the comparisons made, numerical data should be analyzed as seen, rather than converting them to lower the ordinal values prior to analysis. The same holds true for conversion of ordered to categorical values or dichotomous data. Situations in which "lowering" the level of data may be appropriate include the following:

- In a multicenter study in which different methods are used to generate a numerical value (e.g., the antinuclear antibody titer when different substrates are used). In this situation, one may be forced to "dichotomize" patient results, describing them as simply "normal" or "elevated," and conduct the analysis using statistics appropriate for a nominal, rather than a continuous, variable.
- If the experimenter suspects measurement error in the data. An example is adherence with a prescribed drug dosage or with a clinical trial or physical therapy program. It may be necessary to divide the patients dichotomously and classify each as "compliant" or "noncompliant."

Concepts Related to Measurement of Variables: Validity, Variability, and Bias

In clinical research, not all patients treated identically experience an identical response. This is known as the **variability** common to human experimentation. Variability is sometimes called *error*. Error may be broadly classified into nonrandom and random error. *Nonrandom error* is also called *bias* or *systematic error*. It results in a lack of validity of a measure and influences the accuracy of the measure. Variability may arise among individuals from numerous factors, including diurnal variation, or age, diet, or exercise. Variability may also arise from measurement characteristic issues, including poor calibration, inherent lack of precision of the instrument, or reading or recording errors of the information provided.

Validity generally is equated with accuracy. *Random error* refers to imprecision. The difference between accuracy and precision is graphically shown in Fig. 6-3.

External validity may be equated with generalizability of the study results. It determines the population settings to which measurement and treatment variables can be generalized.

Internal validity refers to how valid the conclusions are within the patient sample studied; it is a basic minimum requirement without which any study is not interpretable. The question of external validity is meaningless without first establishing whether the study is internally

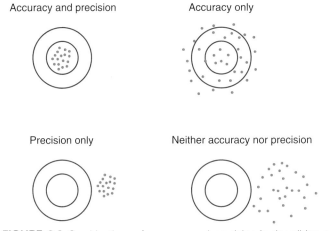

Accuracy and precision   Accuracy only

Precision only   Neither accuracy nor precision

FIGURE 6-3 Combinations of accuracy and precision in describing a continuous variable. Accuracy is impaired by bias or systematic error; precision is impaired by random error.

valid. Both types of validity are important. They may be at odds, however, in that study design features that increase one may tend to decrease the other.

Bias

The concept of **bias** is the lack of internal validity or incorrect assessment of the association between an exposure and outcome in the target population. Bias is distinguished from random error or lack of precision.

Sources of bias that may occur in clinical studies can be categorized in three main groups: selection bias, information bias, and confounding.[65] To complicate matters further, the same type of bias may be known by different names or be a subset of some other bias. A few of the more important types of bias are discussed here.[66]

Selection bias is introduced when the study population does not represent the target population. Selection bias can occur due to the inappropriate definition of study eligibility criteria. Examples include *health care access bias*, when the patients seen in a subspecialty clinic are not representative of the patients seen in the community. Selection bias can also occur due to *lack of accurate sampling*. A convenience sample in which patients are not systematically enrolled in a prospective observational study can lead to bias (e.g., only patients with specific favorable characteristics are enrolled). Post hoc analyses that report on small subgroups can also lead to misleading results. Given that the reports based on post hoc analyses are frequently only reported when significant results are observed, this bias is particularly relevant for meta-analyses of published studies as a manifestation of publication (selection) bias.

Information bias occurs during data collection and can take several forms. *Withdrawal bias* occurs when losses or withdrawals are uneven in both the exposure and outcome categories. There is also bias due to missing information. If participants with complete information do not represent the target population, it can introduce a selection bias. This bias is relevant in studies, mainly retrospective, using data from the clinical chart, in which patients with more complete data have more severe diseases or stay longer at the hospital, or both. *Detection bias* can arise from differing diagnostic procedures in the target population, such as testing for human leukocyte antigen (HLA)-B27 more frequently in boys compared with girls in pediatric rheumatology clinics. This results in a detection bias that will affect the estimate of association between exposure and outcome. Detection bias can also occur if patients are assessed for the outcome differently based upon their

disease management. For example, patients are systematically screened for latent tuberculosis infection prior to starting biologic therapy but not otherwise. It would introduce bias to compare latent tuberculosis rates among children starting biologic therapy to children not initiating biologic therapy and receiving standard care.

Another type of information bias is *misclassification bias*, which occurs when the exposure, the outcome, or other important variables are not determined accurately. This bias may be divided into nondifferential and differential misclassification. Nondifferential misclassification bias occurs when there is no difference in the accuracy of the assessment based on exposure or outcome. An example would be patient self-report of an unacceptable behavior that is not perceived to be associated with the outcome. Inaccurate reporting may be anticipated to affect all patients similarly, irrespective of exposure or outcome status. Therefore, nondifferential misclassification is generally not a threat to the validity of relative measures of association (e.g., relative rates or ORs).

Differential misclassification bias occurs when the inaccuracy in the assessment of outcome varies depending on the exposure status. Differential misclassification bias includes *recall bias*, in which the recall of information about exposure is influenced by whether the person has the disease (e.g., individuals with the disease may have more accurate memory of events prior to disease onset than control individuals (those who did not develop disease during the same time period). *Interview bias* can occur if the circumstances under which different groups of subjects are interviewed are incompatible. These circumstances include time from exposure to interview, setting of the interview, person doing the interview, manner in which questions are asked (prompting), and whether the subject has knowledge of the research hypothesis. Case-control studies are particularly vulnerable to recall and information bias because data are often collected after the outcome is ascertained.

Regression to the mean is the phenomenon that a variable that shows an extreme value on any assessment will tend to be closer to the center of its distribution on a later measurement. The two usual ways of neutralizing this bias are with the existence of an appropriate reference group and a selection based on more than one measurement.

Confounding bias is a distortion of the estimate of the effect of exposure that results from a factor or factors that are associated with both the exposure and the outcome. One of the most common examples of confounding in observational epidemiologic studies of treatment is termed *confounding by indication* or *prescriber channeling*. This occurs when patients with more severe disease preferentially receive a particular treatment, and these patients experience an undesirable outcome more frequently. The association between worse disease and worse outcome confounds the association between treatment and outcome. Brunner and colleagues[67] present an example of confounding bias in pediatric rheumatology. These investigators attempted to identify risk factors for damage in childhood-onset lupus. An association was found between damage and disease duration, indicating a possible (and logical) cause-effect relationship between the two. When the data were corrected for the confounder disease activity over time, disease duration disappeared as a predictor of damage.

Confounding is typically easiest to assess using regression models, as described later. Only established risk factors for the disease should be investigated as potential confounders. In brief, these can be dealt with in the design of the study by matching, restricting enrollment, or randomizing, or can be dealt with in the analysis of the study by stratifying or by adjusting using multivariable analysis (discussion later in this chapter). Another approach that was commonly used in the past to assess the possibility of confounding is to stratify the data by the potential confounder. One looks for an association between the exposure (as a possible causal factor) and the disease; then one compares the subjects who have the confounder with subjects who do not to see whether an association exists.

Propensity score methods are useful to try to minimize *confounding by indication*, when the clinical reason for initiating treatment is itself associated with the outcome of interest. Propensity scores estimate the likelihood of receiving the treatment of interest based on pretreatment variables, whether or not the patient actually received the treatment. One common application of the propensity score is to match patients who were exposed with patients who were not exposed but have similar propensity scores. This matching improves the balance of baseline factors that are thought to be associated with the outcome. An example of the use of propensity scores in pediatric rheumatology is the study by Seshadri and associates of the use of aggressive corticosteroid in juvenile dermatomyositis.[68]

Describing Data and Frequency Distribution of Continuous Variables

Descriptive statistics are commonly used to represent individual data points graphically or to summarize groups of data, regardless of the data level. Many exploratory and epidemiological studies use only descriptive statistics, rather than inferential statistics (tests of hypotheses). Graphs such as dose-response curves represent descriptive statistics. A **rate** (or proportion) implies that the numerator is part of the denominator and is usually associated with a time element (e.g., an annual case-fatality rate of 11/120 implies that the 11 deaths came from a total of 120 cases). The numerator of a **ratio** is not part of the denominator (e.g., the female/male ratio among patients with oligoarticular JIA is 6:1).

Statisticians employ many **types of distributions** for describing and analyzing data. These include the binomial (Bernoulli), geometric, chi-square, Poisson, *t*, and F distributions. The **frequency distribution of continuous variables** is most commonly referred to in the medical literature and is the only distribution discussed in detail in this chapter. Its parameters form the basis of much of the descriptive statistics used in the reporting of data from clinical investigations.

A frequency distribution of a continuous variable is simply an *x-y* plot of the possible values that a variable can take (*x* axis) versus the number of observations having the particular values (*y* axis). If the frequency distribution is normally distributed, it is called a *Gaussian distribution* (Fig. 6-4).

Measures of Central Tendency and Skewness

Every distribution of continuous variables has an **arithmetic mean** (average), which is calculated by adding the observations and dividing the sum by the number of observations. The **median** of any distribution is the centermost value. If the distribution has an even number of observations (i.e., there is no center value), the median is calculated by averaging the two most center values. The median is also the 50th percentile. The **mode** is the most frequently observed value. A distribution has only one mean and one median, but numerous modes are possible; this leads to forms such as *bimodal* and *multimodal* distributions.

The *mean*, *median*, and *mode* are called measures of *central tendency*. In a normal distribution, the mean, median, and mode are all the same value. Figure 6-5 shows the effect of positive skewing on the measures of central tendency.

The **skewness** is said to be positive because there are more observations in the upper (shaded) tail (i.e., toward the right side of the distribution). This type of skewing typically occurs in distributions that have a fixed lower boundary, but no upper boundary (e.g., results of

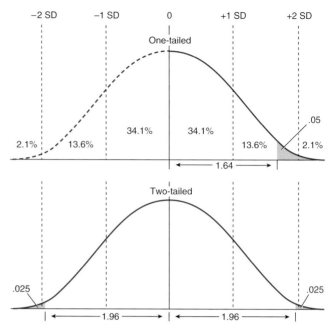

FIGURE 6-4 Normal or Gaussian distribution (bell-shaped curve), showing the approximate percentage of observations expected to be found within 1 and 2 standard deviations (SD) from the mean value. Also note the critical values for one-tailed and two-tailed tests of hypotheses.

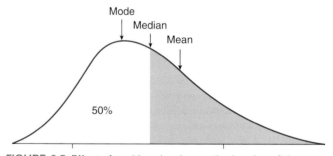

FIGURE 6-5 Effect of positive skewing on the location of the mean, median, and mode. (The mean and median are skewed to the right.) The effect of negative skewing is the mirror image of this figure.

liver function tests). *Negative skewing* is the mirror image and has the opposite effect on central tendency measures. An example is the age at onset of disease among patients with oligoarticular JIA.

Measures of Spread or Variation

The frequency distribution of continuous variables can be described by its **mean** and its **standard deviation (SD)**. The SD is a measure of the spread of values. Abbreviations in common use for the mean include $\bar{x}$ for the sample mean and μ for the underlying population mean from which the sample was drawn. The SD in a formula is designated *s* for the sample SD and σ for the population SD; it is the square root of the variance of the distribution. **Variance** is calculated by subtracting the mean from each of the individual values in the distribution, squaring the differences (to eliminate the negative sign), summing the squares, and dividing the result by the number of observations minus 1. The sample variance is abbreviated s^2, and the variance of the population from which the sample was drawn is σ^2.

If a frequency distribution is normally distributed, the distance ± 1 SD from the mean includes 68.3% of the observations, ± 2 SD includes 95.8% of the observations, and ±3 SD includes 99.7% of the values.

Z Scores: Placing a Single Value Within a Distribution of Values

Frequently, it is useful to locate exactly where an individual patient's value for some variable lies within a distribution of values. Because the normal distribution depends on two parameters, the mean and the SD, there is an infinite number of normal curves, based on the variable being measured. All tables of the normal distribution are for the distribution described by a mean of 0 and SD of 1. Any variable with a mean not equal to 0 and SD equal to 1 must be rescaled so that these parameters are met. The solution is to convert the variable to a standard normal variable, Z (also called a *standard normal deviate*).

A **Z score** can be calculated by subtracting the population mean from the measured value in the individual and dividing the result by the SD of the population: $Z = (x_i - \mu)/\sigma$, where x_i is the individual's value. One may transform the Z scale back to the original scale. A Z score also can be calculated using the sample mean and SD. In addition, two means can be compared to determine whether they are statistically significant via the Z test if the sample size is large. Any continuous numerical variable can be converted to the Z scale.

The **standard error of the mean (SEM)** represents a different concept from the SD. Mathematically, it is expressed as $SEM = SD/\sqrt{n}$, where n is the sample size. Because samples drawn from an underlying population do not each produce the same mean value (but tend to cluster around the same value), one must calculate the range of where the true (unknown) population mean lies. From the formula, it can be seen that the greater the n (i.e., the larger the denominator), the smaller the SEM. The SEM gives the clinical investigator an idea of how "tightly" the estimated mean from the sample represents the true, underlying mean.

Investigators often ask statisticians what should be plotted when presenting the data as a mean and its accompanying measure of variability, the SD or SEM. Because the SEM is always less than the SD, investigators tend to plot it rather than SD. A rule of thumb is that the SD should be used when comparing values from individual subjects with a population distribution. The SEM is used when plotting mean values of two groups of subjects.

As stated earlier, the SD encompasses the variability of individual observations, and the SEM indicates the variability of means. The mean ± 1.96 SD estimates the range of values within which 95% of the observations from subjects can be expected to fall (see Fig. 6-4). Similarly, the mean ± 1.96 SEM estimates the range in which 95% of the means of repeated samples from the same population should fall. If the mean and the SEM are known, 95% **Confidence Intervals (CIs)** can easily be estimated. These limits indicate the range of values within which the investigator is 95% sure that the true mean of the underlying population lies. One can easily calculate any CI level (e.g., 90% CI, 99% CI) based on the SD.

Describing Nonnormal or Nonparametric Distributions

Not all parameters used to describe normal distributions are helpful when one is attempting to describe distributions that are non-Gaussian (i.e., do not follow a bell-shaped curve or reasonable approximation). Although the median, mode, and range (described earlier) are helpful, the mean and SD may be quite meaningless in this situation.

A commonly used method is to group the ranked values in a nonnormal distribution into **quartiles,** which are similar to percentiles, but with only four categories: Q1 = 25%, Q2 = 50%, Q3 = 75%, and Q4 = 100%. The spread, or dispersion, of a nonnormal distribution is described in terms of the **interquartile range.** This is the difference between the highest value in the third quartile (i.e., the 75th percentile) and the highest value in the first quartile (i.e., the 25th percentile). Alternatively, some authors may report the numerical values corresponding to the 25th and 75th percentiles.

STATISTICAL TESTS OF INFERENCE COMMONLY USED IN CLINICAL INVESTIGATIONS

This section does not attempt to describe comprehensively the myriad statistical procedures that are readily available to the clinical investigator through such computer programs as Statistical Analysis System (SAS), the Statistical Package for Social Sciences (SPSS), R, or Bayesian Inference Using Gibbs Sampling (BUGS) for Bayesian analysis. Rather, a basic introduction to statistical concepts is provided, followed by a description of the inferential and other procedures found most commonly in the literature. Formulas are not stressed, because virtually all statistical procedures are now conducted with the use of computer programs. The reader is referred to Table 6-5 for a short summary of what type of test is most appropriate in which setting.

Basic Concepts Relevant to Analysis

Statistical approaches may be divided into frequentist methods and Bayesian approaches. Frequentist methods refer to *P* values and CIs, which can be interpreted as the frequency of specific outcomes from the same experimental situation if it is repeated many times. That is, what are the chances of this outcome (and outcomes even more extreme) if one repeats the experiment many times? Bayesian analysis permits a calculation of the probability that a treatment is superior according to the observed data and prior knowledge.[69] This chapter emphasizes the frequentist school because most statistics in today's literature follow this approach. For more details on Bayesian analysis the reader is referred to Carlin and Louis's popular textbook, *Bayesian Methods for Data Analysis.*[70]

The types of variables in the study and the number of variables analyzed determine the choice of the appropriate statistical approach. Step 1 is to determine which variables are *independent (predictor* or *explanatory)* variables and which are *dependent (outcome* or *response)* variables. An *independent variable* is the parameter that is the explanatory factor or thought to be the cause. A dependent variable is one whose value is the outcome in the study or the response or is thought to be the effect. Step 2 is to determine the measurement scale of the variable: categorical (nominal), ordinal (ranked), or continuous (interval) numeric (the definitions of these terms were provided earlier). Step 3 is to determine whether the study observations are independent of each other.

In the design of a clinical study, one must determine whether the groups to be compared are **independent** or **paired.** Samples in which the values of one group cannot be predicted from the values of the other group are said to consist of independent groups. In other words, the patient group and the control group represent different individuals, rather than the same individual measured at two different times. With paired (matched) groups, the values of one group may be predicted from values of the other. In a paired experiment, a patient may be measured before and after therapy, in which case the patient acts as her or his own control, or a patient may be paired with another individual who has been matched with respect to all of the independent variables (e.g., age, duration of disease) that may affect the dependent variable (response). In animal studies, in which genetically identical animals are frequently used in research, paired experiments are the rule. In human clinical studies, it is rare that two groups can be matched for all of the independent variables that may influence the outcome

TABLE 6-5 Summary of Statistical Tests

NUMBER OF DEPENTENT VARIABLES	NUMBER OF INDEPENTENT VARIABLES	TYPE OF DEPENTENT VARIABLE(S)	TYPE OF INDEPENTENT VARIABLE(S)	MEASURE	TEST(S)
1	0 (1 sample)	Continuous normal Continuous nonnormal Categorical	Not applicable (none)	Mean Median Proportions	One-sample t test One-sample median Chi-square goodness-of-fit, binomial test
	1 (2 independent samples)	Normal Nonnormal Categorical	2 categories	Mean Medians Proportions	2 independent sample t test Mann Whitney, Wilcoxon rank sum test Chi-square test Fisher's Exact test
	0 (1 sample measured twice) or 1 (2 matched samples)	Normal Nonnormal Categorical	Nonapplicable/categorical	Means Medians Proportions	Paired t test Wilcoxon signed rank test McNemar, chi-square test
	1 (3 or more populations)	Normal Nonnormal Categorical	Categorical	Means Medians Proportions	One-way ANOVA Kruskal Wallis Chi-square test
	2 or more (e.g., 2-way ANOVA)	Normal Nonnormal Categorical	Categorical	Means Medians Proportions	Factorial ANOVA Friedman test Log-linear, logistic regression
	0 (1 sample measured 3 or more times)	Normal	Not applicable	Means	Repeated measures ANOVA
	1	Normal Nonnormal Categorical	Continuous Categorical or continuous Continuous		Correlation simple linear regression Nonparametric correlation Logistic regression Discriminant analysis
	2 or more	Normal Nonnormal Categorical Normal Nonnormal Categorical	Continuous Mixed categorical and continuous		Multiple linear regression Logistic regression Analysis of covariance general linear models, general estimation equations (regression) Logistic regression
2	2 or more	Normal	Categorical		MANOVA
2 or more	2 or more	Normal	Continuous		Multivariate multiple linear regression
2 sets of 2 more	0	Normal	Not applicable		Canonical correlation
2 or more	0	Normal	Not applicable		Factor analysis

variable. An investigator may wish to match the groups as closely as possible, to eliminate bias but still treat the groups as if they were independent, improving the overall quality of the experimental design as described earlier.

The nature and distribution of the values of the variables also determine whether **parametric** or **nonparametric tests** can be used. The use of a parametric test is based on certain assumptions. The major assumption is that the variable of interest follows a *normal distribution*. It may be possible to transform variables that are not normally distributed. This technique expresses the values of observations on another scale, such as a natural log scale. This may allow the use of parametric statistical tests when the actual values obtained in the study do not follow a normal distribution. Another alternative is

to use a nonparametric test. Nonparametric methods are based on weaker assumptions in that they do not assume a normal distribution or equality of variance between the different groups. There are nonparametric procedures for most statistical needs, but because they are not based on the assumption of normality, nonparametric tests provide more conservative estimates of differences between groups than their parametric counterparts.

Types of Statistical Error and P Values

A *type I error* is the probability of rejecting a null hypothesis when it is true—that is, concluding that there is a difference when there is none. The probability of committing a type I error is abbreviated as α (alpha error) and set by the investigator at a specific level; by

TABLE 6-6 **Outcome of Study**		
TRUE SITUATION	ACCEPT H_0	REJECT H_0
H_0	Correct	Type I error
H_a	Type II error	Correct

H_0, Null hypothesis; H_a, alternative hypothesis.

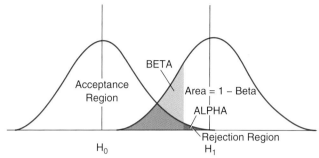

FIGURE 6-6 Theoretical visual representation of acceptance and rejection regions, alpha (α) and beta (β) error regions, and power. There are four possibilities when one compares the means (or other summary descriptors of a distribution of values) of two (or more) populations or samples. (1) One may correctly conclude that there is no difference between the two means (i.e., correctly accept, or fail to reject, the null hypothesis [H_0] of no difference). In this case, the mean of the treated group would fall within the distribution on the left anywhere in the acceptance region *(white)*, but not in the rejection region *(dark red)*, and also not in the stippled region (β). This implies that the second mean arose from a population having the same underlying mean as the population that gave rise to the first mean, and the experimenter correctly recognized this situation. (2) One may correctly conclude that there is a difference between the two means (i.e., correctly reject H_0 in favor of the alternative hypothesis [H_1] that there is a difference between the two means). In this case, the mean of the treated group would fall within the rejection region *(dark red)*, or farther to the right. This implies that the second mean arose from a population with a different underlying mean from that of the population that gave rise to the first mean, and the experimenter correctly recognized this fact. (3) The investigator may incorrectly conclude that there is a difference between the two means when there is not a difference (i.e., incorrectly reject H_0 in favor of H_1 when it should not be rejected). In this case, the value of the second mean happened to fall into the rejection, or α region, even though it arose from the same population as the first mean. This is known as a type I error, and its probability of occurrence is based on the α error level set by the experimenter (typically set at 0.05). This determines the area of the rejection region. (4) The investigator may incorrectly conclude that there is no difference between two means when there is a difference (i.e., incorrectly accept, or fail to reject, H_0 when it is actually false). In this case, the second mean fell somewhere in the β region, leading the experimenter to believe, incorrectly, that the second mean came from the same population that gave rise to the first mean. This is known as a type II error, and its probability of occurrence is based on where the experimenter sets the power (1 – β error level) of a test (typically set at 0.8 or 0.9). Power determines the size of the β area on the graph and is usually heavily dependent on sample size.

convention, this is typically equal to 0.05. The *P* value is the calculated type I error level based on the data; it is defined as the likelihood that a difference at least as large as the observed difference could have occurred by chance alone. It is analogous to a false-positive result in diagnostic tests (discussed earlier). *P* values that are larger than the predefined type I error are called *not statistically significant*; values at or below the preset type I error are called *statistically significant.*

The debate about when and how to adjust *P* values to deal with the issue of multiplicity, or multiple hypothesis testing, seems far from resolved; a spirited debate continues, particularly in new technologies, such as microarray data.[71,72] When one is conducting exploratory studies not aimed at establishing definite cause-effect relationships, *P* values need not be corrected for fear of missing a possible true association or difference. False-positive results can be discarded later in confirmatory, pivotal studies. In confirmatory studies aimed at adding pivotal evidence to a cause-effect relationship, there is no need to correct the *P* value for the main test of hypothesis (i.e., that on which sample size was based). Results of secondary, exploratory hypotheses should present uncorrected and corrected *P* values, however. An alternative to correcting the *P* value is to set α lower (e.g., at 0.01 instead of 0.05) in anticipation of conducting multiple hypothesis testing. There are numerous techniques for correcting *P* values for multiple comparisons; the most widely used is the *Bonferroni correction.* To adjust a *P* value using the Bonferroni correction, the *P* value obtained is multiplied by the number of statistical tests. A *P* value of 0.05 obtained in a series of 10 tests of hypotheses becomes 0.05 × 10, or 0.5. Alternatively, when the experiment is designed, the α error level can be divided by the number of anticipated tests (in the example, 0.05 ÷ 10 = 0.005), with values of *P* value greater than this level referred to as *nonsignificant.*

A *type II error* is the probability of failing to reject a false null hypothesis in favor of the alternative hypothesis—that is, concluding that there is no difference when there is a difference. It is commonly abbreviated as β (beta error) and is equivalent to the false-negative rate. Table 6-6 summarizes the types of decision errors, illustrating the concepts of the null hypothesis and α and β errors.

Traditionally, type I error levels are set lower than type II error levels (e.g., 0.05 for type I and 0.2 for type II). In other words, the experimenter is more willing to make a type II error than a type I error. The conventional rationale for this approach is that type I errors are more serious because they can result in the abandonment of an established, beneficial therapy in favor of a new therapy when no such change is warranted.

Power, the ability of a statistical test to identify a true difference if one exists, is expressed mathematically as (1 – β). It is a consideration in the design of an experiment because the power of the test is affected by the sample size. The distribution of the test statistic is divided into two areas: acceptance and rejection. These concepts are graphically shown in Fig. 6-6. If the null hypothesis is rejected, one concludes that the evidence supports a significant difference between the groups. If the null hypothesis is not rejected, one concludes that there is no such difference. The lower the *P* value, the higher the level of significance.

Sample Size

The estimation of sample size requires statistical skill and knowledge of the underlying basic assumptions being made by the investigator. It involves some guesswork, and the resulting calculation may not always yield the correct sample size needed to answer a specific question. This problem occurs when the investigator's assumptions do not hold true for the sample that is actually enrolled in the study. Sample size should always be calculated during the development of the clinical investigative protocol.

Sample size is most frequently calculated with the use of computer programs, based on specific assumptions including an estimate of the magnitude of effect (i.e., how much difference can one expect between a control group and a treated group in terms of the primary outcome), the desired type I (α) error level (usually 0.05), and the type II (β) error level (i.e., 1 – power) (usually 0.1 or 0.2).

The *effect size* is the deviation from the null that the investigator wishes to be able to detect. The effect size should be clinically meaningful. It may be based on the results of prior or pilot studies. For example, a study might be powered to be able to detect a relative risk of 2 or greater.

Sometimes a standardized effect size is given (i.e., the effect size divided by the standard deviation). This is a unitless value. If power is calculated in this manner, the standardized effect size is usually between 0.1 and 0.5, with 0.5 meaning the alternative hypothesis (H_1) is 0.5 standard deviation away from the null hypothesis (H_0).

To calculate the sample size needed for a parametric test, such as the *t* test, one must also estimate the variance in the variable of interest. The variance estimate may come from published data or from a pilot study that was designed to assess preliminarily the question under consideration.

Because many sample size calculations result in the requirement of an unrealistic number of patients, the statistician is often asked to find ways to decrease the number of patients needed. Besides increasing the tolerated type I and/or type II error of the experiment, the most common approaches are improving the precision of the measurements of the outcome variable, using better equipment, and repeatedly measuring the outcome.

Post Hoc Power Analysis

In the event that an investigation yields nonsignificant differences between groups, the concern is that the investigator has committed a type II error. One option to address this situation is the calculation of the sample size that would be necessary to find the observed difference statistically significant. Another option is the calculation of the size of the difference one could detect as statistically significant with sufficient power (e.g., 80%), given the sample size and variance obtained in the study; this is termed the ***minimum detectable difference.*** If the minimum detectable difference is much larger than would be considered clinically significant, the investigator may conclude that the investigation did not include a sufficient number of patients to detect a clinically meaningful difference as statistically significant. If the minimum detectable difference is smaller than the difference that is considered clinically important, the test was adequately powered, and the investigator may conclude that there is no important difference between the samples.

Confidence Intervals (Limits) on Statistical Tests of Inference

Confidence intervals are frequently calculated around the estimates from statistical hypothesis tests. They may be calculated for the *t* test, chi-square test, analysis of variance, regression, and most other tests of inference. A 95% CI is a range of values within which 95% of the results of repeated samples from the overall population would lie; this is the most frequently reported CI level. The confidence limits are related to the *P* value. If one calculates the 95% CI of the difference in means between two samples, and zero is within the range of the 95% CI, then the *P* value will not be significant at the level less than 0.05.

Statistical Versus Clinical Versus Biological Significance

An important concept that is frequently overlooked is that a statistically significant difference may not indicate clinical significance. Particularly if the sample size is large, many statistical tests may result in *P* values that are less than 0.05 when there is a relatively small degree of clinically significant difference between the two groups. For example, a difference of 1 mm Hg in systolic blood pressure is unlikely to be clinically significant but could be found to be statistically significant given a sufficiently large sample size.

One-Sample Tests

Statistical hypothesis testing may be completed on studies involving one or more groups. The most frequent approach to analyzing data from a clinical investigation that involves only one group is to compare that group with a known population or expected value.

Binomial Test of Proportions

Perhaps the most frequently used test for comparing one sample with a known population is the binomial test. This test asks the question, "What is the probability of *x* number of successes in *N* independent trials, given that the probability of success on any one trial is *y*?" The binomial test has limited applicability in describing the statistical probability that a therapy is beneficial because the odds of success typically are unknown. In pediatric rheumatology, the question may be, "What is the probability that 50 patients with JIA treated with methotrexate will experience improvement as determined by a given index or measure?" The problem is that one is typically unsure of the exact probability of a success in a single-arm independent trial. In some situations, the probability of success is arbitrarily given the value of 0.5 (i.e., 50% chance), and the binomial test is done either to confirm or to fail to confirm that level of probability of success.

Goodness-of-Fit Chi-Square Test

The goodness-of-fit chi-square test is related to the Pearson chi-square test (which is discussed later in the chapter), in which observed proportions are compared with expected values. The goodness-of-fit chi-square test can be used to test the significance of a single proportion or the significance of a theoretical model, such as the mode of inheritance of a gene. A reference population is often used to obtain the expected values. Suppose the frequency of an allele that is thought to produce risk for polyarticular JIA is known to be 2 in 100 in the general population. The observed frequency of the allele in a sample of patients with polyarticular JIA is found to be 10 in 100, however. To assess whether this much deviation from the expected value is significant, the goodness-of-fit chi-square test can be used.

One-Sample *t* Test

When a statistical inference is desired on a single mean, the one-sample *t* test may be used. The test is similar to the Student *t* test for comparing two means, described later. If one wishes to determine whether the mean height of 9- to 10-year-old girls with SLE is significantly less than that of the general population of 9- to 10-year-old girls, a one-sample *t* test would be appropriate.

Two-Sample Tests

The two-sample test to be used is determined by the level of the data and by certain other assumptions, as defined later.

Chi-Square Test with One Degree of Freedom

For categorical (nominal) data and ordinal data with very few ranks, the most frequently used hypothesis test is the Pearson chi-square (χ^2) test. This nonparametric statistical test of inference is for assessing the association between the two variables. It is most commonly performed on contingency tables such as a 2×2 cross-tabulation, which has one degree of freedom (1 df). The significance of the resulting chi-square statistic is determined from a table of critical values.

Most tables of critical values report two-tailed probabilities; the *P* value is divided by 2 to find the one-tailed probabilities. Chi-square analysis with greater than 1 df (i.e., tables larger than 2×2) requires larger values to be significant; the *Yates continuity correction* is used to compensate for deviations from the theoretical (smooth) probability distribution if the total N assessed in the contingency tables is less than 40.

Fisher Exact Test

The Fisher exact test is used as a replacement for the chi-square test when the expected frequency of one or more cells is less than 5. This test is commonly used in studies in which one or more events are rare.

McNemar Test

The chi-square test assumes independence of the cells, as noted earlier. Experimental designs exist for observing categorical outcomes more than once in the same patient. The McNemar test (also known as the *paired* or *matched chi-square*) provides a way of testing the hypotheses in such designs. An example for the use of this statistic may be to test two different concentrations of an analgesic lotion that are given to 51 patients in sequence. The null hypothesis is that the proportion of patients who experience relief when they apply analgesic lotion 1 is the same as the proportion of patients who experience relief when they apply lotion 2. Alternatively, the McNemar test would be used when comparing the effects of the two analgesic lotions in two groups of patients that are matched for independent variables that may influence the dependent variable (i.e., the proportion of patients with pain relief).

Mantel-Haenszel Chi-Square Test

The Mantel-Haenszel chi-square test is known as a stratified chi-square test and is frequently used to detect confounding variables. The procedure involves breaking the contingency table into various strata and then calculating an overall relative risk, with the results from each stratum being weighted by the sample size of the stratum.

Common Errors with Chi-Square Tests

Perhaps because of its frequent use, the chi-square test is often employed or interpreted inappropriately. Common mistakes include unnecessary conversion of continuous or ordinal level data to categorical data to use the chi-square test, nonindependence of the cells in the table (an exception is when the McNemar chi-square test is used); use of the chi-square rather than Fisher exact test when expected cell frequencies are lower than 5; and confusion of statistical significance by chi-square values with clinical or biological importance.

Student *t* Test

What the chi-square test is to categorical data, the *t* test is to continuous data. This test is used for comparing two sample means from either independent or matched samples. The matched *t* test is more efficient (i.e., more powerful) than the Student *t* test for independent groups.

Nonparametric Tests

The *t* tests described earlier are parametric tests. That is, they make assumptions about the underlying distributions, including normality and equality of variances between groups. The *t* test is a very robust test; it is still valid even if its assumptions are substantially violated. If the violations are severe, the investigator may transform the data using either natural logarithms (described earlier) or nonparametric tests. Nonparametric tests ignore the magnitude of differences between values taken on by the variables and work with ranks; no assumptions are made about the distribution of the data. For two-group comparisons, either the Mann-Whitney U test (also known as the *Wilcoxon rank sum test*) is used for independent data or the Wilcoxon signed rank test is used for paired data.

K-Sample Tests

Clinical investigations involving more than two samples (groups) require that modifications be made to the analysis plan to accommodate the need for multiple comparisons.

Chi-Square Test with More Than One Degree of Freedom

When categorical data are analyzed, there may be more than two categories for one or both variables (i.e., the table may be larger than 2×2). If the chi-square test statistic is found to be significant in a table larger than 2×2, it is frequently difficult to determine which proportions were different. One must attempt either to collapse the number of cells in the table or break the table up into several smaller tables. The degrees of freedom of contingency tables larger than 2×2 are equal to the number of rows minus 1 plus the number of columns minus 1.

Analysis of Variance

The use of repeated *t* tests to detect differences among more than two means is considered unacceptable because the resulting P value does not accurately describe the chance one has taken of committing a type I error.

The ***one-way analysis of variance (ANOVA)*** is used for the purpose of comparing more than two sample means. ANOVA divides the total variance among all subjects into two portions: the amount of variance that is a result of the difference between the groups of subjects, and the amount of variance that results from differences within each group. The ratio of the amount between and the amount within each group is known as the **F ratio.** The corresponding test of significance is known as the *F test*. If statistical significance is achieved, the investigator must go one step further. The significance may have arisen because just two means were different from one another, or perhaps all the means were different from one another. To determine exactly which means were different, tests must accommodate the fact that multiple comparisons are being made. This is determined by applying a multiple comparison. Commonly used multiple comparison tests include Tukey honest significant difference test, the Newman-Keuls test, Scheffé multiple contrasts test, and, if one wishes to make multiple comparisons to only one group, the Dunnett test.

ANOVA procedures have an additional capability that can increase the efficiency of analyses when one wishes to compare the influence of two or more independent variables on one dependent variable simultaneously. Suppose one wished to test the effects of methotrexate and a physical therapy program on the disease status of a group of patients with polyarticular JIA. One could carry out two separate studies, conduct *t* tests for treatment effects on the methotrexate-treated patients and the physical therapy–treated patients, and compare each with placebo or no physical therapy. This approach requires substantial numbers of patients to meet sample-size requirements for each study.

A ***two-way ANOVA*** factorial design could make much more efficient use of the available subjects, however, and provide information about the interaction (effect modification) between methotrexate and physical therapy. In this situation, patients could be randomly assigned to both treatments, yielding four groups (methotrexate alone, physical therapy alone, methotrexate and physical therapy, and neither methotrexate nor physical therapy). In addition to providing information about the effect of each treatment alone (i.e., the two main effects), a two-way ANOVA factorial design examines the effect of the interaction between the two treatments. ANOVA techniques can be extended to three-way, four-way, and beyond, provided the sample size is large enough.

Repeated measures ANOVA tests the equality of means among various groups when all subjects are measured for the dependent variable under numerous conditions or levels of the independent variables. Use of the standard ANOVA is inappropriate because it does not account for the correlation between repeated measures of the same variable. It is used frequently in longitudinal research when subjects are measured repeatedly in regard to some outcome.

ANOVA procedures discussed to this point are parametric tests and, as such, make various assumptions about the underlying distribution. If these assumptions are substantially violated, the nonparametric equivalent of ANOVA, the **Kruskal-Wallis test,** can be used. This test is subject to the same sample-size limitations as the chi-square test. If the sample size in any group is less than 5, one must use the Fisher exact test and exact probabilities, as described earlier.

Correlations and Analyses of Association

One of the most important measures of statistical correlation is the **Pearson product-moment correlation.** This statistic is appropriate for estimating the relationship between two variables, x and y, both of which are measured along a continuous scale. Correlation is a two-way model that does not require assumptions of causality. The correlation (r) can range between -1 and $+1$. The magnitude of the correlation shows the strength of the relationship between the two variables. The larger the absolute value of the correlation coefficient, the more strongly associated are x and y. In the extreme, where $r = +1$ or -1, all the data values fall perfectly on a straight line. The sign of the correlation indicates the direction of the relationship. A positive sign means that the two variables are directly related (i.e., they tend to increase or decrease together). A negative sign for r indicates that the two variables are inversely related (i.e., the value of one tends to decrease as that of the other increases). Correlation assumes that the joint distribution of x and y is bivariate normal; that is, their joint probability distribution must be normal. If this assumption is violated substantially, the nonparametric **Spearman rank correlation,** which yields a Spearman rho (r_s), is used. Because Spearman rank correlation deals with ranks, it can be used with continuous variables that violate assumptions and with ordinal data.

Pearson and Spearman correlation coefficients can be interpreted as follows: Variables are unrelated if the r (or r_s) is less than 0.2; values between 0.2 and 0.4 represent weak correlations; and values between 0.41 and 0.6 represent moderate correlations. Coefficients larger than 0.8 constitute strong correlations between the x and y variables tested.

Regression Analysis

Regression analysis is a one-way model in which predictor or explanatory independent (x) variables are thought to affect the dependent outcome (y) variables, but not vice versa. In simple regression models (i.e., models that include only a single predictor), and in multiple regression models, the direction of the effects must be prespecified. The simple linear regression equation is $y = a + bx$, where a is the intercept and b is the beta coefficient (or slope). By using various values of x in the equation, the predicted value of y for a given x can be determined. Simple regression models serve as building blocks for the larger, more complex, and more realistic models, including polynomial regression models and structural equation models.

In **multiple linear regression,** a multitude of independent variables (e.g., x_1, x_2, x_3) can be simultaneously investigated for their influence on a continuous dependent variable (y). The method models the dependent variable as a linear function of all the (k) independent variables.

This method is particularly helpful in evaluating additional variables as possible confounders of the linear relationship between two continuous variables. In other words, linear regression permits the investigator to assess the separate unconfounded effects of several independent variables on a single dependent variable. The x_i terms can be continuous or categorical variables. The b_i (beta coefficients) terms are the regression coefficients. Each b_i is "corrected" simultaneously for the linear relationship between its associated x_i and all the other x_i's and for the linear relationship between the other x_i's and y. In addition to the beta coefficients that estimate the associations between the dependent variable and each independent variable, an overall r^2 value is calculated for the model. It represents the percentage of the total variance of y that is accounted for by the linear relationship with all the x_i's.

A common mistake is to refer to multiple linear regression as a multivariate technique; technically it is not because it deals with multiple independent variables, rather than multiple dependent variables.

Multiple logistic regression is distinguished from multiple linear regression in that the outcome variable (dependent variable) is dichotomous (e.g., diseased or not diseased). Its aim is the same as that of all model-building techniques: to derive the best-fitting, most parsimonious (smallest or most efficient), and biologically reasonable model to describe the relationship between an outcome and a set of predictors. Here, the independent variables are called *covariates.* Importantly, in multiple logistic regression, the predictor variables may be of any data level (categorical, ordinal, or continuous). A major use of this technique is to examine a series of predictor variables to determine those that best predict a certain outcome.

Multiple logistic regression is also very useful to identify potential confounders. A confounder can be defined as a variable that, when added to the regression model, changes the estimate of the association between the main independent variable of interest (exposure) and the dependent variable (outcome) by 10% or more.

A pediatric rheumatology example of the use of this technique can be found in the article by Ruperto and associates,[7] in which predictor variables that are measurable during the very early stages of JIA (e.g., number of active joints during the first 6 months of illness, erythrocyte sedimentation rate [ESR]) were tested to determine their relative predictive ability for either a favorable or a less favorable outcome (i.e., a dichotomous dependent variable) at least 5 years later.

Analysis of Covariance

Analysis of covariance (ANCOVA) combines the principles of ANOVA with the principles of regression. A chief advantage of this technique is that, in contrast to ANOVA, the independent variables can be of any data level. ANCOVA is often used to adjust for initial (baseline) differences between or among groups. In other words, one of its chief purposes is to eliminate systematic bias. Suppose two groups of patients had unequal numbers of swollen joints at baseline (even though the study may have been randomized). The initial number of swollen joints is used as the covariate. ANCOVA adjusts the posttreatment means of the groups to what they would have been if all groups had started out equally on the covariate.

The other purpose of ANCOVA is to reduce the within-group (or error) variances, making the test more efficient (powerful). Suppose a clinical trial investigates the effect on the ESR of a biological agent and an active comparator. Subjects are randomly assigned to receive one or the other treatment, and the change in ESR is observed. Within each treatment group, there is considerable variation in ESR, reflecting individual differences among patients in the degree of active inflammation. In other words, ESR and active inflammation are covarying (covariates). If one could statistically remove this part of the within-group variability by allowing the degree of inflammation to be the covariate in the analysis, a smaller error term would result, and the test would gain power. ANCOVA provides a method to do this.

Survival Analysis

Survival (life table) analysis was developed primarily for the study of how long a particular cohort of subjects survives. The term *survival* is now used in a broader sense for data that involve time to a certain event, such as time to failure of a drug or time to achieve disease remission.[73] There are two basic types of life table analysis: the fixed-interval (actuarial) model and the Kaplan-Meier survival analysis. The latter is used much more frequently in medicine than the former. In **actuarial analysis,** the lengths of each interval shown on the *x* axis all are equal (e.g., 1 year). This is the technique used by life insurance companies to estimate the probability of a person's surviving to a certain age. In the **Kaplan-Meier analysis,** the end of an interval is demarcated by an event. The horizontal components of the lines are unequal, as they are in the actuarial technique. An example of the actuarial method in pediatric rheumatology can be found in a study by Giannini and colleagues[74] of the time to occurrence of eye disease among patients with certain major histocompatibility complex alleles. An example of the Kaplan-Meier approach can be found in the study by Lovell and associates,[48] in which time to failure in subjects given placebo was compared with time to failure in subjects given etanercept. Methods exist for comparing the difference of the life table graphs; the most frequently used is the generalized Wilcoxon test. Figure 6-7 is a graphic representation of a comparison between the characteristic lines of an actuarial model and a Kaplan-Meier analysis. Lee and Wang[75] provide an outstanding reference for survival analysis techniques.

Time-to-event analyses can be performed using regression modeling to adjust for variables of interest. The most commonly used method in clinical epidemiology is the Cox proportional hazards model, which estimates the association of exposure and outcome in terms of a *hazard ratio*. Cox models assume that the relative hazard associated with the exposure is constant over time and thus may not always be the most appropriate choice for analysis.

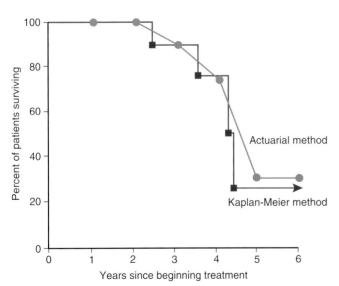

FIGURE 6-7 Comparison of the Kaplan-Meier and actuarial survival curves, showing a theoretical example of the percentage of patients surviving after 0 to 6 years of treatment. (Modified from M.S. Kramer, Clinical Epidemiology and Biostatistics: A Primer for Clinical Investigators and Decision-Makers, Springer-Verlag, Berlin, 1988.)

Measures of Agreement Among and Within Raters

It is often necessary to express in statistical terms how well various raters agree with one another (interrater agreement) or with themselves (intrarater agreement). These are commonly referred to as *measures of reliability* or *reproducibility*. Lack of agreement, either among or within raters, indicates that the values for the measure are nonreliable or nonreproducible. This has dire consequences for the interpretation of the results and for statistical interpretation. Various tests exist for expressing the degree of agreement between and within raters.

The most frequently used test to express rater agreement when the outcome is dichotomous is the **kappa test ratio** (known also as the Cohen kappa, or κ). The κ scores range between 0 and 1 and are often expressed as percentages: less than 20% is considered negligible agreement; 20% to 40%, minimal; 40% to 60%, fair; 60% to 80%, good; and greater than 80%, excellent. Data with three or more categories (i.e., ordinal data) require the use of the more complex weighted kappa test; *Kendall W* or *coefficient of concordance* can also be used. W values range from 0, which indicates poor agreement, to +1, which indicates perfect agreement among all raters.

If more than two raters are to be compared for reliability in numeric outcomes, the **intraclass correlation coefficients (ICCs)** are more appropriate than conducting repeated two-way comparisons between pairs of raters (there is a correction for correlation between raters that becomes apparent when the range of measurement is large). The ICC evaluates the level of agreement among all raters, and the measures (scores) must be parametric in nature. The ICC represents the amount of agreement with an ICC of 1 representing perfect agreement, and an ICC of 0 being no agreement. Conversely, ANOVA on the matrix produces an F value (described previously) and tells the investigator whether the raters are significantly different from one another.[76]

Multivariate Analyses

Multivariate analysis deals with the statistical analysis of data collected on more than one dependent variable. These variables may be correlated with each other, and their statistical dependence is often taken into account when analyzing such data. This consideration of statistical dependence makes multivariate analysis different in approach and considerably more complex than the corresponding univariate analysis, when there is only one response variable under consideration. Interested readers are referred to the text by Stevens for in-depth discussions of the concepts and tests involved.[77]

The response variables considered are often described as *random variables,* and because their dependence is one of the things to be accounted for in the analyses, these response variables are often described by their joint probability distribution. Multivariate normal distribution is one of the most frequently made distributional assumptions for the analysis of multivariate data. If possible, any such consideration should ideally be dictated by the particular context. Also in many cases, such as when the data are collected on a nominal or ordinal scale, multivariate normality may not be an appropriate or even viable assumption. In the real world, most data collection schemes or designed experiments result in multivariate data. A rule of thumb is that there should be at least 10 subjects for each dependent variable investigated in the study. A study in which the subject/variable ratio is smaller is likely to be unreliable.

Classification Tree Analysis

The **classification and regression tree (CART)** is a method of data mining. In these tree structures, CART is related to discriminant analysis. The tree end points represent classifications, and branches represent conjunctions of features that lead to the classifications. CART trees need to be discriminated from decision analysis trees constructed to help with making decisions. CART allows for recursive partitioning iteratively and selects variables that split the sample into progressively purer groups. It has a theoretical advantage over techniques such as logistic regression, in that the structure of the classes in relation to the predictor variables is not assumed—that is, different combinations of the predictor variables may identify subgroups. An example for the use of CART analysis may be the attempted development of new classification criteria for psoriatic arthritis.[78]

Factor Analysis

Factor analysis is used for data exploration to reveal patterns of interrelationships among variables that are not readily apparent, for confirmation of hypotheses, and for reducing the number of variables to a manageable level. In situations involving many different observations concerning the same patient or groups of patients, factor analysis can be used to determine whether it is possible that some of these observations are a result of just a few underlying factors. That is, the correlation among many dependent variables may be explained by some underlying factor or factors.

When groups of patients are studied, the symptoms tend to "load" on the underlying factors differentially. Factor loading is expressed in a factor-loading matrix, in which each row of the matrix is a variable, and each column is a factor. Such a matrix examines how highly each variable correlates with, or loads on, each factor. Each variable may load onto one or more variable. Next, one must decide which factors are most important to keep and which can be discarded as not contributing enough to the explanation of the variables. This is done by calculating an *eigenvalue,* which is the amount of variance in the data that is explained by a particular factor. The procedure to this point is called *principal component analysis.* Additional steps in factor analysis include rotation of axes to determine which are general factors (most variables load significantly on the axes) and which are bipolar factors (some variables load positively and some load negatively on the axes). Factorial complexity is determined by observing how many variables load significantly onto two or more factors.

Item Response Theory and Rasch Analysis

Item response theory (IRT), also known as *latent trait theory,* is used for statistical analysis and the development of outcome measures. Among other things, the purpose of IRT is to provide a framework for evaluating how well questionnaires or outcome measures work and how well individual questions that are part of the questionnaire work. A special type of IRT is the so-called *Rasch analysis,* which has been used in recent years to assess the usefulness of common rheumatology outcome measures.[79-81] Questionnaires or outcome measures developed by and adhering to IRT or Rasch principles function like a common ruler and can be used to describe accurately within-patient and between-patient differences and change over time.

JUDGING THE QUALITY OF A REPORT CLINICAL INVESTIGATION

The most helpful and up-to-date series of guides to the reader of clinical reports was published in the *Journal of the American Medical Association.* These "Users' Guides to the Medical Literature" were subsequently published in book form and provide logical checklists of questions for readers attempting to weigh the evidence from many different types of clinical studies.[38] Although the Users' Guides contain information for judging clinical trials, more detailed guides are available.

In 1995, a group of medical journal editors, clinical epidemiologists, and statisticians developed a consensus statement about how randomized controlled trials should be reported—the Consolidated Standards of Reporting Trials (CONSORT) Statement. The CONSORT Statement comprises a 25-item checklist and a flow diagram, along with some brief descriptive text. The checklist items focus on reporting how the trial was designed, analyzed, and interpreted; the flow diagram displays the progress of all participants through the trial.

Considered an evolving document, the CONSORT Statement is subject to periodic changes as new evidence emerges. The current CONSORT Statement and up-to-date information on extensions to the CONSORT Statement to provide guidance on the reporting of specific trials and patient reported outcomes is provided at http://www.consort-statement.org/.

STROBE is an international collaboration aimed at STrengthening the Reporting of OBservational studies in Epidemiology (http://www.strobe-statement.org/). STROBE provides guidance in form of checklists on how to report observational research well with focus on cohort, case-control, and cross-sectional studies.

REFERENCES

1. D.L. Sackett, Evidence-based medicine and treatment choices, Lancet 349 (1997) 570, author reply 572–573.
4. L.E. Moses, Statistical concepts fundamental to investigations, N. Engl. J. Med. 312 (1985) 890–897.
5. O. Arguedas, A. Fasth, B. Andersson-Gare, A prospective population based study on outcome of juvenile chronic arthritis in Costa Rica, J. Rheumatol. 29 (2002) 174–183.
6. B.A. Gare, A. Fasth, The natural history of juvenile chronic arthritis: a population based cohort study. II. Outcome, J. Rheumatol. 22 (1995) 308–319.
7. N. Ruperto, A. Ravelli, J.E. Levinson, et al., Long-term health outcomes and quality of life in American and Italian inception cohorts of patients with juvenile rheumatoid arthritis. II. Early predictors of outcome, J. Rheumatol. 24 (1997) 952–958.
8. K. Murray, S.D. Thompson, D.N. Glass, Pathogenesis of juvenile chronic arthritis: genetic and environmental factors, Arch. Dis. Child. 77 (1997) 530–534.
9. G.N. Glass, DN, Juvenile rheumatoid arthritis as a complex genetic trait, Arthritis Rheum. 42 (1999) 2261–2268.
10. J.N. Jarvis, I. Dozmorov, K. Jiang, et al., Novel approaches to gene expression analysis of active polyarticular juvenile rheumatoid arthritis, Arthritis Res. Ther. 6 (2004) R15–R32.
11. S. Prahalad, M.H. Ryan, E.S. Shear, et al., Juvenile rheumatoid arthritis: linkage to HLA demonstrated by allele sharing in affected sibpairs, Arthritis Rheum. 43 (2000) 2335–2338.
12. A. Savolainen, H. Saila, K. Kotaniemi, et al., Magnitude of the genetic component in juvenile idiopathic arthritis, Ann. Rheum. Dis. 59 (2000) 1001.
13. H.M. Saila, H.A. Savolainen, K.M. Kotaniemi, et al., Juvenile idiopathic arthritis in multicase families, Clin. Exp. Rheumatol. 19 (2001) 218–220.
14. O. Forre, A. Smerdel, Genetic epidemiology of juvenile idiopathic arthritis, Scand. J. Rheumatol. 31 (2002) 123–128.
15. W. Thomson, R. Donn, Juvenile idiopathic arthritis genetics—what's new? What's next?, Arthritis Res. 4 (2002) 302–306.
16. A.D. Askanase, D.J. Wallace, M.H. Weisman, et al., Use of pharmacogenetics, enzymatic phenotyping and metabolite monitoring to guide treatment with azathioprine in patients with systemic lupus erythematosus, J. Rheumat. 36 (2009) 89–95.
17. H.I. Brunner, N.M. Ruth, A. German, et al., Initial validation of the Pediatric Automated Neuropsychological Assessment Metrics for childhood-onset systemic lupus erythematosus, Arthritis Rheum. 57 (2007) 1174–1182.
18. J.B. Harley, M.E. Alarcon-Riquelme, L.A. Criswell, et al., Genome-wide association scan in women with systemic lupus erythematosus identifies

susceptibility variants in ITGAM, PXK, KIAA1542 and other loci, Nat. Genet. 40 (2008) 204–210.

19. A. Bohan, J.B. Peter, Polymyositis and dermatomyositis (second of two parts), N. Engl. J. Med. 292 (1975) 403–407.

20. F. van den Hoogen, D. Khanna, J. Fransen, et al., 2013 classification criteria for systemic sclerosis: an American College of Rheumatology/European League against Rheumatism collaborative initiative, Arthritis Rheum. 65 (2013) 2737–2747.

21. E.H. Giannini, N. Ruperto, A. Ravelli, et al., Preliminary definition of improvement in juvenile arthritis, Arthritis Rheum. 40 (1997) 1202–1209.

22. H.I. Brunner, D.J. Lovell, B.K. Finck, E.H. Giannini, Preliminary definition of disease flare in juvenile rheumatoid arthritis, J. Rheumatol. 29 (2002) 1058–1064.

23. J.C. Wasmuth, B. Grun, B. Terjung, et al., ROC analysis comparison of three assays for the detection of antibodies against double-stranded DNA in serum for the diagnosis of systemic lupus erythematosus, Clin. Chem. 50 (2004) 2169–2171.

24. S. Magni-Manzoni, N. Ruperto, A. Pistorio, et al., Development and validation of a preliminary definition of minimal disease activity in patients with juvenile idiopathic arthritis, Arthritis Rheum. 59 (2008) 1120–1127.

25. C.H. Hinze, M. Suzuki, M. Klein-Gitelman, et al., Neutrophil gelatinase-associated lipocalin is a predictor of the course of global and renal childhood-onset systemic lupus erythematosus disease activity, Arthritis Rheum. 60 (2009) 2772–2781.

28. R.D. Inman, M.E. Johnston, M. Hodge, et al., Postdysenteric reactive arthritis. A clinical and immunogenetic study following an outbreak of salmonellosis, Arthritis Rheum. 31 (1988) 1377–1383.

29. C.A. Peschken, S.J. Katz, E. Silverman, et al., The 1000 Canadian faces of lupus: determinants of disease outcome in a large multiethnic cohort, J. Rheumatol. 36 (2009) 1200–1208.

30. S.T. Angeles-Han, C.F. Pelajo, L.B. Vogler, et al., Risk markers of juvenile idiopathic arthritis-associated uveitis in the Childhood Arthritis and Rheumatology Research Alliance (CARRA) Registry, J. Rheumatol. 40 (2013) 2088–2096.

31. R.E. Gliklich, N.A. Dreyer (Eds.), Registries for Evaluating Patient Outcomes: A User's Guide, second ed., AHRQ Publication No.10-EHC049, Agency for Healthcare Research and Quality, Rockville, MD, 2010.

33. P. Juni, L. Nartey, S. Reichenbach, et al., Risk of cardiovascular events and rofecoxib: cumulative meta-analysis, Lancet 364 (2004) 2021–2029.

35. T. Beukelman, J.P. Guevara, D.A. Albert, Optimal treatment of knee monarthritis in juvenile idiopathic arthritis: a decision analysis, Arthritis Rheum. 59 (2008) 1580–1588.

36. B.L. Strom, S.E. Kimmel, S. Hennessy, Pharmacoepidemiology, fifth ed., John Wiley & Sons, Oxford, UK, 2012.

37. T. Beukelman, F. Xie, L. Chen, et al., Rates of hospitalized bacterial infection associated with juvenile idiopathic arthritis and its treatment, Arthritis Rheum. 64 (2012) 2773–2780.

38. G. Guyatt, Users' Guides to the Medical Literature: Essentials of Evidence-Based Clinical Practice, McGraw-Hill Medical, New York, 2008.

39. J.A. Singh, D.H. Solomon, M. Dougados, et al., Development of classification and response criteria for rheumatic diseases, Arthritis Rheum. 55 (2006) 348–352.

40. H.I. Brunner, A. Ravelli, Developing outcome measures for pediatric rheumatic diseases, Best Pract. Res. Clin. Rheumatol. 23 (2009) 609–624.

43. R. Temple, Current definitions of phases of investigation and the role of the FDA in the conduct of clinical trials, Am. Heart J. 139 (2000) S133–S135.

45. D. Nakagomi, K. Ikeda, A. Okubo, et al., Ultrasound can improve the accuracy of the 2010 American College of Rheumatology/European League against rheumatism classification criteria for rheumatoid arthritis

to predict the requirement for methotrexate treatment, Arthritis Rheum. 65 (2013) 890–898.

48. N. Ruperto, H.I. Brunner, P. Quartier, et al., Two randomized trials of canakinumab in systemic juvenile idiopathic arthritis, N. Engl. J. Med. 367 (2012) 2396–2406.

49. P.J. Hashkes, S.J. Spalding, E.H. Giannini, et al., Rilonacept for colchicine-resistant or -intolerant familial Mediterranean fever: a randomized trial, Ann. Intern. Med. 157 (2012) 533–541.

50. D.J. Lovell, E.H. Giannini, A. Reiff, et al., Etanercept in children with polyarticular juvenile rheumatoid arthritis. Pediatric Rheumatology Collaborative Study Group, N. Engl. J. Med. 342 (2000) 763–769.

51. V.E. Honkanen, A.F. Siegel, J.P. Szalai, et al., A three-stage clinical trial design for rare disorders, Stat. Med. 20 (2001) 3009–3021.

52. N. Duan, R.L. Kravitz, C.H. Schmid, Single-patient (n-of-1) trials: a pragmatic clinical decision methodology for patient-centered comparative effectiveness research, J. Clin. Epidemiol. 66 (2013) S21–S28.

53. D.M. van der Heijde, M. van 't Hof, P.L. van Riel, L.B. van de Putte, Development of a disease activity score based on judgment in clinical practice by rheumatologists, J. Rheumatol. 20 (1993) 579–581.

58. D.T. Felson, J.J. Anderson, M. Boers, et al., American College of Rheumatology. Preliminary definition of improvement in rheumatoid arthritis, Arthritis Rheum. 38 (1995) 727–735.

59. A. Larsen, K. Dale, M. Eek, Radiographic evaluation of rheumatoid arthritis and related conditions by standard reference films, Acta Radiol. Diagn. (Stockh) 18 (1977) 481–491.

60. J.T. Sharp, D.Y. Young, G.B. Bluhm, et al., How many joints in the hands and wrists should be included in a score of radiologic abnormalities used to assess rheumatoid arthritis?, Arthritis Rheum. 28 (1985) 1326–1335.

61. C.A. Wallace, E.H. Giannini, B. Huang, et al., American College of Rheumatology provisional criteria for defining clinical inactive disease in select categories of juvenile idiopathic arthritis, Arthritis Care Res. 63 (2011) 929–936.

63. J.W. Varni, M. Seid, P.S. Kurtin, PedsQL 4.0: reliability and validity of the Pediatric Quality of Life Inventory version 4.0 generic core scales in healthy and patient populations, Med. Care 39 (2001) 800–812.

65. D.G. Kleinbaum, L.L. Kupper, H. Morgenstern, Epidemiologic Research: Principles and Quantitative Methods, Lifetime Learning Publications, Belmont, Calif., 1982.

67. H.I. Brunner, E.D. Silverman, T. To, et al., Risk factors for damage in childhood-onset systemic lupus erythematosus: cumulative disease activity and medication use predict disease damage, Arthritis Rheum. 46 (2002) 436–444.

68. R. Seshadri, B.M. Feldman, N. Ilowite, et al., The role of aggressive corticosteroid therapy in patients with juvenile dermatomyositis: a propensity score analysis, Arthritis Rheum. 59 (2008) 989–995.

69. J.M. Brophy, L. Joseph, Placing trials in context using Bayesian analysis, JAMA 273 (1995) 871–875.

70. B.P. Carlin, T.A. Louis, Bayesian Methods for Data Analysis, third ed., CRC Press, Boca Raton, FL, 2009.

73. N. Ruperto, A. Ravelli, K.J. Murray, et al., Preliminary core sets of measures for disease activity and damage assessment in juvenile systemic lupus erythematosus and juvenile dermatomyositis, Rheumatology (Oxford) 42 (2003) 1452–1459.

74. E.H. Giannini, C.N. Malagon, C. Van Kerckhove, et al., Longitudinal analysis of HLA associated risks for iridocyclitis in juvenile rheumatoid arthritis, J. Rheumatol. 18 (1991) 1394–1397.

75. E.T. Lee, J.W. Wang, Statistical Methods for Survival Data Analysis, J Wiley, New York, 2003.

Entire reference list is available online at www.expertconsult.com.

7 CHAPTER

Assessment of Health Status, Function, and Quality of Life Outcomes

Ciarán M. Duffy, Brian M. Feldman

Pediatric rheumatic diseases influence many, if not all, aspects of a child's life—not only physical, but also social,[1] emotional,[2] educational, and economic.[3] The impact of pediatric rheumatic disease is not only on the child but extends to the entire family.[4] Conversely, the family's functioning can have a significant impact on the outcome of the child's illness.[4] This chapter describes the instruments that have been developed to assess this web of influence in a quantitative fashion and specifically focuses on the measurement of functional status and quality of life (QoL), with an emphasis on measures developed or used for juvenile idiopathic arthritis (JIA). Some brief discussion is included on measures in use for systemic lupus erythematosus (SLE) and juvenile dermatomyositis (JDM). eTable 7-1 presents a glossary of terms pertinent to assessment of outcomes.

BACKGROUND

Why Quality of Life Is Measured

Today, most pediatric rheumatic diseases are not fatal. They affect children and their families by interfering with normal health, however, and they may have an impact on the enjoyment of life. Many of these diseases are not curable; in situations in which there is no cure, it is important to know that treatments, at least, make patients feel better.[5] In the field of rheumatology, QoL has gained wide popularity because it has been shown to measure outcomes that are of direct interest and importance to patients, to provide effective measurements of patient status, to be predictive of patient outcome, and to produce reliable and effective measures of treatment impact.[6-9]

Concepts of Structure and Function, Activity Limitation, Participation Restriction, Health, and Quality of Life

The terms used to describe the consequences of chronic health conditions have been unclear and overlapping.[10] For this reason, the World Health Organization (WHO) developed the International Classification of Functioning and Health (ICF). The ICF provides a common vocabulary for the consequences of disease.[11,12] This work followed from the WHO description of health as a biopsychosocial construct[13] and the definition of QoL as an "individual's perceptions of their position in life in the context of the culture and value systems in which they live and in relation to their goals, expectations, standards and concerns."[14] The ICF framework is particularly applicable to rheumatic diseases.[15-19]

According to the ICF model (Fig. 7-1), a health condition affects an individual in three domains: (1) structures and functions (anatomy and physiology), (2) activities (e.g., activities of daily living), and (3) social participation. Each of these domains affects the others. For example, JIA might lead to muscle atrophy, weakness, cartilage erosion, joint contracture, and pain (structure and function domain). In addition, a child with JIA may not be allowed by his or her parents to run (activities domain) and not be allowed by his or her teacher to participate in school games (participation domain). In this example, joint pain, weakness, and contracture may also limit the ability to run, and this inability to run may be another reason why the child cannot participate in school games.

In the ICF model, each of the domains may be affected by personal factors and by environmental factors. Given the same level of anatomic and physiological damage, one child may be unable to attend school, whereas another more highly motivated child may be trying out for the basketball team. An example of environmental modification is the building of a ramp or other accessibility modifications so that a child who is a wheelchair user would be able to participate in a school dance.

QoL—which had been considered an additional domain in older models of health outcomes[20]—is not defined in the ICF model. It is a term used ubiquitously in daily language and was originally applied by sociologists to try to determine the effect of material affluence on people's lives. This sociological approach was developed in the United States during World War II. The concept broadened so that it eventually included education, social welfare, economics, and industrial growth.[21] This broad societal approach was also incorporated into questionnaires that were developed to assess the status of an individual within this broad framework of concern.

Many of these areas of concern or domains, although important to an individual, are well outside the influence of disease and health care interventions. Also, QoL is considered to be a highly subjective construct, one that can be determined only by an affected individual based on the individual's own goals and expectations[10,22,23] and their personal evaluation of their current situation in many domains of life.[23,24] For this reason, other terminology was developed to describe QoL, e.g., health-related quality of life (HRQoL), life satisfaction, self-esteem, well-being, general health, functional status, and life adjustment.[21]

The earliest published uses of the term HRQoL date from the early 1980s.[25,26] At that time, it was appreciated that medical interventions might only rarely have an impact on overall QoL, and thus HRQoL has been the term used most often to describe this construct. Tools purporting to measure HRQoL mostly measure symptoms (i.e., according to the patient) related to the ICF domains of structure and function, activities, and participation, and value these symptoms according to normative expectations (i.e., the values of groups of individuals rather than one individual).[10,27-29] HRQoL can be defined as patient-reported "perceptions of health."[30]

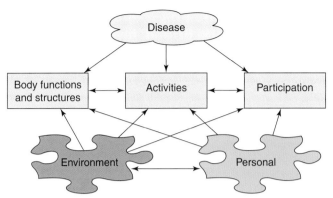

FIGURE 7-1 International Classification of Functioning and Health (ICF).

For the purpose of this chapter, discussion of QoL is mostly restricted to HRQoL. HRQoL is a complex concept that contains numerous subcomponents. Experts differ as to what constitutes HRQoL, and consequently various instruments have been developed to measure it. These instruments may be divided into generic and disease-specific measures.[27] Generic HRQoL measures are measures that purport to be broadly equal across different types and severity of disease, across different medical treatments or health interventions, and across different demographic or cultural subgroups. They are designed to capture aspects of health and disease that cross broad diagnostic categories and social or demographic subgroups. Disease-specific HRQoL measurements are designed to assess specific diseases or patient populations; such instruments are usually more responsive to changes in individual subject status. The past 30 years have seen the development and validation of various instruments to measure the various ICF domains and generic and disease-specific HRQoL. These instruments were first developed in adult rheumatology, but in the past 25 years tools specifically designed to be used in pediatric rheumatic diseases have been developed.

Hierarchy of Outcomes

The ICF framework can be used to structure a hierarchy of outcomes. The first level of outcome assessment is within the domain of structure and function. Most measures of "disease activity" fit in this domain. Disease activity measures include parameters most familiar to clinicians, such as joint counts, morning stiffness, and erythrocyte sedimentation rate. The major drawback to measures in this area is that they are not directly what the patient is interested in. Measures of disease activity are still widely used in clinical trials, however, because inhibition of the disease process or activity is an essential component of an effective therapeutic intervention. At this time, measurement of disease activity is a necessary but insufficient approach to measuring patient outcome. When the performance characteristics of the traditional disease activity measures used in rheumatology were scientifically assessed, many instruments have been found to be unreliable, redundant, insensitive to change, or not correlated with long-term patient outcome.[7] For example, even experienced clinicians often disagree when assessing joint count.[31,32]

The next level up the hierarchy is the measurement of activity and activity limitation and social participation. This domain reflects physical function and disability and social handicaps. The focus here is on measuring the ability of the person to perform physical activities of daily life, such as dressing, walking, climbing stairs, and self-care, and to participate meaningfully in society. This is an area of more relevance to the patient and reflects the view of the WHO that health is a state of physical, mental, and social well-being.[33] Disease-specific HRQoL measures, such as the Health Assessment Questionnaire (HAQ)[7] and the Arthritis Impact Measurement Scale (AIMS),[34] were developed to incorporate the broad WHO concept of health. Despite concerns regarding the ability to measure QoL in children,[35] major advances have been made in the development and validation of disease-specific HRQoL tools for children with rheumatic diseases. These instruments are discussed later.

The highest level in the hierarchy is the measurement of overall QoL. Overall QoL is affected by many life issues and events that do not clearly relate to health.[24] According to the WHO, QoL "reflects the view that quality of life refers to a subjective evaluation, which is embedded in a cultural, social, and environmental context."[36] Because a QoL measure "focuses upon respondents' 'perceived' quality of life, it is not expected to provide a means of measuring in any detailed fashion symptoms, diseases or conditions, nor disability as objectively judged, but rather the perceived effects of disease and health interventions on the individual's quality of life. [It] is, therefore, an assessment of a multi-dimensional concept incorporating the individual's perception of health status, psycho-social status and other aspects of life."[36]

Although overall QoL can be measured,[37] it is unclear how its measurement can contribute to health care. With this in mind, the development of a core set of measures for application in clinical trials in pediatric rheumatic diseases (JIA,[38] SLE,[39-41] and JDM[39,42-44]) has been very influential. These core sets incorporate the types of instruments already alluded to, but focus largely on the measurement of disease activity (Table 7-2).

PROCESS OF INSTRUMENT DEVELOPMENT

The development and validation process for activity limitation assessment or HRQoL instruments has been well established.[45] The development of a new instrument is labor intensive, requires sequential studies, entails input from a wide range of individuals, and needs frequent revisions of the original tool before completion; it may take several years.[46-55] There are several compendia of measuring scales. If one or more existent scales are found in the area of interest, these scales need to be evaluated. If the conclusion is that no existing questionnaire is satisfactory, much work awaits the brave souls who choose to develop a new tool (Table 7-3). The rest of this chapter describes the various tools available in pediatric rheumatology. For a more complete description of these instruments, the reader is referred to the instruments themselves or to published reviews.[9,56,57]

BACKGROUND ON AVAILABLE INSTRUMENTS FOR CHILDHOOD RHEUMATIC DISEASES

As discussed previously, there is an increasing need to incorporate estimates of physical, social, and mental functioning into health assessment, particularly in the assessment of chronic diseases,[10,27,58,59] in an attempt to provide an all-encompassing measure of HRQoL. These aspects have been considered in the development of measurement tools for adult rheumatic diseases[34,60,61] and have been shown to be reliable, valid, and responsive in various conditions.[62-67] They are now believed to be required for inclusion in clinical trials.[68,69]

Since 1986, various groups have attempted to develop the definitive measure for application in JIA. The ideal instrument should be practical and easy to use. It should be capable of completion by the parent or the child within a short time and should measure activity limitation and participation restriction. As suggested by Singsen,[70] the instrument should measure psychological and social function, including school, family, and behavioral issues. It should include a measurement of pain

TABLE 7-2   Core Set Measures and the Definition of Improvement of Disease Activity for Juvenile Idiopathic Arthritis (JIA), Systemic Lupus Erythematosus (SLE), and Juvenile Dermatomyositis (JDM)

JIA	SLE	JDM (PRINTO)	JDM (IMACS)
CORE SET	**CORE SET**	**CORE SET**	**CORE SET**
Physician global assessment	Physician global assessment	Physician global assessment	Physician global assessment
Patient/parent global assessment	Patient/parent global assessment	Patient/parent global assessment	Patient/parent global assessment
Active joint count	Global Disease Activity Tool (ECLAM, SLEDAI, SLAM)	Global Disease Activity (disease activity status)	—
Joints with limited range of motion	—	Muscle strength (manual muscle testing or CMAS)	Muscle strength (manual muscle testing)
Acute phase reactant (ESR or CRP)	Renal involvement (24-hour proteinuria)	Muscle enzymes (CK, LDH, AST, ALT, aldolase)	Muscle enzymes (at least 2 of CK, LDH, AST, ALT, aldolase)
HRQoL or measure of physical function (e.g., CHAQ)	—	Functional ability (e.g., CMAS or CHAQ)	Functional ability (e.g., CMAS or CHAQ)
—	HRQoL (CHQ–Physical Summary Score	—	—
—	—	—	Extramuscular disease
DEFINITION OF IMPROVEMENT	**DEFINITION OF IMPROVEMENT**	**DEFINITION OF IMPROVEMENT**	**DEFINITION OF IMPROVEMENT**
≥30% improvement in 3 of 6 measures with no more than 1 showing >30% worsening	≥50% improvement in 2 of 5 measures with no more than 1 showing >30% worsening	See "Hierarchy of Outcomes" in text	≥20% improvement in 3 of 6 measures with no more than 2 showing ≥20% worsening (muscle strength excluded)

Data from Giannini et al.[38]; Ruperto et al.[39-41,44]; Rider et al.[42,43]
IMACS, International Myositis Assessment and Clinical Studies group; *PRINTO,* Pediatric Rheumatology International Trials Organization.

TABLE 7-3   Comparison of Properties of the Instruments Used for Juvenile Idiopathic Arthritis*

PARAMETER	CHAQ	JAFAR	JASI	JAQQ	CAHP	QOMLQ	CHQ	PEDS QL
Reliability	Strong[†]	Strong	Strong	Strong	Moderate	Strong	Strong	Strong
Validity	Strong	Strong	Strong	Strong	Moderate	Strong	Strong	Strong
Responsiveness	Moderate	Weak	Moderate	Very strong	NA	Strong	Moderate	Strong
Discriminative ability	Moderate	Moderate	Strong	Strong	Moderate	NA	Moderate	Strong
Applicable to a wide range	Very strong	No	No	Very strong	Moderate	Strong	Strong	Very strong
Applicable to a heterogeneous population	Very strong	Strong	No	Very strong	NA	NA	Very strong	Strong
Measures physical function	Moderate	Moderate	Very strong	Strong	Strong	No	Moderate	Moderate
Measures health-related quality of life	No	No	No	Strong	Strong	Strong	Strong	Strong
Measures pain	Moderate	Moderate	No	Strong	No	No	Moderate	Moderate
Tested widely	Very strong	Moderate	No	Strong	No	No	Strong	Strong
Easy to use	Strong	Strong	No	Strong	No	Very strong	Moderate	Strong

*Although most instruments have been developed using patients defined as having juvenile rheumatoid arthritis based on the criteria of the American College of Rheumatology, they are probably equally applicable to patients defined by the International League of Associations for Rheumatology as having juvenile idiopathic arthritis.
[†]*No,* Property absent; *Weak,* property present but weak; *Moderate,* property present and moderately strong; *Strong,* property present and strong; *Very strong,* property present and very strong; *NA,* not applicable.
CAHP, Childhood Arthritis Health Profile; *CHAQ,* Childhood Health Assessment Questionnaire; *CHQ,* Child Health Questionnaire; *JAFAR,* Juvenile Arthritis Functional Assessment Report; *JASI,* Juvenile Arthritis Self-Report Index; *JAQQ,* Juvenile Arthritis Quality of Life Questionnaire; *Peds QL,* Pediatric Quality of Life Inventory; *QoMLQ,* Quality of My Life Questionnaire.

(eBox 7-1). None of the instruments developed to date meets all of these criteria. Each instrument has unique characteristics that make it distinct, however, and each one may have different indications for use. In the following sections, each instrument is discussed with an emphasis on its development, its measurement properties, and the settings in which it might be used.

Most instruments developed to date for childhood rheumatic diseases have their application in JIA (eBox 7-2). Some instruments have been developed or have been modified for use in other pediatric rheumatic diseases such as SLE or JDM. The most relevant measures are discussed here with an emphasis on those applicable to JIA.

INSTRUMENTS FOR JUVENILE IDIOPATHIC ARTHRITIS

Disease-specific measures of functional status developed for JIA include Childhood Arthritis Impact Measurement Scales (CHAIMS),[71] Childhood Health Assessment Questionnaire (CHAQ),[47] Juvenile

Arthritis Functional Assessment Scale (JAFAS) and Report (JAFAR),[48] and Juvenile Arthritis Self-Report Index (JASI).[55,72] Disease-specific measures of HRQoL include Juvenile Arthritis Quality of Life Questionnaire (JAQQ)[50] and Childhood Arthritis Health Profile (CAHP).[51,52] More recently, there has been a greater focus on the use of generic instruments to assess HRQoL in children with JIA. Such measures include the Quality of My Life Questionnaire (QoMLQ),[73] Child Health Questionnaire (CHQ),[74] and Pediatric Quality of Life Inventory (Peds QL)[75] (eBox 7-2). All of these instruments are discussed briefly here, and Table 7-3 summarizes their comparative properties.

Childhood Arthritis Impact Measurement Scales

CHAIMS was the first disease-specific measure developed for JIA.[71] This was a modification of the AIMS.[34] Its measurement properties were poor, however, except for the pain dimension, and, as a result, it has not been used widely.

Childhood Health Assessment Questionnaire

The CHAQ[47] was derived from the adult HAQ.[7,60] It comprises two indices: Disability and Discomfort. The Disability Index assesses function in eight areas distributed among a total of 30 items: (1) dressing and grooming, (2) arising, (3) eating, (4) walking, (5) hygiene, (6) reach, (7) grip, and (8) activities. In each functional area, there is at least one question that is relevant to children of all ages. Each question is rated on a 4-point scale of difficulty in performance, scored from 0 to 3. The Disability Index is calculated as the mean of the eight functional areas. Discomfort is determined by the presence of pain, as measured by a 100-mm visual analog scale (VAS). In the original validation study, mean scores for patients were 0.84 for the Disability Index and 0.82 for the Discomfort Index. Reliability was very good. Convergent validity was also very good, with excellent correlations with Steinbrocker's functional class, active joint count, disease activity index, and degree of morning stiffness. Mean scores for parents and children were not significantly different from one another and were highly correlated, suggesting that parents can reliably report for their children. CHAQ was completed by parents in all cases and by children 8 years and older in a mean of 10 minutes. Responsiveness was established later.[76]

CHAQ has been shown to be a useful instrument for outcome evaluation in longitudinal studies.[77-91] It has also been used in a variety of settings, translated into many different languages and undergone modifications in attempts to improve it while still maintaining excellent reliability, validity, and parent–child correlations.[92-106] Although one study suggested that it had poor responsiveness,[107] good responsiveness has been shown in other studies, including several longitudinal studies of etanercept.[108-112] Several studies have shown its usefulness in the evaluation of rehabilitative interventions.[113-118] Other studies suggest that it is highly predictive of the presence of significant pain,[119,120] and to be highly predictive of short-term outcomes in a large cohort of Canadian children.[121] Scores of 0.13, 0.63, and 1.75 represent mild, mild to moderate, and moderate disability,[122] whereas the minimum clinically important change score (MCID) for improvement is −0.188; for deterioration it is +0.125.[123] A recent study suggests that removal of aids or devices from the scoring does not alter the interpretation of the Disability Index, and thus removal of the aids and devices provides a simplified questionnaire that is a more effective alternative.[124] A digital form developed and validated in a Dutch population was declared to be user friendly.[125]

CHAQ has excellent reliability and validity and reasonable responsiveness. It also has good discriminative properties and can be administered to children of all ages; it is of great use in the clinical setting for long-term follow-up of children with JIA. CHAQ is valuable for longitudinal studies and clinical trials and has become the preferred

measure in both settings. Some attempts have been undertaken to modify it, but the original version is still used in most studies.

Juvenile Arthritis Functional Assessment Scale and Report

JAFAS[26] is an observer-based scale, whereas JAFAR[46] is completed by the patient or parent. Items for both instruments were derived from the AIMS, HAQ, and McMaster Health Index Questionnaire.[127]

JAFAS requires standardized simple equipment and can be administered in about 10 minutes by a health professional who times the child's performance on 10 physical tasks. Good reliability and convergent validity have been shown. JAFAR comprises one dimension and contains 23 items that assess ability to perform physical tasks in children older than 7 years on a 3-point scale scored from 0 to 2; the score range is 0 to 46, with the lower score indicating better function. Two separate versions are available, one for the child (JAFAR-C) and one for the parents (JAFAR-P). Reliability is good for both versions. Construct validity is also good, with predictable correlations among JAFAR-C, JAFAR-P, JAFAS, and pain, and moderate correlations with measures of disease activity. Similar measurement properties were found in an English study.[128] A Dutch translation of JAFAR also showed good measurement properties.[95] Responsiveness was shown in a small trial of intravenous immunoglobulin in polyarticular JIA.[129] JAFAR has also proved to be a useful measure of functional ability in studies on osteopenia[130,131] and sleep disturbance[132] in JIA.

JAFAR has excellent reliability and validity, but limited responsiveness. It cannot be administered to children younger than 7 years, and this prohibits its use in children with early-onset of JIA. Nonetheless, it is a practical instrument that is useful in the clinical setting and in the longitudinal follow-up of most children with JIA.

Juvenile Arthritis Self-Report Index

JASI[55] was developed with a specific focus on physical activity in children older than 8 years with JIA. Its emphasis is on responsiveness, and it is aimed primarily at evaluation of rehabilitation interventions. Through a detailed process, an instrument with 100 items was developed, divided into five categories of physical function: (1) self-care, (2) domestic, (3) mobility, (4) school, and (5) extracurricular. In JASI Part 2, patients identify up to five tasks that are most problematic, and these tasks are evaluated on subsequent follow-up. This maneuver makes this component of JASI potentially more responsive and patient specific. In a validation study, JASI was shown to have good measurement properties.[72] There was reasonable spread of scores, suggesting that JASI has discriminative ability. Reliability was shown with excellent intraclass correlations. Construct validity was established by demonstration of predicted correlations with other measures used.

Although JASI is an excellent instrument, it cannot be administered to children younger than 8 years of age. Also, it takes a long time to complete, and this may make it less attractive for routine clinical use. Nonetheless, JASI is a comprehensive instrument with excellent measurement properties whose greatest value is probably as a research tool for longitudinal studies or to help identify specific goals in a rehabilitation setting.

Juvenile Arthritis Quality of Life Questionnaire

JAQQ[50] was developed by following standard principles of item generation,[54] a process that has demonstrated a very high level of agreement between patients and parents over a wide array of perceived difficulties.[133] Additional items on psychosocial function were added by the incorporation of a previously developed psychosocial instrument.[134]

Generated items were subsequently reduced and categorized into four dimensions, each with approximately 20 items: (1) gross motor function, (2) fine motor function, (3) psychosocial function, and (4) general symptoms. Respondents score all items and are asked to identify up to five items in each dimension with which they are having difficulty; they may also volunteer their own items for each dimension. The mean score for the five highest scoring items in each dimension is computed as the Dimension Score (range, 1 to 7); the Total JAQQ Score is computed as the mean of the four Dimension Scores (range, 1 to 7).

After this initial study, the item number was reduced to 74: gross motor function, 17 items; fine motor function, 16 items; psychosocial function, 22 items; and general symptoms, 19 items. A pain dimension was added as a supplement.[135] Face, content, and construct validity were clearly established.[136] Responsiveness was established after the start of new drug therapy.[137] Responsiveness was also shown to be maintained over time[138] and to be at least as good as responsiveness of CHAQ, CHQ, or Peds QL.[139] Enhancement of responsiveness was shown by a reduction in the number of items scored, and in this study MCID was shown to be 0.35.[140]

JAQQ has been translated into several languages and has been shown to maintain its measurement properties in several different cultural settings.[141-143] In an English study of adolescents with JIA, JAQQ was shown to have excellent reliability and validity.[143] In a further study, the same group showed improvement in JAQQ scores, with excellent responsiveness, after the introduction of a transitional care program.[144] A high level of agreement between the perception of children with JIA and their parents concerning HRQoL was shown in a Canadian study.[145] Another more recent Canadian study showed that JAQQ was highly predictive of several short-term outcomes in a large cohort of children with JIA.[121]

JAQQ has been developed in a detailed fashion, resulting in excellent measurement. It can be administered to children of all ages and disease onset types in a reasonable time with minimal assistance, and it can be scored quickly by hand; this makes it practical for use in the clinical setting.

Childhood Arthritis Health Profile

CAHP[51] is a parent report that is self-administered and consists of three modules: (1) generic health status measures, (2) JIA-specific health status measures, and (3) patient characteristics. Three functional scales were determined for the JIA-specific scales: (1) gross motor function, (2) fine motor function, and (3) role activities (play, family, friends). Internal reliability was shown by good inter-item correlations within scales and minimal item scale variation. Correlation coefficients for the JIA-specific scales with one another ranged from 0.84 to 0.97, whereas those for the generic functioning scales were 0.73, showing validity of these scales and further suggesting that the JIA-specific scales provide additional information beyond that of the generic functioning scales. In a follow-up report,[52] the discriminative ability of CAHP was demonstrated.

Quality of My Life Questionnaire

QoMLQ was developed in an attempt to distinguish between difficulties resulting from the disease itself and difficulties that are more generic.[73] It comprises two separate 100-mm VAS, anchored with the descriptors "worst" and "best," that direct respondents to indicate their "quality of life," in aspects caused by the disease itself (HRQoL) and those caused by overall difficulties not directly related to the disease (QoL). In a further study[37] that included 131 parent–child pairs, there was a high level of agreement between parents and children for QoL and moderate agreement for HRQoL. In this study, there were good correlations for components with pain and disease severity, establishing its convergent construct validity. Also, MCID for improvement in

QoL and HRQoL were 7 mm and 11 mm, and for deterioration were −33 mm and −38 mm, respectively, providing the opportunity for clinicians to interpret changes in scores.

QoMLQ is a short and easy-to-use generic instrument that has been shown to be highly reliable and valid. Given these qualities, it is likely to see more widespread use.

In further work from the same group, a novel approach was used in attempting to measure the gap between an individual's current situation and their expectations, in some respects an extension of the work alluded to earlier. Contemporary measures of QoL tend not to take this "gap" into consideration. This study attempted to measure these gaps for a whole series of domains in children with rheumatic diseases. The result was the development of a measure with 72 items distributed among 5-gap scales (GapS). The GapS are currently undergoing further development.[24]

Child Health Questionnaire

CHQ[74] is a generic instrument that comprises numerous different forms. The form used most commonly in children with JIA is the Parent Form 50 (PF 50), which contains 50 items distributed in several dimensions: global health, physical activities, everyday activities, pain, behavior, well-being, self-esteem, general health, and family. These sections are complemented by general questions about the child and the caregiver. Two separate scores can be computed that estimate physical and psychosocial function; both are scored from 0 to 100, with the higher score indicating better function.

In a study of short-term outcome in 116 children with JIA observed for less than 2.5 years, Selvaag and colleagues[146] showed poorer physical status but minimal psychological impairment in JIA patients relative to controls using CHQ. Numerous studies from the Pediatric Rheumatology International Trials Organization (PRINTO), which has validated CHQ for use in 32 languages,[99] disagree with this study, however. In one study that included 6639 participants (one half had JIA, and one half were healthy), mean scores for physical and psychosocial summary scores were significantly lower for JIA patients relative to controls.[147] In a further study that included three distinct geographical regions (Eastern Europe, Western Europe, and Latin America), determinants of poor HRQoL were similar across all regions, with physical well-being affected by the level of disability and psychosocial well-being affected by the intensity of pain.[148] CHQ was used in combination with CHAQ in a trial of methotrexate, in which it was shown to be highly responsive[109]; this was further confirmed in a follow-up study of the same study group.[149] One study suggested, however, that JAQQ may be at least as responsive as CHQ for studies in JIA.[139] Because of its generalizability, CHQ has become the preferred measure of QoL for JIA trials.

Pediatric Quality of Life Inventory

Peds QL is a modular instrument designed to measure HRQoL in children and adolescents 2 to 18 years old.[75] It contains a generic core integrated with a disease-specific core. The generic core has undergone various iterations, the most recent of which—the Peds QL 4.0 Generic Core Scales—contains 23 items distributed in four scales: (1) physical, (2) emotional, (3) social, and (4) school functioning. The Peds QL 3.0 Rheumatology Module contains 22 disease-specific items distributed in five scales: (1) pain, (2) daily activities, (3) treatment, (4) worry, and (5) communication. It is completed by children and their parents, and consists of developmentally appropriate forms for varying age groups. When it is completed separately, parent–child concordance has been shown to be good. The module takes approximately 15 minutes to complete. Each item is scored on a 5-point scale (0 to 4), with a higher score indicating worse function. A mean Scale Score is computed based on the number of items scored. This score is extrapolated in a reverse fashion to a scale of 0 to 100, with a higher score indicating better function. Total Scale Scores are computed as the mean across all items scored in that scale. This process is the same for the Generic Core Scale and the Rheumatology Module.

This instrument was shown to have excellent reliability, validity, and responsiveness in a study of 271 children with various rheumatic diseases (91 of whom had JIA) and their parents.[150] Reliability varied with the age of the child, being less for younger children. Reliability was also not as good for the Rheumatology Module.

Lower HRQoL, as exemplified by lower Peds QL generic and rheumatology module scores, was noted in one study, despite minimal symptoms or little or no disease activity,[151] whereas another study showed significantly reduced scores in children with polyarticular JIA, particularly in fatigue scores.[152] A further study showed lower Peds QL scores for Medicaid patients even when correcting for health care use and degree of disease activity.[153]

Responsiveness has not been tested in a trial setting. Nonetheless, this instrument represents an important addition to the pool of outcome measures available for use in JIA, and further studies are being followed with interest.

NEWER INSTRUMENTS

Pediatric Rheumatology Quality of Life Scale (PRQL)

The PRQL is a recently developed, simple, 10-item questionnaire that focuses on HRQoL in both physical health and psychosocial health. The short questionnaire is intended for use as a proxy and self-report with a proposed age range of 7 to 18 years. The PRQL underwent preliminary validation in approximately 470 children with JIA and 800 healthy children in one study at one Italian center.[154] The PRQL was found to have good measurement properties and is reported to be a valid instrument for clinical and research assessments of HRQoL in children with JIA. Further study with this instrument is needed to determine if the validity holds across multiple rheumatic diseases and in different cultural environments.

Juvenile Arthritis Multidimensional Assessment Report (JAMAR)

JAMAR was recently developed as an instrument that combines the traditional patient-reported outcomes used in clinical evaluation of children with JIA with other outcome measures not addressed by conventional instruments. There are a total of 15 measurements on JAMAR that include assessments of overall well-being, pain, functional ability, and HRQoL, as well as an evaluation of morning stiffness, overall level of disease activity, rating of disease activity and course, proxy or self-assessment of joint involvement and extraarticular symptoms, description of side effects from medications and assessment of therapeutic compliance and satisfaction with the outcome of the illness. JAMAR is proposed for use as both a proxy report for parents of patients aged 2 to 18 and a patient self-report with the suggested age range of 7 to 18 years old.

JAMAR was validated in a study of parents and children with JIA over 2563 visits.[155] It was noted to be user friendly, easy to understand, and quick to complete. Because JAMAR was designed to be completed in a clinical setting and focuses on information needed for care, the VAS for pain, well-being, and disease activity are presented as 21 numbered circles, instead of the conventional 10-cm horizontal line, to facilitate scoring without a ruler. This approach was shown to increase the precision of the parent/patient ratings.[156] The main limitation to the validation study of JAMAR is that the instrument was tested only in Italian parents and patients at a single center. However, research with

this instrument is ongoing and will be followed with interest given its multidisciplinary nature.

Composite Disease Activity Scores for Juvenile Idiopathic Arthritis

The American College of Rheumatology (ACR) JIA core set and pediatric response criteria focus on change in disease state and assess improvement or deterioration in disease activity. Individually, these measures are incomplete, however. A composite disease activity score for JIA, Juvenile Arthritis Disease Activity Score (JADAS),[157] includes four of the measures included in the core set: (1) active joint count, (2) physician's global assessment of disease activity, (3) patient and parent global assessment of overall well-being, and (4) erythrocyte sedimentation rate. Joint count is modified based on evaluation of 10, 27, or 71 joints in three different versions of the instrument. JADAS has been shown to have good measurement properties, including responsiveness, and is a very useful addition. The literature indicates its use is increasing.[158]

INSTRUMENTS AVAILABLE FOR USE IN RHEUMATIC DISEASES OTHER THAN JUVENILE IDIOPATHIC ARTHRITIS

There has been considerable recent international effort to develop appropriate measures for use in JDM and SLE in adults and children. This effort has culminated in the development of measures of disease activity and damage[159] and a core set of measures for childhood-onset and adult-onset diseases.[160,161] The core set for JDM was conducted simultaneously with a similar effort for juvenile SLE (see Table 7-2).[161]

Through an initial survey of 267 physicians worldwide, followed by a nominal group technique process, 37 response variables for JDM were examined. Ultimately, a core set for JDM was arrived at comprising six measures (see Table 7-2). This instrument has undergone validation testing in an attempt to define improvement in the core set.[162] Such improvement is defined as a minimum of 15% improvement in the domains of muscle strength and physical function, a minimum of 20% improvement for physician and patient global assessments and overall global assessment, and a minimum of 30% reduction in the serum level of muscle enzymes. To complement this core set, which focuses predominantly on myositis, a measure has been developed to measure activity of the skin in JDM—the Cutaneous Assessment Tool (CAT).[163] This tool has excellent measurement properties, which have been maintained even with a modification of the scoring method.[164]

In addition to the core set and CAT, a specific outcome measure has been developed to assess physical function in JDM—the Childhood Myositis Assessment Scale (CMAS).[165] This is a therapist-administered assessment of muscle strength, endurance, and function with excellent measurement properties. It is scored on a scale of 0 to 52, based on the ability of the child to perform specific tasks scored by an observer. CMAS has been shown to have outstanding intraobserver and interobserver reliability, as well as good validity and good correlations with manual muscle testing.

CHAQ has also been validated for use in JDM patients. It was shown to have excellent test–retest reliability, validity, and responsiveness,[166-168] and to be valuable as a measure of outcome.[167] CHQ was used in combination with CHAQ in a study of 272 children with JDM.[169] It performed well and showed that there was a significant reduction in HRQoL as evidenced by decreased physical and psychosocial summary scores.

As a component of the initiative discussed for JDM, a similar effort was conducted for juvenile SLE.[161] In this component of the study, 41 response variables were tested. Ultimately, measures of disease activity were those depicted (see Table 7-2) and included specific SLE immunological tests and renal function measures, as well as physician and parent/patient global assessments, an overall global assessment, a measure of growth and development, and a measure of HRQoL (most likely CHQ, but this has not been finalized). Brunner and associates[170] previously validated the Systemic Lupus Erythematosus Disease Activity Index (SLEDAI) for juvenile SLE and in a more recent study showed the responsiveness of European Consensus Lupus Activity Measurement (ECLAM) for juvenile SLE, suggesting that it might be more sensitive than SLEDAI in this population.[171] Two studies described the extent of damage in juvenile SLE[172,173] using the Systemic Lupus International Collaborating Clinics (SLICC)/ACR Damage Index. A Canadian study showed reduced fitness, increasing fatigue, and reduced HRQoL, measured by CHQ, in a group of 15 adolescents with SLE.[174] Neither fatigue nor fitness correlated with disease activity, disease damage, or HRQoL, however. Similar findings were observed in 24 children using Peds QL.[175]

Finally, a new instrument to measure HRQoL in SLE has been developed—the Simple Measure of the Impact of Lupus Erythematosus in Youngsters (SMILEY).[176] It contains four domains that address patient perceptions of HRQoL: (1) effect on self, (2) limitations, (3) social, and (4) burden of SLE. In the initial validation study, SMILEY was shown to have excellent reliability and validity. Further work with this instrument has been an international effort to provide a cross cultural adaptation with translation to 13 different languages.[177] Further studies to validate the translated and adapted versions of SMILEY are ongoing and will be of interest.

OTHER ISSUES

Instrument Usage and Electronic Applications

The majority of instruments discussed here, and HRQoL assessments in general, have been used mainly within a clinical research setting. However, the use of patient reported outcomes in daily clinical practice has been the topic of much recent discussion. This encompasses self-assessment of functional status, as well as symptoms or other concerns, such as patient needs and satisfaction with care. The use of these instruments in a clinical setting may be of use in the early detection of HRQoL problems and may allow for a tailored intervention prior to an escalation of the issue. For example, the effects of childhood disease and its treatment often increase the child's dependence on adults and decrease the child's participation in peer- and school-based activities. This could have an adverse effect on the accomplishment of developmental tasks, resulting in an impaired QoL. A questionnaire designed to capture pertinent information given to the clinician prior to or at the time of consultation might be of use to identify, monitor, and discuss particular HRQoL issues faced by children with JIA. The choice of instrument is dependent upon the extent, impact, and type of pediatric rheumatic disease.

A survey conducted by one of the authors of this chapter, C.M. Duffy, previously determined that although pediatric rheumatologists are aware of this form of measurement and have participated in studies that have included such measures, in general, clinicians tend not to use them in clinical practice (unpublished data). It is possible that these instruments have been slow to infiltrate the clinical picture due to logistical issues around completing the forms and having the information available to the clinician in a timely fashion. New technology and the availability of Web-based platforms may facilitate the use of HRQoL assessments in clinical practice by allowing the clinician to access the data at the time of a clinic visit. In the future, these instruments could potentially become an integral part of complete patient care as we move increasingly to a complete electronic health record.

The concept of using technology to make clinical assessment of HRQoL more efficient is expected to gain momentum across all fields in the coming years. To overcome the practical issues around completing HRQoL forms in the clinic for clinical assessment, a group in the Netherlands has developed a novel and innovative Web-based application called the KLIK PROfile for patient-reported outcome measures.[178] This program is tailored to general daily pediatric clinical practice, and specifically targets children with chronic diseases. The authors envision parents and children completing the HRQoL measure at home up to 3 days prior to the consultation and clinicians retrieving the patient-reported outcomes directly from the website. It will be of interest to follow the KLIK PROfile and its evaluation for ease of implementation and use. This type of program may promote the widespread use of HRQoL instruments in daily clinical practice, as well as facilitate collaborative research between centers.

CHALLENGES FOR THE FUTURE: HOW CAN WE IMPROVE OUR ASSESSMENTS?

There has been a great deal of development in the field of outcome assessment in pediatric rheumatology. There remain, however, a number of areas in which we can improve the quality of these assessments. We will describe four such challenges.

I. Developing Scoring Summations That Are More Theoretically Correct

Insensitivity of many of the tools described in this chapter may be the result of using summative and item scores that are too simplistic. Each of the 30 items of the CHAQ, for example, is scored on a 4-point ordinal scale.[47] These item scores, though, are dealt with as though each response category was evenly spaced on a ratio scale. "Without any difficulty" is scored 0, "with some difficulty" is scored 1, "with much difficulty" is scored 2, and "unable to do" is scored 3. However, we have no reason to believe that "with much difficulty" is twice as bad as "with some difficulty," nor that it is infinitely worse than "without any difficulty." The overall score of the CHAQ is the average of the domain scores (with each domain taking the score of the most impaired item); as a consequence there are many ways that different patients may have the same score. A child with "some difficulty" tying shoelaces, cutting her own meat, and scribbling with a pencil will have the same score as another child who is completely "unable to" walk on flat ground; however, it is not at all clear that these are equivalent states.

This issue applies to many of the assessments described previously.

The CHAQ comprises 30 ordinal scores; there are 4^{30} unique ways of responding to the CHAQ questionnaire. Each of these ~1,150,000,000,000,000,000 unique ways of responding to the CHAQ may, in theory, describe a functional state of different value.

Likewise, we may be oversimplifying the way we score visual analog scales (e.g., used to measure pain, or global well-being). Although these are *analog* scores, we give them values as though they were *digital* scores; we measure where the patient places a mark on the VAS and give it a number score.

It seems, however, that most people don't respond to a VAS as though it is linear and yields ratio data. Instead, most of us value changes at the extremes of the scale differently from the middle. We are also often influenced by where the anchor points are placed on the line (e.g., a hash mark at each end, or in the middle), and we tend to group our responses closer to these anchors.

These are difficult challenges to solve, but not impossible, e.g., using multiattribute utility theory,[179] choice experiments,[180] and prospect theory.[181,182] This should be an important area for research in the future.

II. Valuing Change More Appropriately

Most of the response criteria for the above listed core sets use "percent" (relative) change as a way of determining whether important improvement or flare occurs. Theoretically, we should only use relative change for numbers with ratio properties. Ratio numbers have a zero that is meaningful and true. However, most of the items that make up our core sets have arbitrary zero scores. This can lead to inconsistencies and can make understanding improvement difficult.

For example, the Fahrenheit and Celsius temperature scales both have arbitrary 0° temperatures. If, in Canada, the temperature changes from 10°C to 20°C, we often (but incorrectly) state that the temperature has doubled. However, this change in temperature is exactly the same as a change in the United States from 50°F to 68°F. It is absurd to say that the same temperature change is a 100% increase in Canada, but only a 36% increase in the United States.

Future research must help us understand how to better score change in our core sets.

III. Incorporating Individual Patient Subjectivity in Quality of Life Measures

QoL, at least as defined by the WHO, is a highly individual and subjective construct.[183] Yet most of the (so-called) measures of QoL used in pediatric rheumatology use questions that a panel of experts, sometimes with the help of *groups* of patients has determined. The value (score) associated with each item in a QoL measure is usually determined by the developer, not the patient. We will probably improve our determinations of patient *important* outcomes if we allow patients to determine which questions are important to them, and we allow them to value their responses individually.

Some of the questionnaires discussed above attempt to do this, either by using global scores (e.g., global well-being VAS, QoML) or by allowing respondents to add additional items of particular importance to themselves (e.g., JASI, JAQQ).

Future research should explore new ways to use true, individual, and subjective patient values in our measurement tools, if, in fact, we really want to measure QoL/HRQoL.[184] As an example, we might consider the gap between expectation and realization[185]—perhaps in many dimensions[23]—as a way, based on theory, of determining individual, subjective values of life quality.[24]

IV. Changing Our Ontogeny (Philosophy) of Assessment and Measurement.

All of the measurement/health outcome tools that have been discussed in this chapter appear to be based on the assumption that there is a "real" construct (concept) being measured. This "philosophic realism" underlies the classic psychometric approach.[186] This approach posits that quality of life, for example, is a real thing that exists. We can't directly observe it (it is a "latent variable") so we use imperfect measures (e.g., items on a QoL scale) that when combined give us a good indication of QoL.

This approach to measurement implies that all the items that measure the (latent) construct of QoL should be highly correlated and interchangeable (because they are all measuring the same thing). (This argument applies equally well to other constructs, such as disease activity, health, well-being, damage, function, etc.) In addition, if QoL is a "real" thing, all validated measures of QoL should give, within measurement error, the same result. Assessment tools developed with this philosophy are called *reflective* measures; all the items and domains *reflect* an underlying, *real*, latent construct.

However, when studied, we sometimes find that different tools used to assess the same construct give very different answers—sometimes not even correlated with each other.[187,188]

It is more likely that constructs such as QoL, function, disease activity, disease damage, health, etc., don't exist as real and independent entities; instead it is likely that they are constructed by human minds (we define them). This approach has been called *philosophic constructivism*.[186] Assessment tools developed with this philosophy are called *formative* measures; the items that we choose to measure *form* the construct, by definition. If we were to use different items (say, in two different questionnaires) we might get two different answers (which is what we often see empirically).

The constructivist ontogeny implies that patients do not walk around with a formed idea of QoL in their heads (e.g., "today I am 7 out of 10"); rather, they construct their idea of QoL depending on how they are asked about it.

We have become very good at assessing the physical properties associated with inanimate objects such as velocity, mass, temperature, etc. It is not clear, though, that we can measure multidimensional and complex human constructs such as QoL, intelligence, health, etc., in such simple terms and quantify them with simple numbers. The professor of financial engineering at Columbia University, Emmanuel Derman, described this quandary using the term *pragmamorphism*.[189]

We must explore how constructivism should be considered when determining the validity of health outcome assessments, and when choosing measures for care or research; this is an important research agenda.

CONCLUSION

In this chapter, we have highlighted the ICF framework (see Fig. 7-1) as suggested by WHO and have illustrated how it might be used to structure a hierarchy of outcomes. We have also discussed the measurement of disease activity, HRQoL, and QoL in relation to pediatric rheumatic diseases. Although measures have been developed that apply to all of these areas, measurement of QoL has proved most difficult, and although it can be measured, it is unclear how its measurement can contribute to health care. For this reason, the greatest focus of clinicians has been on measures of disease activity and HRQoL.

Measures of disease activity have been discussed briefly for JIA, JDM, and SLE. The major development has been the adoption of a core set of measures for each of these diseases (see Table 7-2).

We have focused our attention on measures of HRQoL with a particular emphasis on JIA. The properties of these various instruments were compared (see Table 7-3). They differ significantly from one another and have been developed with different objectives in mind, so each has unique qualities. Attempts to develop better measures for JDM and SLE continue.

The past several years have been a very exciting and active time of research and much has been accomplished. However, genuine concerns exist regarding the current approach to this type of measurement, and here we have suggested that it is perhaps time to reflect on what it is we are measuring and to delve further into describing the real "constructs" of this type of measurement. Ongoing research will add to our knowledge and understanding of this complex process of measurement, not only in JIA, but also in other pediatric rheumatic diseases.

REFERENCES

5. C. Eiser, R. Morse, The measurement of quality of life in children: past and future perspectives, J. Dev. Behav. Pediatr. 22 (2001) 248–256.

6. P. Tugwell, C. Bombardier, W.W. Buchanan, et al., Methotrexate in rheumatoid arthritis: impact on quality of life assessed by traditional standard-item and individualized patient preference health status questionnaires, Arch. Intern. Med. 150 (1990) 59–62.

7. J.F. Fries, Toward an understanding of patient outcome measurement, Arthritis Rheum. 26 (1983) 697–704.

9. C.M. Duffy, Measurement of health status, functional status, and quality of life in children with juvenile idiopathic arthritis: clinical science for the pediatrician, Rheum. Dis. Clin. North Am. 33 (2007) 389–402.

10. T.M. Gill, A.R. Feinstein, A critical appraisal of the quality of quality-of-life measurements, JAMA 272 (1994) 619–626.

12. World Health Organization, WHO International Classification of Functioning, Disability and Health (ICF) (website). (<http://www.who.int/classifications/icf/en/>).

16. G. Stucki, A. Cieza, The International Classification of Functioning, Disability and Health (ICF) in physical and rehabilitation medicine, Eur. J. Phys. Rehabil. Med. 44 (2008) 299–302.

17. G. Stucki, A. Cieza, The International Classification of Functioning Disability and Health (ICF) Core Sets for rheumatoid arthritis: a way to specify functioning, Ann. Rheum. Dis. 63 (Suppl. 2) (2004) ii40–ii45.

18. G. Stucki, T. Ewert, How to assess the impact of arthritis on the individual patient: the WHO ICF, Ann. Rheum. Dis. 64 (2005) 664–668.

23. A.C. Michalos, Multiple discrepancies theory (MDT), Soc. Indic. Res. 16 (1985) 347–413.

24. G.W. Gong, M. Barrera, J. Beyene, et al., The Gap Study (GapS) interview—developing a process to determine the meaning and determinants of quality of life in children with arthritis and rheumatic disease, Clin. Exp. Rheumatol. 25 (2007) 486–493.

27. G.H. Guyatt, S.J. Veldhuyzen Van Zanten, D.H. Feeny, et al., Measuring quality of life in clinical trials: a taxonomy and review, CMAJ 140 (1989) 1441–1448.

28. G.H. Guyatt, D.H. Feeny, D.L. Patrick, Measuring health-related quality of life, Ann. Intern. Med. 118 (1993) 622–629.

29. G.H. Guyatt, Insights and limitations from health-related quality-of-life research, J. Gen. Intern. Med. 12 (1997) 720–721.

30. M.A. Testa, D.C. Simonson, Assessment of quality-of-life outcomes, N. Engl. J. Med. 334 (1996) 835–840.

37. G.W. Gong, N.L. Young, H. Dempster, et al., The Quality of My Life questionnaire: the minimal clinically important difference for pediatric rheumatology patients, J. Rheumatol. 34 (2007) 581–587.

38. E.H. Giannini, R. Ruperto, A. Ravelli, Preliminary definition of improvement in juvenile arthritis, Arthritis Rheum. 40 (1997) 1202–1209.

45. G.H. Guyatt, C. Bombardier, P.X. Tugwell, Measuring disease-specific quality of life in clinical trials, CMAJ 134 (1986) 889–895.

46. S. Howe, J. Levinson, E. Shear, et al., Development of a disability measurement tool for juvenile rheumatoid arthritis. The Juvenile Arthritis Functional Assessment Report for children and their parents, Arthritis Rheum. 34 (1991) 873.

47. G. Singh, B.H. Athreya, J.F. Fries, et al., Measurement of health status in children with juvenile rheumatoid arthritis, Arthritis Rheum. 37 (1994) 1761–1769.

50. C.M. Duffy, L. Arsenault, K.N. Duffy, et al., The Juvenile Arthritis Quality of Life Questionnaire–development of a new responsive index for juvenile rheumatoid arthritis and juvenile spondyloarthritides, J. Rheumatol. 24 (1997) 738–746.

54. B. Kirshner, G. Guyatt, A methodologic framework for assessing health indices, J. Chron. Dis. 38 (1985) 27–36.

55. V.F. Wright, M. Law, V. Crombie, et al., Development of a self-report functional status index for juvenile rheumatoid arthritis, J. Rheumatol. 21 (1994) 536–544.

59. A.R. Feinstein, B.R. Josephy, C.K. Wells, Scientific and clinical problems in indexes of functional disability, Ann. Intern. Med. 105 (1986) 413–420.

61. P. Tugwell, C. Bombardier, W.W. Buchanan, et al., The MACTAR patient preference questionnaire: an individualized functional priority approach for assessing improvement in clinical trials in rheumatoid arthritis, J. Rheumatol. 14 (1987) 446–451.

70. B.H. Singsen, Health status (arthritis impact) in children with chronic rheumatic diseases. Current measurement issues and an approach to instrument design, Arthritis Care Res. 4 (1991) 87–101.

72. V.F. Wright, J.L. Kimber, M. Law, et al., The Juvenile Arthritis Functional Status Index (JASI): a validation study, J. Rheumatol. 23 (1996) 1066–1079.

73. B.M. Feldman, B. Grundland, L. McCullough, et al., Distinction of quality of life, health-related quality of life, and health status in children referred for rheumatology care, J. Rheumatol. 27 (2000) 226–233.

74. J.M. Landgraf, L. Abetz, J.E. Ware, Child Health Questionaire (CHQ): A User's Manual, The Health Institute, New England Medical Center, 1996.

75. J.W. Varni, M. Seid, C.A. Rode, The PedsQL: measurement model for the Pediatric Quality of Life Inventory, Med. Care 37 (1999) 126–139.

79. N. Ruperto, A. Ravelli, J.E. Levison, et al., Long term health outcomes and quality of life in American and Italian inception cohorts of patients with juvenile rheumatoid arthritis. II. Early predictors of outcome, J. Rheumatol. 24 (1997) 952–958.

82. M. Zak, F.K. Pedersen, Juvenile chronic arthritis into adulthood: a long-term follow up study, Rheumatology 39 (2000) 198–204.

85. K. Oen, P. Malleson, D. Cabral, et al., Disease course and outcome of juvenile rheumatoid arthritis in a multicenter cohort, J. Rheumatol. 29 (2002) 1989–1999.

89. S. Bowyer, P.A. Roettcher, G.C. Higgins, et al., Health status of patients with juvenile rheumatoid arthritis at 1 and 5 years after diagnosis, J. Rheumatol. 30 (2003) 394–400.

90. K. Oen, P. Malleson, D. Cabral, et al., Early predictors of long-term outcome in patients with juvenile rheumatoid arthritis: subset-specific correlations, J. Rheumatol. 30 (2003) 585–593.

91. S. Magni-Manzoni, A. Pistorio, E. Labò, et al., A longitudinal analysis of physical functional disability over the course of juvenile idiopathic arthritis, Ann. Rheum. Dis. 67 (2008) 1159–1164.

99. N. Ruperto, A. Ravelli, A. Pistorio, et al., Cross-cultural adaptation and psychometric evaluation of the Childhood Health Assessment Questionnaire (CHAQ) and the Child Health Questionnaire (CHQ) in 32 countries. Review of the general methodology, Clin. Exp. Rheumatol. 19 (4 Suppl. 23) (2001) S1–S9.

110. F.H. Prince, L.M. Geerdink, G.J. Borsboom, et al., Major improvements in health-related quality of life during the use of etanercept in patients with previously refractory juvenile idiopathic arthritis, Ann. Rheum. Dis. 69 (2010) 138–142.

111. M.G. Halbig, G. Horneff, Improvement of functional ability in children with juvenile idiopathic arthritis by treatment with etanercept, Rheumatol. Int. 30 (2009) 229–238.

118. T. Takken, J. van der Net, P.J. Helders, Relationship between functional ability and physical fitness in juvenile idiopathic arthritis patients, Scand. J. Rheumatol. 32 (2003) 174–178.

121. K. Oen, L. Tucker, A.M. Huber, et al., Predictors of early inactive disease in a juvenile idiopathic arthritis cohort: results of a Canadian multicenter, prospective inception cohort study, Arthritis Rheum. 61 (2009) 1077–1086.

122. H. Dempster, M. Porepa, N. Young, B.M. Feldman, The clinical meaning of functional outcome scores in children with juvenile arthritis, Arthritis Rheum. 44 (2001) 1768–1774.

123. H.I. Brunner, M.S. Klein-Gitelman, M.J. Miller, et al., Minimal clinically important differences of the childhood health assessment questionnaire, J. Rheumatol. 32 (2005) 150–161.

124. C. Saad-Magalhães, A. Pistoria, A. Ravelli, et al., Does removal of aids/devices and help make a difference in the Child Health Assessment Questionnaire disability index?, Ann. Rheum. Dis. 69 (2010) 82–87.

125. L.M. Geerdink, F.H. Prince, C.W. Looman, et al., Development of a digital Childhood Health Assessment Questionnaire for systemic monitoring of disease activity in daily practice, Rheumatology (Oxford) 48 (2009) 958–963.

142. B. Amine, S. Rostom, K. Benbouazza, et al., Health related quality of life survey about children and adolescents with juvenile arthritis, Rheumatol. Int. 29 (2009) 275–279.

143. K.L. Shaw, T.R. Southwood, C.M. Duffy, et al., Health-related quality of life in adolescents with juvenile idiopathic arthritis, Arthritis Rheum. 55 (2006) 199–207.

144. J.E. McDonagh, T.R. Southwood, K.L. Shaw, The impact of a coordinated transitional care program on adolescents with juvenile idiopathic arthritis, Rheumatology (Oxford) 46 (2007) 161–168.

145. K.T. April, D.E. Feldman, R.W. Platt, C.M. Duffy, Comparison between Children with Juvenile Idiopathic Arthritis and their parents concerning perceived Quality Of Life, Qual. Life Res. 15 (2006) 655–661.

150. J.W. Varni, M. Seid, T. Smith Knight, et al., The PedsQL in pediatric rheumatology: reliability, validity and responsiveness of the Pediatric Quality of Life Inventory Generic Core Scales and Rheumatology Module, Arthritis Rheum. 46 (2002) 714–725.

152. S. Ringold, C.A. Wallace, F.P. Rivara, Health-related quality of life, physical function, fatigue, and disease activity in children with established polyarticular juvenile idiopathic arthritis, J. Rheumatol. 36 (2009) 1330–1336.

153. H.I. Brunner, J. Taylor, M.T. Britto, et al., Differences in disease outcomes between Medicaid and privately insured children: possible health disparities in juvenile rheumatoid arthritis, Arthritis Rheum. 55 (2006) 378–384.

155. G. Filocamo, A. Consolaro, B. Schiappapietra, et al., A new approach to clinical care of juvenile idiopathic arthritis: the Juvenile Arthritis Multidimensional Assessment Report, J. Rheumatol. 38 (2011) 938–953.

172. H.I. Brunner, E.D. Silverman, T. To, et al., Risk factors for damage in childhood-onset systemic lupus erythematosus: cumulative disease activity and medication use predict disease damage, Arthritis Rheum. 46 (2002) 436–444.

187. H.I. Brunner, D. Maker, B. Grundland, et al., Preference-based measurement of health-related quality of life (HRQL) in children with chronic musculoskeletal disorders (MSKDs), Med. Decis. Making 23 (2003) 314–322.

188. L. Sung, N.L. Young, M.L. Greenberg, et al., Health related quality of life (HRQL) scores reported from parents and their children with chronic illness differed depending on utility elicitation method, J. Clin. Epidemiol. 57 (2004) 1161–1166.

189. E. Derman, Pragmamorphism, in: J. Brockman (Ed.), This Will Make You Smarter, Harper Perennial, NewYork, 2012.

Entire reference list is available online at www.expertconsult.com.

Pain and Its Assessment

Michael Rapoff, Carol B. Lindsley

Chronic or intermittent pain is a primary symptom of many pediatric rheumatic diseases, especially arthritis. Patients often report mild to moderate pain.[1-4] About 25% to 30% report moderate to severe pain,[5,6] and most children with arthritis report at least some pain lasting from 30 minutes to 24 hours a day, with a mean of 4.3 hours per day.[7] A 2-month daily diary study showed that children with arthritis report pain on an average of 73% of the days, with the majority (76%) reporting pain on more than 60% of the days.[8] A 2-week electronic pain diary study showed that adolescents with arthritis reported, on average, mild pain intensity, whereas 9.2% reported no pain, and 17.1% reported pain on every diary entry.[9] About 60% of children with juvenile rheumatoid arthritis (JRA) report joint pain at disease onset, 50% report pain at their 1-year follow-up, and 40% continue to report pain 5 years later.[10] Moreover, adults who as children were diagnosed with JRA report significantly more pain, fatigue, and disability than gender-matched healthy controls.[11] Thus, pain is a significant problem for many children with juvenile idiopathic arthritis (JIA) that persists into adulthood and is associated with greater disability. Pain affects multiple areas of their lives, and its effect is not fully explained by disease activity alone.

The purpose of this chapter is (1) to outline a biobehavioral model of pain, including nociceptive, emotional, cognitive, and behavioral aspects of arthritis-related pain and implications for treatment based on the model; (2) to review cognitive-behavioral treatments for chronic pain, including arthritis-related pain; and (3) to describe measures of pain.

BIOBEHAVIORAL MODEL OF PAIN

A comprehensive understanding of pain and its treatment requires a multidimensional approach that goes beyond nociceptive activity associated with the disease. A model that acknowledges this complexity of pain is needed as a foundation for development of effective pharmacological and nonpharmacological treatments. The most widely accepted definition of pain ("an unpleasant sensory and emotional experience associated with actual or potential tissue damage") views it as simultaneously a physiological and psychological experience.[12] Beginning with the *gate control* theory of pain,[13] researchers have advanced a biobehavioral model focused on the unique and interactive components of nociceptive activity, emotions, cognitions, and behavior.[14,15]

Nociceptive Activity. Nociception describes the physiological, anatomical, and chemical properties of the nervous system that contribute to the perception of pain.[16] Noxious mechanical, thermal, or chemical stimuli generate neuronal impulses conducted along peripheral (afferent) nerve fibers that synapse in the dorsal horn circuitry of the spinal cord and project to the thalamus and cortex via the spinothalamic tract. Neural projections also descend from the brain and synapse with neurons in the spinal cord (Fig. 8-1). The dorsal horn circuitry is an important site within the central nervous system, where modulation (excitatory or inhibitory) of neuronal impulses takes place. The inhibition of spinal nociceptive transmission can diminish the experience of pain, as when endogenous opioids (such as endorphins) are released during stress and produce analgesic effects.[16,17] This descending pain modulation system, first proposed in the gate control theory of pain,[13] provides a neurochemical and anatomical basis for considering the pain-enhancing or pain-inhibiting effects of psychological factors, such as cognitions and emotions.[16,17] Nociceptors may be modality specific or polymodal (respond to multiple types of stimuli). Activation occurs only with intense, potentially damaging stimuli, and generally there is no spontaneous activity.[18] The cell bodies of the afferent nociceptive fibers are in the dorsal root ganglia and terminate over several spinal segments in the dorsal horn of the spinal cord.[19]

The thalamus is the center of integrations of nociceptive information and plays a dominant role in pain modulation.[20] In addition, there are four cortical areas identified as important in the pain experience: (1) the prefrontal cortex, (2) anterior cingulate cortex (ACC), (3) sensory cortex (both primary and secondary), and (4) the insula.[21] The prefrontal cortex is thought to be site of executive function, cognitive aspects of pain, and such beneficial skills as coping. The ACC is part of the limbic system and considered the site of activity related to affective/emotional and motivational aspects of pain. The sensory cortex is where sensory information is processed and the secondary area neurons are some of the first to receive nociceptive input. The insula is another part of the limbic system and possibly functions as a sensory component regarding the body's overall sense of physical well-being as it related to pain.

In rheumatic disease–related pain, nociceptive afferents in the joint are located in the joint capsule and ligaments, bone, periosteum, articular fat pads, and perivascular sites.[16] They are activated by joint motion or any noxious movement or stimuli such as inflammation or injury. Two nociceptive neuropeptide neurons dominate: the isolectin-positive and the calcitonin gene-related peptide-containing neurons. Both spatial and temporal summation in a population of nerve fibers results in the sensation of pain and correlates with the magnitude.[22] The enhanced pain associated with arthritis is probably due to the response of joint afferents to the mechanical and heat stimulation present during inflammation, and chemical mediators of joint inflammation such as prostaglandins, which sensitize joint afferent fibers.[23] This inflammation-induced sensitization of articular afferents likely contributes to hyperalgesia (an increased sensitivity or response to painful stimuli), and allodynia (pain due to stimuli that do not

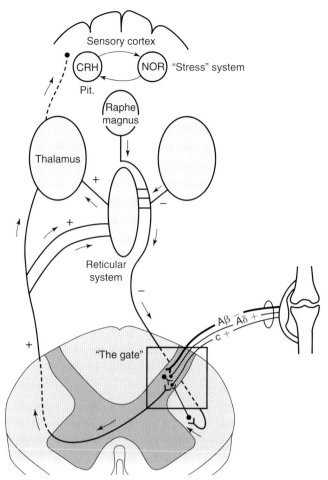

FIGURE 8-1 Diagram showing overview of pain pathways from the peripheral sensory nerves to the cerebral cortex. *CRH,* corticotropin-releasing hormone; *NOR,* norepinephrine.

typically provoke pain).[24] Also, studies of experimentally induced pain found reduced pain threshold in inflamed and noninflamed joints of children with active arthritis and to a lesser degree in the joints of children in remission.[25-27] A recent study showed significantly lower pain threshold among children with JIA, leading the authors to conclude JIA alters pain perception, leading to a continued lower pain threshold.[28] The persistence of a lowered pain threshold, even after nociceptive input to the joint might be expected to cease, suggests a role for long-lasting structural and functional changes or "neuroplastic alterations" due to "central sensitization."[29,30] Thus, peripheral and central sensitization mechanisms may be operative in arthritis-related pain.

Emotions. Pain is an emotional, as well as a sensory, experience.[31-34] There is strong correlational support for the link between negative emotions, particularly anxiety and depression, and increased pain intensity and interference in the lives of children with JRA.[1-5,8,35,36] Also, daily stressful events and negative mood have been linked to increased pain, stiffness, and fatigue in children with polyarticular JRA.[37,38] In addition, pain often varies throughout the day, especially in children with more severe disease, leading to a lower quality of life.[39] Although causality studies examining the link between emotional distress and pain have yet to be conducted, emotional distress and pain may share common etiological factors; they are reciprocally linked and can occur concurrently.[31,40] Increased anxiety can induce muscle tension, thereby

directly inducing or exacerbating musculoskeletal pain, or increased pain can induce anxiety about future prognosis or interference with life activities. Also, substance P, a neuropeptide, has been implicated in the pathophysiology of inflammatory disease, depression and anxiety, and pain, thus possibly sharing a common mediating factor.[41]

Cognitions. Cognitive factors refer to how people attend (or not) to pain and how they evaluate their pain experience. The focus in the pain literature has been on maladaptive rather than adaptive thinking. Cognitive processing of pain can be maladaptive in at least two ways: (1) people can fail to attend to information or fail to generate self-talk that might be helpful in coping with pain, or (2) people can engage in dysfunctional thinking that leads to maladaptive coping and greater pain (such as wishful or catastrophic thinking). Catastrophizing may be the most "toxic" type of dysfunctional thinking related to pain.[42,43] Catastrophizing is thought to include three components: (1) rumination (preoccupation with pain-related thoughts); (2) magnification (exaggeration of the threat value of pain); and (3) helplessness (adopting a helpless orientation to cope with pain).[43]

Several studies have investigated cognitive coping strategies in children with arthritis. Studies in Denmark have found that catastrophizing is associated with higher pain intensity during a cold pressor paradigm[44] and clinically over a 3-week period.[45] Reid and colleagues[46] found that "emotion-focused avoidance" coping (catastrophizing and expressing negative emotions) was associated with greater pain intensity, pain duration, and anxiety. Varni and colleagues[47] found that "cognitive self-instruction" (primarily wishful thinking) was related to greater emotional distress and that "cognitive refocusing" (engaging in activities as a distraction from pain) was related to less pain intensity and emotional distress. Another study found that "pain control and rational thinking" (controlling and decreasing pain while avoiding catastrophizing) predicted lower pain intensity.[6]

Behaviors. When children are in pain, they exhibit a wide variety of pain behaviors, such as limping, grimacing, crying, resting, or asking for medication. How others respond to these pain behaviors can be adaptive or maladaptive for the child experiencing pain. Pain behaviors such as guarding and malpositioning of affected joints may be maladaptive for children with arthritis. Caregivers' responses to children's pain-related behaviors may also be maladaptive, such as when parents allow children to avoid attending school, which results in low academic performance and missed opportunities for social interactions. Conversely, if children engage in "well" behaviors (e.g., positive coping strategies) and parents reinforce adaptive behaviors, children would be expected to experience less pain and disability from pain. This operant behavioral perspective is well supported in the pediatric pain literature, mostly with respect to chronic abdominal pain or headache.[48] For instance, one study found that children with JRA who reported resting more and withdrawing from activities showed higher levels of pain and emotional distress.[47] Another study found that children with JRA who engaged in "approach" coping (which included talking to a friend or family member about how they felt) showed less functional disability.[46] There is some evidence that mothers of children with more severe arthritis engage in overprotective behaviors that can impede children's autonomy and management of their pain and other symptoms.[49]

Treatment Implications. A biobehavioral model of pain would suggest a number of treatment options.[15] Early identification and aggressive pharmacological treatment of chronic arthritis could lead to enhanced pain relief and improved function, both in the short term and long term, via a reduction in peripheral and central sensitization mechanisms. Adequate control of the inflammatory disease is of utmost importance in the overall approach to pain management. Adherence to effective pharmacological therapies (see Chapters 12 and

13) can be less than optimal, and strategies for improving and maintaining adherence need to be routinely implemented in pediatric rheumatology practice.[50]

There are neurochemical mechanisms that suggest the value of nonpharmacological therapies in the treatment of arthritis-related pain, such as cooling and resting inflamed joints (to control nociceptive inputs and avoid peripheral sensitization) and relaxation or other psychological treatments to control pain by influencing "central" mechanisms.[29]

Psychological interventions that reduce negative emotional states would be expected to directly or indirectly reduce pain intensity and pain interference. Helping children to manage disease-related stressors (e.g., relaxation and problem-solving techniques) should result in concomitant reductions in negative emotions and pain. Enlisting the social support and reinforcement of family and friends should foster greater participation in social and recreational activities by patients, thereby reducing emotional distress and preoccupation with pain and suffering. Psychopharmacological agents (such as the serotonin-specific reuptake inhibitors, or SSRIs) could help reduce depression and pain through common biological pathways.

For children who are not "mindful" or fail to attend to their thoughts about pain, increasing their awareness of these thoughts (by using "thought diaries" to record thoughts when their pain is bothersome) may be a useful first step in learning to cope with their pain. However, without additional coping strategies, just making children mindful of their pain-related thoughts could lead to nonadaptive thinking.

Cognitive "restructuring" may be helpful in countering nonadaptive thinking about pain. This involves having children identify negative thoughts (e.g., "I can't do anything to make my pain better"), challenge or question these thoughts, and substitute more helpful thoughts (e.g., "I can distract myself or do relaxation exercises to reduce my pain"). There may be a role for distraction in the management of pain, such as encouraging children to engage in behaviors that divert their attention from their pain. Imagery techniques (e.g., vividly imagining a relaxing place or experience) combined with relaxation exercises are often helpful in diverting attention from pain and reducing muscle tension, thereby reducing pain.

Parents are important role models for their children and need to be made aware of how they cope with their own pain (such as headaches) and thereby influence how their children cope with pain. One may need to directly assist parents in learning more adaptive strategies for coping with pain so they can model these strategies for their children (e.g., not avoid responsibilities because of pain and use effective medical or psychological therapies to control pain). Providers also need to teach family members (especially parents) and friends to respond in adaptive ways to children's pain behaviors. This would include not being overly solicitous and attentive to pain behaviors and, instead, reinforcing alternative and adaptive coping strategies. Children require assistance in finding ways (in spite of their pain) to do what they want and need to do. Also, cautioning parents to avoid being overly protective will help their children develop autonomy and self-management skills. Pain beliefs are influential on the longitudinal course of pain in JIA, and parents' pain beliefs obviously have an impact on the child's. Dysfunctional health beliefs in patients with high pain persist over time.[51]

COGNITIVE-BEHAVIORAL TREATMENTS FOR PAIN

Cognitive-behavioral therapy (CBT) approaches to chronic pediatric pain typically involve teaching children to use deep breathing, guided imagery, and relaxation, and to replace maladaptive thinking (such as

catastrophizing) with adaptive thinking (such as focusing on what can be done to control pain and encouraging oneself to engage in more effective coping). Parents are taught to encourage their children to stay as active as possible and to engage in positive coping. Parents are also taught to avoid reinforcing pain behaviors (such as allowing children to avoid school or other responsibilities). A CBT approach, in conjunction with standard pharmacological treatments, is consistent with the biobehavioral model of pain and is empirically supported as a treatment for chronic pediatric pain.[52-54] A recent meta-analysis of CBT interventions for chronic pediatric pain (mostly on chronic headaches) found large positive effects on pain reduction and that self-administered versus therapist-administered programs showed similar benefits in pain reduction.[55]

Two published studies have tested CBT for children with JRA. Lavine and colleagues[56] used a multiple baseline design with eight children with JRA to evaluate a six-session treatment that included relaxation and biofeedback training. They showed significant reductions in pain intensity and pain-related behaviors at follow-up. Walco and colleagues[57] used a single-group pretest-posttest design with 13 children with JRA to evaluate an eight-session treatment that included progressive muscle relaxation, deep breathing, and guided imagery. Parents were seen for two sessions to review how they could reinforce "well" behaviors and avoid reinforcing pain behaviors. There were significant reductions in pain intensity at immediate follow-up as well as maintenance of gains at 6-month and 12-month follow-ups. Although these studies are promising, they involved small samples and no control or alternative treatment comparison groups. There is a need for well-controlled, multisite pain intervention trials for children and adolescents with arthritis.

There is one study that has shown the benefits of daily massage for children with juvenile rheumatoid arthritis.[58] Children who were massaged 15 minutes a day for 30 days by a trained parent experienced less pain (frequency and severity) and pain-limiting activities relative to a control group. However, the sample size was small (N = 20) and the children were not randomized to conditions. More studies are needed to demonstrated the efficacy of this adjunctive mode of treatment for pain, as well as other complementary and alternative medicine approaches patients and their caregivers use without informing their pediatric rheumatologist.[59]

PAIN MEASURES

As with adults, self-report measures of pain are considered the gold standard for assessing pain intensity, duration, and location in children 3 years of age and older.[60] There have been at least six pain measures that have been validated for use with children and adolescents with arthritis.[61] The most widely used and validated self-report measure of pain for patients with JRA is the Pediatric Pain Questionnaire (PPQ) developed by Varni and colleagues.[62] The PPQ contains a visual analog scale (VAS), which is a 10-cm horizontal line, anchored with the descriptors "not hurting" or "no pain" and "hurting a whole lot" or "severe pain." The patient makes a vertical line on the VAS for present pain and the VAS for worst pain for the previous week. The PPQ also contains a body gender-neutral outline that shows the front and back sides of the body. There are four boxes underneath descriptive categories of pain intensity ("none," "mild," "moderate," "severe"). Patients are given a standard set of eight colors. From these they select colors to match pain intensities (coloring the four boxes with selected colors), and they apply these colors to the appropriate place on the body outline with the color intensity match. Children younger than 7 years will usually need to be read instructions for completing the PPQ.[63] The PPQ VAS is useful in documenting the intensity of pain, and the body outline allows patients to localize their pain, as well as rate its intensity.

Investigators should consider using electronic pain measures (such as e-diaries), rather than pencil and paper ones, because electronic measures have been validated with patients with arthritis, they are feasible, and they result in fewer errors and omissions compared with paper ones.[9,60,64] Stinson and colleagues have developed a comprehensive electronic measure of pain for young people with rheumatic disease.[65,66] It is similar to the PPQ but can be used on computers,

handheld devices, and eventually suitable for use in electronic medical records. It has a faces pain scale for children 4 to 7 years of age and a 10-point VAS for patients 8 to 16 years of age to rate pain intensity (Fig. 8-2). It also has a body outline to identify pain location (Fig. 8-3) and a summary report that is given to providers (Fig. 8-4).

Observational measures of pain behaviors need to be further developed for children with arthritis, particularly those children who are preverbal or have limited verbal capacity.[67] Jaworski and colleagues have developed an observational measure for patients with JRA.[68] This

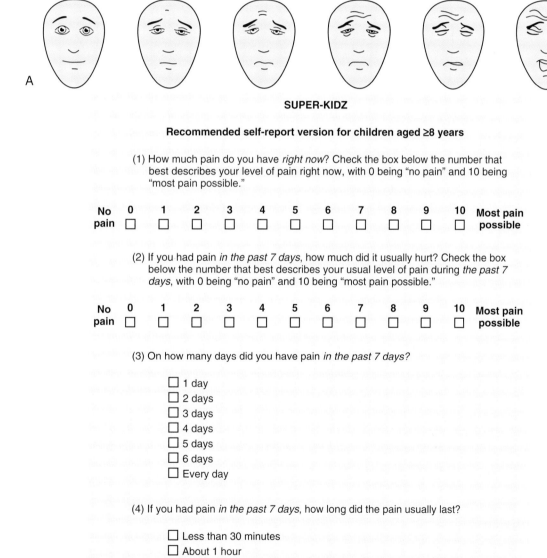

SUPER-KIDZ

Recommended self-report version for children aged <8 years

(1) These faces show how much something can hurt. This first face shows no pain. The faces show more and more pain up to the last face – it shows very much pain. Select the face that shows how much you hurt right now.

A

SUPER-KIDZ

Recommended self-report version for children aged ≥8 years

(1) How much pain do you have *right now*? Check the box below the number that best describes your level of pain right now, with 0 being "no pain" and 10 being "most pain possible."

No pain   0 1 2 3 4 5 6 7 8 9 10   Most pain possible

(2) If you had pain *in the past 7 days*, how much did it usually hurt? Check the box below the number that best describes your usual level of pain during *the past 7 days*, with 0 being "no pain" and 10 being "most pain possible."

No pain   0 1 2 3 4 5 6 7 8 9 10   Most pain possible

(3) On how many days did you have pain *in the past 7 days*?

☐ 1 day
☐ 2 days
☐ 3 days
☐ 4 days
☐ 5 days
☐ 6 days
☐ Every day

(4) If you had pain *in the past 7 days*, how long did the pain usually last?

☐ Less than 30 minutes
☐ About 1 hour
☐ Between 1 and 3 hours
☐ About half the day
☐ All day or longer
☐ No pain in the past 7 days

B

FIGURE 8-2 Pain scales for children 4 to 7 years **(A)** and 8 to 16 years **(B)**. (Reprinted with permission from Dr. Jennifer Stinson, The Hospital for Sick Children, Toronto, Ontario, Canada.)

Select all the parts of your body where you have had pain in the past 7 days.

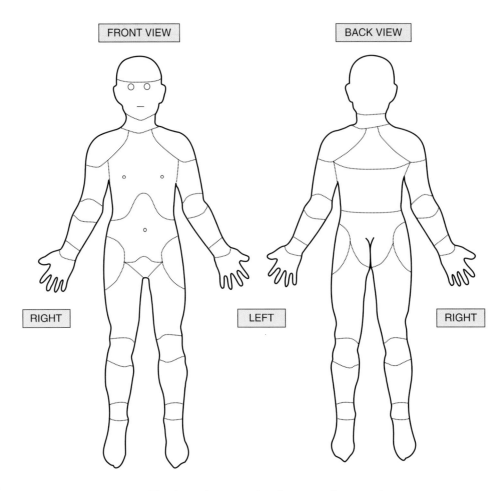

Thank you for answering these questions.

FIGURE 8-3 Body outline to identify pain location. Select all the parts of your body where you have had pain in the past 7 days. (Reprinted with permission from Dr. Jennifer Stinson, The Hospital for Sick Children, Toronto, Ontario, Canada.)

measure contains six pain behaviors (guarding, bracing, active rubbing, rigidity, single flexing, and multiple flexing) that are coded by observers who view a videotape of a 10-minute session during which children perform a series of maneuvers that include sitting, walking, standing, and reclining in a standardized sequence. This measure has been found to be reliable and valid, but it requires fairly extensive training of observers and has been used in only one study thus far.[63] Observational measures can supplement self-report measures and document functional limitations.

FUTURE DIRECTIONS

More work is needed for developing usable, reliable, and valid measures of pain and preferable in an electronic format that can be part of electronic medical records. Patients and/or caregivers can complete these electronic measures in clinic as part of routine assessments. The other exciting development in CBT pain interventions is the use of "e-health formats," such as Internet-based and phone apps. One example is an Internet-based self-management program ("Teens Taking Charge: Managing Arthritis Online") for adolescents with

arthritis, developed by Stinson and colleagues,[69] which resulted in significant lower pain intensity compared to a control group. E-health formats offer several advantages: (1) they can be highly structured, thus enhancing treatment fidelity; (2) they can also be tailored to the specific issues affecting patients and families; (3) more patients and families can have access to pain interventions from their homes, which is particularly beneficial for rural families who would have to travel many miles to receive face-to-face interventions; (4) engaging elements such as audio, animation, and interactivity can be built into these programs to make them more attractive and encourage adherence to the pain interventions; (5) with Web-based programs, outcome assessments can be made online and use of the treatment and assessment programs can be monitored in real time.[70] Finally, many patients with JA are doing well with advancements in pharmacological treatment, and the need for CBT adjunctive interventions specifically for pain might be useful for smaller and smaller numbers of patients. This speaks to the importance of assessing and enhancing adherence to pharmacological treatments that are effective in reducing pain, stiffness, and limiting joint damage and disease-related disability.[50]

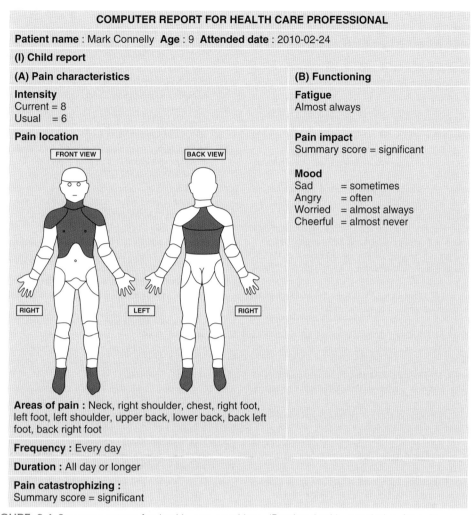

COMPUTER REPORT FOR HEALTH CARE PROFESSIONAL

Patient name : Mark Connelly **Age** : 9 **Attended date** : 2010-02-24

(I) Child report

(A) Pain characteristics

Intensity
Current = 8
Usual   = 6

Pain location

FRONT VIEW   BACK VIEW

RIGHT   LEFT   RIGHT

Areas of pain : Neck, right shoulder, chest, right foot, left foot, left shoulder, upper back, lower back, back left foot, back right foot

Frequency : Every day

Duration : All day or longer

Pain catastrophizing :
Summary score = significant

(B) Functioning

Fatigue
Almost always

Pain impact
Summary score = significant

Mood
Sad   = sometimes
Angry   = often
Worried   = almost always
Cheerful   = almost never

FIGURE 8-4 Summary report for health care providers. (Reprinted with permission from Dr. Jennifer Stinson, The Hospital for Sick Children, Toronto, Ontario, Canada.)

REFERENCES

1. R.A. Gragg, M.A. Rapoff, M.B. Danovsky, et al., Assessing chronic musculoskeletal pain associated with rheumatic disease: further validation of the Pediatric Pain Questionnaire, J. Pediatr. Psychol. 21 (1996) 237–250.
2. K.J. Hagglund, L.M. Schopp, K.R. Alberts, et al., Predicting pain among children with juvenile rheumatoid arthritis, Arthritis Care Res. 8 (1995) 36–42.
3. K.L. Thompson, J.W. Varni, V. Hanson, Comprehensive assessment of pain in juvenile rheumatoid arthritis: an empirical model, J. Pediatr. Psychol. 12 (1987) 241–255.
4. J.W. Varni, M.A. Rapoff, S.A. Waldron, et al., Chronic pain and emotional distress in children and adolescents, J. Dev. Behav. Pediatr. 17 (1996) 154–161.
5. C.K. Ross, J.V. Lavigne, J.R. Hayford, et al., Validity of reported pain as a measure of clinical state in juvenile rheumatoid arthritis, Ann. Rheum. Dis. 48 (1989) 817–819.
6. L.E. Schanberg, J.C. Lefebvre, F.J. Keefe, et al., Pain coping and the pain experience in children with juvenile chronic arthritis, Pain 73 (1997) 181–189.
7. B. Benestad, O. Vinje, M.B. Veierød, et al., Quantitative and qualitative assessments of pain in children with juvenile chronic arthritis based on the Norwegian version of the Pediatric Pain Questionnaire, Scand. J. Rheumatol. 25 (1996) 293–299.
8. L.E. Schanberg, K.K. Anthony, K.M. Gil, et al., Daily pain and symptoms in children with polyarticular arthritis, Arthritis Rheum. 48 (2003) 1390–1397.
9. J.N. Stinson, B.J. Stevens, B.M. Feldman, et al., Construct validity of a multidimensional electronic pain diary for adolescents with arthritis, Pain 136 (2008) 281–292.
10. D.J. Lovell, G.W. Walco, Pain associated with juvenile rheumatoid arthritis, Pediatr. Clin. North Am. 36 (1989) 1015–1027.
11. L.S. Peterson, T. Mason, A.M. Nelson, et al., Psychosocial outcomes and health status of adults who have had juvenile rheumatoid arthritis, Arthritis Rheum. 40 (1997) 2235–2240.
12. [No authors listed], Pain terms: a list with definitions and notes on usage: recommended by the IASP subcommittee on taxonomy, Pain 6 (1979) 249–252.
13. R. Melzack, P.D. Wall, Pain and mechanisms: a new theory, Science 150 (1965) 971–979.
14. R.J. Gatchel, Y.B. Peng, M.L. Peters, et al., The biopsychosocial approach to chronic pain: scientific advances and future directions, Psychol. Bull. 133 (2007) 581–624.
15. M.A. Rapoff, C.B. Lindsley, The pain puzzle: a visual and conceptual metaphor for understanding and treating pain in pediatric rheumatic disease, J. Rheumatol. 58 (Suppl.) (2000) 29–33.
16. A. Randich, Neural substrates of pain and analgesia, Arthritis Care Res. 6 (1993) 171–177.

17. P.A. McGrath, Pain in Children: Nature, Assessment and Treatment, Guilford, New York, 1990.

18. H.G. Schaible, B.D. Grubb, Afferent and spinal mechanisms of joint pain, Pain 55 (1993) 5–54.

19. H.G. Schaible, R.F. Schmidt, Effects of an experimental arthritis on the sensory properties of fine articular afferent units, J. Neurophysiol. 54 (1985) 1109–1122.

20. S. Marchand, The Phenomenon of Pain, International Association for the Study of Pain, Seattle, WA, 2012.

21. M.P. Jensen, A neuropsychological model of pain: research and clinical implications, J. Pain 11 (2010) 2–12.

22. D.T. Felson, The sources of pain in knee osteoarthritis, Curr. Opin. Rheum. 17 (2005) 624–629.

23. R.A. Meyer, J.N. Campbell, S.N. Raja, Peripheral neural mechanisms of nociception, in: P.D. Wall, R. Melzack (Eds.), Textbook of Pain, third ed., Churchill Livingstone, Edinburgh, 1994.

24. J. Levine, Y. Taiwo, Inflammatory pain, in: P.D. Wall, R. Melzack (Eds.), Textbook of Pain, third ed., Churchill Livingstone, Edinburgh, 1994.

25. J.A. Hogeweg, A.C.J. Huygen, C. De Jong-De Vos Van Steenwijk, et al., The pain threshold in juvenile chronic arthritis, Br. J. Rheumatol. 34 (1995) 61–67.

26. J.A. Hogeweg, W. Kuis, R.A.B. Oostendorp, et al., General and segmental reduced pain thresholds in juvenile chronic arthritis, Pain 62 (1995) 11–17.

27. M. Thastum, R. Zachariae, M. Schøler, et al., Cold pressor pain: comparing responses of juvenile arthritis patients and their parents, Scand. J. Rheumatol. 26 (1997) 272–279.

28. A. Leegarrd, J.J. Lomholdt, M. Thastum, T. Herlin, Decreased pain threshold in juvenile idiopathic arthritis: a cross-sectional study, J. Rheumatol. 40 (2013) 1212–1217.

29. W. Kuis, C.J. Heijnen, J.A. Hogeweg, et al., How painful is juvenile chronic arthritis?, Arch. Dis. Child. 77 (1997) 451–453.

30. T.J. Coderre, J. Katz, Peripheral and central hyperexcitability: differential signs and symptoms in persistent pain, Behav. Brain Sci. 20 (1997) 404–419.

31. S.M. Banks, R.D. Kerns, Explaining high rates of depression in chronic pain: a diathesis-stress framework, Psychol. Bull. 119 (1996) 95–110.

32. J.W. Burns, P.J. Quartana, S. Bruehl, Anger inhibition and pain: conceptualizations, evidence, and new directions, J. Behav. Med. 31 (2008) 259–279.

33. L.C. Campbell, D.J. Clauw, F.J. Keefe, Persistent pain and depression: a biopsychosocial perspective, Biol. Psychiatry 54 (2003) 399–409.

34. C.R. Chapman, The psychophysiology of pain, in: J.D. Loser (Ed.), Bonica's Management of Pain, third ed., Lippincott, Williams & Wilkins, Philadelphia, 2001.

35. A.L. Hoff, T.M. Palermo, M. Schluchter, et al., Longitudinal relationships of depressive symptoms to pain intensity and functional disability among children with disease-related pain, J. Pediatr. Psychol. 31 (2006) 1046–1056.

36. J.W. Varni, M.A. Rapoff, S.A. Waldron, et al., Effects of perceived stress on pediatric chronic pain, J. Behav. Med. 19 (1996) 515–528.

37. L.E. Schanberg, M.J. Sandstrom, K. Starr, et al., The relationship of daily mood and stressful events to symptoms in juvenile rheumatic disease, Arthritis Care Res. 13 (2000) 33–41.

38. L.E. Schanberg, K.M. Gil, K.K. Anthony, et al., Pain, stiffness, and fatigue in juvenile polyarticular arthritis: contemporaneous stressful events and mood as predictors, Arthritis Rheum. 52 (2005) 1196–1204.

39. S.M. Tupper, A.M. Rosenberg, P. Pahwa, J.N. Stinson, Pain intensity variability and its variability and its relationship with quality of life in youths with juvenile idiopathic arthritis, Arthritis Care Res. 65 (2013) 563–570.

40. A. Gamsa, Is emotional disturbance a precipitator or a consequence of chronic pain?, Pain 42 (1990) 183–195.

41. M.A. Rosenkranz, Substance P at the nexus of mind and body in chronic inflammation and affective disorders, Psychol. Bull. 133 (2007) 1007–1037.

42. F.J. Keefe, M.E. Rumble, C.D. Scipio, et al., Psychological aspects of persistent pain: current state of the science, J. Pain 5 (2004) 195–211.

43. M.J.L. Sullivan, S.R. Bishop, J. Pivik, The Pain Catastrophizing Scale: development and validation, Psychol. Assess. 7 (1995) 524–532.

44. M. Thastum, R. Zachariae, M. Schøler, et al., A Danish adaptation of the Pain Coping Questionnaire for children: preliminary data concerning reliability and validity, Acta Paediatr. 88 (1998) 132–138.

45. M. Thastum, T. Herlin, R. Zachariae, Relationship of pain-coping strategies and pain-specific beliefs to pain experience in children with juvenile idiopathic arthritis, Arthritis Care Res. 53 (2005) 178–184.

46. G.J. Reid, C.A. Gilbert, P.J. McGrath, The Pain Coping Questionnaire: preliminary validation, Pain 76 (1998) 83–96.

47. J.W. Varni, S.A. Waldron, R.A. Gragg, Development of the Waldron/Varni Pediatric Pain Coping Inventory, Pain 67 (1996) 141–150.

48. L.M. Dahlquist, M.S. Nagel, Chronic and recurrent pain, in: M.C. Roberts, R.G. Steele (Eds.), Handbook of Pediatric Psychology, fourth ed., Guilford Press, New York, 2009, pp. 153–170.

49. T.G. Power, L.M. Dahlquist, S.M. Thompson, R. Warren, Interactions between children with juvenile rheumatoid arthritis and their mothers, J. Pediatr. Psychol. 28 (2003) 213–221.

50. M.A. Rapoff, Adherence to Pediatric Medical Regimens, 2nd ed., Springer, New York, 2010.

51. M. Thastrum, T. Herlin, Pain-specific beliefs and pain experience in children with juvenile idiopathic arthritis: a longitudinal study, J. Rheumatol. 38 (2011) 155–160.

52. C. Eccleston, S. Morley, A. Williams, et al., Systematic review of randomized controlled trials of psychological therapy for chronic pain in children and adolescents, with a sub-set meta-analysis of pain relief, Pain 99 (2002) 157–165.

53. E.W. Holden, M.M. Deichmann, J.D. Levy, Empirically supported treatments in pediatric psychology: recurrent pediatric headache, J. Pediatr. Psychol. 24 (1999) 91–109.

54. D.M. Janicke, J.W. Finney, Empirically supported treatments in pediatric psychology: recurrent abdominal pain, J. Pediatr. Psychol. 24 (1999) 115–127.

55. T.M. Palermo, C. Eccleston, A.S. Lewandowski, et al., Randomized controlled trials of psychological therapies for management of chronic pain in children and adolescents: an updated meta-analytic review, Pain 148 (2010) 387–397.

56. J.V. Lavigne, C.K. Ross, S.L. Berry, et al., Evaluation of a psychological treatment package for treating pain in juvenile rheumatoid arthritis, Arthritis Care Res. 5 (1992) 101–110.

57. G.A. Walco, J.W. Varni, N.T. Ilowite, Cognitive behavioral pain management in children with juvenile rheumatoid arthritis, Pediatrics 89 (1992) 1075–1079.

58. T.F. Field, M. Hernandez-Reif, S. Seligman, et al., Juvenile rheumatoid arthritis: benefits from massage therapy, J. Pediatr. Psychol. 22 (1997) 607–617.

59. K. Zebracki, K. Holzman, K.J. Bitter, et al., Brief report: use of complementary and alternative medicine and psychological functioning in Latino children with juvenile idiopathic arthritis or arthralgia, J. Pediatr. Psychol. 32 (2007) 1006–1010.

60. J.N. Stinson, G.C. Petroz, G. Tait, et al., e-Ouch: usability testing of an electronic chronic pain diary for adolescents with arthritis, Clin. J. Pain 22 (2006) 295–305.

Entire reference list is available online at www.expertconsult.com.

CHAPTER 9

Imaging in Pediatric Rheumatic Diseases

Andrea S. Doria, Johannes Roth, Paul S. Babyn

Imaging often plays a key role in establishing the presence, severity, and extent of joint disease. It can also help monitor for disease complications, exclude other diagnoses, and assess treatment response. Imaging can provide early diagnosis and visualization of inflammatory abnormalities including synovitis and osteochondral damage. This chapter provides an approach to the imaging investigation of the child with inflammatory arthritis and juvenile idiopathic arthritis in particular. The distinct advantages and disadvantages of the available imaging modalities are initially reviewed as this forms the basis for rational imaging evaluation (Box 9-1).[1-9]

A variety of imaging modalities aid in the assessment and diagnosis of a multitude of inflammatory disorders, as well as their complications. Examples include the use of angiography for the vasculitides, high-resolution chest computerized tomography scans for lung disease of systemic sclerosis, and magnetic resonance imaging for the inflammatory myopathies, as well as sonography for enthesitis, vasculitis, myopathies, and localized scleroderma. Some of these indications, such as the sonographic assessment of localized scleroderma and myositis, are still being evaluated. Other indications and techniques are well established and are covered in the disease-specific chapters.

AVAILABLE IMAGING MODALITIES

Radiography

Radiography remains a frequently used means used to evaluate joint abnormalities. Radiography is typically used for assessment of symptomatic and often contralateral joints. Intraarticular soft tissue components have very similar radiographic densities and cannot be clearly differentiated from each other or from adjacent muscles, fascia, tendons, ligaments, nerves, or vessels by radiography. Displacement of adjacent periarticular fat deposits help determine joint effusions of the elbow, knee, and ankle. However, the relationship of these radiolucent fat stripes in other joints is more complex, making accurate determination of joint effusions—for example, about the hip and shoulder—more difficult radiographically. Radiographic features of joint disease are described in Box 9-2.

In neonates and young children, radiography demonstrates wide apparent joint spaces representing immature unossified epiphyses. These chondroepiphyses will eventually ossify, reducing the apparent joint space to the thickness of the opposing layers of articular cartilage and any intervening joint fluid.

Occasionally, intraarticular gas can be seen as a normal finding, but it can also be seen following infection, trauma, or invasive procedure. Radiographically, normal intraarticular gas appears as an intraarticular crescentic lucency and is caused by sudden lowering of intraarticular pressure by muscle pulls or external traction (Fig. 9-1). In the presence of a significant joint effusion, this phenomenon

cannot normally be produced; however, its presence cannot be relied upon to exclude effusion. Intraarticular gas can also be identified with sonography or magnetic resonance imaging (MRI). On MRI, intraarticular gas may simulate meniscal tears, intraarticular loose bodies, or chondrocalcinosis.

The presence of a large amount of fluid (effusion or hemarthrosis) in an elbow joint may generate a "sail sign" that describes the elevation of the anterior fat pad to create a silhouette similar to a billowing spinnaker sail from a boat (Fig. 9-2).

Although radiography should be used initially in the evaluation of joints, the introduction of the cross-sectional imaging techniques has provided a significant improvement in anatomical delineation and diagnosis.

Sonography

Recent advances in sonography, including better transducers and more pediatric musculoskeletal experience, have stimulated increased use of this modality in the assessment of pediatric joint disease. Sonography is ideal for assessing the pediatric musculoskeletal system, largely because of its ability to visualize intraarticular structures such as cartilage and thickened synovium without the need for radiation (Fig. 9-3). Sonography is very sensitive in detecting joint effusions. Multiple joints can be assessed at the same time, and even very young children can be examined without sedation. It can also be used to guide joint aspiration or injection (Fig. 9-4).[11] Intraarticular masses may also be detected with sonography, although their appearance is often nonspecific. Tendons and ligaments can be assessed with higher frequency transducers.[12] Normal tendons have an echogenic fibrillar appearance on ultrasound. Fluid within the synovial sheath appears as an anechoic halo surrounding the tendon, whereas synovial thickening appears as a hypoechoic thickening around the tendon (Fig. 9-5). Sonography has the highest spatial resolution of the commonly used imaging techniques, thereby allowing for a detailed view of even very small structures such as the pulleys of the flexor tendons or entheses of the extensor tendons and collateral ligaments of the fingers (Figs. 9-6 and 9-7). Visualization of these structures has enhanced our understanding of the complexity of the musculoskeletal system in these areas, including, for example, pathology in dactylitis. Vascular anatomy can be assessed by combining sonography with Doppler effects. Synovial hyperemia, for example, leads to increased Doppler signal. Sonography can also be used to assess for other periarticular soft tissue abnormalities including popliteal cysts or other soft tissue masses.

Currently, the major limitation for a more widespread use of sonography has been a lack of standardization in the sonographic assessment of the pediatric joint as well as a lack of normative data.[13] The latter is of great importance in order to reliably distinguish pathological findings from normal sonoanatomy.

BOX 9-1　Commonly Used Imaging Modalities in Pediatric Rheumatology

Conventional Radiography

Traditional standard for assessment of established joint damage including bone erosions, joint space narrowing, joint subluxation, misalignment, or ankylosis

Advantages: Low cost, high availability, helpful in differential diagnosis, reasonable reproducibility, validated assessment methods.

Disadvantages: Not sensitive in detecting early bone disease or soft tissue manifestations, projectional superimposition, use of ionizing radiation.

Ultrasound

Ultrasound can assess joint effusion and synovitis by detecting synovial thickening of inflamed joints, bursas, or tendon sheaths. Vascularity can be assessed with Doppler sonography. Follow-up studies have shown improvement of ultrasound measures of synovitis following successful treatment.

Ultrasound can be used to guide punctures of joints, bursas, and tendon sheaths, improving the success rates of diagnostic or therapeutic aspirations.

Advantages: Noninvasive, relatively low cost, lack of ionizing radiation, ability to visualize both inflammatory and destructive disease manifestations, easy repeatability, possibility of examining several joint regions at one session, potential for guiding interventions.

Disadvantages: Not all joint areas are accessible, operator dependence, time for examination.

Magnetic Resonance Imaging (MRI)

MRI directly visualizes both inflammatory and destructive aspects of arthritic disease. It has potential for accurate monitoring of treatment efficacy, and allows assessment of all structures in arthritic disease including synovial membrane; intraarticular and extraarticular fluid collections; cartilage; bone erosions and edema; ligaments, tendons, and tendon sheaths.

Advantages: Multiplanar tomographic imaging, excellent soft tissue contrast, lack of ionizing radiation, bone marrow edema visualization and direct visualization of cartilage. It is more sensitive than clinical and radiographic examination for detection of inflammatory soft tissue changes and early bone changes.

Two novel MRI techniques, whole-body MRI and high-resolution MRI, have a promising role in imaging enthesitis. Multichannel scanners using accelerated imaging techniques (parallel imaging), a whole-body surface coil system, and a freely moving table enables imaging of the entire body in a single head-to-toe scan in a relatively short period of time. This technique is useful in detecting multiple sites of enthesitis in patients with spondyloarthropathies in one single imaging session. High-resolution MRI enables assessment of small joints such as finger joints, where tendon insertions typically have low spatial resolution.[7]

Disadvantages: Potential allergic contrast reactions, higher cost/lower availability compared with radiography, longer examination times, and evaluation of only a few joints per session, possible need for sedation/general anesthesia, safety concerns with ferromagnetic materials.

Despite a high reported sensitivity of MRI in detecting enthesitis, it lacks specificity. Thus, differentiating between the different etiologies of enthesitis on the basis of their MRI characteristics is difficult and not always possible.[7]

MRI and/or ultrasound can be used in evaluation of suspected but not definite inflammatory joint disease to determine presence of synovitis, tenosynovitis, enthesitis, or bone erosions. Both may be helpful in verifying inflammatory disease response to therapy or choosing appropriate follow-up.

Computed Tomography (CT)

CT is a very good method to demonstrate early and already established bone changes in spondyloarthropathies.

Advantages: For detection of early bone changes such as erosions and regional ankylosis, CT seems to be the best method. It can also be used to guide intraarticular corticosteroid injection into inflammatory sacroiliac (SI) joints, although ultrasound-guided imaging is more frequently used.[8]

Disadvantages: Although CT is superior to conventional radiography in the diagnosis of sacroiliitis, sclerosis and ankylosis can easily be overdiagnosed by CT, as shown in a study of healthy controls.[9] Also, CT is inferior to MRI in the detection of early inflammation. Because of the radiation exposure of CT other techniques are preferred nowadays.

Data from Refs. 1-9

BOX 9-2　Radiographic Features of Inflammatory Joint Disease

Osteopenia
Joint effusion
Joint space narrowing with focal or diffuse cartilage thinning
Bone erosions, subchondral cysts, and bone resorption
Changes in size of ossification centers
Subchondral sclerosis and osteophyte formation
Periosteal new bone formation
Malalignment, subluxation, dislocation
Joint ankylosis
Joint disorganization and destruction
Soft tissue swelling, atrophy, and calcification
Spinal manifestations

Data from K. Johnson, J. Gardner-Medwin, Childhood arthritis: classification and radiology, *Clin Radiol* 57 (2002) 47–58.[10]

Normal Sonoanatomy

The principal difference between the pediatric and adult joint relates to the skeletal development. This is important as the articulating bones will usually serve as a reference point in musculoskeletal sonography. Whereas the skeleton of an adult is completely ossified except for the articular cartilage portion, a varying degree of hyaline cartilage, and in some locations fibrocartilage, is present in children in addition to articular cartilage (Fig. 9-8).[14] At birth, the primary ossification centers in the diaphysis of the long bones are already present, whereas the secondary ossification centers in some epiphyses will only develop subsequently.[15] In some locations, for example the humeral head, multiple secondary ossification centers will develop, and the irregular appearance (as well as the interruptions between these ossification centers) should not be misinterpreted as pathology (Fig. 9-9). The same principle applies to the short bones with one or several ossification centers appearing over time. In some joints, for example the wrist joint, a significant range of ages at which these ossification centers will appear and develop can be observed in the various carpal bones.[16] The ossification progress will also be influenced by the individual progress of maturation.

The presence of variable amounts of cartilage can present significant challenges for the interpretation of radiographs.[17] In contrast,

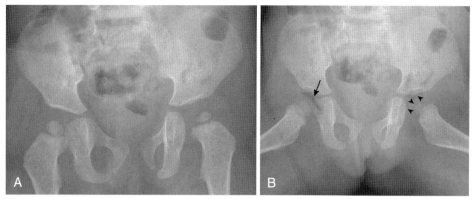

FIGURE 9-1 Two-year-old girl with left developmental hip dysplasia. **A,** Small ossification centers and wide apparent joint space from unossified epiphyseal cartilage. **B,** Normal intraarticular gas seen from traction during frog-leg radiography (*arrow*). The smaller ossification center of the left hip (*arrowheads*) compared with the normal right hip in this child reflects underlying left developmental hip dysplasia.

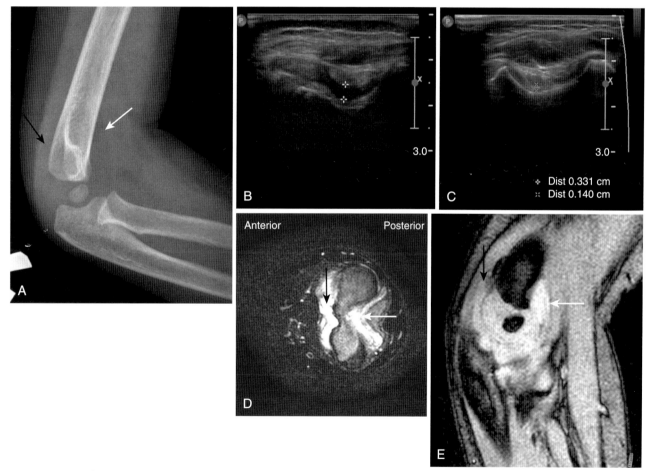

FIGURE 9-2 Right elbow hemarthrosis in a 2-year-old boy with JIA who had a traumatic injury. There is satisfactory alignment of the right radius and capitellum on lateral view and moderate joint effusion. Note the "sail sign" (*white arrow*) as a result of the elevation of the anterior fat pad of the elbow and a thin radiolucent line along the posterior synovial recess (*black arrow*). Corresponding right (**B**, pathological) and left (**C**, control) gray-scale ultrasound images of the posterior elbow show the presence of joint effusion in the right elbow posteriorly. Axial T2-weighted (**D**) and gradient echo (**E**) MR images show mild to moderate amount of hemarthrosis in the right elbow both anteriorly (*black arrow*) and posteriorly (*white arrow*).

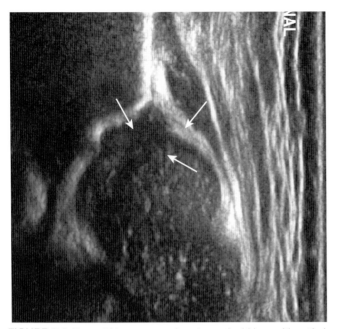

FIGURE 9-3 Normal hip sonogram in a 1-month-old boy with entirely cartilaginous femoral head. The image has been rotated for ease of visualization. The acetabular labrum composed of fibrocartilage is echogenic (*upper right arrow* of figure) on sonography. The hyaline cartilage of the acetabulum is not echogenic (*upper left arrow*). The cartilaginous femoral head and the internal vessels identified within the femoral head are normal (*lower arrow*).

sonography can delineate the cartilage outline very well. Depending on the age of the child, anechoic or hypoechoic cartilage will define the bone contour in a joint as opposed to the hyperechoic outline of the fully ossified bone seen in adults (Fig. 9-10). A careful scanning technique is essential to ensure the clear differentiation of cartilage from the possible presence of fluid in the joint, which may also appear anechoic or hypoechoic. Cartilage is also not compressible by the ultrasound probe, whereas fluid is. Finally, the anatomic location and shape of the anechoic area will help to distinguish between fluid and cartilage.

The growth plate is seen as an anechoic or hypoechoic line separating the epiphyseal from the metaphyseal bone. The cartilage itself may display hyperechogenic spots that represent vascular channels.[18] These spots or vascular channels are physiological in children and should not be interpreted as pathological (Fig. 9-11). The Outcome Measures in Rheumatoid Arthritis Clinical Trials (OMERACT) Ultrasound Group has recognized the importance of a clear description of the sonographic findings in healthy children and has recently published a set of definitions (Box 9-3).[19]

Cartilage Thickness

Joint damage, and especially cartilage loss, is one of the most important radiographic outcome parameters in inflammatory arthritis. The ultrasound assessment of cartilage has traditionally been done by measuring cartilage thickness,[20] but it is not clear if this is the best method to assess cartilage damage.

Even in adults the measurement of cartilage thickness is difficult, and careful scanning technique, as well as knowledge of ultrasound

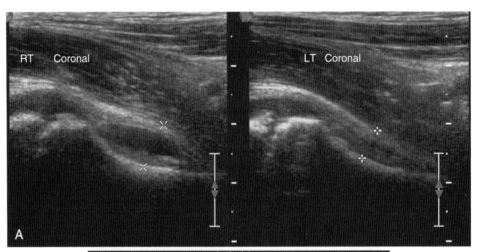

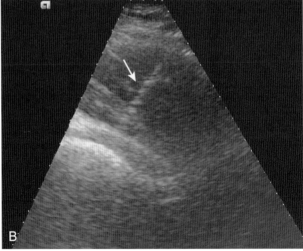

FIGURE 9-4 Ultrasound performed for question of hip joint effusion. **A,** A right hip effusion with widened joint space *(x-x)* compared with normal left hip *(+-+)*. **B,** Needle placement *(arrow)* under ultrasound guidance.

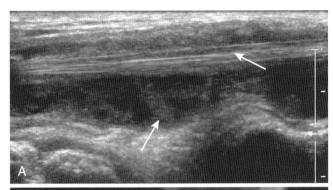

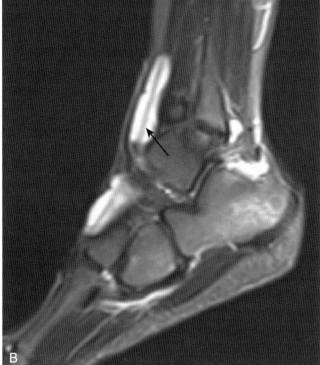

FIGURE 9-5 **A,** Longitudinal sonogram showing extensive tenosynovitis. The *upper arrow* demarcates the tendon with adjacent hypoechoic fluid and the *lower arrow* shows synovial proliferation. **B,** Corresponding sagittal T2-weighted MRI with the *arrow* showing the tendon surrounded by high signal fluid.

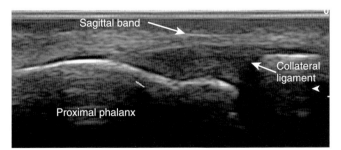

FIGURE 9-6 Longitudinal scan of the medial aspect of the PIP joint showing the medial collateral ligament as well as the sagittal band that includes fibers originating from the lumbrical as well as the interosseous muscles.

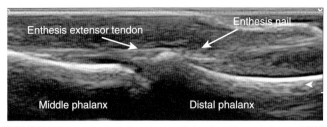

FIGURE 9-7 Longitudinal dorsal scan of the distal interphalangeal (DIP) joint showing the enthesis of the extensor tendon as well as the enthesis of the nail (*arrow*).

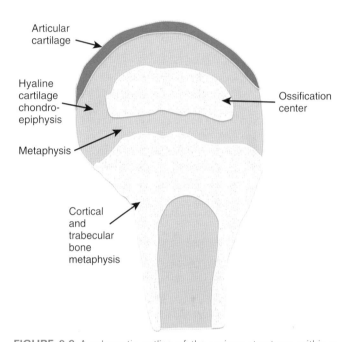

FIGURE 9-8 A schematic outline of the various structures within a bone forming a joint are shown.

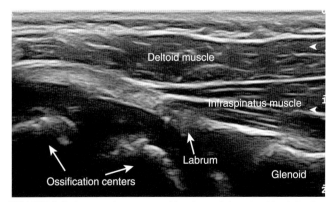

FIGURE 9-9 A posterior sonographic view of the shoulder joint in a 5-year-old girl shows the presence of various hyperechoic ossification centers with anechoic interruptions between them. This finding is normal and does not represent damage to the bone.

BOX 9-3   Definitions for the Sonographic Components of the Normal Pediatric Joint

Definition 1
The hyaline cartilage will present as a well-defined anechoic structure (with/without bright echoes/dots) that is noncompressible. The cartilage surface can (but does not have to) be detected as a hyperechoic line.

Definition 2
With advancing maturity, the epiphyseal secondary ossification center will appear as a hyperechoic structure, with a smooth or irregular surface within the cartilage.

Definition 3
Normal Joint Capsule: A hyperechoic structure that can (but does not have to) be seen over bone, cartilage, and other intraarticular tissue of the joint.

Definition 4
Normal Synovial Membrane: Under normal circumstances, the thin synovial membrane is undetectable.

Definition 5
The ossified portion of articular bone is detected as a hyperechoic line. Interruptions of this hyperechoic line may be detected at the growth plate and at the junction of two or more ossification centers.

Data from Ref. 19

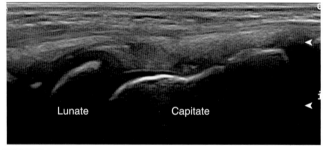

FIGURE 9-10 A longitudinal sonographic view of the wrist joint shows a partially ossified lunate bone with the outline of the future bone being defined by anechoic cartilage. The capitate bone is also partially ossified but in its proximal part the cartilage surface is seen as a thin white hyperechoic line because the cartilage surface is parallel to the ultrasound probe, which results in this reflection.

physics, is essential in order to obtain precise measurements.[21] Depending on the location, the presence of irregular ossification centers in the epiphysis will result in significant challenges to obtain precise measurements in pediatrics. Studies assessing cartilage thickness in healthy children have therefore resulted in very high coefficients of variation especially in the wrist, which limits the utility of cartilage thickness assessments, particularly in younger children.[22] Instead of assessing cartilage thickness, the assessment of the cartilage surface might be an alternative. Studies in adults have demonstrated that the earliest sign of cartilage damage is a blunting of the cartilage surface.[23]

Doppler Sonography

The metabolic activity in the musculoskeletal system of children during growth coincides with significant blood flow into and within bones as well as the joints. This blood flow can be detected with Doppler sonography and needs to be distinguished from pathological blood flow, which is an important sign of active synovitis. Increased Doppler flow has also been shown as the strongest predictor of structural damage in adults.[24,25] As discussed below in the context of inflammatory arthritis, a significant degree of Doppler signals can be detected within the joint but not within the synovial recess. In many joints such as the elbow, wrist, knee, or ankle, the intracapsular space includes connective tissues that are located within the capsule but outside the synovium. Doppler signals within these tissues should not be interpreted as a sign of synovitis because they can be physiological (Fig. 9-12). The same applies to nutrient vessels directly entering bones and thereby crossing the synovial space (feeding vessels).

Computed Tomography

Multidetector computed tomography (CT) scanners generate detailed high-resolution images of bone and can be used to evaluate the joint space and detect adjacent bone abnormalities including tarsal coalitions, bone erosions, subchondral cysts, or primary osseous lesions such as osteoid osteoma. Current-generation CT scanners are fast, and sedation is generally not required for all but the youngest patients. Intravenous contrast may be required for soft tissue assessment. Because MRI provides better soft tissue contrast without need for radiation, CT is primarily used to provide detailed assessment of osseous structures.

Magnetic Resonance Imaging

MRI provides exquisite multiplanar images with superb tissue contrast. It can define vascular anatomy, often without the need for intravenous contrast. However, high cost, limited availability, and the frequent need for sedation have limited its more widespread use. It is

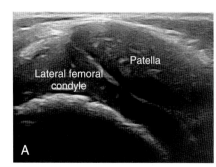
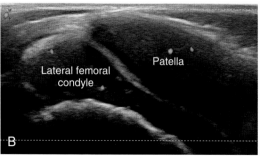

FIGURE 9-11 This ultrasound image of the knee and femoral condyle in a 3-year-old child shows hyperechoic spots within the hyaline cartilage that correspond to vascular channels. In **A** the gray-scale image and in **B** the corresponding Doppler image (*orange dots* indicating blood flow within the channels) are shown.

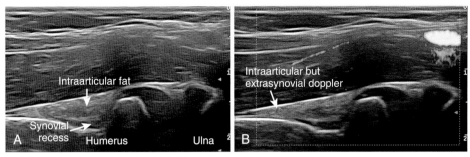

FIGURE 9-12 A, In this longitudinal image of the elbow joint a small amount of (physiological) fluid is shown in the humeroulnar joint recess. **B,** The intracapsular space that includes the intrasynovial space but also connective tissue, which is intracapsular but extrasynovial. This shows a Doppler signal that is, therefore, extrasynovial and does not indicate synovitis. Note in both **A** and **B** the unossified portion of the distal humerus and proximal ulna.

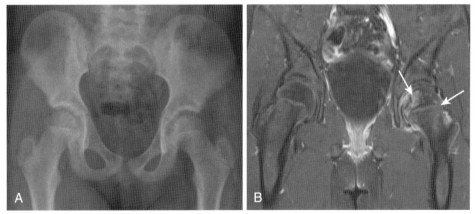

FIGURE 9-13 A, Pelvic radiograph of a 10-year-old girl with left hip pain following a fall. No abnormality is identified on plain film. **B,** Coronal T1-weighted fat-suppressed image following contrast administration with mild synovial thickening of left hip and abnormal femoral head enhancement (*arrows*). The right hip is normal.

the best modality to examine all joint components (perhaps excepting cortical bone), including bone marrow, hyaline and fibrocartilage, ligaments, menisci, synovium and joint capsule, joint fluid, and the unossified cartilaginous skeleton.[26]

MRI provides multiplanar evaluation with a combination of available imaging sequences—T1-weighted and fast spin echo T2–weighted sequences, gradient echo sequences, and postcontrast studies—all tailored to the specific clinical problem.[1,2,27] MRI uses the resonance of the protons (H[1], hydrogen) to generate images. Protons are excited by a radiofrequency pulse of an appropriate frequency and then emit energy in the form of a radiofrequency signal as they return to their original state. The radiofrequency signal decays with an exponential curve characterized by a parameter T1 (spin-lattice relaxation time). T1-weighted images can be obtained by setting short repetition time (TR) [less than 500 ms] and echo time (TE) [less than 30 ms] values in conventional spin echo sequences, whereas in gradient echo sequences they can be obtained by using flip angles of greater than 50 degrees while setting echo time (TE) values to less than 15 ms. T2-weighted (spin-spin relaxation time) images can be obtained by setting long repetition time (TR) [more than 1,500 ms] and TE [more than 90 ms] values in conventional spin echo sequences. On T1-weighted images water components (from tissue edema, joint effusion, cerebrospinal fluid, etc.) appear as "dark" (reduced) signal and on T2-weighted images they appear as "bright" (increased) signal. Because most pathological tissues appear with increased water content at least, T1- and T2-weighted images are required in the assessment of

the joint or muscle pathology. Conversely to fluid, fat presents as "bright" signal on T1-weighted images and as "intermediate to bright" signal on T2-weighted images. Because gadolinium-enhancing tissues may be hidden by the surrounding fat, and due to artifacts (ghost and chemical shift) that can be generated from fat. Fat is usually suppressed on T1-weighted images after the administration of gadolinium. Short tau inversion recovery (STIR) and spectral presaturation with inversion recovery (SPIR) sequences that are applied in whole body MRI also provide fat suppression. Although very useful clinically the use of fat suppression methods increase the scanning time.

In summary, therefore, T1-weighted MRI has a short TE and short TR, which appears with dark fluid and bright fat. T2-weighted MRI has a long TE and long TR, which appears with bright fluid and intermediate-bright fat.

Three-dimensional (3D) sequences can also be obtained, making it possible to reformat images in any desired plane.[28] Cartilaginous structures, including the growth plate, are evident when using gradient-recalled echo techniques or fat-suppressed fast proton density sequences. Gadolinium-enhanced MRI can help differentiate physeal from unossified epiphyseal cartilage and can visualize normal vessels present within the chondroepiphysis.[29] MRI is very helpful in detecting synovial abnormalities within the joint.[30] The normal synovium appears as a thin line on MRI with minimal enhancement following contrast administration (Fig. 9-13). MRI can be used to assess changes in the synovium as a result of therapy.[31] A small amount of joint fluid may normally be seen with MRI.

Pannus is seen as masses of low- to intermediate-signal intensity on T1- and T2-weighted sequences with contrast enhancement following gadolinium infusion. Subchondral cysts and bone erosions appear as low-signal areas on T1 sequences.[27]

MRI can also be used to demonstrate muscle pathology, typically demonstrating nonuniform increased signal intensity on T2-weighted images and normal signal on T1-weighted images. These findings are not specific but may help in selection of a biopsy site.

A number of novel MRI techniques are under evaluation for improved assessment of synovial, cartilaginous, or osseous abnormalities. These MRI techniques include diffusion-weighted and perfusion imaging, delayed gadolinium-enhanced cartilage imaging, and T2 quantification.

Diffusion-weighted imaging evaluates the translational movement (Brownian motion) of water molecules that occurs in all tissues. Alteration of normal diffusion can occur in some diseases, including infection, inflammation, and infarction.[32]

Perfusion imaging assesses blood flow using intravenously administered paramagnetic contrast agents and may be helpful in characterizing ischemic or hyperemic areas.[17] Potential uses of this technique include recognition of epiphyseal ischemia and quantification and monitoring of synovial inflammation.[33,34] Delayed gadolinium-enhanced MRI cartilage imaging (dGEMRIC) is a sensitive technique for assessing cartilage proteoglycan content using the negative charge of the intravenously administered paramagnetic MRI contrast agent.[17,35] The contrast agent distributes into cartilage inversely to the fixed-charge density of negatively charged glycosaminoglycan. T1 relaxation time in the presence of gadolinium agent is approximately linearly related to the glycosaminoglycan content. dGEMRIC may be used to assess early cartilage injury with depletion of glycosaminoglycans.

Cartilage assessment can also be provided by mapping T2 relaxation time measurements. These may help characterize the structural integrity of the cartilaginous tissue and quantitatively assess the degree of cartilage degeneration.[36,37]

Arthrography

Currently, arthrography is rarely indicated. Intraarticular contrast injection may, however, be combined with CT or (now more frequently) with MRI to better delineate joint detail including the evaluation of intraarticular loose bodies or labral tears within the shoulder or hip joint.

Bone Scintigraphy

Bone scintigraphy can help differentiate osseous causes of joint pain from other causes, including synovial, neuromuscular, or periarticular soft tissue disorders. Bone scintigraphy has been used to assess whether an osseous lesion is solitary or multifocal and can reveal increased activity across the joint in arthritis or infection. Specialized adjuncts to routine scintigraphic imaging include magnification scintigraphy, single photon emission (SPECT), and more recently, positron emission tomography (PET/CT).[38] Dual energy X-ray absorptiometry (DEXA) scanning is used in the assessment of bone density.

Radiographic Features of Joint Disease

A variety of radiographic features can be encountered with joint disease. Specific joint findings will depend on the underlying abnormality, chronicity of disease, and response to therapy. Potential radiographic features that can be encountered in juvenile idiopathic arthritis (JIA) are listed in Box 9-4. A systematic approach to interpretation of any joint imaging is highly recommended. This will ensure that the salient radiographic features are considered. One popular approach is

---

BOX 9-4   Radiographic Features of Juvenile Idiopathic Arthritis

Alignment
Atlantoaxial subluxation
Coxa valga or varus
Finger deformities including boutonniere or swan neck deformity
Knee valgus
Hallux valgus

Bone Density
Juxtaarticular osteoporosis
Diffuse osteoporosis (late)
Metaphyseal lucent band (rarely)
Periosteal reaction adjacent to affected small joints

Cartilage and Joint Spaces
Erosions (late), may appear corticated
Cartilage space narrowing (late)
Ankylosis (especially spine, wrists)

Distribution
Monoarticular, oligoarticular, or polyarticular

Growth Abnormalities
Affected small bones are shorter than normal
Overgrowth (lengthening) of affected long bones
Advanced maturation of affected epiphyses
Large epiphyses
Micrognathia (may have mandibular notching)
Protrusio acetabuli
Small fused cervical vertebrae
Angular carpal bones
Square patella
Intercondylar notch widening (also a feature of hemophilia)

Soft Tissues
Effusions and joint distension
Nodules
Periarticular calcification (probably due to corticosteroid injections)

Data from Ref. 10.

---

the **ABCDs** of joint disease, in which one assesses joint **A**lignment, **B**one density and other bone changes, **C**artilage loss, **D**istribution of joint disease (whether monoarticular, oligoarticular, or polyarticular), and **S**oft tissue abnormalities.

INFLAMMATORY ARTHRITIS

Juvenile Idiopathic Arthritis

In JIA, synovial infiltration by inflammatory cells leads to synovial proliferation and thickening, increased secretion of synovial fluid, and pannus formation. Inflammatory changes can also involve the synovial sheaths of tendons and bursae and can give rise to periostitis. With prolonged inflammation, more extensive joint changes, including cartilage destruction, bone erosions, and joint malalignment, are often present.

Radiography

Radiographs of symptomatic areas should be obtained at initial presentation to assist in the diagnosis. The earliest abnormalities are

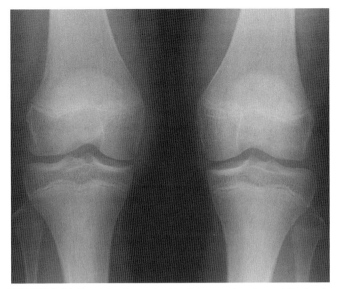

FIGURE 9-14 Frontal radiograph of both knees showing subtle demineralization of the right knee.

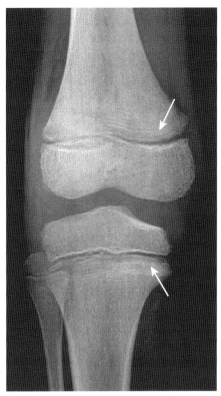

FIGURE 9-15 Frontal knee radiograph of a child with several weeks of knee pain initially suspected of having juvenile inflammatory arthritis. Note a linear subphyseal lucency (arrows), which suggested leukemia that was confirmed by bone marrow biopsy.

nonspecific and include soft tissue swelling, osteopenia, and effusions; periosteal reaction may occasionally be seen. These changes, however, are not always present. Radiography is often of limited value because inflamed soft tissues are not well delineated from adjacent normal soft tissues. Typically, the osteopenia is initially periarticular, becoming more diffuse with time. It may be subtle and better recognized by comparing to the contralateral (if unaffected) extremity (Fig. 9-14). With long-standing disease there may be uniform bone loss with a thin cortex. Although uncommon, linear subphyseal demineralization can be observed, but this is more often seen in leukemia (Fig. 9-15).[39]

Joint effusions can be seen in both inflammatory and noninflammatory joint disease. Signs of knee effusions include fullness in the suprapatellar region, best seen on the lateral view. In the elbow, knee, and ankle, there is displacement of adjacent fat lines and fat pads (Fig. 9-2).

Periosteal reaction, when present, is commonly seen in the phalanges, metacarpals, and metatarsals, but can occasionally also be seen in the long bones.

Joint space narrowing suggests cartilage loss caused by synovitis. In JIA, the joint space narrowing is usually uniform. Chondrolysis can also be seen in slipped capital femoral epiphysis, with joint infection, or following joint surgery; occasionally no cause is found.

Joint space narrowing and bone erosions are later radiographic findings typically noted 2 or more years after disease onset. However, in some patients with rheumatoid factor (RF)-positive polyarthritis or systemic arthritis, erosive disease can develop even earlier.

Bone erosions are typically located at joint margins in the bare areas (not covered by articular cartilage) but may also occur at tendinous insertions. Bone erosions can also be seen in septic arthritis, especially with chronic infections, or in hemophilia as a result of hemorrhage. Growth of granulation tissue into bone can also give rise to an erosive appearance. Pigmented villonodular synovitis may cause well-marginated erosions on both sides of the joint, often with preserved joint width and bone density. Large erosions can be seen in the camptodactyly-arthropathy-coxa vara-pericarditis (CACP) syndrome.[40]

Deformity of the fingers—whether "boutonniere" deformity or "swan neck" deformity—can be seen in a variety of disorders including JIA, CACP syndrome, or systemic lupus erythematosus (SLE). Enlarged or irregular epiphyseal ossification centers can be seen in hemophilia, JIA, and tuberculosis arthritis. Atlantoaxial subluxation may be noted in JIA, the arthropathy of Down syndrome, dysostosis multiplex, and SLE.

Changes in bone growth and maturation, with changes in the normal size of ossification centers and alteration of normal bone modeling, can be seen in JIA but also in joint infections and hemophilia. Enlargement of ossification centers, contour irregularity, and squaring (typically of the patella) can also be seen, as well as trabecular changes. Tibiotalar slant can also be noted in JIA.

Late sequelae of JIA include epiphyseal deformity, abnormal angular carpal bones (Fig. 9-16), widening of the intercondylar notch of knees, and premature fusion of the growth plate with brachydactyly. Growth disturbances are more frequent if disease onset is early. Joint space narrowing as well as osseous erosions are usually late manifestations. At the hip, protrusio acetabuli, premature degenerative changes, coxa magna, and coxa valga can be seen. Joint space loss can progress to ankylosis, particularly in the apophyseal joints of the cervical spine and wrist. Ankylosis can also be seen, however, in larger joints, including the hips, although rarely. Subluxation of the joints, especially at the wrist, may be evident, and atlantoaxial subluxation may also occur. Growth disturbance of the temporomandibular joint (TMJ) may lead to micrognathia and temporomandibular disk abnormality.

Sonography

Although radiography in JIA will mostly demonstrates chronic changes and damage occurring as a consequence of the disease, sonography may be very sensitive in assessing disease activity and useful in monitoring response to treatment. This is important for early diagnosis, the detection of subclinical disease, as well as the reliable demonstration

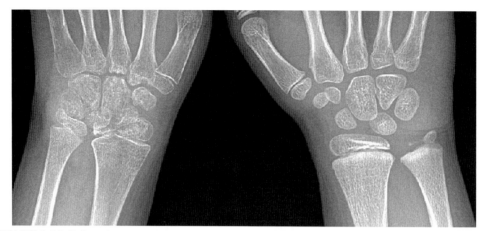

FIGURE 9-16 Unilateral carpal arthritis with marked involvement on the left (left side of the figure). Note the joint space narrowing, carpal bone erosions and irregularity, and overall demineralization.

of remission. New treatment modalities have greatly improved outcomes, including the possibility for long-term remission. The reliable diagnosis of active synovitis as well as its remission is of utmost importance, increasing the need to employ imaging modalities such as ultrasound to refine the clinical assessment. Doppler sonography has especially been shown to correlate well with histological evidence of inflammation in adults[25] and is predictive of structural deterioration.[24] Preliminary data also suggest that ultrasonography in children suffering from JIA can demonstrate subclinical synovitis.[41,42] The limitations of sonography include the paucity of normative data in children, the lack of definition of pathology, as well as the use of semiquantitative scores that have not been validated in children. This might in part explain why, for example, the presence of Doppler signals was not predictive of arthritis flares in one prospective study.[43] On the other hand a reliable diagnosis can be achieved with the application of a careful scanning technique together with the appropriate depiction of synovial recesses and the interpretation of Doppler signals within these recesses.

The knowledge of the location of synovial recesses in the various joints is essential and gray-scale ultrasound can then demonstrate synovial fluid within these recesses as an anechoic (or sometimes hypoechoic) structure that is compressible. Synovial hypertrophy will appear as a hypoechoic structure lining the recess, and the presence of Doppler signals within the synovial hypertrophy will indicate active inflammation.

Figure 9-17 illustrates the complexity of the various synovial recesses and the differentiation of intraarticular versus intrasynovial Doppler signals for the wrist joint. Another example of complex joint anatomy and resulting diversity of inflammatory involvement is the ankle joint. Rooney et al. described findings of ankle swelling in JIA patients.[44] Up to 50% of children showed tenosynovitis only, with no involvement of the tibiotalar or subtalar joints. The sonographic assessment complements the clinical assessment for a precise documentation of inflammatory activity within the joint. This is especially important in preparation for interventions such as joint injections, which themselves will benefit greatly from ultrasound guidance.

Currently only a few standard scan planes have been defined for pediatric rheumatology applications.[22,45-50] It is reasonable, though, to apply standard scanning planes that have been developed for adults, for the time being.[49] Although some of these planes might not be as relevant for the pediatric patient as they are for adults (e.g., rotator cuff pathology), they will still provide a complete assessment of the joint.

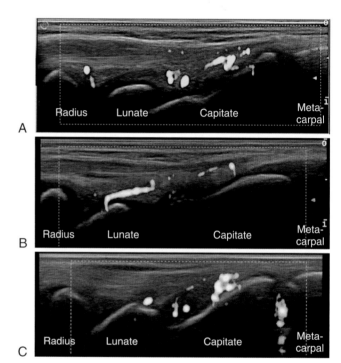

FIGURE 9-17 **A,** A longitudinal scan in midline of the wrist shows a normal wrist with intracapsular Doppler signals but no distension of the synovial recesses. **B,** A blood vessel is noted crossing the synovial recess and directly entering the lunate bone, which represents a feeding vessel. **C,** Distension, especially of the midcarpal recess with Doppler signals within the synovial recess, indicating synovitis. The carpometacarpal joint is affected by synovitis as well.

Assessment of Joint Damage: Cartilage and Erosions. Whereas cartilage can be assessed very well with sonography, the progress of ossification poses distinct challenges in the precise measurement of cartilage in children. In addition, characteristic changes of ossification patterns can be observed in JIA with acceleration of maturation in an affected joint while also showing, at the same time, growth limitation and deformities of bones. A comparison of cartilage thickness measurements with normative data is therefore challenging, especially in younger children.

Ultrasonography is more sensitive than radiographs in the detection of erosions and can be equally as sensitive as MRI, but this depends

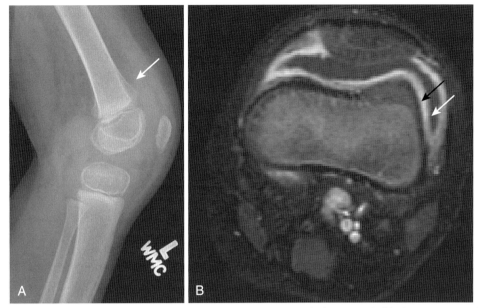

FIGURE 9-18 A 3-year-old girl with persistent effusion and knee pain for 1 month. Moderate suprapatellar joint effusion is present on lateral radiograph (*arrow*). **A,** Fat-suppressed T1-weighted axial MR image of joint effusion after intravenous administration of contrast. **B,** Low T1 signal effusion (*white arrow*) and moderate uniform synovial thickening and enhancement (*black arrow*).

on the location of assessment. A study by Wakefield et al.[50] has illustrated this for finger joints: Ultrasonography was as sensitive as MRI for erosions in the second finger because the joint can be almost completely assessed by sweeping the ultrasound probe around the entire finger. This is more challenging in the third and fourth fingers, where it is more difficult for the metacarpophalangeal joints to be completely assessed medially and laterally with sonography.

Despite all the important information provided by sonography, it is important to emphasize that like any other imaging method or laboratory test it cannot and should not replace clinical exam and review of the patient's history. In fact, it is most useful with the background of a detailed clinical history and exam, which will add useful information supporting the diagnostic process and therapeutic plan.

Magnetic Resonance Imaging

Without contrast, proliferating synovium on MRI appears as thickened synovium of intermediate soft tissue density on T1- and T2-weighted sequences. It may have slightly higher signal intensity than adjacent fluid on unenhanced T1-weighted images. Pannus appears as thickened intermediate to dark signal intensity on T2-weighted images and is best seen when outlined by bright signal joint fluid. Its variable signal intensity reflects the relative amount of fibrous tissue and hemosiderin. Intravenous administration of gadolinium-based contrast agents improves visualization of thickened synovium, especially with the use of fat suppression techniques (Fig. 9-18). Proliferating synovium appears as enhancing linear, villous, or nodular tissue. Images should be obtained immediately after contrast injection because diffusion of contrast material from the synovium into joint fluid occurs over time: Hypervascular inflamed pannus is enhanced significantly, whereas fibrous inactive pannus shows much less enhancement. Quantitative techniques have been developed for synovial volume. MRI is more sensitive than clinical evaluation in detecting some specific joint involvement—including the TMJ, which often demonstrates inflammatory change in the absence of clinical symptoms.

The development of a variety of fast-imaging methods with increased signal-to-noise ratio provides greater cartilage–synovial fluid contrast and has improved the MRI evaluation of cartilage morphology. Fat-suppressed 3D spoiled gradient-recalled echo imaging provides excellent contrast because cartilage is of bright signal compared with adjacent structures. Other sequences that are valuable in cartilage assessment include driven equilibrium Fourier transform, dual-echo steady-state imaging, Dixon water and fat separation technique, and steady-state free precession.

Hemosiderin deposition can occur in JIA but is more frequently seen in other disorders, including pigmented villonodular synovitis, hemophilic arthropathy, synovial hemangioma, and posttraumatic synovitis.[51-53] Gradient echo sequences are most sensitive in detecting hemosiderin deposition within the synovium, with signal loss occurring due to increased magnetic susceptibility. Hemosiderin-containing synovitis appears very low in signal (black) on all MRI sequences, and this is accentuated on gradient echo sequences (Fig. 9-19).

With prolonged synovial inflammation well-defined intraarticular nodules termed *rice bodies* may be present. Rice bodies likely arise from detached fragments of hypertrophied synovial villi. On MRI, rice bodies have dark signal on T2-weighted images owing to their fibrous tissue composition and are associated with joint effusion, synovial hypertrophy, and synovial enhancement after gadolinium administration (Fig. 9-20). Rice bodies may develop in JIA and also in tuberculosis.[54]

Because cartilage is one of the earliest sites of damage in JIA, this is an important area to be evaluated with MRI. Cartilage is of bright signal on both fast spin echo and fat-suppressed proton density sequences, with hyaline cartilage having the highest intensity. Articular cartilage should be assessed for areas of altered signal, thinning, erosions, or deep cartilage loss that may extend to the subchondral bone (Fig. 9-21).

Imaging in the Assessment of Response to Therapy

Once therapy has begun for patients with JIA, imaging can be a helpful adjunct, along with clinical and laboratory parameters, to assess disease activity and response to therapy. To date, several studies have looked

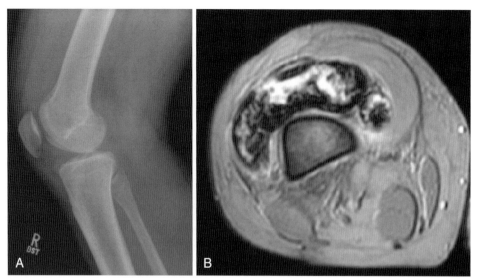

FIGURE 9-19 A 14-year-old boy with right knee swelling for 1 year. **A,** Lateral knee radiograph shows suprapatellar joint effusion. **B,** Axial gradient echo MR image shows low signal intensity margins of suprapatellar bursa due to pigmented villonodular synovitis and hemosiderin deposition.

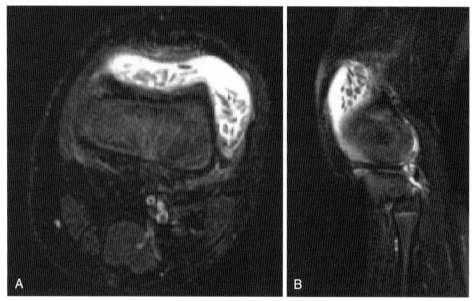

FIGURE 9-20 Axial **(A)** and sagittal **(B)** fat-suppressed T2-weighted MR images show moderate joint effusion and multiple intraarticular low signal intensity rice bodies.

at radiographic changes before and after initiation of therapy. Recent studies have used CT and/or MRI to describe joint changes and have also begun to use more quantitative measures of disease activity, including measurement of synovial volume.

Radiography

Radiography can be helpful in monitoring for the presence of joint distension, epiphyseal overgrowth, osteopenia, joint space narrowing, erosions, subchondral cysts, and periostitis. Sparling and colleagues[55] showed that intraarticular therapy was able to prevent further radiographically detectable joint damage over time. A smaller study using radiography, sonography, and MRI[56] showed that, following the injection of intraarticular triamcinolone hexacetonide, radiography was the best method to use to demonstrate epiphyseal overgrowth and osteopenia.

Carpal length is another parameter that has been used in follow-up. Carpal length is defined as the radio-metacarpal length plotted against the length of the second metacarpal bone on a chart with normal growth carpal scores, as described by Poznanski and colleagues.[57] The values were compared before and after treatment with an increase in carpal length (a positive change) indicating improvement. Three studies have shown improvements in carpal length in clinical responders to methotrexate[58,59] and etanercept.[60] Improved carpal length may be due to the halting of the disease process along with possible articular cartilage regeneration in these growing children.

Sonography

Studies in adults have shown excellent responsiveness of sonographic findings to changes in therapy and disease activity, but few prospective pediatric trials exist at this point. Eich and colleagues[56] used ultrasound

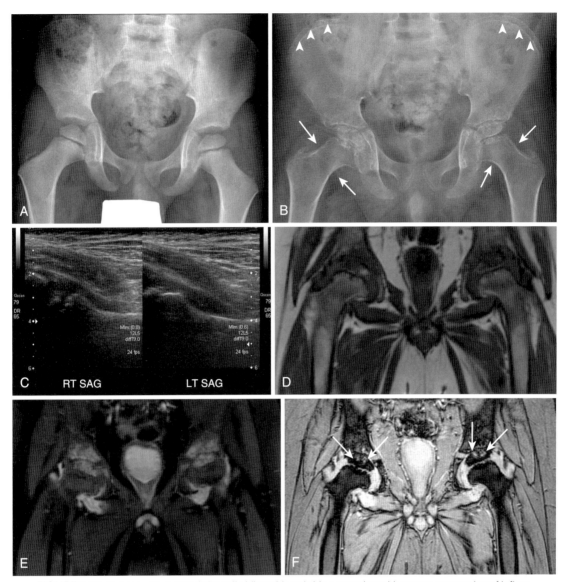

FIGURE 9-21 Patient with systemic juvenile idiopathic arthritis presenting with severe progression of inflammatory arthritis. **A,** At the age of 4 years the femoroacetabular joint spaces are preserved bilaterally. **B,** At the age of 11 years, extensive erosive changes are seen in the femoral heads and acetabula with further joint space loss at the hips bilaterally as seen on X-rays. Interval increased sclerosis is noted along the acetabular roof bilaterally. Nonspecific periosteal reaction is seen along femoral necks bilaterally (*arrows*). Sclerotic lines are shown along the iliac wings (*arrowheads*) compatible with previous bisphosphonate therapy. **C,** Gray-scale ultrasound images obtained at the age of 11 years demonstrate moderate left (LT) hip joint effusion and mild right (RT) joint effusion. **D-E,** On unenhanced coronal T1 **(D)**, contrast-enhanced coronal T1 spectral presaturation inversion recovery (SPIR) and **(E)** multiplanar gradient recalled acquisition (MPGR). **F,** MR images at the age of 11 years. Markedly thickened, lobulated, heterogeneously enhancing synovium is seen in both hip joints. Subchondral cysts (*arrows*) and surface irregularity are seen along the superior compartment of the hip joints. There is marked reduction in the hip joint spaces bilaterally with flattening of femoral heads. Bilateral secondary avascular necrosis of the femoral heads is noted.

and MRI to determine the presence of effusion, pannus, popliteal cysts, and lymphadenopathy in 10 children with JIA affecting 15 joints (11 knee and 4 hip joints) before and after intraarticular therapy. Clinical and ultrasound examinations were performed at 1 week and 1 month, and MRI at 1 month. By comparing the diagnostic accuracy of ultrasound and MRI to assess response to therapy these authors concluded that ultrasound was as sensitive as MRI in demonstrating joint effusion and/or pannus. Nevertheless, the differentiation between the two was difficult, particularly in the hip joint. Collado et al. have suggested that,

in patients with polyarthritis starting therapy for active arthritis, assessment of a smaller number of joints by gray-scale and Doppler ultrasonography was more sensitive to change than assessing a large number of joints.[61]

Computed Tomography

In one study of the TMJ, CT was used to assess disease activity before and after therapy. Ringold and colleagues[62] studied arthritis of the TMJ in 25 children who underwent intraarticular steroid injection with either triamcinolone acetonide or triamcinolone hexacetonide. Twenty-five patients underwent 74 total injections with a mean follow-up of 26 months (range, 5 to 52 months). The most common findings on baseline CT were joint space narrowing, erosions, and condylar flattening. Overall, 10 of 15 patients showed worsening radiological changes, 3 showed stable changes, and 2 showed improvement. The authors commented that the poor outcome was likely a result of selection bias, because only 15 of 25 patients underwent posttreatment imaging.

Magnetic Resonance Imaging

MRI is the modality of choice to document changes before and after therapy. MRI can be used to monitor cartilage and bone erosions, effusion, pannus, and synovial volumes.[17] Huppertz and colleagues[63] examined 21 children with arthritis of the knees and ankles who received intraarticular injection with triamcinolone hexacetonide. MR imaging was done immediately before the injection and at a median period of 49 days and 13 months after injection. Intraarticular steroid therapy had a long-lasting beneficial effect, with suppression of synovial inflammation and reversion of pannus formation. Similarly, Niedel and colleagues[64] assessed joint changes in 50 children undergoing 67 hip injections using unenhanced and gadolinium-enhanced MRI. Joints that continued to demonstrate synovitis after injection had more significant radiographic deterioration than those with minimal postinjection synovitis. These findings demonstrate that triamcinolone hexacetonide is able to reduce synovitis and joint effusion.[1]

Researchers have used MRI to quantify synovial volumes and disease activity.[65,66] Using this approach, Workie and colleagues[67] imaged the small joints of the hands and wrists of 10 JIA patients at baseline, 6 weeks and 3 months after starting therapy, using MRI. The authors demonstrated that total synovial volume averaged 3.7 ml (range, 2.3 to 12.4) at initial examination and 2.2 ml at final examination. Synovial volume calculated from MRI correlated well with the total hand swelling score and total number of active joints at each time point. Workie and colleagues[67] examined the utility of quantitative dynamic contrast-enhanced MRI based on pharmacokinetic (PK) modeling to evaluate disease activity in the knee. The authors demonstrated that PK parameters and synovial volumes were significantly decreased at 12 months after intraarticular steroid therapy; however, improvement in synovial volume appeared to lag behind dynamic parameters, reflecting delay or subclinical synovitis. The authors postulated that patients who exhibit improvement in PK parameters but have an elevated synovial volume may have less active synovial inflammation and a more inactive fibrotic synovium. Thus, dynamic PK parameters may be able to provide additional information concerning disease activity.

Of all the imaging modalities, MRI has been shown to be the most sensitive modality in the assessment of TMJ arthritis in children (Figs. 9-22, 9-23, 9-24). However, according to a recent systematic review on the value of MRI for assessment of axial joints in JIA, there is fair (grade B) evidence that MRI is an accurate diagnostic method for evaluating early and intermediate changes in the TMJ in JIA, and there is insufficient evidence to indicate MRI is an accurate diagnostic method for detecting JIA in the spinal (grade I) and sacroiliac (grade I) joints.[68]

Cahill and colleagues injected TMJs in 15 children with JIA and performed MRI scans 6 to 12 months after contrast injection.[69] Joint changes (effusion, meniscal abnormalities, and loss of normal joint space) and bone changes (erosions and mandibular condyle abnormalities) were present in all joints before injection. Follow-up imaging showed improvement in 11 of 15 (73%) patients. The authors found

good correlation between the lack of acute findings on MRI and improvement in clinical findings, and proposed their grading scheme as a useful tool for future trials.

A critical appraisal of radiological scoring systems for assessment of juvenile idiopathic arthritis is discussed in the paper by Doria et al.[70]

Postinfectious Arthritis

The most common form of inflammatory arthritis in children is postinfectious arthritis. Although this type of arthritis often has a rapid resolution and may not necessarily come to the attention of the rheumatologist, sonography can play a useful role especially when certain joints, such as the hip joint, are involved. Transient synovitis of the hip is very common. Robben et al.[71] demonstrated that ultrasonography of the hip in these children will show distension of the capsule with an increased anterior-posterior diameter but that this distension is exclusively due to fluid and not due to hypertrophy of the synovium. Sonography may therefore be very helpful in the appropriate clinical setting to support the diagnosis of transient arthritis. The differential diagnosis of infectious arthritis as well as other pathology such as a slipped capital femoral epiphysis should also be considered, especially in the slightly older child, and may warrant the performance of additional imaging modalities.

Joint Injections

Despite the availability of effective systemic therapies, joint injections are still an important therapeutic measure either for very limited disease in oligoarthritis or for treatment of residual synovitis in polyarticular and systemic patients. In addition to the precise determination of joint involvement before injection, sonography allows for reliable and precise access to almost any joint recess. Tendon sheaths can be injected without risking an intratendinous application of glucocorticoids, and joints such as the subtalar and hip joint, which would be difficult to access without imaging guidance, are relatively easy to inject under sonographic guidance. Publications have demonstrated increased precision in accessing the respective synovial recess.[72] The ability to document the correct deposition of the medication is an added advantage. For TMJ and sacroiliac joints imaging guidance through other modalities such as CT can be an option.

ENTHESITIS-RELATED ARTHRITIS

Appendicular Skeleton

Radiography

Radiographic findings of enthesitis-related arthritis (ERA) and other spondyloarthropathies are similar to those encountered in other forms of JIA, with the exception of sacroiliitis and enthesitis, which are more specific for spondyloarthropathy (Box 9-5).[73,74] Radiography typically shows asymmetric involvement of the large joints of the lower limb (i.e., hip, ankle, knee, and tarsal joints). The interphalangeal joint of the hallux is also frequently involved. Radiographs may be normal initially or can demonstrate soft tissue swelling, effusion, ossification and epiphyseal overgrowth, erosions, osteopenia, joint space narrowing, or, rarely, fusion. Bone erosions may be associated with irregular bone apposition at joint margins referred to as "whiskering." With hip involvement, these proliferative changes are noted at the junction of the femoral head and neck. Dactylitis may be seen with soft tissue swelling and periosteal reaction along the shaft of metacarpals, metatarsals, or phalanges.

Enthesitis can involve the calcaneus and tibial tuberosity with soft tissue swelling at tendon insertions, localized osteopenia, and bone erosion and/or spur formation, particularly at the site of insertion of

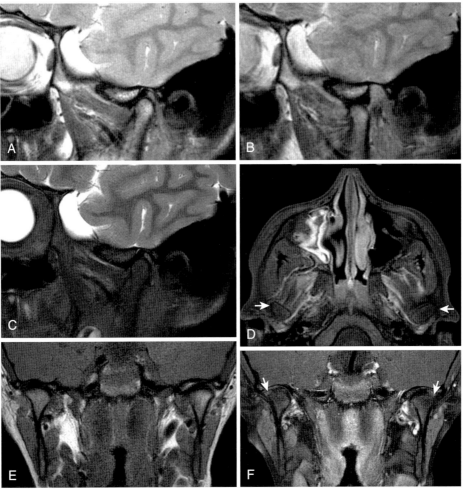

FIGURE 9-22 Nine-year-old boy with juvenile idiopathic arthritis without temporomandibular joint (TMJ) involvement. The shape of the intraarticular disc has the normal bow-tie configuration on sagittal views and has low signal intensity on both proton density **(A, B)** and T2-weighted **(C)** images. Upon a maneuver to open the mouth **(B)**, there is normal anterior translation of the mandibular condyle on the corresponding disc. Please compare **(A)** closed and **(B)** open mouth proton density images. No joint effusion is seen on T2-weighted image **(C)**. Note the absence of substantial synovial enhancement (arrows) after intravenous administration of gadolinium on **(D)** axial and **(F)** coronal T1-weighted fat-saturated images. Precontrast coronal T1-weighted **(E)** image is available for comparison. Right maxillary sinusopathy is noted.

the Achilles tendon into the calcaneus, plantar aponeurosis, or patella (Fig. 9-25). Periostitis may also be seen.

Sonography
Enthesitis
The enthesis is a relatively complex structure presenting with several components, including the tendon itself, fibrocartilage, subtendinous bursae, and insertion of tendon fibers into bone.[75] All these structures can be shown very well with sonography[76] (Fig. 9-26). This has increased our understanding of this important structure in rheumatic diseases.

Sonographic findings of enthesitis include loss of the normal fibrillar echotexture of the tendon and irregular fusiform thickening.[77] Sonography has added interesting information on the pathological processes that occur in enthesitis in adults, for example, by demonstrating distinct topographic locations of enthesophytes at the distal insertion of the Achilles tendon, and erosions in a more proximal location, probably as a consequence of tensile and compressive forces

occurring in these two locations.[78] In adults, Doppler signals very close to bone cortex are thought to be very specific for spondyloarthropathies,[79] although they can be observed in activity-related injuries as well. Using power Doppler sonography, Tse and colleagues[80] demonstrated the ability of color Doppler sonography to show improvement in increased vascularity at the cortical bone insertion of enthesis and along the adjacent synovium in children with ERA, suggesting that this technique may add valuable information to gray-scale sonography. Several pediatric studies have also found a significantly higher percentage of entheseal sites with increased Doppler activity compared with active entheseal sites on clinical exam in children with ERA.[81] The clinical significance of these findings is not entirely clear at this point, as prospective trials are missing. The definition of enthesitis in the growing skeleton should also be clarified because Doppler signals close to the bone cortex can be normal in certain entheseal sites in children. From a practical point of view Doppler signals are very sensitive to compression that may also occur during tendon strain. Sonographic assessment of an enthesis should be done at various angles of the joint.

Left

Right

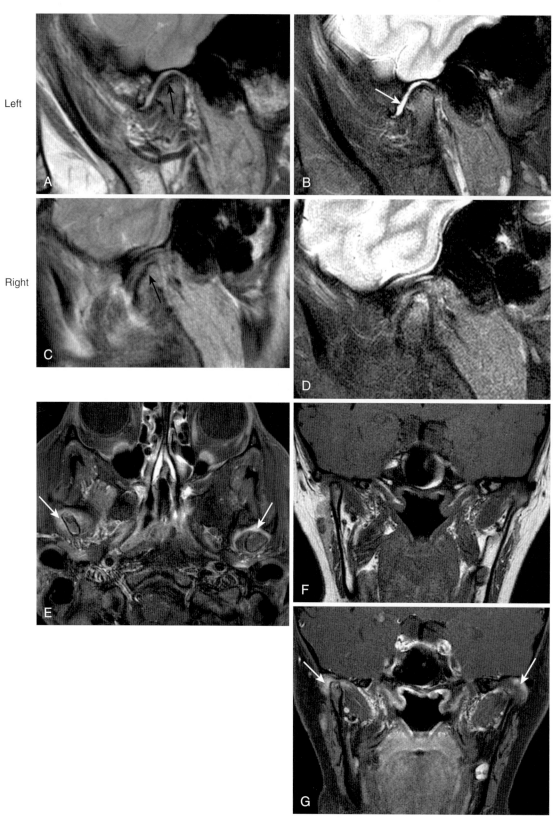

FIGURE 9-23 A 16-year-old girl with juvenile idiopathic arthritis with TMJ involvement. **A,** In the left TMJ incipient condylar flattening and erosions (*arrow*) are noted on the sagittal proton density-weighted image. **B,** Mild joint effusion (*arrow*) is seen on the sagittal T2-weighted image. **C,** In the right TMJ there is severe destruction of mandibular condyle and deep erosions (*arrow*) on the sagittal proton density-weighted image. **D,** No obvious joint effusion is noted on the sagittal T2-weighted image. **E** and **G,** Following intravenous administration of gadolinium marked synovial thickening/enhancement (*arrows*) are noted in both TMJs on **(E)** axial and **(G)** coronal T1-weighted fat-saturated images. **F,** Precontrast coronal T1-weighted image is available for comparison.

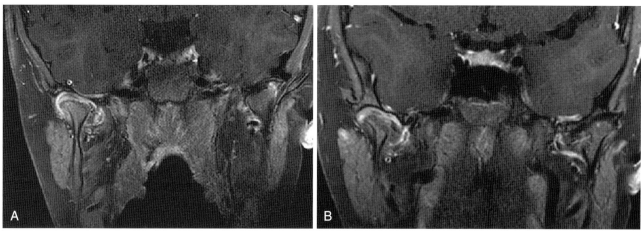

FIGURE 9-24 T2-weighted coronal MRI images of the TMJ in a 6-year-old female patient with JIA before and after intraarticular steroid injection. **A,** Increased synovial enhancement of the right TMJ before injection. **B,** Mild decrease in synovial enhancement 1 year after the injection.

BOX 9-5   Radiographic Features of Enthesitis-Related Arthritis and Spondyloarthropathies

Peripheral Joints
Asymmetrical involvement of the large lower limb joints
Involvement of the interphalangeal joint of the hallux
New bone at the margins of erosions
Affected joints show swelling, effusion, epiphyseal overgrowth, erosions, osteopenia, cartilage space narrowing, and, rarely, fusion
Dactylitis: swelling and periosteal new bone of fingers or toes
Periosteal new bone, e.g., metatarsals, proximal femur

Entheses
Especially tibial tubercle and posterior aspect of calcaneus
Swelling, erosion, new bone formation

Sacroiliitis
Radiographic changes generally delayed until late teens
Asymmetrical involvement may occur early, then become symmetrical
Erosions occur first on the iliac side of sacroiliac joint
Pseudowidening occurs due to erosion
Sclerosis and finally ankylosis develop

Data from E.M. Azouz, C.M. Duffy, Juvenile spondyloarthropathies: clinical manifestations and medical imaging, *Skeletal Radiol* 24 (1995) 399–408.

Finally, sonography might be the most sensitive technique to demonstrate tendon damage in addition to bony changes in enthesitis, as shown in Fig. 9-27 with the partial rupture of the deep portion of the Achilles tendon in the area of an erosion at the posterior calcaneus.

Apophysitis

A particular type of pathology that occurs at certain entheseal sites during growth is apophysitis. The apophysis is a site of bony protuberance at which ligaments or tendons such as the tibial tuberosity or the posterior calcaneus insert. It is built on cartilage matrix in the young child, with the subsequent appearance of a separate ossification center that finally results in complete ossification of the insertion site. Periods

of maximum growth coincide with the time of maximum development of these secondary ossification centers. The increased forces that relate to the growth of the extremities are transmitted through the tendons. Pathology occurs if there is an insertion that is weakened because of the transformation of cartilage into bone cells lacking a firm union of the secondary ossification center with the main bone.[82,83] This can result in pathology, for example, Sinding–Larsen–Johannson disease, which occurs at the insertion of the proximal patella tendon (Fig. 9-28), Osgood–Schlatter disease occurs at the insertion of the distal part of the patella tendon, and Sever disease occurs at the insertion of the Achilles tendon in the posterior calcaneus. Sonography has shown that these diseases do not only result in the fragmentation of the secondary ossification center but also lead to tendon thickening with increased local vascularity and the presence of bursitis. The term *traction apophysitis*, therefore, seems more appropriate to describe this pathology. Figure 9-29 gives an example of Osgood–Schlatter disease as seen on sonography.

Magnetic Resonance Imaging

With MRI one may see bone marrow edema, tenosynovitis, granulation tissue, or cortical erosion at the site of enthesitis.[16]

Axial Skeleton
Radiography

In ERA, changes in the spine and sacroiliac joints are generally not seen until the latter part of the second decade or even adulthood. There may be localized osteitis, erosions, and sclerosis, particularly at the vertebral margins. Syndesmophytes and atlantoaxial subluxation are rarely seen in children.

Radiographs may demonstrate unilateral or bilateral sacroiliitis with indistinct articular margins (also known as *pseudowidening*), erosions, and reactive sclerosis, particularly on the iliac side of the joint. Radiography shows asymmetrical sacroiliac joint space widening initially, but eventually the classic bilateral symmetrical joint involvement can be seen with joint space narrowing and ankylosis. Radiographic evaluation of the sacroiliac joints is often especially difficult in teenagers. Diffuse osteopenia of the pelvic bones is also seen as a late change.

Magnetic Resonance Imaging

MRI can demonstrate early inflammatory changes in the sacroiliac joints and spine and is especially sensitive for evaluation of

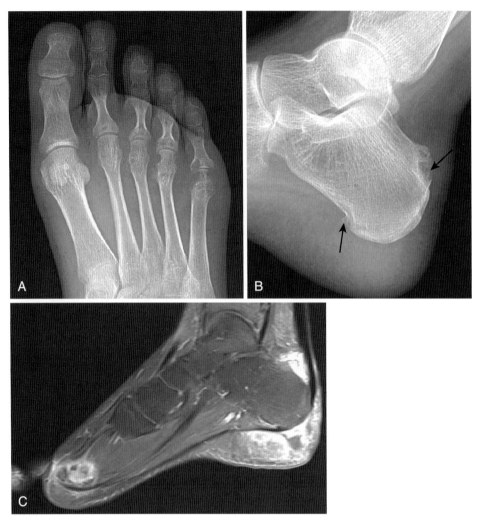

FIGURE 9-25 A 17-year-old girl with ERA. **A,** The forefoot radiograph shows joint space narrowing and extensive bone erosions involving multiple metatarsophalangeal joints, especially the fifth metatarsophalangeal joint. **B,** A spur is noted in the hindfoot radiograph at the insertion of the plantar fascia (*white arrow*) and erosive changes at the calcaneal tendon insertion (*black arrow*). **C,** Sagittal contrast-enhanced fat-suppressed T1-weighted MR image shows intense enhancement adjacent to the calcaneal tendon, heel, and metatarsophalangeal joint.

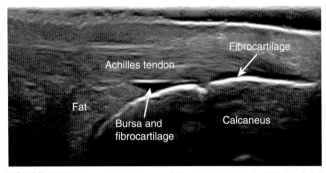

FIGURE 9-26 A longitudinal scan of the posterior heel with the Achilles tendon insertion shows the various structures of the enthesis, including fibrocartilage, retrocalcaneal fat pad, and bursa, as well as the tendon with its enthesis itself.

subchondral bone marrow edema not shown on other types of imaging (Fig. 9-30).[84] The administration of gadolinium contrast improves the detection of early sacroiliitis. On MRI, periarticular low signal may be seen on T1-weighted images, with high signal on T2-weighted images from inflammatory changes in bone marrow. Low signal on both sequences is seen with bone sclerosis. MRI may also demonstrate erosions in the articular cartilage.

Because of efforts of clinicians to treat spondyloarthropathies in the early preradiographic stage of the disease with tumor necrosis factor (TNF) blockers and thereby prevent long-term consequences,[85] there has been a growing utilization of MRI for the detection of sacroiliac and vertebral inflammation.

Whole-body MRI has been recently used as an outcome measure in clinical trials of treatment effectiveness in adult spondyloarthropathies.[86,87] Inflammation of subchondral bone marrow (bone marrow edema) can be demonstrated by the STIR sequence of MRI (Fig. 9-31), whereas chronic changes are better seen on T1-MRI sequence.[88] This technique appears useful in demonstrating the presence of multiple sites of enthesitis-related disease in children.

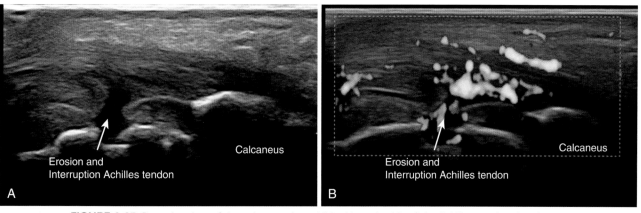

FIGURE 9-27 Posterior view of the calcaneus in a child with enthesitis of the Achilles tendon showing an interruption of the deep portion of the Achilles tendon (partial rupture) with an underlying erosion and increased Doppler signals.

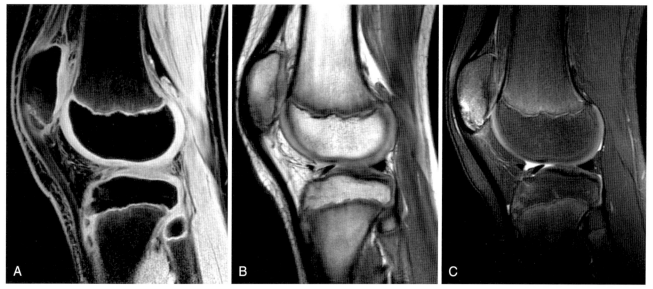

FIGURE 9-28 Magnetic resonance (MR) images of a 12-year-old boy with bilateral knee pain and no history of acute trauma. **A-C,** Sagittal 3D gradient recalled echo (GRE) **(A),** proton-density (PD) **(B),** and T2-weighted **(C)** MR images of the knee show fragmentation of the distal aspect of the patella (**A,** *arrow*) associated with bone marrow edema (low signal on PD **[B]** and high signal on T2-weighted **[C]** images) characterizing the Sinding–Larsen–Johansson disorder.

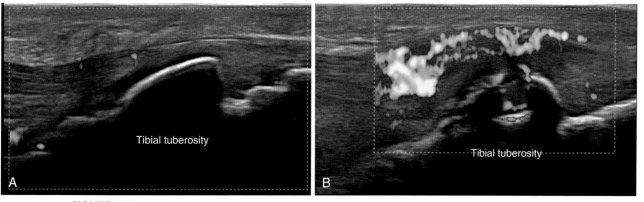

FIGURE 9-29 Longitudinal Doppler sonographic scan of the tibial tuberosity in a child. The **(A)** unaffected and **(B)** affected side show the fragmentation of the tibial tuberosity, as well as the distortion of the regular fibrillar pattern of the tendon with tendon thickening, focal hypoechoic areas and increased Doppler signals, representing Osgood-Schlatter disease.

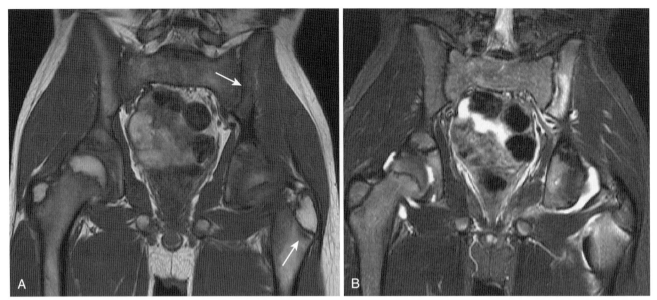

FIGURE 9-30 An 11-year-old boy with ERA. **A,** MRI showed bilateral hip joint effusions and abnormal bone signal adjacent to the left sacroiliac joint and left greater trochanter (*arrows*). Whereas the coronal T1-weighted image **(A)** shows low signal in these regions (*arrows*), the coronal short-tau inversion recovery image **(B)** shows increased signal intensity.

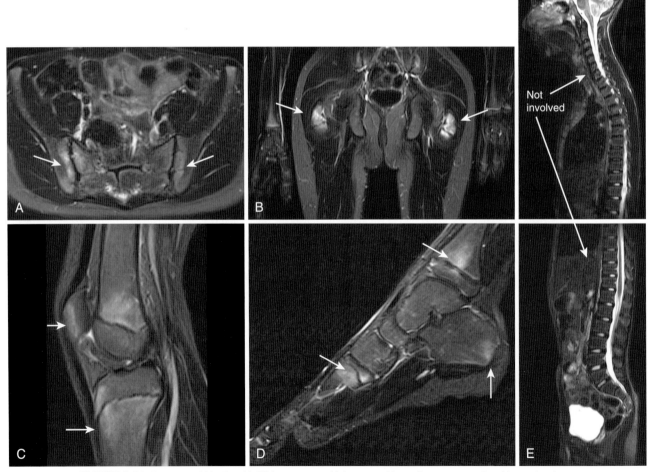

FIGURE 9-31 A 12year-old body with ERA presents with increased inversion recovery signal intensity along both sides of the sacroiliac joints (**A,** *arrows*), right greater than left; around the growth plates of greater trochanter apophyses (**B,** *arrows*); at the distal attachment of the patellar tendon (**C,** *arrow*) and along the anterior aspect of patella (**C,** *arrow*); and at the distal tibial metaphysis (**D,** *arrow*), at the calcaneal insertion (**D,** *arrow*), and within the second right metatarsal (**D,** *arrow*). Note that the spine was not involved **(E)**.

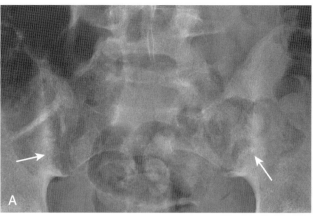 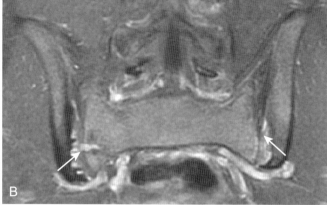

FIGURE 9-32 A 14-year-old boy with arthritis and long-standing history of limping and abnormal gait. **A,** Pelvic radiograph shows sclerosis and irregularity *(arrows)* adjacent to the sacroiliac joints. **B,** Finding confirmed on MRI with multiple erosions evident *(arrows)*.

Computed Tomography

Sacroiliitis may be demonstrated on either CT or MRI at an earlier stage compared with radiography (Fig. 9-32). A CT scan of the sacroiliac joints is useful in demonstrating sclerosis or erosive disease not evident on radiographs. Although MRI is preferable, if CT is used, angled scans through the sacroiliac joint should be used to lower the radiation dose.

Scintigraphy

Bone scintigraphy can overcome the difficulty in recognizing early unilateral sacroiliac abnormalities on radiography. However, there is normally a higher concentration of physiological activity in pediatric sacroiliac joints. Mild to moderate increases in the radioisotope uptake, especially when bilateral, may make assessment difficult. Asymmetric uptake is more common in childhood spondyloarthropathies, other than juvenile ankylosing spondylitis.

PSORIATIC ARTHRITIS

Radiography

Radiographs obtained in the initial phase of the disease may be normal or show juxtaarticular osteoporosis. Findings are often identical to those of oligoarticular or polyarticular JIA. Characteristic radiographic features of psoriatic arthritis (especially in adults) include asymmetric involvement, sausage digits, joint erosions, joint space narrowing, bony proliferation (including periarticular and shaft periostitis enthesitis), osteolysis (including "pencil-in-cup" deformity), acroosteolysis, spur formation, and ankylosis. The bone erosions tend to be larger and more asymmetric than those seen in JIA. The characteristic changes seen at the distal interphalangeal joints are uncommon in children (Fig. 9-33).

Sonography

Sonography may also be a useful tool in the assessment of psoriatic arthritis. Sonography with Doppler evaluation is more sensitive than clinical examination for detection of abnormalities in the hands and wrists, along with calcaneal enthesitis of adults with psoriatic arthritis, and is a reliable tool for assessment of joint response to therapy with biological agents. Given its excellent resolution, sonography is well positioned to analyze very small structures, including the entheses of the extensor tendons of the fingers and collateral ligaments. Recent research in psoriatic arthritis has yielded interesting results on the morphological correlates of the dactylitis observed in this group.[89]

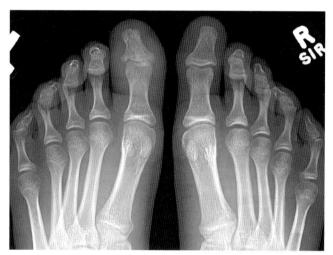

FIGURE 9-33 Dactylitis of the left great toe in a child with psoriatic arthritis. There is diffuse soft tissue swelling of the digit along with narrowing of the first metatarsophalangeal and interphalangeal joints. Irregularity of the base of the distal phalanx is present.

Ultrasonographic findings in the fingers include, besides synovitis and tenosynovitis, the paratenonitis of the extensor tendon as well as enthesitis of the extensor tendons and collateral ligaments.[89]

Magnetic Resonance Imaging

In psoriatic arthritis, MRI demonstrates erosive changes, joint space narrowing, ligament disruption, and tenosynovitis. Sausage digits are seen in patients with psoriatic arthritis and reactive arthritis. These swollen fingers or toes result from tenosynovitis, soft tissue edema, and synovial proliferation.[90] MRI may also be used to evaluate the responsiveness of therapy, as can be noted by a significant reduction in gadolinium uptake following treatment with infliximab.[91]

Axial Skeleton

Sacroiliitis and vertebral involvement typically manifest later on during the progression of the disease. The sacroiliitis of juvenile psoriatic arthritis is usually asymmetric and resembles that of reactive arthritis. Syndesmophytes, paraspinal calcification, and atlantoaxial subluxation are rare in children. Currently there is insufficient evidence to indicate that MRI is an accurate diagnostic method for detecting JIA in the spinal and sacroiliac joints.[68]

CT may be useful in assessing spine disease but has little role in the assessment of peripheral joints. Previous studies have shown that CT is as accurate as MRI for assessment of erosions in the sacroiliac joints but is not as effective for identifying synovial inflammation. CT can be used guide sacroiliac joint injection.

ACKNOWLEDGMENT

The authors would like to acknowledge the contributions of Nasir A. Khan, medical student, University of Toronto.

REFERENCES

1. S. Lamer, G.H. Sebag, MRI and ultrasound in children with juvenile chronic arthritis, Eur. J. Radiol. 33 (2000) 85–93.
3. W. Grassi, E. Filippucci, P. Busilacchi, Musculoskeletal ultrasound, Best Pract. Res. Clin. Rheumatol. 18 (2004) 813–826.
4. M. Østergaard, A. Duer, U. Møller, B. Ejbjerg, Magnetic resonance imaging of peripheral joints in rheumatic diseases, Best Pract. Res. Clin. Rheumatol. 18 (2004) 861–879.
7. A.L. Tan, A.J. Grainger, S.F. Tanner, et al., High resolution magnetic resonance imaging for the assessment of hand osteoarthritis, Arthritis Rheum. 52 (2005) 2355–2365.
11. M. Backhaus, Ultrasound and structural changes in inflammatory arthritis: synovitis and tenosynovitis, Ann. N. Y. Acad. Sci. 1154 (2009) 139–151.
12. M. Ruhoy, K.L. Tucker, R.G. McCauley, et al., Hypertrophic bursopathy of the subacromial-subdeltoid bursa in juvenile rheumatoid arthritis: sonographic appearance, Pediatr. Radiol. 26 (1996) 353–355.
14. R.M. Acheson, Maturation of the skeleton, in: F. Falkner (Ed.), Human Development, W. B. Saunders, Philadelphia, 1966, pp. 465–502.
18. R.W. Haines, The pseudoepiphysis of the first metacarpal of man, J. Anat. 117 (Pt 1) (1974) 145–158.
20. B. Möller, H. Bonel, M. Rotzetter, et al., Measuring finger joint cartilage by ultrasound as a promising alternative to conventional radiograph imaging, Arthritis Rheum. 61 (2009) 435–441.
22. A.H. Spannow, M. Pfeiffer-Jensen, N.T. Andersen, et al., Ultrasonographic measurements of joint cartilage thickness in healthy children: age- and sex-related standard reference values, J. Rheumatol. 37 (2010) 2595–2601.
23. D. Sureda, S. Quiroga, C. Arnal, et al., Juvenile rheumatoid arthritis of the knee: evaluation with US, Radiology 190 (1994) 403–406.
27. V.M. Gylys-Morin, MR imaging of pediatric musculoskeletal inflammatory and infectious disorders, Magn. Reson. Imaging. Clin. North Am 6 (1998) 537–559.
28. H. Cakmakci, A. Kovanlikaya, E. Unsal, Short-term follow-up of the juvenile rheumatoid knee with fat-saturated 3D MRI, Pediatr. Radiol. 31 (2001) 189–195.
31. M. Ostergaard, M. Stoltenberg, P. Gicteon, et al., Changes in synovial membrane and joint effusion volumes after intraarticular methylprednisolone. Quantitative assessment of inflammatory and destructive changes in arthritis by MRI, J. Rheumatol. 23 (1996) 1151–1161.
36. B.J. Dardzinski, T.J. Mosher, S. Li, et al., Spatial variation of T2 in human articular cartilage, Radiology 205 (1997) 546–550.
38. A. Shammas, Nuclear medicine imaging of the pediatric musculoskeletal system, Semin. Musculoskelet. Radiol. 13 (2009) 159–180.
39. I. Spilberg, G.J. Meyer, The arthritis of leukemia, Arthritis Rheum. 15 (1972) 630–635.
49. M. Backhaus, G.R. Burmester, T. Gerber, et al., Guidelines for musculoskeletal ultrasound in rheumatology, Ann. Rheum. Dis. 60 (2001) 641–649.
55. M. Sparling, P. Malleson, B. Wood, R. Petty, Radiographic followup of joints injected with triamcinolone hexacetonide for the management of childhood arthritis, Arthritis Rheum. 33 (1990) 821–826.
57. A.K. Poznanski, R.J. Hernandez, K.E. Guire, et al., Carpal length in children—a useful measurement in the diagnosis of rheumatoid arthritis and some congenital malformation syndromes, Radiology 129 (1978) 661–668.
58. L. Harel, L. Wagner-Weiner, A.K. Poznanski, et al., Effects of methotrexate on radiologic progression in juvenile rheumatoid arthritis, Arthritis Rheum. 36 (1993) 1370–1374.
64. J. Neidel, M. Boehnke, R.M. Küster, et al., The efficacy and safety of intraarticular corticosteroid therapy for coxitis in juvenile rheumatoid arthritis, Arthritis Rheum. 46 (2002) 1620–1628.
73. E.M. Azouz, C.M. Duffy, Juvenile spondyloarthropathies: clinical manifestations and medical imaging, Skeletal Radiol. 24 (1995) 399–408.
74. A.M. Prieur, Spondyloarthropathies in childhood, Baillieres Clin. Rheumatol. 12 (1998) 287–307.
79. M.A. D'Agostino, R. Said-Nahal, C. Hacquard-Bouder, et al., Assessment of peripheral enthesitis in the spondyloarthropathies by ultrasonography combined with power Doppler: a cross-sectional study, Arthritis Rheum. 48 (2003) 523–533.
82. J.A. Ogden, R.F. Hempton, W.O. Southwick, Development of the tibial tuberosity, Anat. Rec. 182 (1974) 431–435.
83. J.A. Ogden, W.O. Southwick, Osgood-Schlatter's disease and tibial tuberosity development, Clin. Orthop. Relat. Res. 116 (1976) 180–189.
91. S.1. Weckbach, S. Schewe, H.J. Michaely, et al., Whole-body MRI imaging in psoriatic arthritis: additional value for therapeutic decision making, Eur. J. Radiol. 77 (2011) 149–155.

Entire reference list is available online at www.expertconsult.com.

CHAPTER 10

Laboratory Investigations

Jonathan Akikusa, Sharon Choo

INTRODUCTION

Over the past 80 years, the role of laboratory investigation in rheumatic diseases has progressed from reports of curious *in vitro* phenomena in diseases defined purely on clinical grounds to sophisticated immunopathology testing that provides information now essential for disease diagnosis. A corollary of this progress is that rheumatology practice has increasingly involved the clinical interpretation of an expanding array of immunopathology tests. To be proficient at this requires two things: a basic understanding of the statistical concepts underlying diagnostic testing and an understanding of the tests themselves.

The statistical concepts commonly referred to in diagnostic testing are *sensitivity, specificity,* and *positive* and *negative predictive values* (see Chapter 6). The sensitivity of a test is defined as the proportion of people with disease (true positives) correctly identified by the test. The specificity of a test is defined as the proportion of people without the disease (true negatives) correctly identified by the test.[1] These are fixed characteristics of a test related to its performance in a population where disease status is known and the test result is in question. The positive and negative predictive values of a test are the probability of the disease being present or absent given a positive or negative test, respectively.[2] These deal with the "real life" situation in which the test result is known and the disease status is in question. They are not fixed test characteristics and are heavily influenced by the prevalence of the condition in the test population. In mathematical terms this can be thought of as the probability of the disease being present before testing or the "pretest" probability of disease. Increasing the prevalence or pretest probability of disease in a sample population increases the positive predictive value of a diagnostic test, as demonstrated in eFig. 10-1. In clinical medicine, this is best achieved by testing only those with a significant likelihood of having the disease based on thorough clinical assessment informed by meticulous attention to history taking, physical examination, and a detailed knowledge of its clinical features.

The second requirement for proficient interpretation of laboratory investigations is a basic knowledge of the assays used and an understanding of the basis and characteristics of the tests themselves, including their strengths, weaknesses, and clinical associations. This chapter will concentrate primarily on immunopathology testing, providing a brief overview of assays commonly used in the immunopathology laboratory and then will review immunopathology tests frequently encountered in rheumatology practice. It will also cover the laboratory assessment of the acute phase response, synovial fluid and urine, and briefly review key issues in diagnostic genetic testing in the evaluation of rheumatic diseases.

Laboratory Methods

Immunofluorescence

The use of immunofluorescence (IF) microscopy for the detection of antibodies in patient serum was one of the first techniques developed in immunopathology. The principle of the test is straightforward. A substrate is mounted on a glass slide and antibodies labeled with a fluorescent tag are used to identify the presence of either antigen *in the* substrate (direct IF) or of antibody *on* the substrate (indirect IF) using a fluorescence microscope (eFig. 10-2). Direct IF requires fluorescent-tagged antibodies of known specificity, whereas indirect IF requires fluorescent-tagged antibodies to human immunoglobulin (Ig). The substrate used in either technique can be tissue sections, cultured cells, or even microorganisms (e.g., *Crithidia luciliae*). IF has several disadvantages; the most important of these are as follows: it is time consuming, labor intensive, requires skilled operators, and has a subjective component that may cause significant variation in results. For these reasons there has been interest in trying to automate the process.[3]

Enzyme-Linked Immunosorbent Assay

Enzyme-linked immunosorbent assay (ELISA) is a commonly used method for detecting the presence of antibody or antigen in a sample. Although there are multiple forms of ELISA, all rely on high specificity antibody–antigen interactions and the use of an automated reader to detect a color change in wells containing a sample and an enzyme-labeled antibody that causes the color change when mixed with an appropriate substrate (eFig. 10-3). Signal strength (color intensity) is related to the amount of labeled antibody present, which in turn is proportional to the amount of antigen or antibody in the sample. The wells used in this assay are contained on a polystyrene plate in large numbers, allowing for the simultaneous testing of numerous samples.

The most basic form of this assay is the direct ELISA, in which a sample containing an antigen to be detected is coated onto the plate wells and labeled antibody of known specificity is added (eFig. 10-4, *A*). This method is useful if the presence of a particular antigen in a sample is in question.

Indirect ELISA is the most common method and involves adding sample to wells coated with a known antigen. Antibodies in the sample that bind to the antigen are detected using enzyme-labeled antihuman Ig antibodies (eFig. 10-4, *B*). This method is useful if it is the presence of a particular antibody in the sample that is in question.

A third variant is the sandwich (or "capture") ELISA, in which the plate wells are coated with a "capture" antibody targeting a specified antigen. This method may be used to identify the presence of a specific antigen or antibody using direct and indirect detection methods, respectively (eFig. 10-4, *C, D*). In a *direct* sandwich ELISA the presence of "captured" sample antigen is detected by the addition of an enzyme-labeled antibody targeting an epitope on the same antigen that does not overlap with that of the capture antibody. In an *indirect* sandwich ELISA the "captured" antigen is bound by an intermediate-unlabeled antibody, the presence of which is then detected using an enzyme-labeled antihuman antibody. An advantage of this method is that it avoids the potential disruption of conformational epitopes on sample antigen that may occur in indirect ELISA.

A final variant, the inhibition ELISA, utilizes competition for labeled antibody between sample and well wall antigen. The resulting reduction in antibody binding to the well wall is an indirect measure of antigen in the sample (eFig. 10-4, *E*).

The advantages of ELISA methodology are as follows: it is rapid, objective, able to analyze multiple samples simultaneously, and can be fully automated. It can also provide quantitative results and is highly sensitive. Its main disadvantage is that it tends to be less specific than other assays.[4,5]

Radioimmunoassay

Radioimmunoassay (RIA) is a highly sensitive way to measure the concentration of antigen in a sample. In this assay, a quantity of the antigen of interest is tagged with a radioactive isotope (typically of iodine-125 or iodine-131) and mixed with a known amount of its cognate antibody. Sample is then added and any antigen in the sample matching the radiolabeled antigen will compete for binding to the added antibody—effectively drawing antibody away from the labeled antigen. Bound and unbound antigen are separated, and the amount of radioactivity in the unbound fraction measured. The level of radioactivity in this fraction is proportional to the amount of antigen in the sample. A variant of this, the Farr assay, is used for the detection of high-avidity anti-double stranded DNA (anti-dsDNA) antibodies that have a higher specificity for the diagnosis of systemic lupus erythematosus (SLE) than low avidity antibodies.[6] With the availability of newer methods of antibody identification, RIA techniques have fallen out of favor because of the need to use and dispose of radioactive material.

Immunoblotting (Western Blotting)

In immunoblotting (Western blotting), protein antigens—typically nuclear and cytoplasmic extracts—are separated according to molecular weight by using electrophoresis on a polyacrylamide gel. The separated antigen "bands" are transferred ("blotted") to a nitrocellulose membrane (or strips) that is then incubated with patient or control serum. Bound antibody is identified by use of labeled antihuman IgG.[7] Antibody present in the patient serum is identified by comparison with the control serum results.

The use of cellular extracts as the source of antigen in immunoblotting has the advantage of not requiring purified antigen for testing, and the separation of proteins by molecular weight allows for the determination of the fine specificities of antibody responses to multisubunit antigens.[5] The disadvantages of this technique are that it is time consuming, relatively expensive, requires the denaturing of proteins prior to gel electrophoresis—and will therefore not detect antibodies against conformational epitopes—and has a poor sensitivity for detecting antibodies against Ro and Scl-70 antigens.[4,5]

Immunodiffusion and Counterimmunoelectrophoresis

These techniques involve the detection of antibody–antigen binding as a "precipitation band" of immune complexes within a gel, which is most often composed of agar. In immunodiffusion, a known antigen and a sample of patient serum are placed in separate but closely approximated wells in the gel and allowed to passively diffuse toward one another. Radial immunodiffusion is a related technique in which

the agar gel incorporates antibody of known specificity and a sample containing antigen is placed in a well within the gel. Antigen diffuses from the sample into the gel and will precipitate as a ring if bound by the gel antibody. The diameter of this ring is a function of the concentration of the antigen in the sample.

The process in counterimmunoelectrophoresis (CIEP) is similar to immunodiffusion. However, the pH of the gel is adjusted such that antigen will diffuse toward the anode and antibody toward the cathode when an electrical field is placed across the gel. The wells are situated so that antigen and antibody will diffuse through each other when the electric field is active. The role of the electric field is to accelerate movement of antigen and antibody and thereby shorten the time to a result.

The materials required for CIEP are relatively inexpensive, and both CIEP and immunodiffusion have high specificity for clinical diagnoses.[4] However, in comparison with other methods (e.g., ELISA) they have a lower sensitivity, their performance and interpretation are more labor intensive and skill dependent, and their turnaround time is longer.[4,5]

Nephelometry and Turbidimetry

Nephelometry and turbidimetry are techniques designed to measure the turbidity of a fluid sample as a gauge of the amount of particulate matter (e.g., immune complexes) it contains. Turbidimetry measures the amount of light able to pass directly through the sample, whereas nephelometry measures the amount of light scattered by the sample. In both techniques, comparison with standard samples of known turbidity is required. These techniques may be used to identify either antibodies or antigens. Both are automated and relatively simple to perform but are less sensitive than other techniques.

Laser Microbead Arrays

Laser microbead arrays are one of a number of emerging "multiplex" immunodiagnostic techniques that allow the assay of multiple analytes (e.g., autoantibodies) from a single sample.[8,9] This technique shares some of the principles of ELISA in that it involves the use of labeled "reporter" antibodies to detect the binding of patient antibodies to a known antigen.[10] However, rather than being bound to a well wall on a plastic plate, in the most common form of this assay the antigen is bound to a "microbead" color coded to indicate the antigen it carries, and the "reporter" antibody is labeled with a fluorescent tag rather than an enzyme.[10] Multiple beads bound to different antigens are then mixed with patient serum. Antibodies in the serum will bind to relevant bead-bound antigens, which in turn will be bound by fluorescent-tagged antihuman antibodies. The microbeads are then "read" by lasers of two different wavelengths: one identifying the color of the bead (and hence the antigen it carries) and the other determining the presence or absence of fluorescent-tagged antibody (Fig. 10-5).

The advantages of this method are the number of antibodies that can be measured in parallel, the small volume of sample required, and the speed with which this can be done.[8] The main disadvantage of this method is its reduced sensitivity for some applications.[11,12]

Tests
Antinuclear Antibodies

The term *antinuclear antibodies* (ANA) refers to any of a large group of autoantibodies that recognize cellular antigens found predominantly, although not always exclusively, in the cell nucleus. These antibodies are associated with numerous autoimmune diseases, most importantly SLE, but may also be found in infectious diseases, malignancies, and apparently healthy individuals (eTable 10-1). The first observation hinting at the existence of ANA was made in 1948 in a

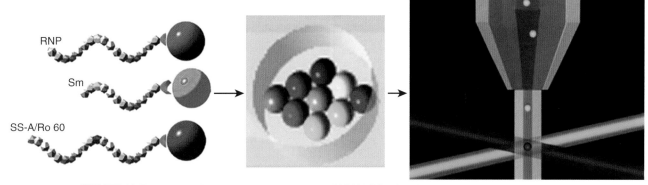

FIGURE 10-5 Addressable laser bead immunoassay (ALBIA). Microbeads are color coded according to the antigen they carry (panel on left) and mixed in wells to which patient serum and a fluorescent tagged antihuman IgG or IgM "reporter" antibody are added (middle panel). The beads are then passed through a chamber and read by lasers of two different wavelengths: one to detect the color of the bead and the other to detect the presence of the reporter antibody. Up to 100 different autoantibodies may be simultaneously tested in a single sample. (From M.J. Fritzler, Lupus 15 (7) (2006) 422–427, copyright © 2006 by SAGE. Reprinted by Permission of SAGE.)

series of patients with SLE.[13] It came in the form of what was termed the *LE cell:* a bone marrow granulocyte that had apparently ingested nuclear material from another cell. Subsequent investigations *in vitro* revealed that this phenomenon could be induced in bone marrow from healthy subjects by the addition of plasma from patients with SLE, and that it resulted from an element in the globulin fraction of serum with an affinity for cell nuclei.[14-16] For several decades, demonstration of LE cells retained a role in the diagnosis of SLE, remaining part of the American College of Rheumatology (ACR) classification criteria for SLE until the 1997 revision.[17]

Detection. Indirect immunofluorescence (IIF) was the technique first used to identify the presence of ANA on the nuclei of cells in tissue sections; it remains the gold standard for their detection.[14,44,45] Early studies noted that ANA could be detected in any cellular tissue but were most easily shown in those tissues in which the cells were arranged in orderly patterns.[46] For this reason early assays used a variety of tissues in which cells were so arranged, including rat and mouse liver and kidney.[47] The use of these tissues, however, was problematic, as their nuclei were small, did not contain all clinically important antigens—particularly Ro/SSA—and rarely contained mitotic cells required for the expression of some antigens, all of which reduced their sensitivity for the detection of ANA in human disease.[45,47] Modern IIF techniques use monolayers of cultured human epithelial cells derived from laryngeal carcinoma (HEp2) as the substrate.[47] This cell line addresses many of the shortfalls of rodent tissue, although the detection of Ro/SSA antibodies in some preparations remains poor.[48,49] For this reason a modified version of these cells, in which the Ro/SSA 60 kDa antigen is hyperexpressed—the HEp-2000 cell line—is used in some laboratories.[50,51] ELISA and other newer methods, such as multiplex bead-based assays, can also be used for the detection of ANA. As they can only offer testing against a limited number of antigens they have a lower sensitivity for the detection of ANA than IIF and are not currently recommended for ANA screening.[44,45]

Immunofluorescence patterns. The cell nucleus contains thousands of antigens, any one of which could theoretically be the target of an ANA. In SLE alone, more than 100 different ANA-target antigens have been reported.[52] The pattern of immunofluorescence produced by ANA in IIF assays is determined in large part by the location of the target antigen within the cell. A recent attempt to harmonize the nomenclature used to describe ANA IF patterns on HEp2 cells divides

them into five broad groups based on the location of the target antigen.[53] Within each of these groups there are between two and nine descriptors based on the immunofluorescent appearance. In this nomenclature, any antibody that binds to HEp2 cells is considered to be an "ANA," although some of the responsible antigens are located exclusively in the cytoplasm (e.g., mitochondria), and therefore their cognate antibodies are not strictly "antinuclear."[44,53] Many laboratories report these cytoplasmic patterns as an addendum in reports of ANA assays on HEp2 cells.[54] eTable 10-2 outlines the proposed nomenclature along with the disease association of each pattern and the responsible target antigen. Updated consensus recommendations regarding the assessment of autoantibodies using HEp2 cells take a slightly different approach by dividing the patterns according to those commonly and less commonly seen but the pattern descriptors themselves and their associations are largely the same.[44] Figure 10-6 demonstrates some of the more common IIF patterns seen in clinical practice.

One of the difficulties of the use of ANA IF patterns in the diagnosis of rheumatic diseases is their lack of disease specificity, as evident in eTable 10-2. This derives largely from the fact that, with few exceptions, the patterns are not specific for a particular antigen; multiple antigens may cause the same pattern and the same antigen may give different patterns in different patients.[55] For this reason, in clinical practice once the presence of one or more ANA have been identified using a screening method, the elucidation of their antigen specificity is generally performed using more targeted assays (see the sections on antibodies to extractable nuclear antigens and anti-DNA antibodies).

Presence in healthy individuals. Although a hallmark of many autoimmune diseases, ANA may be found at low titers (e.g., 1:40) in up to 32% of healthy adults and at higher titers (e.g., 1:160) in 5%.[56] The titer of ANA required before a sample is considered "positive" varies between laboratories and depends on factors such as the technique and materials used. For IIF, titer cut points of 1:80 or 1:160 are commonly used. An increased prevalence of ANA in the adult population has been noted in women, the elderly, and in first-degree relatives of those with autoimmune disease.[57-60] In healthy children, ANA have a prevalence of between 5% and 18%.[57,61-64] Most of these are at titers in the range of 1:80 to 1:320; however, higher titers may occur. In general, they do not have specificity against antigens associated with autoimmune disease, and over time a proportion will decrease in titer or disappear completely.[61-63,65-67] Some may be related to intercurrent

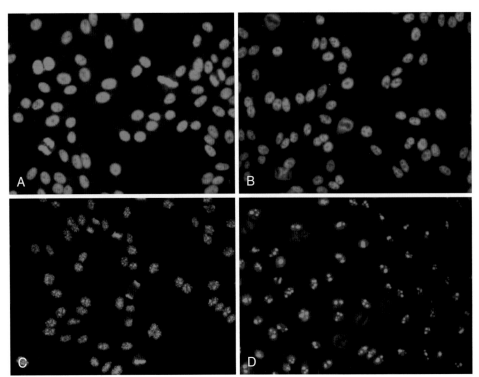

FIGURE 10-6 Common ANA immunofluorescence patterns on HEp2 cells. **A,** Homogenous. **B,** Speckled. **C,** Nucleolar (with occasional speckling). **D,** Centromere.

infection, which can induce transient autoantibodies.[68] Nonetheless a significant number will persist, raising concern about the possibility of autoimmune disease in evolution; studies in adults have found that circulating autoantibodies may be found several years before symptom onset in SLE[69,70] (eFig. 10-7). Reassurance regarding this issue is provided by reports of a combined total of over 50 ANA-positive children referred for assessment in whom rheumatological evaluation did not identify inflammatory or immune-mediated disease.[65,71] In these reports ANA titers were generally less than or equal to 1:320, although titers as high as 1:2560 were occasionally seen. Over a follow-up period ranging between 3 and 5 years only one child developed autoimmune disease, and that child had features at presentation that were suspicious for such an outcome.[71]

Antibodies to Extractable Nuclear Antigens

Extractable nuclear antigens (ENA) are a group of over 100 antigens derived from ribonucleohistone and nonhistone proteins that can be extracted from the saline soluble fraction of cells.[72-74] They are important as they encompass a significant proportion of the antigens to which ANA form in rheumatic diseases; the presence of ANA directed toward these antigens is more concerning for underlying clinically significant autoimmune disease than those for which no antigen specificity can be found. Antibodies against some of these antigens are highly specific for particular conditions (e.g., Scl-70 and systemic sclerosis) or associated with particular clinical phenotypes within a disease group (e.g., the myositis specific autoantibodies; see Chapter 26), whereas others may be found in a range of diseases. As with any test, their relevance is ultimately determined by the clinical context in which they occur. The nomenclature of ENAs is confusing, as a standard approach to their naming was not used. Some are named according to their function (e.g., RNP), others according to the name of the patient for which they were first described (e.g., Sm, Ro, La), and still others according to the disease in which they are most commonly

found (e.g., Scl-70).[73] eTable 10-3 outlines the major clinically relevant ENAs and the disease associations of ANA directed against them.

Detection. Anti-ENA antibodies may be detected by gel precipitation assays such as double immunodiffusion; CIEP; solid phase methods such as ELISA; Western blot-based techniques such as immunoblotting; and by multiplex assays; each has advantages and disadvantages. Although the overall concordance between many of these is satisfactory, there are differences in their sensitivity and specificity for detection of particular antigens.[5,82,83] Reasons for this include differences in the source of antigens used in the assays and loss of conformational determinants of some antigens during their preparation or the running of the assays.[76,80] As no single method can be guaranteed to detect all relevant anti-ENA antibodies, current recommendations are that two methods be used.[5,84,85] Whichever approach is adopted, it is essential for the clinician to be aware of the strengths and weaknesses of locally used methods and, in particular, to follow up with the laboratory if there is a discrepancy between the clinical picture and anti-ENA antibody result.

Anti-DNA Antibodies

Antibodies to DNA are another clinically important group of ANA. They may be directed toward antigens on double-stranded (ds) or single-stranded (ss) DNA, be IgG or IgM in isotype, and be of high or low avidity. *Avidity* describes the net strength of the interaction between an antibody and antigen and is determined by several factors, including the individual affinity of antibody-binding sites for their specific epitopes, the charge carried by the antibody and antigen, and the actual physical interaction between the two. High-avidity IgG anti-dsDNA antibodies are the most clinically useful of this group as they have a high specificity for SLE (97.1% in children[86]) and are associated with an increased risk of development of lupus nephritis in adults, although this association was not confirmed in children in a large cohort study.[87,18] They are present in 60% to 90% of adults and 72%

to 93% of pediatric SLE patients, making them a more sensitive marker of this disease than anti-Sm antibodies, which have a high specificity but low sensitivity for the diagnosis of SLE[18,19,88,89] (eTable 10-3). In addition, antibodies to dsDNA are one of the few autoantibodies whose levels fluctuate with disease activity; rising levels are frequently associated with disease flares.[90,91] Although high-avidity antibodies are relatively specific for SLE, lower-avidity anti-dsDNA antibodies may be found in a range of other conditions including Sjögren's syndrome, rheumatoid arthritis, and autoimmune hepatitis.[92,93] Antibodies to ssDNA have little diagnostic specificity and are rarely used in clinical practice.

Detection. One of the principal determinants of the avidity of the antibodies detected in laboratory testing is the assay used. Those available for the detection of anti-dsDNA antibodies include radioimmunoassay (i.e., Farr assay), IF assay using *Crithidia luciliae* (a flagellate parasite containing circular dsDNA without other nuclear antigens in the kinetoplast), ELISA, and multiplex assays. Of these, *Crithidia luciliae* and Farr assay detect higher-avidity antibodies, with the greatest specificity for the diagnosis of SLE.[94] Most laboratories, however, use ELISA or multiplex assays, which are less labor intensive, faster, more sensitive, and do not involve the use of radioactive materials. However, they detect lower-avidity antibodies with less specificity for the diagnosis of SLE.

Antinucleosome Antibodies

Chromatin is the main form in which DNA is found within the nucleus. At its most basic level it comprises negatively charged DNA wound tightly around positively charged histone protein octamers in conjunction with a linker histone protein in a repeating pattern that gives chromatin a "beads on a string" appearance on electron microscopy.[95] These macromolecular "bead" subunits are known as *nucleosomes* and can be the target of ANA. These may be directed toward epitopes on the individual components of the nucleosome (i.e., dsDNA and histones) or to conformational epitopes derived from interactions between these components on the intact subunits only (so-called nucleosome-restricted autoantibodies).[96] In the past 10 years there has been interest in the diagnostic use of antinucleosome antibodies (ANuAs) for the diagnosis of SLE.[97,98] In adults, ANuAs have similar specificity for the diagnosis of SLE as anti-dsDNA antibodies but greater sensitivity.[86] Although it has been suggested that in the future ANuAs may supplant anti-dsDNA testing in the diagnosis of SLE,[86] their acceptance as a valid diagnostic test is not universal.[99]

Antineutrophil Cytoplasmic Antibodies

Antibodies directed toward antigens in the cytoplasm of neutrophils were first described in 1982 in a series of eight patients with a generalized illness in which necrotizing glomerulonephritis and severe arthralgia or myalgia occurred in all and respiratory symptoms occurred in half—some with pulmonary hemorrhage.[100] These are now recognized as common clinical findings in a group of conditions characterized by predominantly small vessel inflammation and the presence of antibodies directed toward specific neutrophil cytoplasmic antigens—the antineutrophil cytoplasmic antibody (ANCA)-associated vasculitidies (AAVs). The AAVs encompass the following clinical entities: granulomatosis with polyangiitis (GPA, previously known as Wegener granulomatosis); microscopic polyangiitis (MPA); eosinophillic granulomatosis with polyangiitis (EGPA, previously known as Churg–Strauss syndrome); and idiopathic necrotizing crescentic glomerulonephritis (INCGN). As with antinuclear antibodies, the term *ANCA* does not refer to a single antibody but to a family of antibodies, each directed toward a specific antigen. In the case of ANCA, these antigens are contained within granules in the neutrophil cytoplasm and include

proteinase 3 (PR3); myeloperoxidase (MPO); lactoferrin; elastase; cathespin G; and bactericidal/permeability-increasing protein, among others.[101,102] ANCA directed toward PR3 and MPO are the most clinically relevant as they are strongly associated with the AAVs.

Detection. IIF was the method by which ANCA were first identified and remains the recommended method for their initial detection.[100,102] Ethanol-fixed neutrophils are the substrate used and in the presence of ANCA, one of two main IF patterns will be observed: predominant cytoplasmic fluorescence with central interlobular accentuation (c-ANCA) or perinuclear fluorescence, frequently with nuclear extension (p-ANCA)[102] (Fig. 10-8). The p-ANCA pattern is actually an artifact caused by movement of the relevant antigens, which are distributed throughout the cytoplasm *in vivo*, to a perinuclear position during ethanol fixation.[101] This redistribution does not occur with formalin fixation and may be difficult to discern if ANA are also present.[102-104] Patterns lacking the typical fluorescent features of c- or p-ANCA (atypical ANCA) may also occur.

As with ANA, the IIF pattern of ANCA provides some guidance regarding their possible antigen specificity. In patients with AAVs, c-ANCA and p-ANCA patterns are generally associated with antibody specificity for PR3 and MPO, respectively, although occasionally the reverse is seen.[102] In unselected patients, these associations are not as strong, particularly for p-ANCA and atypical ANCA, which may occur with ANCA directed toward a number of antigens other than MPO.[101,102,104] A positive test for ANCA on IIF therefore requires further assessment to determine the antigen specificity of the antibodies.[101,102] ELISA assays are commonly used in this situation. Sandwich ELISA and a related assay, the anchor ELISA—in which a protein rather than antibody binds the antigen to the well—may have particular clinical utility in this setting, offering increased sensitivity without loss of specificity.[105,106] Bead-based multiplex assays have also been developed for this purpose.[12]

Disease associations. ANCA are the serological hallmark of active AAVs. They are found in approximately 90% of adult patients with active GPA, 75% with MPA, and 30% with EGPA.[107-109] The prevalence of ANCA during periods of remission or in localized forms of GPA is lower. In GPA the typical finding is that of a PR3-specific c-ANCA with just 10% to 25% having an MPO-specific p-ANCA.[102,109] This pattern is the converse of that seen in the other AAVs in which PR3-specific c-ANCA is the less common specificity. The prevalence and pattern of specificities of ANCA in pediatric GPA is similar to that in adult disease.[110,111] As with anti-dsDNA antibodies, ANCA titers tend to fluctuate with disease activity.[112] Although some studies have shown them to be useful in predicting disease flares, a recent meta-analysis found their predictive level to be only modest.[113-115]

ANCA may be found in a range of conditions other than AAVs, though their low prevalence and lack of correlation with clinical phenotype mean they have little value for their diagnosis. These conditions include inflammatory bowel disease, autoimmune hepatitis, antiglomerular basement membrane disease, rheumatoid arthritis, juvenile idiopathic arthritis, and various infectious diseases, particularly tuberculosis and hepatitis C.[116,117] Drugs may also induce the formation of ANCA and in some cases lead to the development of AAVs.[118] In general, the ANCA identified in these conditions demonstrate atypical features on IIF, usually with a p-ANCA pattern, and have specificity for antigens other than PR3 or MPO. However, this cannot be relied upon as a distinguishing feature from AAV, as PR3- or MPO-specific ANCA may also occur.[104,119,120]

Antiglomerular Basement Membrane Antibodies

Antibodies directed toward the glomerular basement membrane (GBM) were first shown to be pathogenic in humans in 1967.[121] In

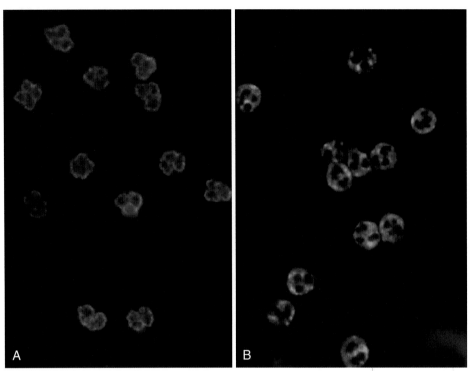

FIGURE 10-8 The two common ANCA immunofluorescence patterns on ethanol-fixed neutrophils. **A,** p-ANCA. **B,** c-ANCA.

most cases these antibodies are of the IgG1 subclass and are directed toward the noncollagenous (NC1) domain of the α3 chain of type IV collagen (α3[IV]NC1), found in the kidney basement membrane, lungs, cochlea, and retina.[122-124] Collectively, the clinical syndromes with which they are associated are termed *anti-GBM disease,* and they consist of the following: isolated rapidly progressive glomerulonephritis (RPGN); pulmonary hemorrhage or the combination of the two—eponymously known as Goodpasture syndrome.[125] By definition, anti-GBM antibodies can be detected in 100% of patients with anti-GBM disease using a combination of serum and tissue diagnostics. Unlike many autoantibodies, they are not detectable in the serum of healthy subjects, although there are reports of their isolation using specialized techniques for identifying low levels of low-avidity antibodies.[126] They may, however, be detectable using standard assays in the context of polyclonal B cell activation in human immunodeficiency virus (HIV) and hepatitis C infection without evidence of pulmonary or renal disease.[127] They can also be found in up to 10% of patients with AAVs, and may portend a more guarded renal prognosis.[128,129]

Detection. Although anti-GBM antibodies can be identified by IIF using normal human or primate kidney as substrate, this method is relatively insensitive—as low as 60% for those with isolated RPGN—and is rarely used.[130,131] The most commonly used method is ELISA, using bovine or recombinant human α3(IV)NC1.[123] Multiple commercial ELISA kits are available for this purpose, with sensitivities and specificities greater than 90%.[130] It is important to be aware, however, that up to 5% of patients with anti-GBM disease will not have circulating antibodies that can be detected by using commercial assays.[130] Reasons for this include the disruption of conformational epitopes during assay preparation; differences in the epitopes recognized by the antibodies of some patients, rendering them unreactive with bovine preparations; and the predominance of IgG4 subclass or other Ig isotype (e.g., IgA or IgM) antibodies in some cases.[132-134]

Demonstration of antibodies *in situ* on the glomerular basement membrane by direct immunofluorescence is considered the diagnostic gold standard, and, where practical, a renal biopsy is recommended in all patients in whom the diagnosis of anti-GBM disease is suspected.[134,135]

Rheumatoid Factor

The report in 1940 of an "agglutination activating factor" in serum from patients with rheumatoid arthritis (RA) that caused clumping of sheep red blood cells (RBCs) sensitized with rabbit anti-sheep corpuscle serum was the first description of the effect of antibodies in RA subsequently known as rheumatoid factor (RF).[136] RF is not a single antibody but a family of antibodies directed toward the Fc portion of IgG. They may be of either low or high affinity.[137] Low-affinity RFs are IgM antibodies that play a role in the clearance, B-cell uptake and complement fixation of immune complexes in the normal immune system and may be seen in the context of infection and in otherwise healthy subjects.[137-140] High-affinity RF can be of any isotype and is frequently associated with autoimmune disease. High-affinity IgM-RF is the most clinically significant, being the predominant isotype in both RA and the RF-positive polyarticular subtype of juvenile idiopathic arthritis (JIA), and the only type considered in the current classification criteria for these two conditions.[141-144] The presence of IgM-RF in both is associated with an increased risk of progressive disease, joint damage, and disability.[139,144] In RA, it is also associated with a greater risk of extraarticular disease.[140] Similar associations have been reported for IgA-RF in both adults and children.[140,144,145] Other conditions in which IgM-RF may be found include other rheumatic diseases, notably Sjögren's syndrome—in which titers of RF are typically very high—and infections, particularly if chronic, secondary, or latent (eTable 10-4).[139,146]

Detection. The agglutination of sheep RBCs to detect RF, known as the Waaler–Rose test after the investigators who described the phenomenon, has largely been replaced by more sensitive detection methods including latex agglutination, nephelometry or turbidimetry, and ELISA.[156] The first two both use human IgG-coated artificial particles rather than sheep RBCs as the reagent, which agglutinate in the presence of RF. Latex agglutination requires visual assessment of the reaction and is at best semiquantitative. In contrast, nephelometry or turbidimetry and ELISA can be automated and provide quantitative results. Nephelometry or turbidimetry and latex agglutination detect mainly IgM-RF, as the other isotypes are poor agglutinins.[157] ELISA is more sensitive than these methods and can be used to detect isotypes other than IgM.[139,144,158]

Anticitrullinated Peptide Antibodies

Anticitrullinated peptide antibodies (ACPA) are a group of autoantibodies that share the property of targeting protein epitopes containing the nonstandard amino acid citrulline. They include antiperinuclear factor (APF), antikeratin antibodies (AKA), and anti-Sa antibodies.[140,159] Although APF and AKA were described in the context of RA as far back as 1964 and 1979, respectively, they did not come into common clinical use because of difficulties with the assays used for their detection.[147,160] An ELISA utilizing a synthetic cyclic citrullinated peptide (CCP) derived from the sequence of filaggrin—the protein recognized by APF and AKA—was the first commercially available assay for determining the presence of ACPA.[159] The use of a single cyclic peptide allows for the detection of a number of different ACPA[160] such that the anti-CCP antibody assay has become the standard test in clinical practice for this purpose. More recent versions of this assay, with alterations in the cyclic peptide to improve sensitivity, are commonly designated anti-CCP2 and anti-CCP3.[161,162]

The primary clinical relevance of ACPA is their association with RA. As they are rarely found in other conditions or in healthy subjects they have a high specificity for this diagnosis. A recent meta-analysis calculated the pooled specificity of anti-CCP antibodies for the diagnosis of RA to be 95%.[163] Their sensitivity, however, is in the range of that for IgM-RF: 67% in the same meta-analysis.[163] As with RF, anti-CCP antibodies are associated with more severe articular disease and in fact may be a stronger predictor of radiographic progression than RF.[140,163] Unlike RF, anti-CCP antibodies are not associated with an increased risk of extraarticular disease.[164] Similar to RA, anti-CCP antibodies are highly specific for the diagnosis of JIA (approximately 98%), but their sensitivity is much lower than that for RA—just 14% in typical cohorts.[155] In most studies they have been found predominantly in the RF-positive polyarticular subgroup, in which their prevalence approaches that of adult RA (~59%).[155] The presence of anti-CCP antibodies in patients with JIA may confer a worse prognosis,[144] although caution is required when interpreting studies to date because of their relatively small sample sizes and confounding by the concurrent presence of RF in most patients.[165-169] At the present time their role in the diagnosis and management of JIA is unresolved.

Antiphospholipid Antibodies

Antiphospholipid antibodies (APLA) are a large heterogeneous group of autoantibodies targeting epitopes not just on phospholipids but also phospholipid-binding proteins and phospholipid-protein complexes.[170,171] A subset of these antibodies predisposes to pregnancy morbidity and thrombosis in what has been termed the antiphospholipid syndrome (APS). This subset currently consists of lupus anticoagulants (LAC), anticardiolipin (aCL) antibodies, and anti-β_2-glycoprotein 1 (anti-β_2GP1) antibodies.[172] The terms aCL and LAC are confusing and reflect early laboratory and clinical observations rather than the current understanding of these antibodies. The target of aCL

is not cardiolipin per se but a complex of the phospholipid-binding protein β_2GP1 and cardiolipin, and LAC are not restricted to patients with lupus nor is their primary clinical effect anticoagulation.[173,174] More confusing still, some LAC are directed toward β_2GP1[175] and some aCL have LAC activity.[176,177] Thus, although the terms LAC, aCL, and anti-β_2GP1 antibody can refer to distinct types of antibodies, they may also refer to different characteristics of the same antibody. The mechanism by which any of these antibodies predispose to thrombosis is not well understood.[178,179] Anticardiolipin antibodies and LAC are found in up to 5% of healthy adults and up to 30% of patients with SLE.[180] They may also occur in the context of infections, malignancies, and drug therapy.[181-183]

LAC are IgG and IgM antibodies directed toward β_2GP1 or prothrombin that, by definition, cause prolongation of phospholipid-dependent assays of coagulation.[184] Of all APLA, those demonstrating this activity carry the highest thrombosis risk.[185] Their presence is proven indirectly by demonstrating the following three attributes in functional tests of coagulation: prolongation of two phospholipid-dependent coagulation assays based on different principles (typically the activated partial thromboplastin time [APTT] and dilute Russell viper venom time [DRVVT]); the presence of an inhibitor (i.e., no correction when mixed with normal plasma); and phospholipid dependence of the inhibitor effect (i.e., partial correction with the addition of phospholipid).[179,186] Measures to exclude other coagulopathies should also be taken. Although unexpected prolongation of the APTT is a widely recognized clue to the presence of LAC, it is important to be aware that not all APTT assays in routine use are sensitive to this effect.[187] The assays used for detection of LAC typically include reduced concentrations of phospholipid to increase their sensitivity.[174,184] In general, it is recommended that testing for LAC be performed before starting anticoagulation.[172,186] However, not all anticoagulant therapies interfere with LAC testing, and some assays incorporate neutralizing agents for certain anticoagulants.[173,184] Discussion with the testing laboratory is therefore recommended in this situation.

Anticardiolipin and anti-β_2GP1 antibodies may be of IgG, IgM, or IgA isotypes; however, only moderate to high titer IgG and IgM antibodies are included in current diagnostic criteria for APS.[172,179] Of these, the IgG isotypes are thought to be the most clinically relevant.[174,175] These antibodies are less strongly associated with thrombosis risk than LAC.[174,185,188] However, when both are present in association with LAC the risk of thrombosis is higher than for any single positive test.[173,189] These antibodies are most commonly detected by ELISA. Unlike those for LAC, assays for these antibodies are generally unaffected by anticoagulation.[179] More information on APLA and associated clinical findings may be found in Chapter 24.

Complement

Complement is a cascading system of more than 30 proteins that account for 10% to 15% of the globulin fraction in serum.[190,191] Although nominally part of the innate immune system it also plays an integral role in adaptive immunity.[191,192] It is divided into three early pathways: (1) classical, (2) mannose-binding lectin (MBL), and (3) alternative, which feed into a common terminal pathway resulting in the generation of a membrane attack complex and cell lysis[190,193] (eFig. 10-9). Among other things, complement is involved in protection against infection, removal of immune complexes and apoptotic cells, regulation of the adaptive immune response, and tissue regeneration.[192,194] An absence of, or reduction in, either amount or function of complement components can be genetic in origin and may be associated with clinical sequelae ranging from none to significant predisposition to bacterial infection or autoimmune disease, depending on the component involved. A reduction in components can also be the result of excessive consumption, as frequently occurs in active SLE, and the detection of such a reduction may be helpful in the diagnosis or monitoring of conditions in which this is seen.

There are two broad screening techniques for investigating the complement system. The first is immunochemical analysis of individual components based on immune complex formation using techniques including radial immunodiffusion, nephelometry or turbidimetry, and ELISA.[193] This type of analysis is most commonly used in the detection of C3 and C4 but can be used to identify other components such as C1 esterase inhibitor. This "antigenic" method does not provide information about the functional status of the protein and may give a misleading picture regarding the true state of the complement cascade in the context of acute inflammation as most components, including C3 and C4, are acute phase reactants.[195,196]

The second means of investigating the complement system are functional assays, in which the ability of whole pathways or individual components to lyse RBCs is determined. The most common measurement methods used are the CH50/CH100 assays that test the integrity of the classical and terminal pathways (components C1-9; eFig. 10-9) and are a function of the dilution at which test serum lyses 50% or 100% of a sample of antibody-bound sheep erythrocytes, respectively.[193] Low or absent lysis implies a reduction in, or absence of, the presence or function of one of the components in the pathways tested. The AH50 is based on a similar principle but tests the alternative and terminal pathways (factors D, B, H, I, properdin, C3, C5-9; eFig. 10-9)[193] and typically uses rabbit erythrocytes. The function of the MBL pathway can be tested by ELISAs in which plate wells are coated with a specific activator of this pathway, and the reagents detect products uniquely generated during pathway activation.[196,197] Similar ELISAs for testing the function of the classical and alternative pathways[193] have also been developed and are now replacing the CH50/CH100 and AH50 assays. Functional tests of individual components may be performed by adding patient serum to samples known to be deficient in single complement proteins to determine if activity is restored.[197]

OTHER LABORATORY INVESTIGATIONS

Measures of the Acute Phase Response

The term *acute phase response* (APR) refers to the increase in specific plasma proteins—collectively known as *acute phase proteins* (APPs)—triggered by infection, inflammation, tissue damage, and neoplasia.[198,199] The APR is integral to the maintenance of an intact organism, acting to neutralize infective and inflammatory agents, reduce tissue damage, and assist in tissue repair.[200] Indeed, some aspects of this response can be considered as the innate immune system analog of humoral immunity in the adaptive immune system in which the recognition of pathogen-specific epitopes has been replaced by a broader recognition of molecular patterns and chemical constituents associated with microorganisms and tissue damage.

The majority of APPs are synthesized in the liver in response to tumor necrosis factor (TNF)-α, interleukin (IL)-1 and IL-6, the key cytokine mediators of the APR.[200,201] Based on the degree to which they increase during the APR, APPs can be divided into three broad groups. Those with the largest increase (1000-fold or more) are the C-reactive protein (CRP) and serum amyloid A (SAA). The next group (with increases of twofold to threefold) include fibrinogen and haptoglobin. The third group (with increases of approximately 50%) include ceruloplasmin and C3.[201,202] Of these, only CRP and SAA are specifically measured in clinical practice as a gauge of the APR.

Erythrocyte Sedimentation Rate

The erythrocyte sedimentation rate (ESR) is a nonspecific measure of the APR, the principles of which were described as far back as 1918.[203] It is defined as the rate at which RBCs settle though plasma to form a sediment in whole blood suspended in a vertical glass tube. It is measured as the distance between the meniscus at the top of the tube and the top of the red cell mass below after 1 hour and is expressed in millimeters/hour (mm/hr).

RBCs have a net negative charge and tend to repel each other, falling as individual cells in suspended whole blood. Under normal circumstances the factors that impede red cell sedimentation—such as plasma viscosity—almost balance the effect of gravity on red cells, and the sedimentation rate is low.[204] The mechanism by which the APR produces an increase in the ESR is not completely understood but may be thought of simplistically as the production of positively charged APPs—of which fibrinogen is the most important—that bind red cells and effectively reduce their negative charge.[203] This allows their aggregation in stacks known as *rouleaux*, increasing their effective mass-to-surface area ratio and therefore the rate at which they sediment.[198,203,204] Two methods are available for ESR measurement: Westergren and Wintrobe.[198] These differ in the type of glass tube used and the mechanism by which coagulation of the blood sample within the tube is prevented, but they rely on the same general principles and are measured in the same way.

The ESR is increased in any condition in which the APR causes an increase in APPs that affect the net charge on red cells, in particular fibrinogen. It is therefore elevated in many infectious and immune-mediated inflammatory conditions. The nonspecific nature of the ESR limits its diagnostic usefulness. A common clinical application for its use is to measure underlying disease activity and monitor treatment response in situations in which the diagnosis is known, although as the proteins that contribute to the ESR generally have half-lives measured in days, it tends to be slow to respond to reductions in the APR.

It is important to be aware that not all APPs cause an increase in ESR, most notably CRP and SAA.[198] It is also important to be aware that ESR may be elevated by plasma proteins other than fibrinogen (e.g., gamma globulins), which may result in marked elevation of the ESR in the absence of an APR, as occurs in hypergammaglobulinemia. Conversely, factors that reduce fibrinogen will cause the ESR to fall, even in the context of ongoing inflammation, a situation commonly seen in macrophage activation syndrome complicated by hypofibrinogenemia. The ESR may also be affected by technical factors and alterations in the physical properties of red cells.[205,206] eTable 10-5 provides an overview of factors that may influence ESR.

C-reactive Protein

CRP was first identified in 1930 in the serum of patients acutely unwell with pneumococcal pneumonia.[198] Although named for the fact that it binds the C-polysaccharide of the pneumococcus, it is now known to be one of the major APPs in humans and is elevated in most diseases where there is active inflammation or tissue destruction.[200,204] The techniques traditionally used for the detection of CRP are radial immunodiffusion, nephelometry, immunoturbidimetry, and ELISA.[198]

Although used clinically as a simple measure of the acute phase response, the physiological function of CRP—a cyclic pentamer of five identical polypeptide subunits—is as a pattern recognition protein.[199,204,208] These proteins serve to identify pathogen-associated molecular patterns (PAMPs) and damage-associated molecular patterns (DAMPs) and direct immune responses toward them.[209] The ligand to which CRP binds with the highest affinity is phosphocholine, a residue common to many prokaryotes and all eukaryotes.[199] It also binds other ligands, including histones, chromatin, and small nuclear ribonuclear proteins.[199,200] Ligand binding induces a conformational change in CRP allowing it to interact with C1q and activate the classical complement pathway.[199,204] In this way CRP plays an important role in directing the immune response to pathogens and damaged and apoptotic cells.

In healthy subjects, CRP is found at very low circulating levels. Increases occur within hours of the onset of the APR, with levels peaking between 1 and 3 days.[199,204] The plasma half-life of CRP is 19 hours, making it a more responsive marker of reductions in the APR than the ESR.[199] In most diseases, CRP levels reflect the degree of inflammation and/or tissue damage more accurately than ESR.[199] A curious and as yet unexplained exception to this general rule occurs in several rheumatic diseases including SLE, juvenile dermatomyositis/ polymyositis, scleroderma, and Sjögren's disease, in which the CRP is typically normal or minimally elevated despite concurrent increased ESR.[198,199] This discrepancy may be useful diagnostically; in SLE a significantly elevated CRP is suggestive of infection, serositis, or arthritis.[210]

Serum Amyloid A

The term *serum amyloid A* (SAA) refers to a family of apolipoproteins synthesized in the liver of which one class—acute phase SAA— constitutes one of the major APPs in humans.[211] As with other APPs, SAA is thought to play an important role in initiating and regulating host immune defense.[211,212] Although an important APP, in clinical practice SAA is not routinely used to monitor the APR. A specific indication for its measurement to assist in titrating colchicine dose has been suggested in patients with familial Mediterranean fever (FMF), in whom chronic elevation of SAA between episodes of clinically overt inflammation may lead to the development of secondary amyloidosis, the fibrils of which are largely composed of SAA.[204,213]

Ferritin

Ferritin is a widely distributed intracellular protein that functions to store, release, and transport iron.[214] The most common clinical indication for its measurement is to gauge body iron stores; it is decreased in iron deficiency and significantly increased in the setting of iron overload. It is also an APP—with levels typically remaining below 1000 ng/mL—although not routinely used to measure the APR. There are two clinical situations, however, in which the finding of significant hyperferritinemia (typically greater than 1000 ng/mL and often much higher) may assist in diagnosis: systemic juvenile idiopathic arthritis or adult-onset Still disease,[215] and macrophage activation syndrome (MAS) or hemophagocytic lymphohistiocytosis (HLH).[215-217] Other conditions in which significant hyperferritinemia has been reported include hepatocellular disease, renal failure, and malignancy.[215,218] In rare instances, elevated ferritin may occur in the context of genetic diseases without underlying iron overload or inflammation (e.g., hyperferritinemia-cataract syndrome).[214]

Synovial Fluid

Examination of synovial fluid in clinical practice is primarily used to determine the presence of either infection or crystals.[219] As crystal arthopathy is extremely rare in the pediatric age group, the majority of synovial fluid examinations requested in children are to exclude infection.

There are three laboratory tests useful in the evaluation of synovial fluid for infection. The first is the synovial fluid white cell count (sWCC); its usefulness for the diagnosis of joint sepsis has been derived from studies of predominantly adult patients. These ranges should be considered a broad guide only because there is significant overlap between the inflammatory (noninfectious) and septic categories. The

use of likelihood ratios for cell count ranges provides a more nuanced view of the use of sWCC in the diagnosis of joint sepsis. In two recent systematic reviews that evaluated the utility of tests in the diagnosis of nongonococcal septic arthritis, sWCC greater than 50,000/mm^3 had positive likelihood ratios of 4.7 (95% confidence interval [CI], 2.5-8.5) and 7.7 (95% CI, 5.7-11.0), which increased to 13.2 (95% CI, 3.6-51.1) and 28 (95% CI, 12.0-66.0) for counts greater than 100,000 mm^3, respectively.[220,221] A predominance of polymorphonuclear leukocytes (i.e., greater than 90%) may also increase the likelihood of infection.[221] It is important to be aware that inflamed synovial fluid will clot, making cell counts unreliable, so measures must be taken to prevent this if they are required. The use of tubes containing ethylenediamine-tetraacetic acid (EDTA) has been shown to allow for reliable cell counts in specimens analyzed up to 48 hours after removal.[222]

The second test that may be of value in the evaluation of possible joint sepsis is a Gram stain, which is performed on a concentrated pellet of synovial fluid debris after centrifugation. Although theoretically a test of high specificity in this situation, there have been no formal studies to confirm this.[220] The reported sensitivity of synovial Gram stains for joint sepsis range from 50% to 70% and 10% to 25% for nongonococcal and gonococcal arthritis, respectively.[223]

The third test of value in the assessment for joint sepsis is culture. The sensitivity of culture for nongonoccoal and gonoccocal joint sepsis in the absence of prior antimicrobial therapy is 75% to 95% and 10% to 50%, respectively.[223] The reduced sensitivity of culture for gonococcal infection may be due in part to the fastidious nature of the organism.[223] In addition to organisms that typically cause septic arthritis in adults, young children are at particular risk of infection from *Kingella kingae*. The inoculation of a sample of synovial fluid directly into a blood culture bottle at the time of collection will greatly increase diagnostic yield.[224] Culture of synovial fluid may not be possible in the context of prior antibiotic therapy. In this situation, molecular techniques such as polymerase chain reaction (PCR) may be used to target the gene for 16S ribosomal RNA with the potential to confirm eubacterial infection and even identify the pathogen.[225,226] Such techniques, with reported sensitivities and specificities of greater than 95%,[226] may become the primary method by which septic arthritis is confirmed in the future.

Although not usually considered in the evaluation of joints for infection with typical bacterial pathogens, when infection with mycobacterium tuberculosis is suspected the sampling of synovial tissue for histology and culture is essential; the reported rate of identification of the organism by these methods is greater than 90%, compared with 20% for Ziehl–Neelson staining of synovial fluid pellets and 60% to 80% for synovial fluid culture alone.[223,227-229]

Urinalysis

The detection of protein, blood, and formed elements that may appear in the urine in the context of glomerulonephritis is the main focus of urinalysis in rheumatological practice. There are four investigations commonly used for this purpose: (1) dipstick analysis, (2) microscopy, (3) protein-to-creatinine ratio (Pr : Cr), and (4) 24-hour collections.

Dipstick analysis is commonly used in the clinic as a guide to the presence of urinary protein and/or blood. In the detection of proteinuria, however, the performance of dipstick testing is relatively poor, with a sensitivity and specificity for proteinuria greater than 300 mg/24 hours (normal less than 150 mg/24 hours) ranging between 60% and 80% and 67% and 95%, respectively.[230] A particular issue is that dipstick reagent squares react to concentrations of protein (in particular albumin) and may miss clinically relevant proteinuria in the presence of dilute urine.[231] Furthermore, within a proteinuria range of 200 to 3000 mg/L, dipstick readings correlate poorly with formal measures of urinary protein loss.[232,233] The reported sensitivity and specificity of dipstick analysis for hematuria is between 91% and 100% and 65% and 99%, respectively.[234] As dipstick reagent squares register the peroxidase activity of hemoglobin, they will also be positive in the setting of hemoglobin and myoglobinuria.

Microscopy of the sediment formed in urine after centrifugation (eFig. 10-10, A) provides information about the presence of RBCs, leukocytes, and formed elements such as casts. More than five RBCs per high-powered field is considered abnormal, and the morphology of the cells may provide information regarding their likely origin (glomerular or nonglomerular).[235-237] The presence of hyaline casts (eFig. 10-10, B) may be a normal finding in concentrated urine or after the administration of diuretics or heavy exercise.[238-240] They are composed mainly of Tamm–Horsfall protein, a glycoprotein derived from cells in the thick ascending loop of Henle important in the prevention of crystal formation.[239,241] Granular and cellular casts (eFig. 10-10, C) are abnormal and indicate leakage of cells through the glomerulus. In addition to Tamm–Horsfall protein, the matrix of these casts frequently includes immunoglobulins, complement components, and fibrin.[239]

Two common methods of quantifying urinary protein loss are by measuring the Pr:Cr ratio on a spot urine or the protein content of a 24-hour urine collection. Although the latter remains the gold standard for assessing proteinuria, the process is cumbersome and samples are often incomplete, resulting in an inaccurate determination. The Pr:Cr ratio (or albumin-to-creatinine ratio) relies on the relatively constant loss or excretion of protein and creatinine that occurs in the context of a stable glomerular filtration rate.[242] It is not affected by urine volume or concentration, is more convenient to obtain than a 24-hour urine collection, and has both a high negative predictive value and high positive predictive value for threshold proteinuria.[233,243,244] It is therefore useful in excluding significant proteinuria and for detecting proteinuria above a range of abnormal threshold values. In the normal population the urinary Pr:Cr ratio is less than 0.2 mg/mg.[242] Although it has a strong correlation with measurements of 24-hour urinary protein, its accuracy at predicting 24-hour protein excretion at higher ranges of proteinuria is poor.[233] Caution should therefore be exercised in using it as the sole means of monitoring response to treatment in patients with heavy proteinuria.

Genetic Assessment of Rheumatic Diseases

Since the discovery of the gene responsible for FMF in 1997, there has been a dramatic increase in the understanding of the genetic basis of an expanding array of conditions collectively known as autoinflammatory diseases.[245,246] A detailed review of the clinical features and genetics of these conditions may be found in Chapter 47.

One of the consequences of the increased understanding of the genetic basis of these conditions has been the development of genetic testing for their diagnosis. A frequent issue that arises in such testing is whether an identified sequence variant within a gene is a single nucleotide polymorphism (SNP) or a disease-causing point mutation. At its simplest, an SNP is the substitution of one nucleotide within a gene for another that is common within a population (>1%) and has no deleterious effect on the organism. Disease-causing point mutations also involve a single nucleotide substitution but by definition are rare in the population (<1%) and in general have a deleterious impact on the production or function of the gene product, resulting in disease. Mutations may also be due to the insertion or deletion of nucleotides within a gene or due to large-scale changes in chromosomal structure; however, these are unlikely to be confused with SNPs. The distinction between SNPs and point mutations typically requires reference to databases in which SNPs and known mutations are cataloged. In practice, commercial diagnostic genetic laboratories routinely perform this

"filtering" step and generally only report identified known mutations within a gene. There are occasions, however, when novel sequence variants or polymorphisms of uncertain significance (i.e., with unclear pathogenicity) may be identified in which case regular reassessment of the diagnosis may be warranted.[246]

The diagnostic genetic testing referred to previously generally requires the targeted sequencing of selected exons of the relevant gene to detect known disease-causing mutations. It is not useful in situations in which the gene responsible is unknown, and it is expensive if there are multiple candidate genes that might equally explain an observed phenotype. In the past 10 years, technology that allows the parallel sequencing of massive numbers of DNA fragments (so-called next-generation sequencing) has made it possible to examine all known coding regions (i.e., exons) of the genome of an individual—whole exome sequencing—in a time frame and at a cost that makes its clinical use in these situations feasible.[247] Although the exome is only 2% of the whole genome, it is thought to contain 85% of pathogenic mutations that cause Mendelian disorders,[248] making it a good starting point for the study of disease genetics. The recent identification of the genetic basis for a number of inflammatory phenotypes by using whole exome sequencing in a relatively small number of kindreds is a testament to the power of this technology.[249-251] Although the bioinformatic challenges in managing the volume of data that exome sequencing produces is significant—a single individual may have upwards of 20,000 single nucleotide variants in their exome—and the scientific challenges of converting that data into clinically relevant information is considerable, efforts to establish "genomic medicine" clinics that incorporate the myriad of clinicians, scientists, and bioinformaticians required to bring the benchside to the bedside are under way.[252] The principles on which they have been established may become an important model for investigating the genesis of many rheumatic diseases in years to come.

THE FUTURE

A review of major textbooks of rheumatology over the past 30 years makes obvious the great advances in the understanding and laboratory investigation of rheumatic diseases that have occurred over this period. With these advances, large sections of text devoted to "current" laboratory tests have become obsolete, and the present example will be no different. In the same way that the LE test is now looked on as being of historical interest only, so may future generations regard the present text's devotion to autoantibody assays and profiles. Current research is providing insights into the mechanisms of immune-mediated diseases that may one day allow precise, individualized analyses of inflammatory pathways and the genetic contributors toward illness that surpass present-day diagnostic labels and allow a more targeted approach to therapy and follow-up. However, although the nature of laboratory investigations for rheumatic diseases may change, their necessity and the need for the clinician to understand their basis, clinical utility, and limitations will remain.

REFERENCES

1. D.G. Altman, J.M. Bland, Diagnostic tests. 1: sensitivity and specificity, BMJ 308 (6943) (1994) 1552.
2. D.G. Altman, J.M. Bland, Diagnostic tests 2: predictive values, BMJ 309 (6947) (1994) 102.
5. T.G. Phan, R.C. Wong, S. Adelstein, Autoantibodies to extractable nuclear antigens: making detection and interpretation more meaningful, Clin. Diagn. Lab. Immunol. 9 (1) (2002) 1–7.
9. R. Tozzoli, C. Bonaguri, A. Melegari, et al., Current state of diagnostic technologies in the autoimmunology laboratory, Clin. Chem. Lab. Med. 51 (1) (2013) 129–138.

18. L.T. Hiraki, S.M. Benseler, P.N. Tyrrell, et al., Clinical and laboratory characteristics and long-term outcome of pediatric systemic lupus erythematosus: a longitudinal study, J. Pediatr. 152 (4) (2008) 550–556.

19. B. Bader-Meunier, J.B. Armengaud, E. Haddad, et al., Initial presentation of childhood-onset systemic lupus erythematosus: a French multicenter study, J. Pediatr. 146 (5) (2005) 648–653.

25. L. Berntson, B. Andersson Gare, A. Fasth, et al., Incidence of juvenile idiopathic arthritis in the Nordic countries. A population based study with special reference to the validity of the ILAR and EULAR criteria, J. Rheumatol. 30 (10) (2003) 2275–2282.

27. P.J. Gowdie, R.C. Allen, A.J. Kornberg, et al., Clinical features and disease course of patients with juvenile dermatomyositis, Int. J. Rheum. Dis. 16 (5) (2013) 561–567.

29. A.M. Sallum, M.H. Kiss, S. Sachetti, et al., Juvenile dermatomyositis: clinical, laboratorial, histological, therapeutical and evolutive parameters of 35 patients, Arq. Neuropsiquatr 60 (4) (2002) 889–899.

32. Y. Inamo, K. Harada, Antinuclear antibody positivity in pediatric patients with autoimmune thyroid disease, J. Rheumatol. 24 (3) (1997) 576–578.

35. M.E. Kaplan, E.M. Tan, Antinuclear antibodies in infectious mononucleosis, Lancet 1 (7542) (1968) 561–563.

39. O. Elkayam, D. Caspi, M. Lidgi, et al., Auto-antibody profiles in patients with active pulmonary tuberculosis, Int. J. Tuberc. Lung Dis. 11 (3) (2007) 306–310.

43. N.H. Heegaard, M. West-Nørager, J.T. Tanassi, et al., Circulating antinuclear antibodies in patients with pelvic masses are associated with malignancy and decreased survival, PLoS ONE 7 (2) (2012) e30997.

45. P.L. Meroni, P.H. Schur, ANA screening: an old test with new recommendations, Ann. Rheum. Dis. 69 (8) (2010) 1420–1422.

53. A.S. Wiik, M. Høier-Madsen, J. Forslid, et al., Antinuclear antibodies: a contemporary nomenclature using HEp-2 cells, J. Autoimmun. 35 (3) (2010) 276–290.

55. I. Peene, L. Meheus, E.M. Veys, et al., Detection and identification of antinuclear antibodies (ANA) in a large and consecutive cohort of serum samples referred for ANA testing, Ann. Rheum. Dis. 60 (12) (2001) 1131–1136.

57. W.Y. Craig, T.B. Ledue, A.M. Johnson, et al., The distribution of antinuclear antibody titers in "normal" children and adults, J. Rheumatol. 26 (4) (1999) 914–919.

62. J. Forslid, Z. Heigl, J. Jonsson, et al., The prevalence of antinuclear antibodies in healthy young persons and adults, comparing rat liver tissue sections with HEp-2 cells as antigen substrate, Clin. Exp. Rheumatol. 12 (2) (1994) 137–141.

73. J. Wenzel, R. Gerdsen, M. Uerlich, et al., Antibodies targeting extractable nuclear antigens: historical development and current knowledge, Br. J. Dermatol. 145 (6) (2001) 859–867.

74. R. Yoshimi, A. Ueda, K. Ozato, et al., Clinical and pathological roles of Ro/SSA autoantibody system, Clin. Dev. Immunol. 2012 (2012) 606195.

75. C.H. To, M. Petri, Is antibody clustering predictive of clinical subsets and damage in systemic lupus erythematosus? Arthritis Rheum. 52 (12) (2005) 4003–4010.

80. F. Franceschini, I. Cavazzana, Anti-Ro/SSA and La/SSB antibodies, Autoimmunity 38 (1) (2005) 55–63.

81. D. Basu, J.D. Reveille, Anti-scl-70, Autoimmunity 38 (1) (2005) 65–72.

84. S.M. Orton, A. Peace-Brewer, J.L. Schmitz, et al., Practical evaluation of methods for detection and specificity of autoantibodies to extractable nuclear antigens, Clin. Diagn. Lab. Immunol. 11 (2) (2004) 297–301.

86. N. Bizzaro, D. Villalta, D. Giavarina, et al., Are anti-nucleosome antibodies a better diagnostic marker than anti-dsDNA antibodies for systemic lupus erythematosus? A systematic review and a study of metanalysis, Autoimmun. Rev. 12 (2) (2012) 97–106.

94. P. Riboldi, M. Gerosa, G. Moroni, et al., Anti-DNA antibodies: a diagnostic and prognostic tool for systemic lupus erythematosus? Autoimmunity 38 (1) (2005) 39–45.

95. A. Annunziato, DNA packaging: nucleosomes and chromatin, Nat Educ 1 (1) (2008) 26.

96. H. Chabre, Z. Amoura, J.C. Piette, et al., Presence of nucleosome-restricted antibodies in patients with systemic lupus erythematosus, Arthritis Rheum. 38 (10) (1995) 1485–1491.

97. O.A. Gutiérrez-Adrianzén, S. Koutouzov, R.M. Mota, et al., Diagnostic value of anti-nucleosome antibodies in the assessment of disease activity of systemic lupus erythematosus: a prospective study comparing anti-nucleosome with anti-dsDNA antibodies, J. Rheumatol. 33 (8) (2006) 1538–1544.

100. D.J. Davies, J.E. Moran, J.F. Niall, et al., Segmental necrotising glomerulonephritis with antineutrophil antibody: possible arbovirus aetiology? Br. Med. J. (Clin. Res. Ed) 285 (6342) (1982) 606.

103. A. Radice, M. Vecchi, M.B. Bianchi, et al., Contribution of immunofluorescence to the identification and characterization of anti-neutrophil cytoplasmic autoantibodies. The role of different fixatives, Clin. Exp. Rheumatol. 18 (6) (2000) 707–712.

105. E. Csernok, J. Holle, B. Hellmich, et al., Evaluation of capture ELISA for detection of antineutrophil cytoplasmic antibodies directed against proteinase 3 in Wegener's granulomatosis: first results from a multicentre study, Rheumatology (Oxford) 43 (2) (2004) 174–180.

115. G. Tomasson, P.C. Grayson, A.D. Mahr, et al., Value of ANCA measurements during remission to predict a relapse of ANCA-associated vasculitis—a meta-analysis, Rheumatology (Oxford) 51 (1) (2012) 100–109.

121. R.A. Lerner, R.J. Glassock, F.J. Dixon, The role of anti-glomerular basement membrane antibody in the pathogenesis of human glomerulonephritis, J. Exp. Med. 126 (6) (1967) 989–1004.

126. Z. Cui, H.Y. Wang, M.H. Zhao, Natural autoantibodies against glomerular basement membrane exist in normal human sera, Kidney Int. 69 (5) (2006) 894–899.

128. J.B. Levy, T. Hammad, A. Coulthart, et al., Clinical features and outcome of patients with both ANCA and anti-GBM antibodies, Kidney Int. 66 (4) (2004) 1535–1540.

132. X.Y. Jia, Z. Qu, Z. Cui, et al., Circulating anti-glomerular basement membrane autoantibodies against alpha3(IV)NC1 undetectable by commercially available enzyme-linked immunosorbent assays, Nephrology (Carlton) 17 (2) (2012) 160–166.

136. E. Waaler, On the occurrence of a factor in human serum activating the specific agglutintion of sheep blood corpuscles, APMIS 115 (5) (1939) 422–438, discussion 439.

137. D.N. Posnett, J. Edinger, When do microbes stimulate rheumatoid factor? J. Exp. Med. 185 (10) (1997) 1721–1723.

139. Y. Renaudineau, C. Jamin, A. Saraux, et al., Rheumatoid factor on a daily basis, Autoimmunity 38 (1) (2005) 11–16.

140. Y.W. Song, E.H. Kang, Autoantibodies in rheumatoid arthritis: rheumatoid factors and anticitrullinated protein antibodies, QJM 103 (3) (2010) 139–146.

141. D. Aletaha, T. Neogi, A.J. Silman, et al., 2010 Rheumatoid arthritis classification criteria: an American College of Rheumatology/European League Against Rheumatism collaborative initiative, Arthritis Rheum. 62 (9) (2010) 2569–2581.

143. R.E. Petty, T.R. Southwood, P. Manners, et al., International League of Associations for Rheumatology classification of juvenile idiopathic arthritis: second revision, Edmonton, 2001, J. Rheumatol. 31 (2) (2004) 390–392.

149. M. Harboe, Rheumatoid factors in leprosy and parasitic diseases, Scand. J. Rheumatol. Suppl. 75 (1988) 309–313.

150. C. González-Juanatey, M.A. González-Gay, J. Llorca, et al., Rheumatic manifestations of infective endocarditis in non-addicts. A 12-year study, Medicine (Baltimore) 80 (1) (2001) 9–19.

153. R.L. Carter, Antibody formation in infectious mononucleosis. II. Other 19S antibodies and false-positive serology, Br. J. Haematol. 12 (3) (1966) 268–275.

158. W. Swedler, J. Wallman, C.J. Froelich, et al., Routine measurement of IgM, IgG, and IgA rheumatoid factors: high sensitivity, specificity, and predictive value for rheumatoid arthritis, J. Rheumatol. 24 (6) (1997) 1037–1044.

160. M.A. van Boekel, E.R. Vossenaar, F.H. van den Hoogen, et al., Autoantibody systems in rheumatoid arthritis: specificity, sensitivity and diagnostic value, Arthritis Res. 4 (2) (2002) 87–93.

163. K. Nishimura, D. Sugiyama, Y. Kogata, et al., Meta-analysis: diagnostic accuracy of anti-cyclic citrullinated peptide antibody and rheumatoid

factor for rheumatoid arthritis, Ann. Intern. Med. 146 (11) (2007) 797–808.

171. R. Willis, S.S. Pierangeli, Anti-β2-glycoprotein I antibodies, Ann. N. Y. Acad. Sci. 1285 (2013) 44–58.

178. G. Espinosa, R. Cervera, Antiphospholipid syndrome, Arthritis Res. Ther. 10 (6) (2008) 230.

179. T.L. Ortel, Antiphospholipid syndrome: laboratory testing and diagnostic strategies, Am. J. Hematol. 87 (Suppl. 1) (2012) S75–S81.

182. J.S. Dlott, R.A. Roubey, Drug-induced lupus anticoagulants and antiphospholipid antibodies, Curr. Rheumatol. Rep. 14 (1) (2012) 71–78.

185. M. Galli, D. Luciani, G. Bertolini, et al., Lupus anticoagulants are stronger risk factors for thrombosis than anticardiolipin antibodies in the antiphospholipid syndrome: a systematic review of the literature, Blood 101 (5) (2003) 1827–1832.

189. V. Pengo, A. Ruffatti, C. Legnani, et al., Incidence of a first thromboembolic event in asymptomatic carriers of high-risk antiphospholipid antibody profile: a multicenter prospective study, Blood 118 (17) (2011) 4714–4718.

191. M.J. Walport, Complement. First of two parts, N. Engl. J. Med. 344 (14) (2001) 1058–1066.

200. D.M. Steel, A.S. Whitehead, The major acute phase reactants: C-reactive protein, serum amyloid P component and serum amyloid A protein, Immunol. Today 15 (2) (1994) 81–88.

204. H. Gewurz, C. Mold, J. Siegel, et al., C-reactive protein and the acute phase response, Adv. Intern. Med. 27 (1982) 345–372.

208. L. Deban, B. Bottazzi, C. Garlanda, et al., Pentraxins: multifunctional proteins at the interface of innate immunity and inflammation, Biofactors 35 (2) (2009) 138–145.

211. C.M. Uhlar, A.S. Whitehead, Serum amyloid A, the major vertebrate acute-phase reactant, Eur. J. Biochem. 265 (2) (1999) 501–523.

212. K.K. Eklund, K. Niemi, P.T. Kovanen, Immune functions of serum amyloid A, Crit. Rev. Immunol. 32 (4) (2012) 335–348.

214. W. Wang, M.A. Knovich, L.G. Coffman, et al., Serum ferritin: past, present and future, Biochim. Biophys. Acta 1800 (8) (2010) 760–769.

215. C. Moore Jr., M. Ormseth, H. Fuchs, Causes and significance of markedly elevated serum ferritin levels in an academic medical center, J. Clin. Rheumatol. 19 (6) (2013) 324–328.

216. S. Davi, A. Consolaro, D. Guseinova, et al., An international consensus survey of diagnostic criteria for macrophage activation syndrome in systemic juvenile idiopathic arthritis, J. Rheumatol. 38 (4) (2011) 764–768.

217. K. Lehmberg, K.L. McClain, G.E. Janka, et al., Determination of an appropriate cut-off value for ferritin in the diagnosis of hemophagocytic lymphohistiocytosis, Pediatr. Blood Cancer 61 (11) (2014) 2101–2103.

221. M.E. Margaretten, J. Kohlwes, D. Moore, et al., Does this adult patient have septic arthritis? JAMA 297 (13) (2007) 1478–1488.

225. A.L. Rosey, E. Abachin, G. Quesnes, et al., Development of a broad-range 16S rDNA real-time PCR for the diagnosis of septic arthritis in children, J. Microbiol. Methods 68 (1) (2007) 88–93.

233. C. Lane, M. Brown, W. Dunsmuir, et al., Can spot urine protein/creatinine ratio replace 24 h urine protein in usual clinical nephrology? Nephrology (Carlton) 11 (3) (2006) 245–249.

238. T. Addis, The number of formed elements in the urinary sediment of normal individuals, J. Clin. Invest. 2 (5) (1926) 409–415.

The entire reference list is available online at www.expertconsult.com.

CHAPTER 11

Managing Children with Rheumatic Diseases

Carol B. Lindsley, Ricardo Alberto Guillermo Russo, Christiaan Scott

Rheumatic diseases are chronic, multisystem disorders characterized by an unpredictable course with periods of exacerbation and remission. Optimal care requires the expertise of many disciplines (Table 11-1, Fig. 11-1); therefore, specialized multidisciplinary teams provide the best approach to the management of these patients. Pharmacologic treatment is discussed in the chapters dealing with individual disease categories. Physical and occupational therapy and rehabilitation are outlined in Chapter 14. This chapter discusses general principles of management applicable to all children with a rheumatic disease, such as team care, adherence, school attendance, and transition to adult care. Because patient care may vary internationally, global issues are discussed.

THE SCOPE OF THE CHALLENGE

There are multiple dimensions to the effects of chronic illness on children and members of their families. The scope of the challenge of managing children and youth with rheumatic diseases goes far beyond medications and therapy. Several early studies suggested that chronic illness has a negative impact on psychosocial development,[1,2] family,[3] school life,[4] and family finances.[5,6] Studies from Sweden and the United States that focused on children with juvenile idiopathic arthritis (JIA) growing up before the availability of modern drugs showed that 30% to 50% entered adult life with active disease[7,8]; it is likely that the percentage is even higher in developing countries. Severe disability was common in this young adult population, with decreased physical functions, poor health perception, and pain.[9,10] All of the psychosocial and physical problems assume greater importance when children reach adolescence[11] or adulthood with continuing disease activity.[12,13]

The current approach to early treatment of JIA, with immune modulators and intraarticular glucocorticoids, has resulted in reduced incidence of severe deformities. However, in one recent study conducted after the introduction of the current therapies, persistent disease activity and impaired functioning were still seen frequently.[14] With the advent of newer, more efficacious therapies, achieving inactive disease and remission is a realistic goal for a significant proportion of children with JIA, and for increasing numbers of children with other rheumatic diseases (systemic lupus erythematosus [SLE], juvenile dermatomyositis, the vasculitides, etc.)

The early observations of poor outcome for children with rheumatic diseases have not been substantiated in recent studies. Even studies that emphasized the negative impacts of growing up with JIA showed that many of these patients completed college, worked full time, and raised children.[9,12,13,15] Recent well-designed studies seem to

indicate that JIA is not necessarily a psychosocial stressor, and families of children with JIA are, in general, resilient.[16,17] Patients with JIA growing into early adulthood were shown to be able to earn a living, live independently, and have a stable spousal relationship, although patients with active disease had poor health-related quality of life in the physical component of the assessment tool.[18] Some children do suffer disabilities, have reduced function and decreased social acceptance,[19] and have overall adjustment problems and internalization of symptoms.[20] For all of these reasons, a program of care for children with rheumatic diseases should be planned for the whole child and the future and should be comprehensive (i.e., family-centered, community-based, coordinated, and cost-effective) (Boxes 11-1, 11-2).[21]

Current research suggests that planning for care of these children should be based on new concepts of disablement, should be evidence-based, and should be individualized. New concepts of the "disablement" process include four distinct constructs: (1) active pathology, (2) impairment, (3) functional limitation, and (4) disability.[22] Each of these stages offers potential for intervention. In addition, there may be other factors, such as coping skills, access to care, economics, comorbidities, and the family's psychosocial climate, that contribute to the disablement process and therefore are appropriate targets for intervention. A tailored program individualized for each patient, considering his or her environment, is thus essential to optimize the efforts of the team providing care and the family. The newer International Classification of Functioning, Disability and Health (ICF) recognizes external factors (physical, social, and attitudinal) that have an impact on disability and impairment.[23] Newer tools for the evaluation of disability include items to measure body function and structure, activities and participation, and environmental and personal factors.[24] Based on this conceptual framework, tools have been developed for use in specific conditions such as rheumatoid arthritis and osteoarthritis[25] and for use in children and youth (ICF-CY).[26]

Based on their well-designed study, Noll and colleagues suggested that "randomly occurring, challenging life events do not alter the child's potential for inclusive fitness by denigrating their social status or emotional well-being."[27] It is important to know why some patients and families are vulnerable to functional and psychosocial disabilities and others are not.[16,17] One concept to explain differences in vulnerability focuses on risk factors that tend to push children with chronic illness and their families to dysfunction and disability, and resilience factors that tend to give them more stability.[28,29] The relative predominance of risk factors or resilience factors influences outcomes (Table 11-2).

In planning for the care of these children, emphasis should be on the child and the family, and efforts should be aimed not only at controlling the disease and managing the current problems, but also at

TABLE 11-1	**Comprehensive Model**			
MODELS OF CARE				
	TEAM MEMBERS	**CARE DELIVERY METHODS**	**PATIENT POPULATION**	**TERTIARY HOSPITAL**
Specialized program	Specialists	Comprehensive care in a multidisciplinary environment	Complex cases	Tertiary hospital
Ongoing management	Rheumatologist, pediatrician	Ongoing monitoring and management—periodic referrals	Rheumatic patients	Community
Outreach clinics	Rheumatologist, pediatrician, general practitioner	Periodic consultant visits to a local clinic where patients are referred by local GP or pediatrician	Rheumatic patients	Rural or isolated places, remote provinces with sparse populations
Telemedicine	Rheumatologist, pediatrician	Linking of patient to specialist through teleconsultation. Usually local pediatrician involved	Rheumatic patients	Tertiary hospital—local hospital

Adapted from C. MacKay, P. Veinot, E.M. Badley, Characteristics of evolving models of care for arthritis: a key informant study, BMC Health Serv. Res. 8 (2008) 147.

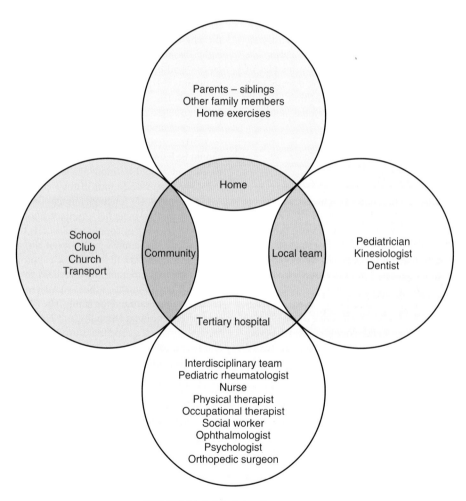

FIGURE 11-1 Models of team care.

planning for the future. Steps should be taken to improve the resilience of patients and families through better education to cope with the vicissitudes of these diseases, and improving social and peer support for the children and their parents. Education in stress management, including family empowerment and self-management to help the child cope better with their disease and disability, is equally important.

THE TEAM

Expertise should be the cornerstone of the care of children with rheumatic diseases. Accurate diagnosis is the first step. Rheumatic diseases may be acute and explosive in onset, or they may evolve over a period of months and years. Only one organ system may be affected, or several

---

BOX 11-1   Components of the Management of Rheumatic Diseases in Children

Medical and surgical management

Family-centered, community-based, coordinated care (school, outreach)

Psychosocial management (social services, mental health services, financial)

Musculoskeletal rehabilitation (physical therapy, occupational therapy, orthopedics)

Well-child care issues (growth and development, nutrition, immunization, anticipatory guidance)

Continuity of care

Cost-effective care

BOX 11-2   Steps in Implementing Family-Centered, Community-Based Care

Recognizing the pivotal roles of the child and the family in the planning of care

Developing resources in the community where the child lives

Recognizing parents and professionals as equals in a partnership of care

Empowering the family with information through education and support

Encouraging pediatricians to assume a greater role in case coordination, become knowledgeable about available local resources, and work with community agencies

Increasing communication among disciplines and between patients and health professionals

Breaking barriers to the development of such a system

TABLE 11-2   Risk and Resilience

RISK FACTORS	RESILIENCE FACTORS
Severity of disease and disability	Family's ability to solve problems
Degree of functional independence	Social support
Daily hassles and struggles	Coping skills

Modified from J.L. Wallender, J.W. Varni, et al: Family resources as resistance factors for psychological maladjustment in chronically ill and handicapped children, J. Pediatr. Psychol. 14 (1989): 157–173.

---

systems may be involved. Rheumatic disease may mimic several other inflammatory and noninflammatory diseases. It may not be possible to place an accurate diagnostic label at first, yet life-threatening complications and functional disabilities may have to be managed. Great skill and patience are required to support the families in managing their problems in the face of uncertainties in diagnosis and prognosis. Therein reside the challenges and pleasures of rheumatology.

Comprehensive treatment centers should be based in tertiary care academic centers. The treatment team (Fig. 11-1) should consist of a pediatric rheumatologist, a nurse specialist, physical and occupational therapists, a social worker, and a psychologist, all working as a team with the child's primary care physician. Consultations with an orthopedic surgeon, ophthalmologist, nutritionist, and dentist should be available when required. Team care is expensive and is not required for every child, particularly with the recent advances in medical management. However, these services should be available when needed. In the developing world, where resources and multidisciplinary tertiary care

centers are scarce or inaccessible, different models of care may have to be considered (Fig. 11-1, Table 11-1). In these situations, for instance, reliance may have to be placed more heavily on less specialized teams for routine follow-up, with less frequent visits to tertiary centers. Communication, possibly assisted by telemedicine, is a central component in ensuring appropriate care in this model. Appropriate outreach training in basic rheumatology and examination techniques for community health care workers, pediatricians, and general practitioners at outreach sites can help to foster trust and facilitate effective communication.[30] Specially trained nurses have fulfilled the contact function effectively in many pediatric rheumatology centers.[31]

PATIENT AND PARENT EDUCATION

Children with rheumatic diseases and their parents require education on several issues. These issues are discussed in detail in publications listed at the end of this chapter. The mode of teaching has to vary to suit the needs and skills of parents. Language barriers, cultural backgrounds, and literacy issues must be kept in mind before such programs are organized. Education about the disease, medications, adverse effects of medications, and therapy programs should be provided both individually by the pediatric rheumatology team and in parent support groups. The belief system of the family should be explored, and all doubts and questions should be addressed. Information required by parents varies with the time that has passed after diagnosis, and also depends on the developmental needs of the child. Therefore, education must be individualized.[32] Services of a translator may also be needed.

Information is readily available on the Internet, where resources are easily accessible. However, families need help to ensure that information is gathered from reliable sources, such as those listed at the end of this chapter, and they will need assistance with interpretation of the information gathered.

COUNSELING

A trusting relationship is the most important requirement for effective counseling. To be trusted, one must be trustworthy. Open, honest communication with the child and the parents is a major component of this relationship.

Collecting information about a child's illness, behavior, and family dynamics may require many visits and observations. Empathic listening and careful observation is the first step, and attention must be paid to nonverbal cues.

Physicians are trained to look for and diagnose weaknesses in the person and the system. It is also important to identify strengths in the patient, family, and the community that can be utilized to counter weaknesses. This strength may lie in the extended family, an interested schoolteacher, or a loving grandparent. Some families grow in strength in the presence of adversity. Factors that contribute to successful coping should be supported and encouraged.[28,33] Referral to a clinical psychologist may be needed.

Children with physical disabilities and deformities and children who look different because of a rash or steroid therapy are bound to feel different and self-conscious. In some parts of the developing world, where adherence to traditional beliefs is strong, this may lead to stigmatization; these afflictions may also be blamed on curses or bewitchment. Children and adolescents who are disabled may be left aside because they may not be considered to be productive individuals in the family. Physical disability and fluctuation in disease activity may make it difficult for these children to participate in social and family activities. Emphasizing what they can do and planning activities in which they can participate helps their sense of self-worth and morale.

The involvement of siblings, friends, and classmates in helping a disabled child during activities should help create a successful experience for everyone, including the healthy children.

ADHERENCE

Children with chronic illness soon tire of taking medicines day after day with no end in sight. They often ask why they have to do mindless exercises that do not appear to help them. Therefore, adherence with medication and therapy programs is a major issue for children with chronic diseases.[34] The word *compliance* implies that the physician gives orders and the patient obeys. But the ideal situation is an informed patient who chooses to follow the treatment prescribed by a trusted physician after being convinced of the benefits and made aware of the consequences of not following the treatment. In other words, the patient chooses to *adhere* to the prescribed program. In pediatrics, one must consider the child, the parent, and the caregiver to ensure the treatment plan is followed. Patient and parent education and including the needs of family members in the planning process are essential. Listening to the specific needs of a child and family and incorporating them into the plan, and designing a plan that accounts for the stresses and strengths of the family and their cultural values, increases the likelihood that the plan will be followed. Factors that affect adherence and strategies to enhance adherence are listed in Table 11-2 and Boxes 11-3 and 11-4.

Meta-analyses show that education and behavioral intervention provide not only improved adherence but better health outcomes overall.[35] Effect sizes ranged from small to large, with particular characteristics such as age, gender, and diagnosis having a significant impact on the effectiveness of interventions. The use of electronic monitors to measure adherence can provide more objective data and enable easy data feedback to parents.[36] Web-based interventions for adherence can also be effective.[37]

SIBLING ISSUES

Stress related to living with chronic illness affects every member of the family, including siblings. The role of siblings and their impact on the developmental needs of the patient may vary with the age and cognitive level of siblings, their perception of the child with chronic illness, parental attitudes, and the demands placed on unaffected siblings.[38] Feelings may range from guilt (that siblings are responsible for the sick child in some magical way), to fear of catching the illness, to embarrassment.[39] Siblings may resent the extra time and attention given to the affected child and perceived favoritism in matters of discipline. Realistically, parents may not be able to provide adequate time to satisfy the developmental needs of the siblings. This is a problem for single parents in particular.

Depending on the parental demands, some siblings may take an important role in the medical treatment of the affected child (such as reminding them about medications and helping with exercises); others may be protected from this role by their parents. Some siblings may take a more protective role of their brother or sister in school and outside the home.

Disease severity, parental functioning, family stress, and family support systems are some of the determinants of the effects of chronic illness on siblings. In spite of ambivalent feelings, siblings of children with arthritis function well in life[40] and can be a great source of extra support, both at home and at school. It is important to evaluate the needs of siblings in caring for children with chronic illness and to help support their needs.[41]

SCHOOL ISSUES

In general, rheumatic diseases do not affect cognition, except for conditions that affect the central nervous system, such as SLE, central nervous system vasculitis, or drug side effects. Children with arthritis can and should attend regular school except in special circumstances. Parents must be advocates for their children and learn both their own rights and responsibilities and those of their children.[39] However, the school system often must institute several adaptations to the standardized schedule.[4] In the United States, children with chronic illness and disabilities must be educated in the "least restrictive environment." Individualized education plans have to be formulated at the parents' request, and there are strong "due process" requirements.[42] Similar requirements are in place in most jurisdictions in the developed world.

BOX 11-3 Factors That Influence Adherence

Cognitive/emotional (e.g., limited ability to understand, depression)
Behavioral (e.g., defiance, adolescent independence)
Cultural (e.g., alternative concepts of disease model)
Social and family issues (e.g., unstable family)
Disease-related (e.g., chronicity)
Medication-related (e.g., side effects)
Organizational (e.g., appointments in the clinic)
Economics (e.g., cost of visit)

From T. Kroll, J.H. Barlow, K. Shaw: Treatment adherence in juvenile rheumatoid arthritis: a review, Scand. J. Rheumatol. 28 (1999) 10–18.

BOX 11-4 Strategies to Facilitate and Promote Adherence

Strategies for improving adherence to pediatric rheumatic disease regimens.

1. Educate early and often about the disease, treatment options, and benefits of consistent adherence.
2. Ensure that patients and families have the requisite behavioral skills to implement regimens. Rehearse these in the clinic (e.g., demonstrate and have patients practice therapeutic exercises).
3. Anticipate and address barriers to adherence (e.g., lack of financial resources).
4. Keep regimens as simple as possible and integrate into family routine.
5. Prevent or minimize negative side effects (e.g., gastrointestinal irritation with NSAIDs).
6. Encourage patients and caregivers to monitor adherence (e.g., use a calendar posted in a prominent place in the home).
7. Teach caregivers positive reinforcement strategies for promoting adherence (e.g., a point system for adhering to regimen components).
8. Review discipline strategies with caregivers for children who are oppositional (e.g., time-out for a younger child who refuses medications).
9. Teach older patients self-management strategies (e.g., problem solving).
10. Refer patients and families to qualified mental health providers if more serious problems exist concurrently with nonadherence or that are directly interfering with adherence.

Adapted from M. Rapoff: Management of adherence and chronic rheumatic disease in children and adolescents, Best Pract. Res. Clin. Rheumatol. 20 (2006) 301–314.

Depending on the medical condition and the nature of the disability, including participation in daily and community life activities,[23-26] one or more of the "related school services" may need to be provided to ensure optimal educational opportunities.[43] Special school services provide physical adaptations in schools for handicapped access and elevators; arrange class assignments on the same floor; and provide a duplicate set of books. Transportation, school counseling, nutrition, adaptive physical education, and homebound instruction are some of the other services that may be needed.[4,43]

Common concerns expressed by children and parents in relation to school, as well as suggested solutions, are given in Table 11-3. The nurse or occupational therapist can provide an individualized checklist for parents that can be shared with the school nurse or teacher. School nurses are some of the best advocates for children with disabilities and special needs. They can work with teachers and physical education instructors to make appropriate modifications within the school. Therefore, communication between the tertiary center staff members (particularly the nurse) and the school nurse is essential. It is important to recognize that teachers and parents tend to emphasize issues

related to activities of daily living as limiting school life, whereas children themselves rate peer acceptance and self-concept as more important.[44] Therefore, these children need more help with peer support and better coping skills.

Finally, if a child is considering vocational training or postsecondary education, early planning beginning in secondary school is essential. It should include visiting prospective campuses, avoiding schedule (credit hours) overload, arrangement for regular meals, and, if the student is leaving home, locating a local pharmacy and physician.

TRANSITION

Growing up through adolescence into young adulthood is a major task for any child. This time becomes a challenge for children with chronic illness and their parents.[11] Adolescents with chronic diseases have to be encouraged gradually to take control of their disease management. This requires preparation of the family and child before adolescence. Preparation of these children requires attention to independent living skills and self-advocacy. Both physicians and parents have to let go of the child in a sensitive and gradual way. The parent has to trust the child, and the child must demonstrate that he or she is capable of taking care of ongoing management and needs. Adolescent support groups with professional leadership may be helpful.

Transition to adult care is a process that should start when a child reaches adolescence.[11,45,46] This requires planning and coordination with participation by the patients, family, the pediatric service team, and the adult service team. It should be comprehensive and responsive to the needs of the patient.[46] Some of the subjects that should be addressed individually or in group sessions are sexuality, alcohol and drug use, and vocational planning. The young person may need coaching in self-management, self-advocacy, communication, and decision making. Barriers may include changing location for college, changing from a well-known care provider to a new one, reluctance of parents to relinquish control, or gaps in insurance coverage.

Box 11-5 lists some strategies that may be useful to achieve successful transition.

FINANCIAL ISSUES

Children with chronic illness account for a large proportion of health care expenditures in the United States.[6,47] Families of children with rheumatic diseases may spend hundreds to thousands of unreimbursed dollars out of pocket per year,[3,5,6] not including time lost

TABLE 11-3 Common School Concerns for Students with Rheumatic Diseases

DIFFICULTY	STRATEGY
Inactivity, stiffness due to prolonged sitting	Sit at side or back of room to allow walking around without disturbing class
	Change position every 20 minutes
	Ask to be assigned jobs that require walking (e.g., collect papers)
Climbing stairs or walking long distances	Request elevator permit
	Schedule classes to decrease walking and climbing
	Request extra time getting to and from classes
	Use wheelchair if needed
Carrying books or cafeteria tray	Keep two sets of books: one in class, one at home
	Have a buddy help carry books
	Get a backpack or shoulder bag for books
	Determine cafeteria assistance plan (helper, reserved seat, wheeled cart)
Getting up from desk	Request an easel-top desk or special chair
Handwriting (slow, messy, painful)	Use "fat" pen/pencil, crayons
	Use felt-tip pen
	Stretch hands every 10 minutes
	Use tape recorder for note-taking
	Photocopy classmate's notes
	Use computer for reports
	Request alternative to timed tests (oral test, extra time, computer)
	Educate teacher (messy writing may be unavoidable at times)
Shoulder movement and dressing	Wear loose-fitting clothing
	Wear clothes with Velcro® closures
	Get adaptive equipment from occupational therapist
Reaching locker	Modify locker or request alternative storage place
	Use lockers with key locks instead of dials
Raising hand	Devise alternative signaling method

From Raising a Child With Arthritis: A Parent's Guide, Arthritis Foundation, Atlanta, 1998.

BOX 11-5 Tips for a Successful Transition Process

1. Start the transition process early during adolescence.
2. Reinforce independence and adherence during the transition years.
3. Address important issues such as alcohol, drugs, and risky sexual behaviors.
4. Take into account the patient's preferences.
5. Consider not only the patient's chronological age but also their maturity level when choosing the right moment to transfer.
6. If possible, wait until the disease is under control or stable to transfer the patient.
7. Establish a fluent, bidirectional, trustworthy, and satisfactory relationship with the adult care provider.
8. Provide adolescents an environment where they can meet other young people in the transition process.

from work. In the current health care competitive environment, children with chronic illness and disabilities are particularly vulnerable. The high cost that goes with chronic illness and the pressures to cut costs may make it difficult to provide adequate and appropriate care for children with chronic illness and disabilities.[47] In the United States and many other countries, families need to be educated about various types of health coverage and how to work with health maintenance organizations, insurance companies, community resources, and government agencies. Both parents and physicians need to work through the political process to bring about changes in financing of medical care that will ensure access to appropriate services for all children with chronic diseases.[48]

NUTRITION

Nutritional abnormalities affect a significant number of children with rheumatic diseases.[49,50] Factors that contribute to these abnormalities include metabolic effects of inflammation, physical inactivity, reduced energy intake, and the effects and side effects of drugs used to treat these diseases. The fact that fasting can have an antiinflammatory effect and that rare patients develop transient arthritis caused by certain foods[50] (e.g., gluten-containing foods) has promoted interest in the relationship between diet and arthritis. The earlier concern regarding relationship of alfalfa sprouts in SLE has generally been disproved.

Patients and parents are also influenced by the publicity for alternative and complementary medicine because scientific medicine cannot promise a cure for rheumatic diseases. Therefore, the following questions are raised often: Can specific food items aggravate or precipitate symptoms of arthritis? If so, what food items should be avoided in the diet? What are the roles of dietary supplements, special diets, and elimination diets?

The physician's main goal should be to control inflammation as rapidly as possible and thus minimize the nutritional abnormalities. The child should be maintained on a well-balanced, healthy diet with adequate vitamins and minerals and should be encouraged to be as physically active as possible. The physician also has to counsel parents on the proper role of nutrition and educate them about fad diets and dietary supplements.

Physicians have to teach parents that at present there is no specific, evidence-based dietary recommendation for the treatment of rheumatic diseases. There are no data to recommend an elimination diet, although rare patients may exhibit altered immune response to items such as milk or gluten. Moreover, an elimination diet should be tried only under strict medical supervision, because there is a danger of precipitating malnutrition and deficiency diseases. Megavitamins and macrobiotic diets should be avoided.

Evidence-based advice should include supplemental calcium and vitamin D, particularly for children on glucocorticoid therapy, folic acid for children on methotrexate, salt restriction and potassium supplementation for children on long-term glucocorticoid therapy, and supplemental iron with or without vitamin C for children with anemia of chronic illness.[51,52]

In previous decades, the main dietary focus for patients with arthritis was increasing caloric consumption. However, as new therapies have been developed, the number of patients with insufficient caloric intake has declined. Today, childhood obesity is becoming an important issue in children with arthritis. Increased body weight adds increased stress on the weight-bearing joints. An individualized weight management plan and consultation with a dietitian are indicated for some patients. Programs that include exercise along with dietary restriction are more likely to be successful. Obesity is often a family problem, and successfully controlling it requires family participation.

Children with rheumatic diseases on chronic glucocorticoid therapy are at increased risk for accelerated atherosclerosis. Therefore, the American Heart Association places children with chronic inflammatory diseases in Tier II in the algorithm for cardiovascular risk reduction.[53] Children in this tier should be screened for additional risk factors. The screenings should include obtaining a family history of early coronary heart disease, assessment of the amount of physical activity, and measurement of blood pressure, body mass index, fasting blood sugar, and a lipid profile. On the basis of this screening, patients may have to be referred to a dietitian or other specialists for further management.

UNCONVENTIONAL REMEDIES

Practitioners of scientific, evidence-based medicine acknowledge that the etiology of rheumatic diseases is not yet known, and a cure cannot be assured. Therefore, it is easy for parents to believe those who promise miracles. This is also the age of alternative medicine.[54,55] There are pressures from well-meaning friends and relatives to try unproven remedies widely advertised in newspapers and on the Internet.

The use of alternative and complementary methods of treatment is increasing even among children, although detailed analyses of available studies do not show any benefit or only limited benefit.[55] One of them (cervical manipulation) is clearly dangerous, particularly in children with arthritis. It is safe to assume that many patients have tried or are trying one or more unconventional remedies. In the developing world in particular, large numbers of patients make use of traditional medicine systems before seeing a doctor. This is particularly true of parents who use such remedies themselves and those who grew up in other cultures. It is better to keep an open and noncritical relationship with patients and their family members so that they feel comfortable talking about their use of these remedies. It is important for pediatric rheumatologists to be aware of the currently available alternative and traditional remedies so they can provide proper guidance when patients ask about such methods. This is an opportunity to educate parents on the conduct of scientific studies and to explain to them the difference between controlled trials and testimonials. It is better to let them try some remedies that are innocuous (acupuncture), caution about some potentially dangerous treatments (e.g., megavitamins, cervical manipulation), and refuse to be part of certain other approaches (e.g., beesting therapy, auto-urine therapy). It is always wise not to make parents feel guilty or ashamed and allow room for them to come back without losing face and feeling humiliated. It is also important to remind them that the use of complementary or alternative medicines should not replace evidenced-based, prescribed medicines.

IMMUNIZATION

There are two major questions related to immunization and rheumatic diseases: (1) Is there any relationship between immunization and onset or exacerbation of these diseases? (2) What are the recommendations for children with rheumatic diseases who are taking immune modulators and the newer biologic agents?

Although some reports suggest that immunization may exacerbate or initiate an arthritic or vasculitic disorder,[56-58] other studies do not support this association.[59,60] Recent studies in adults and children who received immune modulators and the newer biologics showed no exacerbation of the underlying diseases following immunization with inactivated influenza virus vaccine.[60-62] Although there are variations in response between patients on methotrexate as compared with those on tumor necrosis factor (TNF) inhibitors, there is overall good response to immunization with influenza vaccine. It appears that the benefits of yearly immunization of adults and children with rheumatic diseases against influenza far outweigh any risk in most situations.[61,63]

In areas where human immunodeficiency virus (HIV), tuberculosis (TB), and malaria are prevalent, adequate screening, counseling, and prevention programs should be implemented.

Children who receive chronic salicylate therapy and all children considered immunocompromised, including those with SLE, dermatomyositis with significant muscle weakness, systemic scleroderma with cardiopulmonary or renal disease, or systemic vasculitis, may benefit from a yearly influenza virus (inactivated virus) vaccination. Studies also indicate that patients taking glucocorticoids and immunosuppressive drugs respond to influenza,[60,64] measles-mumps-rubella,[65] meningococcal,[66] human papillomavirus,[67] and pneumococcal vaccines[68] with adequate antibody titers. Children with SLE and potential splenic hypofunction should receive the pneumococcal vaccine.[68] However, such immunizations should not give rise to a false sense of security, because immunity is not guaranteed, particularly in patients on biologic treatments who may exhibit accelerated fall in antibody titers and might therefore benefit from vaccine boosters.[66]

Adherence to national vaccination guidelines for live-attenuated vaccines is recommended unless patients are on high-dose disease-modifying antirheumatic drugs (DMARDs) or high-dose corticosteroids or biologic agents. However, vaccination can be considered on a case-to-case basis, weighing the risk of infections against the hypothetical risk of inducing infections by vaccination.[69]

Ideally, children should have received the routine recommended immunizations and antibody status confirmed before the start of immunosuppressive therapies and biologic immune modulators. It is best to advise families to keep the regular schedule of immunizations while cautioning them about the possibility of a flare-up. Following are a few special circumstances, exceptions, and precautions:

1. *Active disease:* Children with severe, active rheumatic disease should not receive any immunization.
2. *Varicella-zoster (VZV):* Varicella can be a major problem for children receiving immunosuppressive therapy, glucocorticoids, methotrexate, and/or biologic agents. For all of these children, a suggested management strategy for the prevention of disease is given in Box 11-6. Ideally, the antibody level against VZV should be known before the start of therapy. Varicella and other live virus and bacterial vaccines are generally contraindicated in children taking glucocorticoids in doses of 2 mg/kg/day of prednisone or its equivalent, to a total of 20 mg/day of prednisone or equivalent for children who weigh more than 10 kg when given for longer than 14 days.[70] For children receiving smaller doses, the risk/benefit ratio must be assessed. Salicylate should not be used for at least 6 weeks after varicella vaccine administration. The potential for Reye syndrome in children treated with salicylates in association with varicella or influenza has been widely discussed.[71]

3. *Children on immunosuppressive therapy and on biological immune modulators:* Children undergoing immunosuppressive therapy, receiving biological immune modulators, or undergoing glucocorticoid therapy should not receive any live virus or bacterial vaccine. If glucocorticoids and cytotoxic drugs have been stopped, live virus vaccines may be given after a minimum of 3 months. It is also important to remember that the new nasal spray vaccine for influenza contains live virus and is therefore contraindicated in immunocompromised patients and their contacts. Only the inactivated parenteral form of the influenza vaccine should be used. Recommendations made by the Committee on Infectious Diseases of the American Academy of Pediatrics should be followed for children.[70] The British Society of Rheumatology recommends the use of influenza A, meningococcus C, *Haemophilus* b, hepatitis B, and tetanus toxoid, but warns that the response may be suboptimal.[63]
4. *Intravenous immunoglobulin:* Children receiving intravenous immunoglobulin should wait at least 3 months after the last dose to ensure an adequate immune response.[72]

OUTREACH

Outreach services beyond the large academic medical centers have been shown to improve access to subspecialty care, particularly in areas with large rural populations and sparse subspecialty workforce[73] (Box 11-7). The improved access also reduces the families' out-of-pocket expenses and work and school absences. It facilitates communication with community physicians.

More recently, telemedicine has made distance access more feasible, but it requires a skilled health professional examiner to assist in the evaluation. The benefits of improved access, reduced cost, and improved communication are balanced by the challenge of assessing quality of care, patient satisfaction, and legal and technological considerations. An Australian study found a mix of both face-to-face and virtual consultation was likely the best solution.[74] In a Canadian study, videoconferencing was preferred to face-to-face or email consultation.[75] A study of adult subspecialties suggested that physician-to-patient communication during teleconferencing was not inferior to communication during face-to-face consultation.[76]

GLOBAL ISSUES

Care of patients with rheumatic diseases in developing countries poses several challenges to families, physicians, and health professionals. Different social, cultural, and economic factors affect the provision of quality health care services, impede the achievement of goals in disease control and quality of life, and may result in a disease course that

---

BOX 11-6   Varicella Prevention Strategy for Children Taking Glucocorticoids, Immunosuppressives, and Biologic Agents

Document successful vaccination in the past; measure serum antibody level.

If seronegative (susceptible), immunize with varicella vaccine 3 weeks before starting therapy.

Susceptible children exposed to varicella should receive varicella-zoster immunoglobulin within 72 hours after exposure.

If chickenpox develops, treat with oral or parenteral acyclovir depending on severity and spread. Stop Enbrel and methotrexate temporarily but continue glucocorticoids.

BOX 11-7   Building an Outreach Network

Goals

Early detection of patients with rheumatic diseases

Initial management of patients with recently diagnosed rheumatic diseases

Timely referral

Monitor disease activity and drug toxicity

Assistance in maintaining continuing care plans

Liaise with local medical and allied health workers, and community members

Creation/promotion of local teams

Provision of information and counseling to patients

Promotion/facilitation of telehealth assessments

closely resembles that of the natural history of untreated disease. Priorities led by the more prevalent and life-threatening infectious diseases usually leave care for rheumatic diseases underserved. In general, public awareness of the existence and specific needs of rheumatic conditions in children is low in the developing world.[77]

The shortage of specialized medical expertise and insufficiently equipped centers that offer limited inpatient care (most often based in the public, state-run hospitals) that serve the majority of the population contrast with the modern and efficient private clinics and hospitals, where a few patients receive world-class, state-of-the-art care. This asymmetry in health care provision frequently leads to a wide range of complications, such as disease flares when treatment is abruptly suspended due to supply cuts.[78]

The following factors are among the most important issues affecting care for children with rheumatic diseases in the developing world.

Epidemiology

Knowledge of disease prevalence is limited. As in the industrialized world, JIA is the most commonly encountered rheumatic disease in childhood, although the relative percentages of patients in different categories of JIA treated by pediatric rheumatologists differ from the ones documented in the developed countries: Polyarticular and systemic JIA are most commonly seen in the developing world, whereas oligoarticular JIA is most common in the developed world.[79-94] This may be due to the fact that most studies in developing countries are done in tertiary hospital populations, where children with more severe disease would be encountered. Moreover, in some parts of the world, access to health care may be more difficult for girls.[93] This may explain the nearly equal sex ratio reported in patients in the Western Cape, South Africa,[94] in contrast to the predominance of girls in studies from Europe and North America. Population-based studies and studies in outreach clinics may correct these distortions.[95] Well-designed and well-maintained databases and registries can increase knowledge of the epidemiological particularities of a given community and provide rapid access to data for use in clinical and public health decision making.[96]

Infectious Diseases and Diseases of Poverty (TB, HIV, Malnutrition)

The overwhelming burden of infectious diseases in some countries of the developing world not only consumes most public health resources but also contributes to the complexity of diagnosis and poses significant problems with respect to the use of antirheumatic drugs such as corticosteroids, methotrexate, and biologics. A significant proportion of patients with rheumatic diseases in some areas of the developing world are also infected with HIV, TB, and parasitic or so-called tropical disease agents, which may confound diagnosis or alter the disease presentation, screening, response to medications, and disease course.[97-100] On the other hand, patients infected with these agents may suffer from multiple rheumatologic complications that mimic diseases such as JIA.[77]

Additionally, the high prevalence of rheumatic fever in many parts of the developing world may lead to erroneous diagnosis of other, clinically similar rheumatic conditions in children. The prevalence of rheumatic fever is maintained by predisposing environmental factors such as low socioeconomic status and large household sizes in both developing and developed countries.[100] To minimize these diseases and their confusion with other rheumatic diseases, physician education and close liaison with infectious disease specialists are absolutely necessary.

Shortage of Specialized Manpower

The number of pediatric rheumatologists is insufficient—even for patient care alone—in most developing countries, and this is more so in remote territories.[101] In a typical developing country, the few pediatric rheumatologists are usually based in metropolitan tertiary hospitals, usually poorly equipped and funded by the state, with no community-based programs. Whereas these hospitals provide low-budget health care to the majority of the population, private hospitals may serve a small, wealthy proportion of the inhabitants. Distribution disparities in workforce supply within a country or region are common. Different barriers (cultural, geographical, administrative) may impede access to health care providers and may cause delay in consultation, and long and inappropriate care pathways—which often include alternative health practitioners—which finally result in substandard quality care and worse disease outcomes. Moreover, teaching and research in pediatric rheumatology are also limited by insufficient numbers of academic specialists. The training of more specialists may eventually solve this problem, but that can take years or decades. Teaching of the basics of musculoskeletal (MSK) examination to undergraduate students and postgraduate pediatricians may help bridge the gap until there are enough specialists to cover the needs in each country. Specific screening MSK examinations, such as pediatric gait arms legs spine (pGALS) or pediatric regional examination of the musculoskeletal system (PREMS), are useful tools that can be easily taught to undergraduate students, interns, and pediatricians.[102,103] The expansion of the roles of pediatricians working in underserved areas may also help provide timely diagnosis, referral, and continuous care for patients living in remote, geographically distant communities.[104,105] Outreach clinics led by the pediatric rheumatologist are an effective option for providing the essential care and shortening the delay in consultation in remote, sparsely populated areas.[100] Telemedicine is another way of bringing patients and scarce human resources together.[106] It may aid consultation and care coordination for collaborative monitoring of the continued care of children with rheumatic diseases. Networking between pediatric rheumatologists and local pediatricians or family doctors is central to maintain a continuous flow of information, provide continuous medical education to pediatricians, and monitor the continued care of rheumatic disease patients. Ideally, training should be tailored to the individual physician or health agent to meet individual abilities and expectations, increase competencies, and match the specific needs of her or his community. Alliance with adult rheumatologists or immunologists may be necessary in some scenarios to expand patient care provision as well as research and teaching activities.[9,10]

Long Disease Duration before Access to Specialized Care

The aforementioned conditioning factors (poor awareness of rheumatic conditions; cultural and geographical barriers in access to health care; saturated public services serving the overwhelming demand of communicable diseases; deficit in training in MSK examination and basics of rheumatology in generalists, family doctors, and pediatricians[107,108]; and the shortage of pediatric rheumatologists) all contribute to inordinate delays in patient access to a pediatric rheumatologist.[85,88,92,109] Use of complementary and alternative medicine may also compete with accessing a timely diagnosis and provision of appropriate health care.[110] Access to pediatric rheumatology care is related to disease outcome and quality of life.[111,112] The use of simple developmental tools to facilitate early referral of potential patients may also shorten time to specialist consultation.[113]

BOX 11-8 Global Challenges in the Management of Children with Rheumatic Diseases

Challenges

Improve the Outcome (QOL) of Children with Rheumatic Diseases

Increase awareness and proper diagnosis

Improve access or shorten the delay in access to specialized care through timely referrals

Optimize integrated care through coordinated teamwork throughout the country

Provide timely, comprehensive, continuing, quality care to rheumatic patients living in remote, underserved communities

Prevent inappropriate care (unnecessary interventions)

Reduce duplication of services

Prevent inequalities in care provision

Improve communication between providers

Set and improve registries and epidemiological information, monitor progress

Reduce hospital costs

TABLE 11-4 Challenges for Developing Countries

Distance	In developing countries, large distances may need to be covered to seek basic medical attention. This may be a huge economic and logistical challenge. The rheumatologist has to be prudent about making decisions that take this major limitation into consideration and may need to work closely with health care workers closer to the patient. The possibility of outreach clinics or telemedicine support has to be investigated.
Poverty	In developing countries, poverty is a frequent barrier to care. Patients struggle to afford regular visits, even for relatively short distances. Patients are frequently unaccompanied by adults, or may be accompanied by neighbors or relatives in cases where parents cannot afford to take time off work.
Traditional medicines	In Africa, up to 85% of children will seek health care from a traditional practitioner. In some African countries, traditional healers far outnumber medical doctors, and up to 70% of patients are reliant on traditional systems for basic health care.[114-116] The WHO recognizes the need for cooperation between allopathic and traditional health care systems.[117] As for other complementary medical beliefs, it is best for the rheumatologist to maintain the trust of the family by not belittling or criticizing these approaches, but rather trying to stay in touch with the alternative therapy regimen. In some cases it is possible to co-opt the traditional career into the multidisciplinary team, for religious and social support.
Access to medicines	Many medicines commonly used in the treatment of rheumatic diseases in the developed world are not accessible in developing countries (e.g., triamcinolone hexacetonide, anti-TNF agents, other biologics). In some areas, even methotrexate may not be available.
Access to expertise	There are fewer than 10 pediatric rheumatologists in sub-Saharan Africa.[118] Models of care therefore need to involve general practitioners and pediatricians.
Infectious risks of medicines	Tuberculosis and other infections are endemic in developing countries, especially sub-Saharan Africa. This must be considered and dealt with when immunosuppressive drugs are required. TB prophylaxis or treatment may be necessary.
Interaction of immunosuppressive drugs with TB treatment or antiretroviral medication.	Liver function derangement of methotrexate or azathioprine may be worsened by TB drugs such as rifampicin and isoniazid (INH), or by antiretroviral drugs.
Rheumatic manifestations of infectious diseases	Infectious diseases such as tuberculosis and AIDS have important rheumatic manifestations. These conditions complicate the diagnosis and treatment of rheumatic diseases in children in the developing world.
Stigma	In areas where traditional beliefs include a prominent role for supernatural forces, stigma around chronic diseases may arise.[119,120] These have to be actively considered and addressed.

Lack of Dedicated Interdisciplinary Teams

Not only is the number of pediatric rheumatologists insufficient to meet the demand, but dedicated interdisciplinary teams are too few or are nonexistent in developing countries. Therefore, the majority of the workload falls on the pediatric rheumatologist, who often is not appropriately trained and equipped to satisfy such demands. Social workers, most frequently overwhelmed by demands from other fields, may be unable to cope with the challenges of chronic patients in an impoverished setting. It is probably in the hands of the public, state-run facilities to provide multidisciplinary care through the assemblage and maintenance of dedicated teams, both in the local community hospital and in the central, metropolitan, tertiary hospitals. The benefit interdisciplinary teams bring to patients with complex, chronic disorders exceeds the sum of individual efforts, often scattered over different appointments, consultation days, and physical environments. This team may agree on diagnostic and therapeutic pathways, adopt and use validated clinical scores in daily practice, and monitor the disease outcome in a rich, stimulating, and multidimensional environment of quality care.

Global management challenges for children with rheumatic disease are listed in Box 11-8. Some special challenges for developing countries to overcome are listed in Table 11-4.

REFERENCES

1. N. Hobbs, J.M. Perrin, Issues in the Care of Children with Chronic Illness: A Source Book on Problems, Services and Policies, Jossey-Bass, San Francisco, 1985.
2. I.B. Pless, C. Power, C.S. Peckham, Long-term psychosocial sequelae of chronic physical disorders in childhood, Pediatrics 91 (1993) 1131–1136.
3. M.C. McCormick, M.M. Stemmler, B.H. Athreya, The impact of childhood rheumatic diseases on the family, Arthritis Rheum. 29 (1986) 872–879.

4. D.A. Lovell, B.H. Athreya, H.M. Emery, et al., School attendance and patterns, special services and special needs in pediatric patients with rheumatic diseases, Arthritis Care Res. 3 (1990) 196.

8. C.A. Wallace, J.E. Levinson, Juvenile rheumatoid arthritis: outcome and treatment for the 1990s, Rheum. Dis. Clin. North Am. 17 (1991) 891–905.

9. L.S. Peterson, T. Mason, A.M. Nelson, et al., Psychosocial outcomes and health status of adults who have had juvenile rheumatoid arthritis: a controlled, population-based study, Arthritis Rheum. 40 (1997) 2235–2240.

10. J.C. Packham, M.A. Hall, Long-term follow-up of 246 adults with juvenile idiopathic arthritis: functional outcome, Rheumatology 41 (2002) 1428–1435.

11. P. Rettig, B.H. Athreya, Leaving home: preparing the adolescent with arthritis for coping with independence and the adult rheumatology world, in: D. Isenberg, J.J. Miller (Eds.), Adolescent Rheumatology, Martin Dunitz, London, 1998.

18. M. Arkela-Kautiainen, J. Haapasaari, H. Kautiainen, et al., Favorable social functioning and health related quality of life of patients with JIA in early adulthood, Ann. Rheum. Dis. 64 (2005) 875–880.

21. E.J. Brewer Jr., M. McPherson, P.R. Magrab, et al., Family-centered, community-based, coordinated care for children with special healthcare needs, Pediatrics 83 (1989) 1055–1060.

22. J. van der Net, A.B. Prakken, P.J. Helders, et al., Correlates of disablement in juvenile chronic arthritis: a cross-sectional study, Br. J. Rheumatol. 35 (1996) 91–100.

26. World Health Organization—WHO Workgroup for Developmental Version of ICF for Children and Youth, International classification of functioning, disability and health—version for children and youth ICF-CY, World Health Organization, Geneva, 2007.

27. R.B. Noll, K. Kozlowski, C. Gerhardt, et al., Social, emotional, and behavioral functioning of children with juvenile rheumatoid arthritis, Arthritis Rheum. 43 (2000) 1387–1396.

28. R.T. von Weiss, M.A. Rapoff, J.W. Varni, et al., Daily hassles and social support as predictors of adjustment in children with pediatric rheumatic diseases, J. Pediatr. Psychol. 27 (2002) 155–165.

33. J.D. Akikusa, R.C. Allen, Reducing the impact of rheumatic diseases in childhood, Best Pract. Res. Clin. Rheumatol. 16 (2002) 333–345.

35. M.M. Graves, M.C. Roberts, M. Rapoff, et al., The efficacy of adherence for chronically ill children: a meta-analytic review, J. Pediatr. Psychol. 35 (2010) 368–382.

36. A.C. Modi, J.R. Rausch, T.A. Glaser, Patterns of nonadherence to antiepileptic drug therapy in children with newly diagnosed epilepsy, JAMA 305 (2011) 1669–1676.

37. S. Naar-King, A.Y. Outlaw, M. Sarr, et al., Motivational Enhancement System for Adherence (MESA): pilot randomized trial of a brief computer-delivered prevention intervention for youth initiating antiretroviral treatment, J. Pediatr. Psychol. 38 (2013) 638–648.

41. P.D. Williams, A.R. Williams, J.C. Graff, et al., A community-based intervention for siblings and parents of children with chronic illness or disability: the ISEE study, J. Pediatr. 143 (2003) 386–393.

42. J.T. Cassidy, C.B. Lindsley, Legal rights of children with musculoskeletal disabilities, Bull. Rheum. Dis. 45 (1996) 1–5.

43. C.H. Spencer, R.Z. Fife, C.E. Rabinovich, The school experience of children with arthritis: coping in the 1990s and transition into adulthood, Pediatr. Clin. North Am. 42 (1995) 1285–1298.

44. J. Taylor, M.H. Passo, V.L. Champion, School problems and teacher responsibilities in juvenile rheumatoid arthritis, J. Sch. Health 57 (1987) 186–190.

45. P.H. White, Success on the road to adulthood: issues and hurdles for adolescents with disabilities, Rheum. Dis. Clin. North Am. 23 (1997) 697–707.

46. J.E. McDonagh, Young people first, juvenile idiopathic arthritis second: transition care in rheumatology, Arthritis Rheum. 59 (2008) 1162–1170.

50. C.J. Henderson, R.S. Panush, Diet, dietary supplements and nutritional therapy in rheumatic diseases, Rheum. Dis. Clin. North Am. 25 (1999) 937–968.

52. D.J. Lovell, D. Glass, J. Ranz, A randomized controlled trial of calcium supplementation to increase bone mineral density in children with juvenile rheumatoid arthritis, Arthritis Rheum. 54 (2006) 2235–2242.

54. K.J. Kemper, S. Vohra, R. Walls, et al., The use of complementary and alternative medicine in pediatrics, Pediatrics 122 (2008) 1374–1386.

56. C.M. Benjamin, G.C. Chew, A.J. Silman, Joint and limb symptoms in children after immunisation with measles, mumps, and rubella vaccine, BMJ 304 (1992) 1075–1078.

57. C.J. Castresana-Isla, G. Herrera-Martinez, J. Vega-Molina, Erythema nodosum and Takayasu's arteritis after immunization with plasma derived hepatitis B vaccine, J. Rheumatol. 20 (1993) 1417–1418.

59. P. Ray, S. Black, H. Shinefield, et al., Risk of chronic arthropathy among women after rubella vaccination. Vaccine Safety Datalink Team, JAMA 278 (1997) 551–556.

60. P.N. Malleson, J.L. Tekano, D.W. Scheifele, et al., Influenza immunization in children with chronic arthritis: a prospective study, J. Rheumatol. 20 (1993) 1769–1773.

63. K. Davies, P. Woo, British Paediatric Rheumatology Group, Immunization in rheumatic diseases of childhood: an audit of the clinical practice of British Paediatric Rheumatology Group members and a review of the evidence, Rheumatology 41 (2002) 937–941.

64. C.L. Park, A.L. Frank, M. Sullivan, et al., Influenza vaccination of children during acute asthma exacerbation and concurrent prednisone therapy, Pediatrics 98 (1996) 196–200.

65. M.W. Heijstek, S. Kamphuis, W. Ambrust, et al., Effects of the live attenuated measles-mumps-rubella booster vaccination on disease activity in patients with juvenile idiopathic arthritis: a randomized trial, JAMA 309 (2013) 2449–2456.

66. S.P. Stoof, M.W. Heijstek, K.M. Siissens, et al., Kinetics of the long-term antibody response after meningococcal C vaccination in patients with juvenile idiopathic arthritis: a retrospective cohort study, Ann. Rheum. Dis. 10 (2013) 2012–2025.

67. M.W. Heijstek, M. Scherpenisse, N. Groot, et al., Immunogenicity and safety of the bivalent HPV vaccine in female patients with juvenile idiopathic arthritis: a prospective controlled observational cohort study, Ann. Rheum. Dis. 73 (2013) 1500–1507 doi: 10.1136/annrheumdis-2013-203429. Epub 2013 May 30.

68. R.N. Lipnick, J. Karsh, N.I. Stahl, et al., Pneumococcal immunization in patients with systemic lupus erythematosus treated with immunosuppressives, J. Rheumatol. 12 (1985) 1118–1121.

69. M.W. Heijstek, L.M. Ott de Bruin, M. Bill, et al., EULAR recommendations for vaccination in paediatric patients with rheumatic diseases, Ann. Rheum. Dis. 70 (2011) 1704–1712.

73. C.B. Lindsley, A. Kunkel, N.Y. Olsen, et al., Outreach clinics provide rural populations access to pediatric rheumatology care, Arth. Rheum. 37 (1994) S419.

74. L.J. Roberts, E.J. Lamont, I. Lim, et al., Telerheumatology: an idea whose time has come, Intern. Med. J. 42 (2012) 1072–1078.

75. M. Jong, M. Kraishi, A comparative study on the utility of telehealth in the provision of rheumatology services to rural and northern communities, Int. J. Circumpolar Health 63 (2004) 415–421.

77. S. Sawhney, C. Saad Magalhaes, Paediatric rheumatology—a global perspective, Best Pract. Res. Clin. Rheumatol. 20 (2006) 201–221.

78. R.A.G. Russo, M.M. Katsicas, Recaídas de la artritis crónica juvenil luego de la suspensión de etanercept, Arch. Argent. Pediatr. 102 (2004) 44–48.

79. F.A. Khuffash, H.A. Majeed, M.M. Lubani, et al., Epidemiology of juvenile chronic arthritis and other connective tissue diseases among children in Kuwait, Ann. Trop. Paediatr. 10 (1990) 255–259.

80. A. Aggarwal, R. Misra, Juvenile chronic arthritis in India: is it different from that seen in Western countries? Rheumatol. Int. 14 (1994) 53–56.

83. A. Stabile, L. Avallone, A. Compagnone, et al., Focus on juvenile idiopathic arthritis according to the 2001 Edmonton revised classification from the International League of Associations for Rheumatology: an Italian experience, Eur. Rev. Med. Pharmacol. Sci. 10 (2006) 229–234.

84. R. Gutierrez-Suarez, A. Pistorio, A. Cespedes Cruz, et al., Health-related quality of life of patients with juvenile idiopathic arthritis coming from

3 different geographic areas. The PRINTO multinational quality of life cohort study, Rheumatology 46 (2007) 314–320.

88. V. Kunjir, A. Venugopalan, A. Chopra, Profile of Indian patients with juvenile onset chronic inflammatory joint disease using the ILAR classification criteria for JIA: a community-based cohort study, J. Rheumatol. 37 (2010) 1756–1762.

90. S. Ringold, T. Beukelman, P.A. Nigrovic, Y. Kimura, Race, ethnicity, and disease outcomes in juvenile idiopathic arthritis: a cross-sectional analysis of the Childhood Arthritis and Rheumatology Research Alliance (CARRA) Registry, J. Rheumatol. 40 (2013) 936–942.

94. K. Weakley, M. Esser, C. Scott, Juvenile idiopathic arthritis in two tertiary centers in the Western Cape, South Africa, Pediatr. Rheumatol. Online J. 10 (2012) 35.

97. I. Colmegna, J.W. Koehler, R.F. Garry, L.R. Espinoza, Musculoskeletal and autoimmune manifestations of HIV, syphilis and tuberculosis, Curr. Op. Rheumatol. 18 (2006) 88–95.

101. M. Henrickson, Policy changes for the pediatric rheumatology workforce: part III, the international situation, Pediatric Rheumatology 9 (2011) 26.

102. H.E. Foster, L.J. Kay, M. Friswell, et al., Musculoskeletal screening examination (pGALS) for school-age children based on the adult GALS Screen, Arthritis Rheum. 55 (2006) 709–716.

103. H. Foster, L. Kay, C. May, T. Rapley, Pediatric Regional examination of the musculoskeletal system: a practice- and consensus-based approach, Arthritis Care Res. 63 (2011) 1503–1510.

104. T.P. Vilet Vlieland, L.C. Li, C. McKay, et al., Current topics on models of care on the management of inflammatory arthritis, J. Rheumatol. 33 (2006) 1900–1903.

105. C. MacKay, P. Veinot, E.M. Badley, Characteristics of evolving models of care for arthritis: a key informant study, BMC Health Serv. Res. 8 (2008) 147.

106. P. Davis, R. Howard, P. Brockway, An evaluation of telehealth in the provision of rheumatologic consults to a remote area, J. Rheumatol. 28 (2001) 1910–1913.

109. N. Tzaribachev, S.M. Benseler, P.N. Tyrrell, et al., Predictors of delayed referral to a pediatric rheumatology center, Arthritis Care Res. 61 (2009) 1367–1372.

111. H.E. Foster, M.S. Eltringham, L.J. Kay, et al., Delay in access to appropriate care for children presenting with musculoskeletal symptoms and ultimately diagnosed with juvenile idiopathic arthritis, Arthritis Care Res. 57 (2007) 921–927.

112. H. Foster, T. Rapley, Access to pediatric rheumatology care—a major challenge to improving outcome in juvenile idiopathic arthritis, J. Rheumatol. 37 (2010) 2199–2202.

113. C.A. Len, M.T. Terreri, R.F. Puccini, et al., Development of a tool for early referral of children and adolescents with signs and symptoms suggestive of chronic arthropathy to pediatric rheumatology centers, Arthritis Care Res. 55 (2006) 373–377.

114. T. Stangeland, S.S. Dhillion, H. Reksten, Recognition and development of traditional medicine in Tanzania, J. Ethnopharmacol. 117 (2008) 290–299.

115. N. Romero-Daza, Traditional medicine in Africa, The Annals AAPSS (Global Perspectives on Complementary and Alternative Medicine) 583 (2002) 173–176.

Entire reference list is available online at www.expertconsult.com.

Pharmacology and Drug Therapy: Nonbiologic Therapies

Mara L. Becker, Dan Lovell, Steven J. Leeder

The principal drugs used in pediatric rheumatology are drugs that suppress the inflammatory and immune responses. This chapter outlines important general principles relating to these medications, particularly as they apply to children. The treatment of specific rheumatic disorders is discussed in detail in the relevant chapters.

CONCEPTS IN PHARMACOLOGY

Optimizing the efficacy and safety of medications used to treat rheumatic disorders in children requires an understanding of the multiple factors involved in drug disposition and response. These include the processes of *drug absorption, distribution, metabolism,* and *excretion* (ADME) characterized mathematically by the pharmacokinetics of the drug as well as the multiple factors that contribute to the pharmacodynamics of drug response. In a simplistic sense, pharmacokinetics describes what the body does to a drug, whereas pharmacodynamics represents what a drug does to the body. Adding to the complexity of drug disposition and response in children is the impact of growth and development ("ontogeny") on the expression of drug metabolizing enzymes, transporters, receptors, and other gene products along the developmental continuum between birth and maturity. There has been considerable interest in the role of genetic variation ("pharmacogenetics") as a determinant of interindividual variability in the clinical response to medications widely used in pediatric rheumatology. The following section provides a brief overview of the general principles of drug disposition and response, and can be supplemented by referring to additional general pediatric texts.[1]

Drug Absorption and Bioavailability

Drugs that are given by the oral route are absorbed through the mucosa of the gastrointestinal (GI) tract, primarily in the small intestine. GI absorption may be influenced by numerous factors, including the presence or absence of food in the gastric lumen, luminal pH, gastric emptying time, and coadministration of other drugs. Drug bioavailability, the net result of these factors, is usually determined by sequential measurement of plasma drug concentrations. Three parameters are routinely considered: (1) peak drug concentration, (2) the time necessary to reach peak concentration, and (3) the area under the time-concentration curve. The area under the curve (AUC) after intravenous administration is considered equivalent to complete absorption after oral administration. Because the effects of drugs that are administered repeatedly are cumulative—with the exception of drugs with extremely short half- lives that are given at infrequent intervals—bioavailability is best determined at the mean steady-state concentration of the drug, that is, the point at which drug intake is equal to drug elimination.

Several physiological processes that contribute to drug absorption undergo changes as children grow and develop. For example, gastric pH is relatively alkaline in neonates, and maturation to adult levels reflects the ontogeny of parietal cells and is not achieved until 3 years of age or older. As a consequence, the bioavailability of acid-labile drugs (e.g., penicillins) is increased and that of weakly acidic drugs (e.g., phenobarbital) is less than expected over this time period. Other factors, such as gastric emptying time, intestinal motility, and intestinal surface area, are also important determinants of drug absorption and all mature over the first year of life.

Volume of Distribution

The volume of distribution is the apparent volume of fluid into which a drug would need to be distributed to achieve a concentration equal to the concentration ultimately measured in plasma. If the drug stays in the plasma, its volume of distribution is essentially the plasma volume—considerably smaller than if the drug is distributed widely in tissues. Body composition changes dramatically between birth and adolescence. Water constitutes approximately 75% of total body mass in newborns and declines to the adult value of 55% by approximately 12 years of age. Body fat is approximately 16% in neonates and increases over the first 10 years of life, but also changes compositionally with age. The consequence of these changes is a decrease in the volume of distribution of hydrophilic drugs, such as aminoglycoside antibiotics.

Drugs in the body are either free or bound to plasma proteins or tissue lipids. The extent and nature of binding affect the volume of distribution of the drug, the rate of renal clearance (because only free drug is filtered by the glomerulus), the drug half-life, and the amount of free drug that reaches the target tissue or receptor. Most acidic drugs are bound to plasma albumin, whereas basic drugs are bound to lipoproteins, α_1-acid glycoproteins, and globulins. In inflammatory states, plasma albumin concentration decreases and α_1-acid glycoproteins increase, although the extent of the decrease usually does not require any change in drug therapy.

Half-Life and Clearance

The half-life of a drug is the time necessary for the serum concentration to decrease by 50% during the elimination phase of the concentration-time curve. *Clearance* is the term used to describe the disappearance of a drug from the systemic circulation and is defined as the volume of body fluid from which a drug is removed per unit of time. Total body clearance represents the sum total of all clearance pathways and generally includes biotransformation to metabolites in the liver as well as elimination of unchanged drug by the kidney or in the bile. Most drugs exhibit *first-order kinetics* whereby the rate of elimination is directly proportional to the concentration in the body. Drugs that are eliminated at a constant rate, independent of concentration, are said to follow *zero-order kinetics*. Salicylates obey capacity-limited kinetics: At low concentrations, first-order kinetics are observed, but at higher concentrations, the enzymes responsible for drug metabolism become saturated, and small increases in dose can lead to disproportionate increases in concentration. Drug clearance determines the relationship between dose administered and concentration achieved, and in general, this relationship is best interpreted after at least five half-lives have passed and steady state has been achieved. Renal clearance changes with age and impacts drug elimination; thus, monitoring of drug levels and attention to the potential for drug toxicity becomes more critical in patients with significant renal disease.

Drug Biotransformation

The process of drug biotransformation is classified into phase I and phase II reactions, which occur sequentially and in most situations serve to terminate biological activity and enhance elimination; some drugs used to treat rheumatic diseases, such as sulindac, prednisone, leflunomide, azathioprine, mycophenolate mofetil (MMF), and cyclophosphamide, require biotransformation to their therapeutically active forms before they exert their principal effects.

Ontogeny

The changes related to ontogeny are critical to understanding the role of drug biotransformation in drug clearance from birth to adolescence. Most genes involved in drug biotransformation and transport are subject to genetic polymorphisms that also then can contribute to interindividual variability in drug disposition. By definition, a pharmacogenetic polymorphism is a heritable trait that involves a single gene locus occurring in more than one form, referred to as an *allele*, in a population, and results in a functional consequence in at least 1% of the population following drug exposure. The frequency of variant alleles, and therefore the prevalence of their functional consequences, differs among populations. In pediatrics, ontogeny factors into the interpretation of pharmacogenetic information as genotype–phenotype associations observed in adults will not occur in children until the gene is fully expressed.

ANTIRHEUMATIC DRUGS

Nonsteroidal Antiinflammatory Drugs

Nonsteroidal antiinflammatory drugs (NSAIDs) provide symptomatic antiinflammatory relief; they are recommended for most patients with juvenile idiopathic arthritis (JIA) and are used in many other rheumatic disorders. NSAIDs that are commonly used in children are presented in eTable 12-1.

Mechanism of Action

NSAIDs inhibit proinflammatory pathways that lead to chronic inflammation. The major antiinflammatory effect of NSAIDs is mediated by inhibition of the cyclooxygenase (COX) enzyme in the metabolism of arachidonic acid to prostaglandins, thromboxanes, and prostacyclins.[2] Currently available NSAIDs (except diclofenac and indomethacin) have little effect on the lipoxygenase pathway, the other major pathway of arachidonic acid metabolism.[3] Individual NSAIDs may have additional specific mechanisms of action.[4-12]

There are two related but unique isoforms of the COX enzyme: COX-1 and COX-2, which are 60% identical in sequence but encoded by distinct genes and differ in their distribution and expression in tissues. COX enzymes catalyze the conversion of arachidonic acid to prostaglandins G_2 and H_2. COX-1 enzyme production is widely distributed and constitutively expressed in most tissues. COX-1 provides prostaglandins that are required for "housekeeping," or homeostatic function resulting in cytoprotection, platelet aggregation, vascular homeostasis, and maintenance of renal blood flow. In contrast, COX-2 is an inducible enzyme that is upregulated at sites of inflammation by various proinflammatory mediators, including interleukin-1 (IL-1), tumor necrosis factor-α (TNF-α), bacterial endotoxins, and various mitogenic and growth factors. However, constitutive COX-2 expression is well recognized in brain, kidney, and the female reproductive tract. COX-2 also seems to have a role in the central mediation of pain and fever. The cardiotoxic effects of COX-2 inhibition also support a constitutive role of COX-2 in maintaining cardiovascular health.

Currently available NSAIDs inhibit both isoforms of COX, but most inhibit COX-1 preferentially, resulting in undesirable adverse effects such as GI toxicity while producing desirable antiinflammatory effects through concurrent inhibition of COX-2.[13] NSAIDs differ in the degree of inhibition of COX-2, compared with COX-1. This difference has been found to correlate with their adverse-effect profiles: NSAIDs that are more selective for COX-2 seem to have more favorable adverse-effect profiles.[14] Celecoxib is the only selective COX-2 inhibitor approved by the FDA for use in JIA.

Pharmacology

The pharmacokinetic evaluation of NSAIDs in children with juvenile rheumatoid arthritis (JRA) or JIA has been variable, ranging from extensive for salicylates to minimal or none with newer agents; the interested reader is referred to reviews on the subject.[15,16] They are weakly acidic drugs that are rapidly absorbed after oral administration, with most absorption occurring in the stomach and upper small intestine. Circadian rhythms in gastric pH and intestinal motility may lead to variability in NSAID absorption.[17]

Most NSAIDs are strongly protein bound, primarily to albumin, leading to a potential for drug–disease and drug–drug interactions. Hypoalbuminemia may be one of the most important factors influencing the pharmacokinetics of NSAIDs in children. Because clinical effects are determined by unbound or free drug levels, states of severe hypoalbuminemia may be associated with a corresponding increase in the unbound fraction and with a potential for increased toxicity. Most studies of NSAID pharmacokinetics in children do not report the level of disease activity, however.[18]

Although the strong plasma protein binding of NSAIDs also makes possible drug–drug interactions with other highly protein-bound drugs, significant clinical interactions are rare.[19,20] NSAIDs may potentially interact with methotrexate (MTX) through several mechanisms, including displacement from plasma protein-binding sites, competition for renal secretion, and impairment of renal function. Although the impact of NSAIDs on MTX clearance varies widely and the potential for clinically significant interactions exists in some children,[21] MTX–NSAID interactions are rarely of clinical significance.

The kinetics of NSAIDs at their antiinflammatory sites of action (e.g., synovial fluid) may be more clinically relevant than their kinetics in plasma. The comparative kinetics of NSAIDs in plasma and synovial fluid are related to the half-life of the drug and to differences in protein binding at these sites.[20] This phenomenon may partially account for the fact that the dosage interval of these drugs is longer than their plasma half-life. In addition, because synovial fluid albumin concentrations are lower than plasma concentrations, the free fraction of NSAIDs in synovial fluid can be significantly higher,[17] resulting in clinical effects observed with relatively low plasma drug levels. Except for naproxen and acetylsalicylic acid (ASA), plasma concentrations correlate poorly with antiinflammatory activity.[22]

NSAIDs are eliminated predominantly by hepatic metabolism; only small amounts are excreted unchanged in urine. Some NSAIDs, such as sulindac or indomethacin, are also secreted in significant amounts in bile and undergo enterohepatic recirculation.[20] Most NSAIDs are metabolized by first-order or linear kinetics, whereas salicylate is metabolized by zero-order or nonlinear kinetics. For this reason, dosage adjustments are frequently required with ASA therapy, and small changes in dose may lead to large fluctuations in serum levels of ASA at the higher end of the therapeutic range.[16] Naproxen may also show nonlinear pharmacokinetics at dosages greater than 500 mg/day in adults because of the saturation of plasma protein-binding sites and associated increase in clearance.[16,17] In children (especially younger children), NSAIDs may be eliminated more rapidly than in adults; children may require more frequent doses to maintain a clinical response.[18,23] Because hepatic metabolism plays a major role in NSAID elimination, it is necessary to assess hepatic function before institution of NSAID therapy; NSAIDs should not be initiated if there is significant elevation of transaminase levels (e.g., three times normal or higher).

General Principles of Nonsteroidal Antiinflammatory Drug Therapy

NSAIDs are generally good analgesic and antipyretic agents and weak antiinflammatory agents. They provide good symptomatic relief but have traditionally not been considered to influence the underlying disease process or to affect long-term outcomes significantly. Nevertheless, there is a suggestion that NSAIDs may change the course of ankylosing spondylitis by preventing syndesmophyte formation.[24] The analgesic effect of NSAIDs is rapid, but the antiinflammatory effect takes longer and can require doses twice as large as those needed for analgesia.[25,26] NSAIDs are relatively safe for long-term use. Although toxicities, especially GI side effects, are frequent, they are seldom serious.[27-29] Given the wide variety of available NSAIDs, a few general principles can be applied in the selection of a particular NSAID for therapy in an individual patient. First, according to empirical evidence from clinical experience and some studies in adults, response to NSAIDs seems to have some disease specificity. Indomethacin may be more useful in treating manifestations of systemic JIA and in managing spondyloarthropathies. Second, individual patient response to NSAIDs is variable and often unpredictable: A child may fail to respond to one drug and yet respond to another,[16] and some NSAIDs, such as ASA or indomethacin, seem to be more toxic than others.[25] An adequate trial of any NSAID should be at least about 8 weeks,[30,31] although about 50% of children who respond favorably to NSAID therapy do so by 2 weeks, and 25% may not respond until after approximately 12 weeks of therapy.[32] Third, additional factors such as availability in liquid form, frequency of dosing, cost, and tolerability of any given NSAID may influence patient preference. A reasonable initial approach is to choose a drug that has a favorable toxicity and efficacy profile; can be taken on a convenient schedule (e.g., once or twice daily); is affordable; and, for young children, is available in a liquid formulation that is palatable.[33,34] Use of multiple NSAIDs concurrently is not recommended because this approach has no documented benefit in terms of efficacy and can be associated with a greater potential for drug interactions and organ toxicity. The dose range and schedule of administration vary with the individual NSAID (see eTable 12-1). Patients who receive long-term daily NSAID therapy should have a complete blood count and liver and renal function tests, including a urinalysis, performed at baseline and every 6 to 12 months.

Toxicity

Serious toxicity associated with the use of NSAIDs seems to be rare in children.[26] Generally, most toxicities are shared to a greater or lesser degree by all NSAIDs, although this can vary in individual patients.[6,27-29,35,36]

Cardiovascular. Data from several clinical trials and observational studies in adults have suggested that there is an increased risk of cardiovascular toxicity associated with several NSAIDs and COX-2 inhibitors. Cardiovascular toxicity not only led to the withdrawal of rofecoxib and valdecoxib from the market but also resulted in more restricted, similar product labels in the United States for celecoxib and traditional NSAIDs.

Meaningful data in children are scarce, so pediatric rheumatologists have traditionally relied on adult data. Consideration of the underlying cardiovascular risk of the patient, including the rheumatic disease being treated, is likely to enter into the calculation. In adults with rheumatoid arthritis (RA) and osteoarthritis, COX-2 inhibitors are recommended to be administered with low-dose aspirin in patients with cardiac risk factors.[37] However, a recent multicenter, prospective, observational registry of 274 JIA patients receiving NSAIDs (55 receiving celecoxib) for a total of 410 patient-years (PY) of observation, revealed no difference in adverse events between nonselective NSAIDs and celecoxib. The two reported cardiovascular events were observed in the nonselective NSAID group.[38]

Gastrointestinal. GI toxicity is common to all NSAIDs. The pathogenesis of gastroduodenal mucosal injury involves multiple mechanisms[39] and ranges from mild epigastric discomfort to symptomatic or asymptomatic peptic ulceration.[40]

The average relative risk of developing a serious GI complication in adult patients exposed to NSAIDs is fivefold to sixfold that of patients not taking NSAIDs.[41] Possible risk factors for GI complications during NSAID therapy include advanced age, past history of GI bleeding or peptic ulcer disease, and cardiovascular disease.[42] Most patients who have a serious GI complication requiring hospitalization have not had prior GI side effects, however.[37,39] Additional risk factors include longer disease duration, higher NSAID dose, use of more than one NSAID, longer duration of NSAID therapy, concomitant glucocorticoid or anticoagulant use, and serious underlying systemic disorders.[39,40] Infection with *Helicobacter pylori* does not seem to play a major role.[43]

The magnitude of this problem in children is poorly documented but has traditionally been thought to be considerably less than in adults, partly because of the absence of the associated risk factors identified in adults. *H. pylori* has not been reported to be an important pathogen in children with JRA treated with NSAIDs.[44] Studies in children confirm that although mild GI disturbances are frequently associated with NSAID therapy, the number of children who develop clinically significant gastropathy is low.[29] A retrospective study of a cohort of 702 children receiving NSAID therapy for JRA who were monitored for at least 1 year found 5 children (0.7%) with clinically significant gastropathy defined as esophagitis, gastritis, or peptic ulcer disease.[45] The retrospective nature of this study may have resulted in underestimation of the prevalence of NSAID-associated gastropathy. A prospective study of a cohort of 203 children found that although 135 children (66.5%) had documented GI symptoms at some point during NSAID therapy, only 9 (4.4%) had endoscopically detected ulcers or erosions.[46] A prospective study reported 45 children (24 of whom who were symptomatic with abdominal pain) who underwent routine endoscopy (in association with general anesthesia for joint injections). Of these children, 19 (42%) had normal gastric and duodenal mucosa, and 20 had histologically mild gastritis. A clear association was seen between abdominal pain and gastroduodenal pathology, but the severity of gastric inflammation did not correlate with the duration of NSAID therapy.[47] The phase IV safety registry of celecoxib and nonselective NSAIDs revealed no evidence of GI ulcer and one report of gastritis in the nonselective NSAID group.[38]

Studies have shown differences in rates of serious GI complications associated with different NSAIDs. Systematic reviews have found ibuprofen to be associated with the lowest risk; indomethacin, naproxen, sulindac, and aspirin with moderate risk; and tolmetin, ketoprofen, and piroxicam with the highest risk.[48,49] GI symptoms can be minimized further by ensuring that NSAIDs are always given with food. The utility of antacids and histamine$_2$-receptor antagonists for prophylaxis against serious NSAID-induced GI complications is controversial. Although these medications suppress symptoms, they do not prevent significant GI events such as endoscopically documented gastric ulcers. Asymptomatic patients on acid-reduction therapies seem to be at greater risk for serious GI complications than patients not taking these medications, so their routine use in asymptomatic patients receiving NSAIDs cannot be recommended.[39,40] Misoprostol, a synthetic prostaglandin E$_1$ analogue, has been shown in adults to be effective in prophylaxis[42,50] and treatment of NSAID-induced gastroduodenal damage, thereby allowing continuation of NSAID therapy while achieving the healing of an ulcer.[51,52] Studies of misoprostol cotherapy in children are limited, but they also suggest that misoprostol may be effective in the treatment of GI toxicity symptoms in children receiving NSAIDs.[53,54] Omeprazole, a proton pump inhibitor, has been shown to be superior to ranitidine and misoprostol for the prevention and treatment of NSAID-related gastroduodenal ulcers in adults.[55-57]

Hepatotoxicity. Hepatitis with elevation of transaminase levels can occur with any NSAID but has most commonly been reported in children with JRA receiving ASA.[27,58] In one retrospective study, transaminase levels were increased in 6% of children receiving naproxen.[27] Elevated transaminase levels are rarely of clinical significance and often resolve spontaneously. However, when they are greater than twice the upper limit of normal, or when present for prolonged periods of time without resolution, it may be necessary to reduce the dose or temporarily stop NSAID therapy. Rarely, hepatotoxicity is severe; NSAIDs have been associated with macrophage activation syndrome (MAS).[59,60] Liver function should be monitored in children taking daily NSAIDs for extended periods, particularly children with systemic JIA.

Renal. Several types of renal complications have been associated with NSAID therapy, including reversible renal insufficiency and acute renal failure; acute interstitial nephritis; nephrotic syndrome; papillary necrosis; and sodium, potassium, and water retention.[61-65] Although more common in adults, cases have been described in children.[64,66-69] A 4-year prospective study of 226 children with JRA treated with NSAIDs found the prevalence of renal and urinary abnormalities attributable to NSAID therapy to be only 0.4%[70]; an even lower prevalence of 0.2% was reported in another cohort of 433 children.[71]

Central nervous system effects. Three general categories of central nervous system (CNS) side effects have been reported in association with NSAID therapy in adults: (1) aseptic meningitis, (2) psychosis, and (3) cognitive dysfunction.[72] The NSAID most commonly reported to cause aseptic meningitis has been ibuprofen; susceptibility seems to be greater in patients with SLE. Indomethacin and sulindac have been reported to induce psychotic symptoms, including paranoid delusions, depersonalization, and hallucinations, in a few patients.[72] More subtle CNS effects, such as cognitive dysfunction and depression, can also occur and are probably underrecognized and underreported. Tinnitus may occur with any NSAID, but particularly with ASA.[26] A prospective study of 203 children with JRA found that CNS symptoms occurred in 55% of patients receiving NSAIDs; the most common symptom was headache, which occurred in about one third of children.[46] Other reported symptoms included fatigue, sleep disturbance, and hyperactivity.

Cutaneous toxicity. A diverse group of skin reactions, including pruritus, urticaria, morbilliform rashes, erythema multiforme, and phototoxic reactions, have been described.[26,73] The syndrome of pseudoporphyria that occurs in association with naproxen therapy in children with JRA[74-79] is a distinctive photodermatitis marked by erythema, vesiculation, and increased skin fragility characterized by easy scarring of sun-exposed skin (Fig. 12-1). In spite of the name, porphyrin metabolism is normal. All findings except scarring resolve with discontinuation of naproxen, but the vesiculation may persist for several months.[80] Children with fair skin and blue eyes are particularly susceptible; one study reported a relative risk of 2.96 if the child had blue-gray eyes and was taking naproxen.[79] In one retrospective and parallel prospective study, young age, JIA itself, duration of therapy, evidence of systemic inflammation, and concurrent antimalarial therapy seemed to be additional risk factors for naproxen-induced pseudoporphyria.[81] It is also rarely reported with other NSAIDs.

Effects of coagulation. NSAIDs decrease platelet adhesiveness by interfering with platelet prostaglandin synthesis. This inhibition is reversible in the case of all NSAIDs except ASA, which irreversibly acetylates and inactivates COX, an effect that persists for the life of the platelet; bleeding time returns to normal only as new platelets are released into the circulation.[26] NSAIDs also displace anticoagulants from protein-binding sites, potentiating their pharmacological effect.

Hypersensitivity and miscellaneous effects. The precipitation of asthma or anaphylaxis with NSAIDs has been reported in adults as a unique syndrome associated with nasal polyps.[13,82] Although this syndrome can theoretically be provoked by any NSAID, it has most commonly been reported with ASA or tolmetin.[26] True hypersensitivity to ASA is exceedingly rare in childhood. ASA hypersensitivity occurs in about 0.3% to 0.9% of the general population, in 20% of patients with chronic urticaria, and in 3% to 4% of patients with chronic asthma and nasal polyps.[83-85]

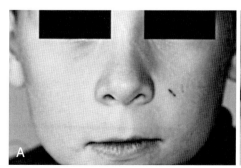
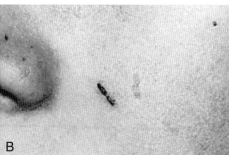

FIGURE 12-1 A and **B,** Distant and close-up views of the face of an 8-year-old boy with pseudoporphyria who was taking naproxen. Note a blistered lesion adjacent to a superficial scar. Superficial scars are also visible on the nose.

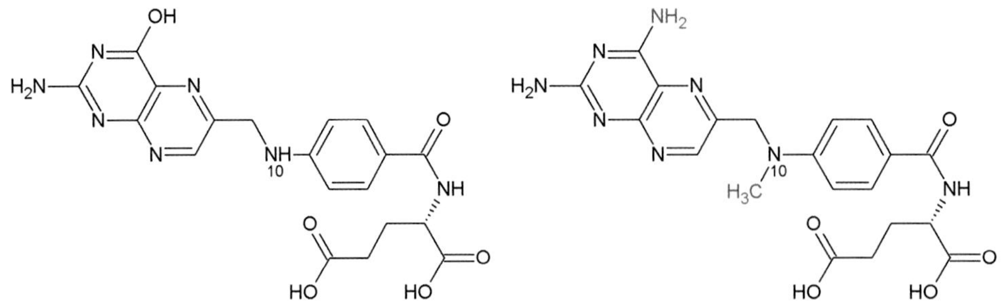

FIGURE 12-2 Structures of folic acid and methotrexate, with notable structural differences in red.

Hematological toxicity, including aplastic anemia, agranulocytosis, leukopenia, and thrombocytopenia, has been reported but is uncommon.[26] Mild anemia occurs in about 2% to 14% of children[27] and may be due partly to hemodilution, hemolysis,[86] or occult GI blood loss secondary to NSAID therapy.[54]

Salicylates

ASA is the oldest NSAID and continues to have a primary role in the management of Kawasaki disease (see eTable 12-1), acute rheumatic fever, and in the treatment of patients who are predisposed to thromboses. The general principles of NSAID mechanism of action and pharmacology and the principles of therapy and the spectrum of known adverse effects have already been addressed with reference to salicylates where relevant.

Pharmacology

The plasma level of salicylate (ASA and salicylate ion) peaks 1 to 2 hours after a single dose, and the drug is virtually undetectable at 6 hours. ASA itself is bound very little to plasma protein, but salicylic acid binds extensively to albumin and erythrocytes. Salicylic acid is found in most body fluids (including cerebrospinal fluid, saliva, synovial fluid, and breast milk), and it crosses the placenta.

Administration

ASA is quickly absorbed from the stomach and proximal small intestine.[87,88] The systemic antiinflammatory effects of ASA are maximal, and in most cases they are achieved only if serum steady-state levels are 15 to 25 mg/dL (1.09 to 1.81 mmol/L).[89,90] At levels greater than 30 mg/dL (2.17 mmol/L), it is likely to be toxic. The dosage necessary to reach these concentrations is the dose used to treat the early acute febrile phase of Kawasaki disease (75 to 90 mg/kg/day, divided into four doses). However, this high dose regimen is only continued until fever is absent for 24 to 48 hours, then a low dose is initiated (3 to 5 mg/kg/day) for antiplatelet effects.

Therapeutic levels are not reliably attained before 2 to 5 days of administration, and most patients with Kawasaki disease have by this point been decreased to low-dose ASA therapy. If prolonged high-dose ASA is required (e.g., for acute rheumatic fever management), serum salicylate and serum liver enzyme levels should be checked 5 days after initiation of therapy or after any dose adjustment.

Toxicity

Salicylism. Symptoms of salicylism include tinnitus, deafness, nausea, and vomiting. Early on, there is CNS stimulation (hyperkinetic agitation, excitement, maniacal behavior, slurred speech, disorientation, delirium, convulsions). Later, CNS depression (stupor and coma) supervenes. There is a narrow margin between therapeutic and toxic

levels.[91,92] In Kawasaki disease, hypoalbuminemia may predispose children to salicylate toxicity due to increased free levels of drug.[93] The reader is referred to the recommendations of Mofenson and Caraccio[94] for details of the management of severe salicylate poisoning.

Disease-Modifying Antirheumatic Drugs

Numerous drugs used to treat JIA and certain other rheumatic diseases exert their beneficial effects weeks to months after initiation of therapy. These compounds—disease-modifying antirheumatic drugs (DMARDs)—currently include MTX, hydroxychloroquine, sulfasalazine, and leflunomide, among others. Recent evidence and experience suggest that early institution of DMARDs for the treatment of JIA is safe and effective, and may likely result in improved outcomes.[95,96]

Methotrexate

Low-dose weekly MTX has emerged as one of the most useful agents in the treatment of rheumatic diseases in children, and it has become the first-choice second-line agent in childhood arthritis, and in some cases arguably a first-line agent. It is also used in many other chronic inflammatory disorders.[97]

Mechanism of action. MTX (Fig. 12-2) is a folic acid analogue and a potent competitive inhibitor of several enzymes in the folate pathway (Fig. 12-3). MTX is absorbed via the proton-coupled folate transporter (*PCFT/ SLC46A1*) in the gut and enters the cells primarily through the reduced folate carrier (*RFC/SLC19A1*) and folate receptors (FOLR) 1 and 2.[98,99] Intracellularly, MTX is bioactivated to a polyglutamated (MTXGlu$_n$) form by folylpolyglutamyl synthase (*FPGS*), which enhances the pharmacological activity and intracellular retention of MTX.[100] The first MTX target to be identified was dihydrofolate reductase (*DHFR*), the enzyme responsible for reducing dietary folates and dihydrofolate to the biologically active tetrahydrofolate. Tetrahydrofolate is the source of one carbon donors supporting the synthesis of thymidylate, purines, and serine, as well as the remethylation of homocysteine to form methionine and subsequently S-adenosylmethionine (SAM), the one-carbon donor for multiple methyltransferase enzymes.[100] Additionally, MTX inhibits thymidylate synthetase (*TYMS*) directly and indirectly via depletion of tetrahydrofolate, leading to inhibition of pyrimidine (thymidylate) biosynthesis with a resultant antiproliferative effect.[101] Importantly, MTX targets aminoimidazole carboxamide ribonucleotide (AICAR) transformylase (gene name, *ATIC*), which inhibits *de novo* purine synthesis and promotes the accumulation of extracellular adenosine.[102-104] Extracellular adenosine is thought to be a large contributor to the site-specific antiinflammatory effects of MTX through inhibition of neutrophil adherence.[104-108] Pharmacogenomic studies in RA and JIA have provided additional support for the involvement of the purine synthesis and adenosine pathways in mediating MTX response.[109,110] Glutamate

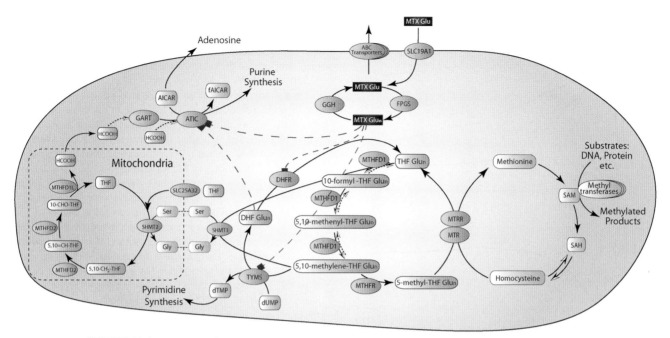

FIGURE 12-3 Intracellular folate pathway. The *red dotted lines* and *squares* denote known enzymes inhibited by methotrexate (MTX). MTX acts as a folate antagonist, entering the cells through the reduced folate carrier (SLC19A1). Once intracellular, MTX is bioactivated to methotrexate polyglutamates (MTXGlun) by folylpolyglutamyl synthase (FPGS). No or low glutamation, facilitated by the deglutamating enzyme g-glutamyl hydrolase (GGH), leads to the efflux of MTX by the ATP-binding cassette (ABC) family of transporters. MTX's initial enzymatic target was identified as dihydrofolate reductase (DHFR), important in the formation of tetrahydrofolate (THF). The list of target genes has been extended to include aminoimidazole carboxamide ribonucleotide (AICAR) transformylase (gene name, *ATIC*, and thymidylate synthetase (TYMS). Additional endogenous enzymes in the folate pathway include methylenetetrahydrofolate dehydrogenase (MTHFD1), methylenetetrahydrofolate reductase (MTHFR), methionine synthase (MTR), methionine synthase reductase (MTRR), S-adenosylmethionine (SAM), S-adenosylhomocysteine (SAH), glycinamide ribonucleotide transformylase (GART), serine hydroxymethyltransferase (SHMT), and folate hydrolase 1 (FOLH1). Folate isoforms and their polyglutamated states are represented as: tetrahydrofolate (THFGlun), 10-formyl-tetrahydrofolate (10-formyl-THFGlun), 5,10-methenyltetrahydrofolate (5,10-methenyl-THFGlun), 5,10-methylene-tetrahydrofolate (5,10-methylene-THFGlun), and 5-methyl-tetrahydrofolate (5-methyl-THFGlun). The mitochondrial folate pathway produces a formic acid for utilization in *de novo* purine synthesis. SLC25A32 is a mitochondrial specific folate transporter. The bifunctional methylenetetrahydrofolate dehydrogenase 2 (MTHFD2) and methylenetetrahydrofolate dehydrogenase 1-like (MTHFD1L) in mitochondria replicate the function of cytosolic MTHFD1.

residues are removed from MTXGlu$_n$ by gamma-glutamyl hydrolase (GGH), allowing efflux of MTX from the cell by the ATP-binding cassette (ABC) family of transporters.[99]

MTX also modulates the function of many of the cells involved in inflammation and affects the production of various cytokines, including the reduction of TNF-α, interferon-γ (IFN-γ), IL-1, IL-6, and IL-8 production, thereby acting as a potent inhibitor of cell-mediated immunity.[111,112] By reducing the expression of adhesion molecules on endothelial cells, MTX may reduce the permeability of the vascular endothelium. In addition, adenosine inhibits adherence of stimulated neutrophils to endothelial cells, protecting the vascular endothelium from neutrophil-induced damage.[113,114] MTX may also have more direct effects in inflamed joints by inhibiting the proliferation of synovial cells and synovial collagenase gene expression.

Pharmacology. There is significant intraindividual and interindividual variability in the absorption and pharmacokinetics of MTX after oral administration.[114] On average, oral bioavailability is about 0.70 (compared with intravenous dosing) and highly variable, ranging from 0.25 to 1.49, with 25% of subjects in one study absorbing less than half their dose.[115] In adults with RA, factors such as age, body weight, creatinine clearance, sex, dose, and fed-versus-fasted state

significantly influenced MTX disposition.[116] The bioavailability of MTX has also been shown to be greater in the fasting state in children with JIA.[117] Oral bioavailability is generally about 15% less than after intramuscular or subcutaneous administration, and oral absorption is saturable (eFig. 12-5).[118,156,157]

After a single dose of MTX, the drug is present in the circulation for a short period before it is redistributed to the tissues (Fig. 12-4). Peak serum levels are reached in approximately 1.5 hours (range 0.25 to 6 hours), with elimination half-life being approximately 7 hours in subjects with normal renal function.[119] Circulating levels diminish rapidly as the drug is distributed into tissue and eliminated. The predominant route of elimination is renal, with more than 80% of the drug eliminated unchanged via glomerular filtration and tubular secretion within 8 to 48 hours. A smaller but significant route of elimination is the biliary tract. The pharmacokinetics of MTX are triphasic. The initial rapid phase represents tissue distribution and renal clearance; the second phase is prolonged because of slow release from tissues, tubular reabsorption, and enterohepatic recirculation; the third phase is flat, reflecting the gradual release of tissue MTX.[119]

Plasma drug levels do not correlate well with clinical effects and are not useful in routine monitoring of MTX therapy.[113] The

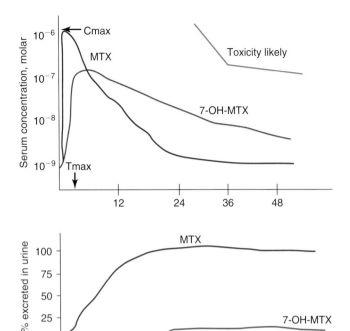

FIGURE 12-4 Time course of methotrexate (MTX) and 7-hydroxymethotrexate (7-OH-MTX) after an oral dose of 15 mg. (Redrawn from J.L. Hillson, D.E. Furst, Pharmacology and pharmacokinetics of methotrexate in rheumatic disease: practical issues in treatment and design, *Rheum Dis Clin North Am* 23: 757–778, 1997.)

pharmacokinetics of oral MTX in JIA seem to be age dependent, with more extensive metabolism of MTX in younger children.[120] This difference may account for the observation that children require higher doses of MTX than adults to obtain similar therapeutic effects.[121,122] As MTX is cleared rapidly from serum, attention has turned to measurement of intracellular concentrations of the therapeutically active polyglutamated forms of MTX ($MTXGlu_n$) as more stable and reliable biomarkers of the effect of MTX.[100,112,119] Higher concentration of $MTXGlu_n$ have been shown to correlate with drug efficacy in patients with RA,[123,124] although similar conclusions have not been consistently seen in children with JIA. $MTXGlu_n$ concentrations have been shown to be quite variable in JIA and are associated with drug dose, route, and duration of MTX therapy.[125] Accumulation of long-chain $MTXGlu_n$ have been shown to be higher in children who experience GI side effects with the drug,[109] and although cross-sectional studies have found no association with drug effectiveness, a recent prospective report has shown that responders to MTX had higher concentrations of long-chain $MTXGlu_n$.[126]

At low doses, MTX is only moderately protein bound (11% to 57%), so the potential for interactions with other protein-bound drugs is small and usually is not clinically significant.[119] Several studies in children have shown an interaction between MTX and NSAIDs that may be clinically significant, particularly in patients with renal dysfunction.[21,127] The combination of MTX and trimethoprim-sulfamethoxazole should be avoided because it may lead to hematological toxicity through the synergistic effects of these drugs on dihydrofolate reductase within the folate pathway.

The effect of genetic variation within the folate pathway upon drug response has been a focus in adult RA, and several review papers have discussed the vast work for the interested reader.[128,129] However, there

has been a lack of reproducibility of results, likely a consequence of several factors including variability in MTX treatment regimens, outcome measurements, and folate supplementation between studies; small sample sizes; the under characterized role of MTXGlu and folate on drug metabolism; and the unknown functional impact of the genetic polymorphisms. In children, recent work has identified clinical outcomes associated with genetic variation in the folate pathway, specifically in genes involved in the purine synthesis portion of the pathway[130-132] as well as cellular transporters of MTX and folate[133,134]; however, these findings have not yet been replicated in larger cohorts.

Efficacy. The efficacy of MTX in controlling the signs and symptoms of JIA is now well established. Benefits reported in countless initial retrospective and uncontrolled studies were subsequently confirmed in a randomized, placebo-controlled clinical trial.[135]

There have been various attempts at identifying the clinical predictors of response to MTX in children with JIA, with regards to the specific JIA subtype. There are data to support MTX as an effective therapy in extended oligoarticular JIA more than several other JIA subtypes.[136,137] Although there have been studies to support its effectiveness in systemic JIA,[138] there are have been others that show no effect, or even worsening in patients on MTX therapy in this subtype of JIA.[139] The utilization of MTX also differs by subtype in clinical practice. In a recent report from the Childhood Arthritis and Rheumatology Research Alliance (CARRA) registry, JIA patients with oligoarticular JIA (53%) and enthesitis-related arthritis (ERA) (63%) were the least likely to ever receive nonbiologic DMARDS such as MTX, compared to RF+ polyarticular (91%) or extended oligoarticular JIA patients (89%).[140] Recently published American College of Rheumatology (ACR) recommendations for treatment of JIA utilize MTX differently by JIA subtype as well. Although in most subtypes a "step-up"/escalation approach is recommended,[141] in patients with high disease activity, poor prognostic, or systemic features, MTX (or biological therapy for systemic JIA) is recommended to be used earlier, and some advocate using it as first-line therapy.[95,96] In fact, with newer cytokine-targeting therapies now available, the most recently updated ACR recommendations for the treatment of systemic JIA suggest MTX primarily for the treatment of mild or moderate arthritis in systemic JIA rather than for the treatment of systemic features or MAS where it has been shown to be less effective.[142]

MTX is also used in many other rheumatic disorders, including systemic lupus erythematosus (SLE),[143] some vasculitides,[144,145] sarcoidosis,[146] systemic sclerosis,[147] localized scleroderma,[148] and uveitis.[149]

Dosage, route of administration, and duration of methotrexate therapy. Standard effective dosing regimens of MTX in children with JIA are 10 to 15 mg/m²/week or 0.3 to 0. 6 mg/kg/week (Table 12-2). Improvement is generally seen by about 6 to 8 weeks on effective doses, but may take up to 6 months to see the full effect. Children seem to tolerate much higher doses than adults, and some series have described using 20 to 25 mg/m²/week or 1. 1 mg/kg/week in children with resistant disease, with relative safety in the short term.[122] Early reports supporting the efficacy of higher dosing regimens (25 to 30 mg/m²/week)[150] for JIA have been followed with studies that do not support additional gains with higher doses.[151,152] However, higher dosages of MTX (1 mg/kg/dose up to 40 mg weekly) have been used in other disease processes such as juvenile dermatomyositis and juvenile localized scleroderma.[153,154]

Many pediatric rheumatologists advocate using parenteral MTX at initiation of treatment to ensure complete absorption and achievement of early disease remission[97,121]; the 2011 ACR recommendations for treatment of JIA assumes MTX dosing to be 15 mg/m²/week administered via the parenteral route.[141] However, there remains variability in clinical practice. F or example, approximately one quarter of the MTX

TABLE 12-2 Dosage and Monitoring of Commonly Use Disease- Modifying Antirheumatic Drugs (DMARDs)

DMARD	DOSAGE AND ROUTE	CLINICAL MONITORING	LABORATORY MONITORING
Hydroxychloroquine	≤6.5 mg/kg/day to a maximum of 400 mg/day, oral	Baseline ophthalmological exam and yearly screening for visual acuity, color vision, visual field, and retinoscopy	None
Methotrexate	10-15 mg/m^2, once weekly, oral (preferably on empty stomach) or subcutaneous. Administer with folic acid or folinic acid (see text)	Improvement seen in 6-12 weeks. Initial evaluation in 2-4 weeks, then monitor every 3-6 months	CBC with WBC count, differential and platelets; MCV; AST, ALT, albumin, (+/− urine pregnancy screening, if appropriate) baseline and in 4-8 weeks initially and with dose adjustments, then every 12 weeks once clinically stable
Sulfasalazine	Initial: 10-15 mg/kg/day (max 500 mg) in two to three divided doses, oral. Increase over course of 4 weeks to 30-50 mg/kg/day in two divided doses (maximum dose 2 g/day)	Improvement seen in 4-8 weeks. Initial evaluation in 2-4 weeks, then every 2-4 months. Discontinue if rash appears	CBC with WBC count, differential and platelets; AST, ALT, creatinine, UA, (consider testing for G6PD deficiency), baseline and every 1-2 weeks with dose increases, then every 3 months while on maintenance doses. Follow immunoglobulins every 6 months
Leflunomide	<20 kg: 10 mg every other day. 20-40 kg: 10 mg daily. >40 kg: 20 mg daily, oral	Improvement seen in 6-12 weeks. Initial evaluation in 2-4 weeks then every 3-6 months	CBC with WBC count, differential and platelets; AST, ALT, creatinine (+/− urine pregnancy screening, if appropriate) baseline and in 2-4 weeks with dose adjustments, then every 3 months while on maintenance doses

users in the CARRA registry received MTX vial the oral route,[140] and in the German Methotrexate Registry over half of patients (63%) received oral MTX exclusively for the first 6 months.[155] Patients in the German registry reported similar rates of ACR Pediatric 30,50, and 70 response, as well as toxicity between routes of MTX administered.[155] It remains agreed upon that parenteral MTX administration should be considered in children who (1) have a poor clinical response to orally administered MTX (this may be due to poor compliance or to reduced oral bioavailability for various reasons); (2) need dosages greater than about 10 to 15 mg/m^2/week to achieve maximum clinical response (oral MTX absorption is a saturable process, whereas subcutaneous administration is not) (eFig. 12-5)[156,157]; or (3) develop significant GI toxicity with orally administered MTX.[97,158] Studies in adult patients with rheumatoid arthritis suggest that oral absorption of MTX is considerably reduced at doses of 15 mg or more, and MTX should be administered parenterally.[159,160] Bypassing the enterohepatic circulation may also reduce hepatotoxicity.

The issue of when, how, and by what criteria to consider withdrawing MTX therapy in JIA remains unclear.[121,137,161] However, the criteria for "remission" or "relapse" have usually not been well defined or standardized among various studies, and the assessment of outcomes has not been the subject of blind studies. Given these limitations, no firm conclusions can be drawn about the optimal time and mode of MTX discontinuation in children with JIA. MTX withdrawal may result in disease flare in more than 50% of patients; this rate may be even higher in younger children.[137,161] Cellular biomarkers such as myeloid-related protein (MRP) 8 (S100A8) and MRP 14 (S100A9) heterocomplex (calprotectin, or MRP8/14)[162] secreted by activated phagocytes at local sites of inflammation[163] may be viable biomarkers to determine the appropriate time to discontinue MTX. Levels of MRP8/14 at the time of MTX discontinuation were significantly higher in patients who subsequently developed flares, compared to those who remained in stable remission.[161]

Safety. Although MTX is associated with many potential toxicities, the documented overall frequency and severity of adverse effects in children with arthritis have been low.[97,165,166] Most side effects are mild and reversible and can be treated conservatively. Although

the precise mechanism of all MTX-related toxicities is not clearly understood, at least some of MTX's adverse effects are directly related to its folate antagonism and its cytostatic effects.[167] This relationship is especially evident in tissues with a high cell turnover rate, such as the GI tract and bone marrow, that have a high requirement for purines, thymidine, and methionine, which may explain why supplementation with folic or folinic acid may diminish these symptoms.

Gastrointestinal toxicity. Abdominal discomfort and nausea, the most frequently reported symptoms, have traditionally been thought to occur in about 12-20%[151] of children with JRA who receive MTX. However, in addition to the physical GI symptoms, in recent years conditioned responses that result in anticipatory and associative GI symptoms with MTX have been recognized and termed *MTX intolerance.*[168] These symptoms have been reported to occur at much higher frequencies (50%),[169] and although previously underreported, they certainly can contribute to MTX dose adjustment and nonadherence, leading to untimely interruption or termination of therapy. Stomatitis or oral ulcers are reported in about 3% of children.[97] MTX-related abdominal discomfort, anorexia, nausea, or oral ulcers usually occur within 24 to 36 hours after administration of the weekly dose and can be diminished by the addition of folic acid supplementation; by dose reduction; or by conversion to subcutaneous MTX administration, although the evidence for the effectiveness of these strategies is only anecdotal.

Liver toxicity. The effect of MTX on liver function and the development of hepatic fibrosis has been extensively reviewed.[170] Mild acute toxicity, with elevations of transaminases, is common, occurring in about 9% to 17% of children with JRA who were treated with MTX[97]; and the majority of these elevations are less than twice normal values.[97,152,171] These elevations are usually transient and resolve without intervention, with lowered dose, or after a brief interval off treatment.[135,166,170] In some of these cases, concurrent administration of NSAIDs may contribute to the elevation in transaminases.[127]

The issue of greatest concern with the long-term use of low-dose MTX in children has been the potential for significant liver fibrosis or cirrhosis. The risk of this complication in children with JIA appears to differ, however, from the risk in adults who have comorbidities that may include heavy alcohol consumption,[172] preexisting liver disease, obesity, insulin-dependent diabetes mellitus, and renal insufficiency.[170,173,174]

In many small studies in children, liver biopsies were performed after cumulative doses of 3000 mg had been reached; none showed cirrhosis.[166,175,176] A cross-sectional study[177] in children exposed to even higher cumulative doses of MTX (>3000 mg or >4000 mg/1.73 m^2 over a mean of 6 years), found no significant fibrosis or cirrhosis on liver histology; however, 13 (93%) of 14 biopsy specimens showed some histological abnormality (with only 1 graded as Roenigk grade II). In addition, higher weekly dosages of MTX (20 mg/m^2/week or more) were not associated with significant hepatic fibrosis in 10 patients who underwent liver biopsy.[178] Only the frequency of biochemical abnormalities and body mass index correlated with the Roenigk grade.[177]

Although these data are encouraging, their interpretation requires some caution. The sample size in these studies is small, and thus the statistical power for detection of infrequent events, such as cirrhosis, is low. Selection bias may have occurred, as not all eligible patients receiving MTX treatment underwent biopsy. There were no control biopsy specimens to help distinguish the effects of disease or concomitant medications on liver histology, and the long-term clinical significance, if any, of the minor histological abnormalities is unknown. Further long-term, prospective studies using greater numbers of children are needed to define more accurately the risk of MTX-related liver fibrosis or cirrhosis and aid in the development of guidelines for monitoring therapy in JIA.

The ACR has suggested guidelines developed by consensus for laboratory monitoring of patients with RA, and traditionally children with JRA/JIA have been monitored via similar guidelines. (Table 12-2).[179] However, based on fewer comorbidities, minimal risk for liver fibrosis, and the low frequency of significantly elevated transaminases,[171] it has been suggested that screening low- risk children for MTX toxicity can be less frequent than adults. In the 2011 ACR recommendations for treatment of JIA and the ACR Top Five for pediatric rheumatology, measurement of serum creatinine, complete cell blood count, and liver enzymes is recommended prior to initiation of MTX, repeated approximately 1 month after MTX initiation or any subsequent increase in MTX dose, and every 3 to 4 months in children receiving stable doses of MTX who do not have recent history of abnormal laboratory monitoring.[141,180]

Infection. Infections reported in patients treated with MTX are usually common bacterial infections (e.g., of the lungs or skin) or herpes zoster. Opportunistic infections associated with MTX treatment are rare,[180] unless there is concurrent treatment with high-dose glucocorticoids.[135,166,181] There have been reports of hypogammaglobulinemia resulting from MTX use in children.[182] A recent study that investigated rates of bacterial infections in hospitalized patients by using U.S. Medicaid administrative claims data revealed a doubling of the background rate of infections in children with JIA, even in the absence of MTX or anti–TNF-α therapy.[183,184] Furthermore, the infection rate in children receiving MTX alone (2,646 person-years of observation) compared with children with JIA without current use of MTX or anti–TNF-α agents (adjusting for age, sex, race, prior bacterial infections, comorbid conditions, and glucocorticoid dose at the start of the study) was similar (adjusted hazard ratio 1.2 [95% CI, 0.9-1.7]). There are no standard guidelines on if and when to withhold MTX administration during a concurrent infection and antibiotic administration. It has been recommended to withhold MTX until a course of antibiotics is completed and perioperatively—specifically 1 week prior and 2 weeks after major surgery. MTX is recommended to be continued uninterrupted for dental work.[185]

Immunization with inactivated vaccines is not contraindicated in children receiving MTX treatment, but immunization with live attenuated vaccines is not currently recommended.[186] However, there are data emerging that support the safety and effectiveness of live vaccine administration without increased risk of flare.[187-190]

Hematological toxicity. Hematological toxicity includes macrocytic anemia, leukopenia, thrombocytopenia, and pancytopenia. In adults with rheumatoid arthritis, pancytopenia has been reported in about 1% to 2%,[191-193] but it has not been reported in children.[97] In patients with mild bone marrow suppression, spontaneous recovery is usually within 2 weeks after withdrawal of MTX. Patients with moderate to severe bone marrow suppression may require folinic acid rescue and supportive therapy (e.g., colony-stimulating factors).[194]

Malignancy. The issue of whether low-dose MTX treatment is an independent risk factor for various malignancies is controversial and remains unresolved. Although *in vitro* studies have shown that MTX has mutagenic and carcinogenic potential, *in vivo* studies in animal models (mice, rats, hamsters) have failed to show any carcinogenicity. In humans, low-dose weekly MTX therapy has not been convincingly linked to malignancy.[195,196] There have been case reports of an association between MTX treatment and lymphoproliferative diseases in adults with RA,[197,198] and several cases of Hodgkin lymphoma[199-201] and non-Hodgkin lymphoma[202,203] have been reported in children with JRA who were treated with MTX ; however, in some of these cases, Epstein–Barr virus (EBV) was implicated.[201,203,204]

It has not been possible to determine whether the development of malignancy while a patient is receiving MTX is merely coincidental or causally linked to MTX or the underlying inflammatory disease process.[196,205] RA is known to be associated with an increased risk of hematological malignancy,[206] and there have been varying reports of an increased incidence of malignancy in JIA, with some reports supporting an increased baseline risk in JIA,[207,208] whereas others do not.[209,210] Using a large U.S. Medicaid claims database from 2000-2005, nearly 8000 JIA patients were compared with large cohorts of children with attention deficit hyperactivity disorder and asthma, and an increased incidence of malignancy was found in children with JIA compared with the control groups, but there was no increased risk of cancer based on MTX or anti–TNF-α use.[207]

Other rare adverse effects

Central nervous system. Various CNS symptoms, including headaches, mood alterations, change in sleep patterns, irritability, fatigue, and impaired academic performance, have been reported to occur transiently in the 12 to 48 hours after the weekly dose of MTX.[97,168]

Teratogenicity. MTX therapy is associated with spontaneous abortions and congenital abnormalities.[211,212] Women of childbearing age should be counseled to practice effective contraception during the course of treatment. They should discontinue MTX therapy at least one ovulatory cycle before trying to conceive. There have not been any reports of azoospermia caused by low-dose MTX treatment of JRA,[97] and a recent study in adult men taking MTX who fathered 113 pregnancies did not show a higher risk of birth defects or spontaneous abortions.[213] MTX is excreted in breast milk in low concentrations, and women taking MTX should be advised not to breast-feed.[214-216]

Rare side effects such as pulmonary toxicity,[217-223] accelerated nodulosis,[224-228] and osteopathy[229-231] have also been reported with MTX.

Folate supplementation. As a potent antifolate drug, the side effects of MTX are also consistent with symptoms of folate deficiency, and it is rational to question how the folate pathway and folic acid supplementation may impact drug efficacy at the expense of minimizing toxicity. Baseline plasma and erythrocyte folate concentrations have been shown to negatively correlate with MTX toxicity scores in RA,[232] and children with historical intolerance to MTX have shown significantly lower cellular folate concentrations in a cross-sectional study.[233] Numerous studies have examined the issue of minimizing MTX toxicities with the use of concurrent folic or folinic acid (leucovorin) supplementation in adults with rheumatoid arthritis.[232,234-236] A Cochrane review of all trials on " low-dose" folic acid (≤7 mg/week) or folinic acid in adults with RA from 1999 through March 2012 revealed a 26% relative risk reduction in the incidence of GI side effects, a 76.9% relative risk reduction in transaminase elevation, and a 60.5% relative risk reduction in MTX withdrawal for any reason, with no observed effect upon efficacy.[237]

However, the effect of folate supplementation upon drug effectiveness is far from clear. Some studies have shown that concurrent folate supplementation may worsen disease activity in psoriasis[238] and RA.[239] A small number of clinical studies that investigated supplemented folic acid in JRA have suggested no substantial effect upon MTX efficacy,[240,241] but higher doses of folinic acid were associated with disease flares.[242] Baseline variability in the endogenous target folate pathway may also be important for drug outcomes, as preliminary data suggest that initiating MTX in a folate replete state may be associated with improved outcomes on MTX, as enhanced cellular folate uptake may also represent enhanced cellular MTX uptake.[243,244]

Based on the data from adult studies and the small trial in children with JRA, it seems that daily (1 mg/day) folic acid supplementation confers a beneficial effect in terms of GI and mucosal toxicities associated with low-dose weekly MTX treatment and does not have any significant detrimental effect on disease control. Without firm data to direct otherwise, folic acid supplementation should be considered at least in symptomatic patients. High-dose folinic acid rescue should be reserved for patients with severe, life-threatening toxicity (e.g., aplastic anemia).

Antimalarials

Hydroxychloroquine sulfate is the first-line antimalarial to treat pediatric rheumatic diseases.[245]

Mechanism of action. The exact mechanism of action of hydroxychloroquine remains unknown, although several physiological effects have been attributed to this drug class that may be pertinent to rheumatic disease. These include the inhibition of neutrophil chemotaxis, nitric oxide production,[246] and phagocytosis.[247] Hydroxychloroquine may also antagonize the action of prostaglandins,[248] interfere with IL-1 release by monocytes[249]; interfere with production of TNF-α, IL-6, and IFN-γ[250]; inhibit natural killer activity[246]; and induce apoptosis.[251,252] It has antiplatelet and antihyperlipidemic effects extremely important in patients with SLE,[253] and antagonistic effects upon Toll-like receptor 7/9.[254,255]

Pharmacology. Hydroxychloroquine is rapidly absorbed from the intestine. Equilibrium concentrations are reached after 2 to 6 months of a constant daily dose, and the half-life exceeds 40 days.[245,256] Tissue levels are much greater than plasma concentrations, and there is increased affinity of the drug for the liver, pituitary, spleen, kidney, lung, adrenals, and specifically for melanin. Excretion is primarily via the kidney.

Dosing/efficacy. The recommended dosage for hydroxychloroquine is less than or equal to 6.5 mg/kg/day to a maximum dosage of 400 mg/day (Table 12-2).[257] Early studies have not shown hydroxychloroquine to be an extremely effective disease-modifying agent in JRA[258-260]; however, it is used commonly in pediatric SLE and cutaneous LE in children,[261] as well as for juvenile dermatomyositis.[262] Although this medication is commonly used, like many older DMARDs, it has been inadequately studied in children. It is used mostly in combination with other medications, or in mild or well- controlled disease. Data from adults has shown an increased risk of lupus flare once their

hydroxychloroquine was withdrawn,[263] and utilizing hydroxychloroquine in addition to MTX and sulfasalazine has been shown to be superior than single or double therapy in adults with RA.[264] Recent data support a protective effect against fetal heart block in neonatal lupus.[265]

Safety. When used at recommended doses, antimalarials are considered extremely safe. At least four young children have died of respiratory failure after accidental ingestion of large doses (1 to 3 g) of chloroquine, however, as there is no antidote.[266]

GI intolerance occurs in 10% of adults, and skin hyperpigmentation,[267,268] myasthenia, and muscle weakness have been described.[269] CNS side effects that include headache, light-headedness, tinnitus, insomnia, and anxiety are common. These side effects may be reversible with dose reduction and may remit spontaneously.

The major concerning side effect is retinal toxicity.[270-272] Retinal toxicity, although rare, can cause blindness, even after the medication has been stopped. Antimalarials accumulate in the pigmented cells of the retina and persist; however, retinitis is sometimes, but not always, reversible.[272] Evidence in adults suggests that retinal toxicity does not occur if the dosage of hydroxychloroquine is maintained at less than 6. 5 mg/kg/day, even for up to 7 years.[273] Routine ophthalmological monitoring can lead to early detection of premaculopathy; vision loss can be prevented if the medication is discontinued. Newly revised recommendations in adults suggest a baseline exam and then annual screening starting after 5 years on therapy.[274] Each examination should include visual acuity, color vision testing, visual field examination,[273,275] and retinoscopy.[276] In addition, newer objective tests including multifocal electroretinogram, spectral domain optical coherence tomography, and fundus autofluorescence have been shown to be more sensitive than visual fields, and at least one is recommended to be performed, if available, in addition to standard testing.[274] Retinal abnormalities or interference with vision, especially with foveal recognition of red,[277] is an absolute indication for discontinuation of hydroxychloroquine. Use of hydroxychloroquine in children younger than 7 years may be limited by difficulty in obtaining satisfactory evaluation of color vision in this age group, and the standard of care in children remains an annual exam until definitive studies in children suggest increasing the frequency of monitoring.

Hydroxychloroquine crosses the placenta but is considered safe to use during pregnancy.[278,279] Hydroxychloroquine does appear in breast milk, but the amount ingested per day by a breast-feeding infant would be very low.[280]

Sulfasalazine

Sulfasalazine is an analogue of 5-aminosalicylic acid linked by an azo bond to sulfapyridine, a sulfonamide. Its development was based on the concept that RA might be an infectious disease and would respond to combination therapy with an antibacterial agent and an antiinflammatory drug.[281,282] Sulfasalazine is used in the treatment of mild to moderate inflammatory bowel disease, and it has been reported to be beneficial in the management of childhood arthritis,[283-291] particularly oligoarthritis,[292] psoriatic arthritis,[293] and reactive arthritis.[293] Its role in ankylosing spondylitis is controversial,[293-295] although it does seem to be effective for the peripheral arthritis associated with this condition.[296]

Mechanisms of action. Several mechanisms of action may explain the antiinflammatory effect of sulfasalazine. Bacterial growth is reduced by sulfasalazine and sulfapyridine, and the bacterial antigenic load delivered to the gut-associated lymphoid tissue may be reduced. This mechanism may be important for patients with spondyloarthropathies, in whom bacteria may gain access through inflamed gut mucosa and stimulate the immune system. Sulfasalazine interferes with many enzymes that are important in inflammation in the formation of leukotrienes and prostaglandins,[297] and it is a potent inhibitor of AICAR transformylase, resulting in an accumulation of extracellular adenosine.[298] There are several additional pharmacological effects reported in the literature.[299-307]

Pharmacology. Sulfasalazine is poorly absorbed from the GI tract.[307-309] Peak serum concentrations are reached after 5 days of therapy. The half-life of the drug is 10 hours. Approximately one third of the dose is absorbed in the small intestine and excreted unchanged in the bile. The remaining 70% enters the colon intact, where the azo linkage is split by bacterial enzymes to sulfapyridine, which is absorbed and excreted in the urine, and 5-aminosalicylate, which reaches high concentrations in the feces. Approximately 90% of sulfapyridine is absorbed from the colon. Sulfapyridine is tightly protein bound and acetylated, hydroxylated, and conjugated with glucuronic acid in the liver. Sulfasalazine and sulfapyridine reach synovial fluid in concentrations comparable with those in serum. About one third of 5-aminosalicylic acid is absorbed, acetylated, and excreted in the urine. The rest is eliminated unchanged in the stool. The small amount of salicylate absorbed is insufficient to reach antiinflammatory levels in the plasma.

Dosing/efficacy. Sulfasalazine is a recommended treatment for ERA following a trial of NSAIDs and/or intraarticular steroid injections.[141] The suggested dosage in children is 30 to 50 mg/kg/day in two to three divided doses, usually taken with food or milk.[283,310] Treatment is initiated at a lower dosage (10 to 15 mg/kg/day) and increased weekly over 4 weeks to achieve maintenance levels. A satisfactory clinical response may occur within 4 to 8 weeks (Table 12-2).

Several studies have investigated sulfasalazine use in children and results have been mixed. A double-blind, randomized, placebo-controlled study of 69 Dutch children with oligoarticular or polyarticular juvenile chronic arthritis showed significant improvement in overall articular severity score, global, and laboratory parameters.[286] A follow-up study showed sustained benefits in these same individuals 7 to 10 years later.[287] Alternatively, in a small, 26-week, randomized, double-blind, placebo-controlled study, no significant differences in active joint count, tender entheses count, pain visual analogue scale, or spinal flexion were seen with sulfasalazine compared with placebo.[291]

Safety. Intolerance and toxic reactions occur in approximately 20% of sulfasalazine-treated adults with rheumatoid arthritis (range 5% to 55%).[299-306,311-334] In a placebo-controlled study of 35 children with JRA, 29% developed adverse effects that led to discontinuation of the drug.[286] Rashes occur in 1% to 5% of patients. A maculopapular rash occurring within 2 days after institution of therapy, especially on sun-exposed skin, is the most common dermatological complication.[317]

Oral ulcers[323] and Stevens–Johnson syndrome[311] are uncommon but important complications. The drug should not be used in infants or in patients with known hypersensitivity to sulfa drugs or salicylates, impaired renal or hepatic function, or specific disease contraindications (e.g., porphyria, glucose-6-phosphate dehydrogenase deficiency). Other rare side effects have been reported and include cytopenias,[324-327] drug-induced SLE,[329] Raynaud phenomenon,[314] interstitial pneumonitis, fibrosis, alveolitis, pulmonary syndromes,[321,334] hepatitis,[333] hypogammaglobulinemia, and IgA deficiency.[286] Serious infections have not been reported, however. Most authors also consider sulfasalazine to be contraindicated in patients with systemic JIA because of an apparent increased risk of toxicity reported in patients with adult-onset Still disease.[288,341]

A reversible decrease in sperm count has been observed,[313] but there are no reports of teratogenicity, and it can be safely used in pregnancy.[335] Sulfasalazine enters breast milk in negligible amounts and thus is not an absolute contraindication to breast-feeding.[336] However,

caution should be exercised because its metabolite, sulfapyridine, is present at significant levels in breast milk,[337] and there has been a single case report of bloody diarrhea in an infant exposed to sulfasalazine through lactation.[338,339] In addition, as sulfapyridine can displace bilirubin, this medication should be avoided in nursing mothers of premature infants, infants who are ill or suffering from hyperbilirubinemia, or glucose-6-phosphate dehydrogenase deficiency.[340]

Leflunomide

Mechanisms of action. Leflunomide is an immunomodulatory agent that, through its active plasma metabolite, A77-1726, inhibits *de novo* pyrimidine synthesis by inhibiting the enzyme dihydroorotate dehydrogenase.[342] As a result of the inhibition, p53 in the cytoplasm translocates to the nucleus and initiates cellular arrest in the G_1 phase of the cell cycle. It also inhibits tyrosine kinase,[343] inhibits leukocyte-endothelial adhesion,[344] affects cytokine production,[345] and decreases serum metalloproteinase activity similarly to MTX.[346] *In vitro*, leflunomide inhibits the production of prostaglandin E_2, matrix metalloproteinase (MMP)-1, and IL-6, and modulates various tyrosine kinases and growth factor receptors.[347]

Pharmacology. Leflunomide is rapidly converted to A77-1726, which is highly protein bound and has a prolonged half-life of up to 18 days.[348] As a result, loading doses have been recommended for the first 3 days of administration to achieve steady state rapidly in RA, although it may increase the frequency of GI toxicity[349]; however, a loading dose has not been adopted consistently in children with JIA.[350]

Dose/efficacy. Dosing guidelines for children are limited and based on studies by Silverman and colleagues (Table 12-2)[349] that compared the safety and efficacy of leflunomide to MTX in patients with polyarticular course JIA. Pharmacokinetic studies were performed. At week 16, 68% of patients receiving leflunomide showed an improvement according to the ACR Pediatric 30 versus 89% of patients treated with MTX; the improvements achieved were maintained at a similar rate in a 32-week extension study. The median time to ACR Pediatric 30 did not differ between the two groups. Body weight was a significant determinant of response, and patients weighing less than 20 kg showed the greatest discrepancy, with the clinically active metabolite notably lower in this group. The incidence of treatment-related adverse events was similar in both groups, although there was an increased frequency of liver transaminase elevations in the MTX group. Furthermore, in a long-term open label study of leflunomide in polyarticular JIA patients who were MTX intolerant or refractory, 52% of patients met ACR Pediatric 30 by 12 weeks, with 65% of those who entered the extension phase maintaining ACR Pediatric 30 status up to 2 years.[351]

An additional retrospective review of 58 German JIA patients treated with leflunomide either alone (n = 48) or in conjunction with MTX (n = 10) were examined over a mean of 1.5 years and found that leflunomide was well tolerated and effective; approximately 30% of patients on leflunomide attained remission.[352]

Safety. Mild and dose-related side effects in adults include GI side effects (abdominal pain, dyspepsia, anorexia, diarrhea, gastritis), allergic rash, reversible alopecia, mild weight loss, and elevated hepatic transaminases.[353,354] Side effects in children have included transiently elevated liver enzymes, abdominal pain and nausea, diarrhea, headaches, mouth ulcers, and alopecia; these symptoms tend to be dose related.[351,352]

Leflunomide is teratogenic.[355] Because of the very long half-life of this drug, it has been recommended that cholestyramine be administered, and that drug levels less than 0.02 mg/L be verified on two separate tests at least 2 weeks apart in men and women before attempting to conceive.[355] Breast-feeding is contraindicated.[355]

Other Disease-Modifying Drugs

Colchicine

The primary use of colchicine in pediatric patients is for treatment of familial Mediterranean fever (FMF), where it has been shown to reduce not only the frequency of attacks, but also prevent the development of amyloidosis. Colchicine is also occasionally used for recurrent aphthous stomatitis, Behçet disease, and cutaneous vasculitis.

Mechanism of action Colchicine's action is thought to depend on binding of two of its rings to cellular microtubules, inhibiting the movement of intracellular granules and preventing secretion of various components to the cell exterior.[356] Interaction between endothelial cells and neutrophils is inhibited by reducing the expression of adhesion molecules on the neutrophil membrane.[357] The drug is present in granulocytes to a much greater extent than in lymphocytes or monocytes.[356]

Pharmacology. Peak plasma levels are reached 1 to 3 hours after oral administration. Colchicine's bioavailability is less than 50%, and its half-life after oral administration is 9 ± 4 hours.[358] It is predominantly eliminated by biliary excretion through the stool. The multidrug transporter molecule ABCB1 (also known as P-glycoprotein and multidrug transporter 1) mediates the extrusion of colchicine into the GI tract, and polymorphisms in *ABCB1* may explain some of the differences in treatment response in patients with FMF.[359] Enteric and hepatic cytochrome P-450 3A4 (CYP3A4) is also important in colchicine metabolism.[360,361] Drug interactions may also occur either at the level of the transporter[362] or through the cytochrome P-450 system, and thus inhibition or competition for CYP3A4 may lead to colchicine accumulation and toxicity. Dose reduction algorithms have been proposed for adults.[363]

The therapeutic dose of colchicine ranges from 0.5 to 2 mg/day as needed to prevent or reduce significantly the frequency of FMF attacks[364] and is administered once or twice daily. Toxicity is extremely rare with oral administration and is generally limited to the GI tract (nausea, vomiting, abdominal pain, diarrhea); this can be helped by administering colchicine in two divided doses and reducing dietary lactose intake. In the case of serious overdose, treatment with colchicine-specific Fab could be considered.[365] Severe toxicity can result in dehydration, multiorgan failure, and a disseminated intravascular coagulation–like syndrome.[356] Colchicine is safe to take during pregnancy and while breast-feeding.[366] Concerns about chromosomal and gonadal aberrations resulting from its effect upon microtubules have not been supported.[367]

Thalidomide and Lenalidomide

Thalidomide (N-α-phthalimidoglutarimide), a major teratogen, has been shown to be effective in various immune-mediated disorders. Its immunosuppressive effects include inhibition of neutrophil chemotaxis,[368] decreased monocyte phagocytosis,[369] decrease in the ratio of T-helper cells to T-suppressor cells,[370] inhibition of expression of TNF-α and IL-6 messenger RNA (mRNA),[371] and inhibition of angiogenesis.[372,373] Mean peak plasma concentrations occur 4.39 ± 1.27 hours after a 200-mg dose.[374] It is metabolized primarily by spontaneous hydrolysis and has an elimination half-life of 3 to 7.3 hours.

Controlled trials have shown the benefits of thalidomide compared with placebo in recurrent aphthous ulcers[375] and in recurrent oral ulceration in men with Behçet syndrome.[376] Several recent small series of children with systemic-onset JIA who have benefited from thalidomide treatment have also been described.[377-379] There are several case reports of its successful use in various other disorders.[380-390]

The dosage of thalidomide ranges from 100 to 400 mg/day administered once or twice daily. Dosages of 2.5 to 5 mg/kg/day have been suggested for children with SLE or systemic-onset JRA.[377,378,391]

Birth control must be practiced due to thalidomide's well-known teratogenic effects. Excellent control is maintained in a postmarketing surveillance program and a restricted distribution program, the System for Thalidomide Education and Prescribing Safety program (STEPS), monitored by Boston University, Celgene Corporation, and the U.S. Food and Drug Administration (FDA).[392] In addition to embryopathy, the major side effects of thalidomide include peripheral neuropathy and drowsiness. Neuropathy is predominantly sensory and manifests as painful paresthesias in a glove-and-stocking distribution.[393] Neuropathy can progress despite discontinuation of thalidomide and may or may not be dose related. Baseline and routine follow-up electrophysiological testing should be performed, and the dose should be reduced or discontinued on detection of abnormalities.[394]

A promising immunomodulatory analogue to thalidomide—lenalidomide—has a better safety profile than thalidomide, with similar immunomodulatory effects.[395] Although there are no published reports on its effects on JIA, there has been a report of successful use in a pediatric patient with refractory complex aphthosis.[396] A risk evaluation and mitigation strategy (REMS) program for lenalidomide has also been developed in conjunction with Celgene and the FDA to prevent the risk for embryo-fetal exposure. Tight regulation requires licensure for prescribers and provides for patient education and monitoring.[397] A recent FDA warning reported an increased risk of secondary malignancies in patients who were treated with lenalidomide to treat multiple myeloma compared to placebo,[398] making a clear risk / benefit analysis imperative prior to prescribing.

Glucocorticoid Drugs

Glucocorticoid drugs are the most potent antiinflammatory agents used the treatment of rheumatic diseases.[399-403] Specific aspects of therapy are discussed in the chapters on individual diseases and in reviews.[404-410]

Pharmacology. Glucocorticoid drugs are structural variants of the naturally occurring glucocorticoid, cortisol. Synthetic compounds, such as prednisone and cortisone, must be hydroxylated to form therapeutically active prednisolone and hydrocortisone. Topical glucocorticoids, such as dexamethasone, or those administered by intraarticular injection (e.g., triamcinolone hexacetonide) already have a hydroxyl group at C11 and are thus in active form. The different relative potencies and durations of biological action of the various synthetic analogues are outlined in Table 12-3.

Orally administered glucocorticoids (prednisone, prednisolone) are rapidly absorbed. Prednisone is converted to prednisolone in the liver and reaches a peak plasma concentration within 2 hours. Hydrocortisone and prednisolone bind to the serum proteins transcortin (high affinity) and albumin (low affinity). Methylprednisolone and dexamethasone are bound primarily to albumin.[411] Prednisolone has a large volume of distribution; about two thirds is taken up by muscle. After metabolism in the liver, excretion occurs principally via the bile.

Physiological and pharmacological effects. Glucocorticoids are unique among pharmacological agents used to treat rheumatic diseases because they are synthetic analogues of endogenous molecules that are produced by the body that perform important physiological and pharmacological functions through glucocorticoid receptors (GRs) and genomic and nongenomic mechanisms.[412-416]

Antiinflammatory and immunosuppressive actions. Glucocorticoids have antiinflammatory and immunosuppressive effects.[404,406,407,417-425] Steroids inhibit the early stages of inflammation (e.g., edema, fibrin deposition, capillary dilation, migration of lymphocytes into inflamed areas, phagocytic activity) and the later manifestations (e.g., proliferation of capillaries and fibroblasts, deposition of collagen).[426] Many of these effects are mediated by inhibition of numerous chemokines and

TABLE 12-3 Relative Doses and Equivalent Potencies of Glucocorticoids (Compared with Hydrocortisone)

GLUCOCORTICOID*	EQUIVALENT DOSE† (mg)	RELATIVE ANTI-INFLAMMATORY POTENCY	RELATIVE SODIUM RETAINING POTENCY
Short Acting			
Hydrocortisone	20	1	1
Deflazacort	6	4	1
Intermediate Acting			
Prednisone	5	4	0.8
Prednisolone	5	4	0.8
Methylprednisolone	4	5	0.5
Long Acting			
Dexamethasone	0.75	25	0

*Biologic half-life, short-acting, 8-12 hours (deflacort, ~1.5 hr); intermediate-acting, 12-36 hours; long- acting, 36-72 hours.
†Oral or intravenous administration only.
Adapted from Goodman and Gilman's (Eds.), Goodman and Gilman's The Pharmacological Basis of Therapeutics, eighth ed., Pergamon Press, New York, 1990. Reproduced with permission of the McGraw-Hill Companies.

cytokines, including arachidonic acid and its metabolites, platelet-activating factor, TNF, IL-1, mitogen-activated protein kinase (MAPK) phosphatase 1, and NF-κB.[424,425,427]

Glucocorticoid effects on the immune system are mediated principally through T lymphocytes.[419] Acute administration of hydrocortisone produces a 70% decline in circulating lymphocytes. T lymphocytes are affected more than B lymphocytes, and T-helper cells are affected more than T-suppressor cells. Lymphopenia is probably a result of sequestration of cells in the bone marrow rather than cell lysis, although drug-induced apoptotic cell death may also be involved.[428] Corticosteroids have been shown to result in a profound and transient lymphocytopenia, maximal at 4 hours after the dose and resolved by 24 hours, due to a redistribution of these cells to the bone marrow.[429] There is also a 90% decline in circulating monocytes within the initial 6 hours. Proliferative T-cell responses to antigens (streptodornase-streptokinase), mitogens (concanavalin A), and cell surface antigens (as in the mixed leukocyte reaction) are reduced by glucocorticoids. IL-2 production by T cells *in vitro* is also reduced.[430] Glucocorticoids cause an increase in the numbers of blood neutrophils by increasing the release of cells from the marginated neutrophil pool, prolonging their stay in the circulation, and reducing chemotaxis of neutrophils to sites of inflammation.[407]

Intravenous glucocorticoid causes a decrease in circulating IgG but has little discernible effect on the serum titer of specific antibodies. The protein catabolic effects of long-term administration may have consequences on the humoral immune system. Endothelial secretion of C3 and factor B of the complement cascade are also inhibited.[431]

Indications for systemic glucocorticoid therapy. When considering glucocorticoid use in children with rheumatic diseases, the risk/benefit ratio must be carefully weighed because these agents are associated with substantial toxicity when used systemically in the long term (eBox 12-1). The overall aim is to limit the dose and duration of steroid therapy as much as possible while achieving disease control.[432]

Adverse effects. Two broad categories of adverse effects are associated with the therapeutic use of systemic glucocorticoids: effects resulting from prolonged use of large doses and effects resulting from withdrawal of therapy. The mechanisms involved in the development of these adverse events are reviewed in detail elsewhere.[414]

Cushing syndrome. Cushing syndrome, a term used originally to identify the effects of idiopathic hypercortisism, may also be

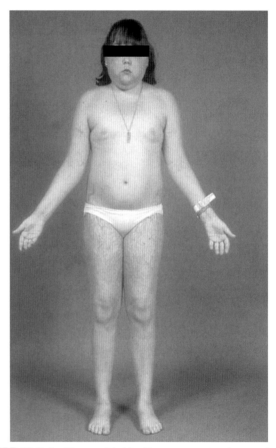

FIGURE 12-6 An 11-year-old girl with severe systemic-onset juvenile idiopathic arthritis requiring high-dose corticosteroid treatment. Cushingoid features shown include moon facies, truncal obesity, and cutaneous striae.

induced by prolonged glucocorticoid administration. It is characterized biochemically by high plasma glucocorticoid levels and suppression of the hypothalamic–pituitary–adrenal axis. It is characterized clinically by many features, including truncal obesity (Fig. 12-6), osteoporosis, thinning of the subcutaneous tissues, and hypertension. The distribution of fat in Cushing syndrome is predominantly in the sub-cutaneous tissue of the abdomen and upper back (buffalo hump) and in the face (moon facies). Weight gain reflects fluid retention and increased caloric intake. Skin changes, in addition to the characteristic purple striae, include hirsutism and acne. Hypertension is usually mild but occasionally requires treatment or reduction of the glucocorticoid dose. With the exception of skin striae, all of these physical features are reversible after cessation of glucocorticoid therapy.

Growth suppression. Growth suppression is one of the most worrisome long-term adverse effects of glucocorticoids. It occurs in young children who receive prolonged therapy[433] in dosages equivalent to 3 mg/day of prednisone, and increases with higher dosages.[434-436] The mechanism of glucocorticoid-associated growth suppression in children with arthritis is controversial. Glucocorticoids have been shown to inhibit cell growth and cell division[434] as well as inhibit production of insulin-like growth factor I (somatomedin C), resulting in decreased chondrocyte proliferation.[437,438] Alternate-day dosing regimens have been shown to minimize this adverse effect.[400,439,440] Although early studies showed that growth hormone did not always improve growth failure in children with glucocorticoid-induced inhibition of growth,[441] more recent reports have shown increased height velocity,[442,443] and catch-up growth in patients who received growth hormone.[444] In fact, achievement of their genetically determined target height was observed in JIA patients randomized to receive growth hormone,[445] with normalization of total bone and muscle cross-sectional area in the treated group.[446] However, the optimal time to initiate growth hormone and the optimal dose to use have yet to be determined.[447] Although considered generally safe, the potential for metabolic complications requires routine monitoring.[448]

Effects on bone: osteoporosis and avascular necrosis. Osteoporosis is one of the most troublesome consequences of long-term, high-dose glucocorticoid therapy,[449] although there are multiple other contributing factors to consider, including inadequate dietary intake of calcium and vitamin D, underlying disease activity,[450] reduced physical activity,[451] and low body weight.[452]

Glucocorticoids are associated with a reduction in bone formation and an increase in bone resorption; the reduction in bone formation seems to be more important and is caused by a direct inhibitory effect on, and apoptosis of, osteoblasts. Glucocorticoids also directly inhibit gut absorption of calcium and cause increased urinary calcium excretion, potentially resulting in secondary hyperparathyroidism and increased bone resorption.[453,454] Additional mechanisms by which glucocorticoids result in bone loss are depicted and detailed in eFig. 12-7. These mechanisms include effects on the production of local growth factors, reduction of matrix proteins, increase in the production of enzymes that break down matrix, increase in apoptosis of osteoblasts and osteocytes, increase in osteoclastogenesis secondary to decreased production of osteoprotegerin, and an increased production of receptor-associated NF-κB ligand (RANK ligand).[455-457]

The extent of bone loss seems to be related to the dose and duration of glucocorticoid therapy, although these factors do not have a consistent relationship with fracture risk. Significant bone loss occurs with dosages of 7.5 mg/day or greater in most adults.[458,459] In adults, bone loss is predominantly trabecular (e.g., spine and ribs) rather than cortical, whereas in children the osteoporotic effects of glucocorticoids are more generalized. Bone loss seems to occur rapidly within the first 6 to 12 months of therapy and then reaches a plateau.[459] Alternate-day glucocorticoid therapy may not be protective.[460] Not all patients exposed to long-term glucocorticoid therapy develop bone loss[461]; there are, however, no reliable biochemical predictive markers.[462] Bone densitometry may be used to screen children who are at high risk for osteoporosis, although there are challenges with misinterpretation due

to adult norms. There are limited guidelines on what frequency to perform densitometry and also controversy on the utility of other types of imaging modalities.[463-465]

High-dose glucocorticoids have also been associated with avascular necrosis of bone (AVN), although the exact mechanism is unknown.[466] Intramedullary vascular compromise may result from increased osteocyte apoptosis induced by glucocorticoids. In the absence of the clearance of these apoptotic osteocytes, reduced blood flow and bony ischemia may result.[387] Glucocorticoids induce adipocyte differentiation via the increased production of PPAR-γ_2, which may result in increased fat in the marrow.[387] Finally, glucocorticoids also increase the expression of endothelin-I, which may also lead to reduced intramedullary blood flow.[467] The most common and clinically significant location for AVN is the femoral head, and the underlying disease process (such as in SLE) can be a contributing factor as well as age.[468]

Infection and immunity. Glucocorticoids interfere with the ability to resist infection through two main mechanisms. They act as immunosuppressives and unpredictably decrease the patient's resistance to viral and bacterial infections. They are also antiinflammatory agents and may mask the signs and symptoms of infection. The minimal dose and duration of systemic steroids that result in immunosuppression in an otherwise healthy child are not well defined.[186] Additional factors that may affect the overall extent of immunosuppression in children with rheumatic diseases include the effects of the underlying disease and concurrent immunosuppressive therapies.

Patients receiving high doses of glucocorticoids for a prolonged period are prone to infections that are associated with defects of delayed hypersensitivity (e.g., tuberculosis). Thus if possible, the Mantoux test (purified protein derivative [PPD], 5 tuberculin units) should be performed before glucocorticoid initiation. The risk of complications of varicella infection must also be considered. A susceptible child being treated with glucocorticoids who is exposed to chickenpox should receive varicella- zoster immune globulin (VariZIG) as soon as possible, but can be given up to 10 days after exposure[469] (this is only effective in prevention or modification of the disease course if administered before the disease is established; therefore, the sooner it is administered the better). If VariZIG is unavailable, intravenous immunoglobulin (IVIG) can also be used at a dose of 400 mg/kg IV up to 10 days after exposure.[470] If acutely infected, IV acyclovir should be used to prevent dissemination,[470,471] as oral acyclovir has poor oral bioavailability.[470]

Central nervous system. The effect of glucocorticoids on the CNS results from changes in the concentration of plasma glucose, circulatory dynamics, and electrolyte balance, reflected by changes in mood, behavior, and electroencephalographic studies.[472] Most glucocorticoid-induced psychoses have an acute onset, are related to high doses, and occur within 96 hours after initiation of medication.[473,474] Early on, there may be euphoria and mania; later, depression tends to predominate. Anxiety and insomnia may occur. Pseudotumor cerebri is rare but may occur after rapid dose reduction.[475] A prospective cohort study of the adverse effects of high-dose intermittent intravenous glucocorticoids in 213 children with rheumatic diseases found behavioral changes in 21 (10%).[476] These abnormalities included altered mood, hyperactivity, sleep disturbance, and psychosis.

Cardiovascular system. The major effects of glucocorticoids on the cardiovascular system result in hypertension and dyslipidemia. The mechanisms by which these undesirable side effects occur are complex,[477] but in part they are thought to be related to the regulation of renal sodium excretion, induction of angiotensin II receptors, increased plasma renin or antidiuretic hormone activity, and glucocorticoid effects upon capillaries, arterioles, and the myocardium.[426] Dyslipoproteinemia and accelerated coronary atherosclerosis[478] have been observed in patients, especially those with SLE, after prolonged administration of glucocorticoids.[479] However, the pathogenesis of coronary artery disease in these patients is multifactorial,[480] as uncontrolled disease activity likely also plays a role.[481,482]

Cataracts and glaucoma. Subcapsular cataracts[475,483,484] can occur with glucocorticoid therapy. The risk of cataract development becomes significant when a dosage of prednisone equal to or greater than 9 mg/m²/day has been maintained for longer than 1 year. These cataracts often do not progress and rarely affect vision. Children should also be monitored for glaucoma.

Muscle disease. Muscle wasting on high-dose glucocorticoid administration is associated with atrophy of muscle fibers, especially type IIB fibers. Myopathy induced by glucocorticoids usually affects proximal muscles, is seldom painful, and is usually associated with normal serum levels of muscle enzymes and an electromyogram suggestive of myopathy. Glucocorticoid-induced hypokalemia may also lead to muscular weakness and fatigue. Recovery from steroid myopathy may be slow and incomplete.[485]

Hematological system. Glucocorticoids decrease the number of circulating lymphocytes, monocytes, basophils, and eosinophils, but increase the number of circulating neutrophils.[486] Excess glucocorticoid may also cause polycythemia.

Other glucocorticoid side effects include glucose intolerance and glycosuria,[487] and peptic ulceration.[488-490]

Minimizing toxicity. The deleterious effects of glucocorticoids can be minimized by choosing a drug with a short half-life (see Table 12-3).[491] Prednisone is the drug most often given for oral therapy, as its prominent glucocorticoid and minimal mineralocorticoid actions give it the lowest risk/benefit ratio of any of the analogues in general use.[492]

The antiinflammatory effect and the toxicity of glucocorticoids increase with larger doses and more frequent administration (Table 12-4).[400,493-495] Short-acting glucocorticoids given in the morning do not suppress the pituitary as much as glucocorticoids given later in the day (which suppress the normal surge of adrenocorticotropic hormone [ACTH] that occurs during sleep) so once daily administration should always be in the morning.[426]

Reduction in glucocorticoid dose must be individualized for the child and the disease, and is often fraught with difficulty because of the adaptation of the patient's metabolism to chronic steroid excess.[496,497] At high dosages (e.g., 60 mg/day), reductions of 10 mg are usually well tolerated; at lower dosages (e.g., 10 mg/day), reductions of only 1 or 2 mg may be possible. An alternate-day regimen should be the goal to minimize toxicity, although some patients do not tolerate this regimen. In some children, steroid pseudorheumatism may result from a rapid dose decrease.[498] These withdrawal effects gradually

resolve over 1 or 2 weeks and are minimized if each decrement in daily prednisone is 1 mg or less per week (at the lower dose levels).

Many approaches for the prevention and treatment of corticosteroid-associated osteoporosis have been studied in adults, and several guidelines have addressed these issues.[499,500] Vitamin D and its analogues, calcitonin, and various bisphosphonates have been used. Calcitriol (vitamin D₃) or cholecalciferol (vitamin D), with or without calcitonin, were shown to prevent bone loss from the lumbar spine better than calcium alone in several randomized controlled clinical trials of adults who started long-term glucocorticoid therapy.[501,502] Treatment with calcium and vitamin D in adults who receive glucocorticoids effectively slows lumbar and forearm bone loss,[503] and treatment with calcium and vitamin D supplementation has become standard practice in most centers for children with rheumatic disease who receive glucocorticoids.[504-507]

Bisphosphonates have also been studied as a potential treatment for glucocorticoid-induced osteoporosis. Etidronate, pamidronate, alendronate, and risedronate have been shown in randomized controlled trials to increase lumbar spine bone mineral density in adults receiving long-term glucocorticoids for various diseases[453,508-511] These trials did not include children, however, and did not show any significant reduction in fracture incidence, which is the most clinically relevant outcome. Bisphosphonates have been studied in children with osteogenesis imperfecta and seem to be beneficial in reducing bone resorption, increasing bone density, and reducing the chronic bone pain associated with this condition.[512-520] In addition, although there are concerns regarding their effects on growth and remodeling, bisphosphonates have been found to be useful and safe in open-label studies of children with idiopathic juvenile osteoporosis,[521] or osteoporosis associated with connective tissue diseases or induced by glucorticoids.[522-525] Binding to bone and prolonged renal excretion (mean 7 years) continues to concern clinicians for long-term safety of these agents in children.[526] This concern necessitates larger, prospective trials to evaluate bisphophonates for the prevention and treatment of glucocorticoid-induced osteoporosis in children.

Preventing acute adrenal insufficiency (addisonian crisis). The use of pharmacological doses of glucocorticoids for a 2-week period may result in transient suppression of endogenous cortisol production,[527] and prolonged therapy may lead to suppression of pituitary–adrenal function that can be slow in returning to normal. This is potentially the most serious and life-threatening adverse effect associated with glucocorticoid therapy. The actual doses and duration of therapy that are associated with suppression and the length of the recovery period after cessation of therapy are not well defined.[528,529] The recovery period may even be affected by the underlying inflammatory process.[530]

If not recognized, suppression of the hypothalamic–pituitary–adrenal axis places a child at risk for vascular collapse, adrenal crisis, and death in situations that demand increased availability of cortisol.[531] Under conditions of stress (e.g., serious infection, trauma, surgery), all children who may be at risk for hypothalamic–pituitary–adrenal axis suppression require additional glucocorticoids.

The "stress dose" regimen is based on the body's requirements for hydrocortisone during stress.[527] Hydrocortisone (6 to 9 mg/m²/day divided three times daily) is needed for physiological maintenance. For febrile or severe illnesses, hydrocortisone requirements increase to 40 mg/m²/day. With induction of anesthesia or in a resuscitation situation, 100 mg/m² IV of hydrocortisone is required initially, and then 25 mg/m² IV every 6 hours for the following 24 to 48 hours.

If the patient is currently receiving glucocorticoids such as prednisone or prednisolone at a dosage equivalent to or greater than 40 mg/m²/day of hydrocortisone (see Table 12-3 for conversion), then the

SCHEDULE	ADVANTAGES	DISADVANTAGES
Divided daily doses	Optimal disease control	More side effects
Single daily dose	Good disease control; fewer side effects	May not control severe disease
Alternate-day dose	Fewer side effects, less chance of developing Cushing syndrome or pituitary suppression	Less disease control
Intravenous pulse therapy	Less long-term toxicity, rapid onset of action	Acute toxicities

TABLE 12-4   Systemic Administration of Glucocorticoid Drugs

current glucocorticoid dose prescribed for disease management may be enough for febrile or severe illnesses. However, as steroids are weaned or discontinued after prolonged use, glucocorticoid replacement may be required to prevent adrenal crisis if the body's corticosteroid needs exceed the dose prescribed for disease management.

High-dose intravenous glucocorticoid therapy. Intravenous glucocorticoid "pulse" therapy is sometimes used to treat more severe, acute, systemic connective tissue diseases.[532-539] The rationale of this approach is to achieve an immediate, profound antiinflammatory effect and to minimize toxicity related to long-term continuous therapy in moderate to high daily doses. Pulse methylprednisolone has been shown to inhibit cytokine generation[540] and dissolve in cell membranes, altering membrane-associated proteins.[416] Differences are seen in the alpha-interferon gene expression signature in pediatric lupus patients receiving pulse methylprednisolone therapy as compared with oral glucocorticoid therapy,[541] which may explain an advantage this dosing regimen may have over oral doses. However, this observation will need further validation, and additional investigation is needed to optimize efficacy and minimize toxicity with this therapeutic modality.

Although oral pulse regimens have been reported,[542] IV methylprednisolone has been the drug of choice, given in a dosage of 10 to 30 mg/kg/pulse up to a maximum dose of 1 g, administered according to various protocols (eBox 12-2): a single administration as clinical circumstances warrant, a pulse each day for 3 to 5 days, or alternate-day pulses for three doses. Intravenous glucocorticoid pulse therapy may be associated with potentially serious complications[476,543-546] (eBox 12-2).

Intraarticular steroids. Injection of long-acting glucocorticoids directly into inflamed joints has emerged as a major advance in the management of various types of arthritis. Although intraarticular steroid (IAS) therapy has not been studied in randomized controlled clinical trials, multiple reports have documented its efficacy and safety in children.[66,199,547-551]

IAS therapy has been used most often in children with oligoarticular disease; indications for use have included lack of response to NSAIDs; significant NSAID toxicity; and the presence of joint deformity, growth disturbance, or muscle wasting, or as an alternative to NSAID therapy in children with oligoarticular disease. In polyarticular disease, multiple IAS injections at one time can be used as a temporizing measure while awaiting response to second-line systemic agents to take effect. IAS may also be useful as an alternative to increasing systemic therapy in children with polyarticular disease who have significant inflammation in only a few joints.

Virtually all patients experience rapid resolution of symptoms and signs of joint inflammation within a few days after injection, resulting in improved physical function.[552] About two thirds achieve remission for at least 12 months after a single injection.[547,548,553] A longer duration of response has been described in children with oligoarticular JIA,[554,555] and in those who are younger, with shorter disease duration,[66] and with higher mean erythrocyte sedimentation rates.[556] Early use of IAS injections have been associated with less leg-length discrepancies in patients with asymmetrical pauciarticular JRA.[557] More recent data suggest the effectiveness of using radiographic assistance to guide IAS injections into involved temporomandibular and subtalar joints.[558-560]

Type of steroid, dosage, and frequency of injection. Various preparations are available for IAS injection. The most frequently studied agents in children are triamcinolone hexacetonide (THA)[66,547,549] and triamcinolone acetonide.[548] These agents are completely absorbed from the site of injection over 2 to 3 weeks. Because of its lower solubility, THA is absorbed more slowly than triamcinolone acetonide, thereby maintaining synovial levels for a longer period and resulting in

lower systemic glucocorticoid levels,[561] and it is preferred by most pediatric rheumatologists. In comparative studies in patients with JIA, at equivalent doses, THA was found to be more effective than triamcinolone acetonide,[562-564] betamethasone,[565] and methylprednisolone.[566]

The dose of THA used in clinical studies has varied: Some data indicate that higher doses (about 1 mg/kg) may be associated with a better response.[66] Generally, children who weigh less than 20 kg receive 20 mg of THA in large joints. Children weighing more than 20 kg receive 30 to 40 mg THA in the hips, knees, and shoulders, and 10 to 20 mg in the ankles and elbows. In smaller joints such as the wrist, midtarsal, and subtalar joints, 10 mg is used. For injections into tendon sheaths and small joints of the hands and feet, 0.25 to 0.50 mL of a combination of methylprednisolone acetate mixed 1:1 with preservative-free 1% lidocaine (Xylocaine) is recommended. The shorter acting steroid is associated with less risk of damage to tendon sheaths or local soft tissue atrophy.

Repeated injections into the same joint are not performed more than three times per year, although there are few data on which to base this recommendation. There are also no controlled studies in children that examine whether postinjection rest has a role. Although full immobilization of the injected joint is common practice in some clinics, the authors' recommendation is to limit ambulation and strenuous activity for the first 24 hours after a joint injection.

Adverse effects. Despite initial reservations about the safety of IAS therapy in children, clinical studies indicate an overall favorable adverse-effect profile. Iatrogenic septic arthritis is always a potential risk, yet it occurs very rarely and can be avoided with appropriate aseptic precautions.[566] Transient crystal synovitis occurs rarely but is self-limited within 3 to 5 days in most cases without any intervention.[199] The most frequent adverse effects are atrophic skin changes at the site of injection, particularly of smaller joints such as wrists, ankles, and interphalangeal joints in young children, and asymptomatic calcifications on radiographs in joints after multiple injections.[555] The frequency of these skin changes differs by joint,[567] and most eventually resolve.[547,567] The skin changes are attributed to leakage of long-acting steroids into subcutaneous tissues and can be minimized by clearing the needle track with injection of saline or local anesthetic as the needle is withdrawn from the joint. Radiographic reviews have shown usually asymptomatic joint calcifications in 6% to 50% of injected joints.[568,569] Nonspecific cartilage changes have been seen in children with multiple IAS injections after long-term monitoring.[566,570-572] Systemic steroid effects can occur in rare instances.[573-575]

Cytotoxic, Antimetabolic, and Immunomodulatory Agents

Cytotoxic drugs prevent cell division or cause cell death. They act primarily on rapidly dividing cells such as cells of the immune system, particularly T lymphocytes, and are immunosuppressive. The cell cycle consists of the G_1 presynthetic phase, the S phase (synthesis of DNA), the G_2 resting (or postsynthetic) phase, and mitosis. Cytotoxic drugs act during various stages of the cell cycle. These agents are maximally effective in inhibiting immunological responses when their administration coincides with the period of proliferation of the specific immunologically competent cells.

Azathioprine

Azathioprine, a purine analogue, is inactive until it is metabolized to 6-mercaptopurine (6MP) by the liver and erythrocytes.[576] After that, 6MP is transported into cells via nucleoside transporters and undergoes intracellular activation: first to thioinosinic acid by hypoxanthine phosphoribosyl transferase and then through several additional steps, which results in the formation of thioguanine monophosphate, which inhibits *de novo* purine synthesis. Azathioprine's immunosuppressive effects are related primarily to inhibition of T-cell growth during the S phase of cell division. A measurable decrease in antibody synthesis occurs with long-term administration.[577-580] Oral bioavailability of azathioprine is approximately 50%, and about one third of absorbed drug is protein bound.[576] The plasma half-life is approximately 75 minutes, with renal excretion being the primary route of elimination for 6MP and its metabolites. Therefore, proportional dosage adjustment for glomerular filtration rate (GFR) of 50 mL/min/1.73 m^2 or lower is recommended.[581]

The use of azathioprine has been reported anecdotally in many pediatric rheumatic diseases and in series of patients with JRA or SLE.[582,583] Starting dosages should be 1 to 1.5 mg/kg/day, increasing as needed and as tolerated to 2 to 2.5 mg/kg/day, with a maximum dose of 150 mg daily (eTable 12-5).

Toxicity to the GI tract (oral ulcers, nausea, vomiting, diarrhea, epigastric pain) is common.[584] Toxicity to the liver, lung (interstitial pneumonitis), pancreas, bone marrow (cytopenias), or skin (maculopapular rash) is uncommonly associated with azathioprine therapy. Use of azathioprine is accompanied by the known risk of idiosyncratic arrest of granulocyte maturation that occurs shortly after initiation of therapy. This bone marrow toxicity has been attributed to genetic variation in thiopurine S-methyltransferase (*TPMT*),[585,586] the enzyme normally responsible for conversion of the active metabolite 6MP to the inactive metabolite 6-methylmercaptopurine.[587] The most common genetic variants (*TPMT*2*, **3A*, and **3C*) account for 98% of low activity phenotypes in Caucasians[588] and are associated with reduced activity of the enzyme, resulting in higher than expected intracellular levels of active 6-thioguanine nucleotide metabolites and subsequent myelosuppression.[589] Approximately 90% of the population possesses two fully active copies of the gene, approximately 10% of the population has one variant allele (heterozygous genotype) and intermediate activity, and approximately 0.03% of the population possess a homozygous variant genotype and are considered to be "TPMT deficient" at highest risk for myelotoxicity with standard azathioprine doses.[591] Lower levels of enzymatic activity have been observed in African Americans,[592] and ontogeny does not appear to contribute to changes in enzyme activity.[593,594] Testing of thiopurine methyltransferase levels, as well as *TPMT* genotype, is available commercially; however, there remains variation in utilization of these tests prior to azathioprine administration across subspecialties.[595] Additional enzymes in the thiopurine metabolic pathway have recently been shown to have an effect on myelotoxicity.[590]

The bone marrow suppressive effects of azathioprine can be increased by concomitant use of trimethoprim.[596] Although the risk of malignancy theoretically increases in patients treated with azathioprine, the long-term data are inconclusive, and in adults with RA treated with azathioprine, there was no increased risk.[597-599] The combination of azathioprine with infliximab is associated with increased hepatosplenic T-cell lymphoma.

Azathioprine crosses the placenta but the fetal liver lacks the enzyme inosinate pyrophosphorylase, which is necessary to convert azathioprine and 6MP to active metabolites, so the fetus should be protected from teratogenic effects.[600] Clinical studies have revealed no association with poor pregnancy outcomes in inflammatory bowel disease patients treated with 6MP.[601,602] Breast-feeding is contraindicated because the drug is transferred into breast milk.[215]

Mycophenolate Mofetil

Mycophenolate mofetil (MMF) is an ester prodrug form of mycophenolic acid (MPA) and has been found to be effective in various autoimmune diseases as a selective noncompetitive and reversible inhibitor of inosine monophosphate dehydrogenase (IMPDH), a key rate-limiting step in the *de novo* synthesis of guanine nucleotide—a pathway in which T and B lymphocytes are primarily dependent.[603] IMPDH exists in two forms: IMPDH1 is ubiquitously expressed in most cell types, whereas IMPDH2 is expressed in activated T cells.[604] MPA exerts more potent cytostatic effects on T cells due to four- to five fold greater inhibition of IMPDH2 relative to IMPDH1.[605]

MMF is rapidly absorbed after oral administration with a bioavailability of approximately 94%. Peak plasma levels occur 1 to 3 hours after a single dose, with a second peak at 6 to 12 hours as a result of enterohepatic circulation. Upon absorption, MMF is hydrolyzed by carboxylesterases in the liver to biologically active MPA.[603] MPA is 97% albumin bound,[606] and because of its extensive binding to albumin, MMF may interact with other albumin-bound drugs. MMF can also be hydrolyzed in the acidic environment of the stomach, and coadministration of proton pump inhibitors that suppress acid production and gastric pH has been reported to result in decreased potency of MMF.[607] Antacids containing aluminum and magnesium decrease absorption and should also not be administered simultaneously. The elimination half-life of MPA is approximately up to 17 hours after oral administration.[608] The major route of elimination is formation of MPA-glucuronide (MPAG) and UDP-glucuronosyltransferases in the liver (UGT 1A9) and intestine (UGT 1A8 and UGT 1A10).[603] Allelic variations in these enzymes have been investigated.[609]

The carboxyl group of MPA can also be glucuronidated by UGT2B7 to form an acyl glucuronide metabolite (AcMPAG), and although a minor pathway, it may contribute to MPA toxicity.[603] MPAG is excreted into bile by the MRP2 (ABCC2) transporter, converted back to MPA by bacterial glucuronidases, and subsequently reabsorbed, giving rise to the secondary peak observed in pharmacokinetic studies. Most MPA (87%) is recovered in the urine as MPAG.

The effective adult dosage in solid organ transplantation is 2 to 3 g/day in two divided doses. The recommended dosage used to prevent solid organ transplant rejection in children 13 months to 18 years of age is 600 mg/m^2/dose twice daily. Cyclosporine and, to a lesser extent, tacrolimus alter the kinetics of MMF so that higher doses may be required when coadministering.[610] In children with autoimmune diseases, initial dosing is recommended at approximately 300 mg/m^2/dose twice daily and then increased to 600 mg/m^2/dose twice day with a maximum daily dose range of 2000 to 3000 mg/day[610-613] (eTable 12-5).

Individual pharmacokinetic profiling is available and can be especially helpful in determining the lowest effective dose in patients who experience side effects,[613,614] and pharmacokinetic and pharmacodynamic (PK/PD) measurements have even been explored to guide dosing in pediatric SLE. Sagcal-Gironella and colleagues reported only a moderate relationship between weight-adjusted MMF dosing and MPA exposure with a large interindividual variability in the AUC.[615] This high interindividual variability in MPA AUC was also seen in adult patients treated with MMF for SLE.[616] Single nucleotide polymorphisms in genes that encode enzymes important in MMF biotransformation are being explored.[617-620]

Adverse effects of MMF include GI toxicity, hematological effects (leukopenia, anemia, thrombocytopenia, pancytopenia), and opportunistic infections. GI side effects are usually improved by giving the dose three or four times a day instead of twice a day or by reducing it. Hematological toxicity usually responds to therapy cessation within 1 week. Pure red blood cell aplasia has been reported in patients treated with MMF, mostly when combined with other immunosuppressing agents after transplantation.[621,622] A large prospective registry of 6751 transplant patients receiving MMF compared with an equal number of matched controls revealed no increased risk of malignancy with MMF.[623]

Several cases of structural malformations have been seen with MMF exposure during pregnancy in renal transplant recipients and others.[624,625] In fact, the FDA has approved a single shared REMS for medications that contain mycophenolate.[626] Breast-feeding is not recommended.

Cyclophosphamide

Cyclophosphamide, an alkylating agent, is a nitrogen mustard derivative. It is well absorbed after oral administration and is also given intravenously (eTable 12-5 and eBox 12-3). It is inactive until metabolized, principally in the liver, by cytochrome P-450 enzymes to inactive intermediates and the active metabolite phosphoramide mustard. Phosphoramide mustard covalently binds to guanine in DNA, destroying the purine ring and preventing cell replication.[627,628] Cyclophosphamide potentially acts on all cells, including cells that are mitotically inactive (G_0 interphase) at the time of administration (e.g., memory T cells).[629,630] Excretion of the drug is primarily by the kidney, and the dose must be reduced in patients with renal impairment (eTable 12-6). As cyclophosphamide is dialyzable, it is important to delay hemodialysis until at least 12 hours after intravenous administration of the drug.[631] The half-life of cyclophosphamide is approximately 7 hours.

Cyclophosphamide exerts antiinflammatory actions by its effects on mononuclear cells and cellular immunity. Alkylating agents cause B- and T- cell lymphopenia. B cells seem to be more sensitive than T cells to the effects of cyclophosphamide.[632] It has been suggested that the route of administration influences the nature of the effects of this drug; daily oral low-dose therapy may affect cell-mediated immunity more profoundly, whereas intermittent high-dose intravenous therapy predominantly affects B-cell immunity.[633,634] In humans, IgG and IgM synthesis is depressed.[629,630]

Cyclophosphamide is administered in one of two ways: either orally each day or by intravenous bolus every 2 to 4 weeks (eTable 12-5 and eBox 12-3). Inpatient and outpatient IV protocols have been developed and vary based on institutional preferences. Intravenous pulse administration is less toxic and at least as efficacious as oral dosing for lupus nephritis[644]; in some systemic vasculitides, it is unclear whether the intravenous route is as effective as oral administration.[634,645] Bladder toxicity (cystitis, fibrosis, transitional cell carcinoma) is a major risk of cyclophosphamide therapy and results from prolonged contact of the metabolite acrolein with the bladder mucosa.[638,639] To prevent cystitis, adequate hydration and frequent voiding must be emphasized for children who receive cyclophosphamide. Prophylactic mesna should be considered a part of any intravenous cyclophosphamide protocol to minimize bladder mucosa contact with acrolein. With the large doses of cyclophosphamide administered by intravenous bolus, children must be encouraged to empty their bladders every 2 hours and must be awakened during the night to do so; if this is impossible, furosemide should be given, and catheterization should be considered to prevent significant contact of the bladder mucosa with acrolein.

Alkylating agents have prominent toxic effects.[635-643] Short-term side effects include anorexia, nausea and vomiting, and alopecia. Alopecia seems to be related to dose and duration of treatment and is usually reversible.

Leukopenia and thrombocytopenia are the most common adverse reactions, although with careful monitoring they are seldom clinically significant. The cyclophosphamide dose should be adjusted to maintain the total granulocyte count at 1500/mm^3 (1.5×109/L) or higher. The nadir of granulocytopenia with intravenous therapy occurs between the first and the second weeks of therapy, and the dose should be adjusted accordingly based on the complete blood count and differential white blood cell count obtained between 7-10 days after

intravenous cyclophosphamide administration. Lymphocyte counts less than 500/mm^3 (0.5×109/L) are also an indication to reduce the dose.

The syndrome of inappropriate antidiuretic hormone secretion has been reported in patients receiving large doses of cyclophosphamide and is exacerbated by the large fluid load that must be administered.[646] Since nausea and vomiting can be a significant problem; prophylactic use of a potent antiemetic (e.g., ondansetron) is encouraged. Pulmonary fibrosis has been reported in a few patients who receive daily cyclophosphamide.[647,648]

An important consideration with the use of alkylating agents is their effect on fertility.[649] The stage of sexual maturity is crucial in inducing gonadal dysfunction; the further beyond puberty, the greater the chance of infertility with an equivalent dose of cyclophosphamide.[650] In female patients with lupus nephritis, amenorrhea and oligomenorrhea occur more frequently with higher total dose and with increased age at administration.[651-654] Use of intravenous bolus administration at currently recommended doses results in a much lower total cumulative dose than daily oral administration and should be the preferred route, presuming equivalent effectiveness. Ovarian destruction attributable to cyclophosphamide has been reported in one child.[635] In children with SLE, amenorrhea more likely results from disease activity and damage than cyclophosphamide treatment.[655]

Luteinizing hormone–releasing hormones may protect the ovary against cyclophosphamide-induced damage, as was shown in a study of women with lymphoma who received gonadotropin-releasing hormone agonist.[656,657] A systematic review concluded that gonadotropin-releasing hormone agonist improved ovarian function and the ability to achieve pregnancy after chemotherapy.[658] Oocyte or ovarian tissue cryopreservation is an option but can be costly. In male patients, sperm cryopreservation may be considered before cyclophosphamide treatment is instituted.

Cyclophosphamide is associated with an increased risk of malignancy in adults with RA, a risk that is dose related and increases with follow-up duration. One case-control study showed a fourfold elevation of myeloproliferative disorders,[641] and there are increased risks of bladder and skin cancer.[659,660] Cyclophosphamide crosses the placenta and is teratogenic. It is contraindicated during breast-feeding.

Chlorambucil

Chlorambucil, similar to cyclophosphamide, is an alkylating agent, but is rarely used due to serious toxicity and can be referenced in previous editions of this textbook and elsewhere.[661-664]

Cyclosporine, Tacrolimus, and Sirolimus

Cyclosporine, a cyclic peptide of fungal origin, and tacrolimus, a macrolide antibiotic, have had a major impact on the prevention of solid organ transplant rejection.[665] The observation that cyclosporine could virtually eliminate mitogen-induced proliferation by T cells but had little effect on other cell types[666] indicated the potential of this drug in the treatment of immunologically mediated disease.

Cyclosporine and tacrolimus have similar downstream immunomodulatory effects, converging and inhibiting the calcium-dependent and calmodulin-dependent serine/threonine protein phosphatase calcineurin.[667] This inhibits the early phase of T-cell activation and IL-2 production. A related drug, sirolimus, binds to the FK-binding protein 12 to form a complex that has no effect on calcineurin but inhibits a key regulatory protein that suppresses cytokine-driven T-cell proliferation.[668]

Cyclosporine inhibits the production of IL-3, IL-4, IFN-γ,[669,670] and IL-15,[671,672] and it enhances the production of transforming growth factor-β$_1$ protein.[673] It is also antiangiogenic, as shown by the inhibition of vascular endothelial growth factor.[674,675] Cyclosporine and tacrolimus may also result in immunosuppression by inhibiting degradation of I-κB,[676] and they may modulate antiinflammatory effects by inhibiting monocyte production of tissue factor, a potential stimulus of the coagulation cascade via inhibition of NF-κB.[677] They may also result in apoptosis of T and B cells.[678]

Cyclosporine is incompletely and variably absorbed from the GI tract, bound principally to serum albumin and erythrocytes, metabolized by the liver, and excreted in the bile. The absorption of cyclosporine, but not tacrolimus, depends on bile salts. Cyclosporine has a half-life of approximately 18 hours; tacrolimus has a half-life of 9 hours. Mean half-life of sirolimus ranged from 26 to 40 hours.[679] A microemulsion formulation of cyclosporine has been developed to improve absorption and bioavailability[680]; this preparation has more consistent interpatient and intrapatient pharmacokinetics.

Several significant drug interactions are associated with cyclosporine,[22] and considerable toxicity is reported, including impaired renal function,[681,682] hypertension,[683] hepatic toxicity,[684] tremor, mucous membrane lesions, and nausea and vomiting. Hypertrichosis, paresthesias, and gingival hyperplasia have been observed. Renal toxicity may result in hypertension from interstitial fibrosis or tubular atrophy. Sirolimus pharmacokinetics display large interpatient and intrapatient variability, and the monitoring of levels is required.[685] Cyclosporine crosses the placenta and is present in breast milk.

Current guidelines for cyclosporine use are outlined in eTable 12-5; these apply to tacrolimus as well. Factors that most commonly limit clinical use of cyclosporine are hypertension and an increase in serum creatinine of greater than 30% from baseline. Long-term renal damage can occur despite normal serum creatinine levels during the course of therapy.[680] In rheumatic diseases, the goal is to achieve a whole-blood trough level between 125 μg/mL and 175 μg/mL. Ingestion of grapefruit juice increases cyclosporine and cyclosporine metabolite levels significantly.[686]

Small Molecules

Advancement in the understanding of the pathophysiology at a cellular level of several rheumatic diseases have led to the identification of key molecules and signaling pathways that are abnormally expressed. Small molecule drugs that inhibit or interfere with these cellular pathways offer hope for rational, effective, less toxic, and less expensive therapy.[687] Because these are oral therapies and the potential list of targets is vast, the development of small molecule drugs will likely represent the next generation of disease-modifying antirheumatic drug (DMARD) therapies.

The focus of small molecule drug development in rheumatology to date has been primarily on drugs that target cytoplasmic kinases. Once a receptor binds to its ligand (e.g., inflammatory cytokine, self-antigen, immune complex), then conformational changes lead to the activation of intracellular kinases that propagate a cascade leading to activation of effector molecules. Three types of kinases have been studied in RA: mitogen-activated phosphokinase p38 (MAP kinase), spleen tyrosine kinase (Syk), and Janus kinases (JAKs).[688] Several MAP kinase inhibitors were promising in preclinical studies but failed to prove sufficiently efficacious in human trials. A Syk-inhibiting agent (fostamatinib) was more efficacious than placebo in RA trials when added to background MTX but failed to demonstrate efficacy in patients who did not respond previously to biologics.[689-691] The JAKs have been the most extensively studied in RA patients. There are four members of the JAK family: JAK1, JAK2, JAK3 and TYK2. JAK2 is known to be associated with hemapoietic cytokine receptors; therefore selected inhibition of JAK2 is generally avoided. Selective inhibitors of JAK1 and JAK3 are in clinical development in RA but the best studied and only JAK inhibitor

with regulatory approval in the United States is tofacitinib (a JAK1 and JAK3, and to lesser extent, JAK2 inhibitor).[692]

Several phase III studies in RA patients who did not respond to MTX and one biologic have demonstrated efficacy superior to placebo.[693,694] In a parallel 12-month study in patients with active RA despite background MTX therapy, patients were randomized to receive tofacitinib 5 mg twice a day ; tofacitinib 10 mg twice a day ; adalimumab 40 mg every other week; or placebo. At 6 months, ACR 20 responses were seen in 52%, 53%, 47%, and 29%, respectively. Both doses of tofacitinib and adalimumab were superior to placebo.[695] In another randomized, placebo-controlled study; tofacitinib monotherapy resulted in responses better than either adalimumab monotherapy or placebo.[696] Response is seen as soon as 2 weeks after initiation of tofacitinib therapy, and there is a reduction in the progression of structural damage in radiographic studies.[697]

Similar side effects have been seen in all trials: diarrhea, abdominal pain, infections, and neutropenia (generally mild); and small increases in creatinine, transaminases, and lipid levels.[698] The long-term safety of tofacitinib is yet to be fully defined, but long-term extension trials have demonstrated an incidence of malignancy and cardiovascular events similar to RA patients who take DMARDs.[688]

Small molecules, including a variety of MAP kinase inhibitors, are currently, and will continue to be, an area of intense clinical development not only for RA but other rheumatic diseases, including SLE.[687]

Antibiotics

The concept that RA was caused by microbial pathogens led to early use of antimicrobial therapy. Gold was first introduced as a treatment for RA for that reason. Sulfasalazine was synthesized to take advantage of its antimicrobial properties.

Penicillin plays a key prophylactic role in preventing the recurrence of acute rheumatic fever and perhaps in preventing poststreptococcal arthritis.[699] Cutaneous polyarteritis nodosa, which may be a streptococcus-related disease, is also often treated with prophylactic penicillin.[700] In granulomatosis with polyangiitis, treatment with trimethoprim-sulfamethoxazole may prevent disease relapses.[701]

Studies in RA have suggested a role for synthetic tetracycline antibiotics.[702] In early disease, minocycline was more effective than placebo[703] or hydroxychloroquine.[704] The mechanism of action may depend more on the biochemical than on the antimicrobial effect of these agents.[705] Antibiotics do not seem to be effective in enteric reactive arthritis, but they may have a role in urogenital reactive arthritis.[706]

PAIN

Many children have pain either as a primary problem or as a component of their rheumatic disease.[707] There are various methods proposed to treat amplified pain in adults and children, and a number of adjunctive medications have been approved for fibromyalgia in adults. Unfortunately, there are no well-controlled studies of these drugs in children. If and when these agents should be utilized in the treatment of pediatric pain remains controversial.

Antidepressants

Amitriptyline is a tricyclic antidepressant that also inhibits reuptake of serotonin and norepinephrine. In a large meta-analysis of six clinical randomized controlled trials in adult fibromyalgia, amitriptyline at a dosage of 25 mg/day was found to have a therapeutic response compared with placebo in the short term in the domains of pain, sleep, fatigue, and overall patient and investigator impression, but not for tender points.[708] Amitriptyline is metabolized primarily through

CYP2D6 and other cytochrome P450 enzymes ; thus plasma levels can be increased by diminished CYP activity secondary to genetic variation or concomitant medications that affect enzyme activity. Higher plasma drug concentrations can increase the risk of toxicity, including prolonged QTc and arrhythmia, and it has been recommended to obtain a baseline ECG before beginning amitriptyline or with any changes in dosing.[709,710] For treating pain in children, it is recommended to start at 0.1 mg/kg at bedtime and titrate to a final dose of 0.5 to 2 mg/kg (maximum dose 25 to 50 mg at bedtime) over 2 weeks.

Duloxetine and milnacipran are selective serotonin and norepinephrine reuptake inhibitors that have analgesic effects by increasing the activity of descending noradrenergic antinociceptive pathways in the brain and spinal cord; both are approved by the FDA for the treatment of fibromyalgia in adults.[711-713] Milnacipran has a higher affinity for the norepinephrine transporter than duloxetine and may be more effective than duloxetine for patient fatigue and difficulty in concentrating. Common adverse events for both agents are somnolence, nausea, and decreased appetite.[714,715] They are excreted primarily in the urine in the conjugated form. The dosage of milnacipran in adults is 100 mg divided into two doses daily, and for duloxetine it is 60 mg twice daily, but some authors recommend starting at lower doses initially and gradually increasing the dose.[713] Case reports of clinical improvement in children on duloxetine are surfacing.[716,717]

All serotonin-activating medications can increase the risk of bleeding, suicidal tendencies, or both, and should be used with caution.

Neuroleptics

Pregabalin is an $\alpha_2\delta$-calcium channel antagonist that limits the neuronal release of excitatory neurotransmitters, with anxiolytic and analgesic activity with a capability to improve slow-wave sleep. It is approved by the FDA for treatment of fibromyalgia in adults.[718,719] Adverse effects include dizziness, somnolence, weight gain, and peripheral edema.[720] The approved dosage is 300 to 450 mg daily divided into two doses, but it is recommended to start at 75 mg twice a day and then increase based on tolerability and effect.[713] It should be discontinued gradually because sudden discontinuation may precipitate seizures in susceptible individuals.

A systemic review of the comparative efficacy and safety of duloxetine, milnacipran, and pregabalin included 17 studies and more than 7700 adult patients.[721] Adjusted indirect comparisons indicated no significant differences among the drugs in achieving 30% reduction of pain, nor were there differences in drop-out rates due to adverse events. However, there were differences in specific symptom reduction and side effects among agents.

REFERENCES

1. K.A. Neville, J.S. Leeder, Pediatric pharmacogenetics, pharmacogenomics and pharmacoproteomics, in: R.M. Kliegman, B.F. Stanton, J.W. St. Geme III, et al. (Eds.), Nelson Textbook of Pediatrics, nineteenth ed., Elsevier Saunders, Philadelphia, PA, 2011 (Chapter 56).

2. J.R. Vane, R.M. Botting, The mode of action of anti-inflammatory drugs, Postgrad. Med. J. 66 (1990) S2.

12. D.E. Furst, Are there differences among nonsteroidal antiinflammatory drugs? Comparing acetylated salicylates, nonacetylated salicylates, and nonacetylated nonsteroidal antiinflammatory drugs, Arthritis Rheum. 37 (1) (1994) 1–9.

21. L.L. Dupuis, G. Koren, A. Shore, et al., Methotrexate-nonsteroidal antiinflammatory drug interaction in children with arthritis, J. Rheumatol. 17 (1990) 1469–1473.

24. A. Wanders, D.V. Heijde, R. Landewé, et al., Nonsteroidal antiinflammatory drugs reduce radiographic progression in patients with ankylosing spondylitis: a randomized clinical trial, Arthritis Rheum. 52 (6) (2005) 1756–1765.

32. D.J. Lovell, E.H. Giannini, E.J. Brewer Jr., Time course of response to nonsteroidal antiinflammatory drugs in juvenile rheumatoid arthritis, Arthritis Rheum. 27 (12) (1984) 1433–1437.

57. N.D. Yeomans, Z. Tulassay, L. Juhasz, et al., A comparison of omeprazole with ranitidine for ulcers associated with nonsteroidal antiinflammatory drugs, N. Engl. J. Med. 338 (1998) 719–726.

104. B.N. Cronstein, D. Naime, E. Ostad, The antiinflammatory mechanism of methotrexate. Increased adenosine release at inflamed sites diminishes leukocyte accumulation in an in vivo model of inflammation, J. Clin. Invest. 92 (6) (1993) 2675–2682.

118. J.W. Jundt, B.A. Browne, G.P. Fiocco, et al., A comparison of low dose methotrexate bioavailability: oral solution, oral tablet, subcutaneous and intramuscular dosing, J. Rheumatol. 20 (11) (1993) 1845–1849.

120. F. Albertioni, B. Flatø, P. Seideman, et al., Methotrexate in juvenile rheumatoid arthritis. Evidence of age dependent pharmacokinetics, Eur. J. Clin. Pharmacol. 47 (6) (1995) 507–511.

124. M.C. de Rotte, E. den Boer, P.H. de Jong, et al., Methotrexate polyglutamates in erythrocytes are associated with lower disease activity in patients with rheumatoid arthritis, Ann. Rheum. Dis. (2013) doi: 10.1136/annrheumdis-2013-203725; [Epub ahead of print].

126. M. Bulatovic Calasan, E. den Boer, M.C. de Rotte, et al., Methotrexate polyglutamates in erythrocytes are associated with lower disease activity in juvenile idiopathic arthritis patients, Ann. Rheum. Dis. (2013) doi: 10.1136/annrheumdis-2013-203723; [Epub ahead of print].

135. E. Giannini, E. Brewer, N. Kuzmina, et al., Methotrexate in resistant juvenile rheumatoid arthritis. Results of the U.S.A.-U.S.S.R. double-blind, placebo-controlled trial. The Pediatric Rheumatology Collaborative Study Group and The Cooperative Children's Study Group, N. Engl. J. Med. 326 (1992) 1043–1049.

141. T. Beukelman, N.M. Patkar, K.G. Saag, et al., 2011 American College of Rheumatology recommendations for the treatment of juvenile idiopathic arthritis: initiation and safety monitoring of therapeutic agents for the treatment of arthritis and systemic features, Arthritis Care Res. (Hoboken) 63 (4) (2011) 465–482.

142. S. Ringold, P.F. Weiss, T. Beukelman, et al., 2013 update of the 2011 American College of Rheumatology recommendations for the treatment of juvenile idiopathic arthritis: recommendations for the medical therapy of children with systemic juvenile idiopathic arthritis and tuberculosis screening among children receiving biologic medications, Arthritis Care Res. (Hoboken) 65 (2013) 1551–1563.

151. N. Ruperto, K.J. Murray, V. Gerloni, et al., A randomized trial of parenteral methotrexate comparing an intermediate dose with a higher dose in children with juvenile idiopathic arthritis who failed to respond to standard doses of methotrexate, Arthritis Rheum. 50 (2004) 2191–2201.

155. A. Klein, I. Kaul, I. Foeldvari, et al., Efficacy and safety of oral and parenteral methotrexate therapy in children with juvenile idiopathic arthritis. An observational study with patients of the German Methotrexate Registry, Arthritis Care Res. (Hoboken) 64 (9) (2012) 1349–1356.

158. K. Alsufyani, O. Ortiz-Alvarez, D.A. Cabral, et al., The role of subcutaneous administration of methotrexate in children with juvenile idiopathic arthritis who have failed oral methotrexate, J. Rheumatol. 31 (1) (2004) 179–182.

164. D. Foell, N. Wulffraat, L.R. Wedderburn, et al., Methotrexate withdrawal at 6 vs 12 months in juvenile idiopathic arthritis in remission: a randomized clinical trial, JAMA 303 (13) (2010) 1266–1273.

171. L. Kocharla, J. Taylor, T. Weiler, et al., Monitoring methotrexate toxicity in juvenile idiopathic arthritis, J. Rheumatol. 36 (2009) 2813–2818.

178. P. Lahdenne, J. Rapola, H. Ylijoki, J. Haapasaari, Hepatotoxicity in patients with juvenile idiopathic arthritis receiving longterm methotrexate therapy, J. Rheumatol. 29 (11) (2002) 2442–2445.

179. K.G. Saag, G.G. Teng, N.M. Patkar, et al., American College of Rheumatology 2008 recommendations for the use of nonbiologic and biologic disease-modifying antirheumatic drugs in rheumatoid arthritis, Arthritis Rheum. 59 (6) (2008) 762–784.

180. K.A. Rouster-Stevens, S.P. Ardoin, A.M. Cooper, et al., Choosing wisely: the American college of rheumatology's top 5 for pediatric rheumatology, Arthritis Care Res. (Hoboken) 66 (5) (2014) 649–657.

184. A. Hurd, T. Beukelman, Infectious complications in JIA, Curr. Rheumatol. Rep. 15 (2013) 327.

191. S. Gutierrez-Ureña, J.F. Molina, C.O. García, et al., Pancytopenia secondary to methotrexate therapy in rheumatoid arthritis, Arthritis Rheum. 39 (2) (1996) 272–276.

208. J.F. Simard, M. Neovius, S. Hagelberg, J. Askling, Juvenile idiopathic arthritis and risk of cancer: a nationwide cohort study, Arthritis Rheum. 62 (12) (2010) 3776–3782.

210. E. Thomas, D.H. Brewster, R.J. Black, G.J. Macfarlane, Risk of malignancy among patients with rheumatic conditions, Int. J. Cancer 88 (2000) 497–502.

238. J. Chladek, M. Simkova, J. Vaneckova, et al., The effect of folic acid supplementation on the pharmacokinetics and pharmacodynamics of oral methotrexate during the remission-induction period of treatment for moderate-to-severe plaque psoriasis, Eur. J. Clin. Pharmacol. 64 (4) (2008) 347–355.

240. P.G. Hunt, C.D. Rose, G. McIlvain-Simpson, S. Tejani, The effects of daily intake of folic acid on the efficacy of methotrexate therapy in children with juvenile rheumatoid arthritis. A controlled study, J. Rheumatol. 24 (11) (1997) 2230–2232.

242. C. Modesto, L. Castro, Folinic acid supplementation in patients with juvenile rheumatoid arthritis treated with methotrexate, J. Rheumatol. 23 (2) (1996) 403–404.

275. D.J. Grierson, Hydroxychloroquine and visual screening in a rheumatology outpatient clinic, Ann. Rheum. Dis. 56 (3) (1997) 188–190.

288. R.J. Sinclair, J.J. Duthie, Salazopyrin in the Treatment of Rheumatoid Arthritis, Ann. Rheum. Dis. 8 (3) (1949) 226–231.

292. C.C. Chen, Y.T. Lin, Y.H. Yang, B.L. Chiang, Sulfasalazine therapy for juvenile rheumatoid arthritis, J. Formos. Med. Assoc. 101 (2) (2002) 110–116.

350. A.C. Alcantara, C.A. Leite, A.C. Leite, et al., A longterm prospective real-life experience with leflunomide in juvenile idiopathic arthritis, J. Rheumatol. 41 (2) (2014) 338–344.

352. I. Foeldvari, A. Wierk, Effectiveness of leflunamide in patients with juvenile idiopathic arthritis in clinical practice, J. Rheumatol. 37 (2010) 1763–1767.

382. O. Bessmertny, T. Pham, Thalidomide use in pediatric patients, Ann. Pharmacother. 36 (2002) 521–525.

414. H. Schacke, W.D. Docke, K. Asadullah, Mechanisms involved in the side effects of glucocorticoids, Pharmacol. Ther. 96 (2002) 23–43.

415. D.Y. Leung, Q. Hamid, A. Vottero, et al., Association of glucocorticoid insensitivity with increased expression of glucocorticoid receptor beta, J. Exp. Med. 186 (9) (1997) 1567–1574.

420. J.J. Rinehart, S.P. Balcerzak, A.L. Sagone, A.F. LoBuglio, Effects of corticosteroids on human monocyte function, J. Clin. Invest. 54 (1974) 1337–1343.

441. H.G. Morris, J.R. Jorgensen, H. Elrick, R.E. Goldsmith, Metabolic effects of human growth hormone in corticosteroid-treated children, J. Clin. Invest. 47 (3) (1968) 436–451.

442. D. Simon, N. Lucidarme, A.M. Prieur, et al., Effects on growth and body composition of growth hormone treatment in children with juvenile idiopathic arthritis requiring steroid therapy, J. Rheumatol. 30 (2003) 2402–2499.

481. P.N. Tyrrell, J. Beyene, S.M. Benseler, et al., Predictors of lipid abnormalities in children with new-onset systemic lupus erythematosus, J. Rheumatol. 34 (2007) 2112–2119.

491. J.G. Gambertoglio, W.J. Amend Jr., L.Z. Benet, Pharmacokinetics and bioavailability of prednisone and prednisolone in healthy volunteers and patients: a review, J. Pharmacokinet. Biopharm. 8 (1) (1980) 1–52.

499. R.A. Adler, M.C. Hochberg, Suggested guidelines for evaluation and treatment of glucocorticoid-induced osteoporosis for the Department of Veterans Affairs, Arch. Intern. Med. 163 (2003) 2619–2624.

510. K.G. Saag, R. Emkey, T.J. Schnitzer, et al., Alendronate for the prevention and treatment of glucocorticoid-induced osteoporosis, N. Engl. J. Med. 339 (1998) 292–299.

523. S. Rudge, S. Hailwood, A. Horne, et al., Effects of once-weekly oral alendronate on bone in children on glucocorticoid treatment, Rheumatology (Oxford) 44 (6) (2005) 813–818.

532. E.S. Cathcart, B.A. Idelson, M.A. Scheinberg, et al., Beneficial effects of methylprednisolone "pulse" therapy in diffuse proliferative lupus nephritis, Lancet 1 (1976) 163–166.

563. B.A. Eberhard, M.C. Sison, B.S. Gottlieb, N.T. Ilowite, Comparison of the intraarticular effectiveness of triamcinolone hexacetonide and triamcinolone acetonide in treatment of juvenile rheumatoid arthritis, J. Rheumatol. 31 (2004) 2507–2512.

565. Z. Balogh, E. Ruzsonyi, Triamcinolone hexacetonide versus betamethasone. A double-blind comparative study of the long-term effects of intra-articular steroids in patients with juvenile chronic arthritis, Scand. J. Rheumatol. Suppl. 67 (1987) 80–82.

593. C. Ganiere-Monteil, Y. Medard, C. Lejus, et al., Phenotype and genotype for thiopurine methyltransferase activity in the French Caucasian population: impact of age, Eur. J. Clin. Pharmacol. 60 (2004) 89–96.

596. R.R. Bailey, Leukopenia due to a trimethoprim-azathioprine interaction, N. Z. Med. J. 97 (766) (1984) 739.

604. Y. Natsumeda, S. Ohno, H. Kawasaki, et al., Two distinct cDNAs for human IMP dehydrogenase, J. Biol. Chem. 265 (1990) 5292–5295.

617. W. Zhao, M. Fakhoury, G. Deschenes, et al., Population pharmacokinetics and pharmacogenetics of mycophenolic acid following administration of mycophenolate mofetil in de novo pediatric renal-transplant patients, J. Clin. Pharmacol. 50 (2010) 1280–1291.

631. M. Haubitz, F. Bohnenstengel, R. Brunkhorst, et al., Cyclophosphamide pharmacokinetics and dose requirements in patients with renal insufficiency, Kidney Int. 61 (4) (2002) 1495–1501.

646. P.J. Harlow, Y.A. DeClerck, N.A. Shore, et al., A fatal case of inappropriate ADH secretion induced by cyclophosphamide therapy, Cancer 44 (3) (1979) 896–898.

655. C.A. Silva, M.O. Hilário, M.V. Febrônio, et al., Risk factors for amenorrhea in juvenile systemic lupus erythematosus (JSLE): a Brazilian multicentre cohort study, Lupus 16 (2007) 531–536.

666. J.F. Borel, C. Feurer, C. Magnée, H. Stähelin, Effects of the new antilymphocytic peptide cyclosporin A in animals, Immunology 32 (6) (1977) 1017–1025.

687. A. Markopoulou, V.C. Kyttaris, Small molecules in the treatment of systemic lupus erythematosus, Clin. Immunol. 148 (3) (2013) 359–368.

689. M.E. Weinblatt, A. Kavanaugh, R. Burgos-Vargas, et al., Treatment of rheumatoid arthritis with a Syk kinase inhibitor: a twelve- week, randomized, placebo-controlled trial, Arthritis Rheum. 58 (11) (2008) 3309–3318.

699. N. Birdi, U. Allen, J. D'Astous, Poststreptococcal reactive arthritis mimicking acute septic arthritis: a hospital-based study, J. Pediatr. Orthop. 15 (1995) 661–665.

Entire reference list is available online at www.expertconsult.com.

CHAPTER 13

Pharmacology: Biologics

Norman T. Ilowite, Ronald M. Laxer

Biologics are different from nonbiologic disease-modifying antirheumatic drugs (DMARDs) in that they are produced by biologic processes rather than chemical syntheses and target specific, well-defined molecules expressed on cells or secreted into the extracellular space.[1,2] The terms "nonbiologic," "conventional," and other descriptors were used to identify the agents discussed in Chapter 12. This chapter focuses on the mechanism of action, pharmacokinetics, pharmacodynamics, dosing, and safety of various *biologic* as well as *targeted synthetic* therapies, also known as "small molecules." For information related to *efficacy* of these agents in pediatric rheumatic diseases, please consult the chapter that discusses the specific disorder.

GENERAL CONSIDERATIONS

In general, affinity is a major determinant of the pharmacokinetic (PK) and pharmacodynamic (PD) profile of monoclonal antibodies (mAbs) and receptors (Cepts).[3] Higher affinity allows efficacy to be maintained at lower serum concentrations. That is why proteins with similar half-lives and sizes can have very different duration of efficacy.[4] Essentially, all biologic agents are immunogenic because they are nonself. Even humanized and fully human mAbs and Cepts can elicit antibody responses.[5] The effects of human antichimeric antibodies (HACAs) or human antihuman antibodies (HAHAs) include reduction in serum levels, neutralization of biologic activity, anaphylactoid reactions, and loss of clinical efficacy. Their generation appears to be related to dose, route, and frequency of administration, as well as host-related factors.[6,7] The interactions with Fc receptors also affect the PD of those mAbs and Cepts that are fusion proteins that include the Fc portion of IgG.[8] The system of naming monoclonal and receptor biologics is shown in Table 13-1. Information (molecule, target, route of administration, dose, and toxicity) regarding the major mAbs and Cepts used in pediatric rheumatology is shown in Table 13-2.

For some biologics, interpretation of safety data is difficult due to the randomized withdrawal study design that results in subjects in both arms of the studies being exposed to the agent with no suitable comparator group of nonexposed subjects. There are concerns that targeting the immune system may result in an increase in serious infections, malignancies, and autoimmune disease, in addition to complications of HACAs and HAHAs. A recent review showed different frequencies of these complications for various biologics and small molecules used in the treatment of juvenile idiopathic arthritis (JIA)[2] (Table 13-3).

Clinical trials powered for efficacy are underpowered to determine whether rare, serious, or adverse events are associated with treatment (e.g., malignancy, serious infections, autoimmune diseases), and thus safety data are difficult to interpret. Large, long-term, multicenter disease-specific registries are more likely to find a significant association of these events with treatment.[2,9,10]

The safety, immunogenicity, and effects of vaccines on the underlying rheumatic disease is of great concern in patients on biologic therapy.[11,12] The 2011 European League Against Rheumatism (EULAR) recommendations state that nonlive vaccines are safe and can be administered to patients on corticosteroids and/or biologic therapy; however, responses may be somewhat lower than in normal children.[13] Live-attenuated vaccines generally have a good safety profile in children with rheumatic diseases who are on biologic therapy, especially with booster doses. It is recommended that an individual without a history of varicella zoster virus infection or vaccination be assessed before the initiation of immunosuppressive therapy and, if possible, vaccination before initiation of therapy be performed when required. In considering the use of biologics, one should weigh the risk of the wild-type infection against the possible side effects of vaccination and the risk of disease flare should treatment be withheld for a period after vaccination. In a study of attenuated measles-mumps-rubella (MMR) boosters in 137 patients, antibody titers were similar in the 15 patients on biologic therapies and the rest of the cohort, and there were no effects on disease activity.[14]

INTRAVENOUS IMMUNOGLOBULIN

Intravenous immunoglobulin (IVIG) is prepared from pooled human plasma. More than 75% of IVIG in the United States is administered to patients with autoimmune or inflammatory conditions.[15] The doses used in inflammatory conditions are many-fold higher than the doses used for replacement therapy in immunodeficient patients, usually 2 g/kg (total dose) administered over a period of 1 to 5 days. Upon intravenous administration, IgG enters the vascular compartment at high concentration, redistributes rapidly into tissue compartments (the α phase involving rapid lysosomal degradation due to saturation of neonatal Fc receptors), and then is slowly catabolized (the β phase when the neonatal Fc receptors are not saturated and IVIG is recycled back to the surface of the cell).[16]

IVIG is relatively safe, but anaphylactoid reactions, thromboembolic events, renal complications including osmotic nephrosis and renal failure, hemolysis, and acute meningeal inflammation do occur.[16,17] Ideally, IgA deficiency should be excluded before administration because of the associated presence of anti-IgA antibodies, but this is not routine practice. Anaphylactoid, thromboembolic, hemolytic, and meningeal (aseptic meningitis) events can be minimized by slower infusion or changing preparations; renal complications can be minimized by better hydration and use of sugar-free stabilizers.[16] Current preparation protocols purify the product so that it is not contaminated

161

TABLE 13-1 Naming of Monoclonal Antibody and Receptor Biologic Therapies (United States Adopted Names System)

All monoclonal antibodies' names end in "mab"
Source identifiers
  u = human (e.g., adalim**u**mab, golim**u**mab)
  o = mouse
  a = rat
  zu = humanized (e.g., tocili**zu**mab, certoli**zu**mab)
  e = hamster
  i = primate
  xi = chimeric (e.g., ritu**xi**mab, infli**xi**mab)
  axo = rat/mouse
  xizu = combination of humanized and chimeric chains
All receptors end in "cept" (e.g., etanercept, rilonacept, abatacept)

with human immunodeficiency virus (HIV), hepatitis C virus, and other known viruses. However, there is always a risk of transmission of as-yet unidentified pathogens. Guidelines for IVIG administration are listed in Table 13-4. The mechanisms whereby IVIG exerts its therapeutic effects are not clear and may differ in each disease state. IVIG has many effects beyond antibody replacement.[15,18] Potential mechanisms are listed in Table 13-5.[19-22]

INHIBITION OF THE COSTIMULATORY PATHWAY

CTLA-4Ig (Abatacept). In order to activate resting T cells, two molecular signals are required: (1) the interaction of the T-cell receptor (TCR) with processed peptide, presented in the appropriate major histocompatibility complex (MHC) setting; and (2) interaction of CD28 on T cells with CD80/86 on the surface of the antigen-presenting cell. Another high-affinity receptor, cytotoxic T lymphocyte–associated antigen-4 (CTLA-4), can also bind to CD80/86 with a higher avidity than CD28, thereby preventing the second signal required for T-cell activation. Abatacept is a fully human, soluble fusion protein comprising the extracellular domain of CTLA-4 and the Fc component of IgG1, which selectively inhibits the costimulatory signal necessary for full T-cell activation[23] (Fig. 13-1). By binding to CD80/86, it can prevent T-cell activation.[24] In an international, multicenter prospective study of 190 subjects with polyarticular course JIA using a randomized, double-blind, placebo-controlled withdrawal design, adverse events were recorded in 37 abatacept recipients (62%) and 34 (55%) placebo recipients ($P = 0.47$). Abatacept was well tolerated in this trial, and there were no serious adverse events.[25] Abatacept is approved by the U.S. Food and Drug Administration (FDA) and European Medicines Agency (EMA) for use in polyarticular course JIA in children age 6 or older. Time to response can be as long as 6 months. In the open-label extension of this study, there were 1.33 serious infections per 100 patient-years among 153 patients.[26] Five patients developed six infections, including dengue fever, erysipelas, gastroenteritis, herpes zoster, bacterial meningitis, and pyelonephritis. Guidelines for abatacept's use in children are shown in Table 13-6.

Subcutaneous dosing of abatacept has been approved by the FDA for rheumatoid arthritis (RA), and studies are under way in JIA.[27] Overall immunogenicity to abatacept is low. Interruption and reintroduction did not affect the safety or efficacy of the drug. The incidence of autoimmune disorders was similar in patients with RA treated intravenously and subcutaneously.[27] In a meta-analysis, abatacept-treated subjects had more serious infections than patients receiving placebo.[28]

In adults with hepatitis B no reactivation occurred if they were on antiviral therapy. Reactivation did occur in patients not treated with antiviral therapy.[29]

B-CELL TARGETED

Rituximab. Rituximab is a chimeric mouse–human monoclonal antibody that binds to the B-cell CD20 receptor, which is present on pre-B and mature B cells but not on stem cells or plasma cells.[30] It was developed initially for the treatment of relapsed Hodgkin's B-cell lymphoma. Rituximab exerts its effect by removing CD20+ B cells from the circulation, both by antibody-dependent and complement-dependent cellular cytotoxicity, and by the induction of apoptosis of B cells. Although the antibody-producing plasma cells are not removed from the circulation, B cells that may act as antigen-presenting cells, produce cytokines, and infiltrate tissues are removed for a prolonged period. Memory B cells, which are also responsible for antibody production, may be removed as well.

Rituximab is theoretically beneficial in diseases in which autoantibodies may be pathogenic. It was first used in patients with idiopathic thrombocytopenic purpura[31] and more recently in a variety of other autoimmune diseases. In lymphoma, a dose of 375 mg/m² administered weekly for four infusions dramatically reduces B cells for a period of 6 to 9 months. This regimen was also used in treatment of antineutrophil cytoplasmic antibodies (ANCAs)-associated vasculitis.[32] Alternative dosing in RA is 1000 mg intravenously in divided two doses, 2 weeks apart. Studies in ANCA-associated vasculitis have shown it to be as effective as cyclophosphamide for remission induction and perhaps better for treatment of disease flares. Rituximab induced a profound depletion of all peripheral blood B-cell populations in patients with RA. Repopulation occurred mainly with naïve mature and immature B cells. Patients whose RA relapsed upon the return of B cells tended to show repopulation with higher numbers of memory B cells.[33,34]

Recommendations for rituximab's use in children are shown in Table 13-7 and are based primarily on adult data, as there is only limited information about the use of rituximab in children. Binstadt and colleagues[36] reported four children with multisystem autoimmune illnesses who received rituximab after the failure of multiple other agents, noting improvement in their neurologic manifestations. Nadirs of IgG levels were seen at 4 to 6 months, and three of the patients required immunoglobulin replacement therapy. Leandro and associates[33] reported improvement in five of six patients with systemic lupus erythematosus (SLE) treated with a combination of two rituximab infusions of 500 mg, two infusions of cyclophosphamide at 750 mg, and high-dose oral corticosteroids. Eleven girls with severe SLE, including eight with class IV or class V lupus nephritis, two with severe autoimmune cytopenia, and one with antiprothrombin antibody with severe hemorrhage, were treated with 2 to 12 intravenous infusions of rituximab (350-450 mg/m²/infusion) and with corticosteroids. Depletion of B cells paralleled remission in seven of eight patients. Severe adverse events were seen, including two patients with septicemia and four with severe hematologic toxicity. The authors concluded that rituximab was effective but noted the incidence of severe adverse events.[37] Treatment with rituximab was reported in 18 patients with lupus who showed improvement in double-stranded DNA antibodies, renal function, and proteinuria, but some patients required repeated courses, and one died of endocarditis. In a study of nine children with SLE manifesting as autoimmune cytopenias, rituximab resulted in complete B-cell depletion, which was seen in all the children in the study. No serious infections occurred, but one patient had an infusion reaction.[38-40] In another study of 19 patients, 5 developed herpes zoster infections.[40]

TABLE 13-2 Molecule, Target, Half-Life, Route of Administration, Indications, Dose, and Major Toxicities of Biologic Agents in Pediatric Rheumatology

BIOLOGIC	MOLECULE	TARGET	T1/2	C/H IV/SC/PO	INDICATION/ OTHER USE	DOSE	MAJOR TOXICITY	COMMENTS
Etanercept	TNFRII/FcIgG1	TNF-α,β	4 d	H / SC	RA, PsA, Ps, AS, JIA	0.8 mg/kg q wk or 0.4 mg/kg twice weekly; max 50 mg	TB, fungal, lymphoma, MS	With or without MTX
Adalimumab	mAb to TNF-α	TNF-α	2 weeks	H / SC	RA, PsA, Ps, AS, JIA, CD, UC/uveitis	15-30 kg-20 mg q2 wk >kg-40 mg q2 wk	rTB, fungal, lymphoma, MS	With or without MTX
Infliximab	mAb to TNF-α	TNF-α	12.4 d (a) 13.2 d (p)	C / IV	RA, PsA, Ps, AS,J IA, IBD/uveitis	6-10 mg/kg q 2 wk-2 mo	Infusion rxns / TB, fungal, lymphoma, MS	With MTX pre-med with corticosteroid, acetaminophen, antihistamine
Golimumab	mAb to TNF-α	TNF-α	2 wk	H / SC	RA, PsA, AS, UC	50 mg q mo adult 30 mg/m² ch	TB, fungal, lymphoma, MS	With MTX
Certolizumab	Peg mAb to TNF-α	TNF-α	14 d	H / SC	CD, RA, PsA	400 mg initially, wks 2 and 4 then 200 mg q2 wk or 400 mg q 4 wks (adult doses)	TB, fungal, lymphoma, MS	With or without MTX
Anakinra	IL-1Ra	IL-1	4-6 h	H / SC	RA/SJIAC, CAPS	1 mg/kg, max 100 mg daily	Injection site rxns, liver	Don't use with other biologics other than abatacept
Rilonacept	IL-1R/IL-1AcP/ FCIgG1	IL-1	7.72 d	H / SC	CAPS/SJIA	4.4 mg/kg (max 320 mg) loading dose then 2.2 mg/kg q week (max 160 mg)	Injection site rxns, liver, lipids	Don't use with other biologics
Canakinumab	mAb to IL-1	IL-1	26 d adults 23-26 d child	H / SC	CAPS/SJIA	150 mg q8 wk (adult dose CAPS) 4 mg/kg q 4 wks SJIA	Injection site rxns, liver, neutropenia	Don't use with other biologics
Abatacept	CTLA4-Ig	CD80/86	13 d IV 14.3 d SC	H / IV SC	RA/JIA, uveitis	<75 kg-10 mg/kg wk 0, 2, 4 then q4 wk 75-100 kg-750 mg >100 kg-1000 mg	Injection site rxns	Don't use with other biologics other than anakinra
Rituximab	mAb to CD20	CD20⁺ B cells	6-62 d	C / IV	RA/RF + polyJIA RF	375-500 mg/m² IV q2 wk × 2 doses	Infusion rxns / Progressive multifocal encephalopathy	With MTX
Tocilizumab	mAb to IL-6 receptor	IL-6	11-13 d	IV	RA, SJIA, pJIA	Poly JIA >2 yr, <30 kg 10 mg/kg q4 wk >2 yr, >30 kg 8 mg/kg SJIA >2 yr, <30 kg 12 mg/kg q2 weeks >2 yr, >30 kg 8 mg/kg q2 weeks	Infection, TB, malignancy, GI perforation, hypersensitivity rxn, anaphylaxis/ anaphylactoidrxns MS lipids	Pre-med with glucocorticoid, acetaminophen, antihistamine With or without MTX; dose interruptions for liver toxicity, neutropenia, thrombocytopenia
Belimumab	mAb to BLyS	B cells	19.5 d	IV	SLE	10 mg/kg q2 wk × 3 then q4 wk	Infections, anaphylaxis, infusion rxns	Observe for 1 hour after infusion is complete
Ustekinumab	mAb to p40 subunit of IL-12 and IL-23	Th17 cells	15-46 d	SC	Ps, PsA	45 mg SC wk 0, wk 4, then q12 wk (PsA; <100 kg) 90 mg SC wk 0, wk 4, then q12 wk (>100 kg)	Infection, malignancy, hypersensitivity rxn, anaphylaxis, PRES, cardiovascular events	With or without MTX
Tofacitinib	Small molecule	Jak 1,2,3	3 hr	PO	RA	5 mg PO BID	Infections, viral reactivation, neutropenia, lymphopenia, anemia, malignancy, GI perforation	Dose adjustments for toxicity; avoid use in severe liver impairment

AS, Ankylosing spondylitis; *C,* chimeric; *CAPS,* cryopyrin-associated periodic syndrome; *CD,* Crohn's disease; *Fungal,* reactivated fungal infection; *H,* humanized; *IV,* intravenous infusion; *JIA,* polyarticular course juvenile idiopathic arthritis; *mAb,* monoclonal antibody; *MS,* multiple sclerosis/demyelinating disease; *MTX,* methotrexate; *P,* pegylated; *PRES,* posterior reversible encephalitis syndrome; *Ps,* psoriasis; *PsA,* psoriatic arthritis; *RA,* rheumatoid arthritis; *rTB,* reactivated tuberculosis; *rxns,* reactions; *SC,* subcutaneous injection; *SJIA,* systemic JIA; *T1/2,* half-life; *UC,* ulcerative colitis.

TABLE 13-3 Rates of Serious Infections Malignancies, Autoimmune Diseases, Antibiologic Antibodies Per 100 Patient-Years Exposed to Biologics in JIA[2]

	SERIOUS INFECTIONS	MALIGNANCIES	AUTOIMMUNE DISEASES	ANTI-BIOLOGIC ANTIBODIES
Normal children	1.0	.032	.0069 new-onset uveitis .0083 IBD .00015 optic neuritis .0001 MS	
JIA without MTX, steroids, or anti-TNF	2.2	.025	2.5 new-onset uveitis	
JIA with MTX	3.3	.033-0.046	.83 uveitis	
JIA with steroids	6.9	ND	ND	
Abatacept	1.3	ND	.22 uveitis flare .22 MS	23 no AEs
Adalimumab	2.9	ND	0	7.6 with MTX within 1 year 25.3 without MTX within 1 year
Anakinra	8.7	ND	ND	75.0 nonneutralizing within 1 year 81.8 after 1 year 6.3 neutralizing within 1 year 0 neutralizing after 1 year
Etanercept	2.7	0.015	.44 new-onset uveitis .57 flares of uveitis .31 new-diagnosis IBD .15 new-onset SLE .64 new-diagnosis sarcoid	2.9 nonneutralizing
Infliximab	1.0	ND	5.1 new-onset uveitis 25.9 new ANA ≥1:320 no symptoms 6.6 new anti-dsDNA no symptoms	36.6 positive 32.4 inconclusive Infusion reaction related
Rituximab	14.5	ND	ND	ND
Tocilizumab	11.6	ND	ND	7.1 1 anaphylactoid reaction

Adapted from J.F. Swart, S. de Roock, N.M. Wulffraat, Arthritis Res. Ther. 15 (2013) 213.

TABLE 13-4 Guidelines for Use of Intravenous Immunoglobulin

Dose
Up to 2 g/kg (max 75 g)
Preparation
Start IV with normal saline
Administration
Give IVIG at rate of 0.5 mL/hr for 30 min, then 1.0 mL/kg/hr for 30 min, then 2.0 mL/kg/hr for the remainder

Clinical Monitoring
Blood pressure and pulse rate every 15 min for first hour, every 30 min for second hour, every 60 min thereafter
Observe
Sudden fall in blood pressure (anaphylaxis)
Headache, vomiting 18-36 hours after infusion (aseptic meningitis)

TABLE 13-5 Antiinflammatory and Immunomodulatory Activities of IVIG[15]

Fab Mediated Activities
Suppression or neutralization of autoantibodies
Suppression or neutralization of cytokines
Neutralization of activated complement components
Restoration of idiotypic, antiidiotypic networks
Blockade of leukocyte adhesion molecule binding
Targeting of specific immune cell-surface receptors
Modulation of maturation and function of dendritic cells

Fc-Dependent Activities
Blockade of the FcRn
Blockade of activating FcγR
Upregulation of inhibitory FcγRRIIB
Immunomodulation by sialylated IgG

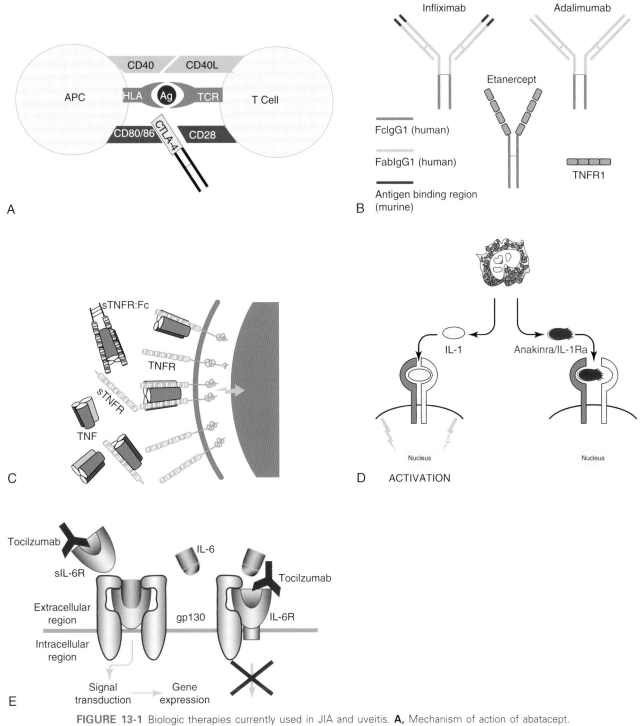

FIGURE 13-1 Biologic therapies currently used in JIA and uveitis. **A,** Mechanism of action of abatacept. Abatacept binds the CD80 and CD86 family of B proteins on antigen-presenting cells, thereby preventing the costimulatory signaling needed to activate T cells via CD28. **B,** Structure of the three anti-TNF biologics used in the treatment of JIA and uveitis. Adalimumab and infliximab are both anti-TNF monoclonal antibodies but differ in that infliximab is a chimeric antibody whose antigen-binding region uses a mouse component. Etanercept is a fusion protein containing a human FcIgG1 linked with a TNF receptor. **C,** Mechanism of action of etanercept. TNF exerts its action on immunoinflammatory cells by binding to cell-bound TNF receptors, resulting in cell activation. Etanercept binds circulating TNF-α, thus preventing cellular binding and cell activation. **D,** Mechanism of action of anakinra. Anakinra binds to the IL-1 receptor and thereby prevents binding of the IL-1 receptor accessory protein (IL-1R-AcP) and subsequent cell signaling. **E,** Mechanism of action of tocilizumab. Tocilizumab is a genetically engineered, humanized, mAb to the IL-6 receptor that is produced by grafting the complementarity-determining region of mouse antihuman IL-6 receptor antibody to human IgG1. Tocilizumab competes with both the soluble and the membrane-bound IL-6 receptor preventing cell signaling.

TABLE 13-6 Guidelines for the Use of Abatacept in the Treatment of JIA[25]

Dose
<75 kg: 10 mg/kg intravenously over 30 minutes on weeks 0, 2, 4 then every 4 weeks
>75 kg: 750 mg intravenously over 30 minutes on weeks 0, 2, 4, then every 4 weeks

Clinical Monitoring
Document absence of latent or active tuberculosis before starting
Improvement should be seen by the third to fourth dose, but may be delayed
Monitor every 1-2 months initially, then every 3-6 months, depending on course
Hold if suspected bacterial infection, varicella

Laboratory Monitoring
CBC with WBCC, differential, and platelet count; AST, ALT, albumin every 4-12 weeks

TABLE 13-7 Guidelines for Use of Rituximab[31,35]

Dose
500 mg/m^2 (maximum 1000 mg) intravenously on weeks 0, 2; or 375 mg/m^2 weekly for 4 doses at 50 mg/hr initially
If no infusion reaction occurs, escalate dose at 50 mg/hr increments every 30 minutes to a maximum of 400 mg/hr. If the first infusion was tolerated well, subsequent infusions can be give over a shorter period of time with an initial rate of 100 mg/hr and every 100 mg/hr increments every 30 minutes.
Premedicate with methylprednisolone 100 mg intravenously 30 minutes prior to infusion
Observe for infusion during therapy. Discontinue and treat with corticosteroids and antihistamines if infusion reaction occurs

Clinical Monitoring
Improvement should be seen within a month of initial infusion
Monitor every 1-2 months initially, then every 3 months, depending on course

Laboratory Monitoring
Screen for hepatitis B virus
Check B-cell numbers before and 1 month after infusion
Quantitative immunoglobulins every 3 months
Follow liver transaminases

In a study of 125 adult and pediatric patients with anti-N-methyl-D-aspartate (NMDA) receptor encephalitis unresponsive to first-line therapy, one anaphylactic reaction and one infection were attributed to rituximab treatment.[41]

Side effects include flushing and itching, usually with the first dose. These manifestations are probably allergic in nature and may be alleviated with pretreatment with an antihistamine and corticosteroids. Infusion reactions, including severe mucocutaneous reactions, are most common with the first infusion. Pretreatment with corticosteroids reduces the incidence and severity.[42] Prolonged reduction of immunoglobulin levels is more common and significant in children than in adults and may require immunoglobulin replacement therapy, especially in patients who have developed serious infection or who are on other immunosuppressive therapy such as cyclophosphamide, mycophenolate, or azathioprine. Reduced baseline immunoglobulin levels may be associated with increased susceptibility to infection. HACAs may develop in one third of patients after treatment and are associated with lower serum levels of rituximab at 2 months, and less effective B-cell depletion.[43] Rituximab is contraindicated in patients with hepatitis B, as reactivation has occurred, resulting in fulminant hepatitis, hepatic failure, and death; thus all patients must be screened for hepatitis B virus prior to treatment. In occult infection with hepatitis B, serum transaminases should be monitored.[44] Rituximab should not be given in the presence of a severe or opportunistic infection. B-cell numbers can be used to time repeated courses of therapy in some diseases.[42]

Patients must be observed closely for development of viral infections, because post-rituximab infections with parvovirus, varicella-zoster virus, cytomegalovirus, and enterovirus have been reported. Serious infections were seen at a rate of 14.5 per 100 patient-years in 55 children with JIA, 46 of whom had systemic juvenile idiopathic arthritis (SJIA).[45] Pneumonias were caused by *Pneumocystis jirovecii*, but the patients were on multiple concomitant medications, including methotrexate, corticosteroids, and cyclosporine, all of which could have contributed to susceptibility to this organism.

A systematic review[46] identified 52 patients with underlying lymphoproliferative disorders who developed progressive multifocal leukoencephalopathy (PML) after treatment with rituximab and other agents (two patients with SLE, one patient with RA, one patient with idiopathic autoimmune pancytopenia, and one with immune thrombocytopenia). Other treatments included hematopoietic stem cell transplantation (7 patients), purine analogs (26 patients), or alkylating agents (39 patients). One patient with an autoimmune hemolytic anemia developed PML after treatment with corticosteroids and rituximab, and one patient with an autoimmune pancytopenia developed PML after treatment with corticosteroids, azathioprine, and rituximab. Median time from the last rituximab dose to PML diagnosis was 5.5 months.[46,47] Four patients with RA treated with rituximab developed PML.[48] Although PML is a rare adverse event associated with rituximab therapy, its devastating nature mandates continued vigilance, particularly in patients with current or prior exposure to an alkylating agent.[49] Baselines screening for JC virus is not required. These data tend to implicate the other treatments as the cause of PML rather than rituximab alone, but further study is necessary. There are insufficient data to require tuberculosis screening, but physicians should be vigilant.[27]

Belimumab. Belimumab is a human IgG1 neutralizing monoclonal antibody against B-lymphocyte stimulating factor (also known as B-lymphocyte stimulator [BLyS]).[50] BLyS, a member of the tumor necrosis factor (TNF) ligand superfamily, is synthesized as a 285-amino acid type II membrane protein and exists in both membrane and cleaved 152-amino acid soluble forms. Expressed on monocytes, macrophages, and monocyte-derived dendritic cells, BLyS is upregulated in response to interferon (IFN)-γ and interleukin (IL)-10, enhancing B-cell proliferation and immunoglobulin secretion. Belimumab binds with high affinity to BLyS and inhibits binding of BLyS to its three receptors, inhibiting BLyS-induced proliferation of B cells and decreasing survival of autoreactive B cells, which are particularly dependent on soluble BLyS.[51,52] Treatment results in decreasing serum anti-double-stranded DNA antibody levels.[53]

Safety data from 1458 adult SLE patients from one phase II study and two phase III studies were analyzed.[53-57] Serious adverse events included infections, hypersensitivity reactions, anaphylaxis, and infusion reactions. Serious cases of pyrexia and anemia occurred more

TABLE 13-8 Guidelines for Use of Belimumab in the Treatment of Systemic Lupus Erythematosus[53]

Dose
10 mg/kg via intravenous infusion via intravenous infusion over 1 hour at 2-week intervals for the first 3 doses, then at 4 week intervals thereafter. Vital signs once at 15 minutes and then at 45 minutes

Laboratory Monitoring
Monitor for leukopenia and elevated transaminases with each infusion

TABLE 13-9 Guidelines for Use of Etanercept in the Treatment of Juvenile Idiopathic Arthritis[65]

Dose
0.4 mg/kg twice weekly or 0.8 mg/kg per week subcutaneously
Max 50 mg/week

Clinical Monitoring
Document absence of latent or active tuberculosis before starting
Improvement should be seen by the third or fourth dose
Monitor every 1-2 months initially, then every 3-6 months, depending on course
Hold if suspected bacterial infection, varicella

Laboratory Monitoring
CBC with WBCC, differential and platelet count; AST, ALT, albumin every 4-12 weeks

frequently in the highest dosage (10 mg/kg) than in the placebo group (approximately 1%). The number of adverse events was similar across the groups on three dosing regimens of belimumab and placebo (between 13% and 20%). Most infusion reactions occurred during the first two infusions and consisted of headache, nausea, pruritus, and rash; these were not dose related. Serious and/or severe hypersensitivity reactions were reported in four patients receiving belimumab. None had anti-belimumab antibodies. Patients should be observed for at least 1 hour after each infusion, particularly early in the course; however, some reactions were seen 3-5 hours after infusion.[27] Three malignancies occurred in the placebo group and three in the 10 mg/kg group. Belimumab has been given continuously for more than 5 years in a minority of patients.[58] A trial in childhood lupus is under way. Recommendations for the use of belimumab are shown in Table 13-8.

INTERFERENCE WITH CYTOKINES

TNF inhibitors

The biologic effects of T cell–derived and monocyte-derived cytokines can explain much of the clinical syndrome of synovitis as well as the systemic manifestations associated with JIA.[59-61] Cytokines are critical in perpetuating and damping the immune response, and as such they are important targets for therapeutic manipulation. TNF inhibitors have now been proven to be effective in the treatment of a number inflammatory conditions, including polyarticular course JIA, psoriatic arthritis, ankylosing spondylitis, and inflammatory bowel disease (Table 13-2).

Anti-TNF agents currently in use or under study in children are etanercept, infliximab, adalimumab, golimumab, and certolizumab (Table 13-2).

Etanercept

Etanercept is a fully human, dimeric protein containing the extracellular domain of the human p75 TNF receptor fused to the Fc region of human IgG1. By binding to trimers of TNF-α in the circulation, etanercept prevents the interaction of TNF-α with its cell surface receptor, thereby preventing cell activation and perpetuation of the inflammatory cascade. It can also modulate biologic responses that are mediated by TNF, such as expression of adhesion molecules, serum concentration of matrix metalloproteinases (MMPs), and cytokines.[62] Although soluble forms of the TNF-α receptor occur naturally, they are generally inadequate to block TNF activity in systemic inflammatory disorders. The dimeric form of the TNF-α receptor is much more efficient at binding TNF because it binds at a much greater affinity (50 to 1000 times higher) than that of the naturally occurring form. Etanercept also binds lymphotoxin (formerly called TNF-β).[63] The role of lymphotoxin in the pathogenesis of arthritis is not as well understood as that of TNF-α. The half-life of etanercept, administered

subcutaneously, is approximately 4 days. Etanercept was initially given twice weekly but is as effective using the same total dose once a week.[64] In adults with RA, steady-state concentrations are achieved in about 2 weeks.[62] Etanercept has been used extensively in children with JIA since the initial report of its effectiveness in 2000.[65] It is currently indicated for children age 2 and above for polyarticular JIA in both North America and Europe. In Europe it is also approved for use in children ages 12-17 with psoriatic arthritis or enthesitis-related arthritis. A study of nearly 600 subjects demonstrated its relative safety over 3 years.[66] Long-term continuous treatment up to 10 years appears to be safe with little evidence of tachyphylaxis.[66-68] Guidelines for the use of etanercept are shown in Table 13-9.

To date, etanercept has been very well tolerated. The placebo-controlled study showed an increase in symptoms of upper respiratory tract infection as well as injection site reactions, although these were generally mild.[65] Injection site reactions may be treated with topical corticosteroids. However, postmarketing studies have reported a variety of unusual side effects; most importantly, systemic infection must be closely watched for. This includes bacterial infection, viral infection such as varicella with or without superimposed bacterial infection, and granulomatous infection. Although these infections are more common in elderly patients, physicians must be attuned to their development in any age group. Two patients in the pivotal trial[65] developed aseptic meningitis secondary to varicella zoster, prompting the recommendation that JIA patients, if possible, be brought up to date with all immunizations in agreement with current immunization guidelines prior to starting etanercept. Patients with a significant exposure to varicella virus should temporarily discontinue etanercept and be considered for prophylaxis with varicella zoster immune globulin. Live virus vaccination is contraindicated, but concurrent methotrexate and etanercept did not appear to decrease the rate of seroconversion to MMR vaccination.[69]

A variety of other side effects have been noted. Although rare enough to be the subject of case reports, there may be an association between treatment with etanercept and the development of vasculitic skin rash,[70] and systemic[71] or drug-induced lupus.[72] The associations with pancytopenia and aplastic anemia are less clear.[73] Several cases of diabetes mellitus after etanercept treatment have been reported in children with JIA.[74] Patients experiencing changes in mood, weight gain, autoimmune hepatitis, thymic enlargement, sterile cholecystitis, tuberculous uveitis, and macrophage activation syndrome[75-79] while being treated with etanercept have been reported.[80]

TABLE 13-10 Guidelines for Use of Infliximab in the Treatment of Juvenile Idiopathic Arthritis[84]

Dose

6-10 mg/kg /infusion over approximately 2 hours on weeks 0, 2, and 6, then every 4-8 weeks thereafter, depending on course; dose may be increased up to 10 mg/kg

Start at 10 cc/hour for 15 minutes, double rate every 15 minutes until 160 cc/hour for 30 minutes, then 250 cc/hour until finished

Usually given with methotrexate

Consider premedication with diphenhydramine, acetaminophen

Clinical Monitoring

Document absence of latent or active tuberculosis before starting

Improvement should be seen by the third or fourth dose

Monitor every 1-2 months initially, then every 3-6 months, depending on course

Hold if suspected bacterial infection, varicella

Laboratory Monitoring

CBC with WBCC, differential and platelet count; AST, ALT, albumin every 4-12 weeks.

TABLE 13-11 Guidelines for Use of Adalimumab in the Treatment of Juvenile Idiopathic Arthritis[101]

Dose

15-30 kg: 20 mg subcutaneously every second week

>30 kg: 40 mg subcutaneously every second week

Can be given with or without methotrexate

Clinical Monitoring

Document absence of latent or active tuberculosis before starting

Improvement should be seen by the second or third dose

Monitor every 1-2 months initially, then every 3-6 months depending on course

Hold if suspected bacterial infection, varicella exposure or infection, hepatitis B infection

Laboratory Monitoring

CBC with WBC count, differential and platelet count, AST, ALT, albumin every 4-12 weeks

Infliximab

Infliximab is a chimeric anti–TNF-α antibody consisting of a mouse Fab' fragment antibody and the constant region of the human IgG1.[82] In contradistinction to Cepts such as etanercept, monomers of infliximab bind not only to monomers of soluble TNF-α but also to membrane-bound TNF-α, leading to both antibody-dependent and complement-dependent cytotoxicity. It seems to be more efficacious than etanercept in granulomatous inflammatory disorders (e.g., sarcoidosis) and uveitis but also seems to be associated with the development of granulomatous opportunistic infections.[83] Administration of infliximab is through the intravenous route (Table 13-10). Dose and frequency vary somewhat with the clinical response. Initial doses in adults usually start at 3 mg/kg and are given at time 0, at 2 weeks, at 6 weeks, and then every 8 weeks depending on clinical response. Starting doses in children should be 6 mg/kg routinely (see the next paragraph). Doses often require escalation, and doses up to 20 mg/kg have been used occasionally in children.[84,85] Alternatively, the length of time between infusions can be shortened. Administration with methotrexate (MTX) is recommended to prevent the development of anti-infliximab antibodies, which seem to correlate with infusion reactions and accelerated clearance of infliximab.[82] It is not certain, however, that these antibodies actually reduce the effectiveness. Similar to etanercept, combination treatment with MTX seems to improve the response to infliximab in patients with RA.[86]

Ruperto et al. reported the results of a randomized, double-blind, placebo-controlled trial of infliximab in patients with polyarticular-course JIA.[87] The clearance of the drug was more rapid in children with juvenile rheumatoid arthritis (JRA) than was observed in adults with RA, resulting in lower trough levels before the next dose. Infliximab was generally well tolerated, but the safety profile of infliximab at a dose of 3 mg/kg appeared less favorable than that of infliximab at a dose of 6 mg/kg, with more frequent occurrences of serious adverse events, infusion reactions, antibodies to infliximab, and newly induced antinuclear antibodies and antibodies to double-stranded DNA observed with the 3 mg/kg dose, perhaps related to the lower trough levels in the 3-mg/kg group.[87,88]

Treatment with infliximab resulted in reduced serum concentrations of interleukin (IL)-6, myeloperoxidase, and soluble adhesion molecules ICAM-1, and E-selectin. TNF-α levels tended to increase while the concentrations of endogenous TNF antagonists (sTNF-RI and sTNF-RII) were reduced.[89-94]

Infection remains the major concern with the use of infliximab. Many more cases of tuberculosis have been reported in patients treated with infliximab than in those treated with etanercept, probably because of the destabilization of previously formed granulomata.[95] Other infections that have occurred with greater than expected frequency include histoplasmosis, coccidioidomycosis, and listeriosis.[82] One case of optic neuritis has been reported in a child.[96] IgA and IgM anti-double-stranded DNA antibodies can occur with infliximab therapy,[97] but only 1 of 156 patients with these antibodies developed lupus.[98] In addition to the side effects noted with etanercept, infusion reactions ranging from mild allergic reactions to anaphylactic reactions may occur, more commonly on the second or third infusions. Therefore, infliximab must be administered under close observation. See Table 13-10 for guidelines regarding administration.

Adalimumab

Adalimumab is a recombinant human IgG1 mAb that acts in a similar fashion to infliximab and golimumab by binding to the TNF both in the circulation and on the cell surface.[99] Therefore, it may result in cell lysis in the presence of complement. Adalimumab, but not etanercept, has been shown to induce immunosuppressive T_{reg} cells.[100,101] It is administered subcutaneously with a half-life of approximately 2 weeks. Initial recommended dosing in children was 24 mg/m[2] every second week. In North America the tendency is to administer 20 mg every second week for patients weighing less than 30 kg, and 40 mg every second week for patients weighing more than 30 kg. As with other anti-TNF agents, the effects are seen quickly, but the dose may need to be given once a week for sustained improvement. Injection site reactions can be problematic. Some practitioners add lidocaine into the syringe. The combination of adalimumab and MTX is safe and results in increased efficacy in RA.[102]

A pivotal study resulted in FDA approval for the use of adalimumab for polyarticular JIA. (Table 13-11).[103] Serious adverse events possibly related to adalimumab occurred in 14 patients; 7 of these patients had serious infections (bronchopneumonia, herpes simplex virus infection, pharyngitis, pneumonia, viral infection, and 2 cases of herpes zoster). Twelve patients discontinued treatment because of adverse events. No deaths, malignant conditions, opportunistic infections, tuberculosis, demyelinating diseases or lupuslike reactions occurred. Sixteen percent of patients (6% on MTX; 26% not on MTX) had at least one positive test for anti-adalimumab antibodies. Development of anti-adalimumab antibodies did not affect the incidence of serious adverse events.

Golimumab

Golimumab is a recombinant human IgG monoclonal antibody to TNF-α. The constant regions of the heavy and light chains of this monoclonal antibody are identical in amino acid sequence to the corresponding constant regions of the human–mouse chimeric mAb infliximab. However, in contrast to infliximab, the heavy and light variable regions are of human sequence. The recommended dosage is 50 mg subcutaneously once a month in combination with MTX. The FDA approved golimumab in 2009 for the treatment of moderately to severely active adult RA, psoriatic arthritis, and ankylosing spondylitis.[104,105] In the pivotal trial, one patient died after developing nausea, diarrhea, ileus, aspiration pneumonia, and sepsis. The most frequent adverse events were infection and injection site reaction. Antinuclear antibodies may occur, and their development may correlate with higher doses of golimumab or the absence of MTX. Antibodies to golimumab were observed in 2.1% of the subjects and were not significantly associated with decreased efficacy or injection site reaction. Pediatric studies are under way, but there are no published pediatric data to date.

Certolizumab

Certolizumab pegol is a pegylated (i.e., conjugated with polyethylene glycol) humanized Fab′ fragment of a monoclonal antibody that binds TNF-α. Pegylation increases its half-life. As opposed to infliximab, adalimumab, and golimumab—which are full-length bivalent IgG mAbs—certolizumab is a monovalent Fab antibody fragment. It has a higher affinity for TNF-α, is devoid of the Fc portion of the antibody, and does not induce complement activation, antibody-dependent cellular cytotoxicity, or apoptosis.[106] Its efficacy and safety in active RA have now been assessed in three phase III, multicenter, randomized, double-blind, placebo-controlled clinical trials.[89,107,108] In the most recent study of 619 subjects, certolizumab pegol plus MTX were more efficacious than placebo plus MTX, rapidly and significantly improving signs, symptoms, and physical function in patients with RA, and inhibiting radiographic progression. The dose was 200 mg or 400 mg subcutaneously every 2 weeks. Five patients developed tuberculosis. Pediatric studies are under way.

Common issues with anti-TNF agents

With the increasing use of anti-TNF agents, a number of common concerns have arisen, one of which is the increased risk of infection, particularly tuberculosis; fungal infections, including histoplasmosis; and other opportunistic infections.[109-112] Children with JIA had a higher rate of opportunistic infections, including an increased rate of coccidioidomycosis, salmonellosis, and herpes zoster.[113,114] Among children with JIA, the rate of infection was not increased with MTX or TNF-inhibitor use but was significantly increased with high doses of corticosteroids.[114] In general, before starting treatment with any of these agents, the following approach is recommended: patients should be screened for the presence of latent tuberculosis with a tuberculosis skin test or a blood-based diagnostic assay (e.g., Quantiferon-Gold). The latter may have higher specificity particularly in patients who have had bacillus Calmette-Guérin (BCG) vaccination.[115] A chest radiograph is probably unnecessary unless the purified protein derivative

(PPD) result is positive. If the skin test or blood-based assay is positive, thorough investigation of the patient and family for active tuberculosis must be undertaken, and the patient must be treated accordingly. If the investigations prove negative, the patient should be given isoniazid (INH).[27] Treatment with anti-TNF agents may be initiated 1 month after starting INH,[116] although some give INH simultaneously with TNF-inhibitor therapy. The FDA advises close monitoring of patients for signs and symptoms of potential fungal infection, especially in endemic areas, both during and after treatment with anti-TNF drugs. Patients in whom fever, malaise, weight loss, sweats, cough, dyspnea, pulmonary infiltrates on chest radiographs, or serious systemic illness develop should undergo a complete diagnostic workup appropriate for immunocompromised patients. The decision to initiate empiric antifungal therapy in at-risk symptomatic patients should be made in conjunction with an infectious diseases specialist, taking into account both the risk for severe infection and the risks of antifungal therapy. TNF inhibitors should be withheld for serious infection or sepsis. Anti-TNF treatment should not be used in patients with active infection and should be discontinued in the case of a serious infection. Mild upper respiratory tract or urinary tract infections are not a reason to stop anti-TNF agents. Patients with hepatitis B who were treated with a TNF inhibitor had worsening symptoms, viral load, or hepatic function,[27] and although hepatitis B reactivation has been added to the label, concomitant antiviral treatment can be given.

Concern remains regarding the development of malignancy, particularly lymphoma.[112] Patients must be observed closely for the occurrence of malignancies. However, any association is difficult to decipher because of the known increased incidence of malignancy in patients with rheumatoid arthritis.[73] Aggressive and fatal hepatosplenic T-cell lymphomas, a rare malignancy, have been reported in patients receiving TNF blockers. Most cases occurred in patients getting infliximab for Crohn's disease or ulcerative colitis who had received concomitant treatment with azathioprine or 6-mercaptopurine; the majority involved adolescent boys and young adult men.

In information obtained from manufacturers of TNF inhibitors approved for use in children (etanercept, infliximab, adalimumab), 48 cases of malignancies in children and adolescents were identified.[117] It was estimated that 14,837 children received infliximab, 9200 received etanercept, and 2636 received adalimumab during the studied period. Approximately half of the malignancies were lymphomas. Others included leukemia, melanoma, and solid organ cancers. Eleven of the patients died (nine from hepatosplenic T-cell lymphoma, and one from T-cell lymphoma). The rates of malignancy were higher with infliximab than expected rates, but the primary use of infliximab was for inflammatory bowel disease in contrast to etanercept, where patients with JIA represented the majority. Eighty-eight percent of cases were in patients taking other immunosuppressive medications such as azathioprine, 6-mercaptopurine, or contradistinction MTX. It was concluded that there is an increased risk of malignancy with TNF-inhibitor exposure, but that the strength of the association, or a definite causal relationship could not be assigned. Some major problems with these conclusions were that the precise denominator for users was not known, and treated patients werc not compared to a control group of JIA patients not treated with biologics. Bernatsky et al., using data from three Canadian centers, did not find an increased incidence of malignancy in patients with JIA.[117] In contrast, Simard et al., using comprehensive administrative data from Sweden, showed that the incidence of malignancy in patients with JIA had increased in the years 1987 to 1999 (before the use of biologics) compared to the preceding two decades.[118] Using national Medicaid data from 2000 through 2005, Beukelman et al. showed that children with JIA in the United States appeared to have an increased incidence of malignancy compared with children without JIA and that the treatment for JIA, including TNF inhibitors, did not appear to be significantly associated with the development of malignancy.[119] Similar data were reported by Nordstrom et al.[120] Thus the role of anti-TNF agents in increasing the risk of malignancy in patients with JIA is not yet clear.[121] A meta-analysis in adults concluded that etanercept is safer than anakinra, adalimumab, or infliximab.[81]

The safety of anti-TNF therapy during pregnancy is unknown, and it is classified as a category B medication, meaning that there is no evidence of risk in humans or if human studies have not been done, no evidence in animals that show risk.[122] Many reports have documented lack of teratogenicity with healthy pregnancy outcomes. Similarly, breast-feeding appears to be safe. Consideration should be given to avoiding live viral vaccines for 6 months in children who have been exposed to biologic therapy during pregnancy.[123]

Similar concerns exist for the development of demyelinating syndromes, especially multiple sclerosis, with anti-TNF therapy. Early postmarketing studies suggested that demyelinating syndromes, including multiple sclerosis, might be more common in patients treated with etanercept. In a trial of lenercept, another TNF antagonist, used to treat patients with multiple sclerosis, those taking the active drug had more exacerbations than those who did not.[124] Patients with JIA have developed demyelinating syndromes, as have adults with RA.[125] Guillain-Barré syndrome developed in 15 patients identified from the FDA database.[126] In children, four cases of optic neuritis have been reported.[127] On the other hand, large studies have failed to demonstrate an occurrence greater than what would have been expected.[128] Patients with previous demyelinating syndromes should not be treated with TNF antagonists, and those with a strong family history should be observed carefully for the development of symptoms that may be suggestive of demyelination. Performing a baseline central nervous system MRI should be considered in patients with a family history of multiple sclerosis.

TNF antagonist therapy has been rarely associated with SLE-like syndromes and antiphospholipid antibody syndrome.[129,130] The development of leukocytoclastic vasculitis had been reported in 35 patients; the disease resolved in the majority after discontinuation of anti-TNF therapy.[131,132] New-onset psoriasis and Crohn disease have been reported.[27]

In trials in patients with congestive heart failure (CHF), neither infliximab nor etanercept was effective, and the drugs may have even worsened the CHF.[133] These agents might exacerbate, or even induce, CHF in patients with no previous risk factors.[134] A meta-analysis in adults with plaque psoriasis found no effect of TNF inhibitors on cardiovascular events.[135] A systematic review showed that TNF inhibition did not lead to significant changes in intima-media thickness, endothelial function, or lipid profiles over 52 weeks.[136,137]

It does not seem that any specific laboratory monitoring is required routinely for any of these agents. Although the induction of antinuclear antibodies is common (up to approximately 15% of patients), screening for them is necessary only if suspicion of a developing autoimmune disease (e.g., drug-induced lupus) is raised.

As with most safety signals from postmarketing surveillance, it is difficult to know whether or not these cases are related to anti-TNF therapy, concomitant therapy, the underlying diseases, or demographics of the patients being treated, but caution is required when considering offering this therapy to candidate patients. It may not be entirely correct to lump all TNF inhibitors together as their mechanisms, pharmacokinetics, and hosts may differ, particularly with the nonmonoclonal antibody etanercept.[27,138]

Guidelines developed for adults suggest withholding biologic DMARDs for at least 1 week before and after surgery.[139] No specific recommendations regarding the use of biologic DMARDs during pregnancy or breast-feeding were made because of conflicting evidence.

IL-1 inhibitors

Anakinra. IL-1 plays a prominent role in RA by stimulating synoviocytes and chondrocytes to produce small inflammatory mediators (e.g., prostaglandins) and matrix metalloproteases (MMPs) that lead to cartilage destruction and bone erosions. IL-1 also increases the expression of receptor-associated NF-κB ligand (RANK ligand), leading to osteoclast differentiation and activation and bone destruction. It exerts its effect by binding to the IL-1 receptor and through cell signaling and production of these various molecules and cytokines. IL-1 receptor antagonist (IL-1Ra), is a naturally occurring, acute phase antiinflammatory protein, part of the IL-1 supergene family.[140] Anakinra is a manufactured IL-1Ra.

IL-1Ra is the most important physiologic regulator of IL-1–induced activity. By binding to the IL-1 receptor on cell surfaces, it prevents the interaction of the receptor with IL-1 and subsequent cell signaling. An imbalance between IL-1 and IL-1Ra can lead to uncontrolled inflammation.

Anakinra is a human recombinant form of IL-1Ra. It has a short half-life of 4 to 6 hours (when given at a dose of 1 to 2 mg/kg in adults with RA[140]) and requires daily subcutaneous injection. Dramatic responses to anakinra in some cases of systemic JIA and cryopyrin-associated periodic syndrome (CAPS), and the deficiency of the IL-1 receptor antagonist (DIRA)[141] provide the evidence for pediatric use (Table 13-12). These responses also provide evidence that this group of disorders are IL-1 driven and autoinflammatory in nature (see below).

Adverse events have, in general, not been serious. The most common are injection-site reactions, which tend to occur within the first 4 weeks and are rare later. They consist of rash, erythema, and pruritus, and may be relieved with ice packs and application of a topical corticosteroid. Rarely are these events severe enough to stop treatment. Although the frequency of serious infections (pneumonia, cellulitis) is increased, no deaths from infection have been reported, and, in contrast with anti-TNF agents, opportunistic infections have not occurred in studies to date. It appears safe to use MTX with anakinra,[143] but etanercept does not seem to add benefit to anakinra in the treatment of JIA, and there was concern about the increased infections, particularly pneumonia, with this combination in patients with RA.[144] This combination has been used in the treatment of hyper-IgD syndrome (HIDS).[145]

TABLE 13-12   Guidelines for the Use of Anakinra in the treatment of Systemic JIA[138,142]

Dose
1-2 mg/kg subcutaneously daily (max 100 mg)
Safe to use with methotrexate but should not be combined with TNF inhibitors

Clinical Monitoring
Although not associated with reactivation of latent tuberculosis, the authors recommend documenting a negative PPD prior to initiation
Improvement most often occurs within 2 weeks
Monitor every 1 month initially then quarterly

Laboratory Monitoring
Neutrophil count prior to initiating, monthly for three months, then quarterly

Due to low enrollment in a double-blind, placebo-controlled trial of anakinra in polyarticular course JIA, the primary end point was changed from efficacy to safety. The incidence and nature of adverse events were similar across all study phases, with the exception of injection-site reactions, which were mild to moderate and decreased with time. Anakinra produced a nonsignificant ($P = 0.11$) reduction in disease flares compared with placebo. When normalized to 1 mg/kg dose, anakinra plasma concentrations were similar to values in adult patients with RA.[146]

Clinical remission after anakinra treatment in systemic JIA (SJIA) patients was associated with a reversal of a gene expression signatures in peripheral blood cells and leukocytes.[147] In a retrospective case series of 35 patients, 1 developed macrophage activation syndrome, and another Epstein-Barr virus (EBV) infection. It was reported that one patient developed visceral leishmaniasis after treatment with anakinra.[148] In a retrospective series, 3 of 46 patients with SJIA treated initially with anakinra developed a serious infection. In both of these retrospective series the majority of patients were also treated with corticosteroids.[149] In a randomized trial involving 24 patients with SJIA, 4 developed a serious infection.[150]

There is no indication that the use of anakinra is associated with an increased incidence of tuberculosis.[27] Anakinra use is associated with an increased incidence of infection, especially with concomitant use of corticosteroids and high-dose anakinra.[151] However, much higher doses than approved for RA have been used seemingly without an increased rate of infections in patients with macrophage activation syndrome (MAS) and CAPS.[149,152,153]

Rilonacept. Rilonacept (also known as IL-1 Trap) is a fully human dimeric fusion protein that incorporates the extracellular domains of both the IL-1 receptor components required for IL-1 signaling (IL-1 receptor type I and Il-1 receptor accessory protein), linked to the Fc portion of human IgG1.[143,154] It has a half-life of approximately 1 week and blocks IL-1 signaling by acting as a soluble decoy receptor preventing its interaction with cell surface receptors. In two consecutive phase III studies of 47 adult patients with CAPS, including familial cold autoinflammatory syndrome (FCAS) and Muckle-Wells (one a 6-week randomized double-blind, placebo-controlled trial, the other a 9-week single-blind withdrawal study), rilonacept at a dose of 160 mg was demonstrated to provide marked and lasting improvement in the clinical signs and symptoms and normalized serum amyloid A (SAA) levels. One serious adverse event (worsening sciatica) was not considered to be related to treatment during the trial, but one elderly patient died after developing sinusitis and *Streptococcus pneumoniae* meningitis. Forty-eight percent of the rilonacept group and 13% of the placebo group reported injection-site reactions. Forty-three percent of patients developed anti-rilonacept antibodies, which did not appear to affect efficacy or safety profile. Increases in total cholesterol, LDL cholesterol, HDL cholesterol, and triglycerides were seen after 6 weeks of open label therapy. In a smaller study, all five patients with FCAS benefited from treatment.[141]

Preliminary data regarding rilonacept treatment in 21 systemic JIA patients enrolled in a double-blind, placebo-controlled study were presented at AXR. Two doses (2.2 mg/kg/week [maximum 160 mg] and 4.4 mg/kg/week [maximum 320 mg]) were studied. Data from an open label phase were published.[155] Discontinuations were due to loss of efficacy or to worsening pancytopenia, mood alteration, and MAS.[155] Seven of the 21 subjects had inadequately responded to anakinra. Fourteen patients with colchicine-resistant familial Mediterranean fever were treated using a novel Bayesian study design of sequential active drug or placebo cycles.[156] Injection-site reactions were more frequent with rilonacept, but no differences were seen in other adverse events. The results of a randomized placebo phase study of rilonacept

---

TABLE 13-13 Guidelines for the Use of Rilonacept in Cryopyrin Associated Periodic Syndrome or Systemic JIA[151,155,158]

Dose

Initiate treatment with a loading dose of 4.4 mg/kg (max 320 mg) delivered as 1 or 2 subcutaneous injections with a maximum single-injection volume of 2 mg. If the initial dose is given as 2 injections, they should be at different sites.

Continue dosing at 2.2 mg/kg (max 160 mg) once weekly

Do not give in combination with TNF inhibitors

Clinical Monitoring

Clinical response is often rapid, sometimes after the first dose

Laboratory Monitoring

Serum lipid monitoring after 2-3 months of therapy (consider use of lipid lowering medication if cholesterol and/or triglycerides are elevated)

Monitor CBC and liver transaminases at baseline, one month after initiating, then every 3 months

---

in SJIA were recently reported.[157] There was not a higher incidence of infection in the rilonacept arm in either phase. Four patients, all in the rilonacept arm, developed elevations in liver transaminases twice the upper limit of normal or higher; two patients developed elevations more than five times the upper limit of normal (one of these was considered a serious adverse event). There were 14 serious adverse events: 9 among patients in the rilonacept arm and 5 in the placebo arm, with the most common being SJIA flare (4 events). The aspartate aminotransferase (AST) liver function test was consistently higher in the rilonacept arm. Guidelines for the use of rilonacept are found in Table 13-13.

Canakinumab. Canakinumab is a fully human IgG1κ monoclonal antibody targeting IL-1β and has no cross-reactivity with other characterized IL-1β family members, including IL-1α and IL-1Ra. Its long half-life of 30 days permitted dosing every 8 weeks in in a three-part, 48-week, double-blind placebo-controlled randomized withdrawal study in 35 patients with CAPS.[159] The dose was 2 mg/kg for patients weighing 40 kg or less, and 150 mg for patients weighing more than 40 kg; doses could be escalated up to 8 mg/kg if necessary. Two patients had serious adverse events (lower urinary tract infection, vertigo with closed-angle glaucoma). There was an increase in the rate of suspected infections in the withdrawal phase in the canakinumab group compared with the placebo group. No serious infections or immunogenicity to canakinumab were detected.

In two randomized trials of canakinumab (dosing every 4 weeks based on modeling studies)[160] in SJIA involving 261 patients, the most common adverse events were infections, and the rates of infection were similar in patients in the canakinumab and placebo arm.[161] Neutropenia and thrombocytopenia were mostly transient, isolated events and were not associated with an increased risk of infection or bleeding. Serious infections did occur: measles, pneumonia, varicella, urosepsis, and gastroenteritis. Elevations in liver transaminases—some dramatic—did occur. Seven episodes of MAS (one with pulmonary hypertension) were reported, with two deaths. This mortality rate is in keeping with that of SJIA in general.[162] However, IL-1 inhibition has been suggested as MAS therapy so one might have expected mortality to be lower in these trials. Injection-site reactions are mild compared to anakinra, and antibodies to canakinumab are uncommon. Recommendations for the use of canakinumab are shown in Table 13-14.

TABLE 13-14   Guidelines for the Use of Canakinumab in the Treatment of Systemic JIA and Cryopyrin-Associated Periodic Syndromes[150,152]

Dose
Cryopyrin-Associated Periodic Syndromes
>40 kg: 150 mg
≥15 kg, ≤40 kg: 2 mg/kg
For children 15 to 40 kg with an inadequate response, the dose can be increased to 3 mg/kg.
Administer subcutaneously every 8 weeks
Systemic Juvenile Idiopathic Arthritis (SJIA)
≥7.5 kg: 4 mg/kg (with a maximum of 300 mg)
Administer subcutaneously every 4 weeks
Monitor CBC and liver transaminases at baseline, one month after initiating, then every 3 months

IL-6 inhibitors

Tocilizumab. IL-6 appears to be an important potential target, particularly in the treatment of systemic-onset JIA, but also polyarticular JIA. An imbalance between IL-6 and its soluble receptor can lead to increased IL-6 binding on cell surfaces with its receptor, binding gp130, on the cell membrane, which can then lead to intracellular signaling and result in cytokine production and release.[163] Elegant studies have produced evidence that levels of IL-6 correlate with fever spikes, thrombocytosis, and joint involvement in patients with SJIA.[164] In mice that are transgenic for IL-6, growth retardation is observed.[165] Therefore, neutralization of IL-6 would be expected to be very beneficial. Tocilizumab is a humanized, mAb to the soluble IL-6 receptor that is produced by grafting the complementarity-determining region of mouse antihuman IL-6 receptor antibody to human IgG1.[163,165] Tocilizumab can bind with both the soluble and the membrane-bound IL-6 receptor. The suggested dose is 4 to 12 mg/kg biweekly intravenously, tailored as the half-life after the third dose of 8 mg/kg biweekly is reached in approximately 10 days.[165]

Thirty-two of 143 adults with RA (22%) in a 5-year, long-term, open-label extension safety study of tocilizumab withdrew from the study due to adverse events and 1 due to an unsatisfactory response; 14 withdrew at the patient's request or for other reasons.[166] The serious adverse event rate was 27.5 events per 100 patient-years, with 5.7 serious infections per 100 patient-years, based on a total tocilizumab exposure of 612 patient-years.

In a preliminary study, 11 children with systemic-onset JIA were treated with tocilizumab in a dose-escalation trial. Three patients received 2 mg/kg, five received 4 mg/kg, and three received 8 mg/kg. No children withdrew due to adverse events or disease flare.[167] In a study of 18 Caucasian SJIA patients treated with a single intravenous infusion of either 2, 4, or 8 mg/kg of tocilizumab, no dose-limiting toxicity was observed, and there were no dose-limiting safety issues. Clinical and laboratory responses were observed within 48 hours after infusion, and these improvements continued well after serum tocilizumab was undetectable.[168] In a randomized, placebo-controlled, withdrawal study in Japan, 56 children were given three 8-mg/kg doses of tocilizumab every 2 weeks during a 6-week open-label lead-in phase. Patients achieving an ACR Pediatric-30 response with a C-reactive protein (CRP) of less than 5 mg/L were randomly assigned to receive placebo or to continue tocilizumab treatment for 12 weeks or until withdrawal for rescue medication in the double-blind phase. Patients who responded to tocilizumab and needed further treatment were

enrolled in an open-label extension phase for at least 48 weeks. Serious adverse events in the open-label run-in and blinded withdrawal phases were an anaphylactoid reaction in a patient who tested negative for IgE-type anti-tocilizumab antibodies (but who had allergic reactions to aspirin and infliximab), gastrointestinal hemorrhage from diffuse acute or chronic colonic ulceration in a patient with chronic diarrhea, and rectal bleeding. One patient developed infectious mononucleosis, hepatitis, and neutropenia. Another developed herpes zoster while receiving placebo. No cases of reactivated tuberculosis occurred. IgE antibodies were noted in 4 of 10 patients with mild infusion reactions. In the extension phase, 13 serious adverse events occurred, including bronchitis, gastroenteritis, or anaphylactoid reaction. Mild increases of alanine aminotransferase (ALT) (12 subjects) and AST (8 subjects) were reported.

In a double-blind, placebo-controlled study of 112 children with SJIA, there were more adverse events and infections in the tocilizumab-treated subjects than those on placebo in the double-blind phase of the study.[169] Serious adverse events, including serious infections, occurred only in the active drug group. Six deaths occurred (tension pneumothorax, traffic accident, streptococcal sepsis, MAS, and two from pulmonary hypertension). Some physicians do regular echocardiography and/or pulmonary function tests routinely in all of their patients who are on tocilizumab.[170] Significant neutropenia associated with infections and elevated liver transaminases were seen exclusively in patients while on tocilizumab. Elevations in LDL cholesterol were also seen.[169]

Preliminary results of a trial of tocilizumab in polyarticular JIA were recently presented.[171] The safety population comprised 188 patients with 307 patient-years. Rates per 100 patient-years of adverse events and serious adverse events were 406.5 and 11.1, respectively; infections were the most common adverse event (151.4) and serious adverse event (5.2). AT and AST elevations three or more times the upper limit of normal occurred in 6.4% and 2.7% of patients, respectively. Grade 3 neutropenia and grade 2/3/4 thrombocytopenia occurred in 5.9% and 1.6% of patients, respectively. Significant low-density lipoprotein cholesterol elevations occurred in 16.2% of patients.

In adults, hypertension and cerebrovascular accidents have been reported. However, in a pooled analysis of five pivotal trials, major cardiovascular events were associated with age, history of coronary artery disease, and disease activity rather than tocilizumab.[172] Tocilizumab should be used with caution in patients with intestinal ulceration or diverticulitis as peritonitis, gastrointestinal perforation, fistulae, and intraabdominal abscesses have been reported.[27] Subcutaneous tocilizumab studies in children are being planned.

Other IL-6 inhibitors in various stages of development include clazakizumab, sarilumab, and sirukumab.[1]

IL-17 inhibition.

Ustekinumab. Ustekinumab is a fully human IgG1κ monoclonal antibody that binds to the p40 subunit common to IL-12 and IL-23, and prevents its interaction with the IL-12 receptor β1 subunit of the IL-12 and IL-23 receptor complexes. Th17 cells are inhibited by IL-23, but the effects may be related to the effects of IL-12 on Th1 cells as well.[173,174] IL-23 has been shown to drive entheseal inflammation in a rodent model.[175] It is given at a dose of either 45 mg or 90 mg depending on weight, subcutaneously at weeks 0,4, and then every 12 weeks. In a phase III trial in 614 adult with psoriatic arthritis, the incidence of adverse events and serious adverse events was similar in both the active drug and placebo groups. The most common adverse events were nasopharyngitis, upper respiratory tract infection, and headache. Concomitant methotrexate use did not affect the number or type of adverse events. No opportunistic infections including tuberculosis, death or malignancies were reported. Cholecystitis occurred in two patients, salpingitis in one, erysipelas in one, and pharyngolaryngeal abscess in one. Three patients had major cardiovascular events including myocardial infarction and stroke. Injection-site reactions were uncommon and mild in intensity. In a meta-analysis of studies performed in adults with plaque psoriasis, major adverse cardiovascular events occurred more often in patients taking the active drug than for those on placebo.[175]

Other IL-17 inhibitors in development include ixekizumab and secukinumab.[1]

Combination Therapies

A number of factors support the use of combination therapies. In adult RA, single agents seem to lose efficacy over time[176]; furthermore, these agents rarely induce sustained long-term remissions. An increased appreciation of the long-term morbidity of both RA and JIA supports a more aggressive approach to medical management.[177] A better understanding of the mechanisms of action of these agents, as well as well-designed studies of combination therapy in adults that demonstrated efficacy without a significant increase in toxicity, supports the use of this approach. There is a suggestion that the combination of leflunomide and infliximab may also be effective.[178] In addition, the improvement noted with biologic therapy can be enhanced by combining it with MTX,[143,179-181] and the combination of etanercept and MTX may also retard structural damage, opening the door to potential long-term remission.[182] However, one combination of the biologic agents anakinra and etanercept was no more effective than either agent alone, and it was more toxic. In JIA, MTX is usually used together with other biologics with no increase in toxicity.[23,75,183,184] In 59 subjects, the efficacy of infliximab plus MTX was compared with that of MTX alone; or MTX, sulphasalazine, and hydroxychloroquine in combination.[185] Twenty-one serious infections occurred. Of those, 18 events occurred in 13 patients receiving MTX. Gastrointestinal symptoms, nausea, loss of appetite, and weight loss seemed to occur more commonly in the combination group than in the other treatment groups. In another randomized controlled trial of etanercept, methotrexate, and corticosteroids versus methotrexate alone, the combination therapy was well tolerated.[186] Both studies demonstrated that clinically inactive disease was achieved in a significant number of patients. In the Trial of Early Aggressive Therapy in Polyarticular Juvenile Idiopathic Arthritis (TREAT) study, patients treated with etanercept had more time in inactive disease states.[186] Rituximab is approved for the treatment of RA with or without MTX.[187] Rituximab in combination with a TNF inhibitor did not result in more serious infections among subjects with RA.[188] A combination of anakinra and abatacept appeared to be safe and effective in four patients with SJIA.[189] Combination therapy would seem particularly appropriate in cases of severe systemic-onset JIA and in patients with MAS (anakinra and cyclosporine). Important questions remaining to be answered include which patients are most at risk for long-term damage and therefore most likely to benefit from combination therapy; whether therapy should be started in combination or medication should be added only after a partial inadequate response; and whether full or reduced doses of each agent should be used.

Stem-Cell Transplantation

In the past 15 years more than 1500 individuals worldwide have received a hematopoietic stem-cell transplant for treatment of autoimmune disease.[190] The principles behind this treatment are that high-dose myeloablative therapy will destroy the autoreactive clones that initiate the autoimmune process, and the marrow can be repopulated with a "naïve" population of stem cells by demonstrating primary responses to vaccination after myeloablation.[191,192] However, many old memory clones survive but are tolerized.[193] As the immune system

redevelops after transplantation, immune cells may become "tolerized" to the putative antigens that are involved in the autoimmune process. In fact, allogeneic matched bone marrow transplantation for patients with rheumatoid factor (RF)-positive RA and associated aplastic anemia has led to remission of the arthritis. However, the length of the remission varied, from as short as 1 year to as long as 13 years.[194,195]

Allogeneic bone marrow transplantation carries a significant risk of both mortality (15% to 35%) and development of graft-versus-host disease (GVHD). The use of an autologous transplant, from either marrow or peripheral blood stem cells (autologous stem-cell transplantation, or ASCT), reduces the mortality from the procedure to 1% to 5% and is not associated with GVHD. Therefore, high-dose immunotherapy with ASCT has become a preferred method that has been used in treating several autoimmune diseases.

Initial studies in patients with autoimmune diseases and associated malignancies who underwent ASCT showed recurrence of disease within 5 weeks to 1 year.[196] In these initial studies, the "retransplanted" stem cells were not manipulated in either a positive way (selection for CD34-positive stem cells) or a negative way (removal of T cells with potential autoreactivity). Relapses may also have occurred because (1) the putative autoantigens responsible for the disease were not eliminated, (2) the human leukocyte antigen (HLA) status of the host did not change and therefore a predisposition to select arthritogenic peptides and a limited number of T-cell developmental pathways persisted, and (3) autoreactive T cells were not completely eliminated before transplantation.

Studies of ASCT have been described in children with JIA, SLE, and scleroderma, with excellent outcomes in most but not all studies.[197-199] An initial mortality rate of 14% raised significant concerns despite remarkable improvement in some patients.[200]

Wulffraat and associates[201] reported the experience with 31 patients with polyarticular-course JIA (25 systemic-onset, 6 polyarticular-onset) treated with ASCT from eight different European pediatric transplantation centers. Bone marrow cells were transfused in 23 cases, and peripheral stem cells, after harvesting with cyclophosphamide (2 g/m^2) and granulocyte colony-stimulating factor, in 8. T cells were selected for CD34 stem cells by either negative or positive selection techniques. Conditioning included 5 days of antithymocyte antiglobulin (ATG) on days −9 through −6 and cyclophosphamide (50 mg/kg) on days −5 through −2; low-dose total body irradiation (TBI) was given to 21 patients on day −1. Frozen stem cells were thawed and infused on day 0. The neutrophil and platelet counts returned to normal by day 35. *In vitro* mitogenic T-cell responses normalized within 6 to 18 months, and T-cell counts were normal by 5 to 9 months. Seventeen patients had a drug-free period of 8 to 60 months. Mild relapses, which were easy to control, occurred in seven patients. Four patients had no response to ASCT at all, and three patients died—two with MAS (one induced by EBV) and one with disseminated toxoplasmosis. Catch-up growth was seen in younger children but not in older children or in those with long disease duration. All patients developed chills, fever, and malaise during the infusion of ATG. In addition to the two patients who died from infection-related causes, infectious complications were common (varicella zoster in seven patients, atypical mycobacteria in one, and Legionella pneumonia in one). A more detailed study reported on 34 children with JIA (29 systemic, 5 polyarticular) treated in nine different European transplant centers.[202] Eighteen of the 34 patients (53%) with a follow-up of 12 to 60 months achieved complete drug-free remission. Seven of these patients had previously failed treatment with anti-TNF agents. Six of the 34 patients (18%) showed a partial response (ranging from 30% to 70% improvement) and seven (21%) were resistant to ASCT. Infectious complications were common. There were three cases of transplant-related mortality (9%) and two of disease-related mortality (6%). The authors recommended that future protocols include elimination of total body irradiation from the conditioning regimen, prophylactic administration of antiviral drugs, and intravenous immunoglobulins until there was a normal CD4[+] T-cell count, to lessen toxicity. A cohort of 22 children (18 systemic, 4 polyarticular) in three centers, representing a subgroup of the above subjects available for long-term follow-up, were shown to have delayed recovery (greater than 6 months) of CD4[+]CD45RA[+] naïve T cells thought to be responsible for the infectious and MAS complications.[203] Five patients relapsed up to 7 years after ASCT. Four new patients who were treated with a fludarabin-containing regimen instead of low-dose TBI had drug-free remission 4 to 5 years later.[204] Additionally, two patients undergoing allogeneic transplant from HLA-matched family donors had drug-free remission in 1- to 2-year follow-up.[204]

In another study, seven children in the UK initially showed dramatic clinical response and in four this was sustained, allowing withdrawal of immunosuppressive and antiinflammatory treatment, significant catch-up growth, and immense improvement of the quality of life in follow-up of 5 to 8 years after transplant.[205] Two patients relapsed within 1 to 12 months, and one died 4 months after transplant. Complications included fatal adenovirus reactivation, hematophagocytic syndrome secondary to EBV, and cytomegalovirus. It has been recommended that a conditioning regimen include antithymocyte globulin and cyclophosphamide, followed by fludarabine and high doses of steroids and cyclosporine to decrease the incidence of MAS.[206]

ASCT has been shown to alter laboratory abnormalities that reflect the immunologic process, including perforin expression,[201] expression of myeloid-related proteins (MRP8/MRP14),[207] and synovial cellularity and cytokine expression.[208] Encouraging reports from the use of ASCT in patients with SLE[209,210] and systemic sclerosis[211] have led to more than 700 patients (50 children) with autoimmune disease undergoing ASCT,[212] mostly patients with systemic sclerosis (scleroderma), multiple sclerosis, RA, JIA, and SLE. A fewer number of patients have received an allogeneic transplant. The authors observed that overall treatment-related mortality of 7% has since decreased, with no further cases being reported in systemic sclerosis or multiple sclerosis in the last 3 years of follow-up at the time of the report. This improvement is thought to be due to more careful patient selection. Although ASCT has not been curative in patients with RA, the disease seems easier to control with DMARDs after the procedure.[213]

Many questions remain regarding this treatment and the crucial variables in the protocols. The intensive immunotherapy required (high-dose cyclophosphamide ± irradiation ± antithymocyte globulin) may itself result in disease remission, as described in several cases of aplastic anemia and SLE.[214,215] It is not clear whether irradiation is necessary, particularly because it may significantly increase the risk of malignancy; it did not seem to improve the outcome in the 31 patients described by Wulffraat and associates.[201] A protocol that includes fludarabine to spare the need for irradiation appears promising.[201] It is likely that manipulation of the "graft" is required before reinfusion. The number of stem cells required must be defined. Other preconditioning regimens may be more effective.[216] Multipotent mesenchymal stromal cells obtained from the bone marrow and expanded *ex vivo* are immune privileged and apparently of low toxicity; they are thought to provide a positive immunomodulatory effect and may be incorporated into future protocols.[212]

Recent reports suggest the potential of autologous mesenchymal stem cell transplantation (more accurately termed *mesenchymal stromal cells*) derived from various tissues, including bone marrow, placenta, umbilical cord, fat, and teeth.[190,217] The exact mode of action

is unknown, but these cells have adipogenic, osteogenic, and chondrogenic differentiation potential and paracrine-mediated antiinflammatory properties with low toxicity.

If ASCT is ultimately proven to be relatively safe and effective, patient selection will be critical to its success. Patients should be chosen whose disease can be predicted to have a severe outcome but who are not yet at the stage of severe, irreversible damage. The development of prognostic markers is critical for proper selection of candidates. The ethical issues of attempting a procedure with a mortality rate of at least 5% in children with chronic diseases but much lower predicted mortality rates are monumental.[218] The long-term risk of immunosuppression is significant, and safer ways to provide immunosuppression need to be developed.

TARGETED SYNTHETIC THERAPIES/SMALL MOLECULES

Protein phosphorylation plays a fundamentally important role in intracellular signal transduction.[219] We now know that there are over 500 human kinases in 8 families. Both Janus kinase (Jak) and spleen kinase (Syk) are tyrosine kinases and appear to be good targets for treatment of inflammatory diseases.

KINASE INHIBITORS

The Jak-stat system involves three components: a receptor, Jak, a signal transducer and activator of transcription (STAT). The receptor is activated by cytokines, growth factors, and other chemical messengers. This results in Jak autophosphorylation turning "on" and "off" switches on proteins. The STAT protein binds to the phosphorylated receptor, where it is phosphorylated by Jak, then dimerizes with another STAT molecule and translocates into the cell nucleus, where it binds to DNA and promotes transcription of genes.

Tofacitinib. Tofacitinib blocks Jak3, Jak1, and to a lesser extent Jak2. It has selectivity remarkably sparing other kinases, resulting in high specificity compared with others. It blocks IL-2, IL-4, IL-7, IL-9, IL-15, and IL-21, all of which signal through Jak3. It blocks IL-6, IL-11, IFN-α/β, IFN-γ, and IL-10 through Jak1. To a lesser extent it inhibits IL-3, GM-CSF, EPO, and IFN-γ through Jak2.[220] Tofacitinib interferes with the differentiation of IFN-γ, producing Th1 cells and pathogenic Th17 cells.[221,222] Jak inhibition with tofacitinib suppresses arthritic joint structural damage through decreased RANKL production in patients with RA.[223] TNF signaling *per se* is not affected, but it blocks autocrine effects of interferons that mediate TNF effects.

Serious bacterial, mycobacterial, fungal, and viral infections have been reported with tofacitinib and other Jak inhibitors.[219,224-226] Increased dissemination of herpes zoster has also been reported. The half-life is short (Table 13-2), so in the face of a serious infection, discontinuation theoretically results in relatively rapid normalization of immune function. Anemia (in some studies, not in others), thrombocytopenia, neutropenia, hypercholesterolemia (including LDL cholesterol), and increased liver transaminases have been shown to be more frequent in subjects on tofacitinib than those on placebo.[227] There are concerns regarding increased cancer risk and gastrointestinal perforation. Recommendations for use are shown in Table 13-15.

Baracitinib. Baracitinib is a Jak inhibitor that inhibits Jak1/Jak2 and looks promising in the treatment of RA but has side effects, which include anemia, neutropenia, and increased LDL and creatinine. Doses of 4 or 8 mg daily appear to be generally well tolerated. ***Ruxolitinib***, another JAK kinase inhibitor that is used for the treatment of myelofibrosis, has been studied in RA and as a topical treatment in psoriasis.[188]

TABLE 13-15   Guidelines for the Use of Tocilizumab for the Treatment of Systemic and PolyarticularJIA[165]

Dose
Polyarticular Juvenile Idiopathic Arthritis
Weight < 30 kg, 10 mg/kg; >30 kg, 8 mg/kg every 4 weeks
Systemic Juvenile Idiopathic Arthritis
Weight < 30 kg, 12 mg/kg; >30 kg, 8 mg/kg every 2 weeks
Infuse over 1 hour
Document absence of latent or active tuberculosis before starting. Do not give if absolute neutrophil count (ANC) below 2000/mm^3, platelet count below 100,000/mm^3, or ALT or AST above 1.5 times the upper limit of normal (ULN). Do not rechallenge if anaphylactoid or anaphylaxis occur
Lab Monitoring
AST, ALT, ANC at baseline, second infusion then every 2-4 weeks
Lipid panel 4-8 weeks after start of treatment, then every 6 months

Spleen kinase, also known as Syk, is a member of the tyrosine kinase family. Syk transmits signals from the B-cell receptor and T-cell receptor. Syk plays a similar role in transmitting signals from a variety of cell surface receptors including CD74, Fcγ receptor, and integrins. Syk inhibition by fostamatinib has been somewhat disappointing as compared with tofacitinib with regard to efficacy in RA, and significant intolerance including diarrhea, upper respiratory tract infections, neutropenia, and hypertension have been reported.[228-230]

VX-509. A selective Jak3 inhibitor (VX-509) has shown promise in the treatment of RA in a phase IIb trial.[231,232] Its high selectivity for Jak3 may spare Jak1- and Jak2-associated toxicities. The most frequent adverse events were headache, hypercholesterolemia, and nasopharyngitis. Serious infections, mild elevation in liver transaminases, and drops in neutrophil and lymphocyte counts did occur.

PHOSPHODIESTERASE INHIBITOR

Phosphodiesterase-4 (PDE4) is the major enzyme class responsible for the hydrolysis of cyclic adenosine monophosphate (cAMP), an intracellular second messenger that controls a network of proinflammatory and antiinflammatory mediators.[233] Hematopoietic cells controlled by PDE4 include dendritic cells, T cells, macrophages, and monocytes. Mesenchymal cells that express PDE4 include keratinocytes within the dermis, smooth muscle, vascular endothelium, and chondrocytes involved in the structure of the joint. Apremilast is an orally administered targeted PDE4 inhibitor that modulates a wide array of inflammatory mediators involved in psoriasis, psoriatic arthritis, and Behçet's disease, including decreases in the expression of inducible nitric oxide synthase, TNF-α, and IL-23, and increases IL-10.[35,143,234] The most frequent side effects in a phase III trial were nausea, diarrhea, and headache, mostly in patients who were receiving the higher dose (20 mg twice per day vs 40 mg twice per day). There were no consistent laboratory abnormalities associated with its use, and the authors do not suggest routine laboratory monitoring.[234-236]

BIOSIMILARS

A biosimilar is a biotherapeutic product that is similar in terms of quality, safety, and efficacy to an already licensed reference biotherapeutic product, with "similarity" defined as the absence of a relevant difference in the parameter of interest.[3] Pediatric rheumatologists have questioned whether biosimilars will have identical biological functions because even minor modifications in manufacturing may alter biological functions, including pharmacokinetic, immunogenetic, glycosylation, sialylation, stability, safety, and efficacy. Differences in these parameters have the capacity to markedly change affinity, which is the key determinant of the pharmacokinetic and pharmacodynamics profile of mAbs and Cepts, thereby influencing dosing regimens.[3] Current guidelines require only PK equivalence to be demonstrated for generic (nonbiologic) drugs. For biologics, extensive nonclinical physiochemical and biological characterization is required to address structural, functional, and immunogenicity concerns prior to efficacy and safety trials.[237] Currently, clinical data requirements differ in the European Union and United States, but both require randomized clinical trials to demonstrate equivalent safety and efficacy to be demonstrated in the short term. Rare events and long-term safety will be assessed through postmarketing safety surveillance studies.[3] It is unclear how the Best Pharmaceuticals for Children Act and the Pediatric Research Equity Act in the United States will be applied to biosimilars.

Extrapolation of clinical data, which enables approval of a biosimilar for a therapeutic indication in which it has not been clinically evaluated, has been advocated by the FDA and EMA, but almost superimposable biological data must be provided. Extrapolation is unlikely to be approved if the mechanism of action for the biosimilar is unknown.

The FDA will likely classify biosimilars as highly similar or interchangeable with only the latter being allowed to be automatically substituted. Physicians prescribing biosimilars should be hypervigilant in identifying and reporting differences they perceive to the "branded" agent.

REFERENCES

The entire reference list is available online at www.expertconsult .com.

Occupational and Physical Therapy for Children with Rheumatic Diseases

Gay Kuchta, Iris Davidson

The goal of occupational and physical therapy in the treatment of children with rheumatic diseases is to enable them to participate in all the activities of everyday life. Integrating cultural norms and developmental stages, therapists help the child develop, maintain, or restore movement and functional abilities. Efficacy in self-management is the ideal.

Despite significant advances in medical management, children with rheumatic diseases continue to have subclinical inflammation and report ongoing pain, fatigue, and functional impairments.[1-14] Occupational and physical therapists are uniquely placed in the management team to identify and quantify these problems and to educate the child about how to manage these issues.[1]

Optimal treatment of rheumatic diseases of childhood requires early and ongoing intervention by an interdisciplinary team of health professionals.[15-19] As the medical management of rheumatic diseases has evolved, the spectrum of problems dealt with by therapists has changed dramatically. Management of significant joint contractures, muscle weakness and mobility, and self-care challenges are less frequently the focus of treatment. Today's therapist must pay attention to both major and subtle functional challenges in physical, emotional, social, and educational spheres. Although the majority of patients seen have juvenile idiopathic arthritis (JIA), therapists are now involved in the treatment of children with the full spectrum of rheumatic diseases.

Whenever possible, therapy interventions are based on evidence. Often, the limited information from studies in childhood rheumatic diseases must be supplemented by information from adult populations with similar diseases, and by personal experience.[20] Occupational and physical therapists are only two components of the therapeutic team. All members must work closely with each other, and the child and family to provide consistent and comprehensive care.

Ideally, therapy assessment and intervention should occur near the time of diagnosis. Initial assessments identify the child's functional impairments in both physical and psychosocial realms. Their functioning as individuals, within families and in their community, is reviewed.[21] Interventions are triaged and negotiated with the patient and family and are discipline specific.[22] Interventions include nonmedicinal methods of controlling and coping with pain, improvement of joint range, muscle strength and length, activity and functional endurance (Can the patient walk across the street before the light turns red? Can they hold a pen and write without pain for 1 hour?), joint and body mechanics, sleep behaviors, and identification of and compensations for environmental barriers (Box 14-1). Periodic reevaluations should occur throughout the disease course, even during disease remission,

since restrictions of function and functional habits often persist beyond the stage of clinically active disease.

Specific indications that prompt referral to a therapist include symptoms of active disease such as pain, stiffness, and fatigue, or changes in function or participation in social or school activities (Box 14-2). Information that will maximize the effectiveness of a referral includes the child's specific diagnosis, the extent of and any restrictions imposed by systemic involvement, comorbidities, medications, and planned medical interventions (Table 14-1).

SYMPTOM ASSESSMENT AND MANAGEMENT

Many symptoms that affect the child's function are common to all of the rheumatic diseases. The timing of symptom management is determined by the disease and the degree to which it is controlled. The intervention goals in early disease are to minimize symptoms (Box 14-3); as the disease is controlled, the goals and interventions change to maximize and normalize function (Boxes 14-4, 14-5, and 14-6).

Pain Management

Pain is the primary issue leading children and their families to seek medical attention.[23,24] Unresolved pain is the reason the great majority of patients seek complementary and alternative medicines.[25] Although many young children with oligoarthritis frequently do not report pain, 70% of children with polyarticular JIA and 50% of those with connective tissue disease recorded pain in the week prior to questioning.[26-28] Pain affects the quality of life in any disease. Even a small decrease in the visual analog pain scale (1 cm) is correlated with a significant improvement in quality of life.[29] The impact of chronic pain is illustrated in Figure 14-1 and ranges from sleep disturbance to joint contractures and psychosocial and educational disturbances.

In the assessment of the child's pain, it is important to determine and record its parameters (location, duration, intensity, frequency, quality, history, and functional impact on sleep, self-care, play, school, and psychosocial development). Developmentally appropriate outcome measures[30-34] are used as required. Recognition of pain behaviors is important, especially in those children who report no pain verbally. Social aggression, withdrawal from usual social or physical activities, irritability, or abnormal movement patterns can all indicate the presence of pain. The impact of pain on movement, posture, and development of gross and fine motor milestones should also be noted.

Teaching children age-appropriate nonpharmacological pain-modifying techniques increases their sense of control over the pain and decreases their overall pain experience.[24,35] Techniques that the child

BOX 14-1   Areas of Occupational and Physical Therapy Intervention

- Assess and teach pain management
- Assess and document impairments, and develop solutions to findings
- Assess, document, and minimize functional restrictions
- Develop consistent, reliable measures of changes in range, muscle strength and length, and function over time
- Develop, upgrade, and negotiate with the child and family an exercise program to address the identified deficits
- Evaluate and teach coping skills for symptom management
- Reinforce education of disease process and management
- Educate on the continued need and safety of physical activity
- Teach ergonomics
- Identify the need for and refer to vocational counseling
- Provide ongoing patient and family support
- Facilitate integration into school and community
- Advocate for the child with the family, school, and community
- Refer to and liaise with community therapists

BOX 14-2   Indications to Refer to Occupational and Physical Therapy

- Active disease
- Significant morning stiffness
- Avoidance of activity or inability to keep up due to pain or weakness
- Overwhelming fatigue
- Restricted/asymmetric movement
- Marked mood or behavioral change, especially isolation from peers
- Regression of age-appropriate development
- Growth abnormalities
- Reduced school attendance or output (>10 days absence in the past 4 months)
- Change in quality of sleep
- Inability to do normal activities in a timely manner

BOX 14-3   Occupational and Physical Therapy Interventions: Uncontrolled Disease

Goal: Minimize Symptoms

- Direct assessment to address patient's stated problems
- Provide frequent reassessment to monitor changes
- Teach pain management and coping skills
- Teach fatigue management—especially with CTD
- Maintain range, strength, and muscle length using exercises, splinting, and positioning
- Reinforce education on disease management
- Intervene at school with all diagnoses
- Provide adaptive devices as indicated by the child
- Teach sleep hygiene
- Teach coping strategies for systemic symptoms (Raynaud's phenomenon, uveitis)
- OT/PT interventions should be minimal until disease is under some control

BOX 14-4   Occupational and Physical Therapy Interventions: Controlled Disease

Goal: Maximize Function

- Full assessment to identify and monitor persisting deficits and their impact on the body mechanics
- Modify pain and fatigue management techniques
- Improve function in self-care
- Increase range, and muscle strength and length
- Increase participation in family, school, and leisure activities, especially physical activities
- Improve exercise tolerance and balance
- Introduce the concepts of self-image and self-efficacy to child and family
- Review and monitor necessary school interventions
- Teach coping skills such as time management and pacing activities
- Review understanding of disease management as the child matures
- Interventions reviewed every 4 to 12 weeks
- Focus for the majority of patients is a home program, with short, specific exercises (10 minutes)
- "Hands-on" interventions (e.g., serial casting) may require three appointments/week
- Occasionally intensive inpatient rehabilitation is needed
- Identify and retrain faulty movement patterns

BOX 14-5   Occupational and Physical Therapy Interventions: Clinical Remission

Goal: Normal Function

- Semiannual to annual full assessment to determine if physical and psychosocial sequelae of previous issues persist
- Focus on:
  - Abnormal movement patterns
  - Mechanical malalignments
  - Risk-taking behaviors
  - Physical and psychological developmental milestones
- Promote physical and emotional independence
- Work on fine motor control, balance, endurance, power
- Integration/participation in activities, sports, and the community
- Reinforce self-image as a healthy, active individual
- Encourage healthy life choices
- Assess for ongoing pain and fatigue issues

BOX 14-6   Occupational and Physical Therapy Interventions: Ongoing Chronic Disease

Goal: Optimize Function within Limitations

- Full assessments with any disease flares
- Annual assessment to monitor deficits
- Assess and plan for preoperative and postoperative interventions
- Address changing pain patterns
- Consider adaptations to the environment of the home and school
- Teach effective adaptive movement patterns
- Assess the need for and teach the use of mobility aids
- Problem solve to maintain independence in self-care, and participation in leisure and work activities
- Teach pain coping skills such as cognitive behavioral therapy
- Refer to vocational assessment
- Provide documentation for financial support

TABLE 14-1	**Red Flags for Therapy Interventions**
Multiple system involvement	• Activity restrictions imposed by other subspecialties • Degree of impaired vision and functional implications • Central nervous system and cognitive restrictions
Comorbidities	• Psychiatric conditions • Developmental delay
At-risk social situation	• Guardianship issues with restricted access • Ability of family to cope with treatment plan • Ability of family to financially cope with treatment recommendations • Social service involvement
Abnormal imaging or lab results	• Bony changes that limit or determine specific therapeutic interventions • Severe anemia that affects function and therapeutic interventions (pool, aerobic activities) • Uncontrolled disease (overwhelming pain and fatigue) • Joint instability, especially of the cervical spine

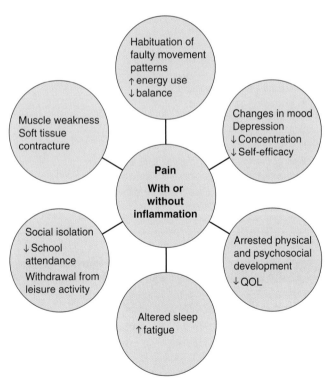

FIGURE 14-1 Impact of pain.

and family can utilize at home are the most useful. These techniques treat pain through peripheral, spinal segmental, supraspinal, and cortical pathways (Chapter 8). The use of thermal modalities, splinting, pacing activities, and ergonomics are particularly suited for home. Heat and cold both reduce pain temporarily. For hot, swollen joints, application of ice over the affected joint until it is erythematous and

numb is recommended. Gentle heat is more effective in reducing muscle spasm and morning stiffness. Superficial joints in the hands and feet often respond better to contrast baths, in which the painful part is alternately submerged in hot and cold water. Thermal modalities must be used with caution and the body's response carefully monitored. Compromised circulation or sensation (e.g., diffuse scleroderma) may contraindicate their use. With rheumatic disease–related Raynaud phenomenon, inappropriate use of thermal modalities can result in tissue damage. Detailed information on thermal interventions and safety issues can be found in the references.[22,36,37] Massage by a parent or caregiver to reduce muscle tension can lessen pain. Massage is particularly useful in desensitizing the affected area in children who have a chronic regional pain syndrome with or without an underlying inflammatory disease. Gentle controlled stretches, performed at home, to both muscular and neural structures can also be used to reduce pain but have not been studied in children with rheumatic diseases.

Specific techniques such as cognitive-behavioral therapy, biofeedback, and electrical modalities can be used on an individual basis as needed. They are only appropriate in older or cognitively competent children who can report responses reliably.

Transcutaneous electrical nerve stimulation (TENS) is useful in treating children with complex regional pain syndromes or localized inflammatory pain (Chapter 52). TENS units can be purchased or rented and parents can be taught to use this modality safely at home. Benefit is established within two treatments in those for whom it is effective. Therapist-applied interferential stimulation is also effective in treating pain. There is some evidence in adults with inflammatory disease[38] that low-level lasers reduce pain and morning stiffness.

Variations of cognitive-behavioral techniques such as controlled breathing, progressive relaxation, visualization, and thought stopping can be used anywhere by the child to gain control over pain, and can be taught to children of all ages.[39] Their effectiveness has been demonstrated in children with JIA,[40,41] and is also useful for children with connective tissue diseases (CTDs) and chronic pain syndromes.[42]

Guidelines for the child's pain management must be disseminated beyond the family to the school-based team and sport/leisure activity coaches. Children are encouraged to continue to participate in leisure activities to the best of their ability and to use changes in their pain levels to indicate when they should temporarily withdraw. Children are often the best judges of their physical limitations, and their decisions should be respected with few exceptions. Activity restrictions imposed because of comorbidities must be adhered to. In the child with JIA, radiographic evidence of cervical instability precludes participation in contact sports. Particular attention should be paid to the child who is involved in high-level competition, as they may feel obliged to continue despite increasing pain and dysfunction. In this instance, the therapist or parent may need to intervene, especially if the child is at risk for injury.

The importance of continued physical activity at an appropriate level needs careful and repeated explanation to both the child and family to ensure that unnecessary constraints are not imposed.[43] Parents are distressed by their child's pain and need mentoring to evaluate if increases in pain are normal responses to increased activity, or a true disease flare. There are numerous advantages of continued involvement in physical activity.[44,45] There is no evidence that exercise results in increased disease activity or damage.

Even after disease control is achieved and pain is no longer a problem, abnormal movement patterns and postures that developed secondary to pain often persist and require a formal retraining program.[6,7] A child's confidence in their body's ability to respond to physical demands may be compromised, and the young child may need encouragement to engage in normal risk behaviors such as jumping and climbing. The older child may require specific physical therapy interventions that target disease-related deficits to successfully return to sports. Sport-specific requirements can be found online.[46] Persistent pain that inhibits function requires reconsideration of the etiology and therapeutic approach.

Fatigue

All rheumatic diseases of childhood are associated with fatigue.[47-50] Some common causes are uncontrolled disease resulting in anemia, pain, nonrestorative sleep,[51,52] antalgic movement patterns requiring increased energy expenditure,[53] depression, poor aerobic fitness, and marked weight gain secondary to corticosteroids. Fatigue is often a silent problem that is poorly recognized but has a major impact on quality of life. The relationship between fatigue, fitness levels, and endurance in rheumatic diseases is not clear.[47] Fatigue issues need to be dealt with early in those children with a diagnosis of systemic lupus erythematosus (SLE), mixed connective tissue disease (MCTD), juvenile dermatomyositis (JDM), or vasculitis because it is often a presenting complaint.

Fatigue can be assessed in a number of ways. Older children can score their fatigue on a verbal or visual analog scale or compare their own energy level to that of their peers or to their pre-illness level. The Kids Fatigue Scale[47,54] is an adapted measurement tool used with children aged 6 to 16. Factors contributing to fatigue can be determined by assessing sleep patterns, looking for abnormal movement patterns or postures, determining endurance for specific activities, and measuring muscle strength. An ergonomic assessment of the home and classroom may indicate environmental contributors to fatigue.

Management of fatigue requires discussion with the child, family, and when appropriate, the school. An understanding of the impact of fatigue on the child's ability to cope with educational demands will aid the school in adapting demands for academic and athletic participation. Ergonomic issues such as the weight of books carried in a backpack, inappropriate seating, the need to climb multiple flights of stairs, and walk long distances between classes all contribute to fatigue. This, in turn, has a negative impact on the child's mood and ability to concentrate. Other issues such as the amount of homework and concurrent assignment deadlines also need discussion. The basic concepts of time management and pacing high- and low-energy activities are introduced to help the child achieve functional goals. Underlying issues that contribute to fatigue must be addressed together with healthy lifestyle coaching.

Nonrestorative Sleep

Sleep disturbances are common at every age and during all disease phases.[49,55]

In the assessment of sleep[22] it is important to know the family norms around sleep times and sleeping arrangements. In the older child and adolescent, inappropriate bedtimes and wake-up times are common, particularly in the child with a pain amplification syndrome. Age-appropriate bedtimes should be encouraged. The interval between bedtime and onset of sleep and the reasons for delay in sleep onset should be determined. The frequency of sleep disruption and the child's subjective evaluation of the quality of sleep should be recorded. Daytime sleepiness and frequency and duration of naps should be monitored; these can indicate a high fatigue level or poor-quality sleep at night. The child's sleeping environment and pre-bedtime activities may contribute to sleep disruptions. Corticosteroids, particularly when given at bedtime, and the use of night splints may interfere with sound sleep.

Activities in the bedroom should be limited to those conducive to initiation of sleep. Bedroom activities that promote restlessness or anxiety (such as doing homework, playing on the computer, or watching television) should be discouraged. Avoidance of foods containing high levels of sugar or caffeine, and limitation of exercise close to bedtime may aid initiation of sleep. In general, vigorous aerobic exercise should be avoided within 2 hours of bedtime. Alterations in the physical environment, such as maintaining a comfortable room temperature and exploring variations in the type and weight of bedcovers and the types and styles of pillows, may make it easier for the child to fall asleep. Judicious use of pillows to decrease weight bearing through painful joints can diminish pain and improve sleep quality. If the child shares the bedroom with others, noise issues and bedtime rituals need to be examined. Cognitive-behavioral techniques similar to those used for pain may be required to reduce anxiety and stress, which can make sleep initiation difficult. Improving sleep patterns is a gradual and prolonged process, often requiring at least a month[30,31] (Fig. 14-2).

Decreased Range of Motion

Restrictions in joint range of motion may reflect intrinsic joint inflammation (increased intraarticular fluid, synovial hypertrophy, pain) or shortening of capsule, ligament, tendon, or muscle.[2,4,56] In children with severe, long-standing joint inflammation, joints may become subluxed or ankylosed, resulting in marked limitation or absence of joint motion. In disorders such as scleroderma, tightening of the periarticular soft tissue leads to joint range restriction. In juvenile dermatomyositis, muscle weakness, atrophy, and disuse may limit functional range of motion. Calcinosis resulting in bony blocks and pain in JDM severely limit motion.

Passive range of motion of all affected joints should be assessed using a goniometer in order to obtain precise and reproducible measurements.[57] Active range should also be recorded when it differs significantly from passive range—for example, when a quadriceps lag exists or there is decreased active finger flexion secondary to tenosynovitis. Particular attention should be paid to the tenodesis effect of muscles that cross two joints, such as the gastrocnemius. If the muscle is on a stretch when joint range is measured, a false "joint restriction" may be recorded. During function, a joint may be restricted due to limitations imposed on it by the overlying short muscles. Normal range of motion varies considerably with age and with each individual, and without knowledge of the normal ranges in each child, the development of minor restrictions can easily be overlooked. Between 8% and 37% of the pediatric population is hypermobile,[58-62] and a decrease in hypermobility may be an important indicator of joint restriction. Loss of hyperextension relative to the opposite side is frequently subtle evidence of a joint effusion in the knee, hip, or elbow. Functional range requirements are related to age and culture. Attention to the quality of movement and the use of compensatory movement patterns is integral to a range assessment. Abnormal motions such as a wrist or knee lateral deviation should also be documented.

A full assessment should be done initially and then at intervals determined by the rate of evolution of the disease and the child's response to therapy. The initial assessment not only defines the extent of the restrictions but establishes a baseline for comparison.

Techniques to improve joint range include active and passive stretching, mobilization, serial casting, and splinting. Most range deficits can be resolved with a specific, active home exercise program. To maximize adherence, this should not exceed 10 minutes per day.[63] Improvements are evident in 4 to 8 weeks. Muscles need retraining to work again in the newly reacquired range. In mildly active or inactive joints with restricted range of motion, passive stretching at end range and mobilizations to gently stretch tight joint capsules[64] are effective.

Functional Implications of Physical Findings (Upper Extremity)

Joint	Physical findings	Functional implications
TMJ 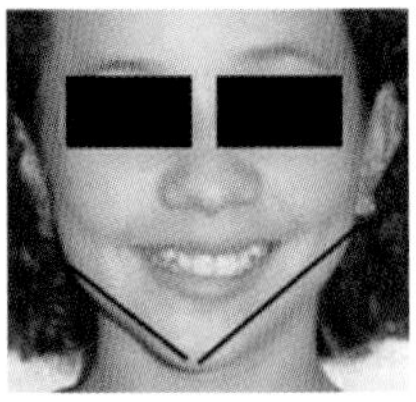	• Unilateral or bilateral TMJ crepitus or pain, resulting in diminished or asymmetric mouth opening and dental malocclusion (open anterior overbite in bilateral disease) • Asymmetric mandibular growth or bilateral undergrowth	• Pain and difficulty biting or chewing • Poor dental hygiene • Sleep disturbance due to pain • Difficulty in intubation for anesthetics • Compromised nutrition • Altered body image with social implications
C Spine 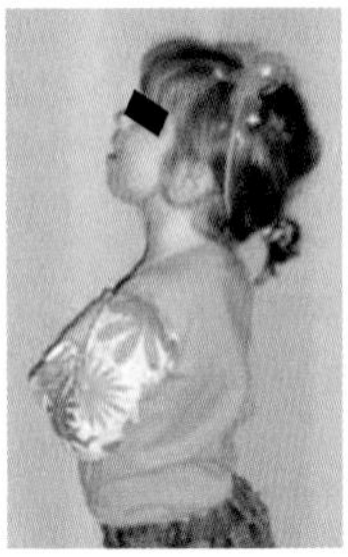	• Range of motion (ROM) decreased in extension (ext) >side flexion (SF)> rotation (rot)> flexion (flex) • Loss of kyphosis and increased lordosis on attempted upward gaze • Atlantoaxial subluxation (rarely symptomatic)	• Impacts on dressing, sleep, school activities (writing, keyboarding, reading, floor sitting, sports, driving, recreation) • No contact sports permitted when C1 and C2 subluxation present • Intubation can be difficult
T Spine and L Spine 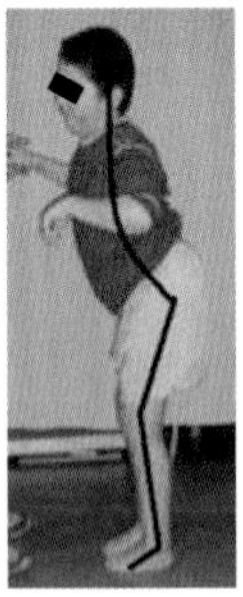	• Poor posture • Limited motion • Marked increase or decrease in thoracic kyphosis +/- scoliosis • Limited thoracic and lumber flexion	• Pain secondary to poor body positioning and mechanics • Abnormal gait • Limited sitting and standing tolerance affect school and leisure activities • Poor sleep
Shoulder 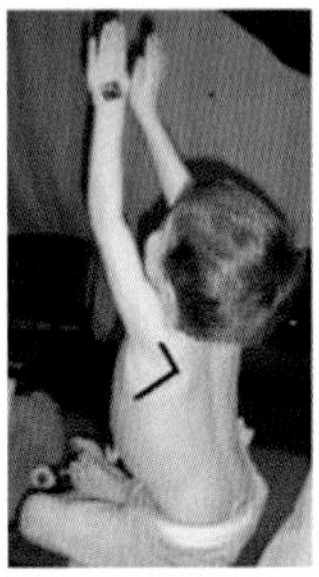 Excessive scapular rotation	• Restricted range leading to adaptive posture or movement patterns secondary to involvement in either glenohumeral, acromioclavicular, or sternoclavicular joints • Weakness/atrophy of rotator cuff muscles and scapular stabilizers	• Donning clothes over head, jackets, bra closures, back packs restricted • Washing/ arranging hair difficult • Sleep disturbance due to increased pain in lying on the side • Any activities that transmit body weight through the joint e.g., climbing frames, crawling, gymnastics, being lifted up by the arms will be affected • Physical education (PE)/ sports that require upper extremity (UE) use will be compromised

FIGURE 14-2 Functional implications of physical findings.

In children with joint restrictions that persist in spite of adequate active exercise and passive stretching, intraarticular corticosteroid injection followed immediately by serial casting in a position of maximal function should be considered. This technique is most effective for contractures at the knees, wrists, elbows, and ankles. Casts are generally changed every 48 hours until a functional range is achieved (i.e., 0° knee extension, 60° wrist extension, 10° ankle dorsiflexion). A bivalved cylindrical cast is worn as a night splint until passive and active ranges are equal. This goal can be obtained in as little as 48 hours or may take as long as 6 months in long-standing deformities. A long-term range and muscle strengthening exercise program is necessary to maintain the gains in range of motion.[65] Tactile or electrical muscle stimulation at end range can be used to regain functional control. When serial casting is ineffective, tendon lengthening or botox injections could be considered. Respecting the child's pain during these interventions improves adherence to the prescribed program and produces faster results.[39] Adaptations to joint restrictions (e.g., rocker bars on shoes, reaching aids) may be required either as a temporary measure during

Functional Implications of Physical Findings (Upper Extremity)

Joint	Physical findings	Functional implications
Elbow	• Flexion deformity (FD) reduces functional length of the arm • Loss of extension and supination most common • Reduced flexion range has the most impact on function • Substitutions by surrounding joints compensate for reduced ROM	• All hand to face activities can be affected (e.g., eating, dental hygiene) • Writing endurance commonly reduced • Carrying even light weights increases pain • Opening doors, especially heavy fire or washroom doors, is difficult • Perineal care may be affected; rarely discussed
Wrists	• Note direction of deviation (ulnar or radial are possible) • Compensatory deviations at the metacarpophalangeal (MCP) joints • Hypomobility or hypermobility in either row of carpal bones • Restricted range • Pain at the end of range • Note abnormal movement patterns	• Most common source of UE disability • Major cause of school issues at all grade levels • Gross and fine motor milestone delay in young children • All sustained UE activities can be affected especially when the dominant side is involved • Grip strength is usually reduced due to wrist posture and pain issues
Hands	• Reduced web space (carpo-metacarpal [CMC] joint of the thumb restricted) • Thumb interphalangeal joint (IP) hypermobility • Reduced tuck and fist positions • MCP flexion loss is common • Proximal interphalangeal joint (PIP) and distal IP extension loss is common • Boutonnière deformity can occur early • Flexor tendon nodules/trigger finger • Tenodesis	• Thumb instability affects prehension in tripod pinch (e.g., buttons, pen, or scissors) • Grasp of large object compromised by CMC restrictions • Trigger finger pain leads to avoidance and UE faulty movement patterns • Delayed developmental milestones if child is unable to explore environment • Reduced dexterity and power affects activities of daily living and self-care • Hand function restrictions have a great impact on school • Hand pain and joint gelling are common causes of sleep disturbance • Perineal care is often affected (seldom reported) • Intimacy can be affected for teens

FIGURE 14-2, cont'd

early or acute disease, or as a permanent intervention for end-stage damaged joints.

Decreased range of motion secondary to muscle shortening is particularly important in children with JDM and scleroderma. This can be seen in all muscle groups but is more pronounced in those muscles crossing two or more joints. Muscles can shorten as a result of the disease process, adaptation secondary to long-term range loss, abnormal posture or movement patterns, or muscle imbalances. Three 30-second stretches, done daily for 2 to 3 weeks, should improve adaptive shortening.[66] Daytime splinting in the stretched position can prevent progression of deformity.[67]

Muscle Weakness

Muscle weakness in children with rheumatic disease may result from muscle tissue disease, pain, disuse, abnormal use, or may develop secondary to adjacent joint inflammation. It is a particularly serious problem for children with JDM, in which muscle weakness may be severe and prolonged.[12,68,69] Generalized muscle wasting and weakness can occasionally be a consequence of the use of high-dose glucocorticoids. Steroid-induced myopathy is predominant in proximal muscles and is usually painless. It can be a confounding factor when assessing patients with JDM, SLE, or vasculitis. Recovery from steroid-induced myopathy can be slow and incomplete.[70]

Functional Implications of Physical Findings (Lower Extremity)

Joint	Physical findings	Functional implications
Hip 	• Loss of extension and internal rotation are most common • Positive Trendelenburg or gluteus medius limp secondary to muscle weakness • Pain on weight bearing • Gait abnormalities	• Compensatory lumbar lordosis with pain • Short stride length • Reduced sitting and walking tolerance • Difficulty climbing stairs • Lower extremity (LE) dressing difficulties • Getting on and off the toilet increases pain • Sitting cross-legged for story time or assembly is difficult • Restricted sexual activity for teens • Impact on ability to continue sports, dance, recreational activities • Increased fatigue
Knee Leg length changes	• Loss of hyperextension • Loss of full flexion • Muscle weakness and wasting • Patellar malalignment • Abnormal gait • Enthesitis • Long bone overgrowth common in JIA • Undergrowth common in linear scleroderma • Scoliosis due to asymmetry of lower extremity (LE) • Changes in posture	• Altered range in adjacent joints • Inability to squat or sit on heels, kneel at school or places of worship • Floor sitting, stairs, rising from ground all difficult • Prolonged sitting in class, movies, airplanes, or car is painful • Difficulty rising due to joint gelling • Self-care related to toileting and showering can be unsafe • Leg length discrepancy $> \frac{1}{8}$" is significant requiring a shoe raise • Increased energy expenditure
Ankle 	• Reduced dorsiflexion > plantar flexion • Tight Achilles tendon • Enthesitis • Tendon sheath inflammation • Muscle wasting • Abnormal gait	• Changes in foot progression angle (in-toe or out-toe) • Shortened stride length • Decreased power for activities such as hopping, jumping, and running • Descending stairs difficult, abnormal patterns common • Early heel rise or no heel strike

FIGURE 14-2, cont'd

Muscle strength should be assessed in all muscle groups. In children with dermatomyositis, muscle weakness is predominantly proximal and usually symmetrical. In 29% to 79% of children with JDM there is weakness of the muscles of respiration and swallowing, which needs specialized assessment.[71] In children with inflammatory joint disease, weakness is usually restricted to muscles affected by the involved joints. In children with systemic scleroderma, weakness of the musculature in the hands may be most evident. In linear scleroderma the muscle tissue underlying the skin lesion is affected.

To obtain reliable, reproducible measures of muscle strength that can be compared over time and between therapists, it is essential that standardized procedures be used. Attention to specific limb positions stipulated in muscle testing methods is essential to ensure reproducibility of results. A 5- or 10-point scale for manual muscle tests is most commonly used, but it is subjective.[72,73] More objective testing devices, such as dynamometers, modified sphygmomanometers, or vigorometers, have age-appropriate norms.[74-77] Functional muscle tests such as the Childhood Myositis Assessment Scale (CMAS) are also age dependent. The CMAS is an efficient, validated outcome measure for monitoring the effects of myositis in children. It has excellent intrarater and interrater reliability, and correlates well with functional abilities as measured with a Childhood Health Assessment Questionnaire (CHAQ), manual muscle testing, and physician global disease assessment.[78-80]

The greatest variable affecting all methods of muscle strength assessment is the child's motivation to exert maximum effort. The degree of effort should be recorded if less than maximum effort is suspected. Loss of muscle bulk is not always consistent with muscle

Functional Implications of Physical Findings (Lower Extremity)

Joint	Physical findings	Functional implications
Subtalar 	• Decreased inversion or eversion • Spontaneous fusion	• Ambulation difficulties on uneven ground (snow, mud, or grass) • Reflex righting mechanism painful and difficult (child falls easily, teen feels vulnerable in crowds) • Inefficient gait patterns increase energy expenditure
Foot and toes 	• Decreased pronation/supination (in conjunction with subtalar motion restriction) • Enthesitis • Decreased extension of MTP1 • Toe deformities (hammer, cock-up) • Dactylitis • Tarsitis	• Ambulation difficulties on uneven ground due to midfoot restriction and pain • Restricted toe off causes decreased stride length on opposite side • Reduces standing tolerance • Avoidance of hopping and running • Antalgic gait • Unable to squat on extended toes
General growth retardation in boy age 12 	• Multiple joint restrictions • Pain limiting motion • Reduced energy for sustained activity • Delayed puberty	• Many difficulties with independence in self-care, work, or leisure • Restricted mobility • Problems with peer pressure, teasing, and social isolation • Limited vocational choices • Interventions in problem solving and coping are required

FIGURE 14-2, cont'd

weakness. In very young children with JIA with sustained joint inflammation, and in those with linear scleroderma, full strength often returns but normal bulk frequently does not.

Aerobic exercise capacity is reduced in children with rheumatic disease when compared with their peers.[81,82] The gold standard for measurement of aerobic capacity is maximal oxygen consumption (VO_2 peak) while on a treadmill or ergonometric bicycle. When this method is not available, the 6- or 9-minute walk test, which measures the distance a child can walk in the prescribed time, is the most commonly used clinical measurement.[83,84] Once a baseline is defined, a child with diminished exercise capacity is instructed to slowly increase the frequency, intensity, type, and duration of moderate to vigorous physical activities. Frequently, a supervised gym program is required to initiate change. Ongoing improvement and maintenance may require a lifestyle change that is supported by the family.[85] Anaerobic capacity is also significantly reduced in children with JIA and CTD.[86,87] The muscle power sprint test[88-90] is a clinical measure of anaerobic capacity.

Assessment of self-care, activities of daily living, and school and leisure activities reflects the impact of pain, weakness, and fatigue on the child. Muscle weakness and decreased endurance can have a direct impact on the ability to participate in activities and may affect self-efficacy. The effort required to keep up can lead to discouragement and mood changes, which in turn can lead to withdrawal from activities.[8] This affects family interactions and expectations. Muscle weakness contributes to fatigue, altered balance, reduced endurance, and vulnerability to physical trauma. For example, teens with significant muscle weakness are at particular risk for injury when negotiating crowded high school hallways. At school, unnecessary physical demands (e.g., climbing three flights of stairs 10 to 15 times a day while carrying a 35-lb backpack) should be minimized.[22] The use of computers with voice recognition and predictive software may be important for the child with significant upper extremity weakness. On rare occasions, mobility aids such as a wheelchair or crutches may be required for generalized weakness.

Physical education teachers and sport coaches need information about the fluctuating nature of rheumatic diseases and the impact of muscle weakness on the child's ability to participate in athletic activities. Subtle strength deficits are particularly evident during endurance activities. Children should be encouraged to participate in physical education activities to the extent of their abilities, but they should be allowed to modify or be excused from participation in activities that are beyond their limit at a particular time. Exercise programs to address specific as well as generalized weakness include a variety of isometric, isotonic, isokinetic, and concentric and eccentric contractions. Muscle strengthening is started as soon as possible. Pain control will improve effective contractions. In children with JDM, the value of early gentle strengthening is supported by recent literature, with no evidence of detrimental effect.[91] Because of the characteristic pattern of muscle weakness in JDM, emphasis is placed on improving core musculature. Neuromuscular electrical stimulation in combination with voluntary contractions may be beneficial in retraining very weak muscles in older children. With all strengthening exercises, muscle substitution and pain should be avoided. Once muscle strength had been regained, balance, agility, higher level skill development, and functional patterns are introduced. Ongoing monitoring is required.

Decreased Function

Normal function can be defined globally as the individual's ability to successfully perform self-care and participate in work or school and leisure activities, and depends on both physical and psychological health.[21] Disruption in either sphere will result in impairment, restrictions or disability. Culture and age-appropriate development determine the norms.

Poor School Attendance and Performance

A primary measure of function in a child with a rheumatic disease is school attendance. School absenteeism has a significant impact on academic achievement[92] and is a major problem for children with rheumatic diseases. School issues are the most common stressors for families, even greater than medication side effects.[93] Common symptoms that affect attendance and classroom participation are pain, fatigue, disrupted sleep, poor concentration, drug side effects (such as weight gain and nausea), and limited mobility. Factors related to treatment, such as medical and therapy appointments, or drug administration, such as hourly eye drops or drug infusions, also contribute to school absences. Physical factors that may affect school attendance and participation include the need for transportation to and from school, the physical environment of the school, and any impediments to access to classrooms, washrooms, activity centers, and recreation facilities.

Early involvement with the school establishes an ongoing collaboration with the staff to alert them to potential issues. Children with systemic CTDs or with pain amplification syndromes are at particular risk for prolonged school absences. Subsequent reentry to school may be difficult academically and socially. It may be complicated by fatigue or by altered body image. An altered physical appearance can also lead to bullying or exclusion. Many children benefit from having an individual education plan early in their disease to allow the staff more flexibility in implementing change. Elevator access, an extra set of textbooks, or the use of a laptop computer may be required. Documentation provided by the therapist will support these changes.

The school staff needs to understand the child's physical and psychological challenges, and the possible safety issues (fracture risk in children with osteoporosis, disease flare due to sun exposure in children with SLE or JDM, and potential tissue damage with cold exposure for children with Raynaud phenomenon). If the child is required to take medications during school hours, discussion with the teacher is necessary, and a plan for the safe storage and administration of medications should be put in place. Teachers frequently identify a change in the child's ability to concentrate. This may reflect pain or a medication side effect. In children with SLE who have a high risk of neuropsychiatric syndromes, a change in ability to concentrate may also indicate a change in disease activity.[94,95] A marked change in concentration should be reported to the rheumatologist. Therapists can teach coping skills to minimize the impact, but a formal psychoeducational assessment is often useful to identify specific problem areas to the school-based team.

Restricted Self-Care

Self-care refers to the age-appropriate activities such as eating, dressing, hygiene, cooking, household chores, and shopping. Pain, reduced muscle strength, joint range, balance, and endurance affect the child's ability to engage in self-care activities in a timely manner. In children with inflammatory joint disease, morning stiffness affects the duration of self-care routines. The timing of medications can make a significant impact on morning activities. A hot shower or bath on first awakening may reduce this stiffness. Additional pain medication may also be of benefit.

A careful history from the child and parent, and observation of the child engaging in self-care activities is useful in determining the degree of difficulty. Validated outcome measurement tools such as the CHAQ, Juvenile Arthritis Functional Assessment Scale, and Juvenile Arthritis Functional Status Index[96,97] are useful in quantifying self-care limitations and allowing comparisons over time.[22,98] However, these measures are not always sensitive to individual patient restrictions (see Chapter 7).

Interventions to improve self-care include improving range of motion, muscle strength, balance, and endurance, and providing alternative techniques or aids and adaptations. Adherence to exercises is better if improvement affects functional abilities that are important to the child.

Inability to Maintain Leisure Activities

Play is the work of childhood and its value to children's physical and psychological development cannot be underestimated.[43] Play activities can be divided into three broad categories: quiet recreation, active recreation, and socialization.[99] All three categories should be included in the patient assessment.

Children with a rheumatic disease have a variety of barriers to play and leisure activities either directly or indirectly related to their disease. These activities are often restricted by pain, decreased range of motion or muscle strength, fatigue, and the time limitations imposed by medical appointments and exercise programs. Discussion with the family and child about the importance of balance between work and play is an ongoing part of therapy. Long-term restrictions to play and leisure can lead to arrested skill acquisition and development, and limit the opportunity to build social relationships.[43] It may be necessary to advocate on behalf of the child with coaches, teachers, and the family to facilitate the child's continued involvement in valued activities. Therapeutic interventions such as exercises should enhance play and leisure activities not replace them. Conversely, play and sport do not eliminate the need for a targeted exercise program.

Decreased Mobility

Impaired mobility results from deficits in one or more of six dimensions: flexibility, strength, accuracy, speed, adaptability, and endurance.[100,101] Pain and inflammation of joints or muscles affects all dimensions. A thorough assessment of each dimension takes into account physical, social, psychological, and environmental factors. Treatment is driven by assessment findings (Box 14-7). Lower-limb retraining for persistent abnormal movement patterns is particularly effective when carried out in a warm pool. The warmth and buoyancy decreases pain and improves flexibility, allowing more normal movement. Splints and orthotics are used to protect, restore, or improve function by reducing pain from the inflammatory process, supporting joints, or correcting alignment.[5] In adults, persistent malalignment is associated with the early onset of secondary osteoarthritis,[102] and it is

---

BOX 14-7 Functional Assessment of Decreased Mobility

Activities are:
- Observed and discussed
- Sustained for a functional length of time

Look for:
- Activities limited by pain
- Completed in a timely manner (walk across a major road with traffic lights)
- Compensations secondary to loss of flexibility or strength:
  - LE examples: Gower or Trendelenburg signs, foot pivot on stair edge
  - UE examples: Weight bearing through MCPs rather than a flat palm, shoulder abduction to augment forearm pronation
- Quality of movement (coordination, symmetry, control)
- Balance
- Functional endurance (able to write for a full exam period)
- Accuracy in fine and gross motor activities

Upper Extremity
- Weight bearing on flat palms
- Reach above head with elbows extended
- Hold a pencil/pen and write for 5 minutes pain free
- Cut with a knife and fork; hold chopsticks
- Lift and pour from a large pitcher into a glass
- Pick up and hold several coins and receive change
- Put on a backpack
- Don and doff a T-shirt, shoes, and socks

Lower Extremity
- Walk a minimum of 50 feet (6-9 minutes preferred)
- Run a minimum of 50 feet
- Hop on one foot or two, depending on age
- Tiptoe walk
- Heel walk
- Climb a minimum of 16 stairs
- Squat with buttocks touching heels
- Sit on floor and return to standing
- Don and doff shoes and socks

---

likely also true in children. This reinforces the need to minimize malalignments and abnormal movement patterns in children.

The need for splinting has diminished dramatically in recent years because of earlier and more effective disease control. Well-designed prefabricated splints are less expensive than custom-made splints and are often more acceptable to teens as their peers associate splints with sports injuries. Splints are usually required only on a temporary basis during flares. However, custom-made splints are better when long-term use is required. Detailed assessment of the foot and ankle will determine if a prefabricated or custom orthoses will improve lower-limb pain and alignment. In conjunction with shoes with a strong heel counter—which provides 50% of the orthotic efficacy—this intervention can improve function and quality of life.[4,103-105]

EFFECTS OF UVEITIS ON FUNCTION

Children with JIA are susceptible to uveitis, which can lead to impaired vision.[106,107] Initial treatment of uveitis usually requires the use of topical corticosteroids, sometimes given as frequently as hourly; this may prevent the child from attending school and interfere with the parents' ability to go to work. Restricted vision may impair safe mobility, lead to poor school performance and social isolation, or precipitate

disruptive behavior at school or home. Attention to the effects of impaired vision on function may identify problems that require referral to a team specialized in vision loss at school or in a health care facility.[108]

Long-Term Considerations
Patient and Family Education

Ongoing education of the child and family underpins all treatment and is the domain of practice of all team members. Families often have misconceptions about rheumatic diseases and face a barrage of advice from well-meaning but often ill-informed friends and relatives. Direction to good information sources helps the child and parents make informed choices about therapy (e.g., websites such as www.printo.it/pediatric-rheumatology/; www.kidswitharthritis.org; www.arthritis.org; www.niams.nih.gov; www.arthritis.ca; www.rheumatology.org.au). It is important that the advice provided by all members of the team is consistent and given in lay language.[109] Education has been shown to improve family coping and reduce stress.[1,110]

Transition

Transition is defined as the "purposeful, planned movement of adolescents and young adults with chronic physical and mental conditions from a child-centered to adult-oriented health care system."[111] The timing of transition is determined, at least in part, by the local health care system and can occur at various times from 13 to18 years of age. The skills necessary for a successful transition are introduced at diagnosis and updated as the child matures.[8,9,112,113]

The goal of transition is to help the child or young adult become more independent in managing health care needs and to assume adult roles such as student, worker, friend, partner, homemaker, and parent. Assessment of physical status and performance of activities of daily living, with the goal of independent living, is critical at this age. Educational and vocational goals should be identified.[114] Specific assessments such as driver training or vocational aptitude are arranged as needed.[115] Documentation of physical limitations and their functional impact may be required to obtain financial assistance for postsecondary education or income assistance. During adolescence, parental supervision of treatment is slowly withdrawn. Responsibility for care is shifted to the young adult. Adherence to recommendations in this stage is variable and compromised by the child's need for autonomy. Adolescents often need coaching in self-management and organizational skills.[116] Parental anxiety about their child's emerging independence must be addressed. The therapist often acts as an advocate for the child within the family. The team member with whom the adolescent is most comfortable should address issues around sexuality. Adolescents have identified continuity of staffing as an important issue for them during the period of transition.[117]

A retreat or camp experience can be a powerful learning environment for both patients and staff. For staff, a retreat is a chance to experience firsthand what it is like to live with a rheumatic disease. In this setting campers witness positive coping skills modeled by both peer counselors and young adults with similar diagnoses and shared experiences. Transition skills are a focus of the camp, and activities integrate education and fun. Campers report feeling less isolated following attendance at a camp as they form new, valued friendships. Knowledge of their disease has been shown to improve significantly as a result of the experience.[118-120]

End-Stage Disease

In children with JIA who have joint damage (end-stage disease), pain secondary to damaged joints is one of the major residual problems requiring occupational and physical therapy.[121] All pain techniques should be reviewed. Splinting for pain is most useful at this stage of the disease. Uncontrolled pain with loss of function is an indication for surgical intervention, especially joint replacement.[122] Joint replacement is very seldom required in children or adolescents, but when indicated it is essential that the patient be psychologically and physically prepared for the procedure. Preoperatively, the patient should become familiar with the postoperative protocol and learn skills such as the use of walking aids or one-handed self-care devices as needed. Occasionally, in order to prepare the child for the rigors of postoperative care, intensive preoperative therapy is required. For example, upper body strength and range may need improvement to allow for effective crutch walking after surgery. A coordinated plan between the surgical and rehabilitation teams is necessary to ensure best results.[123] An intensive postoperative therapy program is often required to maximize the benefits of the surgical intervention.[124]

Despite end-stage disease, children should be expected to progress developmentally toward independent living. To this end, the use of accommodative splinting, compensatory movement patterns to overcome the effects of permanent deformities, adaptive equipment, power mobility, and modifications to the home environment or arrangement of housing designated for people with disabilities should be considered.

Social isolation can be a major problem for the young adult with limited mobility or vision. The ability to drive a car can enhance community access. A driving assessment, driving instruction, and possession of a pass for designated parking areas may be appropriate. A 180° rear view mirror can enhance safety when neck range is compromised. For others, public transportation passes, power mobility, or the acquisition of an assistance or guide dog will improve mobility within the community. The major aim of the rehabilitative process at this stage is to foster independent living. The patients will need to advocate for themselves, so they are socially and psychologically capable of living independently. This may require coaching. Connecting adolescents with others who have overcome similar issues is often helpful. This can be done through groups or social media following consent from both patients and their families. Interventions should be patient driven, time limited, and goal oriented to optimize long-term function. The focus should be on the child's abilities rather than disabilities.

SUMMARY

Recent changes in medical management have led to a paradigm shift in focus for therapists. However, long-term outcome studies show that despite marked improvements in disease control, children continue to report suboptimal health-related quality of life.[8-10,12,125-132] This important area is the focus of occupational and physical therapy as part of a comprehensive team approach for the treatment of children with rheumatic disease.

REFERENCES

1. A. Tong, J. Jones, J. Craig, D. Singh-Grewal, Children's experiences of living with juvenile idiopathic arthritis: a thematic synthesis of qualitative studies, Arthritis Care Res. 64 (2012) 1392–1404.
2. A. Brown, R. Hirsch, T. Laor, et al., Do patients with juvenile idiopathic arthritis in clinical remission have evidence of persistent inflammation on T3 magnetic resonance imaging? Arthritis Care Res. 64 (2012) 1846–1854.
4. G.J. Hendry, J. Gardner-Medwin, M.P.M. Steultjens, et al., Frequent discordance between clinical and musculoskeletal ultrasound examinations of foot disease in juvenile idiopathic arthritis, Arthritis Care Res. 64 (2012) 441–447.
5. S.M. Tupper, A.M. Rosenburg, P. Pahwa, J.N. Stinson, Pain intensity variability and its relationship with quality of life in youth with juvenile idiopathic arthritis, Arthritis Care Res. 65 (2013) 563–570.
6. S. Ringold, T.M. Ward, C.A. Wallace, Disease activity and fatigue in juvenile idiopathic arthritis, Arthritis Care Res. 65 (2013) 391–397.
9. L. Haverman, M.A. Grootenhuis, J.M. van den Berg, et al., Predictors of health-related quality of life in children and adolescents with juvenile idiopathic arthritis: results from a web based survey, Arthritis Care Res. 64 (2012) 694–703.
10. M.T. Apaz, C. Saad-Magalhaes, A. Pistorio, et al., Health related quality of life of patients with juvenile dermatomyositis: results from the paediatric rheumatology international trials organisation multinational quality of life cohort study, Arthritis Care Res. 61 (2009) 509–517.
13. M.H. Bromberg, M. Connelly, K.K. Anthony, et al., Self-reported pain and disease symptoms in juvenile idiopathic arthritis despite treatment advances, Arthritis Rheum. 66 (2014) 462–469.
20. S. Klepper, Exercise and fitness in children with arthritis: evidence of benefits for exercise and physical activity, Arthritis Care Res. 49 (2003) 435–444.
22. G. Kuchta, I. Davidson, Occupational and Physical Therapy for Children with Rheumatic Diseases, Radcliffe, Oxford, 2008.
27. J.E. Weiss, N.J.C. Luca, A. Boneparth, J. Stinson, Assessment and Management of Pain in Juvenile Idiopathic Arthritis, Pediatr Drugs 16 (2014) 473–481.
28. M.H. Bromberg, M. Connelly, K.K. Anthony, et al., Self-reported pain and disease symptoms persist in juvenile idiopathic arthritis despite treatment advances, Arthritis Rheum. 66 (2014) 462–469.
29. S. Dhanani, J. Quenneville, M. Perron, et al., Minimal difference in pain associated with change in quality of life in children with rheumatic disease, Arthritis Care Res. 47 (2002) 501–505.
33. J.W. Varni, K.L. Thompson, V. Hanson, The Varni/Thompson Pediatric Pain Questionnaire. 1. Chronic musculoskeletal pain in juvenile rheumatoid arthritis, Pain 28 (1987) 27–38.
35. F. Zeidan, K.T. Martucci, R.A. Kraft, et al., Brain mechanisms supporting the modulation of pain by mindfulness meditation, J. Neurosci. 31 (2011) 554–5548.
42. K.K. Anthony, L.E. Shanberg, Pediatric pain syndromes and management of pain in children and adolescents with rheumatic diseases, Pediatr. Clin. N. Am. 52 (2005) 611–639.
44. J. Philpott, K. Houghton, A. Luke, Physical activity recommendations for children with specific health conditions: juvenile idiopathic arthritis, hemophilia, asthma and cystic fibrosis, Paediatr. Child Health 15 (2010) 213–218.
45. T. Takken, M. Van Brussel, R.H. Engelbert, et al., Exercise therapy in juvenile idiopathic arthritis: a Cochrane review, Eur. J. Phys. Rehabil. Med. 44 (2008) 287–297.
47. K.M. Houghton, L.B. Tucker, J.E. Potts, et al., Fitness, fatigue, disease activity, and quality of life in pediatric lupus, Arthritis Care Res. 59 (2008) 534–537.
49. Y.B. Aviel, R. Stremler, S.M. Benseler, et al., Sleep and fatigue and the relationship to pain, disease activity and quality of life in juvenile idiopathic arthritis and juvenile dermatomyositis, Rheumatology 50 (2011) 2051–2060.
50. S.B. Sandusky, L. McGuire, M.T. Smith, et al., Fatigue: an overlooked determinant of physical function in scleroderma, Rheumatology 48 (2009) 165–169.
68. M.O. Harris-Love, J.A. Shader, D. Koziol, et al., Distribution and severity of weakness among patients with polymyositis, dermatomyositis and juvenile dermatomyositis, Rheumatology 48 (2009) 134–139.
71. L.J. McCann, S.M. Garay, M.M. Ryan, et al., Oropharyngeal dysphagia in juvenile dermatomyositis (JDM): an evaluation of videofluoroscopy swallow study (VFSS) changes in relation to clinical symptoms and objective muscle scores, Rheumatology 46 (2007) 1363–1366.
73. L.G. Rider, D. Koziol, E.H. Giannini, et al., Validation of manual muscle testing and a sub-set of eight muscles for adult and juvenile inflammatory myopathies, Arthritis Care Res. 62 (2010) 465–472.

76. V. Mathiowetz, D.M. Wiemer, S.M. Federman, Grip and pinch strength norms for 6 to 19 year-old, Am. J. Occup. Ther. 40 (1986) 705–711.

80. A.M. Huber, B.M. Feldman, R.M. Rennebohm, et al., Validation and clinical significance of the childhood myositis scale for assessment of muscle function in juvenile idiopathic inflammatory myopathies, Arthritis Rheum. 50 (2004) 1595–1596.

85. O.T.H.M. Lelieveld, W. Armbrust, M.A. van Leeuwen, et al., Physical activity in adolescents with juvenile idiopathic arthritis, Arthritis Care Res. 59 (2008) 1379–1384.

91. S.M. Maillard, R. Jones, C.M. Owens, et al., Quantitative assessment of the effects of a single exercise session on muscles in juvenile dermatomyositis, Arthritis Care Res. 53 (2005) 558–564.

96. S.E. Klepper, Measures of pediatric function: The Child Health Assessment Questionnaire (CHAQ), Juvenile Arthritis Functional Assessment Report (JAFAR), Juvenile Arthritis Functional Assessment Scale (JAFAS), Juvenile Arthritis Functional Status Index (JASI), and Pediatric Orthopedic Surgeons of North America (POSNA) Pediatric Musculoskeletal Functional Health Questionnaire, Arthritis Care Res. 49 (2003) S5–S14.

98. H.A. Van Mater, J.W. Williams Jr., R.R. Coeytaux, et al., Psychometric characteristics of outcome measures in juvenile idiopathic arthritis, Arthritis Care Res. 64 (2012) 554–562.

105. G.J. Hendry, D. Rafferty, R. Barn, et al., Foot function is well preserved in children and adolescents with juvenile idiopathic arthritis who are optimally managed, Gait Posture 38 (2013) 30–36.

107. S.D. Anesi, C.S. Foster, Importance of recognizing and preventing blindness from juvenile idiopathic arthritis, Arthritis Care Res. 64 (2012) 653–657.

108. <www.uveitis.org>, (accessed January 2014).

112. J.E. McDonagh, Young people first, juvenile idiopathic arthritis second: transition care in rheumatology, Arthritis Care Res. 8 (2008) 1162–1170.

114. A. Malviya, S.P. Rushton, H.E. Foster, et al., The relationship between adult juvenile idiopathic arthritis and employment, Arthritis Rheum. 64 (2012) 3016–3024.

115. L.B. Tucker, D.A. Cabral, Transition of the adolescent patient with rheumatic disease: issues to consider, Pediatr. Clin. North America 52 (2005) 641–652.

119. G. Kuchta, C.J. Green, S.E. Ramsey, et al., Effectiveness of a three day residential educational retreat for children enrolled in a pediatric arthritis program, Arthritis Care Res. 12 (1999) S11–S919.

129. M.T. Apaz, C. Saad-Magalhaes, A. Pistorio, et al., Health-related quality of life of patients with juvenile dermatomyositis: results from the Pediatric Rheumatology International Trials Organisation multinational quality of life cohort study, Arthritis Care Res. 61 (2009) 509–517.

131. J.R.D. Robinson, A. Guilard, M. Schoenwetter, et al., Impact of systemic lupus erythematosus on health, family and work: the patient perspective, Arthritis Care Res. 62 (2010) 266–273.

The entire reference list is available online at www.expertconsult.com

15 | CHAPTER

Juvenile Idiopathic Arthritis

Ross E. Petty, Ronald M. Laxer, Lucy R. Wedderburn

Arthritis is one of the most common chronic diseases of children and youth, and an important cause of short- and long-term disability. There are many causes of chronic arthritis, but the most common are those grouped under the name *juvenile idiopathic arthritis*. Specific information about each category of chronic arthritis is provided in individual chapters. The purpose of this chapter is to summarize general information that relates to all categories of JIA.

CLASSIFICATIONS OF CHRONIC CHILDHOOD ARTHRITIS

Chronic arthritis in childhood is a complex area of study not least because of inconsistencies of classification. Since its introduction in 1995, the term *juvenile idiopathic arthritis* (JIA) has largely supplanted the terms *juvenile chronic arthritis* (JCA) and *juvenile rheumatoid arthritis* (JRA). However, it is necessary to understand the earlier classifications to interpret the older literature on the subject.

In the 1970s, two sets of criteria were proposed to classify chronic arthritis in childhood: those for JRA, developed and later validated by a committee of the American College of Rheumatology (ACR),[1] and those for JCA, published by the European League Against Rheumatism (EULAR).[2] Inconsistencies between these two classifications led to confusion, and a classification proposed[3] and revised[4,5] by the Task Force for Classification Criteria of the Pediatric Standing Committee of the International League of Associations for Rheumatology (ILAR) sought to provide an internationally agreed system of definitions to further the study of childhood arthritis. These three consensus-based classifications are compared in Table 15-1.

ACR Criteria for Classification of Juvenile Rheumatoid Arthritis

The ACR criteria (Box 15-1)[1,6-8] defined an age limit in children, the duration of disease necessary for a diagnosis, and the characteristics of the arthritis and extraarticular disease. The requirement that age at onset of arthritis be less than 16 years is based more on practice patterns than on age-related biological variation in disease. Furthermore, although persistent objective arthritis in one or more joints for 6 weeks is sufficient for diagnosis, a disease duration of at least 6 months is required before the onset type can be confirmed (unless characteristic systemic features are present). When classification depends on the

number of inflamed joints, each joint is counted separately, except for the joints of the cervical spine, carpus, and tarsus; each of these structures is counted as one joint. An affected joint is defined as one with limitation of range of motion with evidence of past or current inflammation (warmth, swelling, pain on motion, or tenderness). Joint swelling or effusion is sufficient to define an actively inflamed joint. The criteria for affected joints are based on physical examination, not imaging.

EULAR Criteria for the Classification of Juvenile Chronic Arthritis

The term *juvenile chronic arthritis* was proposed by EULAR in 1977 for the heterogeneous group of disorders that present as chronic arthritis in childhood of unknown cause (Box 15-2).[2] These criteria differed from the ACR criteria in three ways: (1) arthritis must have been present for at least 3 months (instead of 6 weeks); (2) juvenile ankylosing spondylitis (JAS), psoriatic arthropathy, and arthropathies associated with inflammatory bowel disease are included as separate categories; (3) the term *juvenile rheumatoid arthritis* was applied only to children with arthritis and rheumatoid factor (RF) positivity.

ILAR Criteria for the Classification of Juvenile Idiopathic Arthritis

In 1995, the Classification Taskforce of the Pediatric Standing Committee of ILAR proposed a classification of the idiopathic arthritides of childhood (Box 15-3). This classification[3] and its subsequent revisions[4,5] were developed by consensus with the aim of achieving homogeneity within disease categories to better facilitate clinical and basic research, and to eliminate inconsistencies resulting from the use of the ACR and EULAR classifications. Like its predecessors, this classification system applies to children under the age of 16 years and is based on disease expression during the first 6 months of disease. It differs, however, in the application of exclusion criteria that eliminate overlap and improve homogeneity within the six subtype categories. The designation "undifferentiated arthritis" includes conditions that either do not meet criteria for any other category or meet criteria for more than one category. These criteria have been virtually universally adopted and are the subject of a number of studies.[9-33] They were intended to be modified on the basis of emerging evidence regarding pathogenesis and disease course. Differences in nomenclature require that care be

TABLE 15-1 Comparison of EULAR, ACR, and ILAR Criteria for Classification of Chronic Arthritis of Childhood

CHARACTERISTIC	ACR	EULAR	ILAR
Onset types	3	6	6
Course subtypes	9	None	1
Age at onset of arthritis	<16 yr	<16 yr	<16 yr
Duration of arthritis	6 wk	3 mo	6 wk
Includes JAS	No	Yes	Yes
Includes JPsA	No	Yes	Yes
Includes inflammatory bowel disease	No	Yes	No
Other diseases excluded	Yes	Yes	Yes

BOX 15-2 Criteria for a Diagnosis of Juvenile Chronic Arthritis

1. Age at onset <16 years
2. Arthritis in one or more joints
3. Duration of disease 3 months or longer
4. Type defined by characteristics at onset:
   a. Pauciarticular: <5 joints
   b. Polyarticular: >4 joints, rheumatoid factor negative
   c. Systemic: arthritis with characteristic fever
   d. Juvenile rheumatoid arthritis: >4 joints, rheumatoid factor positive
   e. Juvenile ankylosing spondylitis
   f. Juvenile psoriatic arthritis

From EULAR Bulletin 4, Nomenclature and classification of arthritis in children, National Zeitung AG, Basel, 1977.

BOX 15-1 Criteria for the Classification of Juvenile Rheumatoid Arthritis

1. Age at onset <16 years
2. Arthritis (swelling or effusion, or presence of two or more of the following signs: limitation of range of motion, tenderness or pain on motion, and increased heat) in one or more joints
3. Duration of disease: 6 weeks or longer
4. Onset type defined by type of disease in first 6 months:
   a. Polyarthritis: ≥5 inflamed joints
   b. Oligoarthritis (pauciarticular disease): <5 inflamed joints
   c. Systemic onset: arthritis with characteristic fever
5. Exclusion of other forms of juvenile arthritis

Modified from J.T. Cassidy, J.E. Levinson, J.C. Bass, et al., A study of classification criteria for a diagnosis of juvenile rheumatoid arthritis, Arthritis Rheum. 29 (1986) 274–281.

BOX 15-3 Proposed Classification Criteria for Juvenile Idiopathic Arthritis: Durban, 1997

1. Systemic
2. Oligoarthritis
   a. Persistent
   b. Extended
3. Polyarthritis (rheumatoid factor negative)
4. Polyarthritis (rheumatoid factor positive)
5. Psoriatic arthritis
6. Enthesitis-related arthritis
7. Undifferentiated arthritis
   a. Fits no other category
   b. Fits more than one category

From R.E. Petty, T.R. Southwood, J. Baum, et al., Revision of the proposed classification criteria for juvenile idiopathic arthritis: Durban, 1997, J. Rheumatol. 25 (1998) 199–1994.

taken in interpreting the literature because the terms *JRA*, *JCA*, and *JIA* are often incorrectly used as if they were synonymous.

Criteria for Classification of Spondyloarthropathies

Wright and Moll[34] introduced the concept of the seronegative spondyloarthritis, a grouping of a number of chronic arthritides on the basis of seronegativity for RF, absence of rheumatoid nodules, a tendency to family history of similar diseases, and the frequent involvement of the sacroiliac joints and lumbosacral spine. The later discovery of the association of the human leukocyte antigen HLA-B27 with these diseases further strengthened the legitimacy of the association. Included in the group were ankylosing spondylitis (AS), psoriatic arthritis, reactive arthritis, inflammatory bowel disease, JCA, Whipple disease, Behçet syndrome, and acute anterior uveitis. Currently, the spondyloarthritis concept includes AS, psoriatic arthritis, reactive arthritis, and the arthritis of inflammatory bowel disease. Ankylosing spondylitis is the prototype of the spondyloarthritides, and the other members are quite heterogeneous; some have a strong similarity to AS, others do not, especially in childhood. Criteria[35] for the classification of AS require the presence of radiographic evidence of sacroiliitis as well as a history of pain at the lumbosacral junction or lumbar spine, restriction in range of motion of the spine and limitation of chest expansion. These criteria have limited utility in diagnosing or classifying early disease, or in diagnosing children with AS. Many patients who have some characteristics of AS but do not meet the diagnostic criteria for AS are included in the spondyloarthropathies as defined by Amor

et al.[36] or the European Spondylitis Study Group (ESSG).[37] The ESSG criteria have been studied in children.[38] Children who fall within the category of spondyloarthropathy include those who, by the ILAR criteria, have enthesitis-related arthritis (ERA), or juvenile psoriatic arthritis (JPsA). (See discussions in Chapters 19 and 20). The ESSG criteria also include children with arthritis associated with inflammatory bowel disease, a category not included in the ILAR criteria. There is no question that children with these diseases sometimes have or will develop sacroiliitis, and sometimes they are HLA-B27 positive, but the majority do not have these characteristics and differ significantly from each other clinically. For these reasons the ILAR criteria categorize each separately. The reader is referred to the thoughtful commentary by Colbert.[39]

A Critique of the ILAR Criteria

The ILAR criteria have fulfilled their purpose of providing a common language for investigation and communication concerning chronic childhood arthritis of unknown cause. Some of the parameters of the ILAR criteria are entirely arbitrary in order to retain some continuity with the ACR and EULAR criteria: the age at onset is limited to children under the age of 16; the disease duration (6 weeks), the duration of the onset period (6 months, consistent with the ACR criteria); the number of inflamed joints (less than 5 or greater than 4) that defines

BOX 15-4   **The Yamaguchi Criteria for Diagnosis of Adult Onset Still's Disease**

Major Criteria
  Fever of 39°C of higher, lasting 1 week or longer
  Arthralgia lasting 2 weeks or longer
  Typical rash (nonpruritic macular or maculopapular salmon colored over
    trunk or extremities while febrile)
  Leukocytosis (10,000/mm^3 or greater with 80% or more neutrophils)
Minor Criteria
  Sore throat
  Lymphadenopathy and/or splenomegaly
  Liver dysfunction
  Negative tests for ANA and RF
Exclusions
  Infections, malignancies, and rheumatic diseases

Adapted from Kumar et al.[41]
Diagnosis is made if there are five or more criteria, including at least two major criteria.

oligoarticular and polyarticular JIA, respectively. Inflamed joints are defined clinically, whereas many studies have demonstrated that ultrasound or magnetic resonance imaging are superior to clinical examination for the documentation of joint inflammation.

Systemic JIA. The question arises as to whether systemic JIA should be included in the category of JIA, or whether it is actually an autoinflammatory disease (Chapters 16 and 47). Systemic JIA is probably the same disease as Adult-onset Still's Disease for which the Yamaguchi criteria were developed (Box 15-4).[40] These criteria have been applied to the diagnosis of children who do not meet the ILAR criteria for systemic onset JIA because they do not have arthritis at disease onset.[41] In a study by Kumar and colleagues, of 34 children who eventually fulfilled ILAR criteria for a diagnosis of systemic JIA, 13 did not have arthritis at onset of disease, but developed objective joint disease from 15 days to 1 year later (median 30 days, mean 69.3 days ± 104.6).[41] The ILAR classification is based on the disease characteristics in the first 6 months of disease, and many of the children who did not have frank arthritis when first evaluated did so within 6 months of fever onset, and thus would have fulfilled the ILAR criteria.

Rheumatoid Factor–positive Polyarticular JIA. The presence of RF on two occasions at least 3 months apart was the criterion used to subcategorize polyarticular JIA into RF-positive and RF-negative disease. Anti-cyclic citrullinated peptide (anti-CCP) antibodies, a marker of this disease in adult rheumatoid arthritis (RA), had not been described at the time of the development of the criteria, and have not been considered in the revisions. As noted by Ferrell et al., anti-CCP–positive but RF-negative patients would therefore fail to meet ILAR criteria for RF-positive polyarticular JIA and would be classified as polyarticular JIA RF negative or oligoarticular JIA.[31] The authors suggested that anti-CCP antibodies be included in any future revisions of the ILAR criteria, and proposed prioritizing serology (RF and anti-CCP) over the number of affected joints. According to that proposal, arthritis in any number of joints in the absence of systemic features (characteristic fever and rash), but with either RF or high titer anti-CCP on two occasions, would satisfy criteria for RF-positive JIA. Martini agrees that the number of affected joints should not be a criterion for classification.[20,32] He suggests, further, that with the exception of antinuclear antibody (ANA)-positive arthritis, the other categories all represent childhood onsets of the same diseases that occur in adults, and that the term *JIA* should be abandoned.[32]

The ILAR classification requirement for the presence of two positive tests for RF at least 3 months apart is not always fulfilled. A recent pilot study[33] noted that children in an inception cohort who had only a single positive RF test rarely had polyarthritis. It is possible, therefore, that the requirement for two positive RF tests is an appropriate criterion for definition of RF-positive polyarthritis under the ILAR criteria.

ANA as a Classification Criterion. A number of studies have evaluated the presence of antinuclear antibodies as a classification criterion. Ravelli et al.[42,43] concluded that patients in a group who were ANA positive (titer greater than or equal to 160 on rat liver and HEp-2 cell substrates on at least two occasions) shared many characteristics (early age at onset of arthritis, predominance of girls, asymmetric arthritis, risk of chronic anterior uveitis), irrespective of the number of inflamed joints, and that ANA positivity was a more appropriate classification criterion than the number of affected joints.

Juvenile Psoriatic Arthritis. Probably no category of the ILAR classification has been as difficult to deal with as JPsA. This stems from a number of factors: the onset of arthritis and psoriasis are not always synchronous, psoriasis is quite common in the general population, and the presence of psoriasis in a first-degree relative is difficult to verify. Manners has suggested that this criterion, together with the family history of a human leukocyte antigen (HLA) B27-associated disease in a first-degree relative be discarded for a number of reasons (unknown or uncertain family health status).[22] Berntson et al.[44] recommended eliminating the criterion of psoriasis in a second-degree relative. These recommendations require further testing.

Enthesitis-Related Arthritis. This category grew out of an understanding of the seronegative enthesitis and arthritis syndrome,[45] which frequently eventuates in recognizable AS.[46] Enthesitis has a central role in differentiating ERA from other categories of JIA. As critical as enthesitis is to the diagnosis of ERA, it may be difficult to diagnose clinically with certainty, and it must be noted that enthesitis occurs in other types of JIA, in particular psoriatic arthritis.[47] The presence of imaging changes (sacroiliitis, lumbosacral spine disease) is not required for the diagnosis of ERA.

Undifferentiated JIA. The frequency of categorization of a child as having undifferentiated JIA has varied widely from around 13%[48] to more than 50%,[22] differences which almost certainly reflect differences in the application of the ILAR criteria.

After 20 years, the ILAR criteria are in need of revision; on that most pediatric rheumatologists are agreed. Just how and where the changes should be made remains controversial. Ideally, the application of genetic, transcriptomic, and proteomic analyses of children with chronic arthritis should provide the insight needed to make biologically (and therapeutically) meaningful changes.

HISTORICAL REVIEW

The early descriptions of chronic arthritis in childhood are reviewed in Chapter 1. Although not the first to recognize the disease, George Frederic Still presented the classic description of 22 children with chronic arthritis in 1897.[49] He pointed out that the disease almost always began before the second dentition, was more frequent in girls, and was usually of insidious onset. Still observed that there was often no articular pain and that children exhibited a marked tendency to early contracture and muscle atrophy. The cervical spine was affected in the majority of cases, often during the early stages of the disease. The acute onset of disease in 12 patients who had lymphadenopathy, splenomegaly, and fever was described in detail. Pleuritis and pericarditis were common, although rash was not noted. Still suggested that childhood arthritis might have a different etiology from that of rheumatoid arthritis or that it might include more than one disease. Today, the term *Still's disease* is most often used to describe the adult onset (beyond the age of 16 years) of this acute systemic arthritis. Although suggested by Still, recognition that chronic arthritis in children differed from that in adults took some time. It is now generally acknowledged that chronic arthritis in children differs clinically, often genetically and possibly pathogenically, from adult arthritis, with the exception of RF-positive polyarthritis, which is very similar to adult rheumatoid arthritis, and ERA, which may resemble AS as the disease progresses. Furthermore, the impact of JIA on the growing child is profoundly different from chronic arthritis in the adult.

The interested reader is referred to a number of case series of historic importance.[50-56] These publications described experience with what today would be considered largely untreated patients, and they serve as a reminder of the serious potential long- and short-term effects of childhood arthritis, including death.

EPIDEMIOLOGY

Incidence and Prevalence

JIA is not rare, but the true frequency is not known. It appears to be worldwide in distribution, but the reported incidence and prevalence vary considerably throughout the world. This may reflect the ethnicity, immunogenetic susceptibility, or environmental influences affecting the population under study, or may result from underreporting in the developing world, where data are very sparse and disease recognition and access to specialty care are limited (see Chapter 11). The reports of incidence and prevalence of chronic arthritis of childhood have been recently analyzed by Thierry et al.[57] according to the classification criteria used. All but three reports described children from Europe or North America. Among the 33 prevalence studies, 11 used the EULAR criteria, 15 used the ACR criteria, and 7 used the ILAR criteria. The incidence rates ranged from 1.6 per 100,000 to 23 per 100,000, and the pooled incidence rate in Caucasians was 8.3 per 100,000 (confidence interval [CI] 8.1-8.7). Overall, pooled incidence rates were somewhat higher when the ILAR criteria were used (8.7 per 100,000), than with the ACR criteria (7.8 per 100,000) or EULAR criteria (8.3 per 100,000). Prevalence rates were evaluated in 29 papers (10 using ACR criteria, 11 using EULAR criteria, 7 using ILAR criteria, and 1 using ACR and EULAR criteria.) Prevalence rates ranged from 3.8 per 100,000 to 400 per 100,000, and the pooled prevalence rate was 32.6 per 100,000 (CI 31.3-33.9). Studies using the ACR criteria reported a higher pooled prevalence rate (45 per 100,000) than those using the EULAR criteria (12.8 per 100,000) or the ILAR criteria 30 per 100.000). Incidence rates were lowest in a Japanese study (less than 1 per 100,000),[58] and highest in a Norwegian study (greater than 20 per/100,000).[59] In the report of Danner and colleagues,[60] the ILAR criteria were used in a hospital- or clinic-based population and demonstrated a prevalence of 19.8 cases per 100,000 children under 16 years of age. The difference between referred and community-based study populations in determining prevalence is emphasized by the survey by Manners and Diepeveen,[61] in which a prevalence of 400 per 100,000 was found based on a physical examination by a pediatric rheumatologist of each of the 2241 12-year-old Australian schoolchildren included in the survey. Although this prevalence is considerably higher than that reported in most other studies, Mielants and colleagues[62] found a prevalence of 167 per 100,000 in a similar study of Belgian children.

Estimates of the global frequency of JIA are shown in Table 15-2. Using a range of reference data from European, North American, or Australian studies, an estimated 1.7 to 8.4 million children in the world have chronic arthritis, mostly undiagnosed.

TABLE 15-2 Estimates of the Global Incidence and Prevalence of JIA in Childhood

UNICEF REGION	POP. <18 YR	INCIDENCE	PREVALENCE
East Asia/ Pacific	567,000,000	29,484-56,700	487,620-2,268,000
South Asia	536,000,000	27,872-53,600	444,880-2,144,000
Industrialized	225,000,000	11,700-22,500	186,750-900,000
Latin America	190,000,000	9880-19,000	157,000-760,000
Eastern Europe	138,000,000	7176-13,800	114,540-552,000
West/Central Africa	151,000,000	750-15,000	125,330-604,000
East/Southern Africa	147,000,000	7644-14,700	122,010-588,000
TOTAL	2,105,000,000	109,456-210,300	1,747,150-8,420,000

Incidence ranges and prevalence ranges are based on the range of published estimates.

Proportions of JIA Subtypes

In Europe and North America, oligoarthritis accounts for approximately 50% of patients with JIA in most large series. RF-positive polyarthritis is least common. In clinic-based studies from South Africa,[63] India,[64] and Zambia,[65] oligoarthritis appears to be much less frequently recognized, and ERA and RF-negative polyarticular JIA are more commonly reported

Age at Onset

Quite distinct distributions of age at disease onset characterize each subset (see specific chapters). Disease onset before 6 months of age is distinctly unusual in any category of JIA, however.

Sex Ratio

In North and South America, Europe, and Australasia, twice as many girls as boys are affected. Marked differences in this ratio are apparent in the different onset types. In reports from South Africa,[63] India,[64] and Turkey,[66] however, boys and girls are equally at risk, and in some instances, boys are more frequently affected. These differences may represent differences in the type of JIA that predominates in different areas of the world, or they may reflect biological differences or case ascertainment bias.

Geographical and Racial Distribution

The incidence and prevalence data outlined previously were derived primarily from American or northern European white populations. There are few comparable data for other geographical or racial groups. Nonetheless, suggestions of racial differences in frequency exist.[67-69]

The incidence in Japan was reported to be low (0.83 per 100,000),[58] and lower frequencies of chronic arthritis (identified as JRA) have been reported in children of Japanese, Filipino, or Samoan origin than in white children living in Hawaii.[70] Chronic arthritis may be less common in North Americans of Chinese ancestry than in North American white children,[71,72] but there is a paucity of data describing these children. Schwartz and colleagues[69] concluded that the proportion of African-American children with JRA in a referral clinic population in the United States was consistent with their representation in the population served. However, there was a striking underrepresentation of this ethnic group in young children with oligoarticular and polyarticular onsets. Some reports suggest that chronic arthritis in children and adults is less frequent in African than in European populations. Saurenmann and colleagues[72] compared the frequencies of JIA in children of differing ethnic origin in a multiethnic hospital-based cohort of more than 1000 children living in Toronto. They noted that children of African or Asian origin were underrepresented overall in comparison with their proportion of the healthy population. Children of European origin were more likely to have extended oligoarthritis or psoriatic arthritis than other ethnic groups. Those of Asian origin were more likely to have ERA, and those of African origin were more susceptible to RF-positive polyarticular disease. An analysis of white and First Nations children living in Western Canada suggests that, although the overall frequency of chronic arthritis in aboriginal children is not higher than that for the white population, the frequency of HLA-B27–associated arthritis is appreciably higher in the aboriginal group.[73] Inuit children of northern Canada are reported to have a high overall incidence of chronic arthritis (23.6 per 100,000),[74] and Boyer and associates[75] suggested that the incidence of RF-positive polyarthritis is increased in southeast Alaskan Yupik Eskimo children. The numbers of patients in these studies are small, however, and conclusions with respect to actual incidence and prevalence of chronic arthritis in these groups are tentative.

ETIOLOGY AND PATHOGENESIS

The etiology of JIA is unknown, although it is almost certainly multifactorial, and probably differs from one onset type to another. Systemic arthritis is characterized neither by the presence of autoantibodies nor a strong genetic predisposition and may be more appropriately considered to be an autoinflammatory disease. Autoantibodies are common in oligoarthritis (antinuclear antibodies) and RF-positive polyarthritis (IgM rheumatoid factor). In contrast, ERA, RF-negative polyarthritis, and, to some extent, psoriatic arthritis have less tendency to autoantibody formation but, in the case of ERA, are associated with misfolding of the protein coded for by the genetic marker HLA-B27. The strongest genetic associations with several categories of JIA remain those with genes coded for within the HLA or major histocompatibility complex (MHC) locus on chromosome 6, where a large cluster of immune related genes are found. Recent detailed, large genetic studies of JIA have confirmed these associations with HLA and also indicated several other susceptibility loci, which confirm the autoimmune etiology of JIA.[76] That genetic factors are only part of the puzzle is demonstrated by the fact that, except for ERA and some cases of psoriatic arthritis, familial arthritis is very uncommon, although not unknown.

The fundamental pathological process is chronic inflammation, in which both the innate and adaptive immune systems play critical roles. In all categories of JIA, products of activated T cells and macrophages are involved in pathogenesis of synovitis.

Environmental influences have received little attention. One study suggested that breast-feeding has a protective effect on the development of JIA,[77] especially in oligoarticular disease; however, a strong relationship was not confirmed in another investigation.[78] Maternal smoking during pregnancy has been reported to be a risk factor for the development of arthritis in the first 7 years of life, especially in girls.[79] The possible role played by epigenetic mechanisms is largely unexplored.[80] The increasing understanding of the interactions between the immune system and the microbiome of the gut, and how they play a role in immune health or triggering of autoimmunity, has opened a new field that is likely to be of key importance to our understanding. In addition to polygenic genetic predispositions, disordered immune responses, and putative environmental triggers, any theory of pathogenesis must account for a number of factors: the clinical heterogeneity of the disease; the much higher prevalence of oligoarthritis,

polyarthritis, and psoriatic arthritis in girls, and the strikingly higher incidence of ERA in boys; the narrow peak ages at onset for some types such as oligoarthritis, in contrast to the absence of a peak age at onset for systemic disease; and the association of extraarticular complications such as uveitis in certain disease subsets. There may be multiple etiological events, or the disorder may result from a single pathogenic vector with diverse clinical patterns evolving from interactions with the host. It may be postulated that an environmental agent affecting a child with a particular genetic predisposition, at a point of vulnerability—defined by age, intercurrent illness, prior antigenic experience, trauma, hormonal variations, psychological stress, or immunological maturity—results in a clinical disorder.

Immunopathogenic Mechanisms

A number of observations contribute to the hypothesis that the immune system is intimately involved in pathogenesis. First, there is abundant evidence of altered immunity, abnormal immunoregulation, cytokine production, and polymorphisms of genes involved in the immune response. Second, there is an association between specific immunodeficiencies and rheumatic diseases, including chronic arthritis (see Chapter 46). Third, there is a close relationship between immune reactivity and inflammation, the hallmark of arthritis. Whether it is principally an immunogenetically determined disorder or an antigen-driven immunological response, or the result of interactions between the two, is uncertain. The topics of immunopathogenesis and inflammation are discussed in detail in Chapters 3 and 4, and in chapters discussing specific categories of JIA.

Hormonal Factors

The often striking differences in sex ratio, as well as the characteristic preadolescent or postadolescent peaks in incidence of specific categories of childhood arthritis, suggest that reproductive hormones may play important roles in pathogenesis.[81,82] In one study,[83] levels of progesterone and 17β-estriol were similar in patients with chronic arthritis and age-matched controls, but levels of dehydroepiandrosterone and testosterone were lower. Testosterone synovial fluid levels were lowest in those with disease of the longest duration. Low androgen levels may contribute to pathogenesis because androgens exert a protective effect against cartilage degradation.[84]

Prolactin, produced by cells of the anterior pituitary and other cells, including lymphocytes, is elevated in inflammatory joint disease and inhibits chondrocyte apoptosis and related cartilage loss.[85] Levels were increased in children with chronic arthritis and antinuclear antibody (ANA) positivity.[86-88] The prolactin concentration correlated with levels of IL-6 and with a chronic disease course. Serum and urinary morning cortisol levels were somewhat diminished in children with active JIA.[88]

Infection and Immunizations

Arthritis after viral infections is probably common, although it is usually self-limited. Arthritis in children has been linked to perinatal infection with the influenza virus A2H2N2,[89] and to parvovirus B19.[90-94] Chronic arthritis (especially RF-negative polyarthritis, spondyloarthritis, and oligoarthritis) has been described in children with human immunodeficiency virus infections.[95] The cyclical pattern of incidence of chronic arthritis documented from 1979 to 1992 in Manitoba by Oen and colleagues[96] correlated with the occurrence of infections to *Mycoplasma pneumoniae.*

The relationship between highly conserved bacterial heat shock proteins (HSPs) and chronic arthritis in animal models and humans has been extensively studied.[97,98] Humoral and cellular immune responses to HSPs are present in children with chronic arthritis.[99-105]

TABLE 15-3   Animal Models of Chronic Arthritis

	SPECIES	ANTIGEN	MECHANISM
Adjuvant Arthritis	Mice	Muramyl dipeptide	T cell mediated
Collagen Arthritis	Mice, rats	Native type II collagen	Antibody mediated
Infectious agents	Many species	*Erysipelothrix, Mycoplasma, Chlamydia psittaci*	
Genetically determined	MRL/1 mice		
	K/BxN mice		
	HLA B27 transfected mice, rats		

HSPs have been demonstrated in the serum and synovial fluid.[102,104,105] Van Eden and colleagues[106] postulated that HSP-reactive T cells are part of the normal immune repertoire for TCR V-gene products; self-HSPs and bacterial HSPs may trigger this response. In 13 of 15 children with oligoarthritis, T-lymphocyte proliferative responses to HSP 60 were detected an average of 12 weeks before clinical remission of the inflammatory disease.[102,107] Spontaneous remission was characterized by the presence of CD30+ T cells directed to HSP 60.[108] Albani and associates[105,109] demonstrated immune responses to the dnaJ HSP from *Escherichia coli*, especially in children with polyarticular disease. This protein has five amino acids that are homologous with those in the binding groove of DRB1, which in itself is increased in frequency in these children. Therefore, molecular mimicry may play a role in pathogenesis.[110,111] Intranasal administration of a heat shock peptide suppresses adjuvant induced arthritis in mice.[112] Despite circumstantial evidence, a direct link between infection and chronic childhood arthritis has remained elusive.

Postvaccination arthritis has been described after routine immunizations,[113] and after measles-mumps-rubella vaccine, a persistent arthropathy was documented in one study, predominantly in females.[114] However, a number of recent studies have demonstrated the safety and efficacy of vaccine administration to children with JIA[115] (Chapter 11).

Psychological Factors

High levels of psychological stress are common in families of children with arthritis.[116-118] Psychological factors inherent in the family and child affect their adaptation to chronic illness, but their role in the causation of the disease is controversial. A recent study documented the occurrence of stressful life events preceding the onset of arthritis in many children.[119] Some studies suggest that susceptibility to arthritis is associated with dysregulation of the autonomic nervous system that leads to an inappropriate response of the child's immune system to stimuli[120] and may be influenced by neuroendocrine gene polymorphisms.[121]

Physical Trauma

Chronic arthritis has been reported by parents to follow minor physical trauma to an extremity. Such trauma may serve as a localizing factor, or it may simply call attention to an already inflamed and weakened joint. The fact that certain joints (e.g., the knee) are frequently affected in JIA could be interpreted to suggest that trauma associated with weight bearing in the young child is a factor in initiating chronic inflammation. However, there is no convincing evidence that trauma is a cause of JIA.

Nutritional Factors

To date, there has been no reproducible evidence that nutritional deficiencies or ingestion of particular foods either cause or exacerbate JIA. However, gluten ingestion in children with gluten sensitivity may exacerbate gut disease and as a consequence cause joint inflammation.

Animal Models of Inflammatory Joint Disease

The study of animal models of human disease provides clues about etiology, but these models are, at best, approximations of human disease.[122] Some of these models are listed in Table 15-3.

GENETIC BACKGROUND

Familial JIA

Familial chronic arthritis is uncommon. Over a 10-year period, an American registry identified 200 sets of siblings identified as having JRA, of whom 21 are twins (13 identical).[123] Within any one family, arthritis tends to have the same type of onset, and even the same complication of uveitis.[123,124] In no instance was disease onset simultaneous, although in most cases the *ages* at onset were similar. There is no association between birth order and the development of arthritis.[125]

The development of chronic arthritis in twins has been extensively studied.[126,127] Concordance rates were 44% in identical twins and 4% in dizygotic twins.[128] In a multicenter study[123] of 71 affected sibling pairs and a trio of three siblings in three families, the mean interval between onset of disease in the siblings was 4.4 years. More than three quarters were concordant for onset type and disease course. Among seven sets of twins, the interval between disease onset was shorter (3.3 months) and all were concordant for onset type (six oligoarthritis, one polyarthritis). Uveitis was concordant in only 3 of 16 sibling pairs. There is also an increased prevalence of autoimmunity and of autoantibodies in first-degree relatives of children with chronic arthritis.[129,130] Chronic inflammatory rheumatic diseases are more common in parents of multiple siblings affected by chronic arthritis.[130]

One further association bears attention: the occurrence of JIA and adult RA in the same family. Documentation of this event is scant, and it must be concluded that with the exception of RF-positive polyarticular JIA, JIA and RA uncommonly occur in the same family.

Genetic Associations

Genetic influences on both JIA susceptibility and phenotype are polygenic. Genetic associations have been recently reviewed by Angeles-Han and Prahalad.[131] Until recently, there were five well-established genetic risk factors: HLA class I and class II genes, the PTPN22 and PTPN2 genes, and the IL2RA/CD25 gene. Early studies revealed that specific HLA classes I and II alleles, and whole haplotypes, are associated with particular types of JIA. Some HLA associations parallel those observed in adult disease, such as HLA-DRB1*0401 in RF-positive polyarthritis, whereas others are particular to JIA subtypes such as the associations of HLADRB1*0801, 1101, and 13 with oligoarticular JIA. A recent international effort has led to the largest ever genetic study of JIA, with a focus on oligoarticular and RF-negative polyarticular JIA.[76] This study increased the loci known to be associated with JIA by identifying 14 associated genes at genome-wide significance and a further 11 highly associated loci. Several other genetic associations are JIA subtype specific, such as with the endoplasmic reticulum aminopeptidase-1 (1) gene in ERA and IL-23R in psoriatic arthritis[132]; these associations are considered in subsequent chapters.

There may also be an association of the various types of arthritis with childhood onset with chromosomal abnormalities.[133] Chronic JIA-like arthritis has been observed in patients with IgA deficiency, and with deletion of the short arm of chromosome 18[134] (Chapter 46), 22q11.2 deletion syndrome (also called velocardiofacial or DiGeorge syndrome),[135] and Turner syndrome.[136] In a study of this association,[137] 18 of approximately 500 children with JRA were found to have Turner syndrome (X0 chromosomes); polyarticular disease was present in 7.

It is not entirely clear whether the arthropathy of Down syndrome (trisomy of chromosome 21) differs from JIA.[133] In a community-based survey, chronic arthritis was reported in 0.2% of 440 children with Down syndrome.[138] In some children, the arthritis is more like psoriatic arthritis; and psoriasis is seemingly increased in frequency in children with trisomy 21.[139] Of interest, both RF and anti-CCP antibodies are frequently found in children with Down syndrome even in the absence of arthritis.[140] Arthritis was described in a child with partial trisomy 5q, monosomy 2p.[141]

CLINICAL MANIFESTATIONS OF JIA

Constitutional Signs and Symptoms

Fatigue, anorexia, weight loss, and growth failure occur in many children with active JIA. Significant fatigue is rarely a feature of mild or limited articular disease, but it is a common symptom in children with polyarticular or systemic disease, especially at onset and during periods of poor disease control. Night pain may interrupt sleep and contribute to fatigue. Sleep fragmentation may also exacerbate pain as well as fatigue in these children.[142,143] In a recent study, however, Ward and colleagues[144] could not demonstrate a difference between children with arthritis and healthy subjects with respect to sleep characteristics. Anorexia may result from gastric irritation secondary to nonsteroidal antiinflammatory drug use, or nausea secondary to methotrexate use. Weight loss signifies the presence of active disease or an associated condition such as inflammatory bowel disease or celiac disease. Growth retardation is a frequent consequence of active JIA but is also be contributed to by prolonged corticosteroid use.

Puberty and secondary sexual characteristics are often delayed in children with active inflammation. In a group of Italian girls with JIA, menarche was later than in their mothers or in age-matched normal controls.[145]

MUSCULOSKELETAL MANIFESTATIONS

Pain and Stiffness

Aspects of pain in children with arthritis have been reviewed by Anthony and Schanberg[146] and by LaLouviére et al.[147] It is the rare child who has no pain in the presence of active arthritis. Although a child with chronic arthritis may not complain of pain at rest,[148,149] active or passive motion of a joint elicits pain in the inflamed joint, particularly at the extremes of the range of motion. Pain is usually described as aching or stretching and is of mild-to-moderate severity. In contrast, children with pain-amplification syndromes almost always describe pain as extremely severe (see Chapters 8 and 52). Pain elicited by pressure (tenderness) is usually maximal at the joint line; over hypertrophied, inflamed synovium; or at entheses. Bone pain or tenderness is not characteristic of arthritis, and its presence should alert the

examiner to the possibility of a malignancy or infection involving bone, or chronic nonbacterial osteomyelitis.[150]

Joint stiffness may occur, particularly on arising or after prolonged inactivity. More often, however, evidence of stiffness is provided by the parent, who describes slowness or awkwardness of the gait, most marked in the morning or after a nap or prolonged sitting, which improves with activity or the application of heat to the affected area. The significance of the duration of stiffness has not been extensively examined, but stiffness lasting more than 15 minutes signifies a considerable level of joint inflammation. Stiffness that lasts all day is suggestive of a pain amplification syndrome. The pathophysiology of joint stiffness is unclear.

Characteristics of the Inflamed Joint

An actively inflamed joint exhibits the cardinal signs of inflammation: swelling, pain, heat, loss of function, and sometimes erythema (Fig. 15-1). Swelling of a joint may result from periarticular soft tissue edema, from intraarticular effusion, or from hypertrophy of the synovial membrane. Large synovial cysts are an unusual complication. They may occur in the antecubital area or anterior to the shoulder[151] (Fig. 15-2).When they occur in the popliteal space (Baker cyst) (Fig. 15-3), they may rupture into adjacent muscles, and dissect into the calf.[152] This event is characterized by sudden sharp pain and swelling in the calf, followed by crescentic ecchymoses about the malleoli. They may be the initial or sole manifestation of chronic arthritis and, if unilateral, may be misinterpreted as a tumor or as deep venous thrombosis. A healthy child may occasionally develop a transient popliteal cyst.[153] Ultrasound imaging or magnetic resonance imaging (MRI) aids in making the correct diagnosis. Inflamed joints in children with JIA are often warm but almost never erythematous. In contrast, the joint may be erythematous in septic arthritis or acute rheumatic fever and in some of the other reactive arthritides.

Inflamed joints usually lose range of motion, particularly in extension, because this is usually a position of relative comfort, accommodating shortened soft tissue structures, although to some extent this depends on which joint is involved. Hyperextension is characteristically the first range to be lost in the cervical spine. Elbows, wrists, metacarpophalangeal and interphalangeal joints usually lose range in extension or hyperextension first, but flexion range is also often diminished. The hallmark of intraarticular hip joint disease is loss of internal

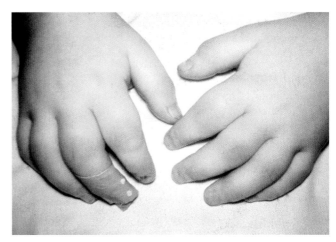

FIGURE 15-1 The joints of the wrists and hands of a 2½-year-old boy with systemic-onset disease are swollen, warm, and painful. The proximal and distal interphalangeal joints are erythematous. There are flexion contractures of the fingers.

rotation and flexion. There is loss of hyperextension or extension, and sometimes flexion in the knees. Loss of ankle dorsiflexion, subtalar eversion, and midfoot supination are characteristic of an inflamed joint. Loss of dorsiflexion of the first metatarsophalangeal joint may be of considerable functional significance.

The Pediatric Gait, Arms, Legs, Spine screen is an excellent tool for the quick evaluation of the child for evidence of musculoskeletal disease.[154] It is most applicable for use by the general physician or pediatrician and does not include the detailed examination that a pediatric rheumatologist would perform.

Distribution of Affected Joints

Any joint may be affected, but large joints (knees, ankles, wrists, elbows, hips) are most frequently involved. Small joints of the hands and feet may also be affected, particularly in polyarticular-onset disease. Disease in the apophyseal joints of the cervical spine occurs at onset in approximately 2% of children and may present as a torticollis.[155] In the pre-methotrexate, prebiologics era, approximately 60% of patients eventually developed involvement of the cervical spine. Instability of this area may occur early, rendering the child at risk for injury in an

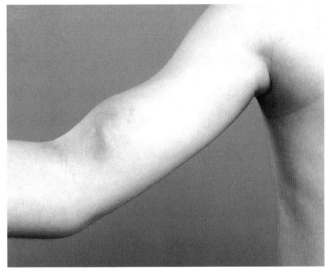

FIGURE 15-2 Brachial synovial cyst. A 6-year-old girl developed this dissecting cyst of her right arm as the first manifestation of chronic arthritis. Later, bilateral effusions developed in both knees.

accident or with attempted intubation before general anesthesia. The sternoclavicular, acromioclavicular, and sternomanubrial joints are infrequently affected. Cricoarytenoid arthritis is unusual but may be responsible for acute airway obstruction.[156] Inflammation of the synovial joints of the middle ear—the incudomalleal and incudostapedial articulations—is rarely appreciated clinically. Tympanometric studies, however, have indicated that subclinical disease may be present in almost two thirds of children with JRA.[157]

Patterns of joint involvement are often quite characteristic. Thus, symmetrical involvement of large and small joints is typical of polyarticular disease. Arthritis predominantly affecting the joints of the lower extremity characterizes ERA. The presence of hip joint disease is not uncommon in ERA, but rarely occurs in oligoarticular JIA. Psoriatic arthritis tends to be somewhat asymmetrical and involves both large and small joints, sometimes including the distal interphalangeal joints.

Tenosynovitis

Tenosynovitis is quite common, but it is generally not a striking or isolated clinical complaint. The most common sites are the extensor tendon sheaths on the dorsum of the hand, the extensor sheaths over the dorsum of the foot, and those of the posterior tibial tendon and the peroneus longus and brevis tendons. If tenosynovitis is very prominent, Blau syndrome should be considered (see Chapter 39). Triggering or loss of extension of the fingers may result from a stenosing synovitis of the flexor tendon sheaths. Clinically recognized carpal tunnel syndrome is uncommon in children. Tenosynovitis of the superior oblique tendon of the eye may cause pain on upward gaze, sometimes with diplopia (Brown syndrome).[158,159]

Bursitis

Bursae are synovial-lined sacs that do not usually communicate with the joint but, when inflamed, may be confused with intraarticular pathology because of their juxtaarticular locations. Trochanteric bursitis, olecranon bursitis, anserine bursitis (between the gracilis and semitendinosus tendons and the tibial collateral ligament), prepatellar bursitis, infrapatellar bursitis,[160] and retrocalcaneal bursitis are typical sites of painful swelling. The Baker cyst, in the popliteal fossa, is usually an expansion of the preexisting gastrocnemius semimembranosus bursa, but in the child with an inflamed knee joint, it may communicate with the intraarticular space or represent a posterior extension of the synovium of the knee.[161] Occasionally, bursitis develops in children from repeated trauma but no underlying rheumatic disease.[162]

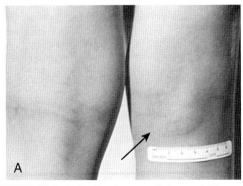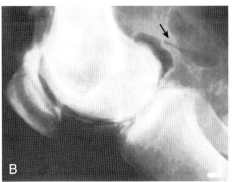

FIGURE 15-3 **A,** Popliteal cyst or Baker cyst. The cyst was associated with pain at the back of the knee, was somewhat tender, and transilluminated. Aspiration yielded clear yellow fluid of low inflammatory activity. **B,** Arthrogram of a popliteal cyst, with contrast medium outlining the communication (*arrow*) between the synovial space and this dissecting cyst in an 18-year-old boy who had had arthritis since the age of 9 years.

Osteopenia

Osteopenia is a potentially major determinant of functional outcome in young adults who have had chronic arthritis as children[163] (see Chapter 53). Children with chronic arthritis have a diminished bone mass and are at increased risk for fractures in adulthood and for an earlier onset of osteoporosis.[164-167] Contributing factors include physical inactivity, high levels of inflammatory cytokines, poor nutrition, and low levels of vitamin D. An important determinant of future fracture risk is the peak bone mass achieved at the end of skeletal maturation, which is almost complete by the late years of adolescence.

Muscle Disease

Atrophy and weakness of muscles around inflamed joints occur frequently and are often accompanied by a shortening of the muscles and tendons that results in flexion contractures. Atrophy of the vastus medialis muscle is characteristic of arthritis in the knee. The calf muscles become atrophic when the ankle joint is involved. Sacroiliitis may be associated with atrophy of gluteal and thigh muscles. Muscles of the forearm become atrophic in children with chronic wrist arthritis. A few children with widespread, prolonged, active arthritis develop progressive muscle atrophy that is most severe and persistent if it occurs before 3 years of age.[168]

Extraarticular Manifestations
Generalized Abnormalities of Growth

Abnormalities of physical growth and development may complicate chronic arthritis. Linear growth is retarded during periods of active systemic disease.[169] Mean weight for age and weight per height are significantly diminished in those with polyarticular disease.[170] Growth retardation (height less than 5th percentile) was documented in 50% of adults who had childhood onset of systemic JIA, 11% of those with oligoarticular onset, and 16% of those with polyarticular onset. Glucocorticoid therapy could only partly explain these observations. In a more recent study, a marked decrease in height velocity (−2 SD) was observed in 56% of children with systemic arthritis.[171] In this study, growth retardation was associated with glucocorticoid administration, nutritional status, bone mineral density, and early disease onset. Each of these studies reflects the effect of disease in a population treated in the pre-methotrexate, pre-biologics era and is an important reminder of the potentially devastating effects of untreated or undertreated JIA on normal growth and development. With better disease control, severe growth retardation is increasingly uncommon. In a recent study of children with oligoarthritis, however, Padeh et al.[172] noted generalized growth retardation in one third.

The mechanisms of growth suppression in JIA involve high levels of proinflammatory cytokines, such as IL-6, IL-1b, and tumor necrosis factor (TNF)-α, seen in children with active arthritis that directly or indirectly influence growth plate chondrocytes and linear bone growth.[173] Levels of growth hormone and IGF-I and -II may be reduced.[174] IGF-I was inversely correlated with IL-6 levels in children with systemic disease.[175]

Localized Growth Disturbances

During early active disease, development of the ossification centers is accelerated, apparently related to the hyperemia of inflammation and local production of growth factors. The result may be either overgrowth of the affected limb or, ultimately (though much less commonly), premature fusion of the involved physes, resulting in diminished length.

If arthritis occurs in one knee only, a discrepancy of leg lengths results. A difference of greater than 1 to 2 cm is probably functionally significant, and differences of 5 cm or more occasionally occur. Apparent leg-length inequality may also result from pelvic rotation and scoliosis. As the child grows, inequalities of minimal to moderate degree may disappear, but they persist in up to two thirds of these children. Significant leg-length inequality was reported to occur much less frequently in a setting in which intraarticular corticosteroids were used to treat inflammation.[176]

Micrognathia and/or retrognathia may result from growth disturbances of the mandible as a consequence of arthritis in the temporomandibular joint (TMJ).[177-179] Early TMJ arthritis is difficult to detect clinically and often not until growth changes are evident.[180,181] Many children with MRI-confirmed TMJ arthritis do not complain of pain, although some have pain on opening the mouth or experience clicking on opening or closing the mouth. In a Swedish survey of 70 children with JIA, 56% had symptoms (crepitus, pain, difficulty opening the mouth) and 41% had radiographic evidence of TMJ pathology attributable to arthritis.[177] In one patient, the disease began in a TMJ. Cannizzarro et al.[182] found that 38.6% of 223 children with JIA had involvement of the TMJ a mean of 4.6 years after disease onset, based on clinical and radiographic evidence. Children with extended oligoarticular JIA were most commonly affected (61%), followed by those with RF-negative JIA (52%), psoriatic JIA (50%), systemic JIA (36%), RF-negative polyarticular JIA, persistent oligoarticular JIA (33%), and ERA (11%). A younger age at onset, a high erythrocyte sedimentation rate (ESR) at diagnosis, upper extremity involvement, and the absence of HLA-B27 were significantly associated with the development of TMJ arthritis. Extreme micrognathia is most likely to occur if arthritis begins before 4 years of age and is poorly controlled.

The mandible ossifies by intramembranous bone production. A number of factors contribute to mandibular growth abnormalities. Pain in the TMJ may inhibit normal masseter muscle development, which in turn retards mandibular bone development, resulting in a shortened mandibular ramus and body. Destruction of the condyle of the mandible causes further diminution of overall mandibular height. In some children, overgrowth of the condyle may contribute to TMJ dysfunction.[179] As demonstrated by MRI, the disease is bilateral in three quarters, but early disease may appear to be unilateral on clinical examination. It is characterized by mandibular asymmetry; deviation to the affected side on opening of the jaw; difficulty in palpating the affected mandibular condyle; and pain, tenderness, or crepitus of one or both TMJs. Heterotopic bone formation has been described in 12 children with severe TMJ arthritis.[183] A report of routine MRI evaluations of the TMJ in children with JIA suggests a high frequency of asymptomatic disease and describes protocols for assessing this joint.[184] Little is understood about the effect of chronic arthritis on dental caries or periodontal disease.[185]

Fitness

There persists a widespread but unsubstantiated assumption by parents and some health professionals that physical activity in children with arthritis should be limited. Children with arthritis tend to be less physically active than their peers.[186-188] Lelieveld and colleagues[186] documented limited physical activity in adolescents with JIA compared to their peers, as measured by a 3-day activity diary and concluded that adolescents with arthritis have low aerobic and anaerobic fitness. Takken and colleagues[189] noted reduced maximal oxygen consumption in children with JIA, compared with controls.

Skin and Subcutaneous Tissue

The classic rash of systemic-onset disease is discussed in Chapter 16. A second cutaneous change, occurring particularly in children with involvement of the hands, is a dark discoloration of the skin over the proximal interphalangeal (PIP) joints.[190] The presence of this finding may reflect disease chronicity. In children with tender joints, retention keratosis may simulate a pigmented lesion and reflects the inability to perform adequate self-care. Nodules occur in a variety of rheumatic diseases in children. Subcutaneous rheumatoid nodules occur in 5% to 10% of children with chronic arthritis, almost always confined to those with RF-positive disease (see Chapter 17). They most commonly occur over the proximal ulna and the Achilles tendon. Tendon-associated nodules may reflect tenosynovitis, especially in the flexor tendons of the fingers.

Asymmetrical lymphedema of the subcutaneous tissues of one or more extremities has been documented in several children with arthritis.[191-193] The swelling is usually painless and may be pitting. The cause is unknown but does not seem to be related to local obstruction caused by joint swelling. The course is chronic but may improve over several years. Cutaneous vasculitis is very rare and occurs most often in the older child with RF-positive polyarthritis.

Ocular Disease

Ocular inflammation may occur at any time in the course of JIA (see Chapter 22). Uveitis is characteristically asymptomatic, except in ERA, where it is usually characterized by a painful pink eye. Reactive arthritis is also associated with symptomatic conjunctivitis and occasionally uveitis. Keratoconjunctivitis sicca occasionally occurs, particularly in RF-positive polyarthritis (see Chapter 30). Scleritis is rare.

PATHOLOGY

The histopathological features of synovitis in patients with JIA are similar to those described in RA. There is villous hypertrophy and hyperplasia of the synovial lining layer (Fig. 15-4). The subsynovial tissues are hyperemic, edematous, and show a dense infiltration by T and B lymphocytes, plasma cells, macrophages, and dendritic cells, and in some cases natural killer (NK) cells. Endothelial hyperplasia is often prominent, likely driven by production of the angiogenic chemokines,

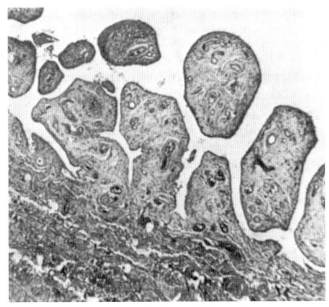

FIGURE 15-4 Photomicrograph of synovial tissue from the knee of a young boy with arthritis. Villous hyperplasia and hypertrophy, edema, proliferation of new blood vessels, and infiltration by mononuclear cells are prominent.

and pro-angiogenic factors including vascular endothelial growth factor (VEGF) and osteopontin, whose production is increased in hypoxic conditions.[194,195] There is a selective accumulation in the synovium of activated T cells, which are clustered around antigen-presenting dendritic cells. Myeloid dendritic cells (mDC) are typically localized to the synovial lining layer, whereas interferon-α secreting plasmacytoid dendritic cells (pDC) are in T and B cell rich aggregates.[196] Both CD4 and CD8 synovial T cells are highly activated. These T cells produce abundant cytokines including tumor necrosis factor (TNF), interferon (IFN)-γ and, as more recently recognized, IL-17 and granulocyte macrophage colony-stimulating factor (GMCSF).[197,198] In parallel, synovial monocytes and tissue macrophages produce cytokines and chemokines that both contribute to local cartilage and bone damage and also to the recruitment of more inflammatory cells. An exuberant synovitis eventually results in progressive erosion and destruction of articular cartilage and, later, of contiguous bone with pannus formation.

Kruithoff et al. have compared the synovial histopathology in adult rheumatoid arthritis with juvenile spondyloarthropathies, juvenile oligoarthritis, and juvenile polyarthritis.[199] There was broad overlap among these disease categories with the exception of hypervascularity, which was less pronounced in juvenile polyarthritis. The inflammatory cell infiltration tended to be higher than in adult arthritis and was frequently characterized by numerous plasma cells and the presence of lymphoid aggregates. A study of 40 JIA synovial biopsies demonstrated that lymphoid neogenesis in JIA synovium was correlated with ANA positivity, although full follicle structures were rare.[200] Two recent studies of synovial tissue histology and specific protein expression have identified clear differences that correlate with JIA subtype.[201,202]

Joint destruction has usually been shown to occur later in the disease course in childhood than in adulthood, and permanent joint damage is absent in many children even after years of chronic inflammation. The greater thickness of juvenile cartilage may offer some protection in this regard. Newer studies with MRI may revise the impression of the extent of joint damage in early disease. The hyaline cartilage of the hip is destroyed in progressive stages during the course of severe disease, and during healing it may be replaced by a fibrocartilaginous layer. Rice bodies may be present and consist primarily of amorphous fibrous material, fibrin, and small amounts of collagen. Viable cells (mainly type B synovial lining cells) are incorporated within this matrix. Residual blood vessels in some of these bodies attest to their former attachment to the synovial membrane.

The rash of systemic disease is characterized by minimal perivascular infiltration of mononuclear cells around capillaries and venules in the subdermal tissues. A neutrophilic perivasculitis resembling that of the rash of rheumatic fever may accompany the more flagrant lesions.

Subcutaneous nodules in RF-positive JIA may be histopathologically typical of rheumatoid nodules, or they may have a looser connective tissue framework resembling that of the nodules of rheumatic fever (see Chapters 17 and 44). Classic rheumatoid nodules consist of three distinct zones: a central area of necrosis and granulation tissue, surrounded by a radially arranged palisade of connective tissue cells, which, in turn, is enveloped by chronic inflammatory cells. In children, the central area of fibrinoid necrosis and the epithelioid palisades may be absent or less structured.

The serosal lining surfaces of the pleural, pericardial, and peritoneal cavities may exhibit a nonspecific fibrous serositis that is characterized by effusion. Enlargement of the lymph nodes is related to a nonspecific follicular hyperplasia that in rare instances may closely resemble lymphoma. Hepatic abnormalities are characterized by a nonspecific collection of periportal inflammatory cells and hyperplasia of Kupffer cells.

LABORATORY EXAMINATION

Although the laboratory may provide support for a diagnosis of JIA, no laboratory test or combination of studies can confirm the diagnosis. The laboratory can be used to provide evidence of inflammation, to support the clinical diagnosis, to predict outcome, to monitor toxicity of therapy, and as a research tool to understand more completely the pathogenesis of the disease. Tests for RF and the HLA-B27 antigen are components of the ILAR classification of JIA. A comprehensive review of the use of the laboratory in pediatric rheumatology is provided in Chapter 10.

TESTS THAT DOCUMENT THE PRESENCE OF INFLAMMATION

Several laboratory tests can be used to detect or monitor inflammation. Leukocytosis, thrombocytosis, elevated ESR, or C-reactive protein (CRP) are indicators of the "acute phase response." There is no unanimity of opinion of the relative value of ESR and CRP in evaluating JIA. A study comparing the clinical evaluation of active synovitis with Doppler ultrasound, CRP, and ESR suggested that the ESR was more sensitive in detection of active disease than CRP.[203] Less commonly, and primarily in research settings, levels of serum amyloid A or calprotectin (MRP8/14) are measured to demonstrate the presence or absence of inflammation and the probability of relapse.[204]

TESTS WITH SOME DIAGNOSTIC SPECIFICITY

Autoantibodies

Rheumatoid Factors

Classic IgM RFs are unusual in a child younger than 7 years of age and are seldom helpful diagnostically at onset of disease. The diagnostic importance of RF positivity in a child with possible chronic arthritis is mitigated by the frequent occurrence of abnormal titers in the other connective tissue diseases of childhood, especially in systemic lupus erythematosus (SLE), and in apparently healthy children. In a study of the diagnostic utility of RF serology in children,[205] RF tests were as likely to be positive in children with diseases other than chronic arthritis as in that disorder. In the diagnosis of JIA, therefore, tests for RFs are of little utility. They are an important component of the ILAR classification criteria, however, and their presence may indicate a poorer prognosis.

RFs are most common in children with later age at onset and polyarticular disease, and in those who are older, have longer disease duration, have subcutaneous rheumatoid nodules or articular erosions, or are in a poorer functional class. They are especially common in the presence of HLA-Dw4 (DRB1*0401) and Dw14 (DRB1*0404) specificities.

Anti-cyclic Citrullinated Peptide Antibodies

Anti-cyclic citrullinated peptide antibodies (ACPA) are also found in children with JIA. Tebo and colleagues evaluated 334 children with JIA and 50 healthy control children[206] and demonstrated IgG anti-CCP antibodies in 73% of children with RF-positive polyarticular JIA, 19% with extended oligoarticular JIA, 13% with systemic JIA, 8% with RF-negative polyarticular JIA, 4% with ERA or persistent oligoarticular JIA, and in 2% of controls. In the group of 23 children with RF-negative, ACPA-positive disease, the ACPA titers were very low. There is evidence that citrullinated fibrinogen is the target antigen for

ACPA in JIA.[207] It is not certain that measurement of ACPA adds appreciably to the diagnosis or management of JIA.

Antinuclear Antibodies

The frequency of ANAs is highest in girls who are younger in age at onset, especially in those with oligoarticular disease, and lowest in older boys and in those with systemic-onset disease and ERA. ANAs reach their highest prevalence (65% to 85%) in young girls who have oligoarthritis and uveitis.[208,209] Therefore, the presence of ANAs supports the diagnosis and is important in identification of children most at risk for chronic uveitis. Persistent ANA positivity can occur in healthy children, and in a small but significant group of children with musculoskeletal complaints in whom no autoimmune or rheumatic disease was found.[210-212] Care must therefore be exercised in interpreting the significance of ANA seropositivity in children who do not have objective evidence of arthritis. ANA determination is, therefore, not a good screening test for JIA. The antigenic specificities of ANAs in JIA have not been identified.

Plasma Lipids

Dyslipoproteinemia occurs *de novo* in children with chronic arthritis, separate from the effects of glucocorticoids.[213-215] Tselepis and colleagues[215] reported that 14 patients with active arthritis had lower plasma cholesterol and high-density lipoprotein cholesterol levels and higher triglycerides than controls or comparable children with another disease. Gonçalves and colleagues[216] found lower levels of both high-density lipoproteins and triglycerides in JIA patients than in controls. Some of these changes may reflect the effects of treatment. However, in the report of Shen and associates,[215] the patients had received neither corticosteroids nor disease modifying agents prior to study and had lower levels of high-density lipoproteins and total cholesterol that normalized with control of inflammation.

Synovial Fluid Analysis

Synovial fluid from patients with JIA is usually inflammatory (Table 15-4). The principal cellular constituents are polymorphonuclear neutrophils and mononuclear cells, including lymphoid dendritic cells. The leukocyte count does not always correlate with the degree of clinical activity. Synovial fluid levels of glucose may be low, as in adult RA. Synovial fluid complement levels are not as uniformly depressed as in adult disease. The concentration of glycosaminoglycans in synovial fluid (hyaluronic acid and chondroitin sulfates) is decreased compared with normal controls, accounting for the low viscosity of inflamed synovial fluid.

GENERAL PRINCIPLES OF TREATMENT

Approach to Management

The British Society for Paediatric and Adolescent Rheumatology (BSPAR) has recently published guidelines for the care of children with JIA.[217] This advocacy statement takes a broad approach to the ideal management of children and youth with JIA, and includes empowering children and their caregivers, facilitating early detection of JIA, prompt referral to a pediatric rheumatology team, prompt access to all necessary pharmacological treatment and to ophthalmological expertise, and regular follow-up and monitoring. Achieving these goals is not yet possible in many parts of the world, but the statement points the way to the goal of providing the best possible care for children and youth with JIA. The treatment team, educational, transition, and psychosocial issues are discussed in Chapter 11. Patient and family education and incorporation of the family's needs into the management program facilitate optimal therapeutic benefit.[211]

TABLE 15-4   Characteristics of Synovial Fluid in Rheumatic Diseases

GROUP AND CONDITION	SYNOVIAL COMPLEMENT FINDINGS	COLOR AND CLARITY	VISCOSITY	MUCIN CLOT	WBC/mm^3 COUNT	PMN (%)	MISCELLANEOUS
Noninflammatory							
Normal	Normal	Yellow and clear	Very high	Good	<200	<25	
Traumatic arthritis	Normal	Xanthochromic and turbid	High	Fair to good	<2000	<25	Debris
Osteoarthritis	Normal	Yellow and clear	High	Fair to good	1000	<25	
Inflammatory							
Systemic lupus erythematosus	Low	Yellow and clear	Normal	Normal	5000	10	Lupus erythematosus cells
Rheumatic fever	Normal to high	Yellow and cloudy	↓	Fair	5000	10-50	
Chronic arthritis	Normal to high	Yellow and cloudy	↓	Poor	15,000-20,000	75	
Reactive arthritis	High	Yellow and opaque	↓	Poor	20,000	80	
Pyogenic							
Tuberculous arthritis	Normal to high	Yellow-white and cloudy	↓	Poor	25,000	50-60	Acid-fast bacteria
Septic arthritis	High	Serosanguineous and turbid	↓	Poor	50,000-300,000	>75	Low glucose, bacteria

Although JIA cannot yet be cured, disease control is often achievable. The goal of therapy should be to induce disease remission, and in the process to control pain and preserve range of motion, muscle strength, and function; to manage systemic complications; and to facilitate normal nutrition, growth, and physical and psychological development (see Chapter 11). Along with advances in therapeutics has come a raised expectation for disease control. An "adequate" response is no longer considered to be acceptable under most circumstances. The total control of inflammation is a goal that should be pursued within the constraints of safety and cost. Although the major focus of medical therapy is on the arthritis, the management of pain as well as other extraarticular complications (e.g., uveitis, serositis, growth retardation, osteopenia) require consideration. Most children with JIA require a combination of pharmacological, physical, and psychosocial approaches.

Pharmacological Management

The more rapidly inflammation can be controlled, the less likely it is that there will be permanent sequelae. Nonsteroidal antiinflammatory drugs (NSAIDs) have been the traditional initial approach. Three developments, however, have fundamentally altered the current therapeutic approach beyond that point: Intraarticular glucocorticoids have proved effective in treating joint disease; low-dose methotrexate (MTX) has substantially changed the choice of treatment options; and new therapeutic modalities such as the anti–TNF-α, anti–IL-1 or anti–IL-6, or costimulation-inhibiting biologics promise even further improvements. Consensus recommendations for the treatment of children with JIA have recently been published.[218,219] Five patient groups were considered (irrespective of ILAR classification): individuals who had a history of (1) oligoarthritis, (2) polyarthritis, (3) sacroiliac arthritis, (4) systemic arthritis with systemic features, and (5) systemic arthritis without active systemic features. In addition, recommendations were made in consideration of the presence or absence of poor prognostic features, and the level of disease activity that was defined

BOX 15-5   Core Set Criteria for Assessing Improvement in JIA

1. Physician's global assessment of disease activity (10 cm visual analog scale)
2. Parent/patient assessment of overall well-being (10 cm visual analog scale)
3. Functional ability (CHAQ)
4. Number of joints with active inflammation
5. Number of joints with limited range of motion
6. Erythrocyte sedimentation rate (mm/hr)

Improvement of at least 30% in three or more criteria, with worsening of not more than 30% in not more than one criterion. Giannini et al.[220]

for each of the five patient groups. The recommendations were made using the RAND/UCLA Appropriateness Methodology and considered the use of NSAIDs, disease-modifying antirheumatic drugs (DMARDs), some biologics, corticosteroid joint injections, and, in systemic disease with active systemic features, systemic corticosteroids. Several of the newer biologics were not considered, and several specific scenarios (macrophage activation syndrome, uveitis, enthesitis) were not evaluated. Specific recommendations for therapy are presented in Chapters 16 to 22. A discussion of the pharmacological aspects of these agents is provided in Chapters 12 and 13.

Evidence of improvement is based on a review of the clinical course, repeated physical examinations, charting of the articular severity index and global responses, and laboratory estimates of inflammation. These evaluations have been systematized in the so-called core set variables[220] (Box 15-5). A minimal clinically significant response is an improvement of at least 30% in at least three of the six variables, with worsening by no more than 30% in not more than one variable. More demanding criteria require 50% 70% or 90% improvement. More recently, the JADAS (Juvenile Arthritis Disease Activity Score) has been proposed, tested, and compared to the core set variables: although still a composite score, this has the advantage of being a numeric score, making it easier to compare disease burden in different cases and groups.[221,222]

Definitions of inactive oligoarticular, polyarticular RF-negative, polyarticular RF-positive, and systemic disease have been proposed by Wallace et al.[223] (Box 15-6). A preliminary definition of disease flare in JIA has also been studied.[224]

It is difficult to be confident of the risk/benefit ratio for many of the therapeutic regimens for children with JIA. Differences in the therapeutic efficacy of antirheumatic drugs in children of different ethnic and genetic background have been largely unexplored,[225] although the results of a genome-wide study have demonstrated genetic traits related to clinical response to methotrexate in JIA.[226] Toxicity is often a foremost concern in the long-term use of glucocorticoids, immunosuppressive agents, or biologics. Because of the relative lack of scientific guidance by appropriately designed studies undertaken in adequate numbers of children with appropriate control of confounding factors such as type of onset and course of the disease, the experience and judgment of the pediatric rheumatologist has become very important.

Alternative and complementary therapies, although of no proven benefit, are widely used by children with chronic arthritis. Their use is often fostered by information or misinformation available through the Internet. Parents should be directed to more objective sources of information, such as the *Arthritis Foundation's Guide to Alternative Therapies*.[227]

As monotherapy, NSAIDs should be continued until all evidence of active disease has disappeared. Methotrexate therapy should probably be continued for up to 6 months after a remission has been achieved. One might also decrease administration of MTX to every 2 weeks for a period of time before discontinuation.[228] In combination therapy, a consensus has not developed on the order of withdrawal of medications. However, discontinuation of corticosteroids, is usually the first goal. NSAIDs can then be discontinued, MTX tapered, and finally, biologics stopped. In children, potentially toxic regimens such as prolonged use of glucocorticoid and immunosuppressive drugs should be employed only in uncontrolled or life-threatening disease.

Nutrition

Several studies have documented varying degrees of undernutrition or obesity in children and adolescents with JIA.[229-233] Assessment of nutritional status should be a component of every patient's evaluation.[230] Growth retardation and impaired bone mineralization almost invariably occur during periods of active disease and are exacerbated by glucocorticoid administration, anorexia, or inanition. Nutritional and

vitamin supplementation (calcium, vitamin D, and folic acid) are often indicated. Management of malnutrition is often difficult in the systemically ill, anorectic child. Specific measures to address osteopenia and osteoporosis are reviewed in Chapter 53. Marked microcytic, hypochromic anemia may not be improved by oral iron supplementation, which often adversely affects appetite. Henderson and Lovell[232] suggested the use of a four-parameter test to screen for protein-energy malnutrition. The presence of any two of the following abnormalities indicates the need for a detailed nutritional assessment: weight below 5th percentile, weight-for-height index below 80th percentile, arm circumference below 5th percentile, and serum albumin less than 2.8 mg/dL (28 g/L).

Physical and Occupational Therapy

The objectives of physical and occupational therapy are to minimize pain, maintain and restore function, and prevent deformity and disability. These aspects of treatment are critically important in the child's total management program and are discussed in Chapter 14.

Orthopedic Surgery

Orthopedic surgery has an important, but limited, role in management of chronic arthritis in young children. In the older child, however, surgical approaches to joint contractures, dislocations, or joint replacement become important components of therapy.

Synovectomy

The long-term outcome of children with joint disease is not altered by prophylactic synovectomy. However, synovectomy may occasionally be useful in some children for relief of mechanical impairment of joint motion related to joint pain or synovial hypertrophy.[234-237] Carl and colleagues[236] reported the results of open hip joint synovectomies in 56 patients with JRA carried out between 1985 and 1997. Synovectomy was performed if, after medical therapy with NSAIDs, systemic glucocorticoids, and disease-modifying antiinflammatory drugs, the patient had persistent synovitis (demonstrated by ultrasound), pain, joint effusion, and a limitation of range of motion of the hip. The authors concluded that at a mean of 50 months after surgery, synovectomy allowed significant improvement in hip function (pain, mobility, and ability to walk) in patients with early or late disease. Five patients required total hip joint replacement at a mean of 39 months after surgery.

Dell'Era and colleagues[237] reported the results of arthroscopic synovectomy at a mean of 5.4 years following surgery performed between 1990 and 2005 on 19 patients (31 knees) with JIA. Disease recurred in 67% of those with oligoarthritis, 95% of those with polyarthritis, and in all with psoriatic arthritis. Recurrence occurred most quickly (0.8 year) in those with polyarthritis. Only 26% of these patients had received MTX. Another 26% had received sulfasalazine, and only two patients had received an anti-TNF agent. The authors concluded that synovectomy of the knee could be useful to "buy time" before systemic therapy became effective." It is difficult to assess if synovectomy of the hip or knee has an important role in the management of children treated appropriately with intraarticular steroids and MTX or biologics.

Soft Tissue Surgery

Soft tissue releases, posterior capsulotomy, and tendon lengthening occasionally are useful in a child with a severe contracture of the knee or hip. Tenosynovectomy may be indicated to reduce the risk of tendon rupture over the dorsum of the wrist or for adhesive flexor tenosynovitis and trigger finger, which sometimes occurs in children who are RF seropositive.

Reconstructive Surgery

Reconstructive surgery for hip or knee arthritis is important in the older patient with marked pain and disability.[238,239] Surgery is usually postponed until bone growth has ceased. Malviya et al.[238] reported the results of hip joint replacement in 25 adults with JIA followed for a mean of 19 years. Eight had RF-positive polyarticular JIA, seven polyarticular RF-negative JIA, seven systemic JIA, and three oligoarticular JIA. Revision was required in 40% of patients at a mean of 11 years after initial arthroplasty. Parvizi et al.[239] reported good results in 25 knees following arthroplasty, although six patients required revision or repeated surgery. Special considerations include the status of the other lower-extremity joints, activity of the rheumatic disease in general, and the anticipated longevity of the prostheses in young active youth and adults.

Counseling the Family

It is of signal importance that the child with arthritis and the parents be educated about the present state of knowledge regarding outcome, and therapy. Counseling should be initiated by the physician at the time of the first visit and reinforced and continued at follow-up by the team. Educational efforts are repeated as needed during the subsequent clinical course, especially in an effort to increase adherence[240,241] (see Chapter 11).

DISEASE COURSE AND OUTCOME

The course of untreated arthritis has probably not changed in the past century. The devastating consequences of prolonged untreated disease are still occasionally encountered in the developed world and are much more common in the developing world (see Chapter 11). Fortunately, the disease course and outcome continue to change dramatically with appropriate early therapy. This makes all long-term outcome studies prior to 1990 of historical, rather than current, importance. To a considerable extent, the outcome with treatment is related to the disease subtype and is discussed in the appropriate chapters. Nonetheless, certain generalizations can be made.

The course of chronic arthritis is especially unpredictable early in the disease. It is impossible to predict the eventual disease outcome in any individual child. Furthermore, "outcome" is a complex concept that can be measured in a number of ways (see Chapter 7).

Functional Disability and Psychosocial Outcome

Wallace and Levinson[242] (Table 15-5) documented outcome at 15 to 20 years after disease onset. Seventeen percent of the patients were in Steinbrocker functional classes III to IV (Table 15-6), and 45% still had active disease (activity of disease was approximately equal for each onset type). Ruperto and colleagues[243] evaluated long-term outcome in a group of 227 patients from Cincinnati and Pavia. This study examined the effect of specific demographic, clinical, and immunological variables that were present during the first 6 months of the illness. The mean duration of disease at assessment was 15 years (range: 5.3 to 36.1 years). With treatment, the best predictor of long-term disability was the initial articular severity score. Early hand involvement was also a strong predictor of future disability, pain, and impaired well-being. ANA positivity was associated with less disability. The long-term outcome, based on quality-of-life scales and health assessment questionnaires, was favorable in most patients 5 years or more after onset of symptoms.[244,245]

The Childhood Health Assessment Questionnaire (CHAQ) has been evaluated for measurement of health status in early and late disease.[246] Oen and colleagues[247] surveyed early predictors of long-term

TABLE 15-5 Functional Outcome of Chronic Arthritis					
AUTHOR (REF. NO.)	FOLLOW-UP (YRS)	STEINBROCKER CLASS (%)			
		I	II	III	IV
Wallace and Levinson[242]	15-20			(17)*	
Oen et al.[247]	0.5			(2.5)*	
Zak and Pedersen[247a]	10		6.1	(7.7)*	
	26		21.5	(10.8)*	
Minden et al.[247b]	7	49	39	10	2
	17	55	33	11	1

*These numbers represent patients in Steinbrocker III and IV.

TABLE 15-6 Functional Classification of Patients with Rheumatoid Arthritis.	
Class I	Complete functional capacity
Class II	Functional capacity adequate to conduct normal activities despite discomfort or limited mobility
Class III	Functional capacity adequate to perform some activities of usual occupation or self-care
Class IV	Largely or totally incapacitated; bedridden or confined to a wheelchair, permitting little or no self-care

Modified from O. Steinbrocker, C.H. Traeger, R.C. Batterman, Therapeutic criteria in rheumatoid arthritis, JAMA 140 (1949) 659–662.

TABLE 15-7 Functional Outcome of Juvenile Rheumatoid Arthritis by the Childhood Health Assessment Questionnaire (CHAQ)			
TYPE OF ONSET (N)	FOLLOW-UP (MEAN YR)	CHAQ SCORE	
		MEAN	RANGE
Systemic (40)	11.6	0.25	0-2.75
Pauciarticular (224)	12.5	0	0-2.13
Polyarticular (RF–) (80)	12.6	0.19	0-2.75
Polyarticular (RF+) (40)	13.9	0.62	0-3.0

Data from K. Oen, P.N. Malleson, D.A. Cabral, et al., Early predictors of longterm outcome in patients with juvenile rheumatoid arthritis: subset-specific correlations, J. Rheumatol. 30 (2003) 585–593.

outcome on the CHAQ in 392 patients with JRA, including 327 white patients, who were 8 years of age or older and had a minimum of 5 years of follow-up (Table 15-7). Worse disability was observed for systemic-onset JIA in males, less disability in patients with RF-negative disease, and a shorter duration of activity in RF-positive polyarthritis. ANA positivity in oligoarthritis was associated with a longer duration of activity, as was a younger age at onset. A subsequent report examined radiologic outcome in children from the same clinics.[248]

More recently, investigators have attempted to avoid the confounding factors of referral-based and clinic follow-up by primarily basing their outcome studies on population surveys. Data from the U.S. Pediatric Rheumatology Disease Registry[249] in 703 patients observed between 1992 and 1997 (before the era of biological therapy) indicated that more than 25% of those with polyarthritis, and almost half of those with systemic onset, had functional limitations affecting school activities. Joint space damage on radiographs was evident at 5 years in two thirds of the polyarticular and systemic-onset groups. Some investigators have also taken the approach recommended by the World Health Organization in 1980 to examine functional adaptation in relation to impairment (based on organ disease), disability (related to personal quality of life), and handicap (related to society's perception of the functioning ability of the individual).[250]

A study by Peterson and colleagues [251] evaluated the physical and psychosocial impacts of disease in a population-based cohort of 44 adults who had experienced onset of the disease during childhood. Controls (n = 102) were matched by age and sex. The average follow-up was 24.7 years, and mean age was 34 years. The patients had greater disability, more body pain, increased fatigue, poorer health perception, and decreased physical functioning, along with lower rates of employment and lower levels of exercise compared with the control group. On the other hand, educational achievement, annual income, health insurance status, and rates of pregnancy and childbirth were similar to those of the controls. Active disease was present in 66%, and 16% were under regular medical care for their arthritis. This study concluded that adults who had had chronic arthritis developed long-term physical and psychosocial impairments that have been often ignored in the evaluation of functional outcome.

Many of the same outcomes and prognostic factors were identified in a study by Flato and colleagues of 268 patients with JRA who were monitored for a median of 14.9 years (range: 11.7 to 25.1 years).[252] Another study from Norway[253] included 53 patients with arthritis and 19 with juvenile spondyloarthropathy. Forty-three (60%) of the 72 patients were in a remission at the time of the study, and 60% reported no disability. This study and subsequent studies[254] supported the conclusion that long-term outcome was more favorable than previously reported, perhaps related to less bias of admission to the study and the early use of more aggressive therapeutic regimens. This group of investigators had previously indicated that poor psychosocial functioning in 22% of the patients on follow-up was associated with premorbid psychosocial dysfunction, chronic family difficulties, and major life events. They also confirmed that approximately 19% of the patients were still suffering from chronic pain without evidence of active arthritis.[252] A chronic pain syndrome may persist in these patients well after their arthritis has gone into remission.[255]

A large detailed study of adults with juvenile onset arthritis by Packham and Hall[256-259] provides important information about the status of adults with JIA with a mean duration of 28.3 years after disease onset. Educational levels were higher than the national average and those of their siblings, although the rate of unemployment was much higher than the national average. Fewer patients were in stable relationships than their siblings. The presence of active disease in 43.3% and Health Assessment Questionnaire (HAQ) scores greater than 1.5 indicating significant disability in 42.9%, supported the need for transitional and ongoing care. MTX had been prescribed in 40.7%, but no patient had received a biologic. Outcome with current therapy is almost certain to yield better outcomes at an equivalent follow-up time.

Malignancy

The risk of malignancy in children with JIA has been the subject of several studies, prompted in large part by the concern that the biologics might be associated with malignancies. Diak et al.[260] reported malignancy in 48 children (19 with JIA) who had received anti–TNF-α treatment together with azathioprine or MTX. The background risk of malignancy in children with JIA was thought to be low.[261] A Swedish study[262] supported this conclusion for patients seen prior to 1987. However, researchers noted an increased rate of lymphoproliferative malignancies in children with JIA seen since 1987, but before the biologics era. Beukelman et al. used registry data and reported an apparent increased incidence of malignancy in patients with JIA that was not increased by the use of TNF inhibitors.[263] Nordstrom et al.[264] demonstrated a threefold increased risk of malignancy in biologics-naïve patients with JIA. The risk that long-term use of biologics might add is not clear. Nonetheless, caution in their use is warranted.[265,266]

Mortality

In early studies of chronic arthritis in children, the overall death rate was 1% to 4%.[267,268] The disease-associated death rate is now probably less than 1% in Europe and less than 0.3% in North America. This mortality represents, however, a fourfold to fourteen-fold increase compared with standardized rates. In a study from England,[269] the standardized mortality ratio was 3.4 for males (95% CI, 2.0 to 5.5) and 5.1 for females (95% CI, 3.2 to 7.8). The majority of the deaths in Europe were previously related to the development of amyloidosis[270]; in the United States, deaths occurred predominantly in children with systemic-onset disease and in many cases were related to infection. Even in Europe, amyloidosis as a complication of chronic arthritis appears to be on the decline.[271]

BURDEN OF DISEASE

The economic burden of any disease including JIA is difficult to measure precisely and depends to some extent on the medical care delivery system. The unreimbursed cost to the family of a child with a chronic rheumatic disease per year is considerable. Allaire and colleagues[272] estimated annual direct medical costs per patient with JIA in the United States in 1992 at $7905. Three studies of economic burden of disease in countries with some form of universal prepaid health care indicate that not only is there is considerable cost in the first year after diagnosis but that this cost continues into adulthood, especially in those with ongoing active disease.

Minden and colleagues[273] studied the economic costs in 215 German patients an average of 17 years after disease onset, using clinical records, a structured interview, and questionnaires. Direct costs (health care, including physician, hospital, and drug costs) accounted for 45% of the total cost. Indirect costs (sick leave, work disability, lost productivity in older patients) accounted for 55%. The authors estimated that the mean annual cost was €3500. The economic burden was greatest in those with active RF-positive polyarthritis (€17,000) and extended oligoarthritis (€11,000), and lowest in those with persistent oligoarthritis (€2700), and active ERA (€1500) (possibly because of later age at onset of arthritis in the last group).

Bernatsky and colleagues[274] studied the economic burden of disease in the families of 155 Canadian children (mean age 10 years) with arthritis, and 181 children (mean age 10.5 years) with other, mainly nonchronic disorders). The annual direct cost medical care, hospitalization, and drugs was estimated to be C$3002 in children with arthritis and C$1315 in the comparison group. Thornton and colleagues[275] studied the economic burden in 297 children in the first year of diagnosis in the United Kingdom. Mean annual economic cost was £1649 (standard deviation [SD] £1093, range £401 to £6967).

PERSPECTIVE

In spite of new insights into causation and considerable advances in treatment, JIA remains an important cause of chronic pain and disability. Delay in recognition and instituting treatment can result in irretrievable damage to joints and other organs, be a significant cause of functional and psychosocial impairment, and pose an economic burden to families and society.

REFERENCES

5. R.E. Petty, T.R. Southwood, P. Manners, et al., International League of Associations for Rheumatology classification of juvenile idiopathic arthritis, second revision, Edmonton, 2001, J. Rheumatol. 31 (2004) 390–392.
6. E.J. Brewer Jr., J. Bass, J. Baum, et al., Current proposed revision of JRA Criteria. JRA Criteria Subcommittee of the Diagnostic and Therapeutic Criteria Committee of the American Rheumatism Section of the Arthritis Foundation, Arthritis Rheum. 20 (1977) 195–199.
30. E.E. Eisenstein, Y. Berkun, Diagnosis and classification of juvenile idiopathic arthritis, J. Autoimmun. 48–49 (2014) 31–33.
31. E.G. Ferrell, L.A. Ponder, L.S. Minor, et al., Limitations in the classification of childhood-onset rheumatoid arthritis, J. Rheumatol. 41 (2014) 547–553.
32. A. Martini, It is time to rethink juvenile idiopathic arthritis classification and nomenclature, Ann. Rheum. Dis. 71 (2012) 1437–1439.
39. R.A. Colbert, Classification of juvenile spondyloarthritis: enthesitis related arthritis and beyond, Nat Rev Rheumatol 6 (2010) 477–485.
41. S. Kumar, D.S. Kunhiraman, L. Rajam, Application of the Yamaguchi criteria for classification of "suspected" systemic onset juvenile idiopathic arthritis (sJIA), Pediatric Rheum 10 (2012) 40.
42. A. Ravelli, G.C. Varnier, S. Oliveira, et al., Antinuclear antibody-positive patients should be grouped as a separate category in the classification of juvenile idiopathic arthritis, Arthritis Rheum. 63 (2011) 267–275.
47. M. Benjamin, D. McGonagle, The enthesis organ concept and its relevance to the spondyloarthropathies, Adv. Exp. Med. Biol. 649 (2009) 57–70.
49. G.F. Still, On a form of chronic joint disease in children, Med. Chir. Trans. 80 (1897) 47. Reprinted in Am. J. Dis. Child. 132 (1978) 193–200.
57. S. Thierry, B. Fautrel, L. Lemelle, F. Guillemin, Prevalence and incidence of juvenile idiopathic arthritis. A systematic review, Joint Bone Spine 81 (2014) 112–117.
59. N. Moe, M. Rygg, Epidemiology of juvenile chronic arthritis in northern Norway: a ten-year retrospective study, Clin. Exp. Rheumatol. 16 (1998) 99–101.
72. R.K. Sauernmann, J.B. Rose, P. Tyrell, et al., Epidemiology of juvenile idiopathic arthritis in a multiethnic cohort, Arthritis Rheum. 56 (2007) 1974–1984.
76. A. Hinks, J. Cobb, M.C. Marion, et al., Dense genotyping of immune loci in juvenile idiopathic arthritis identifies 14 new susceptibility loci, Nat. Genet. 45 (2013) 664–669.
80. N. Bottini, G.S. Firestein, Epigenetics in rheumatoid arthritis: a primer for rheumatologists, Curr. Rheumatol. Rep. 15 (2013) 372.
97. S. Lambrecht, N. Juchtmans, D. Elewant, Heat shock proteins in stromal joint tissues: Innocent bystanders or disease-initiating proteins?, Rheumatology (Oxford) 53 (2014) 223–232.
99. E.R. Graeff-Meeder, W. Van Eden, G.T. Rijkers, et al., Heat-shock proteins and juvenile chronic arthritis, Clin. Exp. Rheumatol. 11 (Suppl. 9) (1993) S25–S28.
112. E. Zonneveld-Huijssoon, S.T. Roord, W. de Jager, et al., Bystander suppression of experimental arthritis by nasal administration of heat shock protein peptide, Ann. Rheum. Dis. 70 (2011) 2199–2206.
115. M.W. Heijstek, S. Kamphuis, W. Armbrust, et al., Effects of the live measles mumps rubella attenuated booster vaccination on disease activity in patients with juvenile idiopathic arthritis: a randomized trial, JAMA 309 (2013) 2449–2456.
117. K.K. Anthony, M.H. Bromberg, K.M. Gil, L.E. Schanberg, Parental perceptions of child vulnerability and parent stress as predictors of pain and adjustment in children with chronic arthritis, Child. Health Care 40 (2011) 53–69.
119. K.M. Neufeld, C.P. Karunanayake, L.Y. Maenz, A.M. Rosenberg, Stressful life events antedating chronic childhood arthritis, J. Rheumatol. 40 (2013) 1756–1765.
122. T. Kobezda, S. Ghassmi-Nejad, K. Mikecz, et al., Of mice and men: how animal models advance our understanding of T-cell function in RA, Nat Rev Rheumatol 10 (2014) 160–170.
131. S. Angeles-Han, S. Prahalad, The genetics of juvenile idiopathic arthritis: What is new in 2010, Curr. Rheumatol. Rep. 12 (2010) (2010) 87–93.
132. A. Hinks, P. Martin, E. Flynn, et al., Subtype specific genetic associations for juvenile idiopathic arthritis: ERAP 1 with enthesitis related arthritis subtype and IL-23R with juvenile psoriatic arthritis, Arthritis Res. Ther. 13 (2010) R12.
138. J. Roizen, C.I. Magyar, E.S. Kuschner, et al., A community cross-sectional survey of medical problems in 440 children with Down syndrome in New York State, J. Pediatr. 164 (2014) 871–875.
147. L. Le Hausse de LaLouvière, Y. Ioannou, M. Fitzgerald, Neural mechanisms underlying the pain of juvenile idiopathic arthritis, Nat Rev Rheumatol 10 (2014) 205–211.
154. H.E. Foster, L.J. Kay, M. Friswell, et al., Musculoskeletal screening examination (pGALS) for school age children based on the adult GALS screen, Arthritis Rheum. 55 (2006) 709–716.
164. C.J. Henderson, B.L. Specker, R.I. Sierra, et al., Total-body bone mineral content in non-corticosteroid-treated postpubertal females with juvenile rheumatoid arthritis: frequency of osteopenia and contributing factors, Arthritis Rheum. 43 (2000) 531–540.
166. J. Thornton, S.R. Pye, T.W. O'Neill, et al., Bone health in adult men and women with a history of juvenile idiopathic arthritis, J. Rheumatol. 38 (2011) 1689–1693.
167. J.M. Burnham, Inflammatory disease and bone health in childhood, Curr. Opin. Rheumatol. 24 (2012) 548–553.
172. S. Padeh, O. Pinhas-Hamiel, D. Zimmermann-Sloutskis, Y. Berkun, Children with oligoarticular juvenile idiopathic arthritis are at considerable risk for growth retardation, J. Pediatr. 159 (2011) 832–837.
179. M. Twilt, A.J.M. Schulten, P. Nicolaas, et al., Facioskeletal changes in children with juvenile idiopathic arthritis, Ann. Rheum. Dis. 65 (2006) 823–825.
180. R. Sauernmann, The difficult diagnosis of temporomandibular joint arthritis, J. Rheumatol. 39 (2012) 1778–1780.
183. S. Ringold, M. Thapa, E.A. Shaw, C.A. Wallace, Heterotopic ossification of the temporomandibular joint in juvenile idiopathic arthritis, J. Rheumatol. 38 (2011) 1423–1428.
184. Y.N. Vaid, D. Dunnavant, S.A. Royal, et al., Imaging of the temporomandibular joint in juvenile idiopathic arthritis, Arthritis Care Res. 66 (2014) 47–54.
186. O.T. Lelieveld, W. Armbrust, M.A. Van Leeuwen, et al., Physical activity in adolescents with juvenile idiopathic arthritis, Arthritis Rheum. 59 (2008) 1379–1384.
187. K. Houghton, Physical activity, physical fitness and exercise therapy in children with juvenile idiopathic arthritis, Physician Sports Med 40 (2012) 77–82.
197. K. Nistala, H. Moncrieffe, K.R. Newton, et al., Interleukin-17-producing T cells are enriched in the joints of children with arthritis, but have a reciprocal relationship to regulatory T cell numbers, Arthritis Rheum. 58 (2008) 875–887.
198. C. Piper, A.M. Pesenacker, D. Bending, et al., T cell FM-CSF expression in juvenile arthritis is contingent upon Th17 plasticity, Arthritis Rheum. 66 (2014) 1955–1960.
201. S. Finnegan, S. Clarke, D. Gibson, et al., Synovial membrane immunohistology in early untreated juvenile idiopathic arthritis: differences between clinical subgroups, Ann. Rheum. Dis. 70 (2011) 1842–1850.
202. S. Finnegan, J. Robson, C. Scaife, et al., Synovial membrane protein expression differs between juvenile idiopathic arthritis subtypes in early disease, Arthritis Res. Ther. 16 (2014) R8.

204. F. Rothmund, J. Gerss, N. Ruperto, et al., Validation of relapse risk biomarkers for routine use in patients with juvenile idiopathic arthritis, Arthritis Care Res. 66 (2014) 949–955.

206. A.E. Tebo, T. Jaskowski, K.W. Davis, et al., Profiling citrullinated peptide antibodies in patients with juvenile idiopathic arthritis, Pediatr Rheumatol 10 (2012) 29.

208. R. Sauernmann, A.V. Levin, B.M. Feldman, et al., Risk factor for development of uveitis differ between girls and boys with juvenile idiopathic arthritis, Arthritis Rheum. 62 (2010) 1824–1828.

209. S.T. Angeles-Han, C.F. Pelajo, L.B. Vogler, et al., Risk markers of juvenile idiopathic arthritis associated uveitis in the Childhood Arthritis and Rheumatology Research Alliance (CARRA) Registry, J. Rheumatol. 40 (2013) 2088–2096.

217. K. Davies, G. Cleary, H. Foster, et al., BSPAR standards of care for children and young people with juvenile idiopathic arthritis, Rheumatology 49 (2010) 1406–1408.

218. T. Beukelman, N.M. Patkar, K.G. Saag, et al., 2011 American College of Rheumatology recommendations for the treatment of juvenile idiopathic arthritis: initiation and safety monitoring of therapeutic agents for the treatment of arthritis and systemic features, Arthritis Care Res. 63 (2011) 465–482.

219. S. Ringold, P.F. Weiss, T. Beukelman, et al., 2013 update of the 2011 American College of Rheumatology recommendations for the treatment of juvenile idiopathic arthritis, Arthritis Rheum. 65 (2013) 2499–2512.

220. E.H. Giannini, N. Ruperto, A. Ravelli, et al., Preliminary definition of improvement in juvenile arthritis, Arthritis Rheum. 40 (1997) 1202–1209.

221. A. Consolaro, N. Ruperto, A. Bazso, et al., Development and validation of a composite disease activity score for juvenile idiopathic arthritis, Arthritis Rheum. 61 (2009) 658–666.

222. F. McErlane, M.W. Beresford, E.M. Baldam, et al., Recent developments in disease activity indices and outcome measures for juvenile idiopathic arthritis, Rheumatology (Oxford) 52 (2013) 1941–1951.

223. C.A. Wallace, E.H. Giannini, B. Huang, et al., American College of Rheumatology provisional criteria for defining clinical inactive disease in select categories of juvenile idiopathic arthritis, Arthritis Care Res. 63 (2011) 929–936.

224. H.I. Brunner, D.J. Lovell, B.K. Finck, E.H. Giannini, Preliminary definition of disease flare in juvenile rheumatoid arthritis, J. Rheumatol. 29 (2002) 1058–1064.

226. J. Cobb, E. Cule, H. Moncrieffe, et al., Genome wide data reveal novel genes for methotrexate response in a large cohort of juvenile idiopathic arthritis cases, Pharmacogenomics J. 14 (2014) 356–364.

230. S.T. Shin, H.H. Yu, L.C. Wang, et al., Nutritional status and clinical characteristics of children with juvenile rheumatoid arthritis, J. Microbiol. Immunol. Infect. 43 (2010) 93–98.

237. L. Dell'Era, F. Facchini, F. Corona, Knee synovectomy in children with juvenile idiopathic arthritis, J. Pediatr. Orthop. B 17 (2008) 128–130.

238. A. Malviya, L.C. Walker, P. Avery, et al., The long-term outcome of hip replacement in adults with juvenile idiopathic arthritis, J. Bone Joint Surg. Br. 93-B (2011) 443–448.

250. T. Hutchison, The classification of disability, Arch. Dis. Child. 73 (1995) 1–93.

257. J.C. Packham, M.A. Hall, Long-term follow-up of 246 adults with juvenile idiopathic arthritis: education and employment, Rheumatology 41 (2002) 1436–1439.

259. J.C. Packham, M.A. Hall, Long-term follow-up of 246 adults with juvenile idiopathic arthritis: functional outcome, Rheumatology 41 (2002) 1428–1435.

260. P. Diak, J. Siegel, L. LaGranade, et al., Tumor necrosis alpha blockers and malignancy in children: forty-eight cases reported to the Food and Drug Administration, Arthritis Rheum. 62 (2010) 2517–2524.

261. S. Bernatsky, A.M. Rosenberg, K.G. Oen, et al., Malignancies in juvenile idiopathic arthritis: A preliminary report, J. Rheumatol. 38 (2011) 760–763.

262. J.F. Simard, M. Neovius, S. Hagelberg, J. Asling, Juvenile idiopathic arthritis and risk of cancer. A nationwide cohort study, Arthritis Rheum. 62 (2010) 3776–3782.

263. T. Beukelman, K. Haynes, J.R. Curtis, et al., Rates of malignancy associated with juvenile idiopathic arthritis and its treatment, Arthritis Rheum. 64 (2012) 1263–1271.

264. B.L. Nordstrom, D. Mines, Y. Gu, et al., Risk of malignancy in children with juvenile idiopathic arthritis not treated with biologic agents, Arthritis Care Res. 64 (2012) 1357–1364.

265. N. Ruperto, A. Martini, Juvenile idiopathic arthritis and malignancy, Rheumatology 53 (2014) 968–974.

Entire reference list is available online at www.expertconsult.com.

CHAPTER 16

Systemic Juvenile Idiopathic Arthritis

Fabrizio De Benedetti, Rayfel Schneider

Systemic arthritis is one of the most perplexing diseases of childhood. Its onset can be quite nonspecific and may suggest bacterial or viral infection, malignancy, or another inflammatory disease. The evolution of the disease eventually confirms the diagnosis, which is entirely clinical. It is unique among the chronic arthritides of childhood, particularly in the range and severity of characteristic extraarticular features that mark this disease as a systemic illness with joint inflammation that ranges from mild to severe.

This disease is defined as *systemic arthritis* by the International League of Associations for Rheumatology (ILAR) classification of juvenile idiopathic arthritis (JIA)[1] based on the following criteria: presence of arthritis and of a documented quotidian fever of at least 2 weeks' duration; plus one of the following: typical rash, generalized lymphadenopathy, enlargement of liver or spleen, or serositis. Criteria and exclusions are shown in Box 16-1.

For almost a century, this disorder bore the name *Still disease,* in recognition of its early description by George Frederic Still.[2] It was classified as *systemic-onset juvenile rheumatoid arthritis* by the 1977 American College of Rheumatology classification. The "onset" terminology has appropriately been abandoned in the ILAR classification because it is not only the onset but also the disease course that is different from other forms of JIA.

EPIDEMIOLOGY

Systemic JIA (SJIA) accounts for 5% to 15% of children with JIA seen in North America and Europe. The exact prevalence of the disease is not known, but studies from Europe indicate an annual incidence for SJIA between 0.3 and 0.8 cases per 100,000 children under 16 years of age.[3-7] At least in Europe, the incidence appears to be higher in northernmost countries compared with Southern European countries. In Asia, SJIA may account for a greater proportion of all childhood arthritis. Of individuals with JIA, 25% of cases in India and 50% in Japan, respectively, appears to be SJIA.[8,9]

The onset of SJIA may occur at any time during childhood, with a broad peak of onset between 1 and 5 years of age.[10-16] It occasionally manifests before 1 year of age, and it also occurs in adolescence. *Adult-onset Still disease* is the term used for patients who develop the disease when they are over the age of 16 years (see below). Males and females are affected with approximately equal frequency. Although one study documented a marked seasonal variation, with no patients having disease onset in the winter months,[11] subsequent studies failed to find clear evidence for seasonal variation in disease onset.[10,13]

ETIOLOGY AND PATHOGENESIS

Although its onset resembles an infectious disease, SJIA has not been consistently associated with any pathogen. The genetic factors associated with SJIA remain largely unclear. SJIA is rarely familial, which is consistent with the hypothesis that the genetic background of the disease is complex and related to multiple susceptibility alleles. In contrast to classic autoimmune diseases, genetic associations with human leukocyte antigen (HLA) class I or II alleles are weak and of uncertain significance. The most consistently reported associations are polymorphisms in the regulatory sequences of genes coding for cytokines of the innate immune response including macrophage-inhibitory factor (MIF), tumor necrosis factor (TNF)-α, interleukin (IL)-6 genes, and the IL-1 and IL-1 receptor loci.[14,17-22] Most of these polymorphisms are functionally relevant, affecting expression levels of the corresponding cytokines. Autoantibodies and autoreactive T cells are not present in SJIA. On the contrary, the number of innate immune cells, such as monocytes and neutrophils, is increased.[23] Studies of gene expression profiles in blood cells provide substantial evidence of a dysregulated innate immune response with consequent increased production of inflammatory cytokines.[24-27] Overexpression of genes of the IL-6 and Toll-like receptor (TLR)/IL-1R pathways has been demonstrated. Moreover, gene pathways related to natural killer cells or T cells are downregulated. The pathways involved appear to be different from those involved in polyarticular JIA,[28] highlighting the unique disease mechanism of SJIA.

Prominent innate immune activation results in elevated levels of several inflammatory cytokines, including IL-1, IL-6, IL-8, IL-18, MIF, and TNF.[29-35] Exaggerated production of these cytokines, generally although not exclusively, produced by monocytes/macrophages and neutrophils, appears to explain many of the features of SJIA. Measurement of up to 30 cytokines, and subsequent cluster analysis, showed that patients with SJIA cluster together and can be distinguished from patients with oligoarticular or polyarticular JIA.[36] Similarly, pathway analysis of plasma proteins in SJIA flares showed a typical signature that distinguished SJIA flares from active polyarticular JIA or from febrile illness.[37]

TNF-α levels, as well as levels of the two soluble TNF receptors, are increased in SJIA,[32,35,38,39] but TNF-α levels do not correlate with fever peaks.[35,40] The clinical response to TNF blockade of patients with SJIA is limited compared with that in other JIA forms, suggesting that TNF does not play a major role in SJIA. A substantial body of evidence supports a major role of increased IL-6 production in mediating signs and symptoms of SJIA.[41] IL-6 is markedly elevated in the blood and synovial fluid.[32,35,42-44] IL-6 levels increase just before fever spikes and correlate with the systemic features of the disease, arthritis, and increase in acute phase reactants.[35,40,42] *In vitro* studies have documented increased production of IL-6 by peripheral blood mononuclear cells from patients with SJIA.[45] In addition to the involvement of IL-6 in animal models of arthritis,[46] studies support a role for prominent IL-6 production in the limitation of growth, systemic osteoporosis, thrombocytosis, and microcytic anemia seen in SJIA.[42,47-49] Studies on serum

BOX 16-1   **Systemic Juvenile Idiopathic Arthritis: International League of Associations for Rheumatology (ILAR) Diagnostic Criteria**

Arthritis in any number of joints together with a fever of at least 2 weeks' duration that is documented to be daily (quotidian) for at least 3 days and is accompanied by one or more of the following:

- Evanescent rash
- Generalized lymphadenopathy
- Enlargement of liver or spleen
- Serositis

Exclusions:

- Psoriasis or a history of psoriasis in the patient or a first-degree relative
- Arthritis in an HLA-B27–positive male beginning after his sixth birthday
- Ankylosing spondylitis, enthesitis-related arthritis, sacroiliitis with inflammatory bowel disease, reactive arthritis, or acute anterior uveitis, or a history of one of these disorders in a first-degree relative
- The presence of IgM RF on at least two occasions at least 3 months apart

HLA, Human leukocyte antigen; *IgM,* immunoglobulin M.

and synovial fluid expression (both proteins and messenger RNA [mRNA] levels) of IL-1β in SJIA have yielded controversial results. Technical difficulties in measuring IL-1β protein levels reliably may account for these findings. Sera from patients with active SJIA induce expression of IL-1β in peripheral blood mononuclear cells (PBMCs) from healthy controls,[50,51] as well as expression of IL-1β inducible genes.[50] The mechanism leading to abnormal production of IL-1β remains unclear. An *in vitro* study of classical inflammasome stimulation, and subsequent caspase 1 activation and IL-1β secretion, failed to find abnormalities.[52] Other proteases in other cell types (e.g., neutrophils) might be involved in processing IL-1.[53] Moreover, the myeloid-related protein 8 (MRP-8) and MRP-14, secreted by neutrophils and monocytes/macrophages, are markedly elevated in the serum of active SJIA patients.[54,55] The MRP-8/MRP-14 complex acts as an endogenous ligand for Toll-like receptor 4 and induces inflammatory cytokines.[56,57] Neutralization of MRP-8/MRP-14 inhibits the stimulatory effect of SJIA sera on IL-1β production,[51] suggesting that MRP-8/MRP-14 may be at least one of the factors involved in inducing IL-1β production.

Although the above-mentioned polymorphisms in cytokine promoters may contribute to excessive cytokine expression, some data also point to defective inhibition of responses. Although classical antiinflammatory mechanisms appear to be stimulated in SJIA, they may not be upregulated to a level sufficient to effectively inhibit responses. These include production of the antiinflammatory cytokine IL-10,[33,39,58] expression of suppressor of cytokine signaling 3 (SOCS3)—which inhibits IL-1 and IL-6 intracellular signaling[27]—activity of the alternatively activated macrophages[24] and number and suppressor activity of regulatory T lymphocytes.[59]

In summary, the available evidence points to a dysregulation of the innate response with a prominent role of cells and cytokines of the innate response. The efficacy of treatment with IL-1 or IL-6 inhibitors provides additional compelling evidence supporting this hypothesis. These observations, together with the absence of autoantibodies and autoreactive T cells, suggest that SJIA should be considered an autoinflammatory disease.

CLINICAL MANIFESTATIONS

Children with SJIA are usually very ill at the time the diagnosis is made. They are fatigued; febrile; in pain with myalgia, arthralgia, sometimes with chest pain and abdominal pain; and frequently they have lost weight. These features predominate early in the course of the disease and may overshadow the arthritis. In a multicenter study of 136 children with SJIA the most common initial clinical features were fever (98%), arthritis (88%), and rash (81%). Only 39% had lymphadenopathy, 10% had pericarditis, and fewer had hepatosplenomegaly.[15] It is noteworthy that many patients did not fulfill the ILAR classification criteria for SJIA, predominantly because they did not meet the strict definition of the quotidian fever or because they did not have arthritis. The interval between the onset of systemic signs and the appearance of arthritis may be as long as 10 years. Nevertheless, the ILAR criteria for SJIA require the presence of arthritis. In contrast, the Yamaguchi criteria for adult-onset Still disease, a disease entity with many similarities with SJIA, do not require the presence of arthritis. Moreover, arthralgia that lasts for at least 2 weeks is only one of the four possible major criteria.[60] The strict application of the requirement for the presence of documented arthritis for the diagnosis of SJIA, early in the disease course, may result in unnecessary delays in initiating appropriate treatment. It is rare for fever to first manifest after the development of arthritis.

Fever

The temperature rises to 39°C or higher on a daily or twice-daily basis, with a rapid return to baseline or below the baseline (Fig. 16-1). This quotidian pattern is highly suggestive of the diagnosis of SJIA, although very early in the course of the disease the classic quotidian fever may not be apparent, and the pattern may be indistinguishable from that of sepsis. In these children, a more typical fever pattern may be seen after treatment with nonsteroidal antiinflammatory drugs (NSAIDs) is initiated. The fever may occur at any time of the day but is characteristically present in the late afternoon to evening in conjunction with the rash. The temperature may be subnormal in the morning. Chills are frequent at the time of the fever, but rigors are rare. These children are often quite ill while febrile but may be surprisingly well during the rest of the day. The fever usually lasts for several months, may recur with flares of disease, and occasionally persists for years.

Rash

The intermittent fever is almost always accompanied by a classic rash that consists of discrete, erythematous macules 2 to 5 mm in size that may appear in linear streaks (Fig. 16-2).[61] This rash is usually described as salmon pink, but very early in the disease it may be more erythematous although never purpuric. It most commonly occurs on the trunk and proximal extremities but may develop on the face, palms, or soles. The macules are often surrounded by a zone of pallor and larger lesions develop central clearing. The rash tends to be migratory and is strikingly evanescent in any one area. Individual lesions disappear within a few hours and leave no residua. The rash may be much more persistent in children who are systemically very ill, and it may reappear with each systemic exacerbation. Individual lesions may be elicited by rubbing or scratching the skin (the *Koebner phenomenon* or *isomorphic response*) or by a hot bath or psychological stress. The rash is sometimes pruritic,[62] particularly in older patients, where it resembles urticaria. Cutaneous vasculitis is rare[63] and has been associated with the use of TNF inhibitors.[64] Persistent pruritic papules and plaques that are violaceous or brownish in color may be seen on the trunk, neck, face, and extensor surfaces of the extremities in adult-onset Still disease and rarely in SJIA.[65,66]

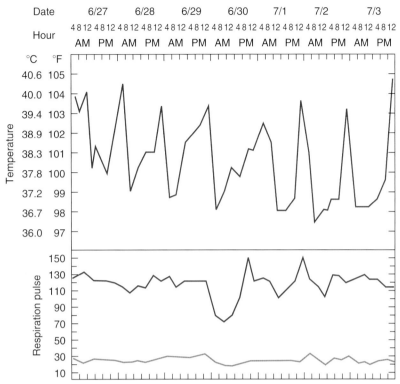

FIGURE 16-1 Intermittent fever of SJIA in a 3-year-old girl. The fever spikes usually occurred daily in the late evening to early morning (quotidian pattern), returned to normal or below normal, and were accompanied by severe malaise, tachycardia, and rash.

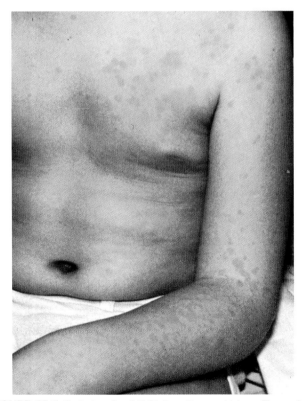

FIGURE 16-2 Typical rash of SJIA in a 3-year-old boy. The rash is salmon colored, macular, and nonpruritic. Individual lesions are transient, occur in crops over the trunk and extremities, and may occur in a linear distribution (Koebner phenomenon) after minor trauma such as a scratch.

Musculoskeletal Disease

Arthritis

Any number of joints can be affected at onset or during the disease course. Monoarthritis is uncommon; the course for those with persistently active disease is characteristically polyarticular. The knees, wrists, and ankles are most commonly involved, but cervical spine and hip disease, as well as inflammation of the small joints of the hands and the temporomandibular joint, occur in more than half of patients. Joint disease usually increases in extent and severity over weeks or months. Some children develop severe polyarthritis that is very resistant to treatment and eventually results in significant disability. Joint damage can ensue rapidly with joint space loss, erosions, and even ankylosis occurring within the first 2 years of onset. In other children, the disease is less severe and eventually goes into clinical remission. Prior to the current biological era, severe destructive polyarticular arthritis was reported in approximately one third of patients after a mean follow-up of 5 years.[67]

Tenosynovitis and Synovial Cysts

Tenosynovitis is frequently seen in children with a polyarticular course. The most common sites involved are the extensor tendon sheaths on the dorsum of the hand, the finger flexor tendon sheaths, the extensor sheaths over the dorsum of the foot, and those of the posterior tibial tendon and the peroneus longus and brevis tendons around the ankle. Some children develop synovial cysts that communicate with shoulder, elbow, wrist, or knee joints. Bicipital synovial cysts may cause acutely painful upper arm swelling.[68]

Myalgia and Myositis

Myalgias are common at onset, during periods of active systemic inflammation and may be more painful than the arthritis. True myositis with muscle pain and tenderness and elevation of muscle enzymes is very rare, and magnetic resonance imaging abnormalities have been reported.[69]

Cardiac Disease

Pericardial involvement is common. In one study, an effusion or pericardial thickening was present in 36% of patients, and 81% of children with active systemic manifestations had abnormal echocardiographic findings.[70] Most pericardial effusions are asymptomatic: They are not accompanied by obvious cardiomegaly or typical electrocardiographic changes and escape recognition except by echocardiography.[70] Chest pain, with or without dyspnea, especially when lying supine, is the classical symptom of acute pericarditis. Tamponade is rare, but some children will require drainage of pericardial fluid.[71-73] Chronic constrictive pericarditis is very rare. Pericarditis should not necessarily be regarded as a poor prognostic sign. Pericarditis is not related to gender or the severity of joint disease but appears to be more common in children with disease onset who are younger than 18 months of age.[74] Pericarditis may precede development of arthritis or occur at any time during the course of the disease, usually accompanied by a systemic exacerbation.

Myocarditis is much less common than pericarditis. Although it is rare, it may occur in the absence of pericarditis and may result in cardiomegaly and congestive heart failure.[75-77] A recent report describes a child with active SJIA, treated with anakinra, who died with isolated inflammatory myocarditis confirmed at autopsy.[78] Although endocarditis in the context of systemic inflammatory disease should prompt exclusion of acute rheumatic fever, valvular disease, seemingly unrelated to other causes, has been documented in at least two patients with SJIA.[79,80] Coronary artery abnormalities have been reported in children with SJIA who are febrile (see differential diagnosis below).[81]

Pleuropulmonary Disease

Pleural effusions, the most common respiratory manifestation, may occur with pericarditis and are commonly asymptomatic, detected only as incidental findings on chest radiographs. Parenchymal pulmonary disease is rare, but diffuse interstitial fibrosis occurs in a small number of children.[82-85] Interstitial lung disease (ILD),[83] pulmonary fibrosis,[82] and isolated cases of pulmonary arterial hypertension (PAH)[86] and alveolar proteinosis (AP) or lipoid pneumonia[87] have been reported. Recently, an international series of 25 patients[88] described 16 patients with PAH, 7 with ILD, and 5 with AP or lipoid pneumonia (some children had more than one of these diagnoses). These children had severe SJIA: most had active systemic manifestations, 44% had serositis, and 60% had suspected or confirmed macrophage activation syndrome (MAS) when the pulmonary disease was diagnosed. These pulmonary complications portended a poor prognosis—two thirds of patients died within a mean of less than 1 year. One patient with severe SJIA and lipoid pneumonia that was unresponsive to multiple medications received a double lung transplant.[89]

Lymphadenopathy and Splenomegaly

Enlargements of lymph nodes and spleen may occur alone or together and are characteristic of SJIA. Marked symmetrical lymphadenopathy is particularly common in the anterior cervical, axillary, and inguinal areas and may suggest the diagnosis of lymphoma. The enlarged lymph nodes are typically nontender, firm, and mobile. Tender lymphadenopathy may reflect necrotizing lymphadenitis associated with Kikuchi disease.[90] Splenomegaly, seen in less than 10% of patients at presentation, is usually most prominent within the first years after onset and may be extreme (Fig. 16-3).

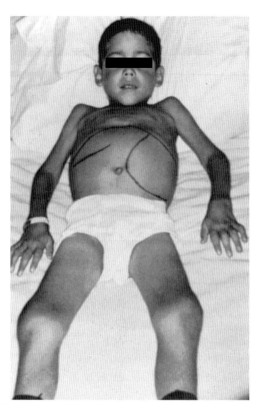

FIGURE 16-3 This 8-year-old boy had onset of SJIA at the age of 4 years. There is symmetrical large and small joint arthritis. Note the axillary lymphadenopathy and marked hepatosplenomegaly.

Hepatic Disease

Hepatomegaly is less common than splenomegaly. Moderate to marked enlargement of the liver is often associated with only mild derangement of functional studies and relatively nonspecific histopathological changes,[91] especially at disease onset. Chronic liver disease generally does not occur, but there are rare reports of hepatic nodular regenerative hyperplasia, which can lead to portal hypertension.[92,93] Progressive hepatomegaly is characteristic of secondary amyloidosis. Occasionally, a fatty liver is associated with glucocorticoid administration. Elevated transaminases occur in approximately 25% of patients at presentation[15] and may also occur with treatment with NSAIDs, disease-modifying antirheumatic drugs (DMARDs) (see Chapter 12) and biological agents, including anakinra,[94] canakinumab,[95] and tocilizumab.[96] The rapid rise of transaminases may be an early feature of MAS. A rare, and apparently benign, transient elevation of serum alkaline phosphatase has been observed in several children with JIA.[97,98]

Central Nervous System Disease

Acute neurological events are rare in children with SJIA, but may carry a significant mortality risk. Encephalopathy, seizures, and intracranial hemorrhages are serious manifestations of central nervous system involvement in MAS.[99] Deaths have been reported with noninfectious meningitis with neutrophilic cerebrospinal fluid pleocytosis[100-103] and cerebral edema associated with the rapid development of hyponatremia, most likely the result of inappropriate antidiuretic hormone secretion.[104] Children with fever and vomiting appear to be most at risk of developing this latter complication and should be carefully monitored with regard to fluid balances and serum electrolytes and should not receive hypotonic intravenous fluid solutions. Some patients develop benign raised intracranial pressure, and epidural lipomatosis causing spinal cord compression has been reported in two patients,[105] possibly as a result of chronic glucocorticoid use.

Other Rare SJIA Features

Nasal septal perforation has been reported in three patients with severe, refractory disease.[63] The most frequent ocular abnormalities in SJIA are cataracts secondary to chronic glucocorticoid treatment. Uveitis occurs in less than 1% of patients[106] and Brown syndrome—inflammatory tenosynovitis of the superior oblique muscle and tendon sheath—has been reported in a small number of patients.[107,108] Renal involvement occurs in MAS associated with SJIA but is otherwise rare. Glomerulonephritis has been reported, including antineutrophil cytoplasmic antibody (ANCA)-associated disease.[109] Persistent proteinuria may be associated with amyloidosis.

Macrophage Activation Syndrome

MAS, the most devastating complication of SJIA, bears close resemblance to hemophagocytic lymphohistiocytosis (HLH). It is associated with serious morbidity and a mortality of 8% in a series of more than 350 patients with SJIA-associated MAS.[110] It occurs in at least 7% of patients during the disease course,[111] although many more show incomplete clinical and laboratory features of the syndrome.

The predisposition of individuals with SJIA to develop MAS may be associated with cytolytic pathway defects that are similar to those seen in primary HLH. These appear to be linked to heterozygous mutations in some of the genes associated with primary HLH, including *PRF1*, *MUNC13-14*, *LYST*, and *STXBP2*, as well as to high levels of proinflammatory cytokines (i.e., IL-6).[112-116] MAS may be triggered by infection, particularly by members of the herpesvirus family, including Epstein–Barr virus.[111,117-119] Many reports have noted the onset of MAS after changes in medications, including NSAIDs, methotrexate, and etanercept.[120-125] Considering the wide array of pharmacological agents that have been reported to be associated with MAS, it seems likely that these events are coincidental, occurring in children who are susceptible to MAS and who require additional therapy for uncontrolled SJIA. MAS most often occurs during periods of active disease, especially early on in the disease course, with approximately 20% of MAS episodes occurring at the time of initial diagnosis.[110,117] Very rarely, it may occur during periods of remission. Even patients whose SJIA is well controlled by IL-1 or IL-6 inhibitors may develop MAS.[95,126]

MAS is characterized clinically by the rapid development of an unremitting fever, hepatosplenomegaly, lymphadenopathy, hepatic dysfunction (sometimes with jaundice and even liver failure), encephalopathy, purpura, bruising, and mucosal bleeding.[99,119,127,128] More severely affected patients develop multiorgan involvement that may progress to respiratory distress, renal failure, disorientation, seizures, reduced level of consciousness, hypotension, and shock.

Laboratory studies indicate hematocytopenia, especially thrombocytopenia. Normal or even elevated neutrophil counts may be seen in the early stages of MAS. Typically, liver enzymes, lactate dehydrogenase (LDH), triglycerides, and ferritin levels are elevated, sometimes with extreme hyperferritinemia above 10,000 μg/L, and serum albumin is low. Markedly elevated levels of D-dimers are present in the plasma. The prothrombin time (PT) and the partial thromboplastin time (PTT) may be prolonged. The erythrocyte sedimentation rate (ESR) may drop sharply in association with hypofibrinogenemia, but C-reactive protein (CRP) is typically elevated. Cerebrospinal fluid may show pleocytosis and an elevated protein concentration but is often difficult to obtain because of the risk of bleeding associated with the coagulopathy. The demonstration of prominent hemophagocytosis in the bone marrow or other tissues such as lymph nodes, liver, or spleen

TABLE 16-1 The Main Clinical and Laboratory Features of Macrophage Activation Syndrome

CLINICAL	LABORATORY
Unremitting fever	Fall in ESR
Bruising, purpura, and mucosal bleeding	Fall in WBC and platelet counts
Enlarged lymph nodes, liver, spleen	Elevated ferritin
Liver dysfunction (jaundice, liver failure)	Elevated liver enzymes and LDH
CNS involvement (disorientation, seizures)	Elevated triglycerides
Multiple organ failure	Fall in fibrinogen and elevated D-dimers Prolonged PT and PTT Bone marrow hemophagocytosis

ALT, Alanine aminotransferase; *AST,* aspartate aminotransferase; *ESR,* erythrocyte sedimentation rate; *LDH,* lactate dehydrogenase; *PT,* prothrombin time; *PTT,* partial thromboplastin time; *WBC,* white blood cell count.

is diagnostic, but florid MAS may occur in the absence of demonstrated tissue hemophagocytosis in up to 40% of patients.[110] Table 16-1 summarizes the main clinical and laboratory features of MAS. Some of these laboratory abnormalities, typically less prominent, occur in children with SJIA in the absence of full-blown MAS.

Prompt diagnosis and treatment of MAS are essential. The guidelines for the diagnosis of HLH[129] have not been validated for the diagnosis of MAS. Strict application of these guidelines may result in unnecessary delays in the diagnosis and treatment. Preliminary criteria for the diagnosis of MAS in patients with SJIA have been suggested by Ravelli but have not been validated.[130] These include a combination of clinical features (central nervous system dysfunction, hemorrhages, and hepatomegaly) and laboratory features (platelets $\leq 262 \times 10^9$/L; aspartate aminotransferase [AST] >59 U/L; white blood cells [WBCs] $\leq 4 \times 10^9$/L or less; and fibrinogen $\leq$.5 g/L). Because patients with active SJIA typically have marked elevation of WBCs, neutrophils, platelets, and fibrinogen, their sudden and sustained reductions, in association with other clinical and laboratory features of MAS, suggest the diagnosis even in the absence of profound cytopenias and hypofibrinogenemia. Indeed, in a recent report, neutrophil count and CRP in SJIA-associated MAS were significantly higher than in primary HLH or viral-associated HLH.[131] The evolution of MAS may be best identified by closely following the trend of changes in laboratory parameters in Table 16-1. Ferritin, platelet count, liver transaminases, LDH, triglycerides, and D-dimers tend to show the most prominent changes.[110] Further international collaborative efforts to identify diagnostic criteria for MAS in SJIA are underway.[132] MAS must be differentiated from active systemic disease and from viral infections and medication toxicities that can result in hematocytopenias and elevated transaminase levels. Cytopenias and elevated transaminases, induced as possible side effects by tocilizumab and less often by IL-1 inhibitors, may be confusing when evaluating a suspected MAS episode. Although treatment with IL-1 or IL-6 inhibitors may modify features of MAS,[133] this has not been reported in all series.[126]

Treatment

MAS must be treated vigorously and rapidly because of the extreme morbidity and high fatality rates. One approach has been to use intravenous methylprednisolone pulse therapy,[99,111,118,127] although half of the patients require additional treatment. Several reports describe the rapid resolution of features of MAS with cyclosporine over the course of a few days.[134-136] Cyclosporine is preferentially used orally, and careful monitoring for toxicity is required, especially if it is administered intravenously. Because MAS often develops during active disease, and because IL-1 inhibitors have been used for active SJIA, some have adopted a newer approach, using anakinra and glucocorticoids, with or without other MAS treatments. Recent case series report the successful use of anakinra in SJIA-associated MAS,[137-139] which may require significantly higher doses of anakinra.[140] There are inconsistent reports of the efficacy of intravenous immunoglobulin, which may be more effective if administered early in the course of MAS.[141] For rapidly progressive disease with multiorgan involvement, early treatment with the combination of systemic glucocorticoids, cyclosporine, and etoposide, as recommended in the HLH-2004 protocol, may be effective.[129] Further details about the pathophysiology and treatment of MAS are discussed in Chapter 49.

Amyloidosis

Secondary amyloidosis as a complication of JIA is exceedingly rare in North America but has been reported in earlier studies in 5% to 7% of children with chronic arthritis in Europe, particularly Northern Europe,[142,143] and in 10% in a Turkish series from the 1990s.[144] It is seen most commonly in SJIA. In Europe, amyloidosis as a complication of chronic arthritis is on the decline, with a decreasing number of deaths.[144-147] A report of 24 children in Finland with JIA-associated amyloidosis, diagnosed over a 30-year period, identified no new cases from 1991 to 2005.[148] Mutations in the familial Mediterranean fever gene (MEFV) may be more frequent in children with SJIA, at least in certain populations,[149] and may result in a higher risk of amyloidosis.[150]

In a United Kingdom JIA series, amyloidosis was, in rare instances, observed as early as 1 year after onset of the arthritis, but it could develop as late as 23 years after onset, and was associated with significant mortality.[143] The outcome of amyloidosis in the Finnish series was also poor, with a mortality rate of 42% and renal insufficiency or renal transplantation required in 25% of survivors, after a mean follow-up of 15 years.[151] In secondary amyloidosis, monitoring of serum amyloid A levels is of utmost importance because it predicts mortality and progression to renal failure.[152] Control of the underlying disease is critical in treating amyloidosis.[153] Treatment with chlorambucil improved survival in JIA-associated amyloidosis,[146] and more recently, treatment with TNF-α inhibitors[154] and anti-IL-6 receptor antibody[155] has been reported to result in regression of amyloidosis in some patients.

DIAGNOSIS AND DIFFERENTIAL DIAGNOSIS

The diagnosis of SJIA is made clinically, supported by typical laboratory findings, and it is a diagnosis of exclusion. In its fully developed state, the clinical characteristics are quite diagnostic. In particular, the presence of a classic rash and quotidian fever are very suggestive of this diagnosis.

The diagnosis of suspected SJIA may be difficult, especially at onset or early in the course of the disease, when the child may have a high, spiking fever and evidence of systemic inflammation but no arthritis and no specific sign or symptom that allows a definitive diagnosis.[156] In such children, the possibilities of malignancy, inflammatory bowel disease, other connective tissue diseases such as systemic lupus erythematosus, or vasculitides such as polyarteritis nodosa or Kawasaki disease, should be considered (Box 16-2). Differentiating SJIA at onset from Kawasaki disease can be difficult because they have many common clinical and laboratory features, particularly when arthritis is

---

BOX 16-2 Differential Diagnosis of Systemic Juvenile Idiopathic Arthritis

Infections
- Bacterial endocarditis
- Acute rheumatic fever
- Cat scratch disease (Bartonella)
- Lyme disease (Borrelia burgdorferi)
- Brucellosis
- Mycoplasma
- Many others

Malignancy

Rheumatic and inflammatory diseases:
- Systemic lupus erythematosus
- Dermatomyositis
- Polyarteritis nodosa
- Kawasaki disease
- Serum sickness
- Sarcoidosis
- Castleman disease

Inflammatory bowel disease

Autoinflammatory syndromes
- Familial Mediterranean fever
- Mevalonate kinase deficiency (mevalonic aciduria/hyperimmunoglobulin D syndrome)
- TNF receptor–associated periodic syndrome (TRAPS)
- Muckle–Wells syndrome
- Chronic infantile neurological cutaneous and articular syndrome (CINCA)/Neonatal-onset multisystem inflammatory disease (NOMID)

---

one of presenting features of Kawasaki disease, when Kawasaki disease is incomplete, or when it is complicated by MAS.[157]

Children with SJIA may be thought to have an acute infectious disease or septicemia. Infectious mononucleosis and other viral illnesses may mimic the disease, but for the most part the arthropathies that occur secondary to viral infections are transient. Fever in children with infectious diseases is typically more hectic, spikes less predictably, and usually does not repetitively return to, or below, a baseline each day, as does the fever of SJIA.

When the constellation of clinical and laboratory findings is not typical for the diagnosis, more extensive investigations, including imaging of the chest and abdomen, examination of bone marrow, and biopsies of lymph nodes or affected organs may be necessary. It is very important to exclude the expanding spectrum of autoinflammatory syndromes (see Chapter 47). Some of them have clinical and laboratory features that may mimic SJIA. In particular, TNF receptor-associated periodic syndrome may manifest with recurrent fever for several weeks, rash, arthralgia or arthritis, and myalgia.[158] Among the cryopyrin-associated periodic syndromes, Muckle–Wells syndrome often presents with fever, urticarial rash, and sometimes arthritis, with the later development of hearing loss.

A sustained or remittent fever is characteristic of acute rheumatic fever and should respond dramatically to NSAIDs. Although many children with SJIA have isolated pericarditis, a pericardial effusion with evidence of endocarditis suggests a diagnosis of rheumatic fever or bacterial endocarditis. The arthritis is characteristically acute and painful, migratory, and asymmetrical, involving the peripheral joints without sequelae. Evidence of a prior infection with β-hemolytic group A streptococci is present; however, the antistreptolysin O titer may be chronically increased to a moderate degree in one third of children with JIA as a manifestation of polyclonal B-cell activation.[159]

Adult-Onset Still Disease

The hallmarks of adult-onset Still disease (AOSD) are similar to those found in individuals whose SJIA begins before the age of 16 years,[160-163] but sore throat is a more common symptom than in SJIA.[164] There is a similar association with MAS and hyperferritinemia, and a very low proportion of glycosylated ferritin has been reported in both adult-onset Still disease and reactive HLH.[165-167] Although controlled studies of biological agents are lacking for AOSD, the efficacy and safety of IL-1 inhibitors[168-171] and IL-6 inhibitors[172-174] appear to be similar in children with SJIA.

PATHOLOGY

The rash of SJIA is characterized by minimal perivascular infiltration of mononuclear cells around capillaries and venules in the subdermal tissues.[61] A neutrophilic perivasculitis may accompany the more flagrant lesions. Prominent expression of endothelial adhesion receptors and proinflammatory S-100 proteins MRP8 and MRP14 is seen.[175]

The serosal lining surfaces of the pleural, pericardial, and peritoneal cavities of the body may exhibit nonspecific fibrous serositis. Enlargement of the lymph nodes is related to a nonspecific follicular hyperplasia. Hepatic abnormalities are characterized by a nonspecific collection of periportal inflammatory cells and hyperplasia of Kupffer cells. Synovitis does not differ histologically from that seen in other types of JIA.

LABORATORY EXAMINATION

Indicators of inflammation are usually strikingly elevated in active systemic JIA. The WBC count is often higher than 30,000 cells/mm^3 with a predominance of polymorphonuclear leukocytes. The platelet count is usually elevated, sometimes to more than 1,000,000/mm^3 (1000×10^9/L), although it is rare that thrombocytopenia occurs early in the disease course.[176] Hemoglobin in the range of 7 to 10 g/dL (70 to 100 g/L) is usual, and occasionally it is even lower. Erythrocytes are characteristically hypochromic but can be normocytic or microcytic. Erythroid aplasia has been reported.[177,178] The ESR is usually very high, except in patients with MAS, in whom it may be normal or low. CRP is elevated, and ferritin, fibrinogen and D-dimer levels are often high, reflecting the extent of inflammatory disease. Complement levels are usually increased as part of the acute-phase response, and increased levels of complement activation products have been reported.[179] The presence of rheumatoid factors or antinuclear antibodies is very uncommon.

Synovial fluid analysis confirms the presence of inflammatory arthritis, with cell counts in the range of 10,000 to 40,000/mm^3, predominantly polymorphonuclear leukocytes. When there is marked systemic inflammation, synovial fluid white cell counts can rise to the 100,000/mm^3 range, mimicking those seen in septic arthritis.

The laboratory profile, although supportive of the diagnosis, is nonspecific and can be seen in other infectious and inflammatory conditions. S100A12, a marker of granulocyte activation, has been reported to be significantly elevated in patients with SJIA.[180] Serum concentrations of MRP8/MRP14 may be useful in differentiating SJIA from infections and other causes of systemic inflammation.[51,55]

RADIOLOGICAL EXAMINATION

Radiographs demonstrate bone and soft tissue changes in a high proportion of children with SJIA. In addition, growth abnormalities may be marked, and generalized delay in bone age is a frequent observation.

Juxtaarticular osteoporosis indicates the effect of active arthritis. In a study of 30 children with SJIA, Oen and colleagues[181] found that radiographs performed within the first 2 years of disease revealed joint space narrowing in 30% of the children, erosions in 35%, and growth abnormalities in 10%. These early changes, which have also been shown to correlate with thrombocytosis and persistently active systemic symptoms in the first 6 months from onset,[67] were most frequently seen in wrist, hip, and shoulder radiographs. In later radiographs (a median of 6.4 years after onset), joint space narrowing was demonstrated in 39% of the children, erosions in 63%, and growth abnormalities in 25%. Changes in the cervical spine and hips were most common in late radiographs. Ankylosis, especially involving the wrist and apophyseal joints of the cervical spine, is seen in severe, refractory disease.[182]

TREATMENT

Approach to Management

The child with new-onset SJIA is often acutely ill and may require hospitalization for diagnosis and management. In addition to the evaluation and treatment of joint inflammation, careful assessment of the extraarticular manifestations, including cardiac and pulmonary status, anemia, and the possibility of MAS must be part of the initial evaluation.

Major advances in the treatment of SJIA in recent years can be attributed to the results of controlled trials conducted specifically in patients with SJIA with agents inhibiting IL-1 and IL-6. Although these trials provide, for the first time in SJIA, convincing evidence of the efficacy of these biological agents, they did not enroll patients with short disease duration and, therefore, do not provide specific information about the most appropriate treatment approach in new-onset SJIA.

It is appropriate to use an NSAID alone as initial therapy for patients who do not have severe disease manifestations, both to aid in control of the systemic inflammatory features (e.g., fever) and to modulate joint pain and inflammation, particularly while the diagnosis is being confirmed. However, NSAIDs alone seldom satisfactorily control systemic symptoms or even arthritis. Subsequent treatment choices should take into account the severity of the systemic features and arthritis and the extent to which MAS features and poor prognostic features are present. Recent treatment recommendations for SJIA have been developed by the American College of Rheumatology (ACR).[183] As with all treatments, the safety profile, tolerance of the route of administration, availability, and cost of each of the therapeutic agents influence physician recommendations and patient/family preferences. The more traditional option is to use oral or intravenous glucocorticoids. Intravenous pulses of methylprednisolone (30 mg/kg/day to a maximum of 1 g/day for 1 to 3 consecutive days) are effective in controlling the systemic and articular features of the disease, and are indicated in the presence of very severe disease, clinically relevant pericarditis, and features of impending MAS. Because the benefits are often short-lived, pulses are usually followed by administration of oral prednisone (1 to 2 mg/kg/day to a maximum of 60 mg/day in one or more doses). Starting with oral glucocorticoids is also appropriate, depending on disease severity.

A second option is the early use of biological agents, particularly anakinra, with or without concomitant glucocorticoids. This is an attractive choice for many patients and families because they may be able to completely avoid using glucocorticoids or at least minimize their use by rapidly tapering down the dosage, if this approach is effective. Concomitant glucocorticoids are still strongly recommended for severe disease or impending MAS. The hypothesis behind the use

TABLE 16-2 Target, Mechanism of Action and Dosing Regimen of the IL-1 and IL-6 Inhibitors Available at Present for the Treatment of SJIA

	MOLECULE	MECHANISM OF ACTION	HALF-LIFE	DOSING*
Anakinra	IL-1 receptor antagonist	Neutralizes effects of IL-1α and IL-1β	3-6 hours	BW >50 kg: 100 mg/day BW >10< 50 kg: 2 mg/kg/day BW <10 Kg: 4 mg/kg/day
Canakinumab	Fully human monoclonal antibody to IL-1β	Neutralizes effects of IL-1β	25 days†	4 mg/kg every 4 weeks
Rilonacept	IgG1 Fc/IL-1 receptor fusion protein f	Neutralizes effects of IL-1α and IL-1β	6 days	Loading dose 4.4 mg/kg, then 2.2 mg/kg/week
Tocilizumab	Humanized monoclonal antibody to the membrane and the soluble IL-6 receptor	Neutralizes effects of IL-6	6 days	BW ≤30 kg: 12 mg/kg every 14 days BW >30 kg: 8 mg/kg every 14 days

*Dosing regimens used in controlled clinical trials and/or recommended based on pharmacokinetic studies.
†Derived from patients with cryopyrinopathies. The half-life in patients with SJIA is not available.
BW, Body weight.

of biological agents early in the disease course is that inhibition of IL-1 (or possibly IL-6) may exploit a window of opportunity to prevent the evolution of chronic, destructive synovitis.[184] This hypothesis, far from being proved, is based on the effects of IL-1 blockade as a first-line treatment, reported in case series. In a retrospective series of 46 patients who were treated with anakinra as part of the initial therapy, approximately 60% achieved inactive disease.[185] A single center observation in 20 patients reported a JIA ACR 90 response in 85% of the patients with 7 of the 20 patients requiring other treatments in addition to anakinra.[186] Although these results appear to be very promising, they may be biased by the inclusion of patients with monocyclic disease, which may spontaneously remit. If the early use of a biological agent results in inactive disease, weaning the biological agent should be attempted (possibly within 6 months) to avoid unnecessary exposure of the patient to the drug. The experience with early use of biological agents is at present largely limited to anakinra, but the possibility exists for other IL-1 and IL-6 inhibitors to be used early in the disease. The recently published Childhood Arthritis and Rheumatology Research Alliance (CARRA) consensus treatment protocols for new-onset SJIA include treatment options with early use of anakinra, canakinumab, or tocilizumab, with or without glucocorticoids,[187] suggesting a willingness among pediatric rheumatologists in North America to adopt this practice.

The general principles of management, outlined in Chapters 11-15, should be applied to the management of SJIA. As mentioned above, systemic glucocorticoids may be part of the initial treatment and are often necessary during the course of the disease. Tapering glucocorticoids to a minimum acceptable dose, or withdrawing them, should always be a major goal. With the presently available inhibitors of IL-1 or IL-6, withdrawal of glucocorticoids is attainable for many patients. While disease activity and occurrence of side effects guide their tapering in the individual patient, plans for tapering glucocorticoids may be adapted from expert consensus recommendations or guidelines for tapering used in controlled clinical trials.[95,96,187,188] DMARDs such as methotrexate have traditionally been used in patients with SJIA, but their efficacy is limited. Biological agents that inhibit IL-1 or IL-6 currently represent the mainstay of treatment. TNF inhibition should not be considered the first-line biological approach in patients with persistently active SJIA. Intraarticular triamcinolone hexacetonide injections may be very effective for active arthritis regardless of concurrent therapy. Benefits from intraarticular corticosteroid injections may be less durable than they are for other subtypes of JIA,[189] especially if performed when the systemic disease is very active.

Pharmacological Therapy
IL-1 and IL-6 inhibitors
Several uncontrolled studies and one controlled clinical trial have reported on the favorable response of SJIA patients to anakinra, an IL-1 receptor antagonist. Anakinra is administered subcutaneously at a starting dosage of 1 to 2 mg/kg/day. The only pharmacokinetic study of anakinra in children, suggests that higher doses should be used in lower-weight children (Table 16-2).[190] Higher dosages of anakinra (up to 5 mg/kg/day) have also been used to treat patients with unsatisfactory responses to standard dose therapy.[185] Heavier patients may require more than a single dose per day. The only controlled trial of anakinra enrolled 24 patients with a mean disease duration of almost 4 years, a mean active joint count of 16, and active systemic features in 37%.[191] In the 1-month randomized phase, anakinra was markedly superior to placebo. Several case series have demonstrated a prompt effect of anakinra on systemic features and laboratory measures of inflammation in 50% to 90% of patients.[50,52,192-194] Anakinra appears to be less effective for arthritis than for the systemic features.[52] In one of the largest reported series, a JIA ACR 50 response was observed in only 25% of the patients,[193] whereas in another large series, a complete response was observed in approximately 40% of the patients.[52] Overall, up to half of the patients with SJIA appear to respond promptly. Some may indeed reach clinical remission. Following a phase II study,[195] a phase III development program with two controlled trials in a total of 190 patients has been recently conducted with canakinumab, a fully human monoclonal antibody to IL-1β.[95] These trials enrolled patients with active systemic features (i.e., presence of fever), a median disease duration of approximately 2 years, and a median active joint count was approximately 10. One trial was a short-term, randomized, placebo-controlled trial with a primary outcome at day 15 after a single injection. The second trial was a randomized withdrawal study performed in the 100 patients who responded to canakinumab and successfully reduced their glucocorticoid dose to a predefined level. In both studies, canakinumab was superior to placebo. Of the 50 evaluable patients at the end of the withdrawal phase, 76% attained a JIA ACR 90 response plus absence of fever. Glucocorticoids were discontinued in one third of the patients.

Rilonacept has also shown to be superior to placebo in a randomized, controlled trial.[188] This trial enrolled 71 patients with a mean disease duration of 2.5 years, a mean active joint count of 11, with fever being present in approximately 20%. In the long-term extension of 6 months' duration, 64% of the 55 patients remaining on treatment attained a JIA ACR 70 response plus absence of fever. One third of patients were able to discontinue glucocorticoids.

The only available IL-6 inhibitor is tocilizumab, a humanized anti-IL-6 receptor antibody. Two small phase I and II studies with tocilizumab in SJIA reported a prompt improvement in clinical and laboratory parameters.[196,197] Subsequently, two phase III studies were conducted in SJIA: a withdrawal design in 56 patients in Japan[198] and a randomized, placebo-controlled trial in 112 patients in Europe, North America, and Australia.[96] In the study performed in Japan, at the end of the 48-week open phase extension, approximately 90% of the patients were still taking tocilizumab, with the great majority of them (90%) having achieved a JIA ACR 70 response. Long-term follow-up (3.5 years) of patients enrolled in the phase II and III studies in Japan showed continuation of treatment in 58 out of 67 patients, with a JIA ACR 90 response in 61% and discontinuation of glucocorticoids in 33%.[199] In Japan, tocilizumab was administered at 8 mg/kg every 2 weeks. In the study performed in Europe, North America, and Australia, a higher dosing regimen, identified through modeling and simulation, was used in children with lower body weight (see Table 16-2) and demonstrated to be the appropriate dose according to drug level profiling and efficacy.[96] In this study, a severe population with established disease was enrolled with a mean disease duration of 5 years, a mean number of active joints approaching 20, and with approximately half of patients having active systemic features. Tocilizumab was clearly superior to placebo in the randomized phase, leading to prompt responses of both systemic and articular features.[96] In the long-term extension, after 2 years 72% of the patients had a JIA ACR 90 response, 55% of them with no active joints; 60% were able to withdraw glucocorticoids.[200] Treatment with tocilizumab was associated with catch-up growth (higher than expected height velocity for age)[201] and halted radiological progression in the majority of patients.[202]

The benefits of long-term inhibition of IL-1 or IL-6 still remain to be determined in a larger number of patients, but preliminary evidence suggests a very favorable outcome. It should be kept in mind that even in the very good responders to IL-1 and IL-6 inhibitors, some joints may remain active. The safe taper and withdrawal of these effective treatments are being evaluated at present and should be considered in patients who have achieved sustained remission and whose glucocorticoids have been withdrawn. It is difficult to evaluate the comparative effectiveness and safety of IL-1 and IL-6 inhibitors, as the analysis of published trials is hampered by differences in the characteristics and disease severity of the enrolled patients, and by the different designs used in the studies. In the tocilizumab and rilonacept trials, previous treatment with anakinra did not appear to affect response. Similarly, a significant portion of patients who failed to respond to anakinra seemed to improve with canakinumab.[203] The interplay between IL-6 and IL-1 in the pathogenesis of SJIA is yet to be clarified. Hopefully, mechanistic studies may help to identify predictors of response to either IL-1 or IL-6 inhibition, allowing a personalized approach to treatment. At present, one possible approach is to use anakinra as the first biological agent. Its short half-life is an advantage from a safety perspective. Moreover, in the absence of a satisfactory response to anakinra, one may choose to switch to tocilizumab or to a longer-acting IL-1 inhibitor within 24 to 48 hours of discontinuing anakinra. If a longer-acting biological agent is used, it may be advisable to wait five half-lives before initiating treatment with an alternative biological agent.

Injection site reactions with significant pain are present in more than half of patients receiving anakinra. These are rarely reported with canakinumab. Infections, including serious infections, have been reported with both IL-1 and Il-6 inhibitors. Neutropenia and liver enzyme elevations can occur with all treatments, although they appear to be more frequent with tocilizumab. It is noteworthy that neutropenia induced by tocilizumab does not appear to be associated with a higher risk of serious and nonserious infections.[204] The treating physician must remain vigilant for the development of MAS, which has been reported in patients treated with both IL-1 and IL-6 inhibitors, even in those with well-controlled disease. These MAS episodes appear to respond to the standard treatment.

TNF Inhibitors

TNF inhibition in SJIA is not as effective as in other JIA subtypes, and there is little evidence for its effectiveness for systemic symptoms. In the original multicenter clinical trial of etanercept in polyarticular course JIA, there were 22 patients with systemic arthritis without systemic features.[205] In the 2-year follow-up study,[206] a JIA ACR 70 response was seen in 47%. Published data from three different national registries of JIA patients on etanercept showed a significantly higher rate of treatment failure and of flares during treatment in SJIA compared to other JIA subtypes.[207-209] The proportion of SJIA patients who continued etanercept after 2 years was approximately 40% compared with more than 80% in non-SJIA patients.[208] A multicenter survey of 82 SJIA patients treated with etanercept in the Unites States showed an excellent response in approximately one third of the patients.[210] Anecdotally, infliximab, or adalimumab have been reported to be effective in some children with SJIA. Experience from a single center in South America reported that of 45 SJIA patients treated with various TNF inhibitors, one fourth reached clinical remission, with half of these patients flaring in the subsequent year.[211]

Other Biologics

A multicenter study of abatacept in polyarticular course JIA included 37 patients who had SJIA without systemic features. Of the 32 patients continuing treatment in the open-label extension up to 1.5 years, 16% attained an ACR 90 response.[212] In one small series, it was reported that patients with refractory SJIA had responded to treatment with a combination of abatacept and anakinra.[213] Because the combined use of TNF and IL-1 inhibitors in rheumatoid arthritis patients was associated with an increase in severe infections, the safety of biological agents used in combination remains a major concern. In an open-label single center study performed in Russia, 55 patients with treatment-resistant JIA (47 with SJIA, none of whom received prior IL-1 or IL-6 inhibitors) were treated with rituximab. At week 96, 93% of patients achieved a JIA ACR 70 response.[214] These results have not been replicated in a clinical trial.

Methotrexate

In children with SJIA, the response rate to methotrexate is not as high as it is for oligoarthritis or polyarthritis, and there is no evidence that it is efficacious for the systemic features. In the only placebo-controlled study, performed specifically in patients with SJIA, there was no significant difference in ACR 30 response rate, systemic feature score, ESR, or CRP compared with placebo.[215] In the phase III study of tocilizumab in SJIA that was conducted in Europe, North America, and Australia, there was no difference in the response rate in patients on background methotrexate compared to those treated with tocilizumab without methotrexate.[216]

Others

A number of other approaches have been used in the era preceding the availability of IL-1 and IL-6 inhibitors. Presently, these approaches may be considered in patients who failed treatment with IL-1 and IL-6 inhibitors because of inefficacy or intolerance.

Intravenous immunoglobulin (IVIG) has been used to treat systemic JIA, although the evidence supporting its use is limited. In small, uncontrolled trials, IVIG was found to be useful for systemic features but not consistently effective for arthritis.[217-220] A controlled, randomized trial of IVIG in children with SJIA failed to recruit sufficient patients but suggested that the drug had little benefit compared with placebo.[221] Cyclosporine A has been shown to be of limited utility in two open-label studies in SJIA,[222,223] although it is important in the treatment of patients with MAS. Some reports support the use of thalidomide in children with treatment-resistant SJIA,[224,225] including a multicenter retrospective review of experience in 13 children who showed improvement in active joint count, with two thirds of patients achieving an ACR 50 response and a reduction in prednisone dose by 6 months. The histone deacetylase inhibitor givinostat has been evaluated in a single phase II, open-label trial.[226] At week 12, JIA ACR 70 response was recorded in 35% of the patients with an evident trend in the reduction of systemic features and number of active joints. Autologous stem-cell transplantation (ASCT) has also been used in patients with resistant SJIA. Long-term follow-up data have been published in 22 patients from the Netherlands and in 7 from the UK.[227,228] Drug-free remission was obtained in 30% to 50% of patients. Significant mortality, however, was, reported by both groups, with fatal MAS being the major complication. If ASCT is considered as a last-resort option, careful attention should be given to T-cell depletion and the conditioning regimen.

COURSE OF THE DISEASE AND PROGNOSIS

The acute manifestations of SJIA are variable in duration. Systemic features such as fever, rash, and pericarditis tend to subside during the initial months but may persist for years. Up to 40% of children with SJIA follow a monocyclic disease course and eventually recover completely after a variable period. A small proportion of children have a polycyclic course of the disease, characterized by recurrent episodes of active disease interrupted by periods of remission without medications. Studies over the past 30 years have consistently shown that more than half of the children with SJIA have a persistent disease course.[229-232] This has resulted in progressive arthritis and moderate to severe functional disability in some studies[67,233,234] but not in others.[235] Those who have a severe, protracted course of disease may have profound morbidity secondary to long-term treatment with systemic glucocorticoids. The eventual functional outcome in these children depends more on the extent and severity of the arthritis than on the nature of the systemic disease.[231] Persistence of systemic symptoms without arthritis is unusual and is seldom a cause of permanent disability. In one long-term follow-up series, 48% of children still had active arthritis 10 years later[236]; more recent studies have reported remission in only approximately 33% of patients.[230,237-239]

The most important early predictors of destructive arthritis are polyarthritis, thrombocytosis, persistent fever, or the need for systemic corticosteroids in the first 6 months after disease onset.[67,233,240,241] Very early onset SJIA, before 18 months of age, may be associated with worse outcomes including more severe, destructive arthritis, greater disability, and more severe growth failure.[16] Early hip arthritis may also be associated with a worse outcome. A polymorphism of the MIF gene is the only reported genetic predictor of poor outcome in SJIA. The MIF-173*C allele results in higher serum and synovial fluid levels of MIF and is associated with poor response to glucocorticoid treatment, persistently active disease, and poor outcome.[21] Persistently elevated levels of fibrin D-dimer may be associated with poor joint and functional outcomes.[242]

In early studies of JIA, the death rate was 2% to 4%.[243,244] Deaths occurred predominantly in children with the systemic subtype. In European children, this was most frequently due to amyloidosis; in North American children, this was due to infections associated with glucocorticoid therapy. The JIA disease-associated death rate is now less than 0.5%, but a disproportionately high percentage of deaths still occur in the SJIA subtype. In a large U.S. study that included 962 children with SJIA diagnosed between 1992 and 2001, the observed death rate was 0.6%, and the standardized mortality ratio was 1.8.[245] MAS remains a serious threat, with a mortality rate as high as 8%, even in the modern era.[110] Deaths have less commonly been reported due to infections and rarely as a result of neurological, cardiac and pulmonary complications.

Although introduced relatively recently, the widespread use of IL-1 and IL-6 inhibitors, possibly together with a personalized approach, will likely lead to a marked improvement in the long-term functional prognosis and in the mortality rate of SJIA.

REFERENCES

1. R.E. Petty, T.R. Southwood, P. Manners, et al., International League of Associations for Rheumatology classification of juvenile idiopathic arthritis: second revision, Edmonton, 2001, J. Rheumatol. 31 (2) (2004) 390–392.

15. E.M. Behrens, T. Beukelman, L. Gallo, et al., Evaluation of the presentation of systemic onset juvenile rheumatoid arthritis: data from the Pennsylvania Systemic Onset Juvenile Arthritis Registry (PASOJAR), J. Rheumatol. 35 (2) (2008) 343–348.

16. R.A. Russo, M.M. Katsicas, Patients with very early-onset systemic juvenile idiopathic arthritis exhibit more inflammatory features and a worse outcome, J. Rheumatol. 40 (3) (2013) 329–334.

21. F. De Benedetti, C. Meazza, M. Vivarelli, et al., Functional and prognostic relevance of the -173 polymorphism of the macrophage migration inhibitory factor gene in systemic-onset juvenile idiopathic arthritis, Arthritis Rheum. 48 (5) (2003) 1398–1407.

23. C. Macaubas, K. Nguyen, C. Deshpande, et al., Distribution of circulating cells in systemic juvenile idiopathic arthritis across disease activity states, Clin. Immunol. 134 (2) (2010) 206–216.

24. M.G. Barnes, A.A. Grom, S.D. Thompson, et al., Subtype-specific peripheral blood gene expression profiles in recent-onset juvenile idiopathic arthritis, Arthritis Rheum. 60 (7) (2009) 2102–2112.

27. E.M. Ogilvie, A. Khan, M. Hubank, et al., Specific gene expression profiles in systemic juvenile idiopathic arthritis, Arthritis Rheum. 56 (6) (2007) 1954–1965.

36. H.J. van den Ham, W. de Jager, J.W. Bijlsma, et al., Differential cytokine profiles in juvenile idiopathic arthritis subtypes revealed by cluster analysis, Rheumatology (Oxford) 48 (8) (2009) 899–905.

37. X.B. Ling, J.L. Park, T. Carroll, et al., Plasma profiles in active systemic juvenile idiopathic arthritis: Biomarkers and biological implications, Proteomics 10 (24) (2010) 4415–4430.

41. F. de Benedetti, A. Martini, Targeting the interleukin-6 receptor: a new treatment for systemic juvenile idiopathic arthritis?, Arthritis Rheum. 52 (3) (2005) 687–693.

48. F. De Benedetti, N. Rucci, A. Del Fattore, et al., Impaired skeletal development in interleukin-6-transgenic mice: a model for the impact of chronic inflammation on the growing skeletal system, Arthritis Rheum. 54 (11) (2006) 3551–3563.

50. V. Pascual, F. Allantaz, E. Arce, et al., Role of interleukin-1 (IL-1) in the pathogenesis of systemic onset juvenile idiopathic arthritis and clinical response to IL-1 blockade, J. Exp. Med. 201 (9) (2005) 1479–1486.

52. M. Gattorno, A. Piccini, D. Lasiglie, et al., The pattern of response to anti-interleukin-1 treatment distinguishes two subsets of patients with systemic-onset juvenile idiopathic arthritis, Arthritis Rheum. 58 (5) (2008) 1505–1515.

55. D. Holzinger, M. Frosch, A. Kastrup, et al., The Toll-like receptor 4 agonist MRP8/14 protein complex is a sensitive indicator for disease activity and predicts relapses in systemic-onset juvenile idiopathic arthritis, Ann. Rheum. Dis. 71 (6) (2012) 974–980.

60. M. Yamaguchi, A. Ohta, T. Tsunematsu, et al., Preliminary criteria for classification of adult Still's disease, J. Rheumatol. 19 (3) (1992) 424–430.

61. E.G. Bywaters, I.C. Isdale, The rash of rheumatoid arthritis and Still's disease, Q. J. Med. 25 (99) (1956) 377–387.

65. J.Y. Lee, C.K. Hsu, M.F. Liu, et al., Evanescent and persistent pruritic eruptions of adult-onset still disease: a clinical and pathologic study of 36 patients, Semin. Arthritis Rheum. 42 (3) (2012) 317–326.

75. J. Goldenberg, M.B. Ferraz, A.P. Pessoa, et al., Symptomatic cardiac involvement in juvenile rheumatoid arthritis, Int. J. Cardiol. 34 (1) (1992) 57–62.

88. Y. Kimura, J.E. Weiss, K.L. Haroldson, et al., Pulmonary hypertension and other potentially fatal pulmonary complications in systemic juvenile idiopathic arthritis, Arthritis Care Res. (Hoboken) 65 (5) (2013) 745–752.

91. J. Schaller, B. Beckwith, R.J. Wedgwood, Hepatic involvement in juvenile rheumatoid arthritis, J. Pediatr. 77 (2) (1970) 203–210.

95. N. Ruperto, H.I. Brunner, P. Quartier, et al., Two randomized trials of canakinumab in systemic juvenile idiopathic arthritis, N. Engl. J. Med. 367 (25) (2012) 2396–2406.

96. F. De Benedetti, H.I. Brunner, N. Ruperto, et al., Randomized trial of tocilizumab in systemic juvenile idiopathic arthritis, N. Engl. J. Med. 367 (25) (2012) 2385–2395.

110. F. Minoia, S. Davi, A. Horne, et al., Clinical features, treatment and outcome of macrophage activation syndrome complicating systemic juvenile idiopathic arthritis A multinational, multicenter study of 362 patients, Arthritis Rheumatol. 66 (2014) 3160–3169.

111. S. Sawhney, P. Woo, K.J. Murray, Macrophage activation syndrome: a potentially fatal complication of rheumatic disorders, Arch. Dis. Child. 85 (5) (2001) 421–426.

115. K.M. Kaufman, B. Linghu, J.D. Szustakowski, et al., Whole exome sequencing reveals overlap between macrophage activation syndrome in systemic juvenile idiopathic arthritis and familial hemophagocytic lymphohistiocytosis, Arthritis Rheumatol. (2014).

118. J.L. Stephan, I. Koné-Paut, C. Galambrun, et al., Reactive haemophagocytic syndrome in children with inflammatory disorders. A retrospective study of 24 patients, Rheumatology (Oxford) 40 (11) (2001) 1285–1292.

129. J.I. Henter, A. Horne, M. Arico, et al., HLH-2004: Diagnostic and therapeutic guidelines for hemophagocytic lymphohistiocytosis, Pediatr. Blood Cancer 48 (2) (2007) 124–131.

130. A. Ravelli, S. Magni-Manzoni, A. Pistorio, et al., Preliminary diagnostic guidelines for macrophage activation syndrome complicating systemic juvenile idiopathic arthritis, J. Pediatr. 146 (5) (2005) 598–604.

134. R. Mouy, J.L. Stephan, P. Pillet, et al., Efficacy of cyclosporine A in the treatment of macrophage activation syndrome in juvenile arthritis: report of five cases, J. Pediatr. 129 (5) (1996) 750–754.

139. P.M. Miettunen, A. Narendran, A. Jayanthan, et al., Successful treatment of severe paediatric rheumatic disease-associated macrophage activation syndrome with interleukin-1 inhibition following conventional immunosuppressive therapy: case series with 12 patients, Rheumatology (Oxford) 50 (2) (2011) 417–419.

140. P.J. Kahn, R.Q. Cron, Higher-dose Anakinra is effective in a case of medically refractory macrophage activation syndrome, J. Rheumatol. 40 (5) (2013) 743–744.

148. K. Immonen, H.A. Savolainen, M. Hakala, Why can we no longer find juvenile idiopathic arthritis-associated amyloidosis in childhood or in adolescence in Finland?, Scand. J. Rheumatol. 36 (5) (2007) 402–403.

151. K. Immonen, A. Savolainen, H. Kautiainen, et al., Longterm outcome of amyloidosis associated with juvenile idiopathic arthritis, J. Rheumatol. 35 (5) (2008) 907–912.

152. H.J. Lachmann, H.J. Goodman, J.A. Gilbertson, et al., Natural history and outcome on systemic AA amyloidosis, N. Engl. J. Med. 356 (23) (2007) 2361–2371.

168. C. Giampietro, M. Ridene, T. Lequerre, et al., Anakinra in adult-onset Still's disease: long-term treatment in patients resistant to conventional therapy, Arthritis Care Res. (Hoboken) 65 (5) (2013) 822–826.

170. A. Kontzias, P. Efthimiou, The use of Canakinumab, a novel IL-1beta long-acting inhibitor, in refractory adult-onset Still's disease, Semin. Arthritis Rheum. 42 (2) (2012) 201–205.

172. F. Ortiz-Sanjuán, R. Blanco, V. Calvo-Rio, et al., Efficacy of tocilizumab in conventional treatment-refractory adult-onset Still's disease: multicenter retrospective open-label study of thirty-four patients, Arthritis Rheumatol. 66 (6) (2014) 1659–1665.

180. H. Wittkowski, M. Frosch, N. Wulffraat, et al., S100A12 is a novel molecular marker differentiating systemic-onset juvenile idiopathic arthritis from other causes of fever of unknown origin, Arthritis Rheum. 58 (12) (2008) 3924–3931.

181. K. Oen, M. Reed, P.N. Malleson, et al., Radiologic outcome and its relationship to functional disability in juvenile rheumatoid arthritis, J. Rheumatol. 30 (4) (2003) 832–840.

182. B.A. Lang, R. Schneider, B.J. Reilly, et al., Radiologic features of systemic onset juvenile rheumatoid arthritis, J. Rheumatol. 22 (1) (1995) 168–173.

183. S. Ringold, P.F. Weiss, T. Beukelman, et al., 2013 update of the 2011 American College of Rheumatology recommendations for the treatment of juvenile idiopathic arthritis: recommendations for the medical therapy of children with systemic juvenile idiopathic arthritis and tuberculosis screening among children receiving biologic medications, Arthritis Rheum. 65 (10) (2013) 2499–2512.

184. P.A. Nigrovic, Review: is there a window of opportunity for treatment of systemic juvenile idiopathic arthritis?, Arthritis Rheumatol. 66 (6) (2014) 1405–1413.

185. P.A. Nigrovic, M. Mannion, F.H. Prince, et al., Anakinra as first-line disease-modifying therapy in systemic juvenile idiopathic arthritis: report of forty-six patients from an international multicenter series, Arthritis Rheum. 63 (2) (2011) 545–555.

186. S.J. Vastert, W. de Jager, B.J. Noordman, et al., Effectiveness of first-line treatment with recombinant interleukin-1 receptor antagonist in steroid-naive patients with new-onset systemic juvenile idiopathic arthritis: results of a prospective cohort study, Arthritis Rheumatol. 66 (4) (2014) 1034–1043.

188. N.T. Ilowite, K. Prather, Y. Lokhnygina, et al., Randomized, double-blind, placebo-controlled trial of the efficacy and safety of rilonacept in the treatment of systemic juvenile idiopathic arthritis. Arthritis Rheumatol. 66 (9) (2014) 2570–2579.

190. S. Urien, C. Bardin, B. Bader-Meunier, et al., Anakinra pharmacokinetics in children and adolescents with systemic-onset juvenile idiopathic arthritis and autoinflammatory syndromes, BMC Pharmacol. Toxicol. 14 (2013) 40.

191. P. Quartier, F. Allantaz, R. Cimaz, et al., A multicentre, randomised, double-blind, placebo-controlled trial with the interleukin-1 receptor antagonist anakinra in patients with systemic-onset juvenile idiopathic arthritis (ANAJIS trial), Ann. Rheum. Dis. 70 (5) (2011) 747–754.

198. S. Yokota, T. Imagawa, M. Mori, et al., Efficacy and safety of tocilizumab in patients with systemic-onset juvenile idiopathic arthritis: a randomised, double-blind, placebo-controlled, withdrawal phase III trial, Lancet 371 (9617) (2008) 998–1006.

199. S. Yokota, T. Imagawa, M. Mori, et al., Longterm safety and effectiveness of the anti-interleukin 6 receptor monoclonal antibody tocilizumab in patients with systemic juvenile idiopathic arthritis in Japan, J. Rheumatol. 41 (4) (2014) 759–767.

206. D.J. Lovell, E.H. Giannini, A. Reiff, et al., Long-term efficacy and safety of etanercept in children with polyarticular-course juvenile rheumatoid arthritis: interim results from an ongoing multicenter, open-label, extended-treatment trial, Arthritis Rheum. 48 (1) (2003) 218–226.

207. G. Horneff, H. Schmeling, T. Biedermann, et al., The German etanercept registry for treatment of juvenile idiopathic arthritis, Ann. Rheum. Dis. 63 (12) (2004) 1638–1644.

211. R.A. Russo, M.M. Katsicas, Clinical remission in patients with systemic juvenile idiopathic arthritis treated with anti-tumor necrosis factor agents, J. Rheumatol. 36 (5) (2009) 1078–1082.

212. N. Ruperto, D.J. Lovell, P. Quartier, et al., Long-term safety and efficacy of abatacept in children with juvenile idiopathic arthritis, Arthritis Rheum. 62 (6) (2010) 1792–1802.

215. P. Woo, T.R. Southwood, A.M. Prieur, et al., Randomized, placebo-controlled, crossover trial of low-dose oral methotrexate in children with

extended oligoarticular or systemic arthritis, Arthritis Rheum. 43 (8) (2000) 1849–1857.

228. D.M. Brinkman, I.M. de Kleer, R. ten Cate, et al., Autologous stem cell transplantation in children with severe progressive systemic or polyarticular juvenile idiopathic arthritis: long-term follow-up of a prospective clinical trial, Arthritis Rheum. 56 (7) (2007) 2410–2421.

231. C. Lomater, V. Gerloni, M. Gattinara, et al., Systemic onset juvenile idiopathic arthritis: a retrospective study of 80 consecutive patients followed for 10 years, J. Rheumatol. 27 (2) (2000) 491–496.

232. D. Singh-Grewal, R. Schneider, N. Bayer, et al., Predictors of disease course and remission in systemic juvenile idiopathic arthritis: significance of early clinical and laboratory features, Arthritis Rheum. 54 (5) (2006) 1595–1601.

233. L.R. Spiegel, R. Schneider, B.A. Lang, et al., Early predictors of poor functional outcome in systemic-onset juvenile rheumatoid arthritis: a multicenter cohort study, Arthritis Rheum. 43 (11) (2000) 2402–2409.

240. C. Modesto, P. Woo, J. García-Consuegra, et al., Systemic onset juvenile chronic arthritis, polyarticular pattern and hip involvement as markers for a bad prognosis, Clin. Exp. Rheumatol. 19 (2) (2001) 211–217.

245. P.J. Hashkes, B.M. Wright, M.S. Lauer, et al., Mortality outcomes in pediatric rheumatology in the US, Arthritis Rheum. 62 (2) (2010) 599–608.

Entire reference list is available online at www.expertconsult.com.

Polyarticular Juvenile Idiopathic Arthritis

Alan M. Rosenberg, Kiem G. Oen

DEFINITIONS

Chronic childhood arthritis affecting five joints or more during the first 6 months of disease is defined as polyarthritis.[1,2] The International League of Associations for Rheumatology (ILAR) classification system for juvenile idiopathic arthritis (JIA)[2] further categorizes polyarthritis as rheumatoid factor (RF) negative if tests for RF are negative, and RF positive if RF is detected on two occasions at least 3 months apart (Table 17-1). RF-negative and RF-positive JIA subsets have distinguishing clinical features, disease courses, and outcomes; therefore, in this chapter RF-negative and RF-positive polyarthritis JIA subsets are considered separately as distinct clinical entities.

RHEUMATOID FACTOR NEGATIVE POLYARTICULAR JIA

Epidemiology

Polyarthritis accounts for approximately 20% of JIA patients; of these, approximately 85% have negative tests for RF,[3,4] although RF frequencies vary in accord with ethnicities.[5-7]

Incidence and Prevalence

Incidence and prevalence data vary widely because of differences in case ascertainment, diagnostic and classification criteria applied, accessibility to care, and genetic and ethnic characteristics of the respective populations.[8] The estimated incidence of chronic childhood arthritis varies from 7 to 21 per 100,000 in North American and Northern European studies.[9-14] Prevalence rates of 121 to 220 per 100,000 have been reported; meta-analysis indicates a chronic childhood arthritis prevalence of 132 (95% confidence interval [CI] 119 to 145) per 100,000 from population studies.[15] Estimating that 20% of JIA populations have polyarthritis and 85% of the polyarthritis populations are RF-negative, the annual incidence and prevalence for RF-negative polyarthritis can be estimated as 1 to 4 per 100,000 and 21 to 37 per 100,000, respectively.

Age at Onset and Sex Ratio

RF-negative polyarticular JIA can begin at any age before 16 years, but onset age displays a biphasic trend with a peak at ages 1 to 3 years and another encompassing later childhood and adolescence.[16] RF-negative polyarthritis affects girls four times more frequently than boys.[5] The predominance of females is greater in those with an onset during adolescence (female-to-male ratio, 10:1) compared with those with a younger onset age (female-to-male ratio, 3:1). Younger onset RF-negative polyarthritis patients are more likely to be antinuclear antibody (ANA) positive and are at greater risk for iridocyclitis.[17] A young onset age of RF-negative polyarthritis is associated with a less favorable long-term outcome.[18-20] Greenwald et al.[16] found 2-year outcomes in an older onset, RF-negative JIA subgroup to be generally favorable even prior to the era of biological therapies.

Geographic and Racial Distribution

JIA occurs worldwide but prevalence varies widely among geographic regions. Oen and Cheang[15] reported that polyarthritis accounted for a higher proportion of East Indian (61%) and North American Indian (64%) children with chronic arthritis, compared with white children (27%). Saurenmann et al.[4] analyzed ethnicity as a risk factor for JIA in a multiethnic cohort; among 223 children with RF-negative polyarthritis, no significant differences among European and non-European patients were found. However, the North American Indian population had a high relative risk (3.2) of developing RF-negative polyarthritis.

Etiology and Pathogenesis

The etiologies of the respective JIA subtypes are unknown but are thought to have complex origins that include interactions among an array of susceptibility genes and as yet unidentified exogenous factors. Environmental and lifestyle influences have been proposed as factors promoting arthritis in the context of genetic vulnerability.

There are no cytokine or chemokine response patterns in either blood or synovial fluid that are unique to RF-negative polyarthritis.[21] De Jager and colleagues[22] noted comparable plasma level increases in interleukin (IL)-6 and -12, and chemokines C-C motif ligand (CCL3), C-X-C motif ligand (CXCL)9, and CXCL10 were found in a small group of children with RF-negative polyarthritis (10 patients) and oligoarthritis with a polyarticular course (5 patients).[22,23] Increased levels of IL-17 found in seronegative polyarthritis are considered to be of potential pathogenic importance because IL-17 promotes other proinflammatory cytokines and enhances matrix metalloproteinase production, leading to cartilage degradation.[24] CCL20 derived from synovial fluid mononuclear cells was increased in children with polyarthritis (including those with extended oligoarticular JIA); the enhanced production was attributed to the hypoxic synovial environment.[25] The hypoxic synovial environment has also been suggested as a factor that promotes increases in intraarticular vascular endothelial growth factor and osteopontin, which enhance angiogenesis in synovial tissue in children with RF-negative polyarthritis and extended oligoarthritis JIA subsets.[26]

Genetic Background

A genetic influence in the pathogenesis of JIA is indicated by ethnic variability in the incidence of certain JIA subsets, female

TABLE 17-1 ILAR Criteria for Classification of the Polyarthritis JIA Subtype

RF-Negative Polyarthritis

Arthritis affecting five or more joints during the first 6 months of disease; a test for RF is negative

Exclusions:
- Psoriasis or a history of psoriasis in the patient or first-degree relative
- Arthritis in an HLA-B27–positive male beginning after the sixth birthday
- Ankylosing spondylitis, enthesitis-related arthritis, sacroiliitis with inflammatory bowel disease, Reiter's syndrome, or acute anterior uveitis or a history of one of these disorders in a first-degree relative
- IgM RF on at least two occasions at least 3 months apart
- The presence of systemic JIA in the patient

RF-Positive Polyarthritis

Arthritis affecting five or more joints during the first 6 months of disease; two or more tests for RF at least 3 months apart during the first 6 months of disease are positive

Exclusions:
- Psoriasis or a history of psoriasis in the patient or first-degree relative
- Arthritis in an HLA-B27–positive male beginning after the sixth birthday
- Ankylosing spondylitis, enthesitis-related arthritis, sacroiliitis with inflammatory bowel disease, Reiter's syndrome, or acute anterior uveitis or a history of one of these disorders in a first-degree relative
- The presence of systemic JIA in the patient

IgM, Immunoglobulin M; *ILAR*, International League of Associations for Rheumatology; *JIA*, juvenile idiopathic arthritis; *RF*, rheumatoid factor.

preponderance, increased sibling recurrence rates, and associations with both human leukocyte antigen (HLA) and non-HLA genes.[27,28]

HLA Genes

Genes both within and outside the major histocompatibility complex (MHC) contribute to genetic susceptibility to JIA. The HLA class I A2 allele confers susceptibility in RF-negative polyarthritis as do the class II alleles DRB1*08, DQAI*04, and DPB1*03.[29] These HLA-related profiles are distinct from those characterizing RF-positive polyarthritis,[29] supporting the view that children without RF have a disease different, at least genetically, from children with RF. Further, certain HLA alleles that confer susceptibility to RF-negative polyarthritis (A2, DRB1*08, and DQA1*04) also confer susceptibility to the oligoarthritis JIA subtype,[29] suggesting that RF-negative polyarthritis is more allied genetically with oligoarticular JIA than with RF-positive polyarthritis. The association of HLA-DRB1 is similar between oligoarticular JIA and the younger onset subgroup of polyarticular JIA; the HLA-DRB1*1103/1104 haplotype is found in the oligoarticular cohort and the younger polyarticular group in contrast with the HLA-DRB1*08 susceptibility haplotype found in the older polyarticular JIA group.[30,31]

In the MHC of children with oligoarticular JIA and, to a somewhat lesser extent with RF-negative polyarticular JIA, a single nucleotide polymorphism (SNP), rs7775055, which tags the HLA-DRB1*0801–HLA-DQA1*0401–HLA-DQB1*0402 haplotypes, is frequently found, again suggesting these two JIA subsets tend to share common genetic influences.[30-32]

Non-HLA Genes

The TRAF1/C5 region on chromosome 9 encodes the tumor necrosis factor (TNF)-receptor-associated factor 1 and the complement component 5.[33] In polyarticular JIA there is an increase in the A allele of an SNP in the TRAF1/C5 region when compared with controls.[33]

The protein tyrosine phosphatase nonreceptor type 22 (PTPN22) gene codes for lymphoid-specific phosphatase, which modulates antibody-mediated T-cell activation. A missense SNP in the PTPN22 gene reduces the ability to downregulate T-cell activation and has been associated with JIA.[34] There is an association of this PTPN22 SNP and RF-negative polyarthritis[35]; however, the association has not been found consistently,[36,37] possibly reflecting ethnic differences in the populations studied. Certain PTPN22 SNPs, although found with significant frequency in RF-negative polyarthritis, are not specific for this JIA subtype, as the same markers are found in RF-positive and oligoarticular JIA.[35,38,39]

Continued mining of JIA genome-wide scans is expected to expose additional susceptibility genes allowing for more precise biologically based categorization of JIA, providing insight into mechanisms of disease and informing new treatment strategies.[27]

Clinical Manifestations

In children with RF-negative polyarticular JIA, joint disease predominates; extraarticular features are infrequent. Variations in onset ages, clinical and serological features, and courses suggest the RF-negative class of polyarthritis comprises different clinical entities. For example, some patients with RF-negative polyarthritis have a young onset age, positive tests for ANA and uveitis, and therefore, apart from the number of involved joints, are similar to the oligoarthritis JIA subtype.

Joint Disease

Onset of arthritis may be acute, but it is more often insidious, with progressive accumulation of additional joints. Morning stiffness, indicative of active arthritis, may persist for hours or occasionally all day. The arthritis may be remittent or indolent. Joint swelling is a result of synovial hypertrophy and/or intraarticular fluid. Joints may be warm but are generally not tender or red. Hot, red, tender joints suggest infection or malignancy rather than JIA. Among children with RF-negative polyarthritis knees, wrists and ankles are most commonly affected. Small joint involvement of the hands or feet may occur early or late in the course of the disease; distal interphalangeal joints are seldom affected at onset (Fig. 17-1).[40] The temporomandibular joint (TMJ) is commonly affected in children with a polyarticular disease course regardless of onset subtype, but those with RF-negative polyarthritis are more likely to have TMJ involvement, particularly at long-term follow-up, than those who are RF-positive.[41,42] The earlier age of onset, when the TMJ might be more vulnerable to damage, is thought to be a reason for the greater prevalence of radiographically evident destruction in the RF-negative group.[41,42] Advances in TMJ imaging, including computed tomography and magnetic resonance imaging (MRI), demonstrate that TMJ arthritis is more common and the severity more variable than can be discerned by clinical assessment alone; TMJ arthritis can be present even in the absence of clinical symptoms or signs.[43-45] In experienced hands ultrasonography can be a suitable method for detecting and monitoring TMJ arthritis.[46] Joint damage associated with TMJ arthritis can result in altered physiognomy, including micrognathia, retrognathia, malocclusion, and facial asymmetry (Fig. 17-2).[47-49]

Cervical spine involvement is not commonly recognized early in the course of RF-negative polyarthritis either clinically or by conventional radiography but with longer term follow-up decreased range of motion can ensue.[50] More sensitive imaging modalities, such as MRI, reveal that cervical spine involvement is more common than is generally appreciated even in asymptomatic patients.[51,52] Atlantoaxial

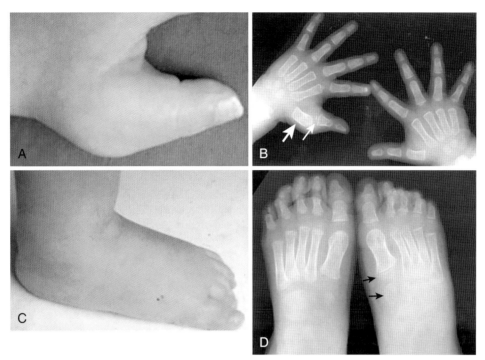

FIGURE 17-1 Images of an 18-month-old boy with seronegative polyarticular JIA. Swelling of the right thumb was associated with clinical signs of intraarticular fluid and synovial hypertrophy (A) and radiographic evidence (B) of soft tissue swelling, bony overgrowth of the first metacarpal (*thick arrow*), and premature ossification of the proximal phalanx growth center (*thin arrow*). Similarly, the right foot and ankle show swelling due to fluid and synovial hypertrophy (C) and accelerated bone growth on the affected side (D; *arrows*).

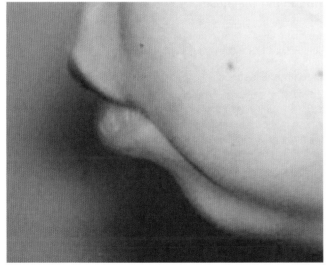

FIGURE 17-2 Retrognathia in a 12-year-old girl who had onset of RF-negative polyarticular JIA at 3 years of age.

subluxation (Fig. 17-3), erosion of the odontoid process, and vertebral ankylosis can occur (Fig. 17-4).

In RF-negative polyarthritis the number of affected joints tends to be less and the pattern of involvement more asymmetric than in RF-positive polyarthritis (Fig. 17-1). In RF-negative disease involvement of wrists and small joints of the hands is less frequent in RF-positive disease. Clinical signs of hip involvement are present in fewer than 20% with RF-negative polyarthritis at first presentation, but progressive hip abnormalities become evident with longer term follow-up.

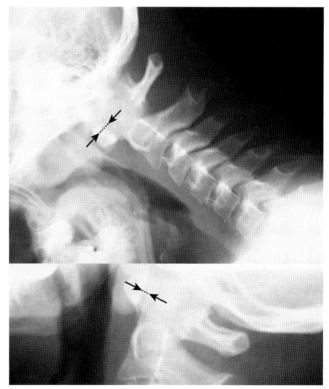

FIGURE 17-3 Flexion (A) and extension (B) radiographs of the cervical spine of a child with RF-negative polyarthritis. The increased distance between the posterior surface of the anterior arch of the first cervical vertebra and the anterior margin of the odontoid (*arrows*) in flexion suggest mild atlantoaxial subluxation in this patient.

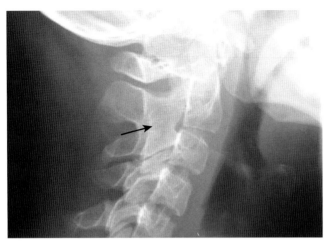

FIGURE 17-4 Lateral radiograph of the cervical spine of a child with RF-negative polyarthritis showing bony ankylosis of the second and third cervical vertebrae.

Oen et al.[50] reported that radiological signs of hip joint involvement during childhood were more likely to occur in RF-negative than RF-positive polyarthritis; the tendency for RF-negative polyarthritis to have its onset at a younger age compared with RF-positive disease might be a factor contributing to the higher frequency of abnormalities identified during childhood in the seronegative group. Wrist and ankle involvement at first presentation has been suggested as a predictor of progression to polyarthritis in those first presenting with oligoarthritis.[53]

A small subset of RF-negative children have "dry synovitis," a condition characterized by polyarthropathy, minimal or absent clinical signs of joint effusion or synovial hypertrophy, joint stiffness, limited range of motion, and joint contractures associated with laboratory indicators of inflammation.[54] This uncommon subset of polyarthritis can be considered a variant of RF-negative polyarthritis although it has also been suggested to be a *forme fruste* of scleroderma.[54]

Systemic Manifestations

Systemic manifestations in seronegative polyarticular JIA are unusual but can include fatigue and growth failure. Fever seldom occurs and when present is low grade.

Fatigue in children with polyarthritis can be present even in the absence of active joint disease.[55] Ringold et al.[56] studied fatigue in 60 children with polyarthritis, of whom 24 (61.2%) were RF negative, using a survey tool that includes assessment of general fatigue, sleep/rest fatigue, and cognitive fatigue domains. Both JIA children and their parent/proxies reported lower scores in all domains compared with controls.[56] Fatigue in JIA is significantly associated with poor functional ability.[57] Factors contributing to fatigue can include pain and stress, decreased muscle mass, low aerobic and anaerobic capacity, and anemia.[55,57-59] Sleep disturbance does not appear to be a common factor contributing to fatigue in JIA.[60]

Growth disturbances are common in JIA.[61-64] In children with polyarthritis height-for-age Z scores (reflecting the number of standard deviations from the normal mean) may decline in the first several years of disease but tend to return to normal.[62] In those children without RF, the negative deviation is less marked and less prolonged than those with RF, particularly with longer disease duration.[62] Low growth velocity tends to correlate with disease severity and activity and with the number of involved joints.[61,63,64]

Extraarticular Manifestations

Subcutaneous nodules. Subcutaneous nodules are rare in RF-negative polyarthritis. Among 131 children with RF-negative polyarticular JIA from a Canadian JIA inception cohort, only 1 (0.7%) had subcutaneous nodules at initial presentation.

Uveitis. Next to oligoarticular JIA (which accounts for more than half of JIA patients affected by uveitis), chronic asymptomatic uveitis is most common in the RF-negative polyarthritis group.[65,66] Approximately 15% to 20% of children with RF-negative polyarthritis have uveitis and account for approximately 20% of all JIA uveitis patients.[65,67,68]

Sabri and colleagues[65] reported that 32 of 142 JIA patients (22.5%) with uveitis had RF-negative polyarthritis; none with RF-positive JIA had uveitis. As with the oligoarthritis, JIA subgroup uveitis in RF-negative polyarthritis tends to be associated with younger onset age and ANA positivity. Greenwald et al.[16] reported that only 2% of patients with older onset RF-negative polyarticular JIA had uveitis despite the fact that 47% were ANA positive.

Cardiovascular and pulmonary disease. RF-negative polyarthritis is not typically associated with overt cardiovascular pathology. Bharti et al.[69] reported that children with arthritis, regardless of onset subtype, had significantly greater left ventricular volumes and other abnormalities suggesting abnormal left ventricular diastolic relaxation. Knook et al.[70] demonstrated lower 1-second forced vital capacity and peak expiratory flows in a group of 31 children with chronic arthritis, of whom more than two thirds had RF-negative polyarthritis. These abnormalities were attributable to impaired respiratory muscle strength rather than intrinsic restrictive or obstructive lung disease.[70]

Differential Diagnosis

The differential diagnosis for a child with polyarthritis includes other rheumatic diseases, infections, other inflammatory conditions, malignancies, and metabolic and genetic disorders.

Rheumatic Diseases

The onset of polyarthritis in a girl later in childhood or during adolescence could suggest the possible diagnosis of systemic lupus erythematosus (SLE). The arthritis of SLE may mimic that of JIA, although it is nonerosive and less likely to be deforming; the presence of other clinical hallmarks and a positive test for anti-double stranded DNA (anti-dsDNA) antibodies establishes the diagnosis of SLE. Ragsdale and colleagues[71] described nine children (six of whom were RF negative) who developed SLE years after an initial diagnosis of polyarticular juvenile arthritis.

The differential diagnosis of RF-negative polyarthritis also includes enthesitis-related arthritis (ERA). Predominant involvement of large joints of the lower extremities and the presence of enthesitis supports the diagnosis of ERA although enthesitis can occur, albeit uncommonly, in other types of JIA.[72]

Scleroderma begins insidiously with joint contractures of the small joints of the hands mimicking features of polyarthritis but ordinarily without associated signs of intraarticular swelling. Children with dermatomyositis may have polyarthritis, but they can be distinguished from those with JIA by clinical manifestations such as typical rash and muscle weakness.

Infections

Septic arthritis affecting multiple joints is unusual; only 3% of the 65 children with septic arthritis reported by Al Saadi et al.[73] had more than one involved joint. Lyme disease may be polyarticular, but it can usually be differentiated from RF-negative polyarthritis by its intermittent pattern of arthritis activity and accompanying extraarticular abnormalities. Arthritis caused by *Neisseria gonorrhoeae* may have an early migratory polyarticular phase.[74]

Reactive polyarthritis in response to infection in the respiratory, gastrointestinal, or genitourinary tracts ordinarily can be distinguished from polyarticular JIA by a limited duration of the disease and associated clinical manifestations. Acute rheumatic fever following group A beta-hemolytic streptococcal pharyngitis is characterized by acute, painful, nonerosive, migratory polyarthritis (see Chapters 43 and 44).

Malignancy

Malignant infiltration of bone or synovium can mimic polyarthritis, although in most instances the malignant focus is in juxtaarticular bone rather than in the joint. However, joint swelling can occur in lymphoblastic leukemia as a result of leukemic infiltration of the synovium. Joint involvement in malignancy tends to be oligoarticular rather than polyarticular and associated with systemic manifestations of malignancy.[75]

Other Inflammatory Conditions

Arthritis associated with inflammatory bowel disease or sarcoidosis should be considered in the differential diagnosis of RF-negative polyarthritis. Sickle cell disease causes diffuse, symmetrical swelling of the hands and feet that may mimic true arthritis. Hypermobility syndromes, mucopolysaccharidoses, familial hypertrophic synovitis,[76,77] familial arthritis and camptodactyly,[78] familial osteochondritis dissecans,[79] Stickler's syndrome,[80] velocardial facial syndrome,[81] Turner's syndrome,[82] and relapsing polychondritis[83] are rare causes of disease that may suggest polyarticular JIA. Scurvy should be considered in the differential diagnosis of polyarthropathy in children at risk for nutritional deficiencies, including those with autism and other developmental disorders.[84]

Laboratory Examination

Laboratory tests can provide evidence of inflammation, are useful in excluding other diagnoses, and important in classification, prognostication, and guiding therapy (see Chapter 10).

Indicators of Inflammation

Children with polyarthritis typically have moderate elevations of the erythrocyte sedimentation rate (ESR) and C-reactive protein, and may have elevated white blood cell and platelet counts and a normocytic, hypochromic anemia associated with chronic inflammation.

Autoantibodies

Rheumatoid factors. Applying ILAR criteria, discrimination between RF-positive and RF-negative polyarthritis is based on at least two positive RF results as determined by an accredited laboratory. RFs are antibodies that bind to the CH2 and CH3 domains of the Fc portion of IgG. Customarily, RF is detected by agglutination assays that preferentially detect pentameric IgM RF. Approximately one third of children with polyarthritis who do not have IgM RF detectable by agglutination methods have IgM RF detected by more sensitive enzyme immunoassays (EIAs). RF detected by either technique is associated with deforming and erosive joint disease.[85,86] Further, children with IgM RF-negative polyarthritis, determined by conventional methods, can have "hidden RFs." Hidden IgM RF is 19S IgM RF that, because it is bound to IgG in the serum being tested, cannot generate a response in a standard agglutination assay until it is acid eluted from the IgG. Up to 85% of children with polyarticular disease have been reported

to have such antibodies associated with active disease.[87-89] IgA RF, alone or in combination with IgM RF, has been associated with active disease, disability, and radiographic joint space narrowing and bone erosions in polyarthritis.[86,90]

Anticitrullinated peptide/protein antibodies (ACPA) have been reported to occur in 0% to 17% of children with RF-negative polyarthritis.[91]

Antinuclear antibodies. ANAs are present in approximately half of children with RF-negative polyarthritis.[92] The group of ANA-positive RF-negative polyarthritis patients is generally not substantially different from the group with oligoarthritis with respect to age at first presentation, sex ratio, or prevalence of uveitis, suggesting that ANA positivity, irrespective of JIA onset subtype, distinguishes a relatively homogeneous group characterized by early onset, female predominance, asymmetric arthritis, and risk of uveitis.[93] The antigenic specificities of ANA in JIA are generally unknown[94]; antibodies to individual histones and to histone-histone and histone-DNA complexes are occasionally, but inconsistently, found.[95]

Synovial fluid analysis. Synovial fluid analysis in RF-negative polyarthritis reveals a nonspecific inflammatory reaction that is indistinguishable from characteristics found in other JIA subtypes. In children with polyarthritis (including those with extended oligoarthritis) polymorphonuclear neutrophils tend to be higher in synovial fluid compared with persistent oligoarticular disease but not significantly different from findings in systemic JIA.[96,97] Cytokine, chemokine, and proteome profiles in synovial fluids have been explored in JIA but not sufficiently elucidated to be of clinical utility.[22,25,26,98]

Radiological Examination

Radiographic evidence of joint space narrowing (decreased joint space, ankylosis, and carpal collapse) was demonstrated in 12% of 39 children at 2 years after onset and in 43% by 6 years after onset in the RF-negative JIA subset.[50] Erosions and growth abnormalities likewise increased with time.

Pathology

The limited information about synovial pathology indicates that the histological appearance of the synovium is similar for all JIA subtypes although there is greater vascularity in the polyarthritis group compared with enthesitis related arthritis, psoriatic arthritis, and oligoarthritis.[99] Finnegan et al.[100] reported knee joint synovial membrane histopathological and immunopathological features among 42 children with JIA of whom 8 had seronegative polyarthritis. All subjects were within 2 years of diagnosis (mean 5.3 months) and had not been treated with steroids or disease-modifying antirheumatic drugs (DMARDs). When compared with persistent oligoarticular JIA pathology, subjects with polyarthritis (RF positive, RF negative, and extended oligoarthritis) had more inflammatory infiltrates and synovial hypertrophy, and more abundant CD3, CD4, and CD20 cells. The adhesion receptor $\alpha V\beta 3$ integrin, which is upregulated on endothelial cells during angiogenesis,[101] was significantly more prominent in the polyarticular subjects than in either oligoarticular or extended oligoarticular patients.

Treatment

As with all forms of chronic childhood arthritis, RF-negative polyarthritis requires a multifaceted approach to management. The mainstays of treatment include early and judicious use of pharmacotherapy, physical and occupational therapy, and the promotion of healthy lifestyles, including optimal nutrition, physical activity, and reduction of stress. Achieving and sustaining complete disease control is now an attainable objective.

Medical Management

An initial trial of nonsteroidal antiinflammatory drugs (NSAIDs) is appropriate. The trend to more aggressive treatment at first presentation of polyarthritis has resulted in the early use of a disease-remitting agent, usually methotrexate, often in combination with an NSAID; earlier initiation of biological therapies has also been advocated.[102]

American College of Rheumatology (ACR) guidelines for treating JIA promote early treatment of JIA with rapid escalation of therapies as required in accord with responses.[103] In RF-negative polyarthritis the aggressiveness of therapy can be guided by prognostic and disease activity indicators. Unfavorable prognostic indicators, which would prompt more aggressive early treatment, include hip and cervical spine involvement, radiographic evidence of joint space narrowing and/or bone erosions, and the presence of ACPA. Indicators of moderate to severe disease activities, judged by the number of active joints, levels of inflammatory markers, and poor physician and patient/parent global assessments would also prompt aggressive, early treatment.

There are no established guidelines for stopping drug therapy in JIA. Once disease remission is induced with a remittive agent, NSAIDs can often be discontinued without exacerbation of disease activity. In any event, even in polyarthritis with a favorable prognostic profile and low disease activity score, failure of NSAIDs to control the disease within 6 weeks should prompt the addition of methotrexate. Methotrexate is usually given by mouth initially, in doses of 10-15 mg/m^2/week. In the absence of an adequate response the dose can be increased to 15-20 mg/ m^2/week, preferably administered subcutaneously. The response to methotrexate is usually excellent.[104-106] Nonresponse to methotrexate in RF-negative polyarthritis, as in other JIA subtypes, might be predicted by considering SNPs of genes involved in methotrexate metabolic pathways.[107] For patients who are unresponsive to or intolerant of methotrexate, leflunomide is an option, although there is insufficient information to evaluate leflunomide's role in RF-negative polyarthritis specifically.[108] Treatment approaches that include use of biologically based anti-TNF agents at first presentation either in combination with a DMARD or alone have been suggested.[109]

Anti-TNF agents are effective in treating children with polyarthritis who are unresponsive to methotrexate or leflunomide alone although there is little information to indicate that RF status correlates with responsiveness.[110-116] Anti-TNF therapy should be considered in any child with polyarticular JIA with moderate or high disease activity who has not responded to methotrexate or leflunomide by 3 months or, for those with low disease activity, by 6 months.[103] Biologically based therapies targeting proinflammatory cytokines other than TNF, including IL-6 as an example (tocilizumab), are emerging as treatment options. When patient-specific biomarker profiling becomes more clinically accessible, the selection of specific anticytokine therapies can be more biologically based.

Glucocorticoids are important as intraarticular therapy. Breit and colleagues[117] reported a longer median duration of response to intraarticular triamcinolone hexacetonide in children with juvenile chronic arthritis who were RF negative (105 weeks) than in those who were RF positive (63 weeks). Glucocorticoids have a limited role as systemic therapy in polyarthritis although judicious use of systemic steroids as a bridging agent can be considered until disease-modifying agents become effective.[118] Gold compounds and penicillamine are seldom used since the advent of generally safer and more efficacious pharmacotherapeutic options. Although hydroxychloroquine is at times used in RF-negative polyarthritis as an adjunctive and relatively safe agent, often in combination with methotrexate, there is no substantive evidence reported to support its efficacy.

There are no established guidelines to direct when pharmacotherapies can be safely discontinued in RF-negative polyarthritis. Although there is no evidence-based rationale for continuing treatment beyond the point of clinical remission, there is accumulating concern that clinical remission might not always reflect actual biologic remission. Both magnetic resonance and ultrasound imaging indicate that synovial inflammation can persist even in patients in whom clinical remission is achieved.[119,120] Undetected, subclinical inflammation leads to joint damage and disability. Persistent biologic activity is evidenced by expression of TNF-α and IL-4-regulated genes and elevated levels of S100 proteins in patients in apparent clinical remission.[121,122] In the future it is expected that incorporation of clinical, imaging, and biomarker indicators will be possible and will help identify true disease remission and thus guide the timing of when to safely stop treatment.[123]

Exercise and Physical and Occupational Therapy

Regular participation in physical activity by children with JIA is beneficial.[124] Functional impairment generally correlates with the extent and severity of articular disease, but poor fitness also occurs even in those with mild symptoms and persists even after disease remission.[58] Both aerobic and anaerobic exercise capacity are decreased in children with polyarthritis compared with those with oligoarticular disease; those with RF-positive polyarthritis are somewhat more limited than those with RF-negative disease.[58] Notwithstanding the advantages of active exercise, it is important to have a carefully designed passive therapy program. Children tend to function within the range of motion they have, not the range they should be trying to achieve. Focused physical therapy should be instituted as soon as inflammation subsides sufficiently to facilitate the child's cooperation. Physical therapy aimed at restoration of range of motion can be facilitated by pretreatment with an analgesic or application of heat. Major contractures are often more amenable to therapy after intraarticular triamcinolone hexacetonide (see Chapter 14).

Surgery

The need for surgical management is now less common as a consequence of more effective medical management. Nonetheless, some children with resistant or untreated disease will require joint replacement of hips, knees, or, less commonly, other joints. Prior to surgical procedures the child with polyarthritis should be evaluated for conditions that might present added anesthesia and surgery risk, including cervical spine and TMJ damage, immunosuppression that heightens infection risk, and poor bone quality that can compromise the integrity of joint implants.

Course of the Disease and Prognosis

RF-negative polyarticular JIA is a chronic disease, lasting years or decades. Oen et al.[125] reported that only 25% of 80 children with RF-negative polyarthritis diagnosed between 1977 and 1994 and followed for at least 5 years had gone into remission by the age of 16. Children who had not remitted by this age were likely to have ongoing active arthritis into their late 20s or early 30s. These earlier data indicate that RF-negative polyarticular JIA was associated with substantial morbidity in most affected children. More recent studies, reflecting advances in treatment, suggest more favorable short-term outcomes. However, based on results of a prospective study, Oen et al.[126] reported that only 19% of RF-negative polyarthritis patients achieved clinical remission within 6 months of enrollment. One third to half of patients with a severe polyarticular disease course who fail treatment with methotrexate achieve ACR Pedi 70 criteria response to an anti-TNF agent within 12 months.[127-129] Greenwald et al.[16] studied an older onset subset of patients with polyarticular JIA and found almost 50% had a favorable functional outcome at 2 years even before the era of biological therapies. By 6 months after initial diagnosis, almost half of the patients had fewer than five active joints and by 24 months all patients had fewer than five active joints, regardless of how many active joints they had at diagnosis. More favorable medium- and long-term outcomes are anticipated in the RF-negative polyarthritis group as a result of treatment advances.

Most children with RF-negative polyarthritis will retain their classification category; however, manifestations of psoriasis or inflammatory bowel disease, as examples, might first manifest months or years following the onset of arthritis, thereby necessitating reclassification.[130]

RHEUMATOID FACTOR POSITIVE POLYARTHRITIS

RF-positive polyarticular JIA shares a similar clinical phenotype, serology, and immunogenetic profile to that of adult rheumatoid arthritis, and both can occur in the same family. Because of these features, RF-positive polyarthritis is generally accepted to be equivalent to RF-positive adult rheumatoid arthritis (RA) but with onset at younger than 16 years of age. The association with ACPA emphasizes this relationship.

Epidemiology
Incidence and Prevalence
There is limited published information about incidence and prevalence rates for the RF-positive polyarthritis onset subtype. Estimated incidence rates of 0.3 to 0.7 per 100,000 person-years at risk have been reported or can be calculated from publications from Europe and the United States.[9,10,131-133] In comparison, incidence estimates as high as 12.3 can be calculated from published data for East Coast Alaskan Indian children, and 8.1 per 100,000 person-years at risk for Native Canadian Indian children in Manitoba.[5,134] Similarly, estimates of point prevalence of 0 to 6.7 per 100,000 in Europe and the United States, and 54 per 100,000 at risk for Manitoba Canadian Indian children, can be calculated from published data.[15,133,135-137]

Age at Onset and Sex Ratio
The mean age at juvenile onset of RF-positive polyarthritis is 9 to 11 years, and the range is 1.5 to 15 years.[6,131,138,139] Affected girls outnumber boys from 4 : 1 to 13 : 1 in large series.[4,6,131,138,140,141]

Geographic and Racial Distribution
RF-positive polyarthritis is one of the least frequent JIA subtypes in white children but occurs at higher relative frequencies in non-white children. Reported frequencies range from 51% in a series of Native Canadian Indian children to 18% of Hispanic-American children, 7% to 17% of East Indian children, 14% of African-American children, and 12.5% of Japanese children, and 0.2% to 6% in European and US children and adolescents with chronic arthritis.[3,4,6,9,131-133,135,136,140,142-144]

Etiology and Pathogenesis
ACPA occur in 60% or more of patients with RF-positive polyarthritis,[91,145-150] and may have a role in disease pathogenesis. ACPA are directed against citrullinated peptides that are formed in dying cells by deimination of arginine by peptidylarginine deiminases. It is postulated that these modified peptides are exposed to the immune system if clearance does not occur.[151] Moreover, peptidylarginine deiminases leak from dying cells, allowing citrullination of peptides in tissues such as the synovium.[151] It has been shown that shared epitope–bearing

HLA-DR alleles have increased binding affinity for citrulline.[151,152] This phenomenon is a most likely explanation for the association of the SE specifically with ACPA-positive JIA and RA.[91,148,151,153-155] Further, a pathogenic role of ACPA is suggested by their presence prior to clinically evident RA, the increased severity of erosive disease in ACPA-positive patients with RA or JIA, and the induction of arthritis by ACPA in experimental animals.[146,149-151,156-160] ACPA immune complexes can activate complement *in vitro*, and therefore complement activation through complexes of ACPA and their tissue targets may be a mechanism of disease.[151,157] These postulates likely apply to ACPA-positive RF-positive polyarticular JIA as much as they do to ACPA-positive RA.

Although disease initiation may differentiate RF-positive polyarthritis, it shares inflammatory pathways with other JIA subtypes. These include chemokine and cytokine secretion, angiogenesis, the infiltration of inflammatory cells into the synovium, synovial cell hyperplasia, and finally secretion of matrix metalloproteinases (see Chapters 3 and 4).

Genetic Background
HLA Genes
Distinct from RF-negative polyarticular JIA, RF-positive polyarticular JIA shares genetic predispositions with adult RA. The shared epitope (SE), a specific sequence present on a number of HLA-DRB1 antigens, is associated with increased risk of both RF-positive polyarthritis and adult RA. The SE is found on HLA-DRB1*04 (0401, 0404, 0408, or 0405), DRB1*01 (0101), and DRB1*14 (1402) alleles.[161] Population frequencies of the SE and particular SE-bearing HLA alleles vary in different ethnic groups. Thus, RF-positive polyarthritis and RA are associated with DRB1*04 alleles, mainly DRB1*0401 and *0404, in white populations. The relative risk of RF-positive polyarthritis attributable to DRB1*0401 is 3.2 to 7.2, and to DRB1*0404, 3.8 to 8.9.[32,162-168] Double doses of the SE further increase the relative risk of the disease.[166,167] The associated allele is DRB1*0405 in Asian (i.e., Japanese, Chinese, Korean) populations.[161,169] In Native North American Indian tribes the SE is represented by DRB1*04 alleles and DRB1*1402 and is associated with RA.[170-173] In some tribes the population frequency of DRB1*1402 is so high that no significant increase is found in patients with RA.[173] In Native Canadian Indian children, the situation is more complex when both the SE and DRB1*0901 occurring together as a genotype are associated with RF-positive polyarthritis.[6,7,170,174] This dual association supports the suggestion that earlier age at onset is associated with a greater genetic influence.

Population frequencies of the SE tend to correlate with frequencies of RA and RF-positive polyarticular JIA. For example, the frequency of the SE in white populations is 27% to 36%, whereas Native North American Indian populations with high incidence and prevalence rates of RA and RF-positive polyarthritis have frequencies of 66% to 98%.[32,162,171,174] As discussed above, the SE is associated specifically with ACPA-positive, rather than RF-positive, disease.[91,148,151,153-155]

Non-HLA Genes
HLA-DR alone accounts for 17 % of the genetic risk for juvenile rheumatoid arthritis (JRA)[175] and provides the greatest risk with odds ratios (OR) ranging from 3 to 12.[167] Moreover, HLA associations are specific for JRA or JIA subtypes. In contrast, although the remaining genetic risk is large, it is contributed by multiple genes, each providing only modest probabilities with OR values less than 1.5, with the exception of PTPN22.[31,35,39,176] Many associations with non-HLA genes are shared by a number of autoimmune conditions, suggesting common immunopathogenic pathways. The associated genes are often called autoimmune genes and many are involved in T-cell activation and

differentiation.[39,177] Autoimmune genes with replicated associations with JIA include SNPs of TNF-α–induced protein 3 (TNF AIP3), STAT-4, IL-2RA, PTPN22, and PTPN2 genes, whereas associations with TRAF1/C5, IL2RA gene variations are controversial.[39,176-180] Not all studies have included patients with RF-positive polyarthritis, and few have stratified patients by JIA subtype. One study showed a suggestive association of RF-positive polyarthritis with a STAT4 SNP[180] and another with a SNP in the MVK gene, the gene for hyper-IgD syndrome.[181] However, as with HLA, it is likely non-HLA gene associations for RA are shared with RF-positive polyarthritis. These associations include all the autoimmune genes mentioned above. In contrast to shared autoimmune genes, the peptidylarginine deiminase 4 (PADI4) gene association is specific for RA, particularly for ACPA-positive RA, but this association is strongest in East Asian populations.[182-185] The PADI4 genes code for PAD enzymes. There is a possible functional correlation as the associated PADI4 haplotype stabilizes PADI4 messenger RNA (mRNA), allowing increased citrullination.[183] An association of PADI4 polymorphisms specifically with RF-positive polyarthritis has not been investigated.

Clinical Manifestations
Joint Disease
Upper and lower extremity large and small joints are affected, as well as the cervical spine and TMJs. The thoracic and lumbar spine and sacroiliac joints are spared. Although large joints are commonly involved, the characteristic pattern is symmetrical arthritis affecting the metacarpophalangeal (MCP) and proximal interphalangeal (PIP) joints of the hands, the wrists, and the metatarsophalangeal (MTP) and PIP joints of the feet. In contrast to RF-negative polyarthritis, micrognathia (TMJ involvement) does not usually occur because of the individual's older age at onset. Early limited range of motion occurs at the wrists and can eventually progress to more substantial debility and deformity. Deformities that develop at the hands include ulnar drift at the wrists and the MCP joints, and boutonnière and swan neck deformities at the fingers (Fig. 17-5). Deformities that develop at the feet include hallux valgus deformity at the first MTP joints, hammertoe, and cock-up toe deformities.

Systemic Manifestations
Fatigue and weight loss may occur with active disease. Fatigue may persist even if disease is inactive.[56] Fever is rare in RF-positive polyarthritis, and a rash does not occur.

Extraarticular Manifestations
Other than nodules, uveitis or extraarticular disease manifestations associated with adult RA (described below) rarely occur in patients with RF-positive polyarthritis, whether during childhood, adolescence, or adulthood.

Uveitis. Frequencies of uveitis of 1.4 and 4.5% in children with RF-positive polyarthritis have been reported in large series.[67,186]

Subcutaneous nodules. The most common extraarticular signs in patients with RF-positive polyarthritis are rheumatoid nodules. In Ansell's series, 30% of patients with polyarticular RF-positive arthritis had rheumatoid nodules during the first year of disease.[187] Nodules often occur distal to the olecranon and at other bony prominences and pressure points, on flexor tendon sheaths, Achilles tendon, and on the soles of the feet. They are firm, mobile, and nontender; however, pressure of the nodule against soft tissues or bone may cause pain. The presence of rheumatoid nodules indicates a poor prognosis. Accelerated nodulosis may occur in patients on methotrexate. In this case the nodules are multiple, develop over a short time, tend to occur on the hands, and regress on discontinuation of methotrexate. This

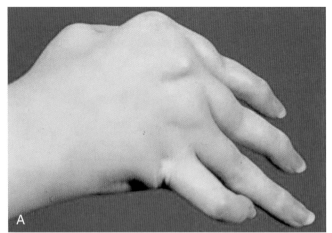

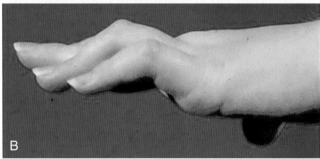

FIGURE 17-5 Hands of children with RF-positive polyarthritis. **A,** Swan neck deformities in digits 2, 3, and 4 displaying characteristic extension at the proximal interphalangeal joints and flexion at the distal interphalangeal joints. Ulnar deviation at the metacarpophalangeal joints is also demonstrated. **B,** Boutonnière deformities at digits 4 and 5 displaying characteristic flexion at the proximal interphalangeal joints and extension at the distal interphalangeal joints.

complication has been described in two children with RF-positive polyarthritis and four with systemic JIA.[188-190] Methotrexate-induced nodulosis is associated with minimal discomfort and may stabilize with use of hydroxychloroquine. Nodulosis associated with methotrexate does not necessarily preclude continuation of methotrexate therapy.[188,190,191]

Rheumatoid nodules must be distinguished from subcutaneous nodules of rheumatic fever, which are smaller; so-called benign rheumatoid nodules that are not associated with chronic arthritis; granuloma annulare, which are small nodules arranged in a circular pattern; erythema nodosum; and nodules seen in cutaneous polyarteritis nodosa.

Vasculitis. Rheumatoid vasculitis is rarely described in RF-positive polyarticular JIA during childhood or adolescence. In 1978, Ansell noted nailfold and extensive cutaneous vasculitis in several patients during prolonged follow-up.[192] However, the lack of reports of this complication in recent literature may reflect improved therapies for arthritis or less severe disease, as vasculitis in adults with RA tends to occur in those with the most severe disease.

Felty syndrome. Felty syndrome consists of persistent neutropenia, splenomegaly, and RA, and is associated with frequent infections. The bone marrow is normocellular, and the mechanism of neutropenia is complex, involving both antigranulocyte antibodies and decreased granulopoiesis.[193] In adults, Felty syndrome occurs in RF-positive patients with long disease duration. It has been reported rarely in adolescents with RF-positive polyarthritis and in adults who had juvenile onset disease.[194,195]

Cardiovascular and pulmonary disease. Valvular heart disease has been reported in at least eight patients with childhood-onset RF-positive polyarthritis.[196-203] Aortic insufficiency is the most common lesion. Patients present with sudden onset of congestive heart failure or may deteriorate suddenly after a variable period of stability following the detection of cardiac murmurs. Valve replacement is almost always required. Cardiac symptoms may start during childhood, adolescence, or adulthood, at intervals varying from 4 to 17 years from onset of JIA. However, pathological murmurs may be detected as early as 1 year after onset. Patients with JIA who have organic cardiac murmurs should be evaluated for valvular insufficiency and monitored carefully.

Pulmonary parenchymal disease, so-called rheumatoid lung, has been reported in seven cases of RF-positive polyarthritis.[204-208] Two types of pulmonary involvement have been reported: lymphoid interstitial pneumonitis, and bronchiolitis obliterans or bronchiolitis obliterans organizing pneumonia (BOOP). These pulmonary complications may occur during childhood and adolescence or in adulthood. The time interval between the clinical presentation of pulmonary disease and onset of JIA has ranged from 10 years before to 20 years after onset of JIA. Symptoms include tachypnea, dyspnea, a nonproductive cough, and fever. On auscultation, crackles and an end-inspiratory squeak are often heard. Diagnosis is based on clinical history and findings, pulmonary function tests, chest radiographs, and high-resolution computed tomography (HRCT). Bronchoalveolar lavage and/or lung biopsy may be necessary. Pulmonary function tests show reduced lung volumes and decreased diffusion capacity. A restrictive pattern is seen when interstitial pneumonitis is present, and an obstructive pattern is seen in BOOP. Chest radiographs may be normal or may show interstitial infiltrates. HRCT abnormalities include ground glass changes suggesting inflammation, bronchiectasis, or bronchiolectasis (suggesting BOOP), and honeycombing (suggesting fibrosis). The differential diagnosis includes drug-induced pulmonary toxicity and infection. The prognosis of rheumatoid lung is variable in children and adolescents. Although a few patients have improved with corticosteroid therapy, others have deteriorated despite corticosteroid and immunosuppressive therapy.

Differential Diagnosis

The differential diagnosis of polyarthritis is discussed above. Specific diagnoses to be considered in the context of RF-positive polyarthritis are connective tissue diseases, reactive arthritis, and infections, in which polyarthritis and a positive test for RF may occur concurrently. Among the connective tissue diseases, SLE and overlap syndromes, including mixed connective tissue disease, are diagnostic considerations in the child or adolescent with polyarticular arthritis who has a positive test for RF. RF is positive in 10% to 30% of children with SLE and in approximately 66% of children with mixed connective tissue disease. RF may be present in cases of acute rheumatic fever. Tuberculosis and subacute bacterial endocarditis can be associated with arthritis accompanied by a positive test for RF.

Laboratory Investigations
Indicators of Inflammation

These are identical to those in RF-negative polyarthritis discussed earlier.

Autoantibodies

Rheumatoid factor. The classification of RF-positive polyarthritis is based on the presence of two positive tests for RF performed at least 3 months apart during the first 6 months of disease.[2] Patients with RF-positive polyarthritis are characterized by persistently positive IgM RF, generally in high titer.

Antinuclear antibodies. Approximately 42% to 56% of children with RF-positive polyarthritis have antinuclear antibodies.[4,209]

Anticitrullinated protein antibodies (ACPA). ACPA are much more prevalent in RF-positive polyarthritis than in other JIA subtypes; however, as in adults with RA, the concordance with RF positivity is not complete. The frequency of ACPA in RF-positive polyarthritis varies from 57% to 90% (mean 74%); but up to 17% of children with RF-negative polyarthritis, and 6% of children with subtypes other than RF-positive polyarthritis, have positive ACPA tests.[91,145-148,150,210-213] ACPA correlate with disease severity and joint damage evidenced by radiographs, suggesting that ACPA have a prognostic significance in JIA as in RA.[146,148-150]

Synovial fluid analysis. Synovial fluid analyses from patients with RF-positive polyarthritis show an inflammatory fluid not clearly differentiated from that found in other forms of JIA. Synovial fluid cell counts and proportions of neutrophils may be higher in RF-positive polyarthritis than in those with oligoarticular arthritis.[96]

Radiological Examination

Most information on joint damage in RF-positive polyarthritis comes from a limited number of studies of plain radiographs of patients treated before the introduction of biological therapies. Joint space narrowing and erosions occur within the first 1 to 2 years after onset and are most frequent at the wrists, hands, feet, and shoulders (Fig. 17-6). At the wrist, cartilage loss occurs at the proximal wrist joint and in the intercarpal joints, resulting in carpal ankylosis and shortening.[50,214] Both erosions and cartilage loss occur more frequently in RF-positive polyarthritis than in other forms of JIA.[20,50,215,216] Atlantoaxial subluxation of the cervical spine is more frequent in patients with RF (36% frequency) than in other patients with JRA (16%).[217] In patients with long disease duration extending into adulthood, radiographic damage at the hands and feet is more frequent in RF-positive (91%) than RF-negative polyarthritis (55%), but hip damage is more frequent in RF-negative polyarthritis (20% vs 50%); the frequency of all radiographic lesions at the cervical spine is similar, at 65%.[51,218]

Pathology
Synovium

Despite similarities in overall appearance, the cellular infiltrates in the synovium may differ among various types of JIA. As detailed above, B- and T-lymphocyte infiltrates, vascularity, and synovial hyperplasia are all more pronounced in both RF-negative and RF-positive polyarthritis compared with persistent oligoarticular JIA, and there is a greater predominance of CD4 over CD8 T cells compared with oligoarticular JRA or juvenile spondyloarthropathies.[100,219]

Rheumatoid Nodules

The mature rheumatoid nodule consists of characteristic zones.[220] The innermost zone is a core of necrotic tissue containing cellular material surrounded by fibrinoid, an eosinophilic material composed mainly of fibrin. The next layer is a palisade of radially arranged elongated mononuclear cells, and the outermost connective tissue layer is a vascular region containing a lymphocytic infiltrate. Lymphocytes are found both in a perivascular and/or a diffuse distribution. Immunohistochemical studies have shown that the palisade consists of macrophages and the majority of the lymphocytes are T cells—both CD4 and CD8, in ratios of 1:1 to 3:1.[220-222] B cells and plasma cells are scarce. Dendritic cells are also found in perivascular areas or scattered

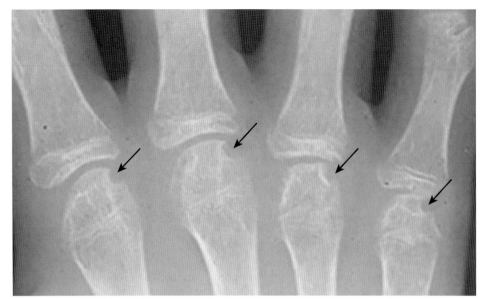

FIGURE 17-6 Bone erosions in a girl with RF-positive polyarticular JIA.

in the periphery of the nodules but are rare and are not found in close proximity to T cells.[222]

Cardiac Valvular Lesions

Excised aortic valves of children with RF-positive polyarthritis who have aortic insufficiency are grossly thickened.[201,203] Granulomatous, nodular lesions are often present on the valve cusps.[200,202,203] Histological findings include destruction of the normal architecture of the valve, granulomas that are histopathologically similar to rheumatoid nodules, nonspecific inflammatory changes, and fibrosis.[196,198,202,203]

Pulmonary Lesions

Lung biopsies of patients with RF-positive polyarthritis who have parenchymal lung disease show typical findings of interstitial pneumonia and bronchiolitis obliterans.[204,206-208,223] In the former the alveolar septa are thickened by a predominantly lymphocytic infiltrate. Lymphoid follicles or germinal centers, plasma cells, and histiocytes are also seen within the septae. Bronchiolitis obliterans is characterized by infiltrates of lymphocytes and plasma cells in the bronchiolar wall, destruction of the respiratory epithelium, occlusion of bronchioles with plugs of inflammatory cells and mucus, and fibrosis and obliteration of bronchioles. In BOOP, granulation tissue extends into the alveolar spaces. Chronic interstitial inflammation is seen concurrently with bronchiolitis obliterans or BOOP.[208,223]

Treatment

Aggressive medical treatment of RF-positive polyarthritis is warranted because of its almost uniformly poor prognosis.[110] Children with this disease should be treated with NSAIDs and a DMARD at the time of diagnosis in the absence of contraindications. Current treatment recommendations for RF-positive polyarthritis include methotrexate as the DMARD of first choice and leflunomide as an alternative.[103,224] Persistence of high or moderate disease activity should prompt an escalation to biological therapy.[103,224] The role of biological therapies as the first treatment of children with polyarthritis is still unclear.[102,225,226] NSAIDs should be used as adjunctive therapy because they can help improve symptoms but do not impact substantially on the disease course. Intraarticular steroid injections should be used, particularly for large, painful joints early in the treatment regimen. Low-dose

prednisone, if used at all, should be limited to a bridging period until DMARD therapy becomes effective. As with patients with RF-negative polyarthritis, the total treatment plan for patients with RF-positive polyarthritis includes patient and parent education, physical and occupational therapy, maintenance of physical activities, and optimal nutrition.

Course of the Disease and Prognosis
Mortality

In 1983 Ansell reported an 8% mortality rate among 85 patients with RF-positive polyarthritis.[187] Renal amyloidosis was the cause of death in two patients and quadriplegia resulting from cervical spine involvement complicated by infection in another. In Finland, the 10-year survival after a diagnosis of amyloidosis in 24 patients with JRA was only 75%.[227] However, patients who died were not identified by onset subtype. No new case of amyloidosis-complicating JIA has been reported since 1991 in Finland, and this complication appears to be increasingly rare worldwide.

More recent data also indicate an increased mortality in patients with JIA.[228,229] In Scotland, the standardized mortality ratio (the ratio of observed to expected deaths), derived from International Classification of Disease codes on hospital records and linkage to national death registers, was 3.39 for males and 5.09 for females with juvenile chronic arthritis.[228] Deaths among patients with musculoskeletal and connective tissue disease were most frequently related to circulatory or respiratory causes, although no details are available. Similarly, in Rochester, Minnesota, a high mortality of 0.27 compared with an expected rate of 0.068 per 100 patient-years was calculated for adults with a history of JRA; however, the causes of death were comorbid illnesses.[229] In contrast, at a relatively short mean follow-up of 8 years, the standardized mortality rate in a cohort of children entered into a registry at diagnosis indicated a reduced mortality for JRA, 0.57 (95% CI 0.34-0.89).[230] Specific rates for RF-positive polyarthritis are not available in these studies.

Remission

Remission is variously defined, but patients with RF-positive polyarthritis have the lowest rates among children with chronic arthritis, varying from no remissions to a 5% frequency of remission off medications during 8 to 10 years of follow-up.[231-233] During their disease course, patients with RF-positive polyarthritis may have active disease for 74% of their follow-up time; but clinical remission on medications can be achieved in 42% to 65% of patients.[20,233]

Disability

Until recently patients with RF-positive polyarthritis continued to have significant disability. The frequency of patients with severe disability or in Steinbrocker functional class III (capable of limited to few or none of activities of usual occupation or self-care) or IV (incapacitated largely or wholly bedridden, capable of little or no self-care) was 15% in 1976 and 1994 publications, and 5% in 2002 after mean or median disease durations of 14 to 20 years.[231,234,235] However, in Childhood Health Assessment Questionnaires (CHAQs), 18% of patients had scores of greater than 1.5, reflecting severe disability.[231] These reports originated from pediatric rheumatology centers, where selection bias may be less and follow-up times shorter than in reports from adult rheumatology clinics. For example, in an adult rheumatology clinic, 38% of adult patients with RF-positive polyarthritis since childhood and with a mean disease duration of 28 years were in Steinbrocker class III or IV, and 53% had a health assessment questionnaire score of greater than 1.5.[236] More recent studies suggest improved functional outcomes in the short term. For example, a cross-sectional study showed a mean CHAQ score of 0.530 for children with RF-positive polyarthritis at a median of 2.6 years follow-up.[56] A prospective cohort study showed a decrease in CHAQ scores from a median of 1.13 (interquartile range [IQR] 0.5-1.5) at diagnosis to 0.56 (IQR 0.13-1.13) a year later, but the proportion of children with moderate to severe disability remained high (64% with CHAQ ≥ 0.75 at diagnosis and 40% at 1 year).[237]

REFERENCES

2. R.E. Petty, T.R. Southwood, P. Manners, et al., International League of Associations for Rheumatology classification of juvenile idiopathic arthritis: second revision, Edmonton, 2001, J. Rheumatol. 31 (2) (2004) 390–392.

4. R.K. Saurenmann, J.B. Rose, P. Tyrrell, et al., Epidemiology of juvenile idiopathic arthritis in a multiethnic cohort: ethnicity as a risk factor, Arthritis Rheum. 56 (6) (2007) 1974–1984.

8. P.J. Manners, C. Bower, Worldwide prevalence of juvenile arthritis why does it vary so much? J. Rheumatol. 29 (7) (2002) 1520–1530.

15. K.G. Oen, M. Cheang, Epidemiology of chronic arthritis in childhood, Semin. Arthritis Rheum. 26 (3) (1996) 575–591.

16. A.G. Greenwald, A. Zakerzadeh, R.M. Laxer, et al., Later-onset rheumatoid factor negative polyarticular juvenile idiopathic arthritis (JIA): a unique patient group? Clin. Exp. Rheumatol. 31 (4) (2013) 645–652.

20. S. Ringold, K.D. Seidel, T.D. Koepsell, C.A. Wallace, Inactive disease in polyarticular juvenile idiopathic arthritis: current patterns and associations, Rheumatology (Oxford) 48 (8) (2009) 972–977.

22. W. de Jager, E.P. Hoppenreijs, N.M. Wulffraat, et al., Blood and synovial fluid cytokine signatures in patients with juvenile idiopathic arthritis: a cross-sectional study, Ann. Rheum. Dis. 66 (5) (2007) 589–598.

27. J.E. Cobb, A. Hinks, W. Thomson, The genetics of juvenile idiopathic arthritis: current understanding and future prospects, Rheumatology (Oxford) 53 (4) (2014) 592–599.

31. A. Hinks, J. Cobb, M.C. Marion, et al., Dense genotyping of immune-related disease regions identifies 14 new susceptibility loci for juvenile idiopathic arthritis, Nat. Genet. 45 (6) (2013) 664–669.

35. A. Hinks, A. Barton, S. John, et al., Association between the PTPN22 gene and rheumatoid arthritis and juvenile idiopathic arthritis in a UK population: further support that PTPN22 is an autoimmunity gene, Arthritis Rheum. 52 (6) (2005) 1694–1699.

39. S.D. Thompson, M. Sudman, P.S. Ramos, et al., The susceptibility loci juvenile idiopathic arthritis shares with other autoimmune diseases extend to PTPN2, COG6, and ANGPT1, Arthritis Rheum. 62 (11) (2010) 3265–3276.

45. R. Saurenmann, The difficult diagnosis of temporomandibular joint arthritis, J. Rheumatol. 39 (9) (2012) 1778–1780.

50. K. Oen, M. Reed, P.N. Malleson, et al., Radiologic outcome and its relationship to functional disability in juvenile rheumatoid arthritis, J. Rheumatol. 30 (4) (2003) 832–840.

55. L.E. Schanberg, K.M. Gil, K.K. Anthony, et al., Pain, stiffness, and fatigue in juvenile polyarticular arthritis: contemporaneous stressful events and mood as predictors, Arthritis Rheum. 52 (4) (2005) 1196–1204.

56. S. Ringold, C.A. Wallace, F.P. Rivara, Health-related quality of life, physical function, fatigue, and disease activity in children with established polyarticular juvenile idiopathic arthritis, J. Rheumatol. 36 (6) (2009) 1330–1336.

58. M. van Brussel, O.T. Lelieveld, J. van der Net, et al., Aerobic and anaerobic exercise capacity in children with juvenile idiopathic arthritis, Arthritis Rheum. 15 57 (6) (2007) 891–897.

59. S.E. Klepper, Exercise in pediatric rheumatic diseases, Curr. Opin. Rheumatol. 20 (5) (2008) 619–624.

67. A. Heiligenhaus, M. Niewerth, G. Ganser, et al., Prevalence and complications of uveitis in juvenile idiopathic arthritis in a population-based nation-wide study in Germany: suggested modification of the current screening guidelines, Rheumatology (Oxford) 46 (6) (2007) 1015–1019.

68. R.K. Saurenmann, A.V. Levin, B.M. Feldman, et al., Risk factors for development of uveitis differ between girls and boys with juvenile idiopathic arthritis, Arthritis Rheum. 62 (6) (2010) 1824–1828.

76. B.H. Athreya, H.R. Schumacher, Pathologic features of a familial arthropathy associated with congenital flexion contractures of fingers, Arthritis Rheum. 21 (4) (1978) 429–437.

77. J. Jacobs, J. Downey, Juvenile rheumatoid arthritis, in: J. Downey, N. Low (Eds.), The Child with Disabling Illness, WB Saunders, Philadelphia, 1974, p. 5.

78. P. Malleson, J.G. Schaller, F. Dega, et al., Familial arthritis and camptodactyly, Arthritis Rheum. 24 (9) (1981) 1199–1204.

79. R.P. Robinson, W.A. Franck, E.J. Carey, et al., Familial polyarticular osteochondritis dissecans masquerading as juvenile rheumatoid arthritis, J. Rheumatol. 5 (2) (1978) 190–194.

80. H. Hakim, M. Elloumi, M. Ben Salem, et al., Polyarthritic manifestations revealing Stickler syndrome, J. Radiol. 83 (12 Pt 1) (2002) 1856–1858.

81. K. Davies, E.R. Stiehm, P. Woo, et al., Juvenile idiopathic polyarticular arthritis and IgA deficiency in the 22q11 deletion syndrome, J. Rheumatol. 28 (10) (2001) 2326–2334.

82. F. Zulian, H.R. Schumacher, A. Calore, et al., Juvenile arthritis in Turner's syndrome: a multicenter study, Clin. Exp. Rheumatol. 16 (4) (1998) 489–494.

83. S.K. de Oliveira, A.R. Fonseca, R.C. Domingues, et al., A unique articular manifestation in a child with relapsing polychondritis, J. Rheumatol. 36 (3) (2009) 659–660.

86. B.E. Gilliam, A.K. Chauhan, J.M. Low, T.L. Moore, Measurement of biomarkers in juvenile idiopathic arthritis patients and their significant association with disease severity: a comparative study, Clin. Exp. Rheumatol. 26 (3) (2008) 492–497.

91. A.E. Tebo, T. Jaskowski, K.W. Davis, et al., Profiling anti-cyclic citrullinated peptide antibodies in patients with juvenile idiopathic arthritis, Pediatr. Rheumatol. Online J. 10 (1) (2012) 29.

92. A. Ravelli, E. Felici, S. Magni-Manzoni, et al., Patients with antinuclear antibody-positive juvenile idiopathic arthritis constitute a homogeneous subgroup irrespective of the course of joint disease, Arthritis Rheum. 52 (3) (2005) 826–832.

98. D.S. Gibson, S. Blelock, J. Curry, et al., Comparative analysis of synovial fluid and plasma proteomes in juvenile arthritis–proteomic patterns of joint inflammation in early stage disease, J Proteomics. 72 (4) (2009) 656–676.

100. S. Finnegan, S. Clarke, D. Gibson, et al., Synovial membrane immunohistology in early untreated juvenile idiopathic arthritis: differences between clinical subgroups, Ann. Rheum. Dis. 70 (10) (2011) 1842–1850.

102. C.A. Wallace, E.H. Giannini, S.J. Spalding, et al., Trial of early aggressive therapy in polyarticular juvenile idiopathic arthritis, Arthritis Rheum. 64 (6) (2012) 2012–2021.

103. T. Beukelman, N.M. Patkar, K.G. Saag, et al., 2011 American College of Rheumatology recommendations for the treatment of juvenile idiopathic arthritis: initiation and safety monitoring of therapeutic agents for the treatment of arthritis and systemic features, Arthritis Care Res. (Hoboken) 63 (4) (2011) 465–482.

104. E.H. Giannini, E.J. Brewer, N. Kuzmina, et al., Methotrexate in resistant juvenile rheumatoid arthritis. Results of the U.S.A.-U.S.S.R. double-blind, placebo-controlled trial. The Pediatric Rheumatology Collaborative Study Group and The Cooperative Children's Study Group, N. Engl. J. Med. 16 326 (16) (1992) 1043–1049.

108. E. Silverman, R. Mouy, L. Spiegel, et al., Leflunomide or methotrexate for juvenile rheumatoid arthritis, N. Engl. J. Med. 352 (16) (2005) 1655–1666.

112. D.J. Lovell, E.H. Giannini, A. Reiff, et al., Long-term efficacy and safety of etanercept in children with polyarticular-course juvenile rheumatoid arthritis: interim results from an ongoing multicenter, open-label, extended-treatment trial, Arthritis Rheum. 48 (1) (2003) 218–226.

120. M. Rebollo-Polo, K. Koujok, C. Weisser, et al., Ultrasound findings on patients with juvenile idiopathic arthritis in clinical remission, Arthritis Care Res. (Hoboken) 63 (7) (2011) 1013–1019.

121. D. Foell, H. Wittkowski, I. Hammerschmidt, et al., Monitoring neutrophil activation in juvenile rheumatoid arthritis by S100A12 serum concentrations, Arthritis Rheum. 50 (4) (2004) 1286–1295.

122. N. Knowlton, K. Jiang, M.B. Frank, et al., The meaning of clinical remission in polyarticular juvenile idiopathic arthritis: gene expression profiling in peripheral blood mononuclear cells identifies distinct disease states, Arthritis Rheum. 60 (3) (2009) 892–900.

124. S.E. Klepper, Exercise and fitness in children with arthritis: evidence of benefits for exercise and physical activity, Arthritis Rheum. 49 (3) (2003) 435–443.

125. K. Oen, P.N. Malleson, D.A. Cabral, et al., Early predictors of longterm outcome in patients with juvenile rheumatoid arthritis: subset specific correlations, J. Rheumatol. 30 (3) (2003) 585–593.

130. E. Nordal, M. Zak, K. Aalto, et al., Ongoing disease activity and changing categories in a long-term nordic cohort study of juvenile idiopathic arthritis, Arthritis Rheum. 63 (9) (2011) 2809–2818.

133. L.R. Harrold, C. Salman, S. Shoor, et al., Incidence and prevalence of juvenile idiopathic arthritis among children in a managed care population, 1996–2009, J. Rheumatol. 40 (7) (2013) 1218–1225.

141. S. Bowyer, P. Roettcher, Pediatric rheumatology clinic populations in the United States: results of a 3 year survey. Pediatric Rheumatology Database Research Group, J. Rheumatol. 23 (11) (1996) 1968–1974.

145. J.M. Low, A.K. Chauhan, D.A. Kietz, et al., Determination of anti-cyclic citrullinated peptide antibodies in the sera of patients with juvenile idiopathic arthritis, J. Rheumatol. 31 (9) (2004) 1829–1833.

148. E.D. Ferucci, D.S. Majka, L.A. Parrish, et al., Antibodies against cyclic citrullinated peptide are associated with HLA-DR4 in simplex and multiplex polyarticular-onset juvenile rheumatoid arthritis, Arthritis Rheum. 52 (1) (2005) 239–246.

151. W.J. van Venrooij, J.J. van Beers, G.J. Pruijn, Anti-CCP antibodies: the past, the present and the future, Nat. Rev. Rheumatol. 7 (7) (2011) 391–398.

153. T.W. Huizinga, C.I. Amos, A.H. van der Helm-van Mil, et al., Refining the complex rheumatoid arthritis phenotype based on specificity of the HLA-DRB1 shared epitope for antibodies to citrullinated proteins, Arthritis Rheum. 52 (11) (2005) 3433–3438.

155. L. Klareskog, P. Stolt, K. Lundberg, et al., A new model for an etiology of rheumatoid arthritis: smoking may trigger HLA-DR (shared epitope)-restricted immune reactions to autoantigens modified by citrullination, Arthritis Rheum. 54 (1) (2006) 38–46.

161. J.D. Gorman, L.A. Criswell, The shared epitope and severity of rheumatoid arthritis, Rheum. Dis. Clin. North Am. 28 (1) (2002) 59–78.

167. B. Nepom, The immunogenetics of juvenile rheumatoid arthritis, Rheum. Dis. Clin. North Am. 17 (4) (1991) 825–842.

175. S. Prahalad, M.H. Ryan, E.S. Shear, et al., Juvenile rheumatoid arthritis: linkage to HLA demonstrated by allele sharing in affected sibpairs, Arthritis Rheum. 43 (10) (2000) 2335–2338.

176. A. Hinks, J. Cobb, M. Sudman, et al., Investigation of rheumatoid arthritis susceptibility loci in juvenile idiopathic arthritis confirms high degree of overlap, Ann. Rheum. Dis. 71 (7) (2012) 1117–1121.

177. S. Angeles-Han, S. Prahalad, The genetics of juvenile idiopathic arthritis: what is new in 2010? Curr. Rheumatol. Rep. 12 (2) (2010) 87–93.

180. S. Prahalad, S. Hansen, A. Whiting, et al., Variants in TNFAIP3, STAT4, and C12orf30 loci associated with multiple autoimmune diseases are also associated with juvenile idiopathic arthritis, Arthritis Rheum. 60 (7) (2009) 2124–2130.

181. A. Hinks, P. Martin, S.D. Thompson, et al., Autoinflammatory gene polymorphisms and susceptibility to UK juvenile idiopathic arthritis, Pediatr. Rheumatol. Online J. 11 (1) (2013) 14.

186. S.T. Angeles-Han, C.F. Pelajo, L.B. Vogler, et al., Risk markers of juvenile idiopathic arthritis-associated uveitis in the Childhood Arthritis and Rheumatology Research Alliance (CARRA) Registry, J. Rheumatol. 40 (12) (2013) 2088–2096.

209. K. Oen, C.M. Duffy, S.M. Tse, et al., Early outcomes and improvement of patients with juvenile idiopathic arthritis enrolled in a Canadian multi-center inception cohort, Arthritis Care Res. (Hoboken) 62 (4) (2010) 527–536.

214. R.A. Williams, B.M. Ansell, Radiological findings in seropositive juvenile chronic arthritis (juvenile rheumatoid arthritis) with particular reference to progression, Ann. Rheum. Dis. 44 (10) (1985) 685–693.

Entire reference list is available online at www.expertconsult.com.

CHAPTER 18

Oligoarticular Juvenile Idiopathic Arthritis

Ross E. Petty, Carol B. Lindsley

DEFINITION

Oligoarticular juvenile idiopathic arthritis (JIA) is defined as a chronic inflammatory arthritis of unknown origin that begins before the age of 16 and persists for at least 6 weeks (Box 18-1).[1] It is further characterized as being either persistent (if no more than four joints are affected during the disease course) or extended (if, after the initial 6-month period, the total number of affected joints exceeds four). The International League of Associations for Rheumatology (ILAR) classification also requires that patients who otherwise fulfill these criteria be excluded from the category if the patient has psoriasis, or if there is a history of psoriasis or a disease associated with the human leukocyte antigen (HLA) allele HLA-B27 in a first-degree relative; if the disease began in a male older than 6 years of age; or if two positive tests for rheumatoid factor (RF) were obtained at least 3 months apart. Such exclusions do not apply to the European League Against Rheumatism (EULAR) criteria for oligoarticular juvenile chronic arthritis[2] or American College of Rheumatology (ACR) criteria for pauciarticular juvenile rheumatoid arthritis,[3] terms that are of historic significance and refer to diseases that are very similar to oligoarticular JIA (see Chapter 15). Oligoarthritis is a distinctly, if not uniquely, pediatric disease, and it is the most commonly diagnosed category of chronic arthritis among children in North America and Europe. In these classifications, the words *oligoarticular* and *pauciarticular* have the same meaning: few joints (≤4).

EPIDEMIOLOGY

Oligoarthritis accounts for 50% to 80% of all children with chronic arthritis, at least in North American and European white populations. Oen and Cheang[4] noted that the proportion of all children with chronic arthritis who had oligoarthritis (ACR or EULAR criteria) was higher in North American and European children (58%) than in East Indian (25%), North American Indian (26%), or other racial groups (31%). A study of a multiethnic cohort of Canadian children with JIA (ILAR criteria) confirmed the relatively low proportion of non-European children with either persistent or extended oligoarticular JIA, compared with children of European ancestry seen in the same clinic.[5] Several reviews of incidence and prevalence studies have been published.[4,6-8]

Incidence

Reports of the incidence of oligoarthritis are difficult to interpret because of the variation in criteria used to classify the patients. Using information from hospitals and community physicians, Andersson-Gare and colleagues[9] determined an annual incidence of oligoarthritis (EULAR criteria) of 7 per 100,000 children younger than 16 years of age in Sweden. Using the same criteria, a Norwegian study[10] reported a somewhat higher incidence of 11.2 per 100,000 per year. It should be noted that 42% of these children were HLA-B27–positive, strongly suggesting that children with enthesitis-related arthritis (ERA) or juvenile ankylosing spondylitis (JAS), which can also present with fewer than four active joints at onset, were included in the group. In studies that used the ACR criteria, estimates of the incidence have ranged from less than 1 per 100,000 per year in Japan[11] to more than 18 per 100,000 per year in Finland.[12]

Prevalence

The prevalence of oligoarthritis in reported studies varies greatly depending on the diagnostic criteria used; whether the study was hospital, clinic, or community based; and the geographic location of the study.[7] Using information from hospitals and community physicians, Andersson-Gare and associates[9] found 146 children with oligoarthritis (EULAR) in a population of 400,600 children younger than 16 years of age, a prevalence of 36 per 100,000. In the study by Manners and Diepeveen,[13] oligoarthritis fulfilling the EULAR criteria for juvenile chronic arthritis (JCA) was found in 9 of 2241 12-year-old school children who were examined by the authors of the study. This prevalence (4 per 1000) is markedly higher than that reported in other studies but may be closest to reality, because it was community based and verified by physical examination by a pediatric rheumatologist. It is possible that this high prevalence is not representative of the disease worldwide, however.

Age at Onset

Oligoarthritis has a striking age at onset distribution, with a peak incidence between 1 and 3 years of age (Fig. 18-1).[14] A small proportion of children with oligoarthritis have disease onset after this time, but when this occurs it raises the possibility of alternative diagnoses, such as ERA, JAS, psoriatic arthritis, or developing polyarthritis.

Sex Ratio

In North America and Europe, oligoarthritis is predominantly a disease of girls, with a female-to-male ratio of approximately 3:1. In children with oligoarthritis and uveitis, the ratio of girls to boys is even higher: 5:1 to 6.6:1.[15-17] In parts of Asia[18] and Africa,[19,20] however, oligoarthritis occurs predominantly in boys, and uveitis is reported to be rare.[18]

GENETICS

Oligoarthritis is seldom familial. When sibling pairs both have arthritis, however, three quarters are concordant for onset type (most

229

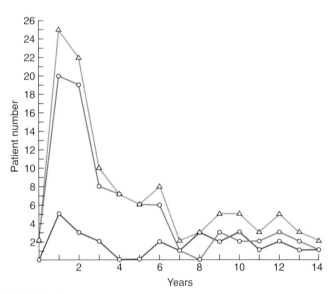

FIGURE 18-1 Age at onset of oligoarticular JRA: total group (*purple*), girls (*blue*), boys (*orange*). Data from D.B. Sullivan, J.T. Cassidy, R.E. Petty, Pathogenic implications of age of onset in juvenile rheumatoid arthritis, Arthritis Rheum. 18 (1975) 251.

commonly oligoarthritis).[21] Early-onset oligoarthritis, particularly if it is complicated by uveitis, appears to be very uncommon in populations of non-European origin. It is likely that oligoarthritis, like other types of childhood arthritis, is a multigenic disease.

HLA Genes

For the sake of clarity, the classification system (ACR—JRA; EULAR—JCA; ILAR—JIA) employed in studies cited in this section is indicated.

There are quite characteristic associations of oligoarthritis, or subsets of oligoarthritis, with some HLA genes. The unusual disease association of an A locus antigen, A2, has been reported and confirmed in children with JRA (ACR criteria) in general and in early-onset pauciarticular JRA in girls in particular.[22-24]

An increase in the HLA-B27 allele in early studies reflects the inclusion of children with juvenile ankylosing spondylitis (similar to ERA of the ILAR classification). Later investigations documented inconsistent increases in the frequency of this antigen in subgroups of children with JRA.[25]

Among the class II alleles, the most consistent association has been with the DRB1*08-DQA1*04-DQB1*04 haplotype encoding DR8 and DQ4. These two alleles are in strong linkage disequilibrium, but Smerdel et al. showed that it was DR8, not DQ4, that was associated with JIA.[26] DR8, DR5, DR6, DPB1*0201, and certain DQ alleles are also reportedly more frequent in children with early-onset oligoarthritis[23,26,27] and in pauciarticular JRA, with relative risks in the range of 2 to 13.[25,27,28-32] Linkage disequilibrium probably accounts for some of the reported associations. The transmission disequilibrium test was used by Moroldo and colleagues[21] to examine linkage and association in 101 white families who had a child with oligoarthritis. DR8 and DR5 (as well as A2, B27, and B35) had significantly higher frequencies of transmission to the affected child; DR4 and DR7 were found less often. These data suggest that these numerous HLA associations partly reflect linkage between the HLA gene region in children with JRA and a population stratification effect. However, age and sex influenced these effects. Prahalad and colleagues[33] studied sibling pairs with arthritis to confirm the linkage of pauciarticular JRA with the HLA-DR region, especially DR8 and DR11. Using restriction fragment length polymorphisms, Morling and colleagues[31] found that children with pauciarticular JRA had increased frequencies of DRB1*08; DRB3*01/02/03 (DRw52); DQA1*0401 and 0501; DQB1*0301; DPA1*0201; and DPB1*02, compared with healthy controls. Both subtypes of DR5 (DR11 and DR12) and DR8 (DRB1*0801) contributed to susceptibility to early-onset oligoarticular disease.[34,35] DR11, DR12, and DR8 haplotypes share similar DQA1 alleles: DQA1*0401, *0501, and *0601.[36,37] These three DQ alleles have a common motif in exon 2 at the 42 to 53 positions, which was present in 86% of children with JCA but in only 36% of controls.[35,36] Haas and colleagues[36] demonstrated that distinct differences in the DQA1 promoter are strongly associated with susceptibility to early-onset disease. Nepom and associates[37] identified a 13-nucleotide region of sequence identity in the first hypervariable region of DR5, DR6, and DR8 alleles, which is a possible "shared epitope" that could be important in antigen recognition.

DR1 and DR4 are present in lower frequency in young girls with *persistent* pauciarticular JRA and antinuclear antibody (ANA) seropositivity, compared with the normal population.[21] However, DR1 is a risk factor for *extended* oligoarthritis as well as for polyarthritis in older children.[38] It is in linkage disequilibrium with DQA*0101, which was associated in one study with progressive erosive disease in children with early-onset pauciarticular JRA and was negatively associated with the presence of uveitis.[39] This DQA gene, although not present in all children with the disease, may be critically important in the development of this onset type.[40] DQA*0101 and A2*0101 are also binding sites for the 45-kD DEK proto-oncogene.[41,42] Anti-DEK antibodies are characteristic of oligoarticular-onset disease (78% positive), especially in children who are ANA positive and have a history of uveitis, and may negate the regulatory function of the gene,[43] or they may simply be a reflection of autoimmunity.[44] One study associated ANA positivity in early-onset disease with DQB1*0603.[45]

Pauciarticular JRA is also associated with DP2 (DPB1*0201),[46-48] which in one study[47] was present in 67% of patients but only 34% of controls. It has been suggested that this DP allele increases the risk conferred by DR alleles but is not sufficient in itself to increase susceptibility to pauciarticular JRA.[49] A number of studies have discussed the role of interactions among alleles at different loci in producing susceptibility to disease.[31,50] Interactions between class I and class II genes led to the hypothesis that at least two genetic loci are involved in the predisposition to oligoarthritis. Zeggini and co-workers[24] demonstrated linkage to HLA-A, -B, and -DRB1 in girls with persistent and extended oligoarticular JIA. They suggested that linkage appeared to

TABLE 18-1 Human Leukocyte Antigen Associations in Oligoarthritis

HLA GENE	CRITERIA	ASSOCIATIONS	REFERENCE NO.
A2	ACR	Young age, female sex	22, 23
B27	ACR	Oligoarthritis	21
DR 6	ACR	Oligoarthritis	21
DRB1*08	ACR	Oligoarthritis	26
	EULAR	Early onset	35
	ACR	Persistent disease	127
DRB3*01/2/3	ACR	Oligoarthritis	23
DPA*0101	ACR	Progressive erosive disease	40
	ACR	Decreased in uveitis	40
DPA1*0201	ACR	Oligoarthritis	40
DPB1*0201	EULAR	Oligoarthritis	47
	ACR	Oligoarthritis	49
DR 1	ACR	Extended oligoarthritis	39
	ACR	Decreased in persistent oligoarthritis	39
DR 4	ACR	Decreased in persistent oligoarthritis	21
DR11 (DR5)	EULAR	Early onset	34, 35, 36
DR12 (DR5)	EULAR	Early onset	35, 36
DQA1*0401	ACR	Oligoarthritis	23
DQA1*0501	ACR	Oligoarthritis	23
DQB1*0301	ACR	Oligoarthritis	23
DQB1*0603	EULAR	Early onset, ANA positive	46

be attributable to preferential maternal transmission of these alleles. HLA associations are summarized in Table 18-1.

Non-HLA Genes

A number of genes involved in antigen presentation or cytokine expression may be important in either a predisposition to JCA or its pathogenesis.[49] IL-1A2, a variant of the IL-1β gene, is associated with early-onset oligoarthritis.[50] Children with extended oligoarthritis (ILAR criteria) were shown to have a high frequency of the interleukin (IL)-1 receptor antagonist gene IL1RN*2; this was also observed, to a lesser extent, in children with ERA.[51] The gene for the cytokine IL-1β, or a gene for which its polymorphism is a marker, may contribute risk for early-onset disease and uveitis.[50,52]

Crawley and colleagues[53,54] found a decrease in the IL-10 phenotype associated with low IL-10 production in children with arthritis affecting fewer than five joints, compared with those with more than four affected joints. The frequency of the tumor necrosis factor (TNF)-α2 microsatellite allele was significantly increased in Latvian children with oligoarticular JCA, and the frequency of TNF-α9 was significantly decreased in this population.[55] The TNF-α2 allele is associated with high TNF-α production.[56] Zeggini and colleagues reported an increased frequency of the intronic +851 TNF single nucleotide polymorphism (SNP) in persistent oligoarticular JIA (odds ratio, 3.86; 95% confidence interval [CI], 1.6 to 9.2).[57] Kaalla et al.[58] have performed a

meta-analysis of data regarding four SNPs in loci that had previously been associated with JIA: MIF (G173C), TNFA (G308A and G238A), and PTPN22 (C1858T). They confirmed the association of the PTPN22 SNP and TNFA G238A, but not MIF G173C with oligoarticular JIA. Genome-wide association studies have been recently published.[59-61]

ETIOLOGY AND PATHOGENESIS

Environmental Factors

The etiology of oligoarticular JIA is unknown. The narrow age-at-onset profile suggests the possibility of exposure at a time of immunological immaturity to a ubiquitous environmental agent, possibly a virus, but none has been consistently identified. In a study of six twin pairs with pauciarticular JRA, there was an average of approximately 3 months (range, 0 to 12 months) separating disease onset in each twin, again raising the question of an environmental agent as an initiating event.[62] One study alleged that breast-feeding has a protective effect on the development of JRA,[63] especially oligoarticular disease; however, a strong relationship was not confirmed in another investigation.[64] Radon et al.[65] found no association of urban versus rural residence or exposure to farm animals or pets with development of oligoarticular JIA. Neufeld and colleagues[66] have reported a significant increase in a serious psychological upset, illness in the family, or difficulties with interpersonal interactions in children prior to the onset of oligoarticular JIA, compared to healthy age-matched controls.

Immunological Factors

T Lymphocytes

Although it is generally agreed that the pathogenesis of oligoarticular JIA involves abnormalities in the adaptive immune system, studies of lymphocytes have yielded inconsistent results. The synovial infiltrate predominantly comprises an oligoclonal population of CD4+ and CD8+ T lymphocytes that differ functionally from those in the peripheral blood. High frequencies of different T-cell receptor alleles (TCR Vβ6.1)[67] and TCR Vβ20 [68] have been reported in some studies but not confirmed in others.[69,70] The degree of activation of synovial T cells (CD3+ IL-2R+) and the CD4/CD8 ratio were significantly higher in oligoarthritis.[71] CD4+ cells that lack CD28 are more frequent in oligoarticular JIA than in polyarticular JIA.[72,73] CD4+CD28[null] T cells are markers of immunological aging and have shortened telomeres consistent with cells that are senescent. Such cells are activated in a TCR-independent manner.

There is a high frequency of the highly proinflammatory Th17 cells in synovial tissue of children with JIA.[74] The importance of Th17 cells in synovial fluid in the pathogenesis of oligoarticular JIA was investigated by Cosmi et al.[75] There was a shift from Th17 to Th17/Th1 or Th1 phenotype in synovial fluid, which correlated with parameters of inflammation.

B Lymphocytes

The high frequency of autoantibodies to nuclear antigens indicates a break in immunological tolerance, but there is no evidence that autoantibodies participate directly in disease pathogenesis. The identity of the specificities of the antigens to which ANAs react in children with oligoarthritis is still largely unknown. Antibodies to an epitope on the high-mobility group (HMG)-17 protein are increased in JRA, and antibodies to an HMG-2 protein are increased in oligoarticular disease.[76,77] In a study searching for IgG antibodies to a large number of autoantigens in children with oligoarticular JIA, Stoll and colleagues[78] identified two groups of patients, one with elevated autoantibody production, who were relatively resistant to therapy, and a second group with lower autoantibody production who were treatment responsive. It is not certain whether the differences reflect predispositions to treatment-resistant disease or the results of effective therapy. Further studies are required to determine the significance of these findings.

Humoral and cellular immune responses to highly conserved bacterial heat shock proteins (HSPs) are present in children with chronic arthritis.[79-83] In 13 of 15 children with oligoarthritis, T-lymphocyte proliferative responses to HSP-60 were detected an average of 12 weeks before remission of the inflammatory disease.[83,84] The investigators hypothesized that induction of tolerance to specific T-cell epitopes of HSP-60 by nasal administration may be a promising route of immunotherapy for childhood arthritis.[85]

Other Factors

Finnegan et al.[86] compared the proteomic profile of synovium from children with oligoarticular JIA (n = 7) and those with polyarticular JIA (n = 8) using two-dimensional (2D) difference gel electrophoresis (DIGE) and matrix-assisted laser desorption ionization tandem time of flight analysis and Western blotting. All patients were studied within 2 years of disease onset, and none had received corticosteroids or disease-modifying agents. Analysis of variance revealed 26 differentially expressed proteins. Proteins overexpressed in the oligoarticular group included type VI collagen alpha 2, integrin alpha 2b, and fibrinogen fragments. These proteins were not overexpressed in the polyarticular group. Some of these proteins are potential autoantigens and may participate in the initiation or perpetuation of joint inflammation.

Serum prolactin levels were increased in children with JRA and were associated with ANA seropositivity.[87] Modest hyperprolactinemia was also identified in prepubertal girls who were ANA seropositive and had oligoarthritis.[88,89] The prolactin concentration correlated with levels of IL-6 and with a chronic course of the disease.

CLINICAL MANIFESTATIONS

The first 6 months of disease is characterized by inflammation in four or fewer joints. These children are not systemically ill, and, except for chronic uveitis, extraarticular manifestations are distinctly unusual. In the child with oligoarthritis, the affected joint is swollen and often warm, but usually not very painful or tender, and almost never red. Varying degrees of effusion may be present involving either the joint space, suprapatellar or prepatellar bursa, or both. The ambulatory child with lower extremity arthritis can usually bear weight but often limps. Oligoarticular JIA is predominantly a disease of the lower extremities. In a study[90] of 64 children with pauciarticular JRA, one or both knees were most commonly affected at disease onset (89%), followed by the ankles (36%). Arthritis affecting small joints of the fingers and toes occurred in only 6% of the children, and arthritis in elbows, hips, wrists, or temporomandibular joints in 3%. Although it is the authors of the study's impression that wrists and small joints of the hands or feet are seldom affected in oligoarticular JIA at onset, others disagree.[91] In at least half of the reported cases, only a single joint is affected (monarticular onset), usually the knee. Uveitis may be present at onset of the disease; it eventually affects up to 20% of children and is usually asymptomatic (see Chapter 22).

Growth abnormalities may be generalized or limited to one limb. Generalized growth retardation is becoming much less frequent with the availability of effective treatment, although Padeh et al.[92] reported short stature in approximately one third of children with oligoarticular JIA. Localized growth abnormalities are particularly common when one knee is affected, with the leg on the affected side usually becoming longer. The opposite effect is seen with unilateral temporomandibular

joint disease in which the ramus of the affected mandible is shorter. Muscles around inflamed joints may quite quickly become atrophic: muscles of the thigh may atrophy in the child with arthritis in the knee, those of the calf in ankle joint disease, and of the forearm when the wrist is inflamed.

LABORATORY EVALUATION

Laboratory indicators of inflammation may be normal in children with oligoarthritis, although mild to moderate elevation of the erythrocyte sedimentation rate (ESR) and elevation of C-reactive protein levels may occur. Hemoglobin levels and white blood cell and platelet counts are usually normal, and the presence of marked abnormalities in these parameters should suggest a diagnosis other than oligoarticular JIA.

Tests for RF are almost always negative, although occasionally children with a single affected joint (often the wrist) have RF. These children may progress to have RF-positive polyarthritis. In contrast, tests for ANAs are positive in low to moderate titer (1 : 160 to 1 : 640) in 62% to 65% of children with oligoarthritis, particularly in girls and in those with uveitis.[93,94] Antibodies to double-stranded DNA and the extractable nuclear antigens are rarely detectable and should raise the possibility of an alternative diagnosis such as systemic lupus erythematosus. Antibodies to histones have been described in 6% of children with oligoarticular JIA, 12% in those with uveitis.[95]

Antibodies that react with citrullinated peptides have rarely been demonstrated in children with oligoarthritis, their frequency depending to some extent on the antigen used. Syed and colleagues noted that IgA anticyclic citrullinated peptide (anti-CCP) antibodies were more common than other isotypes in children with JIA.[96] Anticardiolipin antibodies were reported in up to 46% of children with oligoarthritis.[97] They are usually transient and do not appear to be associated with intravascular thrombosis, however.

Elevated concentrations of activated C3 (C3c, C3d) were demonstrated in about one third of children with active oligoarthritis (a lower frequency than in children with systemic arthritis or polyarthritis),[98] possibly the result of activation of the alternative pathway.[99] Circulating immune complexes are not characteristic of oligoarthritis.

Routine synovial fluid analysis does not distinguish one type of JIA from another. The fluid is usually moderately inflammatory, with a cell count of 5 to 20,000 cells/mm³, mostly polymorphonuclear leukocytes. CD8+ cells constitute the predominant lymphocyte population.[99] Specialized studies of the synovial fluid proteome have identified differences between JIA subtypes[100] with elevations of antichymotrypsin, ceruloplasmin, Apo A-1, and haptoglobin in oligoarthritis, as compared with polyarthritis.

RADIOGRAPHIC EVALUATION

The radiographic changes in oligoarthritis are similar to those seen on other kinds of arthritis, although often less frequent and less severe (see Chapter 9). In a follow-up study[101] of 97 children with pauciarticular JRA, joint space narrowing was present in only 5% of children early in the disease course, increasing to approximately 15% at a median of 6.2 years after disease onset. Erosions were seen in 10% of children with early disease, and in approximately 25% of children 6 years later. Bone overgrowth was more common; it occurred in more than 20% of children early in the disease and slightly more frequently later in the disease course. Not surprisingly, overgrowth was most common at the knee (Figs. 18-2 and 18-3). Advanced maturation, particularly at the wrist, may also occur.

Magnetic resonance imaging with gadolinium confirms the presence of synovitis, increased intraarticular fluid, and occasionally bone

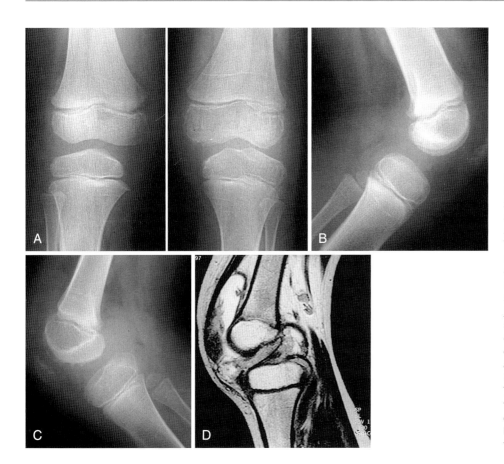

FIGURE 18-2 **A-C,** Anteroposterior and lateral radiographic films of the knees of a 3-year-old girl who developed monarthritis of the left knee at the age of 2 years with an initial flexion contracture of 32 degrees. There is marked joint space narrowing with regional osteoporosis of the left knee and epiphyseal enlargement. **D,** Postgadolinium magnetic resonance imaging sagittal studies of the left knee. There is a large joint effusion with marked inflammatory synovial hypertrophy, demonstrated by enhancement of the pannus throughout all compartments of the joint, and thinning and irregularity of the articular cartilage involving the femur, tibia, and patella. There is almost bone-on-bone apposition of the femorotibial articulation. Asymmetrical enlargements of the epiphyses of the left knee are visible, with relative hypoplasia of the menisci.

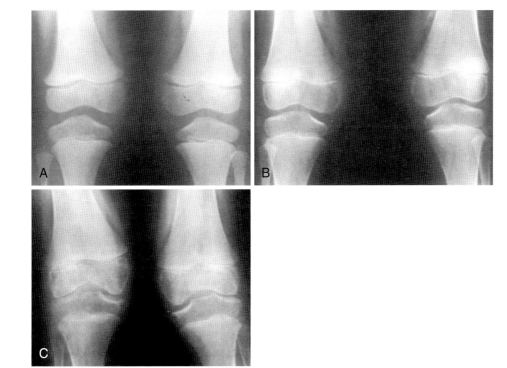

FIGURE 18-3 These radiographs illustrate the 5-year progression of osteoporosis, joint space narrowing, and degenerative changes in the knees of a girl with oligoarticular juvenile rheumatoid arthritis. **A,** In this radiograph, taken 2 years after onset of disease, there is only minimal epiphyseal advancement and osteoporosis. **B,** After 4 years of disease, there is increased prominence of the trabecular pattern secondary to osteoporosis, narrowing of the joint spaces, and remodeling of the normal contours of the articular surfaces. **C,** After 5 years of disease, there is marked narrowing of joint spaces and flattening of the tibial plateaus. Degenerative changes include squaring of the femoral condyles, development of osteophytes at the medial margin of the tibial plateaus, and development of subchondral cysts in the femoral epiphyses.

marrow edema. Its main utility, however, is in differentiating other causes of joint swelling, particularly in the child with monarthritis.[102]

In a study of 32 children with JIA (including 20 with oligoarthritis), it was demonstrated that ultrasound was able to detect subclinical synovitis in 5.5% of clinically normal joints. The authors point out that application of this technique could result in reclassification of some children with clinical oligoarthritis.[103] Ultrasound can also detect early cartilage thickness changes.[104]

PATHOLOGY

There have been few reports of the histopathology of the joints of children with oligoarticular JIA, and most have studied children with chronic arthritis treated with corticosteroids and disease-modifying agents. Finnegan and colleagues[105] compared the immunohistochemical characteristics of children with newly diagnosed, untreated oligoarthritis, polyarthritis and systemic JIA. They subdivided the patients with oligoarthritis in to those with persistent disease, and those who subsequently developed extended JIA ("extended-to-be"). The biopsies, stained with hematoxylin-eosin, were analyzed for degree of synovial hypertrophy, fibrosis, proliferating capillaries, focal cell aggregates, and lymphocytes as a percentage of total inflammatory cells. Immunochemical staining used monoclonal antibodies to T-cell antigens (CD3, CD4, CD8), B-cell antigen (CD20), macrophage antigen (CD68), and endothelial markers factor VIII–related antigen and $\alpha V\beta 3$. The immunohistological characteristics of oligoarticular JIA differed from those of polyarticular JIA; in addition, those of persistent oligoarticular JIA differed from those with extended-to-be oligoarticular JIA. Angiogenesis, focal lymphocytic aggregates, and synovial hyperplasia were significantly more prominent in the extended-to-be and polyarticular groups than in the persistent oligoarticular patients. CD3 and CD4 T cells were also more prominent in the extended-to-be group. Macrophage numbers did not differ among groups.

DIAGNOSIS

Oligoarticular JIA is the most common cause of chronic oligoarthritis, especially in girls younger than 6 years of age. Psoriatic arthritis, which affects large and small joints in an asymmetrical pattern, is also a possibility at this age (see Chapter 20). ERA is a more likely cause of a monarthritis or oligoarthritis of the lower extremities with onset in the older child or adolescent boy.[106] A diagnosis of oligoarticular JIA or psoriatic arthritis may be substantiated by the demonstration of asymptomatic anterior uveitis by slit-lamp examination, although juvenile sarcoidosis (Blau syndrome) also rarely manifests in this way. ANA positivity supports the diagnosis of oligoarticular JIA or psoriatic JIA but may also be found in some healthy children[107] and in some children with noninflammatory musculoskeletal pain.[108] Lyme disease may present as an oligoarthritis (see Chapter 42).

In a child with a single swollen joint (monarthritis) of recent onset (within 72 hours), the differential diagnosis includes trauma (sprain), septic arthritis, hemarthrosis (hemophilia, hemangioma, or intraarticular arteriovenous malformation) and malignancy (Box 18-2).[109] If the monarthritis is long-standing, trauma, malignancy, and infection (except for tuberculosis) are very unlikely. Reactive arthritis usually resolves within weeks. There have been reports of infection with human immunodeficiency virus presenting as oligoarthritis.[110] A painful joint effusion may be associated with an internal structural abnormality such as a discoid meniscus[111] or osteochondritis dissecans, or with recurrent patellar dislocation. Recurrent involvement has been described in occult celiac disease.[112] Rare causes of chronic monarthritis, such as tuberculosis, sarcoidosis, intraarticular hemangioma

or arteriovenous malformation, villonodular synovitis,[113] lipomatosis arborescens,[114] or synovial chondromatosis[115] should also be considered. A migrating monarthritis, sometimes associated with fever and a rash, has been described in children of Assyrian ancestry.[116] The various forms of idiopathic osteolysis may mimic arthritis of a limited number of joints (e.g., wrists) at onset. Rarely, arthritis has resulted from administration of a drug such as isotretinoin[117] or antithyroid medication.[118,119]

If a joint is acutely painful and erythematous, or if the child is febrile, immediate joint aspiration is always indicated to exclude septic arthritis or osteomyelitis. Needle or arthroscopic synovial biopsy is useful in children with chronic monarthritis in whom granulomatous disease is suspected.[120] Culture and microscopic examination of synovial tissue may be more rewarding than culture of the fluid only in the case of tuberculosis. A negative purified protein derivative skin test or negative QuantiFERON TB Gold test virtually excludes the diagnosis of active tuberculosis. A biopsy should not be performed simply to confirm a diagnosis of oligoarticular JIA.

Arthritis of the hip joint or shoulder is exceedingly rare at the onset or during the course of oligoarticular JIA. Onset of apparent arthritis in the hip in a very young child should be considered first to be a septic process or transient synovitis (see Chapters 41 and 43). In children with transient synovitis of the hip, pain may be severe, but the process is self-limited, lasting no more than 1 to a few weeks.

In the older child, osteonecrosis of the femoral head (Legg-Calvé-Perthes disease) is a diagnostic consideration. In the adolescent age

---

BOX 18-2   Differential Diagnosis of Monarthritis

Acute Monarthritis
Early rheumatic disease
  Oligoarthritis
  Enthesitis-related arthritis
  Psoriatic arthritis
Arthritis related to infection
  Septic arthritis
  Reactive arthritis
Malignancy
  Leukemia
  Neuroblastoma
Hemophilia
Trauma
Familial Mediterranean fever

Chronic Monarthritis
Juvenile idiopathic arthritis
  Oligoarthritis
  Enthesitis-related arthritis
  Juvenile psoriatic arthritis
Villonodular synovitis
Sarcoidosis, Blau syndrome
Tuberculosis
Hemophilia
"Pseudoarthritis" (e.g., hemangioma, synovial chondromatosis, lipoma arborescens)
Some autoinflammatory syndromes (mevalonate kinase deficiency, chronic infantile neurocutaneous and articular syndrome, or neonatal onset multisystem inflammatory disease)

group, a slipped capital femoral epiphysis may initially mimic JIA. In older boys, ERA may manifest as unilateral or bilateral hip disease (see Chapter 19).

MANAGEMENT

Prompt and accurate diagnosis is essential to the optimal outcome for treatment of oligoarticular JIA. Because of the subtlety of the signs and symptoms, medical attention may not be sought early in the disease course. At first glance, it might appear that management of the child with oligoarthritis, particularly monarthritis, is straightforward. However, in order to achieve an optimal outcome, prompt, careful treatment by an experienced team of health professionals is necessary. Guidelines for management of oligoarticular JIA have been recently published.[121] The aim of therapy should be to achieve total remission of signs and symptoms of joint inflammation. Initial management of oligoarthritis should include careful clinical general and musculoskeletal assessment. In the child with monarthritis, other possible causes of inflammation in a single joint should be excluded. Evaluation by a physical therapist and occupational therapist to assess joint range, muscle strength, and function should be obtained. A slit-lamp examination by an experienced ophthalmologist is essential to exclude the possibility of asymptomatic uveitis, as soon as possible after the diagnosis of oligoarthritis (see Chapter 22).

In the absence of features of poor prognosis (arthritis of hip, cervical spine, wrist, or ankle; marked or prolonged elevation of ESR or CRP; or radiographic evidence of joint damage), absence of joint contractures and in the presence of mild disease activity (not more than one active joint, normal ESR or CRP, physician global assessment <3/10, parent global assessment <2/10), initial pharmacotherapy usually consists of a nonsteroidal antiinflammatory drug (NSAID) for a period of 8 weeks. Naproxen in a dosage of 15 to 20 mg/kg/day is often the drug of choice because of its twice-daily dosing. The parents and patient should be cautioned to take the medication with food to minimize the risk of gastric upset and be reminded of the risk of naproxen-induced pseudoporphyria. During this time, the physical therapist may recommend passive and active stretching to maintain range of motion. If after 8 weeks inflammation persists, or before 8 weeks if inflammation worsens, intraarticular corticosteroids, preferably triamcinolone hexacetonide (1 mg/kg with a maximum of 40 mg in large joints such as the knee, hip, and shoulder; 0.5 mg/kg in elbow and ankle with a maximum of 20 mg; and a maximum of 10 mg/joint in the wrist), is recommended. In children who have moderate or high disease activity, or in whom poor prognostic factors are present, intraarticular corticosteroids are recommended as initial therapy. Beukelman and colleagues used decision analysis to evaluate optimal initial therapy for monarthritis of the knee in JIA.[122] They compared the three most common approaches to *initial* management: NSAIDs alone, NSAIDs for 2 months followed by intraarticular corticosteroids, and intraarticular steroids alone. This study concluded that the use of intraarticular steroids alone as initial therapy was the optimal strategy. It may be necessary to serially cast joints with restricted range of motion. This can be done at the same time as joint injection using conscious sedation with a drug such as midazolam. Others use propofol as a general anesthetic agent.

The response to NSAIDs and intraarticular glucosteroids is usually very good, and many patients with oligoarthritis respond to this approach. Joint injections can be repeated two or more times, but children who are resistant to such therapy require the addition of a second-line agent. A different NSAID may occasionally be of benefit. The child who has an extended oligoarticular course is known to have a guarded outcome, and such children should be given the benefit of

methotrexate earlier rather than later in the course of disease. Children who do not respond to a course of 8 weeks of NSAIDs and intraarticular steroids on one or two occasions, particularly in those who have wrist or ankle disease, should be started on methotrexate (0.30 to 0.65 mg/kg/week; 15 mg/m^2). Methotrexate can be given orally, or if that is ineffective, by subcutaneous injection in the same dose. If inflammation persists after a methotrexate trial of 6 months (or if disease activity is moderate or high and poor prognostic features are present, 3 months), a TNF inhibitor should be prescribed.

The possible development of a leg-length inequality (in the child with a single affected knee) or contractures of affected joints requires ongoing assessment and physical therapy. Major leg-length inequalities are unusual in the child who is treated early and effectively. Sherry and colleagues[123] demonstrated the effectiveness of intraarticular corticosteroids in preventing this complication. Should a leg-length inequality of greater than 2 cm develop, a lift to partially compensate for the difference should be applied to the sole of the shoe of the shorter leg. Flexion contractures around the knee or ankle are usually much more responsive to physical therapy after corticosteroid injection of the affected joint. An active physical therapy program should be undertaken under the guidance of the therapist (see Chapter 14) with close attention to the presence or development of muscle atrophy and institution of appropriate therapy.

Surgical management of oligoarthritis is rarely necessary. Occasionally, soft tissue releases are required in the child who has not received early treatment and has developed a flexion contracture that is unresponsive to intraarticular corticosteroids and physical therapy.

DISEASE COURSE AND PROGNOSIS

The course of oligoarticular JIA is variable. Some children pursue an oligoarticular course and never have more than four affected joints (persistent oligoarthritis). In such children, the disease often goes into remission, although flares of the disease may occur many years later. In a second group, there is a progressive increase in the number of affected joints after the first 6 months of disease (extended oligoarthritis), so that by 1 or 2 years after onset, they have polyarthritis, although the number of affected joints is often much lower than in children with polyarticular JIA at onset. In this group, the prognosis is somewhat guarded, and fewer children enter remission. Because of the limited extent of the joint involvement, serious functional disability is uncommon. Fixed flexion contractures may persist, however, or osteoarthritis of a weight-bearing joint may eventually develop late in the course of the disease after clinical remission. Four large studies, reported in 2003, have described the outcome of children who were treated for oligoarticular JRA in the late 1980s and early 1990s. Bowyer and colleagues[124] reported on the health status of 232 children with pauciarticular JRA who were monitored for 1 to 5 years. By 1 year after disease onset, half no longer required medications, and 98% were in Steinbrocker functional class I or II. Five years after diagnosis, no patient with pauciarticular JRA was in Steinbrocker class III-IV. Childhood Health Assessment Questionnaire scores were 0 in the majority of patients, but approximately 25% had scores of between 0 and 0.5, and 12% had higher scores. Measures of psychosocial outcome were also evaluated in this study. Educational achievement and employment were comparable to the national norms. There was little negative impact of pauciarticular JRA on school participation: only 6% of the children were unable to participate in a full school program 5 years after diagnosis. Oen and associates[125] studied the outcomes of children with pauciarticular JRA who had been monitored for at least 5 years from disease onset and who were at least 8 years of age. Using stringent criteria for remission (absence of active arthritis, off medications for at least 2 years), these authors found that 47% of children with pauciarticular JRA were in remission 10 years after disease onset. Ninety-four percent of the remissions occurred before the age of 16 years. Although some patients had a monocyclic course, 25% relapsed approximately 5 years after the end of the first episode. An extended pauciarticular course was observed in 20% of children with pauciarticular onset, at a median of 3.9 years after disease onset. Children with pauciarticular JRA were mostly (85%) in Steinbrocker functional class I; 14.5% were in class II, and 0.5% in class III or IV. Radiographic outcome was evaluated in the same population group.[101] Fantini and colleagues[126] reported the follow-up of 420 children with pauciarticular-onset JCA. Mean follow-up for these patients was 8.1 years, with a range of less than 1 year to more than 30 years. At last follow-up, 36% of these patients were in remission, which was defined as absence of clinical or laboratory evidence of active arthritis for a period of at least 6 months in the absence of antirheumatic therapy. Fifty-three percent of children with oligoarticular JCA had never gone into remission, and 13% had remitted but relapsed. Twenty-four percent of these patients had a polyarticular course. Flato and associates[127] compared physical and psychosocial status in patients with pauciarticular JRA—who were monitored for a median of 14.9 years—with those of the healthy population. They found that early age at onset and an elevated ESR on first admission to hospital predicted persistent disease. In addition to these factors, the presence of DRB1*01 predicted joint erosions in these patients. Elevated ESR at onset, early age at onset, and the presence of hip disease in the first 6 months were predictors of disability. Early age at onset has not always been found to be a predictor of poor outcome, however.[128,129] Patients with persistent pauciarticular disease fared better than those with extended pauciarticular disease with respect to development of erosions, Health Assessment Questionnaire scores, and remission rates.[128,129] In a recent study, Nordal et al.[130] reported that 34.7% of children with oligoarthritis developed extended disease by a median of 98 months of follow-up.

The disease course and prognosis in children with oligoarthritis have improved considerably in the past 10 to 15 years. In particular, the frequency of significant joint contractures or leg-length inequalities has diminished, probably as the result of prompt institution of pharmacological and physical therapy, in particular the use of intraarticular steroids. Sequelae from uveitis remain an important issue, although here, too, some centers report decreased frequency and severity of this complication (see Chapter 22).

Clinical characteristics that are predictive of disease extension include ankle or wrist disease, symmetrical joint involvement and an elevated ESR. ANA test positivity correlated with worse outcome in this group of patients.[125] Genetic predispositions (e.g., the presence of HLA-DR1, low production of IL-10), the immunohistochemical characteristics of the synovium,[105] and the characteristics of the synovial fluid at or near disease onset (higher synovial fluid levels of CCL5 and a lower CD4:CD8 ratio)[99] may be very useful in predicting which child is likely to develop extended oligoarticular JIA, thereby enabling earlier and more aggressive therapy in such patients.

PERSPECTIVE

Oligoarthritis is complex. Current understanding recognizes two subcategories (persistent and extended), and further studies may reveal other groups within this disease category. Its early recognition is essential to optimal management, which usually leads to a good functional outcome. Nonetheless, the disease is chronic and is complicated by chronic anterior uveitis, which may further compromise function. An important challenge is to identify those children in whom progression to extended oligoarthritis will occur in order to use disease-modifying or biological therapy early.

REFERENCES

1. R.E. Petty, T.R. Southwood, P. Manners, et al., International League of Associations for Rheumatology classification of juvenile idiopathic arthritis, second revision, Edmonton 2001, J. Rheumatol. 31 (2004) 90–392.
2. European League Against Rheumatism, EULAR Bulletin No. 4: Nomenclature and Classification of Arthritis in Children, National Zeitung AG, Basel, 1977.
5. R.K. Saurenmann, J.B. Rose, P. Tyre, et al., Epidemiology of juvenile idiopathic arthritis in a multiethnic cohort, Arthritis Rheum. 56 (2007) 1974–1984.
7. P.J. Manners, C. Bower, Worldwide prevalence of juvenile arthritis—why does it vary so much? J. Rheumatol. 29 (2002) 520–530.
8. K. Oen, Comparative epidemiology of the rheumatic diseases in children, Curr. Opin. Rheumatol. 12 (2000) 410–414.
13. P.J. Manners, D.A. Diepeveen, Prevalence of juvenile chronic arthritis in a population of 12-year-old children in urban Australia, Pediatrics 98 (1996) 84–90.
21. M.B. Moroldo, M. Chaudhari, E. Shear, et al., Juvenile rheumatoid arthritis affected sibpairs: Extent of clinical phenotype concordance, Arthritis Rheum. 50 (2004) 1928–1934.
22. K. Oen, R.E. Petty, M.L. Schroeder, An association between HLA-A2 and juvenile rheumatoid arthritis in girls, J. Rheumatol. 9 (1982) 916–920.
23. K.J. Murray, M.B. Moroldo, P. Donnelly, et al., Age-specific effects of juvenile rheumatoid arthritis-associated HLA genes, Arthritis Rheum. 42 (1999) 1843–1853.
24. E. Zeggini, R.P. Donn, W.E. Ollier, et al., Evidence for linkage of HLA loci in juvenile idiopathic oligoarthritis: independent effects of HLA-A and HLA-DRB1, Arthritis Rheum. 46 (2002) 2716–2720.
26. A. Smerdel, R. Ploski, B. Flato, et al., Juvenile idiopathic arthritis (JIA) is primarily associated with HLA-DR8, but not DQ4 on the DR8-DQ4 haplotypes, Ann. Rheum. Dis. 61 (2002) 354–357.
33. S. Prahalad, M.H. Ryan, E.S. Shear, et al., Juvenile rheumatoid arthritis: linkage to HLA demonstrated by allele sharing in affected sibpairs, Arthritis Rheum. 43 (2004) 2335–2338.
45. R.P. Donn, W. Thomson, L. Pepper, et al., Antinuclear antibodies in early onset pauciarticular juvenile chronic arthritis (JCA) are associated with HLA-DQB1*0603: a possible JCA-associated human leucocyte antigen haplotype, Br. J. Rheumatol. 34 (1995) 461–465.
54. E. Crawley, S. Kon, P. Woo, Hereditary predisposition to low interleukin-10 production in children with extended oligoarticular juvenile idiopathic arthritis, Rheumatology 40 (2001) 574–578.
55. L. Nikitina Zake, I. Cimdina, I. Rumba, et al., Major histocompatibility complex class I chain related (MIC) A gene, TNFa microsatellite alleles and TNFB alleles in juvenile idiopathic arthritis patients from Latvia, Hum. Immunol. 63 (2002) 418–423.
57. E. Zeggini, W. Thompson, D. Kwiatkowski, et al., Linkage and association studies of single-nucleotide polymorphism-tagged tumor necrosis factor haplotypes in juvenile oligoarthritis, Arthritis Rheum. 46 (2002) 3304–3311.
58. M.J. Kaalla, K.A. Broadway, M. Rehani-Pichavant, et al., Meta-analysis confirms association between TNFA-G238A variant and oligoarticular, RF-polyarticular and RF-positive polyarticular JIA, Pediatr. Rheumatol. Online J. 11 (2013) 10.
59. S.D. Thompson, M.C. Marion, M. Sudman, et al., Genome-wide association analysis of juvenile idiopathic arthritis identifies a new susceptibility locus at chromosomal region 3q13, Arthritis Rheum. 64 (2012) 2781–2791.
60. A. Hinks, J. Cobb, M.C. Marion, et al., Dense genotyping of immune-related disease regions identifies 14 new susceptibility loci for juvenile idiopathic arthritis, Nat. Genet. 45 (2013) 664–669.
61. S. Prahalad, D.N. Glass, A comprehensive review of the genetics of juvenile idiopathic arthritis, Pediatric. Rheum. 6 (2008) 11.

65. K. Radon, D. Windstetter, D. Poluda, et al., Exposure to animals and risk of oligoarticular juvenile idiopathic arthritis: a multi-center case control study, BMC Musculosekeletal Disord. 11 (2010) 73.

66. K.M. Neufeld, C.P. Karunanayake, L.M. Maenz, A.M. Rosenberg, Stressful life events antedating chronic childhood arthritis, J. Rheumatol. 40 (2013) 1756–1765.

73. J.A. Dvergsten, R.G. Mueller, P. Griffin, et al., Premature cell senescence and T cell receptor-independent activation of CD8+ T cells in juvenile idiopathic arthritis, Arthritis Rheum. 65 (2013) 2201–2210.

74. K. Nistala, H. Moncrieffe, K.R. Newton, et al., Interleukin-17-producing T cells are enriched in the joints of children with arthritis, but have a reciprocal relationship to regulatory T cell numbers, Arthritis Rheum. 58 (2008) 875–887.

75. L. Cosmi, R. Cimaz, L. Maggi, et al., Evidence of the transient nature of the Th17 phenotype of CD4+CD161+ T cells in the synovial fluid of patients with juvenile idiopathic arthritis, Arthritis Rheum. 63 (2011) 2504–2515.

77. A.M. Rosenberg, D.M. Cordeiro, Relationship between sex and antibodies to high mobility group proteins 1 and 2 in juvenile idiopathic arthritis, J. Rheumatol. 27 (2000) 2489–2493.

78. M.L. Stoll, Q.Z. Li, J. Zhou, et al., Elevated IgG autoantibody production in oligoarticular juvenile idiopathic arthritis may predict a refractory course, Clin. Exp. Rheum. 29 (2011) 736–742.

80. E.R. de Graeff-Meeder, W. van Eden, G.T. Rijkers, et al., Heat-shock proteins and juvenile chronic arthritis, Clin. Exp. Rheumatol. 11 (Suppl. 9) (1993) S25–S28.

83. A.B. Prakken, M.J. van Hoeij, W. Kuis, et al., T-cell reactivity to human HSP60 in oligo-articular juvenile chronic arthritis is associated with a favorable prognosis and the generation of regulatory cytokines in the inflamed joint, Immunol. Lett. 57 (1997) 139–142.

84. A.B. Prakken, W. van Eden, G.T. Rijkers, et al., Autoreactivity to human heat-shock protein 60 predicts disease remission in oligoarticular juvenile rheumatoid arthritis, Arthritis Rheum. 39 (1996) 1826–1832.

85. B. Prakken, M. Wauben, P. van Kooten, et al., Nasal administration of arthritis-related T cell epitopes of heat shock protein 60 as a promising way for immunotherapy in chronic arthritis, Biotherapy 10 (1998) 205–211.

86. S. Finnegan, J. Robson, C. Scaife, et al., Synovial membrane protein expression differs between juvenile idiopathic arthritis subtypes in early disease, Arthritis Res. Ther. 16 (2014) R8.

89. P. Picco, M. Gattorno, A. Buoncompagni, et al., Interactions between prolactin and the proinflammatory cytokine network in juvenile chronic arthritis, Ann. N. Y. Acad. Sci. 876 (1999) 262–265.

90. C. Huemer, P.N. Malleson, D.A. Cabral, et al., Patterns of joint involvement at onset differentiate oligoarticular juvenile psoriatic arthritis from pauciarticular juvenile rheumatoid arthritis, J. Rheumatol. 29 (2002) 1531–1535.

91. S. Sharma, D.D. Sherry, Joint distribution at presentation in children with pauciarticular arthritis, J. Pediatr. 134 (1999) 642–643.

92. S. Padeh, O. Pinhas-Hamiel, D. Zimmerman-Sloutskis, Y. Berkun, Children with oligoarticular juvenile idiopathic arthritis are at considerable risk for growth retardation, J. Pediatr. 159 (2011) 832–837.

93. K. Oen, C.M. Duffy, S.M.L. Tse, et al., Early outcome and improvement of patients with juvenile idiopathic arthritis enrolled in a Canadian multicenter inception cohort, Arthritis Care Res. 62 (2010) 527–536.

94. S.T. Angeles-Han, C.F. Pelajo, L.B. Vogler, et al., Risk markers of Juvenile idiopathic arthritis-associated uveitis in the Childhood Arthritis and Rheumatology Research Alliance (CARRA) registry, J. Rheumatol. 40 (2013) 2088–2098.

95. E.B. Nordal, N.T. Songstad, L. Berntson, et al., Biomarkers of chronic uveitis in juvenile idiopathic arthritis; predictive value of antihistone antibodies and antinuclear antibodies, J. Rheumatol. 36 (2009) 1737–1743.

96. R.H. Syed, B.E. Gilliam, T.L. Moore, Rheumatoid factors and anticyclic citrullinated peptide antibodies in pediatric rheumatology, Curr. Rheumatol. Rep. 10 (2008) 156–163.

97. T. Avcin, A. Ambrozic, B. Bozic, et al., Estimation of anticardiolipin antibodies, anti β2 glycoprotein 1 antibodies and lupus anticoagulant in a prospective longitudinal study of children with juvenile idiopathic arthritis, Clin. Exp. Rheumatol. 20 (2002) 101–108.

99. P.J. Hunter, K. Nistala, N. Jina, et al., Biologic predictors of extension of oligoarticular juvenile idiopathic arthritis as determined from synovial fluid cellular composition and gene expression, Arthritis Rheum. 62 (2010) 896–907.

100. M.E. Rosenkranz, D.C. Wilson, A.D. Marinov, et al., Synovial fluid proteins differentiate between subtypes of juvenile idiopathic arthritis, Arthritis Rheum. 62 (2010) 1813–1823.

101. K. Oen, M. Reed, P.N. Malleson, et al., Radiologic outcome and its relationship to functional disability in juvenile rheumatoid arthritis, J. Rheumatol. 30 (2003) 832–840.

103. S. Magni-Manzoni, O. Epis, A. Ravelli, et al., Comparison of clinical versus ultrasound determined synovitis in juvenile idiopathic arthritis, Arthritis Rheum. 61 (2009) 1497–1504.

104. D.O. Pradsgaard, A.H. Spannow, C. Heuck, T. Herlin, Decreased cartilage thickness in juvenile idiopathic arthritis assessed by ultrasonography, J. Rheumatol. 30 (2013) 1596–1603.

105. S. Finnegan, S. Clarke, D. Gibson, et al., Synovial membrane immunohistology in early untreated juvenile idiopathic arthritis: differences between clinical subgroups, Ann. Rheum. Dis. 70 (2011) 1842–1850.

109. D.A. Cabral, L.B. Tucker, Malignancies in children who initially present with rheumatic complaints, J. Pediatr. 134 (1999) 53–57.

110. K. Chinniah, G.M. Mody, R. Bhimma, M. Adhikari, Arthritis in association with human immunodeficiency virus infection in Black African children: causal or coincidental, Rheumatology 44 (2005) 915–920.

120. Y.T. Konttinen, V. Bergroth, I. Kunnamo, et al., The value of biopsy in patients with monarticular juvenile rheumatoid arthritis of recent onset, Arthritis Rheum. 29 (1986) 47–53.

121. T. Beukelman, N.V. Patkar, K.G. Saag, et al., 2011 American College of Rheumatology recommendations for the treatment of juvenile idiopathic arthritis: initiation and safety monitoring of therapeutic agents for the treatment of arthritis and systemic features, Arthritis Care Res. 63 (2011) 465–482.

122. T. Beukelman, J.P. Guevari, D.A. Albert, Optimal treatment of knee monoarthritis in juvenile idiopathic arthritis. A decision analysis, Arthritis Rheum. 59 (2008) 1580–1588.

123. D.D. Sherry, L.D. Stein, A.M. Reed, et al., Prevention of leg length discrepancy in young children with pauciarticular juvenile rheumatoid arthritis by treatment with intraarticular steroids, Arthritis Rheum. 42 (1999) 2330–2334.

124. S.L. Bowyer, P.A. Roettcher, G.C. Higgins, et al., Health status of patients with juvenile rheumatoid arthritis at 1 and 5 years after diagnosis, J. Rheumatol. 30 (2003) 394–400.

125. K. Oen, P.N. Malleson, D.A. Cabral, et al., Disease course and outcome of JRA in a multicenter cohort, J. Rheumatol. 29 (2002) 1989–1999.

126. F. Fantini, V. Gerloni, M. Gattinara, et al., Remission in juvenile chronic arthritis: a cohort study of 683 consecutive cases with a mean 10 year followup, J. Rheumatol. 30 (2003) 579–584.

127. B. Flato, G. Lien, A. Smerdel, et al., Prognostic factors in juvenile rheumatoid arthritis: a case-control study revealing early predictors and outcome after 14.9 years, J. Rheumatol. 30 (2003) 386–393.

129. K. Minden, U. Kiessling, J. Listing, et al., Prognosis of patients with juvenile chronic arthritis and juvenile spondyloarthropathy, J. Rheumatol. 27 (2000) 2256–2263.

130. E. Nordal, M. Zak, K. Aalto, et al., Ongoing disease activity and changing categories in a long-term Nordic cohort study of juvenile idiopathic arthritis, Arthritis Rheum. 63 (2011) 2809–2818.

The entire reference list is available online at www.expertconsult.com.

Enthesitis Related Arthritis

Shirley M.L. Tse, Ross E. Petty

DEFINITION AND CLASSIFICATION

Enthesitis-related arthritis (ERA), a term introduced in the International League of Associations for Rheumatology (ILAR) classification of juvenile idiopathic arthritis (JIA),[1,2] is defined according to the inclusion and exclusion criteria shown in Box 19-1. It is predominantly a disease affecting joints and entheses of the lower extremities and can eventually affect the spine or sacroiliac (SI) joints. It is characterized by the absence of rheumatoid factor (RF) and by a strong association with the human leukocyte antigen–B27 (HLA-B27). In many instances, the disease evolves to closely resemble ankylosing spondylitis (AS), although the spine and SI joint involvement at disease onset are seldom present in childhood or adolescence. The progression to juvenile ankylosing spondylitis (JAS) is unpredictable but possible and early identification of individuals with axial disease is important so that appropriate therapeutic interventions can be initiated. ERA's relationship to other subtypes of JIA, such as psoriatic arthritis, is not entirely clear (see Chapters 15 and 20).

JAS is a chronic inflammatory arthritis of the axial and peripheral skeletons, frequently accompanied by enthesitis, characterized by RF seronegativity, paucity of ANA, and having a firm genetic basis. Unlike ERA, radiological evidence of bilateral inflammation of the SI joints is required for a definitive diagnosis. AS in adults is defined by sets of criteria that are based on clinical, laboratory, and radiographic abnormalities. Only a few children or adolescents meet these criteria, principally because of the low frequency of spinal or sacroiliac signs or symptoms in the young patient. In addition, criteria for the diagnosis of AS in adults (see Chapter 15)[3-6] are not applicable to the younger age group for a number of reasons: Normal values for some of the required physical measurements have not been published for children, or, if reported (back range),[7] they have not yet been validated. In addition, limitations of spine and chest motion may reflect disease duration and are therefore of little aid in facilitating early diagnosis.[8] The fact that peripheral joint disease precedes clinical axial involvement by years in many children precludes an early diagnosis by criteria in which abnormalities of spinal mobility or radiological changes are essential diagnostic features. Reasons for these differences between adults and children, whether they have an immunological, genetic, biochemical, or structural basis, are not understood.

The ILAR classification criteria allow most but not all JAS patients to be included into the ERA category because of the requirement to exclude patients with psoriasis, or with a first-degree relative with psoriasis; those with two positive tests for RF at least 3 months apart; or those with signs of systemic JIA in addition to lack of radiological documentation of axial involvement to serve as an inclusion criterion.[1,2] The term *juvenile spondyloarthritis* (JSpA) may be used to represent the full spectrum of arthritis that appears in late childhood and adolescents, and which has a strong association with HLA-B27 and potential axial involvement. ERA and JAS are often referred to as the undifferentiated and differentiated forms of JSpA, respectively.

Historical Review of the Spondyloarthritis Concept

Wright and Moll[9] introduced the term *spondyloarthritis* to include AS, psoriatic arthritis, the arthritis associated with ulcerative colitis and Crohn's disease, juvenile chronic arthritis, Whipple disease, Behçet syndrome, reactive arthritis, and acute anterior uveitis. They observed that these patients were RF seronegative, lacked subcutaneous nodules, and had inflammatory peripheral arthritis. Many had radiological evidence of sacroiliitis. They also observed a tendency toward familial aggregation. In adults, members of this group are currently included the name *seronegative spondyloarthritides*: AS, the arthritides of inflammatory bowel disease (IBD), reactive arthritis, and psoriatic arthritis. In addition to a high frequency of HLA-B27, adults with these diseases often share certain clinical features that are associated with AS, the prototypic disease in this category: inflammation of joints of the axial skeleton and entheses, absence of RF and ANA, and the occurrence of uveitis. Juvenile psoriatic arthritis is classified as a separate category of JIA by the ILAR criteria and differs significantly from AS and ERA (Chapter 20). In children with psoriatic arthritis, ANAs are frequent, and the uveitis is usually asymptomatic, similar to that of oligoarticular JIA, rather than acute like that of AS. The fact that RF is absent does not distinguish psoriatic arthritis from most other categories of JIA, which, with the exception of the RF-positive polyarticular JIA, are RF negative. Most children with arthritis associated with IBD have peripheral joint disease, rather than inflammation of the SI joints and spine and do not have the HLA-B27 antigen (Chapter 21). Arthritis with IBD and reactive arthritis are regarded as separate entities outside the JIA rubric of the ILAR classification.

Recognition of the seronegative enthesitis and arthritis (SEA) syndrome[10] permitted the identification of children who were different from other children with chronic inflammatory joint disease: Although they had enthesitis in addition to peripheral arthritis, they did not satisfy the criteria for adult AS. Children with the SEA syndrome have some of the characteristics of JAS but, at least at onset, lack the SI joint involvement needed to confirm that diagnosis.[10] These children are seronegative (lack RF and ANA), have enthesitis (usually around the heel or knee), and have arthritis of a few joints, particularly the large and small joints of the lower extremities. The SEA syndrome probably represents, for the most part, children with very early JAS or ERA, rather than a separate disease. The absence or rarity of axial spinal involvement in childhood led to the recognition of ERA rather than

BOX 19-1 Enthesitis-Related Arthritis (ILAR Classification) Definition

Arthritis and enthesitis
  Or
Arthritis or **enthesitis** with two or more of the following:
- Sacroiliac joint tenderness and/or inflammatory lumbosacral pain
- Presence of HLA-B27
- Family history of HLA-B27–associated disease (AS, ERA, sacroiliitis with inflammatory bowel disease, reactive arthritis, acute anterior uveitis) in a first-degree relative
- Acute symptomatic anterior uveitis
- Onset of arthritis in a boy after 6 years of age

Exclusions: Psoriasis in patient or first-degree relative, IgM RF, systemic JIA, arthritis fulfilling two JIA categories

ILAR, International League of Associations for Rheumatology. Modified from R.E. Petty, T.R. Southwood, J. Baum, et al., Revision of the proposed classification criteria for juvenile idiopathic arthritis: Durban, 1997, J. Rheumatol. 25 (1998) 1991–1994; and R.E. Petty, T.R. Southwood, P. Manners, et al., International League of Associations for Rheumatology classification of juvenile idiopathic arthritis: second revision, Edmonton, 2001, J. Rheumatol. 31 (2) (2004) 390–392.

BOX 19-2 New York Criteria for a Diagnosis of Ankylosing Spondylitis (AS)

Clinical Criteria
1. Limitation of lumbar spine motion in all three planes
2. Pain or history of pain at the dorsolumbar junction or lumbar spine
3. Limitation of chest expansion to 2.5 cm or less at the level of the fourth intercostal space

Definite AS
Grade 3-4 bilateral sacroiliac arthritis on radiography with at least one clinical criterion
  or
Grade 3-4 unilateral or grade 2 bilateral sacroiliac arthritis on radiography with clinical criterion 1 or clinical criteria 2 and 3

Probable AS
Grade 3-4 bilateral sacroiliac arthritis on radiography without clinical criteria

From P.H. Bennett, P.H.N. Wood (Eds.), Population Studies of the Rheumatic Diseases, Excerpta Medica, New York, 1968, p. 456.

AS in the ILAR classification.[1,2,11] It will take decades of observation and evaluation to determine whether JAS, ERA, and the SEA syndrome are simply earlier or later, milder or more severe, versions of the same disease; it seems highly likely that they are variants of the same disease.

Many of the challenges of classification of RF-negative arthritides remain. In ERA, clinical or radiographic spine and SI joint involvement is infrequent at disease onset, and most children and teens do not meet the modified New York criteria for AS (Box 19-2). Further revisions of the ILAR criteria may help to represent the ERA and AS spectrum of patients.

The Assessment in Spondyloarthritis International Society (ASAS) has developed criteria for adults with SpA and categorized patients into predominantly peripheral and axial forms of SpA (Table 19-1).[12,13] The ASAS classification system, along with its treatment guidelines, has sometimes been applied to the pediatric population and used in conjunction with the ILAR classification system, with ERA and JAS patients best represented by the peripheral and axial forms of SpA, respectively.

EPIDEMIOLOGY

The data examining the epidemiology of ERA are emerging. For this reason, the discussion that follows relies heavily on the study of patients who fulfilled traditional criteria for AS. Where there is sufficient evidence, ERA-specific information is included.

Incidence and Prevalence

Among children with JIA, the proportion with ERA in published studies ranged from 8.6% to 18.9%.[14-18] Increasing awareness of the possibility of the occurrence of ERA in childhood and its clinical and laboratory differentiation from other chronic arthritides of childhood will probably result in an increase in the proportion of children with inflammatory arthritis in this category. In contrast, children with JAS accounted for 1% to 7% of children in national pediatric rheumatic disease registries of the United States,[19] Canada,[20] and the United Kingdom,[21] and from studies in Sweden,[22] Finland,[23] and Croatia.[24]

TABLE 19-1 Assessment in Spondyloarthritis International Society (ASAS) Classification Criteria for Spondyloarthritis (SpA)

AXIAL SpA		PERIPHERAL SpA
In patients with ≥3 months back pain and age at onset <45 years		In patients with peripheral symptoms ONLY
Sacroiliitis on imaging* plus ≥1 SpA feature	or **HLA-B27** plus ≥2 other SpA features	**Arthritis or enthesitis or dactylitis** plus ≥1 SpA feature
SpA features		• Uveitis
• Inflammatory back pain (IBP)		• Psoriasis
• Arthritis		• Crohn's/colitis
• Enthesitis (heel)		• Preceding infection
• Uveitis		• HLA-B27
• Dactylitis		• Sacroiliitis on imaging
• Psoriasis		*Or*
• Crohn's/colitis		≥2 other SpA features
• Good response to NSAIDs		• Arthritis
• Family history for SpA		• Enthesitis
• HLA-B27		• Dactylitis
• Elevated CRP		• IBP ever
		• Family history for SpA

*Sacroiliitis on imaging:
- Active (acute) inflammation on MRI highly suggestive of sacroiliitis associated with SpA.
- Definite radiographic sacroiliitis according to modified NY criteria.

Modified from M. Rudwaleit, D. van der Heijde, R. Landewé, et al., The development of Assessment of Spondyloarthritis International Society classification criteria for axial spondyloarthritis (part II): validation and final selection, Ann. Rheum. Dis. 68 (6) (2009) 777–783; and M. Rudwaleit, D. van der Heijde, R. Landewé, et al., The Assessment of Spondyloarthritis International Society classification criteria for peripheral spondyloarthritis and for spondyloarthritis in general, Ann. Rheum. Dis. 70 (1) (2011) 25–31.

It is estimated that the prevalence of AS in adults is from 0.5% to 1.9%[25,26] with 8.6%[6] to 11%[27] having onset in childhood. However, the occurrence of AS varies among different racial and ethnic groups as demonstrated by population-based studies,[28] with reported prevalence of AS in adults to be 0.24% in Europe, 0.17% in Asia, 0.10% in Latin America, 0.32% in North America, and 0.07% in Africa. On the basis of the prevalence of HLA-B27 and the frequency of sacroiliitis in the HLA-B27–positive population, the prevalence of AS was estimated to be 0.86% to 1%[25,29] and was highest in HLA-B27–positive individuals.[29] Although this estimate includes asymptomatic persons, it also excludes the 8% to 10% of the AS population who do not have HLA-B27, and it may be a more accurate reflection of the prevalence of the entire spectrum of AS.

Age at Onset

In cohorts of ERA patients around the world, the mean age at diagnosis has been reported to be around 10 to 13 years (range 2.8 to 17.6 years),[15-18,30,31] similar to that for JAS. The age distribution appears to be homogeneous and presumably is continuous with that described in adult populations, suggesting that, at least on this basis, the disease as seen in adults is the same or very similar to that as seen in children.

Sex Ratio

In ERA, there is a predominance of boys but variations in the male-to-female ratio can be seen among cohorts from Canada (3.4 to 4.1 : 1),[15,30] United States (1.4 : 1),[18] Taiwan (3.3 : 1),[31] and Spain (8 : 1).[16] JAS has a much higher frequency in boys than in girls: of 247 children with this disorder, 216 were boys, for a male-to-female ratio of 7 : 1.[32-36] This disproportionate representation of boys may not accurately represent the actual occurrence of the disease in girls. The strong correlation of JAS and ERA with HLA-B27 and the equal distribution of this antigen in males and females suggest that JAS and ERA could be as common in girls as in boys. Furthermore, in radiographic surveys of HLA-B27-positive adult blood donors, SI arthritis was as common in women as in men.[37] In a questionnaire survey of members of the National Ankylosing Spondylitis Society in the United Kingdom, the male-to-female ratio was 2.7 : 1.[27] However, in women, manifestations of the disease may occur later[27] and be less severe,[38] and they may have more peripheral and less axial disease.[39] It is possible that these observations contribute to the relative infrequency of the diagnosis in women.

Geographic and Racial Distribution

Few data are specifically related to geographic and racial differences in the frequency of ERA or JAS.[40] The low incidence of AS in African Americans[41] and the Japanese,[42] and the high frequency in the Haida Indians of Pacific Canada,[43] reflect, in part, the frequency of HLA-B27 in these populations. Other factors may be significant, however, because this antigen occurs in only 50% of African Americans with AS[44] and in 65% to 90% of Japanese with the disease.[42] In a multiethnic Canadian population, ERA was twice as common in children of European ancestry as in those of non-European origin.[15] However, among children of non-European ancestry, children of Asian origin were more likely to develop ERA than any of the other categories of JIA.[15,45,46]

ETIOLOGY AND PATHOGENESIS

The cause of JAS or ERA is unknown. The clinical, genetic, and epidemiological similarities of these disorders and diseases such as reactive arthritis, in which enteric or genitourinary tract infections play a triggering role, suggest the possibility of an infectious etiology, although none has been proven. Although no organisms have been isolated from the joints of patients with AS, evidence of a local inflammatory response to antigen is supported by some antibody and cellular immune studies,[47,48] although confirmation of these findings is lacking.

The relationship between gastrointestinal infection and HLA-B27 is complex. The HLA-B27 transgenic rat develops a disease that is remarkably like AS[49-51] in the presence of intestinal bacteria. In humans with IBD, there is a strong association between HLA-B27 and sacroiliitis. Reports of an association between HLA-B27 and gastrointestinal (GI) isolation of *Klebsiella* species in adults with AS[47,48] remain largely unconfirmed.[52,53] Mielants and associates[54,55] described the presence of inflammatory gut changes in adolescents with spondyloarthropathies, supporting a pathogenic relationship between spondylitis and inflammation of the GI tract. Clinical or occult GI inflammation may be related in ERA and AS to the association with HLA antigens[56] as well as to cellular immunity to cartilage proteoglycans.[57]

The mechanisms whereby HLA-B27 is involved in disease pathogenesis have been the subject of much debate. As a class I major histocompatibility complex (MHC) molecule, the role of HLA-B27 is to present endogenous peptides to the T-cell receptor on CD8[+] lymphocytes. It has been proposed that the HLA-B27 molecule or peptides it presents share amino acid sequences with a microbial antigen (molecular mimicry) and thereby become a target for CD8[+] T cells or cross-reacting antibody, resulting in an inflammatory response.[58,59] However, to date no "arthritogenic peptide" has been identified. Misfolding of the HLA-B27 heavy chain in the endoplasmic reticulum may invoke an inflammatory response. One possible mechanism arises due to a unique Cys67 residue in the HLA-B27 heavy chains that leads to self-association, and homodimerization and misfolding, which results in retention in the endoplasmic reticulum. This, in turn, causes induction of the proinflammatory unfolded protein response.[60] Another mechanism suggests that HLA-B27 homodimers are not retained in the endoplasmic reticulum but are in fact expressed on the cell surface and lead to activation of disease relevant immunoreceptors and downstream pathways (i.e., KIR3DL1, KR3DL2, and immunoglobulin-like transcript 4 receptors on synovial and peripheral monocytes, B and T cells).[61] In support of this mechanism, Myles et al. have demonstrated that membrane-bound toll-like receptors are overexpressed in synovial and peripheral blood monocytes in ERA, which leads to increased levels of interleukin (IL)-6 and IL-8 levels compared with healthy controls.[62] The last hypothesized mechanism has no reference to HLA-B27 homodimerization but relates to the inability of HLA-B27–positive persons to clear intracellular pathogens. In fact, carriers of HLA-B27 are defective in the killing of intracellular bacteria such as *Yersinia, Salmonella, Shigella, and Chlamydia*, the same pathogens implicated in triggering reactive arthritis.[63] Furthermore, bacterial antigens or DNA have been identified in the synoviocytes of patients with reactive arthritis supporting the role of infection in the pathogenesis of SpA.[64] Finally, genetic microarray studies are providing new insights into the pathogenesis in ERA. Preliminary studies in the peripheral blood and synovial fluid mononuclear cells of ERA patients compared to healthy controls demonstrate a distinct genetic profile with higher expression of genes associated with antigen presentation, scavenger function, chemotaxis, and proteases, along with a lower expression of genes associated with natural killer (NK) cell function, cell adhesion, and inhibition of apoptosis.[65]

The pathogenesis of enthesitis, the characteristic abnormality of ERA and JAS, has been extensively studied by Benjamin and McGonagle.[66] An inflammatory infiltrate that includes CD8[+] and CD14[+] cells develops at sites of enthesitis in subchondral bone with bone absorption and new bone formation.[58] Tumor necrosis factor-α

(TNF-α) messenger RNA is increased in affected bone.[58] CD2R, a T-cell activation marker, is expressed at high levels in patients with JAS and JRA.[67] A type 1 helper T-cell (Th1) response has been suggested, with lymphocytic and mononuclear cellular infiltrates. Cells of the synovial membrane express TNF-α, TNF-β, and TNF receptors similar to those of children with other types of JIA.[68]

GENETIC BACKGROUND

The major genetic factor in ERA is the association with HLA-B27, as it is with AS. Family studies have indicated that AS is inherited as an autosomal dominant trait with penetrance of about 20%.[69] Although the risk of development of ERA or AS in an HLA-B27–positive person is not precisely known (approximately 1% to 3%), epidemiological studies suggest that AS occurs 10 to 20 times more frequently in relatives of patients with AS (20%) and 50 to 80 times more frequently in their siblings.[70,71] Thus, HLA-B27–positive persons with a family history of AS have a tenfold greater risk of AS than that of HLA-B27–positive persons with no family history of AS.[71] The general risk that an HLA-B27 heterozygous parent with AS will have a male child with the disease is approximately 5% to 10% (20% if the child is also HLA-B27 positive; close to zero if the child is HLA-B27 negative).[71] The risk of having a female child with JAS is lower. Risk may or may not be increased in first-born children.[72] Familial disease may not be concordant for phenotypes in each member. As less than 5% of HLA-B27–positive individuals develop SpA, there are likely other genetic or environmental influences. Other genes make minor contributions to the genetic risk of AS. Reveille has summarized the genetic factors implicated in SpA (Table 19-2).[73]

Family studies, disease concordance in twins, and modeling of genetic risk has implicated genetic factors in AS.[74,75] The strongest association with AS is with HLA-B27. There are at least 105 different HLA-B27 subtypes.[76] The most common subtypes associated with AS are HLA-B27*05 (Caucasians), HLA-B27*04 (Chinese), and HLA-B27*02 (Mediterraneans).[76] Two subtypes, HLA-B*2706 and HLA-B*2709, seem to have no disease association.

Of 247 children with JAS, HLA-B27 was present in 91%, confirming its strong disease association.[32-36] The possibility that homozygosity for HLA-B27 was responsible for the juvenile onset of AS was not supported by data in one small study,[77] and the idea that disease severity is genetically determined is unresolved.[78,79] In 56 Latvian children with JIA (44% ERA patients) who were HLA-B27 positive, 8 HLA-B27 subtypes were identified with HLA-B*2705 being the most commonly associated with ERA.[80] Additionally, the authors suggested that the HLA-B27 subtypes may be useful in predicting the treatment response. Specific single nucleotide polymorphisms (SNPs) of ERAP1 (AS associated gene) and IL23R (AS and PsA associated gene) were studied in JIA patients (N = 1054 including 65 ERA, 76 PsA and 24 undifferentiated patients) and healthy controls (N = 5200).[81] The ERAP1 SNP was most strongly associated with the ERA subtype ($P = 0.005$) while the IL23R SNP was best associated with PsA ($P = 0.04$), although there was a trend toward association in the ERA category. Neither the SNPs of ERAP1 nor IL23R were associated with the other JIA subtypes. There are few known class II associations with JAS. A higher frequency of HLA-DRB1*08 (44.9%) was reported in a Mexican population with JAS than in a control population (25.4%).[82] Maksymowych and colleagues[83] reported that the LMP2A allele frequency in patients with adult- and juvenile-onset AS with uveitis was twice that in those without this complication (odds ratio [OR], 2.51). Ploski and colleagues[84] reported an increase of B*4001, DRB1*08, and DPB1*0301, and the LMP2 b/b phenotype in patients with JAS compared with HLA-B27–positive controls or adults with AS. It is very likely that JAS and ERA are polygenic disorders.

CLINICAL MANIFESTATIONS

The onset of ERA may be insidious and characterized by intermittent musculoskeletal pain and stiffness or objective inflammation of peripheral joints, particularly those of the lower extremities, together with enthesitis at one or more sites around the knee or foot. Occasionally, the disease may have an abrupt onset. Systemic signs are often minimal, but fatigue, sleep disturbances, and low-grade fever may be present. Symptoms related to the back are usually absent at onset but become increasingly evident during the disease course in adolescents. Differing modes of presentation and course may characterize specific population groups.[85,86]

TABLE 19-2   Contribution to Heritability of AS with Confirmed Susceptibility Genes

GENE NAME OR CHROMOSOMAL REGION	MOST HIGHLY ASSOCIATED SNP	ODDS RATIO	OVERALL CONTRIBUTION TO AS HERITABILITY (%)
HLA-B27	rs 4349859	90.4	23.3
IL23R	rs 11209026	1.90	0.31
LTBR-TNFRSF1A	rs 11616188	1.38	0.075
2p15	rs 10865331	1.36	0.54
ERAP1	rs 30187	1.35	0.34
KIF21B	rs 2297909	1.25	0.25
21q22	rs 378108	1.25	0.035
TBKBP1	rs 8070463	1.24	0.054
ANTXR2	rs 4389526	1.21	0.054
PTGER4	rs 10440635	1.20	0.052
RUNX3	rs 11249215	1.19	0.12
IL12B	rs 6556416	1.18	0.11
CARD9	rs 10781500	1.18	0.034
IL1R2	rs 2310173	1.18	0.12
Total			25.39

From J.D. Reveille, Genetics of spondyloarthritis–beyond the MHC, Nat. Rev. Rheumatol. 8 (5) (2012) 296–304.

Enthesitis

Entheses—the sites of attachment of ligament, tendon, fascia, or capsule to bone—are characteristic sites of inflammation, especially in the lower limbs, that occurs in 60% to 80% of ERA and JAS patients. Consequently, many patients with ERA complain of knee, foot, or heel pain. Weiss et al.[87] noted that in 32 newly diagnosed patients with ERA, 66% had at least one tender entheseal site while 44% have more than two sites involved. The presence of an increasing number of tender entheses at presentation was associated with persistence at 6 months (OR 2.18). Although the presence of exquisite, well-localized tenderness at characteristic entheses strongly suggests ERA, it must be noted that enthesitis occurs occasionally in other disorders, including other types of JIA, other rheumatic diseases, and occasionally in children without disease.[88] Osgood–Schlatter disease should also be excluded before making a diagnosis of enthesitis affecting the tibial tuberosities. The presence of enthesitis is, however, the most helpful clinical feature in differentiating ERA from other types of JIA. Enthesitis is a characteristic early manifestation of JAS and occurs with greater frequency in JAS than in adult-onset AS. It frequently produces severe pain and resultant disability, which may be the child's most important complaints.[89]

A careful history and a thorough but gentle palpation of entheses may document evidence of past or present inflammation. The entheseal exam can include any of the anatomical sites shown in Figs. 19-1 and 19-2. Enthesitis is diagnosed clinically from the presence of marked localized tenderness or swelling at the entheseal insertion into the bone. A diagnosis of ERA is strongly supported by enthesitis in the lower extremities especially at insertional sites around the patella (10, 2, and 6 o'clock positions especially), heel, and plantar fascial attachments to the heads of the metatarsals (Fig. 19-2). Less commonly, pain can also be demonstrated at insertional sites around the pelvis (including the origin of adductor longus near the pubic symphysis), over the spinous processes, and at the entheses of the upper extremities. Observation of stance and gait (including walking on the toes and heels), may reveal altered weight bearing as the child avoids pressure on inflamed entheses.

Arthritis

Among 59 Italian ERA patients (66% HLA-B27 positive), the most frequently affected joints at disease onset included knees (65%), midfoot (58%), and ankles (48%).[90] The frequency of specific joint involvement after a mean follow-up of 7.6 years was reported by Shen et al.[91] in a series of 73 Taiwanese children with ERA (82% HLA-B27 positive). During the disease course, the knees (52%), hips (42%), ankles (38%), and lumbosacral spine (48%) were most commonly involved. From the cohort of 74 ERA patients (76% HLA-B27 positive) at The Hospital for Sick Children (SickKids), Toronto, Canada, the most frequently affected joints in descending order at disease onset and during the disease course were hips, knees, ankles, and midfoot. Upper extremity involvement was infrequent and lumbosacral spine involvement at disease onset was noted in only 16%.

The presenting joint symptoms recorded in the largest reported series of patients with JAS are summarized in Table 19-3. Initial musculoskeletal symptoms are often difficult for the child to localize and

Anatomic region	Enthesitis exam
Foot and ankle	Achilles tendon insertion to calcaneus Plantar fascia insertion to calcaneus Plantar fascia insertion to metatarsal heads Plantar fascia insertion to base of fifth metatarsal
Knee	Quadriceps tendon insertion to patella (2 and 10 o'clock) Infrapatellar ligament insertion to patella (6 o'clock) and tibial tuberosity
Pelvis	Hip extensor insertion at greater trochanter of femur Sartorius insertion at anterior superior iliac spine Posterior superior iliac spine Abdominal muscle insertions to iliac crest Gracilis and adduction insertion to pubis symphysis Hamstrings insertion to ischial tuberosity
Spine	5th lumbar spinous process
Upper extremity	Common flexor insertion at medial epicondyle of humerus Common extensor insertion at lateral epicondyle of humerus Supraspinatus insertion into greater tuberosity of humerus
Chest	Costosternal junctions (1st and 7th)

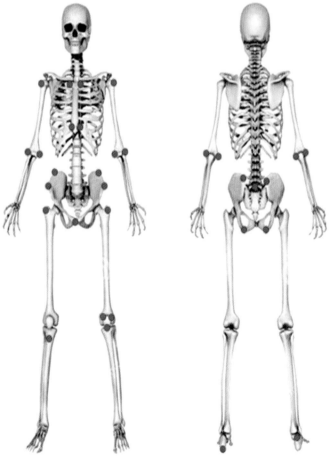

FIGURE 19-1 Anatomical sites for assessment of enthesitis in ERA and JA.

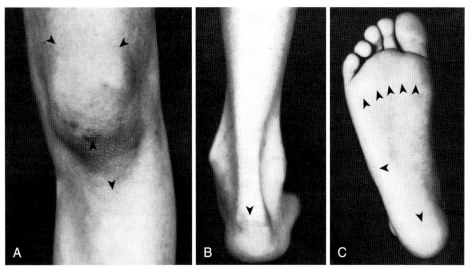

FIGURE 19-2 A, *Arrows* indicate the most common sites of tenderness associated with enthesitis at the insertions of the quadriceps muscles into the patella and the attachments of the patellar ligament to the patella and tibial tuberosity. **B,** *Arrow* indicates the site of tenderness at the insertion of the Achilles tendon into the calcaneus. **C,** *Arrows* indicate the most common sites of tenderness associated with enthesitis at the insertion of the plantar fascia into the calcaneus, base of the fifth metatarsal, and heads of the first through fifth metatarsals. Swelling in this area is best visualized by having the child lie prone on the examining table with the feet over the edge. (*B* and *C* from R.E. Petty, P. Malleson, Spondyloarthropathies of childhood, Pediatr. Clin. North Am. 33 (1986) 1079–1096.)

TABLE 19-3   Musculoskeletal Signs and Symptoms in Juvenile Ankylosing Spondylitis (JAS) at Onset*

CLINICAL EVIDENCE OF JOINT INVOLVEMENT AT ONSET	PERCENTAGE
Arthritis, Painful Limitation of Range of Motion	
Proximal limb joints	35
Distal limb joints	44
Upper limb joints	16
Lower limb joints	82
Axial skeleton joints	24
Joint Involvement During Course	
No peripheral joints affected	3
1 to 4 peripheral joints affected	43
More than 4 peripheral joints affected	54
Sacroiliac involvement[†]	95
Lumbosacral spine affected[†]	90
Cervical spine involvement	—
Enthesitis	
Around the knee[†]	80
Around the ankle and foot[†]	90
Myopathy	
Pain/Wasting[†]	50

*Clinical or radiographic evidence of involvement of the sacroiliac joints, and particularly the lumbosacral spine, may not be evident until adulthood. Data are from published studies.
†Estimate.

include pain in the buttocks, groin, thighs, heels, or around the shoulders. The vague quality and localization of this pain and its frequent spontaneous disappearance early in the disease are recurring sources of delay and confusion in the diagnosis.

PERIPHERAL JOINT ARTHRITIS

The peripheral arthritis in ERA and JAS is often asymmetrical and mainly involves the lower extremities. In most instances, the number of joints involved is limited (four or fewer),[18,30,90] although children may have a polyarticular involvement in up to 25% at disease onset and up to 45% during the disease course.[18] Joints of the lower extremity are affected more frequently than the upper extremity.[91] Unlike other types of JIA, hip involvement at disease onset and during the disease course is common. Isolated hip disease may be the presenting feature.[92] Although involvement of one or both knees is characteristic of both oligoarticular JIA and ERA, the child's age at onset, especially if a boy, is a useful distinguishing feature. Small joints of the foot and toes are commonly involved. The least commonly affected joints are the small joints of the hands. Consequently, symmetrical disease of the small joints of the hands or polyarticular disease, particularly in a girl, is more likely to be another type of JIA. Shoulders are not uncommonly affected, and even the temporomandibular joint may be involved.

Tarsitis (inflammation of the intertarsal joints, overlying tendons, entheses, and soft tissues) is an unique manifestation occurring in up to one third of children with ERA at disease onset (Fig. 19-3).[93] It is accompanied by pain, tenderness, and restriction of movement in the midfoot that, in the presence of disease of the first metatarsophalangeal joint, results in a characteristic forefoot adduction deformity. Burgos-Vargas and associates[94] concluded that a diagnosis of JAS could be

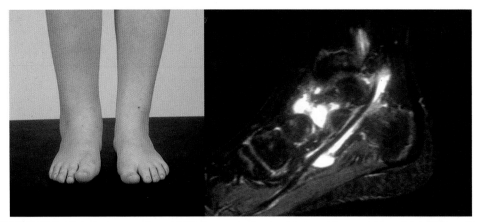

FIGURE 19-3 Clinical photograph and MRI demonstrating tarsitis in a 12-year-old boy (HLA-B27 positive) with ERA.

confirmed or strongly suspected shortly after onset of disease in children who displayed enthesopathy, midtarsal foot involvement, sparing of the hands, and progressive onset of lumbosacral disease.

Pain at the costosternal and sternoclavicular joints and the sternomanubrial joint, often in conjunction with tenderness over the proximal clavicle, may be associated with significant impairment of chest expansion. In the work by Schaller and associates,[35] five of seven patients with JAS had decreased chest expansion. Aside from the number and distribution of the affected joints, there is nothing clinically to distinguish the peripheral joint disease of ERA from that of other types of JIA. Burgos-Vargas and colleagues[95] have identified a subgroup of children with typical adult-type onset of disease. Whether this presentation represents a distinct entity or merely an extreme end of the clinical spectrum is not certain.[96]

Axial Skeleton

Involvement of the joints of the axial skeleton (spine or SI joint), although seldom present at disease onset can occur within 5 to 10 years from disease onset.[97-101] In a population of Mexican children, spinal involvement developed within 3 to 5 years, with some patients reporting axial symptoms within the first year of disease onset.[94,95] Distinct from AS in adults, children seldom have symptoms of axial involvement at disease onset; only 24% of children with JAS are reported to have pain, stiffness, or limitation of motion of the lumbosacral spine or SI joints at presentation. Many children may have difficulty reporting axial symptoms, but it is important to inquire about any pain in the lower back or buttock regions that is worsened by periods of inactivity (i.e., sitting for prolonged periods). Predictors of sacroiliitis or AS include HLA-B27,[10,102] DRB1*04,[100,102] male sex,[102] age at onset of symptoms,[102] family history of AS,[102] arthritis,[10] polyarthritis,[90,95] enthesitis,[90,98,102] tarsitis,[98] hip involvement,[100,102] axial involvement,[95,98,100,102] and psoriasis.[102]

In children with SI arthritis, pain may be elicited by direct pressure over one or both SI joints, compression of the pelvis, or distraction of the SI joints by the Patrick test (FABER test), or Gaenslen's test. Examination of the back may demonstrate abnormalities in contour, such as loss of the normal lumbar lordosis, exaggeration of the thoracic kyphosis, or increased occiput-to-wall distance. The contour of the back on full forward flexion may demonstrate loss of the normal smooth curve in the lower part of the thoracolumbar spine (Fig. 19-4), or there may be restriction of hyperextension, signifying early axial disease. The rigid spine of long-standing AS is rare in children. Cervical

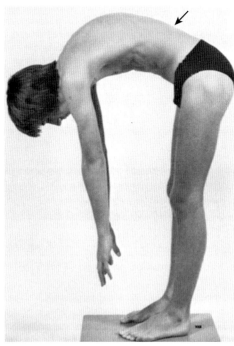

FIGURE 19-4 A 15-year-old boy shown in the position of maximal forward flexion. Note the flattened back (*arrow*). Radiographs demonstrated bilateral sacroiliac arthritis but no abnormality of the lumbosacral spine.

spine involvement is also a late development.[103] Although observations of abnormalities of the contour of the back are often more informative than actual numerical measurements, sequential measurement of thoracolumbar mobility is useful in documenting progression of the disease. Muscle wasting and weakness of the muscles around the hip joints may be quite prominent.

The modified Schober test[104,105] provides one index of abnormality (Fig. 19-5). With the child standing with the feet together, a line joining the dimples of Venus is used as a landmark for the lumbosacral junction. A mark is made 5 cm below (point A) and 10 cm above (point B) the lumbosacral junction. With the patient in maximum forward flexion with the knees straight, the increase in distance between points A and B is used as an indicator of lumbosacral spine mobility. Normal

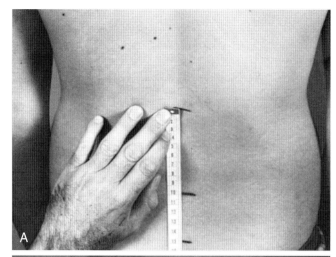

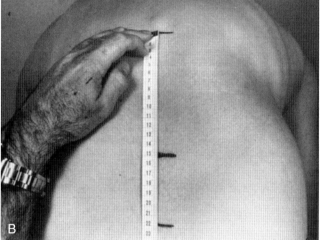

FIGURE 19-5 Schober test. **A,** Measurement 10 cm above and 5 cm below the lumbosacral junction (the dimples of Venus) in the upright position. **B,** Measurement of the distance between the upper and the lower marks when the child is bending forward.

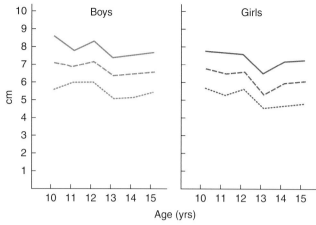

FIGURE 19-6 Normal values for the modified Schober test: mean (*dashed line*) ± 1 standard deviation (*solid line*). (Adapted from H.M. Moran, M.A. Hall, A. Barr, et al., Spinal mobility in the adolescent, Br. J. Rheumatol. Rehab. 18 (1979) 181–185.)

values plus or minus 1 standard deviation are indicated in Fig. 19-6. In general, a modified Schober measurement of less than 6 cm (e.g., an increase from 15 cm to less than 21 cm) should be regarded as abnormal. However, care should be exercised in interpreting this measurement, because there are large normal variations at each age, and the data have not been adequately validated in children with musculoskeletal disease. Measurement of the distance from the fingertips to the floor on maximum forward flexion is often used to quantitate spinal motion but is poorly reproducible and does not correlate with the Schober measurement. Furthermore, finger-to-floor distance reflects hip as well as back flexion.

Thoracic disease may be reflected in limitation of chest expansion. Normal thoracic excursion varies a great deal, and normal age- and sex-adjusted ranges have not been established. However, in a specific child, sequential measurement of thoracic motion may be useful in documenting progressive loss of range. In the adolescent, any thoracic excursion of less than 5 cm (maximum expiration to maximum inspiration, measured at the fourth intercostal space) should be regarded as probably abnormal. Even in the absence of symptoms, chest expansion in children with JAS may be restricted to 1 or 2 cm. Pain and tenderness at the costosternal and costovertebral joints may be elicited by firm palpation. Sternomanubrial tenderness sometimes occurs, but sternoclavicular pain is more common.

Uveitis

The uveitis seen in JAS or ERA is characterized by an acutely red, painful, photophobic eye, and contrasts with the typical asymptomatic anterior uveitis seen in JIA patients with oligoarthritis or polyarthritis. It is usually unilateral, frequently recurrent, and usually, but not always, leaves no ocular residua. It rarely precedes the onset of musculoskeletal complaints.[106] Uveitis has been reported in 3% to 7% of ERA patients from Germany,[107] Canada,[108] the United States,[109] and Taiwan.[34] Polymorphisms in the HLA-linked LMP2 locus was found to be confer a higher risk of developing acute uveitis in a HLA-B27–positive Mexican population of JAS and AS patients.[79]

Gastrointestinal Disease

The presence of gastrointestinal symptoms (chronic abdominal pain, diarrhea, hematochezia) in a child thought to have ERA should raise the question of the possibility of arthritis related to inflammatory bowel disease (see Chapter 21). Poor weight gain and slow growth may often be the first clue for gastrointestinal involvement.

Cardiopulmonary Disease

Overall cardiovascular disease is uncommon in ERA or JAS. However, it can occasionally be severe,[110] and marked aortic insufficiency has been reported in at least seven patients with JAS.[111-117] The apparently low frequency of such complications in children may reflect the fact that follow-up is generally of shorter duration than in adults, in whom cardiac disease (aortic insufficiency, heart block) develops in approximately 5% of patients an average of 15 years after disease onset.[118] However, one study of a Mexican JAS cohort followed for an average of 20 years confirmed that aortic abnormalities are less frequent compared with adult-onset AS.[119] Rarely, cardiac involvement precedes development of SI disease.[120]

None of 36 consecutive patients with JAS who were monitored for a mean of 4.3 years had symptoms related to the cardiovascular system, and only 1 developed the murmur of aortic regurgitation.[121] Echocardiographs documented no structural cardiac abnormalities and electrocardiography no conduction defects, but color Doppler assessment confirmed mild mitral regurgitation in two patients and mild aortic regurgitation in three; systolic ventricular function was impaired in one. In contrast, transesophageal echocardiography in adults with AS demonstrated aortic root abnormalities and valvular disease in 82% compared with 27% in controls.[122] Valve thickening was demonstrable as nodularity of the aortic cusps and basal thickening of the anterior mitral valve leaflet, creating the characteristic subaortic bump. Aortic valve regurgitation was present in almost one half of the patients.

Few data relating to pleuropulmonary disease are available. In a study of 18 children aged 8 to 17 years who fulfilled the Amor criteria,[5] abnormalities of pulmonary function were present in 33%.[123] All patients had normal chest radiographs at baseline and on follow-up at 2 years. No patient had symptoms attributable to the respiratory system, and all had normal chest expansion. Nonetheless, six patients (33%) had abnormal pulmonary function tests. The most common abnormality was reduction in the forced vital capacity (22%); occasionally, increased functional residual capacity (11%) and residual volume (5%) were observed. Restrictive patterns were more common than diffusion defects, and diffusing capacity of the lungs for carbon monoxide was reduced in only 11%. Small airways disease was not present.

In adults, although diminished chest expansion and resultant decreased vital capacity are not infrequent, clinical parenchymal pulmonary disease is rare. In the review by Rosenow and associates,[124] 1.3% of 2080 adults with AS had radiographic evidence of pleuropulmonary disease (apical pleural thickening). In a systematic review, the prevalence of lung abnormalities in AS using high-resolution computed tomography (CT) was found to be 61%. These finding included upper lobe fibrosis (6.9%), emphysema (18.1%), bronchiectasis (10.8%), ground glass attenuation (11.2%), and nonspecific interstitial abnormalities (33%) such as pleural thickening and parenchymal bands.[125] Cor pulmonale can develop secondary to kyphoscoliosis and decreased chest wall movement, characteristic of advanced spondylitis, but it has not been reported in children or adolescents.

Nervous System Disease

Intrinsic central nervous system disease does not occur in ERA, but atlantoaxial subluxation has been reported in three JAS patients (one boy with severe cervico-occipital pain,[126] a 12-year-old boy 8 years after disease onset,[127] and in one HLA-B27–negative girl,[128]), in two boys with SEA syndrome,[129] and in a 12-year-boy with ERA.[130] Additionally, it was also seen in a 10-year-old boy who was diagnosed with polyarthritis affecting only the joints of the lower extremities.[131] Atlantoaxial subluxation has been reported in AS occurring as an initial manifestation or developing during the disease course.[132,133] The cauda equina syndrome, caused by bony impingement on the cauda equina and characterized by weakness of bowel and bladder sphincters, saddle anesthesia, and leg weakness, occurs in adults[134] but has not been reported in children.

Renal Disease

Renal abnormalities are rare. Papillary necrosis, perhaps secondary to nonsteroidal antiinflammatory drugs (NSAIDs), has been reported.[135] Immunoglobulin A (IgA) nephropathy, occasionally with uveitis,[136] was observed in 115 adults with SpA.[137] Most of these patients had elevated serum IgA concentrations; some had impaired renal function and hypertension. Ansell[138] documented amyloidosis in 3.8% of 77 patients with JAS seen before 1980; she noted its association with severe peripheral arthropathy and a persistently elevated erythrocyte sedimentation rate (ESR).

Cardiopulmonary, central nervous system, and renal diseases appear to be very rare in children with ERA. Most of these complications occur after many years of disease in patients with JAS or AS. It is likely that with very long-term follow-up, these rare, but important, complications will be recognized in children with ERA.

PATHOLOGY

The pathology of JAS or ERA has not been studied, but it is probable that abnormalities are similar to those of AS. The synovitis is in general much milder, and the degree of cartilage erosion in peripheral joints much less, in AS compared with adult rheumatoid arthritis (RA).[139] The synovitis itself is otherwise virtually indistinguishable from that of RA, although there may be relatively more polymorphonuclear leukocytes present.

The characteristic pathological changes in the apophyseal and SI joints are enchondral and capsular ossification. The earliest lesion in the SI joints is subchondral inflammation, rather than synovitis, with formation of granulation tissue with few inflammatory cells. The surfaces of the SI joints are minimally affected, and pannus is not present.[140] Enchondral ossification on the iliac side of the joint accounts for the radiographic appearance of erosions. As Ball commented[141]: "As a rule, it seems that in any synovial joint in AS, the outcome represents a balance of erosive synovitis and capsular and/or ligamentous ossification. In joints of low mobility the ossific process tends to be the dominant feature."

Enthesitis is characterized by nonspecific inflammation.[142] Granulation tissue, infiltrated with lymphocytes and plasma cells and causing a localized osteitis, undermines the bony and cartilaginous attachment of the ligament or tendon. Healing of this lesion gives rise to a bony spur, such as a calcaneal spur at the insertion of the plantar fascia into the calcaneus or a syndesmophyte at the attachment of the outer fibers of the annulus fibrosus to the anterolateral aspects of the rim of the vertebral body.

DIFFERENTIAL DIAGNOSIS

At onset, ERA most closely resembles oligoarticular JIA (OJIA). However, whereas OJIA is characteristically a disease of young girls, ERA typically occurs in older boys and adolescents. The presence of enthesitis is the distinguishing clinical feature in children with ERA. ERA may mimic other inflammatory arthropathies, mechanical causes of back or lower extremity pain, or, very occasionally, infection or malignancy. A history of cramping abdominal pain, diarrhea, weight loss, and fever suggests an accompanying IBD in a child who otherwise has typical ERA. A few children with ERA also have psoriasis and would fulfill criteria for psoriatic arthritis. In most instances, however, children with ERA lack SI and back symptoms at onset, but, unlike children with OJIA, may have hip joint involvement.

In older children with established ERA, signs and symptoms of spine and SI arthritis clearly differentiate the child from one with OJIA. The disease then resembles JAS or AS. Arthritis of the cervical spine is infrequent and, when present, mimics that in children with polyarticular JIA. Thoracolumbar pain may reflect Scheuermann disease. Lumbar and lumbosacral pain has a myriad of causes, including spondylolysis, spondylolisthesis, osteoid osteoma, osteomyelitis, diskitis, and (rarely) lumbar disk herniation. Trauma may cause chronic pain in the sacrum and coccyx. SI tenderness and pain occurs in many patients with JAS, but septic SI disease, osteomyelitis, Ewing sarcoma of the ilium, and familial Mediterranean fever[143] also produce pain in and around these joints.

Pain that mimics enthesitis may result from a number of causes, including excessive running or jogging. Usually, the pain of traumatic enthesopathy is less severe and more diffuse than that caused by inflammation. Osteochondrosis of the tibial tuberosity (Osgood–Schlatter disease), of the inferior pole of the patella (Sinding–Larsen–Johansson syndrome), or of the apophysis of the calcaneus (Sever disease) may mimic inflammatory enthesitis at those sites. The coexistence of enthesitis at multiple sites usually eliminates these disorders from consideration. The absence of HLA-B27 positivity also assists in differentiating these disorders from the inflammatory enthesitis of JAS.[144] Pressure over bony prominences, including entheses, may produce pain in children with leukemia or bone tumors. In most instances, however, the pain resulting from such infiltrative diseases is less discrete and more severe than that of inflammatory enthesitis and frequently awakens the child from sleep.

LABORATORY EXAMINATION

There are few distinguishing laboratory features. Anemia is usually mild and characteristic of the anemia of chronic disease. White blood cell counts are usually normal or moderately elevated with normal differential counts. Indices of inflammation may not be a reliable measure of disease activity as they can be normal or minimally elevated even with clinically active disease. Very high values for the ESR (above 100 mm) occasionally occur but should also suggest the possibility of occult IBD.

Elevated immunoglobulin levels reflect inflammation, and selective IgA deficiency has been reported.[145,146] High levels of IgA and C4[147,148] and of circulating immune complexes[149] in adults with AS suggest an immunoreactive state. In a cohort of Chinese JAS patients, significantly higher levels of serum IgA were found compared with adult-onset AS patients and reflected the worse functional outcome and global assessment of disease activity in the JAS patients.[150] Characteristically, RFs are absent. ANAs do not occur in children with ERA more commonly than in a healthy population. Antiphospholipid antibodies have been demonstrated in 29% of adults with AS,[151] but children with ERA have not been studied. Although there are no reports of systematic studies of other autoantibodies in ERA or JAS, experience suggests that they are not common. Fecal calprotectin levels are high in children with ERA compared to those with other types of JIA.[152]

HLA-B27 is present in 90% of children with JAS, 60% to 80% of ERA patients, and in approximately 8% of the overall white population; it does not constitute a diagnostic test but rather an indicator of risk. The diagnosis of ERA rests on clinical characteristics, and the use of HLA typing for diagnosis may lead to misdiagnosis, although typing is important as a criterion to classify patients for study.

There are no specific studies of synovial fluid, but the changes are probably similar to those in adults with AS, in which the differential white blood cell count includes more neutrophils and fewer lymphocytes than in RA.[153] It has been reported that the predominant large mononuclear cell in synovial fluid in RA is lymphocyte derived, whereas that in AS is of macrophage origin.[154] Macrophages containing degenerated neutrophils are more common in the synovial fluid of patients with AS and related diseases such as reactive arthritis than in those with RA.[155] Descriptions of the synovial fluid are otherwise similar to those for RA, except that the complement level is usually normal[156] or increased.[138]

RADIOLOGICAL EXAMINATION

Box 19-3 lists the radiological characteristics seen in ERA and JAS.

Sacroiliac Joints

The SI joint has some unique anatomical characteristics, an understanding of which assists in the interpretation of certain radiological features. The sacral side of the joint is covered by hyaline cartilage, whereas the iliac side is protected by a thin layer of fibrocartilage. These differences may account for the higher frequency of abnormalities on the iliac side. Only the lower one third to one half of each joint is

> **BOX 19-3   Radiological Characteristics of Enthesitis Related Arthritis and Juvenile Ankylosing Spondylitis**
>
> Sacroiliac disease (bilateral)
>   Diffuse osteoporosis of the pelvis
>   Blurring of subchondral margins
>   Erosions (iliac side first)
>   Reactive sclerosis
>   Joint-space narrowing
>   Fusion (late)
> Vertebral column
>   Vertebral epiphysitis with anterior vertebral squaring
>   Anterior ligament calcification
>   "Bamboo spine"
> Enthesitis (e.g., at calcaneus, tibial tuberosity)
>   Soft tissue swelling
>   Erosions or spur formation at insertions
> Peripheral joints
>   Soft tissue swelling
>   Accelerated ossification and epiphyseal overgrowth
>   Periostitis
>   Joint-space narrowing, erosions
>   Ankylosis

diarthrodial and enclosed in a synovial membrane; the upper portion is a fibrous synostosis.[157]

Early radiographic changes in peripheral joints in ERA are like those of any type of JIA (Box 19-3 and see Chapter 9.) Evidence of enthesitis is most commonly seen at the plantar fascia insertion to the calcaneus or the insertion of the Achilles tendon to the calcaneus (Fig. 19-7). Radiographic demonstration of sacroiliitis often follows the onset of peripheral arthritis by years but is the first radiological evidence of inflammation affecting the axial skeleton. Radiological evidence of bilateral sacroiliitis or severe unilateral sacroiliitis is necessary to establish an unequivocal diagnosis of AS, although the classic radiographic changes may not be seen for many years after the onset of ERA.

Radiological evaluation of the SI joints is difficult, and the preferred techniques used vary from one radiologist to another. For radiographs, it is the authors' practice to obtain a standard anteroposterior (AP) view of the pelvis. Dedicated oblique views of individual SI joints result in increased radiation exposure to the pelvis but do not add significantly to information obtained from the standard AP views. Initial radiographic changes include apparent widening of the joint as a result of erosions of the subchondral bone, particularly in the inferior synovial portion of the joint, together with sclerosis of the iliac or sacral sides of the joint (Fig. 19-8). The lesion may appear initially as haziness of the cortical margins, followed by dissolution of the subchondral plate, which results in a punched-out appearance. Although these changes may be unilateral initially, they eventually become bilateral and symmetrical. An osteoblastic reaction occurring on both sides of the joint results in increased density or reactive sclerosis. Late changes may include fusion of the SI joints and regional osteoporosis. A normal or equivocal plain radiograph does not exclude the diagnosis of sacroiliitis and in that circumstance, magnetic resonance imaging (MRI) is helpful.

MRI identifies early changes in the SI joints and the spine, and may be the most sensitive radiological indicator of inflammation (Fig. 19-9).[158] It is critical to establish an early diagnosis in order to determine appropriate therapy, especially the use of TNF inhibitors. From

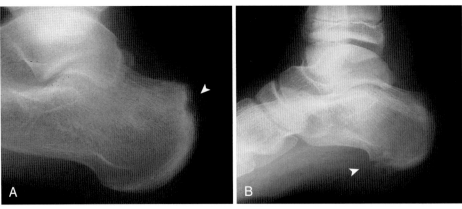

FIGURE 19-7 Lateral radiographs of the calcaneus in ERA. **A**, Erosions at the site of insertion of the Achilles tendon into the calcaneus *(arrowhead)*. **B**, Bony spur formation and erosions at the plantar fascia insertion into the calcaneus *(arrowhead)*.

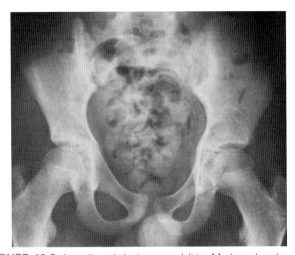

FIGURE 19-8 Juvenile ankylosing spondylitis. Moderately advanced radiographic changes. The widening, erosions, and reactive sclerosis are marked on this anteroposterior view of the pelvis.

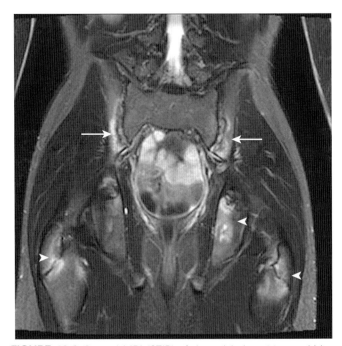

FIGURE 19-9 Coronal MRI (STIR) of the pelvis in a 14-year-old boy with ERA (HLA-B27 positive). Fluid and pathology appear bright; spinal fluid also appears bright. Increased signal abnormality is observed around bilateral triradiate cartilages and greater trochanteric apophyses *(arrowhead)*, common areas of involvement for ERA. Also, signal abnormality appears on the iliac side of the sacroiliac joints bilaterally around more curvilinear dark sclerotic subchondral areas representing erosions and sacroiliitis *(arrows)*. (From S.M. Tse, R.M. Laxer, New advances in juvenile spondyloarthritis, Nat. Rev. Rheumatol. 10 8 (5) (2012) 269–279.)

studies in adults with AS, evidence of bone marrow edema and osteitis was believed to be the MRI abnormality most indicative of active sacroiliitis, although synovitis, enthesitis, and capsulitis were also demonstrated.[159] In one large study,[160] dynamic MRI was used to evaluate 100 children younger than 6 years of age with probable SpA (European Spondylarthropathy Study Group [ESSG] criteria) and 30 control children. Early and chronic SI joint inflammation was detected by contrast-enhanced MRI with higher sensitivity compared with conventional radiographs.[160,161] In 11 juvenile axial SpA (ASAS criteria) patients with normal SI radiographs and a mean duration of back pain of 12 months (73% HLA-B27 positive), sacroiliitis was confirmed in all patients by MRI (short T1 inversion recovery [STIR]).[162] MRI was additionally able to detect multiple sites of enthesitis-osteitis within the pelvis, including pubic symphysis (91%), greater/lesser trochanter (55%), coxofemoral (45%), iliac crest (27%), and ischium pubis regions (27%).[162] Twenty-one of 59 ERA patients (35% with symptoms of inflammatory back pain) had normal pelvic radiographs, but dynamic MRI confirmed sacroiliitis in 81% as early as 1 year after disease onset.[90]

Although CT gives excellent images of the SI joints, its use requires a high radiation dose, and for this reason it is less often used. Scintigraphic study of the SI joint is of limited value in the growing child or adolescent unless there are distinct unilateral abnormalities. Sufficient

experience in the interpretation of radionuclide scans in this age group is required before interpretation of bone scans can be relied on, and even then the yield is limited. Increased uptake in one SI joint can result not only from inflammation or infection but from asymmetrical weight bearing caused by arthritis in a lower extremity joint or from enthesitis around the foot.

Spine

Radiological changes in the lumbosacral spine are less frequent and occur much later than abnormalities in the SI joints.[163] Periostitis with deposition of new bone along the anterior margin of the vertebral border results first in the "shiny" corner, and subsequently toward the flattening of the normally concave anterior margin of the vertebral body. Syndesmophyte formation, the hallmark of advanced disease in adults, is rare in children and adolescents but develops during the adult years in some patients with juvenile-onset disease. Periostitis at the iliac crests or the inferior pubic rami and erosion at the symphysis pubis are uncommon. Arthritis affecting the cervical spine is less commonly symptomatic than that of the lumbosacral spine but can cause severe damage.[164]

Although spinal lesions are infrequent in children and adolescents, spinal MRI is used for the diagnosis of AS and axial SpA in adults. Bone marrow edema and fatty lesions at the vertebral edges (corner lesions) are the most typical findings in SpA (Fig. 19-10). In screening adults for axial involvement, a spinal MRI is scored as positive for inflammation provided there are at least three corner inflammatory lesions on at least two sagittal slices.[165] Studies in adults with normal pelvic radiographs and negative SI joints on MRI indicated that spinal MRI added little incremental value compared with SI joint MRI alone for diagnosing patients with nonradiographic axial SpA, nor did it enhance confidence in this diagnosis.[166] Consequently, dedicated spinal MRIs may not be indicated in the pediatric population, especially in the setting of a normal SI MRI, unless the child is symptomatic and there is a high degree of suspicion for spinal disease. In a lumbar spine MRI study of 58 ERA patients with back pain compared with 21 adolescents with mechanical back pain, apophyseal joint synovitis was seen significantly more frequently in ERA patients (38% vs 5%).[167] Inflammation in the interspinous ligaments was also more common in ERA

patients. Spinal lesions were most common in patients with concurrent sacroiliitis.

Entheses

Radiographic evaluation of entheses around the calcaneus, and rarely the patella, may demonstrate subtle changes in soft tissue density. Loss of the distinct margins at the insertion of the Achilles tendon, together with effacement of the triangular fat shadow, may be an early sign of inflammation. Erosion of bone at the insertion of the Achilles tendon or spur formation at that site is readily evaluated by a lateral radiograph of the calcaneus (see Fig. 19-7). Azouz and Duffy[168] have described changes in the bone marrow subjacent to an inflamed enthesis in children with JAS. A comparison of adult-onset and juvenile-onset AS documented exclusively peripheral joint disease in 26% of those with juvenile-onset AS, compared with 4.6% in adult-onset AS.[169]

Ultrasonography with power Doppler is useful in the early detection of clinically silent enthesis. In 26 JIA patients (35% with ERA) and 41 healthy children, enthesitis was assessed with power Doppler ultrasonography.[170] None of the healthy control patients were found to have evidence of enthesitis. In contrast, power Doppler ultrasonography demonstrated enthesitis in 9.4% of all JIA patients, but in 70% of those with ERA. Furthermore, in one half of the sites with ultrasound evidence of enthesitis, the clinical exam was normal. A comparison of ultrasonography and dolorimetry in evaluation of enthesitis in ERA showed that ultrasonography was superior, and that dolorimetry had poor accuracy and reliability.[171]

Whole-body MRI was used to detect disease activity in the joints, entheses, and axial skeleton in 23 patients with ERA, and the findings

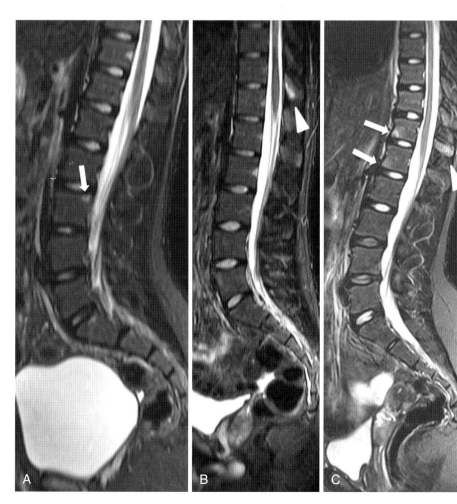

FIGURE 19-10 Sagittal MRI (STIR) of spine in a 17-year-old with JAS (HLA-B27 positive). "Corner lesions": foci of increased STIR signal at the (**A**) posterior aspect of the superior end-plate of L3 and (**C**) anterior aspect of the inferior end-plates of T12 and L1 in three different patients (*arrows*). Spinous process involvement at (**B**) T11 and (**C**) T12 (*arrowheads*).

were correlated to clinical examination.[172] Whole-body MRI was superior to clinical examination for detecting active disease in the hips, SI joints, and spine. The study suggested that clinical examination may overestimate the presence of enthesitis in the periphery. Whole-body MRI may potentially be used as a tool for both early detection as well as objective monitoring of disease activity in this population.

TREATMENT

General Management

Children with ERA have frequently had undiagnosed symptoms for months or years. Explanation of the correct diagnosis, its chronicity, possible complications, and the need for long-term medical treatment, physical therapy, and follow-up facilitates compliance with the therapeutic recommendations. A team of health professionals helps to provide necessary education and care. In the older adolescent, realistic career goals must be discussed along with current means of minimizing work-related stress to the low back and joints of the lower extremities. The patient should be encouraged to participate as fully as possible in age-appropriate social and recreational activities. The relatively good long-term prognosis should be emphasized, particularly in the adolescent, who may regard the diagnosis as marking the end of recreational, social, educational, and career goals.

Management should be individualized according to the patient's specific problems. Current treatments are most successful in controlling the signs and symptoms of the disease; none have been demonstrated to alter the progression of ankylosis. If widespread, severe joint inflammation is the overwhelming problem, systemic medications (NSAIDs, sulfasalazine, glucocorticoids) are appropriate. If the joint disease is localized, it may be more useful to use NSAIDs and intraarticular glucocorticoid in joints that are particularly problematic. Enthesitis, particularly around the foot, is unlikely to respond to systemic antiinflammatory drugs alone; the use of custom-made orthotics often provides relief. In all patients, exercise and maintenance of good posture to minimize loss of range of motion (ROM) in the spine and its articulations are recommended. A firm mattress and thin pillow are important adjuncts to the program. Smoking should be discouraged because of its demonstrated adverse effects on pulmonary function.[173]

Medications

Nonsteroidal Antiinflammatory Drugs (NSAIDs)

NSAIDs are the initial pharmacological management and help to provide symptomatic relief of peripheral and axial symptoms. Although there are no reported trials of NSAIDs in ERA or JAS, studies of adults with AS suggest that continuous NSAID treatment may result in disease remission.[174,175] Any NSAID can be considered but it is probable that children respond best to naproxen or indomethacin. Because of lower toxicity, the use of naproxen (15 to 20 mg/kg/day, maximum 500 mg twice daily) is recommended before indomethacin (1 to 3 mg/kg/day, maximum 50 mg three times per day). Although indomethacin is often effective, toxicity is common, and the drug must be started in low doses, and monitored carefully. Headache, epigastric pain, and inability to pay attention in school occur in 20% to 30% of children taking this drug and frequently necessitate cessation of its use.

Glucocorticoids

Glucocorticoids (oral or intravenous) have a role only in short-term therapy in the severely ill patient,[176] as topical agents in the management of acute uveitis, and for intraarticular administration in children with limited joint disease.[177,178] Short-term treatment with glucocorticoids is preferred to avoid any adverse effects, especially with affecting growth and bone health in children. Triamcinolone hexacetonide is the preferred intraarticular steroid and can be given in a dose of 1 mg/kg to a maximum of 40 mg in large joints (hip, knee, shoulder, SI joint), or 0.5 mg/kg to a maximum of 20 mg smaller joints (wrist, elbow, ankle, midfoot, subtalar) (see Chapter 12). Image guided administration of glucocorticoids into the SI joints has been reported to result in both clinically and radiological (MRI) improvement in ERA[179] and adults with AS.[180] Local injections of glucocorticoids at sites of enthesitis may occasionally be useful but should be used cautiously due to the increased risk of tendon rupture.

Disease Modifying Antirheumatic Drugs (DMARDs)

Sulfasalazine (40 to 50 mg/kg/day, upper limit 2000 to 3000 mg) is effective for the management of peripheral disease activity that is the predominant presenting manifestation in both ERA and JAS patients. Two pediatric randomized placebo-controlled studies have been reported. In one study in JSpA patients, there was a statistically significant improvement in the patient and physician global assessment of disease activity in the sulfasalazine treatment group compared with placebo.[181] In a second study, sulfasalazine in comparison to placebo was found to be efficacious and safe, and the effects were sustained over many years.[182] Several open-labeled studies in children have shown good response, tolerability, and in some cases, achievement of disease remission with sulfasalazine.[183-188] Use of sulfasalazine in children has largely been based on experience in the adult AS, which has shown that although it is ineffective for axial disease, it has been helpful for the management of peripheral disease.[189-194] Beneficial effects of sulfasalazine are usually not evident for several weeks after initiation of treatment. Toxicity to bone marrow and liver must be monitored closely.

No controlled studies of methotrexate therapy in ERA or JAS have been reported, but based on efficacy and safety data from controlled studies in JIA,[195-197] methotrexate is used to treat peripheral arthritis of ERA. In a study of adults with AS who had not responded to NSAIDs and sulfasalazine, modest benefit was demonstrated with the use of methotrexate in a dose of 7.5 to 15 mg/week.[198,199] As the majority of patients with ERA are adolescents, strict counseling that includes avoiding alcohol consumption and pregnancy is mandatory to minimize the risks of methotrexate.

There are no reports of hydroxychloroquine or leflunomide in ERA or JAS. However, based on its efficacy in treatment of polyarticular JIA,[200,201] leflunomide could be considered for treatment of peripheral arthritis in ERA in children intolerant of sulfasalazine or methotrexate.

It is still unclear whether DMARDs have any effect on axial disease in ERA or JAS. However, based on evidence in adults with AS, biological therapies would be indicated in these patients.

Biological Agents

TNF inhibitors are efficacious and safe for the management of arthritis and enthesitis. They are indicated for peripheral disease refractory to DMARDs or when axial disease is present. The selection of a TNF inhibitor should be made based on patient preference and presence of associated extraarticular features of GI or eye inflammation when monoclonal TNF inhibitors are preferable.

Etanercept (0.2 to 0.8 mg/kg twice weekly) led to a rapid and sustained clinical response (up to 1 year) in patients with ERA based on four open-label observational studies, including one prospective, multicenter study (CLIPPER).[202-206] Moreover, a single weekly etanercept dose (0.8 mg/kg) was shown be as efficacious and tolerable in ERA and is the usual recommended dosing frequency.[206] However, at a median follow up of 7.2 years, 50% had flared in no more than two joints after achieving disease remission.[207] Remission of arthritis and enthesitis was documented by MRI and color power Doppler ultrasonography in one patient at 2-year follow-up.[208]

Infliximab (5 mg/kg initial loading every 2 weeks for 3 infusions and then every 8 weeks) was shown to be efficacious and safe in a randomized placebo-controlled trial and two open-label observations studies.[203,204,209,210] The trial showed statistically significant improvement in arthritis, enthesitis, inflammatory markers, pain, and physical function at 3 months, which was sustained in the open-labeled extension phase at 52 weeks.[209] Longer follow-up over a median of 7.2 years showed that 30% had flared with no more than three joints involved.[207] Infliximab did not halt the progression of preexisting hip disease in two patients.

In a phase 3 multicenter study, adalimumab (24 mg/m² every other week), led to a statistically significant reduction in the active joint count enthesitis count and pain at 3 months that was sustained in the open-labeled extension phase at 52 weeks.[211] No serious adverse events were reported.

From the Dutch registry,[212] 22 ERA patients (68% HLA-B27 positive, median follow-up duration 1.2 years) received TNF inhibitors (20 etanercept, 1 adalimumab, 1 infliximab). The rates of inactive disease achieved at 3, 15, and 27 months were 32%, 38%, and 64%, respectively. Although patients improved and tolerated the TNF inhibitors with no adverse events, sustained disease remission was more difficult to achieve, and no patients were able to discontinue their biological agents. In comparison, the German Etanercept Registry[213] followed 112 ERA patients among 787 JIA patients receiving treatment, and over 50% of ERA patients were able to achieve inactive disease. Finally, in a retrospective analysis of 125 JIA patients (42% ERA) treated with

TNF inhibitors (83% etanercept, 6% infliximab, 11% adalimumab) from a single center, inactive disease was achieved in 43% of ERA patients at some time point, but in only 24% at the 1-year follow-up, the lowest rates compared with the other JIA categories. Predictors of failure to achieve inactive disease included a CHAQ>1, and active enthesitis at baseline.[214]

The 2011 treatment guidelines for JIA recommended by the American College of Rheumatology (ACR) propose treatment algorithms based on clinical parameters including disease activity, features of poor prognosis, and treatment response (Fig. 19-11).[215] In patients with high disease activity and poor prognostic factors, a TNF inhibitor is recommended if a 1- to 2-month trial of NSAIDs has failed to induce remission. It is recommended that patients with isolated high disease activity or persistent moderate disease activity should escalate to a TNF inhibitor after 3 months of methotrexate or sulfasalazine. Patients with persistent low disease activity and poor prognostic factors following 6 months of sulfasalazine treatment should receive a TNF inhibitor. In patients without active sacroiliitis (i.e., predominantly peripheral involvement), TNF inhibitors are not recommended until an adequate trial of 3 to 6 months of methotrexate or sulfasalazine in addition to 1 to 2 months of NSAIDs and glucocorticoid joint injections.

The adult SpA treatment recommendations for use of TNF inhibitors may be applied to the pediatric population (Fig. 19-12). Both guidelines support early use of TNF inhibitors in the presence of any inflammation of the SI joint or spine by any imaging modality and are not reliant solely on radiographic evidence as described in the JIA treatment guidelines. Secondly, patients with axial involvement can

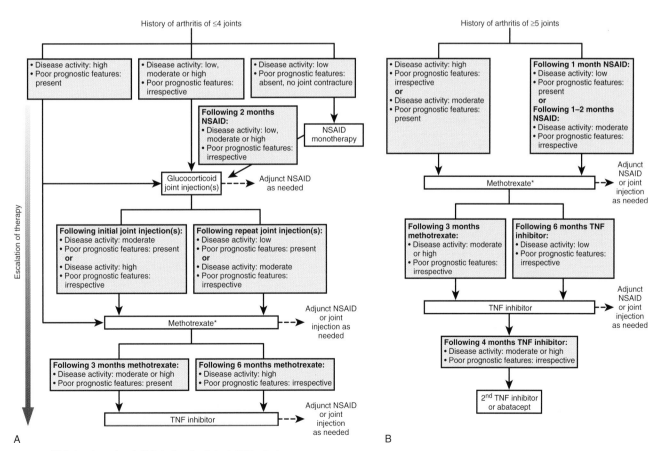

*Methotrexate can be substituted with sulfasalazine in ERA patients.

FIGURE 19-11 The 2011 ACR treatment recommendations for JIA applied to the JSpA and ERA patient populations. (Modified from S.M. Tse, R.M. Laxer, New advances in juvenile spondyloarthritis, Nat. Rev. Rheumatol. 10 8 (5) (2012) 269–279.)

proceed to a TNF inhibitor after failing 4 to 6 weeks of NSAIDs, a shorter course compared with the 1 to 2 months of NSAID monotherapy needed in the pediatric guidelines. Both adult guidelines also use the Bath Ankylosing Spondylitis Disease Activity Index (BASDAI) to define disease activity whereby a score of greater than 4 reflects high disease activity. Although the BASDAI needs to be formally validated in the ERA/JAS population, preliminary studies has confirmed it is reliable and valid in this patient group.[216,217] The Canadian Rheumatology Association–SPARCC (Spondyloarthritis Research Consortium of Canada) recommendations does not limit peripheral inflammation only to the presence of arthritis but also includes enthesitis. This is relevant to children and may allow earlier and appropriate access to TNF inhibitors to those with refractory peripheral arthritis and enthesitis.

Physical and Occupational Therapy

Physical therapy should be directed at preventing loss of ROM and poor functional positioning in the spine and chest, as well as stabilizing or regaining lost ROM in peripheral joints. Attention to posture and daily active ROM exercises for the back, and deep-breathing exercises for the chest help to preserve range. Some young patients with JAS breathe predominantly with the diaphragm and have to relearn to use the intercostal muscles. Strengthening of abdominal and back muscles should be undertaken cautiously. Swimming is an ideal form of physical activity that can be encouraged to augment these specific exercises. (See Chapter 14) In general, while children and adolescents with JIA have reduced aerobic fitness,[218,219] participation in exercise does not exacerbate disease.[220] Indeed, exercise can improve physical function and quality of life measures.[221,222] In adults with AS, home-based or supervised exercise programs were found to improve aerobic capacity.[223,224]

In one randomized trial in JIA patients, custom-made foot orthotics improved pain, speed of ambulation, and reduced disability in comparison with off-the-shelf inserts or athletic shoes.[225] Painful

enthesitis in the feet may be additionally be relieved by the use of custom-made orthotics, fitted to support the fat cushion under the heel and to take pressure off the plantar aspects of the heel and metatarsophalangeal joints. If the Achilles enthesis alone is involved, the use of a slightly higher heel may help to reduce stress at this site. Therapeutic ultrasound and transcutaneous nerve stimulation are sometimes useful in the management of pain caused by enthesitis around the foot. Enthesitis can be quite resistant to therapy and may be the most functionally limiting aspect of the disease.

Surgery

Orthopedic surgery has a very limited role in management of ERA in childhood or adolescence. Later in life, joint reconstruction and replacement are invaluable contributions to function and quality of life in the patient with severely damaged joints. The outcome of total hip replacement in young adults who were monitored for up to 30 years indicates that the probability that both components of low-friction arthroplasty will survive 10 years is 91%; this figure was 70% at 20 years.[226,227] Advances in total joint replacement will undoubtedly continue to improve long-term outcome. Bony ankylosis as a result of exuberant overgrowth of bone around the prosthesis has been reported after hip joint replacement as an almost unique complication related to AS. This complication may be amenable to the prophylactic use of medication.[138]

COURSE OF THE DISEASE AND PROGNOSIS

The disease course of ERA is highly variable, with disease remission reported in up to 44% of patients.[100,101,228,229] The variations in prognosis and outcomes are largely attributed to differences in case definition and clinical outcome measure (Table 19-4).

The majority of current studies show a worse prognosis with poorer physical function, higher pain scores, and ongoing disease activity in

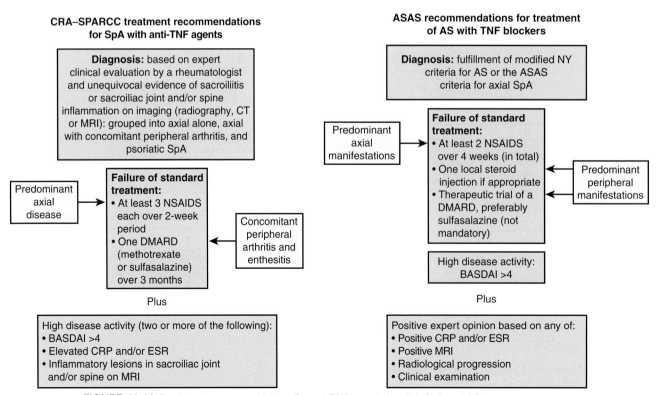

FIGURE 19-12 Treatment recommendations for anti-TNF agents in adult SpA and AS.

TABLE 19-4   Outcomes in JSpA

STUDY	POPULATION	HLA-B27 POSITIVE (%)	MEAN FOLLOW-UP (YEARS)	SUMMARY OF OUTCOMES FOR THOSE WITH JUVENILE SPA
Undifferentiated Juvenile SpA				
Minden et al. (2002)[101]	ERA (n = 33) versus JIA (n = 182)	24	16.0	Better HAQ Disease remission rate in 18% (2nd lowest); 39% developed AS (NY criteria); 36% with probable AS
Flato et al. (2006)[100]	ERA (n = 55) versus JIA (n = 205: oligoarthritis or polyarthritis)	85	15.3	Worse HAQ Poorer physical health and increased body pain (SF-36) Disease remission in 44% 35% developed AS (NY criteria), 75% had decreased spinal mobility
Selvaag et al. (2005)[230]	JSpA (n = 12: 3 JAS [NY criteria], 4 SEA, 5 PsA) vs JRA (n = 185)	50	3.0	Worse CHAQ (physical function) Highest pain scores and patient/physician global assessment of disease
Qen et al. (2010)[30]	ERA (n = 36) vs JIA (n = 318)	59	0.5	50% ongoing active arthritis (median AJC = 1) 31% ongoing active enthesitis Inactive disease activity in 19% (2nd lowest)
Pagnini et al. (2010)[90]	ERA (n = 59)	66	3	66% inactive disease, disease remission in 20% 36% decreased spinal mobility 29% developed AS (axial-SpA)
Aggarwal et al. (2008)[231]	ERA (n = 49)	53	6.0 (median)	Abnormal HAQ in 75% (49% moderate to severe disability) 62.6% ongoing active enthesitis Disease remission in 8% 35% had evidence of radiological damage (especially hips) 65.3% experienced lost years of education 28.6% had decreased spinal mobility
Olivieri et al. (2012)[233]	JSpA (n = 14 : 9 ERA, 4 PsA, 1 dactylitis)	100	5	None with radiographic signs of SI disease 79% doing well with self-limited disease 21% active disease (all responded to TNF inhibitors)
Weiss et al. (2012)[18]	ERA (n = 268) vs JIA (n = 2303)	53	NA (convenience sample)	More and higher pain intensity More with impaired physical function (64% abnormal CHAQ) Poorer health status
Hugle et al. (2014)[207]	JSpA (n = 16: 4 JAS [NY criteria], 8 ERA, 1 PsA, 2 U-SpA, 1 IBD associated arthritis) all receiving TNF inhibitors	93	7.2 (median)	38% flare in arthritis after achieving clinical remission 12% flare in enthesitis after clinical remission 13% required hip replacement Disease remission in 6% 50% progression of radiological damage in SI (NY grading) Majority of patient with good physical function
Juvenile-Onset AS				
Calin et al. (1988)[232]	Juvenile-onset AS (n = 135) vs adult-onset AS (n = 135)	NA	Juvenile = 24.5 Adults = 23.5	Better employment rate More hip replacement
Stone (2005)[234]	Juvenile-onset AS (n = 326) vs adult-onset AS (n = 2,021)	NA	Juvenile = 18.3 Adult = 13.4	Greater delay in diagnosis Worse BASFI Outcome worse in females than in males Age and income status correlated to worse functional outcome
O'Shea (2008)[169]	Juvenile-onset AS (n = 84) versus adult-onset AS (n = 183)	Juvenile = 75 Adult = 81	Juvenile = 14.7 Adult = 16.7	More peripheral and less axial features (spinal mobility impairment, radiographic involvement) Better BASFI, HAQ and quality of life (SF36), and less fatigue Disease remission in 11%

AJC, Active joint count; AS, ankylosing spondylitis; BASFI, Bath Ankylosing Spondylitis Functional Index; CHAQ, Childhood Health Assessment Questionnaire; ERA, enthesitis-related arthritis; HAQ, Health Assessment Questionnaire; NA, not applicable; PsA, psoriatic arthritis; RA, rheumatoid arthritis; SpA, spondyloarthritis.

Modified from S.M. Tse, R.M. Laxer, New advances in juvenile spondyloarthritis, Nat. Rev. Rheumatol. 8 (5) (2012) 269–279.

ERA patients compared with other JIA subtypes.[18,100,230,231] Persistent enthesitis is common. Additionally, a large proportion (35%) have damaged joints, with the hip being the most common joint affected (29%).[231] As none of the patients in this cohort were treated with TNF inhibitors, it is possible that earlier treatment with biological agents could have altered the disease course. Up to 40% of ERA patients eventually develop AS (New York criteria), typically within 10 years of disease onset.[100,101] However, in a cohort of Mexican children, early evolution to AS occurred within 3 to 5 years.[95,97]

Poor prognostic factors in ERA associated with a failure to achieve remission include presence of AS in a first-degree relative, HLA-DRB1*08, ankle or hip arthritis within the first 6 months of onset, development of sacroiliitis, and persistently elevated inflammatory markers within the first 6 months of onset.[100] Prognostic factors in ERA associated with poor physical health include female sex, family history of AS, and high numbers of affected joints within first 6 months of onset.[100] Moreover, high disability as measured by the CHAQ and poor well-being within the first 6 months were also associated with poor outcome at follow-up.[230]

In comparison with adult AS, JAS patients had more severe hip disease and required more total hip replacements (17% vs 4%, $P < 0.01$).[232] Despite this, they had good physical function and had significantly better full-time employment rates (74% vs 56%, $P < 0.01$) compared to adult AS patients.[232] The majority of JAS studies reported better physical function and quality of life measures compared to adult AS. Although uveitis is less common compared to the other JIA subtypes, uveitis in JAS occurred twice as likely over the disease course compared with adult-onset AS and highlights the importance of ongoing eye are in JAS patients.[169]

Current assessments of outcomes in ERA and JAS are limited as there are currently no disease activity measures specific to this population. Modification of the juvenile arthritis damage index (JADI) with the addition of tarsal joints and lumbar spine has been shown to improve articular damage assessment in ERA.[235] Application of adult SpA disease activity measures, core sets, and definitions for improvement[236] is challenging, as all adult measures are weighted to axial signs and symptoms that are not prevalent in the pediatric population. New insights with the use of biomarkers in the determination of disease activity in ERA are underway. Preliminary work suggest that serum myeloid-related proteins (MRPs), in particular MRP 8/14,[237] as well as matrix metalloproteinase-3 (MMP-3),[238] correlate to disease activity in ERA. Further work needs to be done to develop new or adapt current activity measures to more accurately assess disease activity in this population.

Life expectancy in AS is reduced compared with the US population as a whole. Cardiopulmonary and cerebrovascular diseases are the leading causes of death. At least during the years of childhood and adolescence, functional outcome probably remains good.[193] In one study,[194] however, outcome in JAS was worse than in AS. Peripheral joint disease may be more common in children than in adults, and persistent hip disease, in particular, is associated with a poor functional outcome.[195,196] Acute uveitis seldom leaves significant residua, even if recurrent, but, uncommonly, it can be severe. Aortitis is rare but, if present, contributes to late morbidity and mortality. Although amyloidosis may develop in adults with AS, little information is available in children.[37]

REFERENCES

2. R.E. Petty, T.R. Southwood, P. Manners, et al., International League of Associations for Rheumatology classification of juvenile idiopathic arthritis: second revision, Edmonton, 2001, J. Rheumatol. 31 (2) (2004) 390–392.

10. A.M. Rosenberg, R.E. Petty, A syndrome of seronegative enthesopathy and arthropathy in children, Arthritis Rheum. 25 (9) (1982) 1041–1047.

12. M. Rudwaleit, D. van der Heijde, R. Landewe, et al., The development of Assessment of SpondyloArthritis international Society classification criteria for axial spondyloarthritis (part II): validation and final selection, Ann. Rheum. Dis. 68 (6) (2009) 777–783.

13. M. Rudwaleit, D. van der Heijde, R. Landewe, et al., The Assessment of SpondyloArthritis International Society classification criteria for peripheral spondyloarthritis and for spondyloarthritis in general, Ann. Rheum. Dis. 70 (1) (2011) 25–31.

18. P.F. Weiss, T. Beukelman, L.E. Schanberg, et al., Enthesitis-related arthritis is associated with higher pain intensity and poorer health status in comparison with other categories of juvenile idiopathic arthritis: the Childhood Arthritis and Rheumatology Research Alliance Registry, J. Rheumatol. 39 (12) (2012) 2341–2351.

50. J.D. Taurog, Immunology, genetics, and animal models of the spondyloarthropathies, Curr. Opin. Rheumatol. 2 (4) (1990) 586–591.

55. H. Mielants, E.M. Veys, C. Cuvelier, et al., The evolution of spondyloarthropathies in relation to gut histology. III. Relation between gut and joint, J. Rheumatol. 22 (12) (1995) 2279–2284.

58. J. Braun, M. Bollow, L. Neure, et al., Use of immunohistologic and in situ hybridization techniques in the examination of sacroiliac joint biopsy specimens from patients with ankylosing spondylitis, Arthritis Rheum. 38 (4) (1995) 499–505.

60. R.A. Colbert, M.L. DeLay, G. Layh-Schmitt, D.P. Sowders, HLA-B27 misfolding and spondyloarthropathies, Adv. Exp. Med. Biol. 649 (2009) 217–234.

66. M. Benjamin, D. McGonagle, The enthesis organ concept and its relevance to the spondyloarthropathies, Adv. Exp. Med. Biol. 649 (2009) 57–70.

68. A.A. Grom, K.J. Murray, L. Luyrink, et al., Patterns of expression of tumor necrosis factor alpha, tumor necrosis factor beta, and their receptors in synovia of patients with juvenile rheumatoid arthritis and juvenile spondylarthropathy, Arthritis Rheum. 39 (10) (1996) 1703–1710.

73. J.D. Reveille, Genetics of spondyloarthritis–beyond the MHC, Nat Rev Rheumatol. 8 (5) (2012) 296–304.

76. M.A. Khan, Polymorphism of HLA-B27: 105 subtypes currently known, Curr. Rheumatol. Rep. 15 (10) (2013) 362.

81. A. Hinks, P. Martin, E. Flynn, et al., Subtype specific genetic associations for juvenile idiopathic arthritis: ERAP1 with the enthesitis related arthritis subtype and IL23R with juvenile psoriatic arthritis, Arthritis Res. Ther. 13 (1) (2011) R12.

87. P.F. Weiss, A.J. Klink, E.M. Behrens, et al., Enthesitis in an inception cohort of enthesitis-related arthritis, Arthritis Care Res. (Hoboken) 63 (9) (2011) 1307–1312.

89. R. Burgos-Vargas, C. Pacheco-Tena, J. Vazquez-Mellado, A short-term follow-up of enthesitis and arthritis in the active phase of juvenile onset spondyloarthropathies, Clin. Exp. Rheumatol. 20 (5) (2002) 727–731.

90. I. Pagnini, S. Savelli, M. Matucci-Cerinic, et al., Early predictors of juvenile sacroiliitis in enthesitis-related arthritis, J. Rheumatol. 37 (11) (2010) 2395–2401.

91. C.C. Shen, K.W. Yeh, L.S. Ou, et al., Clinical features of children with juvenile idiopathic arthritis using the ILAR classification criteria: a community-based cohort study in Taiwan, J. Microbiol. Immunol. Infect. 46 (4) (2013) 288–294.

93. C. Alvarez-Madrid, R. Merino, J. De Inocencio, J. Garcia-Consuegra, Tarsitis as an initial manifestation of juvenile spondyloarthropathy, Clin. Exp. Rheumatol. 27 (4) (2009) 691–694.

95. R. Burgos-Vargas, J. Vazquez-Mellado, N. Cassis, et al., Genuine ankylosing spondylitis in children: a case-control study of patients with early definite disease according to adult onset criteria, J. Rheumatol. 23 (12) (1996) 2140–2147.

98. R. Burgos-Vargas, J. Vazquez-Mellado, The early clinical recognition of juvenile-onset ankylosing spondylitis and its differentiation from juvenile rheumatoid arthritis, Arthritis Rheum. 38 (6) (1995) 835–844.

99. D.A. Cabral, K.G. Oen, R.E. Petty, SEA syndrome revisited: a longterm followup of children with a syndrome of seronegative enthesopathy and arthropathy, J. Rheumatol. 19 (8) (1992) 1282–1285.

100. B. Flato, A.M. Hoffmann-Vold, A. Reiff, et al., Long-term outcome and prognostic factors in enthesitis-related arthritis: a case-control study, Arthritis Rheum. 54 (11) (2006) 3573–3582.

101. K. Minden, M. Niewerth, J. Listing, et al., Long-term outcome in patients with juvenile idiopathic arthritis, Arthritis Rheum. 46 (9) (2002) 2392–2401.

102. B. Flato, A. Smerdel, V. Johnston, et al., The influence of patient characteristics, disease variables, and HLA alleles on the development of radiographically evident sacroiliitis in juvenile idiopathic arthritis, Arthritis Rheum. 46 (4) (2002) 986–994.

110. H. Huppertz, I. Voigt, J. Muller-Scholden, K. Sandhage, Cardiac manifestations in patients with HLA B27-associated juvenile arthritis, Pediatr. Cardiol. 21 (2) (2000) 141–147.

123. G. Camiciottoli, S. Trapani, M. Ermini, et al., Pulmonary function in children affected by juvenile spondyloarthropathy, J. Rheumatol. 26 (6) (1999) 1382–1386.

129. H.E. Foster, R.A. Cairns, R.H. Burnell, et al., Atlantoaxial subluxation in children with seronegative enthesopathy and arthropathy syndrome: 2 case reports and a review of the literature, J. Rheumatol. 22 (3) (1995) 548–551.

150. H.A. Chen, C.H. Chen, H.T. Liao, et al., Clinical, functional, and radiographic differences among juvenile-onset, adult-onset, and late-onset ankylosing spondylitis, J. Rheumatol. 39 (5) (2012) 1013–1018.

160. M. Bollow, T. Biedermann, J. Kannenberg, et al., Use of dynamic magnetic resonance imaging to detect sacroiliitis in HLA-B27 positive and negative children with juvenile arthritides, J. Rheumatol. 25 (3) (1998) 556–564.

162. M.H. Yilmaz, M. Ozbayrak, O. Kasapcopur, et al., Pelvic MRI findings of juvenile-onset ankylosing spondylitis, Clin. Rheumatol. 29 (9) (2010) 1007–1013.

167. K. Vendhan, D. Sen, C. Fisher, et al., Inflammatory changes of the lumbar spine in children and adolescents with enthesitis-related arthritis: magnetic resonance imaging findings, Arthritis Care Res. (Hoboken) 66 (1) (2014) 40–46.

168. E.M. Azouz, C.M. Duffy, Juvenile spondyloarthropathies: clinical manifestations and medical imaging, Skeletal Radiol. 24 (6) (1995) 399–408.

169. F.D. O'Shea, E. Boyle, R. Riarh, et al., Comparison of clinical and radiographic severity of juvenile-onset versus adult-onset ankylosing spondylitis, Ann. Rheum. Dis. 68 (9) (2009) 1407–1412.

170. S. Jousse-Joulin, S. Breton, C. Cangemi, et al., Ultrasonography for detecting enthesis in juvenile idiopathic arthritis, Arthritis Care Res. (Hoboken) 63 (6) (2011) 849–855.

171. P.F. Weiss, N.A. Chauvin, A.J. Klink, et al., Detection of enthesis in children with enthesitis-related arthritis: dolorimeter examination compared to ultrasonography, Arthritis Rheum. 66 (1) (2014) 218–227.

172. A.C. Rachlis, P.S. Babyn, E. Lobo-Mueller, et al., Whole body magnetic resonance imaging in juvenile spondyloarthropathy: will it provide vital information compared to clinical exam alone? Arthritis Rheum. 63 (10S) (2011) S292.

175. A. Wanders, D. Heijde, R. Landewe, et al., Nonsteroidal antiinflammatory drugs reduce radiographic progression in patients with ankylosing spondylitis: a randomized clinical trial, Arthritis Rheum. 52 (6) (2005) 1756–1765.

179. J. Fritz, N. Tzaribachev, C. Thomas, et al., Evaluation of MR imaging guided steroid injection of the sacroiliac joints for the treatment of children with refractory enthesitis-related arthritis, Eur. Radiol. 21 (5) (2011) 1050–1057.

180. J. Braun, M. Bollow, F. Seyrekbasan, et al., Computed tomography guided corticosteroid injection of the sacroiliac joint in patients with spondyloarthropathy with sacroiliitis: clinical outcome and followup by dynamic magnetic resonance imaging, J. Rheumatol. 23 (4) (1996) 659–664.

181. R. Burgos-Vargas, J. Vazquez-Mellado, C. Pacheco-Tena, et al., A 26 week randomised, double blind, placebo controlled exploratory study of sulfasalazine in juvenile onset spondyloarthropathies, Ann. Rheum. Dis. 61 (10) (2002) 941–942.

203. S.M. Tse, R. Burgos-Vargas, R.M. Laxer, Anti-tumor necrosis factor alpha blockade in the treatment of juvenile spondylarthropathy, Arthritis Rheum. 52 (7) (2005) 2103–2108.

205. M. Sulpice, C.J. Deslandre, P. Quartier, Efficacy and safety of TNFalpha antagonist therapy in patients with juvenile spondyloarthropathies, Joint Bone Spine 76 (1) (2009) 24–27.

206. G. Horneff, R. Burgos-Vargas, T. Constantin, et al., Efficacy and safety of open-label etanercept on extended oligoarticular juvenile idiopathic arthritis, enthesitis-related arthritis and psoriatic arthritis: part 1 (week 12) of the CLIPPER study, Ann. Rheum. Dis. 73 (6) (2014) 1114–1122.

207. B. Hugle, R. Burgos-Vargas, R.D. Inman, et al., Long-term outcome of anti-tumor necrosis factor alpha blockade in the treatment of juvenile spondyloarthritis, Clin. Exp. Rheumatol. 32 (3) (2014) 424–431.

208. S.M. Tse, R.M. Laxer, P.S. Babyn, A.S. Doria, Radiologic Improvement of juvenile idiopathic arthritis-enthesitis-related arthritis following anti-tumor necrosis factor-alpha blockade with etanercept, J. Rheumatol. 33 (6) (2006) 1186–1188.

209. R. Burgos-Vargas, J. C-V, R. Gutierrez-Suarez, A 3-month, double-blind, placebo-controlled, randomized trial of infliximab in juvenile-onset spondyloarthritis (SpA) and a 52-week open extension, Clin. Exper Rheumatol. 26 (4) (2008) 745.

210. H. Schmeling, G. Horneff, Infliximab in two patients with juvenile ankylosing spondylitis, Rheumatol. Int. 24 (3) (2004) 173–176.

211. R. Burgos-Vargas, S.M.L. Tse, G. Horneff, et al., Efficacy and safety of adalimumab in pediatric patients with enthesitis related arthritis, Arthritis Rheum. 65 (10S) (2013) S336.

212. M.H. Otten, F.H. Prince, M. Twilt, et al., Tumor necrosis factor-blocking agents for children with enthesitis-related arthritis–data from the dutch arthritis and biologicals in children register, 1999-2010, J. Rheumatol. 38 (10) (2011) 2258–2263.

213. V. Papsdorf, G. Horneff, Complete control of disease activity and remission induced by treatment with etanercept in juvenile idiopathic arthritis, Rheumatology (Oxford) 50 (1) (2011) 214–221.

214. K.J. Donnithorne, R.Q. Cron, T. Beukelman, Attainment of inactive disease status following initiation of TNF-alpha inhibitor therapy for juvenile idiopathic arthritis: enthesitis-related arthritis predicts persistent active disease, J. Rheumatol. 38 (12) (2011) 2675–2681.

215. T. Beukelman, N.M. Patkar, K.G. Saag, et al., 2011 American College of Rheumatology recommendations for the treatment of juvenile idiopathic arthritis: initiation and safety monitoring of therapeutic agents for the treatment of arthritis and systemic features, Arthritis Care Res. (Hoboken) 63 (4) (2011) 465–482.

228. K. Minden, U. Kiessling, J. Listing, et al., Prognosis of patients with juvenile chronic arthritis and juvenile spondyloarthropathy, J. Rheumatol. 27 (9) (2000) 2256–2263.

229. B. Flato, A. Aasland, O. Vinje, O. Forre, Outcome and predictive factors in juvenile rheumatoid arthritis and juvenile spondyloarthropathy, J. Rheumatol. 25 (2) (1998) 366–375.

230. A.M. Selvaag, G. Lien, D. Sorskaar, et al., Early disease course and predictors of disability in juvenile rheumatoid arthritis and juvenile spondyloarthropathy: a 3 year prospective study, J. Rheumatol. 32 (6) (2005) 1122–1130.

231. P.K. Sarma, R. Misra, A. Aggarwal, Outcome in patients with enthesitis related arthritis (ERA): juvenile arthritis damage index (JADI) and functional status, Pediatr. Rheumatol. Online J. 6 (2008) 18.

232. A. Calin, J. Elswood, The natural history of juvenile-onset ankylosing spondylitis: a 24-year retrospective case-control study, Br. J. Rheumatol. 27 (2) (1988) 91–93.

234. M. Stone, R.W. Warren, J. Bruckel, et al., Juvenile-onset ankylosing spondylitis is associated with worse functional outcomes than adult-onset ankylosing spondylitis, Arthritis Rheum. 53 (3) (2005) 445–451.

The entire reference list is available online at www.expertconsult.com.

20 | CHAPTER

Juvenile Psoriatic Arthritis

Peter A. Nigrovic, Robert P. Sundel

The association of arthritis with psoriasis was described almost 200 years ago, but it was not reported in children until the 1950s.[1-4] Juvenile psoriatic arthritis (JPsA) is a heterogeneous entity, recognized in patients with frank psoriasis but also in cases in which a psoriatic diathesis is suspected on other grounds. The diagnosis captures certain characteristic phenotypic features of this condition, although clinical overlap with other subtypes of juvenile idiopathic arthritis (JIA) is considerable.

DEFINITION AND CLASSIFICATION

Juvenile psoriatic arthritis, as classified by the criteria of the International League of Associations for Rheumatology (ILAR), is arthritis that has its onset before the 16th birthday, lasts for at least 6 weeks, and is associated with either psoriasis or with two of the following: dactylitis; nail pitting or onycholysis; or psoriasis in a first-degree relative.[5] This definition resembles that defined by the older Vancouver criteria (Table 20-1).[6] However, under ILAR criteria the diagnosis of JPsA cannot be made if the patient has a positive test for rheumatoid factor (RF) on two occasions at least 3 months apart, a first-degree family history of an human leukocyte antigen (HLA)-B27–associated disease, or if the arthritis began in a boy over the age of 6 years who is HLA-B27 positive.

The diagnosis of JPsA is complicated by the presentation of psoriasis in children. Psoriasis in the young child may be subtle, atypical, and transient; initial misdiagnosis as eczema is common.[7-9] Psoriasis occurs in about 0.5% to 1% of children, with a prevalence rising to 2% to 3% in adulthood.[10-12] Although skin disease lags behind arthritis in about half of children with JPsA, sometimes by a decade or more (Table 20-2), diagnosis often relies on the presence of dactylitis or family history.[6-8,13-25] Agents such as methotrexate and tumor necrosis factor (TNF) blockers are effective treatments for cutaneous psoriasis and could potentially forestall its appearance in a child treated for joint inflammation. Finally, not every patient with arthritis and psoriasis has psoriatic arthritis. Typical seropositive rheumatoid arthritis (RA) with coincidental psoriasis is well recognized.[26] Confirming that a particular child does, or does not, have JPsA is therefore challenging, and diagnostic uncertainty is common.

These challenges have been reflected in the evolution of diagnostic criteria for JPsA. Initially, JPsA was limited to children with chronic arthritis who developed classic psoriasis.[3,7,13-16,27] Recognizing that the psoriatic diathesis may be suggested by features beyond the typical eruption, including dactylitis, nail pits, and a family history of psoriasis, Southwood et al. extended the diagnosis of JPsA to patients with such features even in the absence of the typical rash, yielding the Vancouver criteria for JPsA (Table 20-1).[6] These criteria have been validated.[19,23,24] With the development of the ILAR nomenclature, the

definition of JPsA was restricted to make it mutually exclusive with other subtypes of JIA. These definitions remain a work in progress.[5,23,24,28-32] Both Vancouver and ILAR criteria were designed for research, and in practice the diagnosis of JPsA is often used more fluidly, acknowledging that the diagnosis may change as the clinical phenotype evolves.

EPIDEMIOLOGY

Incidence and Prevalence

The incidence and prevalence of JPsA are unknown. Population data, enumerating largely patients with adult-onset psoriatic arthritis (PsA), suggest a prevalence of 0.10% to 0.25% in the United States.[33,34] It can occur in all ethnic groups. The proportion of JIA patients with JPsA varies widely depending on the population studied and the diagnostic criteria employed. Series that recognize patients on the basis of frank psoriasis, or using ILAR criteria, find that JPsA represents approximately 7% (range: 0% to 11.3%) of patients with JIA.[6,8,18,21,24,35-43] Series employing the more inclusive Vancouver criteria find that JPsA represents 8% to 20% of JIA.[6,21,24,44]

Age at Onset and Sex Ratio

In the pediatric population, the age at onset of JPsA is bimodally distributed (Fig. 20-1).[6,21] A first peak (mainly in girls) occurs during the preschool years, and a second is seen during middle to late childhood. JPsA is very uncommon before the age of 1 year. Due to the female preponderance of early-onset JPsA, girls account for 60% of patients in larger series (Table 20-2).[21,45,46]

ETIOLOGY, PATHOLOGY, AND PATHOGENESIS

The cause of JPsA and the reasons for the link between psoriasis and arthritis are unknown.

PATHOLOGY

Synovial Pathology

Pathological data concerning the psoriatic synovium are available largely from adult-onset disease, with rare exception.[47] Gross examination, as performed by arthroscopy, reveals a synovial lining that is less villous than in adult RA but with distinctive tortuous, bushy superficial blood vessels.[48,49] This microvascular pattern resembles that of the psoriatic plaque and is also observed in synovial tissue from the spondyloarthropathies.[48,50] There are histological changes throughout the psoriatic synovium (Fig. 20-2). The lining becomes hypertrophic with expansion of both type A (macrophage-like) and type B (fibroblast-like) synoviocytes.[51] The infiltrate in the loose connective tissue

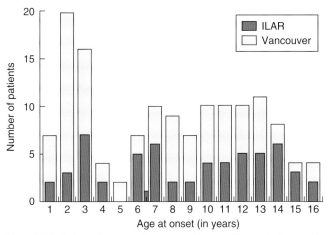

FIGURE 20-1 Age of onset of patents with juvenile psoriatic arthritis. (From: Stoll, et al., Arthritis Rheum. Jan 15; 59 (1) (2008) 51–58.)

beneath the synovial lining is composed principally of lymphocytes and monocyte/macrophage lineage cells, with occasional neutrophils, plasma cells, and mast cells.[52-55] Lymphoid follicles may be observed. Recently, a population of myofibroblast-like cells has been identified in synovium from both psoriatic and non-psoriatic spondyloarthritis, but the identity and significance of these cells remains unknown.[56] Compared with RA, lining hypertrophy and sublining infiltrates are typically less extensive. Infiltrating neutrophils are more prevalent in PsA, but they are not invariably present.[52,53,55] In general, given the variability between patients and within different parts of the same synovium, pathological findings are inadequate to define the diagnosis in an individual patient.

Characterization of the psoriatic synovial infiltrate by immunohistochemistry shows that the majority of infiltrating lymphocytes are T cells that express the memory CD45RO phenotype, with CD4 helper cells predominating over CD8 cytotoxic cells.[52,53,57-59] These cells are present at frequencies similar to that in RA, as are CD20+ B cells, plasma cells and CD68+ macrophages. T-cell oligoclonality suggests

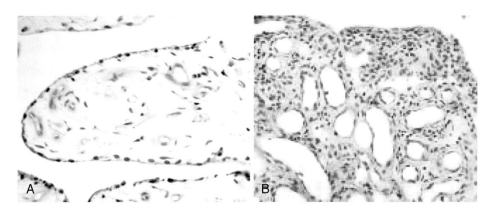

FIGURE 20-2 Synovial pathology in juvenile psoriatic arthritis. **A,** Normal synovium with gracile synovial lining layer supported by a loose connective tissue sublining that contains small blood vessels. **B,** Synovium from a 35-year-old patient with juvenile-onset psoriatic arthritis, demonstrating lining hyperplasia, mononuclear infiltration of the subsynovium, and striking vascular hyperplasia. (Courtesy of D.L. Baeten, University of Amsterdam, The Netherlands.)

TABLE 20-1   Vancouver and ILAR Criteria for Juvenile Psoriatic Arthritis

	VANCOUVER	ILAR (EDMONTON REVISION)
Inclusion	Arthritis plus psoriasis or arthritis plus at least two of the following: Dactylitis Nail pits FHx of psoriasis in a first- or second-degree relative Psoriasis-like rash	Arthritis plus psoriasis or arthritis plus at least two of the following: Dactylitis Nail pits or onycholysis FHx of psoriasis in a first-degree relative
Exclusion	None	1. Arthritis in an HLA-B27–positive male beginning after the sixth birthday 2. AS, ERA, sacroiliitis with IBD, reactive arthritis, or acute anterior uveitis, or a history of one of these disorders in a first-degree relative 3. The presence of IgM RF on at least two occasions at 4. The presence of systemic JIA in a patient 5. Arthritis fulfilling ≥ 2 JIA categories

For both criteria sets, arthritis must be of unknown etiology, begin before the 16th birthday, and persist for at least 6 weeks. Under the Vancouver criteria, "definite JPsA" is arthritis plus psoriasis or arthritis plus three minor criteria, whereas "probable JPsA" is arthritis plus two minor criteria.

AS, Ankylosing spondylitis; *FHx,* family history; *ERA,* enthesitis-related arthritis; *IBD,* inflammatory bowel disease; *RF,* rheumatoid factor.

TABLE 20-2 Clinical Series of Patients with Juvenile Psoriatic Arthritis

YEAR	FIRST AUTHOR	N	% F	DEFINITION OF JPSA	FOLLOW-UP (Y, MEAN)	PSORIASIS %	% ARTHRITIS BEFORE SKIN	% FHX OF PSORIASIS	DACTYLITIS %	% NAIL CHANGES	UVEITIS %
1976	Lambert	43	74	Lambert	11	100	53	40	71	9	0
1977	Calabro	12	58	Arthritis + Psoriasis		100	33		58	92	
1980	Sills	24	71	Lambert*		71*	58			83	8
1982	Shore	60[†]	58	Lambert	10.8	100	43	42	23	77	8
1985	Wesolowska	21	38		4.2		56			86	14
1989	Southwood	35	69	Vancouver	4.4	60	48	88	49		17
1990	Truckenbrodt	48	44	Arthritis + Psoriasis	5	100	50	42	17	67	10
1990	Hamilton	28	57	Arthritis + Psoriasis	8.8	100	21	73	39	71	0
1991	Koo	11	55	Arthritis + Psoriasis		65	36	18		45	18
1996	Roberton	63	70	Vancouver	7		56	85	35		14
2006	Stoll	139	59	Vancouver	2	25	29	53[‡]	37	47[‡]	8
2009	Flato	31	77	ILAR	>15	39	50	75	42	30	19
2013	Butbul Aviel	115	67	Vancouver or ILAR	6.2	83	33	59	31	57	5

Blank = not specified.
*Nail disease counted as cutaneous psoriasis.
[†]Includes 32 from Lambert 1976.
[‡]M. Stoll, P.A. Nigrovic, unpublished data.
Lambert criteria: inflammatory arthritis beginning <16 years, psoriasis preceding or within 15 years of onset, usually negative for rheumatoid factor.

local antigen-driven expansion.[60] CD83[+] dendritic cells are less common than in RA, whereas interleukin (IL)-17–expressing mast cells are more common.[61] Increased numbers of macrophages expressing CD163 are identified in adult PsA and the adult spondyloarthropathies,[53,62] though not as clearly in juvenile-onset disease.[47] CD163 is a scavenger receptor, typically expressed on mature resident tissue macrophages that may help to limit rather than promote inflammation. However, the activity of these cells in the psoriatic synovium is unknown.[62,63]

Complement-fixing immune complexes are not typically found in the psoriatic synovium, and synovial fluid complement levels are usually normal.[64-66] Similarly, citrullinated peptides are observed commonly in the rheumatoid synovium but rarely in PsA.[53]

Entheseal Pathology

Entheseal sites are not readily accessible to biopsy, but small series in adult spondyloarthropathies provide a degree of histological insight.[67-69] A low-grade inflammatory infiltrate is observed, often in association with underlying erosion of bone. This infiltrate is not limited to the surface of the bone and is often more extensive in the bone marrow underlying the enthesis. Such osteitis can be visualized as bone marrow edema by magnetic resonance imaging (MRI).[69-71] Cells observed at the interface include macrophages, lymphocytes (particularly CD8[+] T cells) and occasional neutrophils. A recent studied identified IL-23–responsive T cells in the enthesis, suggesting a key pathway mediating inflammation at these sites.[72] Bone healing is commonly evident, with woven bone filling in the defect left by erosions. This new bone often extends beyond the previous bony surface to interface with the ligament.[67] These observations have given rise to the hypothesis that the new bone formation characteristic of the spondyloarthropathies results from recurrent cycles of injury and healing, perhaps enabled by fluctuations in the degree of inflammation.[67,73] Whether such a mechanism underlies the hypertrophic periostitis observed in some patients with JPsA (see Fig. 20-4, C) is unknown.

PATHOGENESIS

Environmental Contribution

Both psoriasis and psoriatic arthritis exhibit only limited concordance in monozygotic twins, suggesting that environmental contributions play a pivotal role in the development of disease.[74-76] The Koebner phenomenon, in which physical trauma precipitates skin disease, is evident in at least one third of patients with psoriasis[77,78]; there have been reports of psoriatic arthritis being precipitated by physical trauma.[79] Because the entheses are points of mechanical stress, an exaggerated reaction to injury ("deep Koebner phenomenon") could contribute to clinical enthesitis in JPsA, with potential spread to adjacent structures. In adults, the relationship between cigarette smoking and the risk of PsA is controversial.[80,81] Interestingly, in ankylosing spondylitis, smoking correlates with accelerated radiographic progression.[82] Obesity increases the risk of PsA among patients with psoriasis, though the basis of this connection is unknown.[83] Streptococcal infection is a known precipitant for guttate psoriasis, raising the possibility that infection with streptococci or other agents could trigger joint inflammation.[84,85] Indeed, elevated antistreptococcal antibody titers have been observed in adults with psoriatic arthritis compared with other arthritides.[86] In support of a role for bacteria, many rodent arthritis models fail to develop joint disease if deprived of normal bacterial flora. Among these is the rat transgenic for human HLA-B27, which develops features reminiscent of PsA, including synovitis, spondylitis, and nail dystrophy.[87,88] Varicella infection has been reported to precipitate JPsA,[15] but a survey of childhood arthritis found no

correlation between the onset of JPsA and coincident infections with mycoplasma, adenovirus, influenza A or B, parainfluenza, rubella, herpes simplex, or respiratory syncytial virus.[44] Exacerbation of psoriatic arthritis by emotional stress has also been observed in adults[74] and may potentially be modeled by the male DBA/1 mouse, which develops arthritis, dactylitis, and nail dystrophy with aging but only if caged with other mice not originally from the same litter.[89]

Genetic Contribution

There is convincing clinical evidence for a genetic contribution to psoriasis and PsA. More than 50% of patients with childhood-onset psoriasis, with or without JPsA, have a family history of psoriasis (Table 20-2).[9,77,90] The risk for both psoriasis and psoriatic arthritis appears to be transmitted more effectively via the paternal line (genetic imprinting).[91,92] A fiftyfold increased risk for PsA was observed in family members of the adults with PsA, suggesting that a propensity for arthritis is inherited over and above the propensity for psoriasis.[74] Similar results were noted in other studies.[93,94]

Association studies have begun to shed light on the genes that explain these strong familial associations.[75,95] In adults, psoriasis with an onset age of younger than 40 years (type I psoriasis) is more strongly familial than older-onset (type II) disease.[96,97] Type I psoriasis is strongly associated with the major histocompatibility complex (MHC) class I allele HLA-Cw6. This allele is also associated with adult PsA, and possibly with older-onset JPsA in children, but the link appears secondary to risk for psoriasis.[97,98] Certain alleles, including HLA-B27, are overrepresented in patients with PsA compared to psoriasis controls.[99-101] The results of studies of HLA associations in JPsA have been inconsistent, likely because of differences in definitions employed and variability within JPsA across the pediatric age spectrum.[6,7,17,19,98,102]

Beyond the MHC, JPsA has been linked with single nucleotide polymorphisms (SNPs) near genes involved in the autoinflammatory diseases (*MEFV*, *NLRP3*, *NOD2*, and *PSTPIP1*).[103] These associations have not emerged in adult genome-wide association scans and have yet to be replicated. In adult studies, psoriasis and psoriatic arthritis have been associated with SNPs in a range of genes, including *HCP5* (involved with control of viral replication) and genes related to the cytokines TNF, IL-13, and IL-23.[104-106] The association with IL-23R has been corroborated in JPsA.[107] The functional consequences of these SNPs remain to be determined, but the cytokine findings are of particular interest. TNF blockade is markedly beneficial in psoriasis and psoriatic arthritis. IL-23 is involved in the differentiation of proinflammatory Th17 cells, which increase in frequency in the circulation and joints of patients with PsA and are present in psoriatic plaques.[108-111] IL-23–responsive cells are also found in entheses and the aortic root, and IL-23 overexpression in mice can induce a spondyloarthritis phenotype with inflammation at both sites.[72] Genetic studies have linked both psoriasis and PsA to *IL12B*, encoding the common p40 subunit of both IL-12 and IL-23, as well as to the IL-23 receptor *IL23R*. IL-13 suppresses the Th17 axis in favor of differentiation along a Th2 pathway, and the risk allele linked to psoriasis is associated with decreased cytokine production. Murine models suggest that Th17 cells may contribute importantly to arthritis.[112] The implication of these findings is that the Th17 axis may be important in both psoriasis and its associated arthritis. Indeed, the anti-IL-12/IL-23 agent ustekinumab is highly effective for cutaneous psoriasis, although its efficacy for PsA is more modest.[113-115]

Cytokines and Other Mediators

Data on cytokine expression in psoriatic synovium and synovial fluid exhibit considerable variability. The range of mediators expressed is broadly similar to that in other inflammatory arthritides, and includes the classical proinflammatory cytokines TNF, IL-1β, and IL-6, as well as IL-1α; the neutrophil chemoattractant IL-8; the IL-2-like cytokine IL-15; interferon (IFN)-γ; and others.[55,57,58,63,116-119] Proangiogenic factors such as vascular endothelial growth factor (VEGF) are also elevated,[58,120,121] as are matrix metalloproteinases and their inhibitors.[58,63,122] No pattern of mediators has yet emerged as specific for PsA, although compared with RA there are typically higher levels of proangiogenic factors and lower levels of proinflammatory mediators.

Synthesis: Pathogenesis of Juvenile Psoriatic Arthritis

Despite substantial advances in understanding, much remains to be learned about the pathogenesis of psoriatic arthritis. In the proper genetic context, an environmental trigger such as infection or trauma appears to unleash an inflammatory process involving infiltration of lymphocytes as well as neutrophils and other effectors of innate immunity into entheses and synovium. The target of this immune response remains unknown. Lymphocytes likely play a key role, as suggested by clonal expansion of these cells within the synovium and the role of lymphocytes in relevant murine models.[60,72,123] Joint inflammation is accompanied by an exuberant vascular expansion reminiscent of cutaneous psoriasis, with a tendency to promote bone formation as well as injury to cartilage and bone. Whether these principles apply equally to patients with JPsA, including those with early-onset disease, is unknown.

CLINICAL MANIFESTATIONS

Subgroups within JPsA

JPsA is clinically heterogeneous. Age-of-onset data reveal a bimodal distribution, particularly in JPsA defined under the Vancouver criteria (Fig. 20-1).[6-8,21,23] This distribution is similar to that of JIA as a whole, with a peak around ages 2 to 3 years and a second, less prominent peak in adolescence.[22,40,124] Younger patients with JPsA who develop the disease before they are 5 years of age are more commonly female, antinuclear antibody (ANA) positive, and affected by dactylitis, the sausagelike swelling of individual digits.[15,21] This subgroup bears marked clinical and demographic similarity to early-onset oligoarticular JIA, although clinical differences include the tendency to develop dactylitis, to involve the wrists and small joints of the hands and feet, and to progress to polyarticular disease in the absence of effective therapy.[20,24,25,125] The merit of distinguishing these younger patients from oligoarticular JIA is controversial (Box 20-1). By contrast, older children exhibit a gender ratio closer to 1:1, with a tendency to enthesitis and axial disease, more closely resembling adult psoriatic arthritis.[8,15,17,21] The presence of these clinical subgroups helps to explain the long-standing observation that girls with JPsA develop the disease at an earlier age than do boys[7,8,15,19,46] and corroborate data that HLA associations within JPsA depend on the age of onset of disease, as is also true in other subtypes of juvenile arthritis.[98,124]

Peripheral Arthritis

Arthritis in JPsA begins as an oligoarthritis in approximately 60% to 80% of children (Table 20-3). Initial presentation as monoarthritis is relatively common, and in some patients the disease begins with dactylitis in the absence of other joint involvement.[15] The knee is affected most frequently, followed by the ankle; hip arthritis occurs in 10% to 30% (Table 20-3). Even in children in whom arthritis remains oligoarticular, wrists, ankles, and small joints of the hands are more frequently affected than in oligoarticular JIA.[20,24,25] Without effective therapy, polyarticular progression is common.[6,15,19,46] Polyarticular onset is observed in 20% to 40% of cases, though the number of joints

---

BOX 20-1   Psoriatic Arthritis, or Arthritis with Psoriasis?

The recognition of psoriatic arthritis in adults as an entity in its own right emerged gradually out of a number of observations. Inflammatory joint disease is encountered at a rate far higher than expected (10% to 20%) among patients with psoriasis.[34,126,127] This arthritis is often clinically distinctive. Rheumatoid factor is usually absent or present in low titer, distal interphalangeal (DIP) and sacroiliac joints are commonly involved, and radiographs demonstrate new bone formation as well as erosions.[1] Even where psoriatic arthritis is clinically indistinguishable from RA, it appears at a younger age and in males and females equally, often clustered within certain psoriatic families.[26,74] Finally, PsA and RA synovial tissue can be differentiated, to some degree, on the basis of distinctive gross and microscopic features (see the section titled "Pathology"). Taken together, these data provide strong support for the existence of psoriatic arthritis in adults as a distinctive syndrome rather than simply the coincident occurrence of two common diseases.

In contrast, the case for JPsA in children remains controversial. In most respects, patients with JPsA fit somewhere in the spectrum of JIA.[46,128,129] The hallmark psoriatic rash may take years to emerge. Absence of rheumatoid factor does not separate JPsA from most other JIA subtypes. Histopathological data are limited, and interpretation of genetic studies is complicated by issues of definition.[21,23,129,130] Finally, patients with JPsA respond to the therapies used in other JIA patients and generally appear to do equally well.

Nevertheless, there are reasons to suspect that the association between psoriasis and arthritis spans both adults and children.[31] The prevalence of psoriasis in children is 0.5% to 1%, with most showing symptoms in adolescence.[10,11,77] Thus, the identification of a psoriatic diathesis in 7% or more of patients with JIA (of whom 40% or more have the classic rash) is not likely to reflect a chance association. Further, the pattern of arthritis in these children is distinctive in aggregate, if not always in an individual patient. Among younger patients, this includes dactylitis and involvement of small joints in the setting of oligoarthritis; in older patients, it includes an even gender ratio and an appreciable incidence of enthesitis and sacroiliitis.[20,21,25] Disease outcome may also differ.[24] Finally, JPsA (but not other subtypes of JIA) is linked genetically with a single nucleotide polymorphism in the IL-23 receptor that is also associated with PsA in adults.[107]

Although older-onset JPsA patients resemble their adult counterparts, questions remain about arthritis that begins before 5 or 6 years of age.[22,129] Like patients with early-onset oligoarticular JIA, patients showing symptoms of early-onset JPsA are most commonly female, frequently ANA positive, and prone to chronic asymptomatic uveitis.[21] Some share expression of the MHC II antigen HLA-DRB1*0801 (DRw8) associated with early-onset oligoarticular and polyarticular arthritis.[98,131,132] It seems very likely that shared pathophysiological mechanisms underlie these similarities,[22] and it has been proposed that JPsA in this age group is simply early-onset oligoarticular or polyarticular JIA.[129] However, at least under the Vancouver criteria, the proportion of these patients with a recognizable psoriatic diathesis greatly exceeds the less than 0.5% prevalence of psoriasis in this age group.[11] Further, young patients with JPsA manifest changes such as nail pits and dactylitis that are highly specific for psoriatic arthritis in adults, an association noted even before these features were incorporated into the diagnostic criteria.[7,15,133] Therefore, even among younger children, the psoriatic diathesis seems to carry an elevated risk of an arthritis that is phenotypically distinct from other types of JIA. Clarification of the relationship between JPsA and other types of JIA awaits an improved understanding of the biology of these diseases.

TABLE 20-3   Joint Involvement in Juvenile Psoriatic Arthritis

SERIES	SILLS	SHORE	SOUTHWOOD	TRUCKENBRODT	ROBERTON	STOLL	FLATO	BUTBUL AVIEL
YEAR	1980	1982	1989	1990	1996	2006	2009	2013
Oligoarticular onset		73	94	85	73	84	68	55
Cervical spine		32	17		25			2
TMJ			34		40	7		8
Shoulder		23	9	8		3		5
Elbow		43	20	15	30	13	33	14
Wrist	33	62	43	31	43	25	42	22
Small hand joints	88		60	31	62		61	
MCP		53			43			17
PIP		40			51			25
DIP	63	42			27			9
Sacroiliac joint	29		11	17	5	1	0	4
Hip	33	38	23	21	32	11	23	9
Knee	67	77	89	67	84	60	87	67
Ankle		63	63	50	60	51	71	33
Small foot joints	67		46	25	56		42	
Any peripheral small joint	>88	>53	69	>31	>62	57	65	42

All numbers indicate percentage of patients.

involved is often lower than in polyarticular JIA, especially RF-positive disease. As a result, joints affected by JPsA are often asymmetrically distributed.[6,134] Distal interphalangeal (DIP) involvement was identified in 30% to 50% of patients in early JPsA series[16-18] but is less common (10% to 30%) in patients diagnosed according to more inclusive criteria.[6,19,21,46] Fortunately, the highly destructive form of adult PsA known as arthritis mutilans is rare in children.

Axial Arthritis

Unlike most forms of JIA, JPsA is accompanied by an appreciable incidence of sacroiliitis, affecting 10% to 30% of patients in some studies (Table 20-3). Sacroiliitis affects principally patients who were older at the onset of disease.[21,46] These patients exhibit other features reminiscent of the adult spondyloarthropathies, including a balanced gender ratio, a tendency to manifest enthesitis, and an elevated frequency of the HLA-B27 antigen.[21,98] Patients in this older subgroup resemble adults with psoriatic arthritis, in whom definite radiographic sacroiliitis is detected in 30% to 70%.[135-137] Inflammatory disease of the lumbar spine occurs in less than 5% of children with JPsA.[6,19,21] Axial disease in JPsA is generally milder than in ankylosing spondylitis, with a tendency for asymmetric sacroiliac (SI) joint involvement and a failure to progress to spinal ankylosis (Fig. 20-3).[138]

Enthesitis

Enthesitis denotes inflammation localized to the insertion of a tendon, ligament, fascia, or joint capsule into bone. Clinically, enthesitis is diagnosed in children with specific tenderness and occasionally swelling at characteristic sites, in the absence of an alternate (e.g., traumatic) explanation. Using this standard, enthesitis is prevalent in patients within the older subgroup of JPsA, where it was observed in 57%, compared with 22% in younger patients.[21] This finding is in line with adult PsA, where enthesitis is a hallmark feature of the disease and can be documented radiographically in at least one site in many patients[139-142] (see Box 20-2). Typical sites of symptomatic enthesitis include the insertion of the Achilles tendon into the calcaneus and the

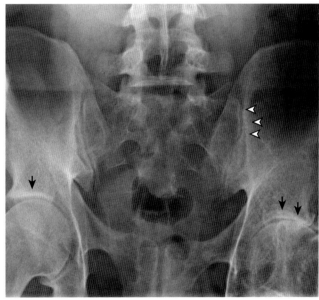

FIGURE 20-3 Sacroiliitis and hip arthritis in juvenile psoriatic arthritis. This radiograph depicts the pelvis and hip joints of a 23-year-old man with psoriasis who developed psoriatic arthritis at age 15. Note sclerosis at the left sacroiliac joint (*arrowheads*) and loss of joint space with reactive sclerosis at the hips, left greater than right (*arrows*).

insertions of the plantar fascia; other sites accessible to examination include the poles of the patellae, the iliac crests, the medial femoral condyles, and lateral epicondyles of the elbow.[140,143] Suspected enthesitis can be confirmed by ultrasound or by MRI.[142,144] Compared with an ultrasound gold standard, entheseal tenderness may overestimate enthesitis; parallel testing of nonentheseal sites is important.[145] Using the ILAR criteria, most children with arthritis and enthesitis are

BOX 20-2   Enthesitis: A Unifying Characteristic of Juvenile Psoriatic Arthritis?

Entheses are subject to substantial mechanical stresses. To dissipate these forces, a number of adaptations have emerged. For example, tendons often become infiltrated with fibrocartilage as they approach the site of insertion into bone, increasing in stiffness to limit the concentration of shear stress at the bone–tendon interface. Because the insertion of the joint capsule into bone is itself an enthesis, and tendons and ligaments frequently insert near joints, the synovial lining is usually in intimate contact with entheses.[146]

MRI studies of adults with psoriatic synovitis have identified edema at periarticular entheses.[70] McGonagle and colleagues have proposed that psoriatic arthritis begins at the enthesis and subsequently extends into the joint.[141] Because entheses are frequent sites of microtrauma, this process may be initiated by mechanical injury.[146]

Entheses in the lower extremities are more prone to inflammation, presumably related to mechanical loading, and this may explain the predilection of PsA for joints of the lower extremity (knee, ankle).[140]

Enthesitis also unifies hallmark features of the psoriatic digit. The finger contains a large number of entheses at sites where intrinsic and extrinsic muscles of the hand insert, as well as all along the shaft of the finger where the fibrous tendon sheath is anchored to prevent "bowstringing" with flexion.[147] Ultrasound and MRI have identified inflammation at these entheses in some but not all studies.[148-152] Such enthesitis may explain why the "sausage digit" is rarely observed in RA despite the occurrence of hand tenosynovitis at least as frequently in RA as in PsA.[153] The DIP joint may be particularly susceptible to inflammation originating at entheses, because the joint capsule is largely replaced by ligaments and tendons residing, therefore, in unusually close proximity to the synovium.[147] These structures become inflamed in PsA of the DIP.[154] Interestingly, the extensor tendon enthesis extends distally along the DIP to interact with the nail bed. By MRI, thickening of the nail bed is present in almost all adults with PsA; more severe thickening is associated with visible changes in the nails, and these patients are prone to DIP synovitis.[155,156] Indeed, flares at the DIP often coincide with worsening psoriatic nail disease, whereas psoriasis and arthritis elsewhere are largely uncorrelated.[26] These results suggest that the primary lesion affecting the distal finger is enthesitis, with "spillover" into DIP synovitis when severe. The connection between finger entheses and the nail bed also explains the otherwise puzzling observation that nail changes may be more common in patients with psoriatic arthritis than in those with isolated skin disease.[1,157,158] (Table 20-2). Further, patients with psoriatic nail changes have been observed to have more enthesitis elsewhere, as determined by ultrasonography.[159] Taken together, these insights suggest that enthesitis could be a distinguishing feature of JPsA not just among older patients but also among younger children in whom dactylitis and nail changes are common presenting features.[21]

classified as enthesitis-related arthritis (ERA) (see Chapter 19), although patients with enthesitis may still be diagnosed with JPsA if they fulfill appropriate criteria.[5,23]

Dactylitis

Dactylitis refers to swelling within a digit that extends beyond the borders of the joints. Such swelling is typically uniform, giving the appearance of a "sausage digit," but can also be fusiform with accentuation around the proximal interphalangeal (PIP) joint (Fig. 20-4, A and B). Radiographically, flexor tenosynovitis is the most evident finding, with or without accompanying synovitis in the nearby joints; edema beyond the tendon sheath is common, suggesting the importance of enthesitis in the full phenotype (Box 20-2).[148-152] Subperiosteal new bone growth can also contribute to the thickness of the digit (Fig 20-4,

C). In children with JPsA, dactylitis is observed in 20% to 40% of patients (Table 20-2). Commonly, only one or a few digits are affected, most commonly the second toe and index finger.[19] Dactylitis may be symptomatic or asymptomatic, and in one series it was the only musculoskeletal finding at presentation in 12% of children with JPsA.[15] Onset after trauma has been reported, and this may explain the predilection for particular digits.[160] The specificity of dactylitis for psoriatic arthritis is incompletely defined. It has been reported in up to 18% of children with non-psoriatic JIA, although some of these children might actually have had JPsA.[6,31,128] Digital swelling also occurs in children with sickle cell disease, tuberculous osteomyelitis, and sarcoid arthropathy, but these are rarely confused with JPsA.

Extraarticular Manifestations

Skin and nail disease. Overt psoriasis occurs in 40% to 60% of patients with JPsA.[6,24] In the large majority of patients, psoriasis presents as the classic vulgaris form, although guttate psoriasis is also observed.[7,8,14,15,17] Pustular and erythrodermic variants are rare.[8] This pattern approximates the presentation of psoriasis in childhood in general.[9] Psoriasis in children tends to be subtle, with thin, soft plaques that may come and go.[9,77] Lesions may be isolated to the hairline, umbilicus, behind the ears, or in the intergluteal crease, and thereby escape ready notice (Figs. 20-5, A and B). Misidentification as eczema is common, and some lesions are in fact ambiguous even to expert examination.[9] There are insufficient data to determine whether psoriasis associated with JPsA differs in age of onset or clinical course from the rest of childhood-onset psoriasis.

One substantial difference between children with JPsA and those with nonarthritic psoriasis is the prevalence of nail changes. Psoriatic changes in the nail surface include pits, onycholysis, horizontal ridging, and discoloration (Fig. 20-5, C). Nail changes accompany childhood psoriasis in up to 30% of cases.[161,162] By contrast, the prevalence of nail changes in JPsA is approximately 50% to 80% of all cases.[8,14,15,21,46] Nail changes are almost uniformly present in both adults and children with DIP involvement, although nail pits are commonly found in the absence of overt DIP arthritis.[157] In adults, the presence of nail pits correlates with a more severe arthritis course, but this association is not obvious in children.[163]

Uveitis

Chronic uveitis, indistinguishable from that in oligoarticular and polyarticular JIA, occurs in 10% to 15% of children with JPsA (Table 20-2).[40,164] As in other JIA subsets, young patients with ANA are at highest risk, and standard uveitis screening guidelines apply (see Chapter 22). Acute anterior uveitis can occur in older children, although chronic uveitis is also observed in this subgroup.[8,18,21,23,165] Acute anterior uveitis is associated with the presence of HLA-B27.[166] In one study, the rate of complications of uveitis was higher in JPsA than in other subtypes of juvenile arthritis.[167]

Other Systemic Manifestations

Children with significant polyarticular JPsA may have the constitutional features of chronic inflammatory disease, including anorexia, anemia, and poor growth. Histological enteritis and occasionally symptomatic colitis are reported.[168] Alternately, psoriasis is associated with obesity, and children with JPsA may exhibit a higher body mass index that places them at risk for metabolic syndrome.[46,169] Fever may rarely occur in very severe cases but should not be ascribed to JPsA without a careful search for alternate causes.[7,26] Amyloidosis is a rare complication of long-standing active disease.[7,16] Adults with psoriasis, and particularly PsA, exhibit an enhanced risk of Crohn's disease.[170] The SAPHO syndrome (synovitis, acne, pustulosis, hyperostosis, and

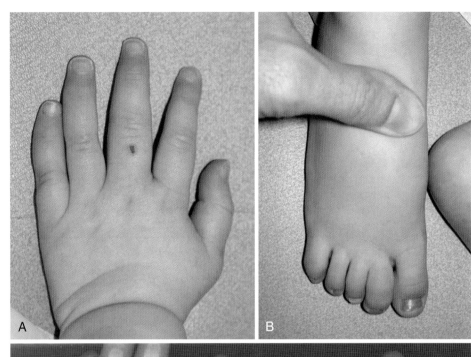

FIGURE 20-4 Dactylitis in juvenile psoriatic arthritis. **A,** Dactylitis of the third finger (with incidental abrasion). **B,** Dactylitis of the second and fifth toes. **C,** Radiograph of the hands from the patient in A, demonstrating periosteal reaction in the affected digit (*arrow*).

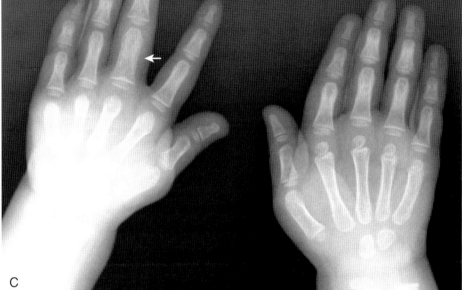

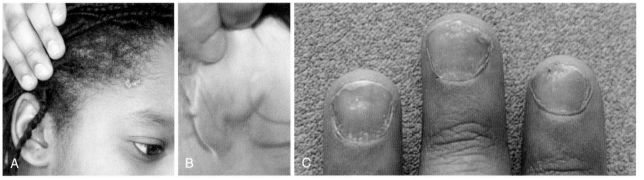

FIGURE 20-5 Cutaneous manifestations in juvenile psoriatic arthritis. **A,** Psoriasis vulgaris on the scalp of a child with polyarticular JPsA. **B,** Scaling behind the retracted ear of a 2-year-old girl with knee monoarthritis and a first-degree family history of psoriasis. This rash is suggestive of psoriasis but not diagnostic. **C,** Nail dystrophy in JPsA. Findings include multiple nail pits, discoloration, and early onycholysis. This example shows florid changes, but more commonly nail findings are subtle and easily missed.

osteitis) and CRMO (chronic recurrent multifocal osteomyelitis) have been associated with psoriasis and may be related to JPsA[171] (see Chapter 48). Other rare complications include lymphedema, aortic incompetence, and mitral valve prolapse.[172-174]

LABORATORY EXAMINATION

Laboratory tests are of limited diagnostic value in JPsA. Inflammatory markers, including the erythrocyte sedimentation rate (ESR) and C-reactive protein (CRP), may exhibit mild to moderate elevation, but they are frequently normal.[15,21] Elevation in the platelet count has been noted in younger patients.[21] ANA is found in low or moderate titer in 60% of younger patients and 30% of older patients; it is helpful primarily to define uveitis risk for the purpose of ophthalmological screening.[21] Antibodies to extractable nuclear antigens are usually absent. RF is typically negative, and indeed its sustained presence excludes a diagnosis of JPsA under ILAR criteria (Table 20-1). The presence of psoriasis may be considered incidental in patients with a clinical presentation otherwise consistent with systemic JIA, or with symmetric polyarthritis positive for RF or anticyclic citrullinated peptide antibodies.[26]

RADIOLOGICAL EXAMINATION

Plain radiographic features of JPsA generally follow a sequence of changes similar to those in other forms of childhood arthritis. In early arthritis, soft tissue swelling around the joint (with or without joint effusion) is the only abnormality. Periarticular osteoporosis may occur

within a few months after the onset of joint swelling, and periosteal new bone formation is common in digits affected by dactylitis (Fig. 20-4, *C*). Joint-space narrowing, indicating significant cartilage loss, and erosive disease of bone are usually late features of JPsA (Fig. 20-6, *A*). Bone remodeling may eventually occur, secondary to persistent periostitis and altered epiphyseal growth, although proliferative new bone formation is less often evident in children than in adults.[71] When it occurs, sacroiliitis is commonly asymmetric (Fig. 20-3).[138] MRI findings in JPsA include synovitis, tendonitis, and bone marrow edema at both articular and nonarticular sites, though the specificity of individual findings for JPsA has not been determined (Fig. 20-6, *B*).[71] Both ultrasound and MRI can be used to assess entheseal involvement. In experienced hands ultrasound may be superior.[144]

TREATMENT

No randomized controlled trials (RCTs) have been conducted in JPsA. Recommendations are therefore extrapolated from RCTs in polyarticular course JIA, from RCTs and clinical practice in adult PsA, and from experience in the treatment of JPsA and other types of JIA.

Peripheral Arthritis

Psoriatic synovitis is potentially destructive of cartilage and bone and like other types of synovitis may compromise bone growth in the immature skeleton. The goal of therapy is remission of symptoms, with normalization of physical findings and laboratory markers of inflammation. Studies, often conducted in adult PsA, support efficacy for nonsteroidal antiinflammatory drugs (NSAIDs); sulfasalazine,

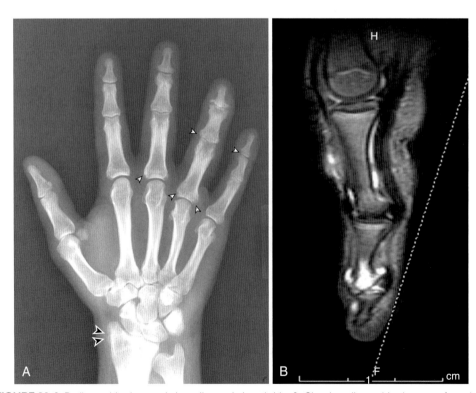

FIGURE 20-6 Radiographic changes in juvenile psoriatic arthritis. **A,** Classic radiographic changes of psoriatic arthritis including soft tissue swelling (dactylitis) of the fourth digit, arthritic and secondary degenerative changes of the fourth DIP joint, joint space loss at fourth and fifth PIP joints, multiple erosions of MCP (metacarpophalangeal), PIP, and DIP joints (solid arrowheads) in the absence of periarticular osteopenia, and fluffy periostitis (open arrowheads) **B,** Sagittal STIR MRI of a finger in JPsA showing DIP synovitis, marrow edema affecting the distal middle phalanx, and possible flexor and extensor tenosynovitis.

methotrexate, leflunomide, or cyclosporine; anti-TNF agents; abatacept; ustekinumab (anti-IL-12/23); and apremilast (phosphodiesterase 4 inhibitor), with some data in favor of secukinumab (anti-IL-17A) and rituximab.[114,115,175-183] No data beyond the case report level are available for tocilizumab (anti-IL-6 receptor).

The basic treatment algorithm for JPsA is similar to that employed in other subtypes of JIA. NSAIDs are often employed initially but typically do not induce remission and are inappropriate as extended monotherapy. Individual large joints can be treated effectively with glucocorticoid injection (see Chapters 12 and 18). In patients with involvement of multiple joints, disease-modifying antirheumatic drugs (DMARDs) such as sulfasalazine or methotrexate are indicated. An inadequate response is addressed by addition of a second DMARD or, more typically, the addition/substitution of anti-TNF therapy. A TNF blockade is particularly useful when there is axial disease, because efficacy for inflammation in the spine and sacroiliac joints is best established for this class of agent (see below). Anti-TNF agents are also the only medications with demonstrated activity against dactylitis and enthesitis. In obese patients, concomitant weight loss may promote a positive therapeutic response to TNF antagonism.[184,185] If one anti-TNF agent has failed, switching to another may prove effective in some patients.[186,187] No specific anti-TNF agent has been shown to be superior in JPsA, however, so both initial and subsequent choices may be made on the basis of convenience, patient preference and tolerability, and cost.

Several specific considerations apply in the choice of agents for psoriatic disease. Based on anecdotal evidence and experience, PsA has been thought to be less responsive to systemic or intraarticular corticosteroids than other types of arthritis. This observation has not been examined rigorously, and both modes of administration are in common use. Substantial doses of systemic corticosteroids can provoke a flare of cutaneous psoriasis when tapered and are avoided when possible. Similarly, antimalarials can worsen cutaneous psoriasis, though the magnitude of this risk is uncertain.[188,189] In any case, evidence for the efficacy of these agents is limited. Methotrexate has been associated in some, but not all, studies with a higher risk of transaminase elevation in adults with PsA than in RA.[175,190,191] It is not clear that this experience is relevant in JPsA, where consequential hepatic injury from methotrexate is extremely rare.

Spondylitis

Treatment of psoriatic spondylitis is based primarily on experience with ankylosing spondylitis (AS).[188] Although axial disease is relatively common in older children and adults with JPsA, it tends to run a milder course. Treatment should be considered in patients who experience axial symptoms or show substantial or progressive limitation of spinal mobility. Continuous treatment with NSAIDs results in measurable radiographic improvement, but the effect is small.[192] Standard DMARDs, including sulfasalazine, methotrexate, and leflunomide are of minimal benefit. Anti-TNF therapy is highly effective for axial disease as assessed both by symptoms and by MRI evidence of inflammation.[188] Early studies in adults failed to show a corresponding reduction in radiographic progression, though a more recent study supports a disease-modifying effect, especially for patients treated early in the course of disease.[73,82,193] Resistant sacroiliitis may be treated with local steroid injections or systemic steroids. Recently, studies in AS have shown efficacy for ustekinumab (anti-IL-12/23) and secukinumab (anti-IL-17A), rendering these agents potential alternatives for resistant axial arthritis.[194,195] By contrast, tocilizumab is ineffective, and IL-1 antagonism with anakinra is of marginal benefit.[196,197]

COURSE AND PROGNOSIS

The long-term outcome of children with JPsA is incompletely defined. Patients followed for at least 15 years demonstrated worse functional outcome than patients with oligoarticular or polyarticular JIA, and 33% still required DMARD therapy.[24] Another study of patients with JPsA followed for at least 5 years demonstrated persistently active disease in 70% and limitations on physical activity in 33%.[19] More recent studies documented achievement of clinical remission (on medication) in approximately 60%, though only a minority achieve remission off medication.[21,46] These data mirror outcomes in adults.[198] Impaired visual function may also occur, especially if uveitis is not discovered promptly.

REFERENCES

1. J.M. Moll, V. Wright, Psoriatic arthritis, Semin. Arthritis Rheum. 3 (1973) 55 78.
5. R.E. Petty, T.R. Southwood, P. Manners, et al., International League of Associations for Rheumatology classification of juvenile idiopathic arthritis: second revision, Edmonton, 2001, J. Rheumatol. 31 (2004) 390–392.
6. T.R. Southwood, R.E. Petty, P.N. Malleson, et al., Psoriatic arthritis in children, Arthritis Rheum. 32 (1989) 1007–1013.
17. M.L. Hamilton, D.D. Gladman, A. Shore, et al., Juvenile psoriatic arthritis and HLA antigens, Ann. Rheum. Dis. 49 (1990) 694–697.
19. D.M. Roberton, D.A. Cabral, P.N. Malleson, R.E. Petty, Juvenile psoriatic arthritis: followup and evaluation of diagnostic criteria, J. Rheumatol. 23 (1996) 166–170.
20. C. Huemer, P.N. Malleson, D.A. Cabral, et al., Patterns of joint involvement at onset differentiate oligoarticular juvenile psoriatic arthritis from pauciarticular juvenile rheumatoid arthritis, J. Rheumatol. 29 (2002) 1531–1535.
21. M.L. Stoll, D. Zurakowski, L.E. Nigrovic, et al., Patients with juvenile psoriatic arthritis comprise two distinct populations, Arthritis Rheum. 54 (2006) 3564–3572.
23. M.L. Stoll, P. Lio, R.P. Sundel, P.A. Nigrovic, Comparison of Vancouver and International League of Associations for rheumatology classification criteria for juvenile psoriatic arthritis, Arthritis Rheum. 59 (2008) 51–58.
24. B. Flato, G. Lien, A. Smerdel-Ramoya, O. Vinje, Juvenile psoriatic arthritis: longterm outcome and differentiation from other subtypes of juvenile idiopathic arthritis, J. Rheumatol. 36 (2009) 642–650.
25. M.L. Stoll, P.A. Nigrovic, A.C. Gotte, M. Punaro, Clinical comparison of early-onset psoriatic and non-psoriatic oligoarticular juvenile idiopathic arthritis, Clin. Exp. Rheumatol. 29 (2011) 582–588.
31. P.A. Nigrovic, Juvenile psoriatic arthritis: bathwater or baby? J. Rheumatol. 36 (2009) 1861–1863.
43. K. Oen, C.M. Duffy, S.M. Tse, et al., Early outcomes and improvement of patients with juvenile idiopathic arthritis enrolled in a Canadian multicenter inception cohort, Arthritis Care Res. (Hoboken) 62 (2010) 527–536.
46. Y. Butbul Aviel, P. Tyrrell, R. Schneider, et al., Juvenile Psoriatic Arthritis (JPsA): juvenile arthritis with psoriasis? Pediatr. Rheumatol. Online J. 11 (2013) 11.
47. E. Kruithof, V. Van den Bossche, L. De Rycke, et al., Distinct synovial immunopathologic characteristics of juvenile-onset spondylarthritis and other forms of juvenile idiopathic arthritis, Arthritis Rheum. 54 (2006) 2594–2604.
53. E. Kruithof, D. Baeten, L. De Rycke, et al., Synovial histopathology of psoriatic arthritis, both oligo- and polyarticular, resembles spondyloarthropathy more than it does rheumatoid arthritis, Arthritis Res. Ther. 7 (2005) R569–R580.
58. A.W. van Kuijk, P. Reinders-Blankert, T.J. Smeets, et al., Detailed analysis of the cell infiltrate and the expression of mediators of synovial inflammation and joint destruction in the synovium of patients with psoriatic

arthritis: implications for treatment, Ann. Rheum. Dis. 65 (2006) 1551–1557.

62. D. Baeten, P. Demetter, C.A. Cuvelier, et al., Macrophages expressing the scavenger receptor CD163: a link between immune alterations of the gut and synovial inflammation in spondyloarthropathy, J. Pathol. 196 (2002) 343–350.

64. T.J. Pekin Jr., N.J. Zvaifler, Hemolytic Complement in Synovial Fluid, J. Clin. Invest. 43 (1964) 1372–1382.

69. D. McGonagle, H. Marzo-Ortega, P. O'Connor, et al., Histological assessment of the early enthesitis lesion in spondyloarthropathy, Ann. Rheum. Dis. 61 (2002) 534–537.

70. D. McGonagle, W. Gibbon, P. O'Connor, et al., Characteristic magnetic resonance imaging entheseal changes of knee synovitis in spondylarthropathy, Arthritis Rheum. 41 (1998) 694–700.

72. J.P. Sherlock, B. Joyce-Shaikh, S.P. Turner, et al., IL-23 induces spondyloarthropathy by acting on ROR-gammat+ CD3+CD4-CD8- entheseal resident T cells, Nat. Med. 18 (2012) 1069–1076.

74. J.M. Moll, V. Wright, Familial occurrence of psoriatic arthritis, Ann. Rheum. Dis. 32 (1973) 181–201.

82. N. Haroon, R.D. Inman, T.J. Learch, et al., The impact of tumor necrosis factor alpha inhibitors on radiographic progression in ankylosing spondylitis, Arthritis Rheum. 65 (2013) 2645–2654.

87. R.E. Hammer, S.D. Maika, J.A. Richardson, et al., Spontaneous inflammatory disease in transgenic rats expressing HLA-B27 and human beta 2m: an animal model of HLA-B27-associated human disorders, Cell 63 (1990) 1099–1112.

88. J.D. Taurog, J.A. Richardson, J.T. Croft, et al., The germfree state prevents development of gut and joint inflammatory disease in HLA-B27 transgenic rats, J. Exp. Med. 180 (1994) 2359–2364.

89. R.J. Lories, P. Matthys, K. de Vlam, et al., Ankylosing enthesitis, dactylitis, and onychoperiostitis in male DBA/1 mice: a model of psoriatic arthritis, Ann. Rheum. Dis. 63 (2004) 595–598.

92. P. Rahman, D.D. Gladman, C.T. Schentag, A. Petronis, Excessive paternal transmission in psoriatic arthritis, Arthritis Rheum. 42 (1999) 1228–1231.

93. A. Myers, L.J. Kay, S.A. Lynch, D.J. Walker, Recurrence risk for psoriasis and psoriatic arthritis within sibships, Rheumatology (Oxford) 44 (2005) 773–776.

96. P. Rahman, C.T. Schentag, D.D. Gladman, Immunogenetic profile of patients with psoriatic arthritis varies according to the age at onset of psoriasis, Arthritis Rheum. 42 (1999) 822–823.

99. R. Winchester, G. Minevich, V. Steshenko, et al., HLA associations reveal genetic heterogeneity in psoriatic arthritis and in the psoriasis phenotype, Arthritis Rheum. 64 (2012) 1134–1144.

100. L. Eder, V. Chandran, F. Pellett, et al., Differential human leucocyte allele association between psoriasis and psoriatic arthritis: a family-based association study, Ann. Rheum. Dis. 71 (2012) 1361–1365.

101. L. Eder, V. Chandran, F. Pellet, et al., Human leucocyte antigen risk alleles for psoriatic arthritis among patients with psoriasis, Ann. Rheum. Dis. 71 (2012) 50–55.

102. W. Thomson, J.H. Barrett, R. Donn, et al., Juvenile idiopathic arthritis classified by the ILAR criteria: HLA associations in UK patients, Rheumatology (Oxford) 41 (2002) 1183–1189.

105. Y. Liu, C. Helms, W. Liao, et al., A genome-wide association study of psoriasis and psoriatic arthritis identifies new disease loci, PLoS Genet. 4 (2008) e1000041.

108. C. Jandus, G. Bioley, J.P. Rivals, et al., Increased numbers of circulating polyfunctional Th17 memory cells in patients with seronegative spondylarthritides, Arthritis Rheum. 58 (2008) 2307–2317.

114. A. Gottlieb, A. Menter, A. Mendelsohn, et al., Ustekinumab, a human interleukin 12/23 monoclonal antibody, for psoriatic arthritis: randomised, double-blind, placebo-controlled, crossover trial, Lancet 373 (2009) 633–640.

115. I.B. McInnes, A. Kavanaugh, A.B. Gottlieb, et al., Efficacy and safety of ustekinumab in patients with active psoriatic arthritis: 1 year results of the phase 3, multicentre, double-blind, placebo-controlled PSUMMIT 1 trial, Lancet 382 (2013) 780–789.

117. C. Ritchlin, S.A. Haas-Smith, D. Hicks, et al., Patterns of cytokine production in psoriatic synovium, J. Rheumatol. 25 (1998) 1544–1552.

123. R. Zenz, R. Eferl, L. Kenner, et al., Psoriasis-like skin disease and arthritis caused by inducible epidermal deletion of Jun proteins, Nature 437 (2005) 369–375.

124. K.J. Murray, M.B. Moroldo, P. Donnelly, et al., Age-specific effects of juvenile rheumatoid arthritis-associated HLA alleles, Arthritis Rheum. 42 (1999) 1843–1853.

133. W. Taylor, D. Gladman, P. Helliwell, et al., Classification criteria for psoriatic arthritis: development of new criteria from a large international study, Arthritis Rheum. 54 (2006) 2665–2673.

134. P.S. Helliwell, J. Hetthen, K. Sokoll, et al., Joint symmetry in early and late rheumatoid and psoriatic arthritis: comparison with a mathematical model, Arthritis Rheum. 43 (2000) 865–871.

135. D.D. Gladman, R. Shuckett, M.L. Russell, et al., Psoriatic arthritis (PSA)–an analysis of 220 patients, Q. J. Med. 62 (1987) 127–141.

137. L. Williamson, J.L. Dockerty, N. Dalbeth, et al., Clinical assessment of sacroiliitis and HLA-B27 are poor predictors of sacroiliitis diagnosed by magnetic resonance imaging in psoriatic arthritis, Rheumatology (Oxford) 43 (2004) 85–88.

139. P.V. Balint, D. Kane, H. Wilson, et al., Ultrasonography of entheseal insertions in the lower limb in spondyloarthropathy, Ann. Rheum. Dis. 61 (2002) 905–910.

141. D. McGonagle, R.J. Lories, A.L. Tan, M. Benjamin, The concept of a "synovio-entheseal complex" and its implications for understanding joint inflammation and damage in psoriatic arthritis and beyond, Arthritis Rheum. 56 (2007) 2482–2491.

142. R.P. Poggenborg, I. Eshed, M. Ostergaard, et al., Enthesitis in patients with psoriatic arthritis, axial spondyloarthritis and healthy subjects assessed by "head-to-toe" whole-body MRI and clinical examination, Ann. Rheum. Dis. (2014 Jan 3) doi:10.1136/annrheumdis-2013-204239; [Epub ahead of print].

149. I. Olivieri, C. Salvarani, F. Cantini, et al., Fast spin echo-T2-weighted sequences with fat saturation in dactylitis of spondylarthritis. No evidence of entheseal involvement of the flexor digitorum tendons, Arthritis Rheum. 46 (2002) 2964–2967.

156. A.L. Tan, M. Benjamin, H. Toumi, et al., The relationship between the extensor tendon enthesis and the nail in distal interphalangeal joint disease in psoriatic arthritis–a high-resolution MRI and histological study, Rheumatology (Oxford) 46 (2007) 253–256.

162. N. Al-Mutairi, Y. Manchanda, O. Nour-Eldin, Nail changes in childhood psoriasis: a study from Kuwait, Pediatr. Dermatol. 24 (2007) 7–10.

165. E.S. Paiva, D.C. Macaluso, A. Edwards, J.T. Rosenbaum, Characterisation of uveitis in patients with psoriatic arthritis, Ann. Rheum. Dis. 59 (2000) 67–70.

177. G. Horneff, R. Burgos-Vargas, T. Constantin, et al., Efficacy and safety of open-label etanercept on extended oligoarticular juvenile idiopathic arthritis, enthesitis-related arthritis and psoriatic arthritis: part 1 (week 12) of the CLIPPER study, Ann. Rheum. Dis. 73 (2014) 1114–1122.

178. P. Mease, M.C. Genovese, G. Gladstein, et al., Abatacept in the treatment of patients with psoriatic arthritis: results of a six-month, multicenter, randomized, double-blind, placebo-controlled, phase II trial, Arthritis Rheum. 63 (2011) 939–948.

179. G. Schett, J. Wollenhaupt, K. Papp, et al., Oral apremilast in the treatment of active psoriatic arthritis: results of a multicenter, randomized, double-blind, placebo-controlled study, Arthritis Rheum. 64 (2012) 3156–3167.

180. I.B. McInnes, J. Sieper, J. Braun, et al., Efficacy and safety of secukinumab, a fully human anti-interleukin-17A monoclonal antibody, in patients with moderate-to-severe psoriatic arthritis: a 24-week, randomised, double-blind, placebo-controlled, phase II proof-of-concept trial, Ann. Rheum. Dis. 73 (2014) 349–356.

186. B. Glintborg, M. Ostergaard, N.S. Krogh, et al., Clinical response, drug survival, and predictors thereof among 548 patients with psoriatic arthritis who switched tumor necrosis factor alpha inhibitor therapy: results from the Danish Nationwide DANBIO Registry, Arthritis Rheum. 65 (2013) 1213–1223.

187. K.M. Fagerli, E. Lie, D. van der Heijde, et al., Switching between TNF inhibitors in psoriatic arthritis: data from the NOR-DMARD study, Ann. Rheum. Dis. 72 (2013) 1840–1844.

190. H. Amital, Y. Arnson, G. Chodick, V. Shalev, Hepatotoxicity rates do not differ in patients with rheumatoid arthritis and psoriasis treated with methotrexate, Rheumatology (Oxford) 48 (2009) 1107–1110.

192. A. Wanders, D. Heijde, R. Landewe, et al., Nonsteroidal antiinflammatory drugs reduce radiographic progression in patients with ankylosing spondylitis: a randomized clinical trial, Arthritis Rheum. 52 (2005) 1756–1765.

195. D. Baeten, X. Baraliakos, J. Braun, et al., Anti-interleukin-17A monoclonal antibody secukinumab in treatment of ankylosing spondylitis: a randomised, double-blind, placebo-controlled trial, Lancet 382 (2013) 1705–1713.

The entire reference list is available online at www.expertconsult .com.

Arthropathies of Inflammatory Bowel Disease

Carol B. Lindsley, Ronald M. Laxer

DEFINITION AND CLASSIFICATION

The arthropathies of inflammatory bowel disease (IBD) may be defined as any noninfectious arthritis occurring before or during the course of Crohn's disease (CD), indeterminate colitis (IC), or ulcerative colitis (UC). Arthritis is the most common extraintestinal complication of these disorders.[1] There are two patterns of joint inflammation that can accompany IBD: peripheral polyarthritis and, less commonly, involvement of the sacroiliac (SI) joints and axial skeleton. Arthritis associated with IBD is not included in the American College of Rheumatology classification of childhood arthritis but is included in both the European League Against Rheumatism and the International League of Associations for Rheumatology criteria (see Chapter 15).

EPIDEMIOLOGY

Incidence and Prevalence

Arthropathy has been reported in 7% to 21% of children with IBD[2-6] (Table 21-1). Passo and colleagues[6] found arthritis in 9% of 44 children with UC and in 15.5% of 58 children with CD. Arthralgia was much more common than arthritis in children, occurring in 32% of those with UC and 22% of those with CD.[6] Differentiation of UC from CD is not always easy, and differences in the reported frequencies of arthritis in each may reflect the accuracy of diagnosis in these types of IBD.[3,4] A recent study showed much lower frequencies of 1% in CD and 2% in UC. These lower frequencies may reflect the current biological therapies for IBD.[7] However, a recent study of adults with spondyloarthropathy showed a fourfold cumulative incidence over 30 years.[8] A Swedish study reported a stable and unchanged rate of UC and CD during the past 30 years.[9] Regional differences may also exist, as shown by a recent study of northeastern Slovenia children, which demonstrated an increased incidence.[10]

Musculoskeletal pain in children with IBD may be related to other causes including bone fractures secondary to osteoporosis (disease and glucocorticoid induced), secondary hypertrophic osteoarthropathy and noninflammatory causes such as hypermobility.

Age at Onset and Sex Ratio

In a study of 136 patients with onset of IBD before the age of 20 years,[5] age at onset did not differ in patients who had arthritis or those who did not. The ratios of boys to girls in those with and without peripheral arthritis were almost identical, although the five children who developed spondylitis were boys.

ETIOLOGY AND PATHOGENESIS

The causes of both IBD and its accompanying arthritis are obscure. The possible roles of gastrointestinal (GI) infections or allergic reactions to foods absorbed across an inflamed mucosa remain speculative. The SI arthritis probably shares its etiology with that of ankylosing spondylitis (AS), and studies of associated enteric species and immunity to them may be relevant.[11] Peripheral arthropathy may involve entirely different immunoinflammatory mechanisms (immune complexes), however, and it is clinically more closely related to the activity of the intestinal disease. Picco and colleagues[12] found increased gut permeability in all subtypes of juvenile arthritis using the lactulose/mannitol test, but IBD patients with spondyloarthropathy had the highest levels. Reciprocally, subclinical gut inflammation in the majority of patients with seronegative spondyloarthropathy has been described.[13]

GENETIC BACKGROUND

There is a pronounced tendency for familial, racial, and ethnic clustering of UC and CD. Hamilton and associates[3] reported that approximately 15% of children with UC and 8% of those with CD had first-degree relatives with IBD. Both diseases are more common in children of Jewish descent, who comprised 21% of the IBD population but only 2% of the general population in one study.[3] Published reports support the view that genes of the major histocompatibility complex are important in determining susceptibility to UC in particular,[14] but inherited predispositions are undoubtedly polygenic. In Japanese[15] and Jewish patients,[16] but not in other ethnic groups, the human leukocyte antigen (HLA) DRB1*1502 (DR2) allele is increased in frequency. It is estimated that SI arthritis is at least 30 times more common in patients with IBD than in the general population,[17] a fact that reflects the high frequency of HLA-B27 in such patients. The peripheral polyarthritis accompanying IBD has no known HLA association.

Studies have identified NOD2/Card 15 variants that are associated with CD in both children and adults, particularly in those with ileal disease and lower weight at time of diagnosis.[18] However, no association has been reported with articular involvement or AS.[19] Recently, genome-wide associations between the IL-23R gene and CD have been shown in the pediatric age group.[20] In a separate study, Leshinsky and colleagues showed that haplotypes without the common disease-associated mutations in the NOD2/Card 15 and Toll-like receptor (TLR) genes are associated with age at onset of the IBD.[21] Epigenetic factors may also play a role, adding complexity to understanding IBD.

CLINICAL MANIFESTATIONS

Arthritis and Enthesitis

Two distinct patterns of joint disease occur. The more common one in patients with IBD is peripheral arthritis. Lower extremity joints, especially ankles and knees, are most frequently affected,[4-6] although upper extremity joints, occasionally also including small joints of the hand

TABLE 21-1 Arthritis in Inflammatory Bowel Disease in Children

AUTHOR AND YEAR	DISEASE	NUMBER OF PATIENTS	NUMBER WITH ARTHRITIS	% WITH ARTHRITIS
Farmer & Michener, 1979[2]	CD	522	39	7
Hamilton et al., 1979[3]	CD	58	11	19
Burbige et al., 1975[4]	CD	58	6	10
Lindsley & Schaller, 1974[5]	CD	50	5	10
Passo et al., 1986[6]	CD	58	9	15
Lindsley & Schaller, 1974[5]	UC	86	18	21
Hamilton et al., 1979[3]	UC	87	8	9
Passo et al., 1986[6]	UC	44	4	9

CD, Crohn's disease; *UC*, ulcerative colitis.

and the temporomandibular joints, may be involved. Lindsley and Schaller[5] reported that four or fewer joints were affected at onset or during the course of the illness in 11 of 18 children; in five children, five to nine joints were affected; in only two children were more than 10 joints affected, including small joints of the hand. Episodes of acute peripheral arthritis are usually brief, lasting 1 or 2 weeks (occasionally longer), and tend to recur.[6] In some children, arthritis may last for several months, particularly if the GI disease is active. If joint inflammation persists for months, permanent functional loss or joint damage is unusual. However, erosive disease has been described in young adults with juvenile-onset disease.[22,23] Whereas the SI arthritis bears little relation to the activity of the gut disease, the peripheral arthritis may reflect the activity and course of the GI inflammation. A clinical flare in a child's arthritis was associated with increased musculoskeletal symptoms in 33% of patients with IBD, and an additional 7% had increased symptoms just prior to an IBD flare.[24]

In adult patients, additional clinical phenotypes have been described in the peripheral arthropathy group (non–HLA-B27 associated): type I, which is similar to the previously described disease and is frequently associated with uveitis and erythema nodosum (EN), and type II, which is a symmetrical polyarthritis that is independent of IBD activity, of longer duration, and rarely associated with EN.[25]

SI arthritis, which may be asymptomatic but often is characterized by pain and stiffness in the lower back, buttocks, or thighs, is a much less common complication of IBD than is polyarthritis. It is sometimes accompanied by enthesitis identical to that occurring in other forms of spondyloarthritis. SI arthritis may also be associated with chronic symmetrical oligoarthritis predominantly affecting the joints of the lower limbs: 5% to 10% of established cases of AS in adults are associated with chronic IBD.[26] Also, an additional category of asymptomatic SI disease (18%) occurs in patients with IBD, most often in those with greater disease duration.[27] This may apply to the pediatric age group as well.

Hypertrophic osteoarthropathy is a relatively rare, very painful musculoskeletal complication of IBD.[28] The pain occurs symmetrically in the limbs (rather than the joints) and may be accompanied by increased sweating and purple discoloration of the affected limbs.

Osteoporosis can be a significant component of articular disease or, rarely, a presenting manifestation when associated with fractures.[29] Patients treated with corticosteroids are especially at high risk. In addition they may develop avascular necrosis, most commonly involving the femoral head. However, patients who were not treated with steroids have about a 12% risk of developing osteoporosis as well.[30] Chronic recurrent multifocal osteomyelitis has been associated with IBD in some patients.[31]

Infantile-onset IBD is a particularly severe form of IBD that appears to be an autoinflammatory disease. It results from mutations in

TABLE 21-2 Gastrointestinal and Other Systemic Diseases in Children with Inflammatory Bowel Diseases

SYMPTOM OR SIGN	ULCERATIVE COLITIS	CROHN'S DISEASE
Diarrhea	++++	++
Hematochezia	++	+
Abdominal pain	++	+++
Weight loss	++	++++
Fever	+	+++
Vomiting	+	++
Perianal disease	+	+++
Finger clubbing	+	++
Erythema nodosum	+	+
Oral lesions	+	+
Uveitis	(+)	(+)
Pyoderma gangrenosum	(+)	(+)

interleukin (IL)-10 or its receptor and has been associated with treatment-resistant colitis, perianal fistula formation, folliculitis, and arthritis. Due to the severe morbidity and mortality, hematopoietic stem-cell transplantation should be considered early in the course of disease and may be curative.[32]

Gastrointestinal Disease and Extraarticular Manifestations
Gastrointestinal Disease

Cramping abdominal pain, often with localized or generalized tenderness, anorexia, and diarrhea, sometimes occurring at night, is characteristic of IBD. Differentiation of UC and CD on the basis of GI symptoms alone is unreliable, although bloody diarrhea is highly suggestive of UC, whereas perianal skin tags and fistulae are typical of CD (Table 21-2). More recent terminology adds the category of IC.[7] Many of these patients will meet criteria for a revised diagnosis, usually UC, within 2 years.[7]

GI symptoms usually precede joint disease by months or years. However, occasionally both systems are affected simultaneously, or joint symptoms can precede intestinal disease. In the latter case, the arthritis resembles that of juvenile idiopathic arthritis (JIA), juvenile AS, or the seronegative enthesopathy and arthropathy syndrome, with a course punctuated by intermittent abdominal pain that may be incorrectly ascribed to the effects of antiinflammatory drugs. Low-grade diarrhea, anemia, unexplained fever, weight loss, growth retardation out of proportion to the extent and activity of the joint disease, or a family history of IBD should alert the physician to the possibility of occult IBD. Mucocutaneous lesions (EN, aphthous stomatitis, pyoderma gangrenosum) seem to be more common in children who have arthritis (especially peripheral arthritis) as a complication of IBD, although this association is not supported by some clinical studies.[6]

Although there are no clear-cut correlations between the extent of GI inflammation and arthritis, most reports support the view that there is a higher frequency of arthritis in children with extensive, as opposed to segmental, bowel disease.[2,3,6] Patients with arthritis usually have active gut disease, although the onset of arthritis is not necessarily related to obvious flare-ups in GI tract inflammation. The occurrence of first-time joint symptoms after proctocolectomy for UC has been associated with the development of "pouchitis."[33]

Erythema Nodosum

The lesions of EN (nodular panniculitis) occur most commonly in the subcutaneous fat of the pretibial region (Fig. 21-1) as erythematous, painful, slightly elevated lesions, 1 to 2 cm in diameter, which erupt in groups and reappear sequentially in new areas after several days. The nodules tend to persist for several weeks and recur in crops for several months. As they heal, they frequently leave pigmented areas that persist for many months. Articular pain and synovitis accompany each exacerbation in approximately two thirds of instances. Erythema nodosum is more likely associated with peripheral arthritis that is of short duration and involving few joints.[25]

Pyoderma Gangrenosum

The lesions of pyoderma gangrenosum may occur alone or in concert with IBD (Fig. 21-2). They often arise after minor trauma, may be single or multiple, and usually begin as a pustule that breaks down and rapidly enlarges to form a chronic, painful, deep, undermined ulcer with a red, raised border. They have rarely been reported in children but may in fact be the initial clinical manifestation. In adults, the lesions occur with IBD, rheumatoid arthritis, or other systemic diseases.[34] A single report, not confirmed, of pyoderma gangrenosum in a 2-year-old boy with joint effusions, but without IBD, was associated with enhanced leukocyte mobility.[35] This may have been an early description of the pyogenic arthritis, pyoderma gangrenosum and acne syndrome (see Chapter 47).

Oral Lesions

Occasionally, painful oral ulcerations are seen, particularly in CD (Fig. 21-3). These may precede the onset of prominent GI symptoms. If recurrent, the patient may be misdiagnosed as having Behçet disease. Lip swelling secondary to cheilitis granulomatosa is a rare presentation of CD.[36]

Vasculitis

Vasculitis of several types has been reported in patients with IBD and arthritis. Involvement of large vessels was found in at least two studies.[37,38] Takayasu arteritis in patients with CD was first described in 1970[39] and has been reported in several other adults and in a 15-year-old boy[40]; it has also been described in a young adult with UC and

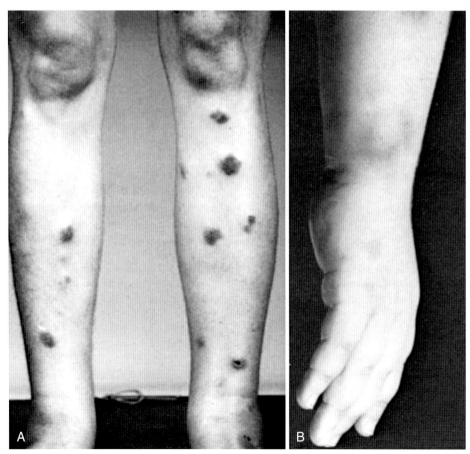

FIGURE 21-1 Erythema nodosum. **A,** This young girl had tender, circumscribed, purple-red nodules on the shins. **B,** Lesions on the forearm of a child.

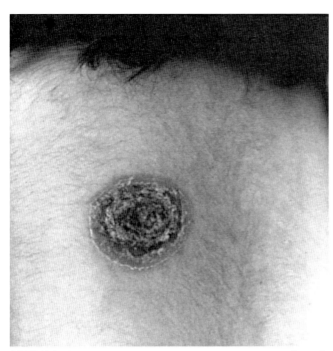

FIGURE 21-2 Pyoderma gangrenosum on the upper back of a child. These lesions begin as nodules but progress to ulcers with considerable loss of subcutaneous tissue.

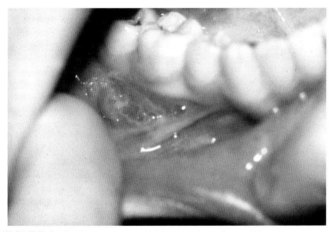

FIGURE 21-3 Oral ulcer in a child with ulcerative colitis.

juvenile AS.[41] It seems unlikely that coincidence could account for the simultaneous occurrence of these rare diseases, but the data are insufficient to allow for certainty. A syndrome of cutaneous vasculitis, glomerulonephritis, and circulating immune complexes was reported in two adults with IBD and spondyloarthritis (one with juvenile-onset colitis).[42] Immunoglobulin A nephropathy has been described in AS and in at least three patients with IBD.[43,44] Cutaneous vasculitis was reported as the presenting feature in a 14-year-old girl with CD.[45] Numerous reports of cerebral vasculitis also exist.[46]

Uveitis

Lyons and Rosenbaum[47] compared the characteristics of uveitis in 17 adults with IBD and 89 patients with spondyloarthritis. Twelve of the 15 patients with uveitis and IBD had CD, and 82% were female. Uveitis accompanying IBD was usually bilateral, posterior, and of insidious onset and chronic duration. The frequency of HLA-B27 was half that in the spondyloarthritis group. Episcleritis, scleritis, and glaucoma were more common among patients with IBD. At least in adults, the

uveitis associated with IBD was frequently complicated by cataract (35%), glaucoma (24%), cystoid macular edema (24%), or posterior synechiae (29%). There are no reported studies of uveitis in children with IBD and arthritis. However, it is known that children with IBD may develop asymptomatic uveitis.[48]

PATHOLOGY

The histopathology of the synovitis of IBD is nonspecific with proliferation of lining cells and infiltration of the synovium with lymphocytes, plasma cells, and histiocytes.[49] Granulomatous synovitis occasionally occurs.[50] For a discussion on the full spectrum of the histopathology of IBD, the reader is referred to current textbooks of gastroenterology.

DIAGNOSIS AND LABORATORY EXAMINATION

Making the diagnosis of arthritis associated with IBD rests on recognition of the significance of this association and on a high level of clinical suspicion. A diagnosis of IBD should be suspected in any child with arthritis who also has lower abdominal pain, hematochezia, unexplained weight loss, anemia, fever, or poor growth. Occult GI blood loss can be verified by repeated stool guaiac examinations.

This suspicion would be supported by laboratory evidence of inflammation (high erythrocyte sedimentation rate, C-reactive protein and other acute phase reactants, low serum albumin), and negative results for rheumatoid factor and antinuclear antibody tests. Antibodies to neutrophil cytoplasmic antigens (pANCA—a perinuclear pattern on immunofluorescence) and anti-*Saccharomyces cerevisiae* antibody (ASCA) are frequently present in the sera of children with IBD.[51] Tests for antineutrophil cytoplasmic antibody (ANCA) were positive in 73% of children with UC and 14% of those with CD.[52] In spite of the known association of this autoantibody with systemic vasculitis, vasculitis does not appear to be more frequent in ANCA-positive patients with IBD.[53] Noninvasive markers of intestinal inflammation in IBD including fecal lactoferrin, calprotectin, and polymorphonuclear neutrophil elastase can be helpful in early diagnosis as they distinguish between active and inactive IBD as well as irritable bowel syndrome.[54]

In addition, early diagnosis can be aided by the use of wireless capsule endoscopy in children presenting with arthropathy in whom traditional endoscopic studies are negative.[55]

Synovial fluid analyses of children with IBD have not been reported, although in adults counts of synovial fluid white blood cells have ranged from 5000 to 15,000/mm³ (5 to 15 × 10⁹/L), with a predominance of neutrophils. Synovial fluid protein, glucose, and hemolytic complement levels have been normal.[56]

RADIOLOGICAL EXAMINATION

Radiographs of peripheral joints document only soft tissue thickening and joint effusions. SI arthritis, when it occurs, is not clearly distinguishable from that associated with juvenile AS. Periostitis may be demonstrable by radiography or by radionuclide scanning (Fig. 21-4). Burbige and co-workers[4] noted erosive lesions secondary to granulomatous synovitis in one child. Although radionucleotide scanning or magnetic resonance imaging is optimal for documenting early changes in SI joints, high-resolution computed tomography is more reliable in detecting erosions.[57]

TREATMENT

Successful management of the peripheral arthritis generally depends on effective treatment of the GI disease: Control of the primary disease

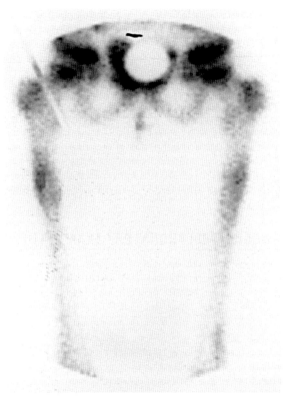

FIGURE 21-4 Bone scan documents increased uptake in the sacroiliac joints and along the femoral shafts, representing sacroiliac joint arthritis and periostitis in a 14-year-old girl with ulcerative colitis.

usually results in remission of the peripheral arthritis. Colectomy in UC may be followed by a striking remission in peripheral joint symptoms, although colectomy for the control of peripheral joint arthritis alone is certainly not indicated. Peripheral arthritis may be managed with nonsteroidal antiinflammatory agents, but there is increasing evidence that these drugs can exacerbate IBD.[58] Selective cyclooxygenase-2 inhibitors may be preferred in this situation. Early use of sulfasalazine or glucocorticoids may provide the best management of the arthropathy of IBD directly by way of a beneficial effect on the GI inflammation, although no therapeutic trials have been published. For persistent arthritis in one or two joints, intraarticular glucocorticoid should be considered. In CD, the use of oral budesonide, predominantly a topically acting steroid, resulted in the remission of joint symptoms in 74% of affected patients.[59]

Methotrexate results in improvement of both GI symptoms and arthritis in CD.[60] Anti–tumor necrosis factor (TNF) therapy, particularly infliximab, produced prompt, substantial improvement of GI symptoms as well as arthritis in CD.[61] Adalimumab may be useful as well, and there is reported improvement in bowel manifestations in patients who failed infliximab and subsequently were treated with adalimumab.[62] As these potent antiinflammatory drugs are used earlier and more aggressively in the treatment of IBD, it is possible that the associated arthropathies will decrease in frequency or severity. However, patients with JIA have developed CD while undergoing anti-TNF therapy, mainly while taking etanercept.[63-65] Patients with enthesitis-related arthritis (ERA), psoriatic arthritis, and extended oligoarticular JIA may have increased risk for developing IBD.[66]

The HLA-B27–associated spondylitis of IBD is much more likely than the peripheral arthritis to persist and progress without remission, independent of the activity of the GI disease and unaffected by procedures such as colectomy. It is therefore much more difficult to manage

in the long term. Sulfasalazine is the initial drug of choice, in a dose of 30 to 50 mg/kg/day to a maximum of 2.5 g/day. Methotrexate and anti-TNF agents may also be helpful in patients who have no response to initial therapy.[67] A physical therapy program with range-of-motion exercises to maintain back and chest motion (as for juvenile AS) may help to prevent or slow the effects of the disease. Custom-made orthotics may be useful to minimize pain secondary to enthesitis around the foot. Vasculitis accompanying IBD should be treated with systemic glucocorticoids. Topical glucocorticoids are used to treat uveitis, at least initially, but more immunosuppression with methotrexate or anti-TNF agents may be required.

COURSE OF THE DISEASE AND PROGNOSIS

The outcome of GI disease is the most important determinant of overall prognosis in the child with IBD and arthritis.[2] Prognosis of the peripheral joint disease is usually excellent, although axial disease may progress independent of the course of the GI inflammation. Permanent changes in the spine and hips are frequent in this group of children. Poor nutrition and accompanying growth retardation may be major problems in poorly controlled disease. Advances in therapeutics will no doubt result in improved short- and long-term outcomes for patients with IBD and associated arthritis.

REFERENCES

1. F.A. Jose, E.A. Garnett, E. Vittinghoff, et al., Development of extraintestinal manifestations in pediatric patients with inflammatory bowel disease, Inflamm. Bowel Dis. 15 (2009) 63–83.
2. R.G. Farmer, W.M. Michener, Prognosis of Crohn's disease with onset in childhood or adolescence, Dig. Dis. Sci. 24 (1979) 752.
3. J.R. Hamilton, M.D. Bruce, M. Abdourhaman, et al., Inflammatory bowel disease in children and adolescents, Adv. Pediatr. 26 (1979) 311–341.
4. E.J. Burbige, H. Shi-Shung, T.M. Bayless, Clinical manifestations of Crohn's disease in children and adolescents, Pediatrics 55 (1975) 866–871.
5. C. Lindsley, J.G. Schaller, Arthritis associated with inflammatory bowel disease in children, J. Pediatr. 84 (1974) 16–20.
6. M.H. Passo, J.F. Fitzgerald, K.D. Brandt, Arthritis associated with inflammatory bowel disease in children: relationship of joint disease to activity and severity of bowel lesion, Dig. Dis. Sci. 31 (1986) 492–497.
7. E.A. Newby, N.M. Croft, M. Green, et al., Natural history of paediatric inflammatory bowel diseases over a two-year follow-up: a retrospective review of data from the register of paediatric inflammatory bowel diseases, J. Pediatr. Gastroenterol. Nutr. 46 (2008) 539–545.
8. B.S. Bensen, B. Moum, A. Ekbom, Incidence of inflammatory bowel disease in children in southeastern Norway, Scand. J. Gastroenterol. 37 (2002) 540–545.
9. R. Shivashankar, E.V. Loftus Jr., W.J. Tremaine, et al., Incidence of spondyloarthropathy in patients with ulcerative colitis: a population-based study, J. Rheumatol. 40 (2013) 1153–1157.
10. D. Urlep, T.K. Trop, R. Blagus, R. Orel, Incidence and phenotypic characteristeris of pediatric IBD in northeastern Slovenia 2002–2010, J. Pediatr. Gastroenterol. Nutr. 58 (2014) 325–332.
12. P. Picco, M. Gattorno, N. Marchese, et al., Increased gut permeability in juvenile chronic arthritides: a multivariate analysis of the diagnostic parameters, Clin. Exp. Rheumatol. 18 (2000) 773–778.
13. M. Devos, C. Cuvelier, H. Mielants, et al., Ileocolonoscopy in seronegative spondyloarthropathy, Gastroenterology 96 (1989) 339–344.
16. H. Toyoda, S.-J. Wang, H. Yang, et al., Distinct association of HLA class II genes with inflammatory bowel disease, Gastroenterology 104 (1993) 741–748.
17. D.A. Brewerton, D.C.O. James, The histocompatibility antigen HLA-27 and disease, Semin. Arthritis Rheum. 4 (1975) 191–207.
18. G. Tomer, C. Ceballos, E. Concepcion, et al., NOD2/CARD15 variants are associated with lower weight at diagnosis in children with Crohn's disease, Am. J. Gastroenterol. 98 (2003) 2479–2484.

19. I. Ferreiros-Vidal, J. Amarelo, F. Barros, et al., Lack of association of ankylosing spondylitis with the most common NOD2 susceptibility alleles in Crohn's disease, J. Rheumatol. 30 (2003) 102–104.

20. D.K. Amre, D. Mack, D. Israel, et al., Association between genetic variants in the IL-23R gene and early-onset Crohn's disease: results from a case-control and family-based study among Canadian children, Am. J. Gastroenterol. 103 (2008) 615–620.

21. E. Leshinsky-Silver, A. Karban, E. Buzhakor, et al., Is age of onset of Crohn's disease governed by mutations in NOD2/caspase recruitment domains 15 and Toll-like receptor 4? Evaluation of a pediatric cohort, Pediatr. Res. 58 (2005) 499–504.

22. A. el Maghraoui, A. Aouragh, M. Hachim, et al., Erosive arthritis in juvenile onset Crohn's disease, Clin. Exp. Rheumatol. 18 (2000) 541.

23. K. Benbouazza, R. Bahiri, H.E. Krami, et al., Erosive polyarthritis in Crohn's disease: report of a case, Rev. Rhum. 66 (1999) 743–746.

24. F. McErlane, C. Gillon, T. Irvine, et al., Arthopathy in paediatric inflammatory bowel disease: a cross-sectional observational study, Rheumatol. 47 (2008) 1251–1252.

25. T.R. Orchard, B.P. Wordsworth, D.P. Jewell, Peripheral arthropathies in inflammatory bowel disease: their articular distribution and natural history, Gut 42 (1998) 387–391.

26. P. Wordsworth, Arthritis and inflammatory bowel disease, Curr. Rheumatol. Rep. 2 (2000) 87–88.

27. K. de Vlam, H. Mielants, C. Cuvelier, et al., Spondyloarthropathy is underestimated in inflammatory bowel disease: prevalence and HLA association, J. Rheum. 27 (2000) 2860–2865.

28. G. Neale, A.R. Kelsall, F.H. Doyte, Crohn's disease and diffuse symmetrical periostitis, Gut 9 (1968) 383–387.

29. M. Thearle, M. Horlick, J.P. Bilezikian, et al., Osteoporosis: an unusual presentation of childhood Crohn's disease, Endocrinol. Metab. 85 (2000) 2122–2126.

30. F. Walther, C. Fusch, M. Radke, et al., Osteoporosis in pediatric patients suffering from chronic inflammatory bowel disease with and without steroid treatment, J. Pediatr. Gastroenterol. Nutr. 43 (2006) 42–51.

33. A. Balbir-Gurman, D. Schapira, M. Nahir, Arthritis related to ileal pouchitis following total proctocolectomy for ulcerative colitis, Semin. Arthritis Rheum. 30 (2001) 242–248.

35. J.C. Jacobs, E.J. Goetzl, "Streaking leukocyte factor," arthritis, and pyoderma gangrenosum, Pediatrics 56 (1975) 570–578.

36. C.W. Wilbur, A long-swollen lip, then daily fever and vomiting: What's the cause?, Consultant for Pediatricians (2013) 518–520.

37. S. Yassinger, R. Adelman, D. Cantor, Association of inflammatory bowel disease and large vascular lesions, Gastroenterology 71 (1976) 844–846.

38. S. Gormally, W. Bourke, B. Kierse, et al., Isolated cerebral thromboembolism and Crohn disease, Eur. J. Pediatr. 154 (1995) 815–818.

39. M. Soloway, T.W. Moir, D.W. Linton, Takayasu's arteritis: report of a case with unusual findings, Am. J. Cardiol. 25 (1970) 258–263.

40. M.O. Hilário, M.T. Terreri, G. Prismich, et al., Association of ankylosing spondylitis, Crohn's disease and Takayasu's arteritis in a child, Clin. Exp. Rheumatol. 16 (1998) 92–94.

41. S. Aoyagi, H. Akashi, T. Kawara, et al., Aortic root replacement for Takayasu arteritis associated with ulcerative colitis and ankylosing spondylitis–report of a case, Jpn. Circ. J. 62 (1998) 64–68.

44. D. McCallum, L. Smith, F. Harley, et al., IgA nephropathy and thin basement membrane disease in association with Crohn's disease, Pediatr. Nephrol. 11 (1997) 637–640.

45. M.H. Kay, R. Wyllie, Cutaneous vasculitis as the initial manifestation of Crohn's disease in a pediatric patient, Am. J. Gastroenterol. 93 (1998) 1014.

46. M. Krasnianski, A. Schluter, S. Neudecker, et al., Serial magnet resonance angiography in patients with vasculitis and vasculitis-like angiopathy of the central nervous system, Eur. J. Med. Res. (2004) 247–255.

47. J.L. Lyons, J.T. Rosenbaum, Uveitis associated with inflammatory bowel disease compared with uveitis associated with spondyloarthropathy, Arch. Ophthalmol. 115 (1997) 61–64.

48. P. Hofley, J. Roarty, G. McGinnity, et al., Asymptomatic uveitis in children with chronic inflammatory bowel disease, J. Pediatric Gastroenterol. Nutr. 17 (1993) 397–400.

49. B.M. Ansell, R.A.D. Wigley, Arthritis manifestations in regional enteritis, Ann. Rheum. Dis. 23 (1964) 64–72.

50. H. Lindstrom, H. Wramsby, G. Ostberg, Granulomatous arthritis in Crohn's disease, Gut 13 (1972) 257–259.

51. K. Khan, S.J. Schwarzenberg, H. Sharp, et al., Role of serology and routine laboratory tests in childhood inflammatory bowel disease, Inflamm. Bowel Dis. 8 (2002) 325–329.

52. J.P. Olives, A. Breton, J.P. Hugot, et al., Antineutrophil cytoplasmic antibodies in children with inflammatory bowel disease: prevalence and diagnostic value, J. Pediatr. Gastrol. Nutr. 25 (1997) 142–148.

53. C. Rosa, C. Esposito, A. Caglioti, et al., Does the presence of ANCA in patients with ulcerative colitis necessarily imply renal involvement?, Nephrol. Dial. Transplant. 11 (1996) 2426–2429.

54. J. Langhorst, S. Elsenbruch, J. Koelzer, et al., Noninvasive markers in the assessment of intestinal inflammation in inflammatory bowel diseases: performance of fecal lactoferrin, calprotectin, and PMN-elastase, CRP and clinical indices, Am. J. Gastroenterol. 103 (2008) 162–169.

55. A. Taddio, G. Imonini, P. Lionetti, et al., Usefulness of wireless capsule endoscopy for detecting inflammatory bowel disease in children presenting with arthropathy, Eur. J. Pediatr. 170 (2011) 1343–1347.

56. T.W. Bunch, G.G. Hunder, F.C. McDuffie, et al., Synovial fluid complement determination as a diagnostic aid in diagnostic joint disease, Mayo Clin. Proc. 49 (1974) 715–720.

57. A.R. Mester, E.K. Makò, K. Karlinger, et al., Enteropathic arthritis in the sacroiliac joint: imaging and different diagnosis, Eur. J. Radiol. 35 (2000) 199–208.

58. J.M. Evans, A.D. McMahon, F.E. Murray, et al., Non-steroidal anti-inflammatory drugs are associated with emergency admission to hospital for colitis due to inflammatory bowel disease, Gut 40 (1997) 619–622.

59. T.H.J. Florin, H. Graffner, L.G. Nilsson, et al., Treatment of joint pain in Crohn's patients with budesonide controlled ileal release, Clin. Exp. Pharmacol. Physiol. 27 (2000) 295–298.

60. D.R. Mack, R. Young, S.S. Kaufmann, et al., Methotrexate in patients with Crohn's disease after 6-mercaptopurine, J. Rheumatol. 132 (1998) 830–835.

61. F. Van den Bosch, E. Kruithof, M. De Vos, et al., Crohn's disease associated with spondyloarthropathy: effect of TNF-alpha blockade with infliximab on articular symptoms, Lancet 356 (2000) 1821–1822.

62. J.D. Noe, M. Pfefferkorn, Short-term response to adalimumab in childhood inflammatory bowel disease, Inflamm. Bowel Dis. 14 (2008) 1683–1687.

63. V. Wiegering, H. Morbach, A. Dick, H.J. Girschick, Crohn's disease during etanercept therapy in juvenile idiopathic arthritis: a case report and review of the literature, Rheumatol. Int. 30 (2010) 801–804.

64. A. Dallocchio, D. Canioni, F. Ruemmele, et al., Occurrence of inflammatory bowel disease during treatment of juvenile idiopathic arthritis with etanercept: a French retrospective study, Rheumatol. 49 (2010) 1694–1698.

65. M. Taarkianinen, P. Tynjala, P. Vahasala, P. Lahdenne, Occurrence of inflammatory bowel disease in four patients with juvenile idiopathic arthritis receiving etanercept or infliximab, Scand. J. Rheumatol. 40 (2011) 150–152.

66. D. Barthel, G. Horneff, Inflammatory bowel disease in juvenile idiopathic arthritis patients on biologics, Arthritis Rheum. 65 (2013) S268.

67. M. Can, S. Aydin, A. Nigdelioglu, Conventional DMARD therapy (methotrexate-sulphasalazine) may decrease the requirement of biologics in routine practice of ankylosing spondylitis patients: a real-life experience, Int.J.Rheum. Dis. 15 (2012) 526–530.

The entire reference list is available online at www.expertconsult.com.

SUGGESTED READINGS

N.T. Ventham, N. A. Kennedy, E. Nimmo, J. Satsanogi, Beyond gene discovery in inflammatory bowel disease: the emerging role of epigenetics, Gastroenterology 145 (2013) 293–308.

Uveitis in Juvenile Idiopathic Arthritis

Ross E. Petty, James T. Rosenbaum

Inflammatory eye diseases comprise some of the most devastating complications of childhood rheumatic diseases, especially juvenile idiopathic arthritis (JIA). Chronic (initially asymptomatic) uveitis accompanying JIA is one of the most common causes of uveitis in childhood. It is predominantly anterior, nongranulomatous inflammation affecting the iris and ciliary body (iridocyclitis) of insidious onset (Fig. 22-1). Acute (symptomatic) anterior uveitis is characteristic of human leukocyte antigen-B27 (HLA-B27)–associated diseases such as enthesitis-related arthritis. The posterior uveal tract—the choroid—is rarely affected in rheumatic diseases of childhood.

CLASSIFICATION OF UVEITIS

It has been customary to classify anterior uveitis as *acute* or *chronic*, terms that are used imprecisely, and often synonymously, with *symptomatic* and *asymptomatic*, respectively. The Standardization of Uveitis Nomenclature (SUN) Working Group has proposed a framework for the classification of uveitis, a standardized grading system, and definitions of other terminology used to describe uveitis[1] (Tables 22-1 and 22-2). The SUN working group suggests the use of the terms *insidious* or *sudden* to describe the onset of uveitis, and *limited* (if the duration is 3 months or less) or *persistent* (if the duration exceeds 3 months) to describe its course (which may be influenced by treatment). It recommends that the term *acute* be applied to those instances in which the onset was sudden and the duration limited (as seen in HLA-B27–associated acute anterior uveitis), and that the term *chronic* be used to describe persistent disease with prompt (within 3 months) relapses after discontinuation of therapy (Table 22-2). Most uveitis in children with oligoarthritis, polyarthritis, or psoriatic JIA has an insidious onset, with a chronic and frequently recurrent course. Intermediate uveitis with inflammation predominantly in the vitreous humor is occasionally described in JIA.

UVEITIS IN JUVENILE IDIOPATHIC ARTHRITIS

The uveitis associated with JIA accounts for 20% to 40% of cases of uveitis in some large series that characterize uveitis in childhood.[2,3] Interpretation of data on this subject is hindered by the use of different classifications to describe chronic arthritis in children (see Chapter 15), different types of uveitis, different definitions of response and remission of uveitis, and different types of study populations. For these reasons, care must be taken in interpreting and generalizing conclusions from published information.

History: The Association of Arthritis and Uveitis

Ohm[4] first described chronic uveitis and band keratopathy in 1910 in a child with arthritis. The association of ocular disease and juvenile arthritis was confirmed by several authors.[5-7] In Sury's large series of children with chronic arthritis,[7] chronic uveitis was found in 15% of the total, and two thirds of those patients with uveitis had band keratopathy. The majority of his patients had an insidious onset of uveitis with little or no early disturbance of vision; diagnosis was often delayed until slit-lamp examination was performed. The occurrence of "chronic, asymptomatic, nongranulomatous anterior uveitis" became recognized as an important complication of what was called juvenile rheumatoid arthritis, particularly the limited joint disease referred to as pauciarthritis, equivalent to oligoarthritis, a subset of juvenile idiopathic arthritis in the International League of Associations for Rheumatology (ILAR) classification,[8] as well as rheumatoid factor (RF)-negative polyarthritis and psoriatic arthritis.

Epidemiology

The reported frequency of chronic uveitis in children with chronic arthritis has varied considerably, from 2% in Costa Rica[9] to 11.6 % in the United States,[10] 13% in Canada,[11] and 16% in the Nordic countries.[12,13] It appears to be particularly uncommon in Asian and African populations but has been reported worldwide. A recent population-based study of 2636 children with JIA in Taiwan reported uveitis in 4.6%.[14] There is some evidence that, although the prevalence of JIA may be increasing, there may be a decreasing frequency of uveitis in children with JIA.[15]

The frequency of chronic uveitis is related to the subtype of JIA: it occurs in 15% to 20% of children with oligoarthritis (in up to 30% of those with extended oligoarthritis), 10% of those with psoriatic arthritis, and 14% of those with polyarthritis (RF negative). It is extremely uncommon in children with systemic JIA or RF-positive polyarthritis.[11,16]

Early studies have consistently shown that the frequency of uveitis in JIA is highest in young girls who have oligoarthritis with an early age at onset (younger than 7 years of age) and who are antinuclear antibody (ANA) positive (Table 22-3).[17-26] However, in a recent study of 1047 patients with JIA, the age-associated risk of uveitis was seen only in young girls but not in young boys.[27] A large study from Germany failed to demonstrate gender as an independent risk factor for the development of uveitis in JIA.[28] In a recent study of 56 Greek children with JIA,[29] the high frequency of ANA positivity in children with JIA, with or without uveitis, limited the value of ANA positivity as an indication of risk for uveitis. Reports from India document a low frequency of ANA positivity in children with JIA, including those with uveitis.[30]

Etiology and Pathogenesis

The pathogenesis of chronic uveitis and the basis of its association with JIA are not known, although it is evident that T lymphocytes and their

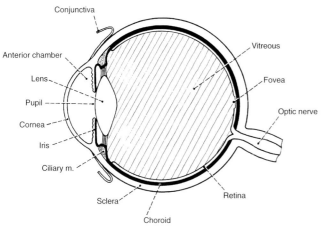

FIGURE 22-1 Schematic view of a sagittal section of the eye. Chronic anterior uveitis (iridocyclitis) involves the iris and ciliary body primarily, but secondary effects occur in the cornea, anterior chamber, lens, vitreous, and (rarely) retina.

TABLE 22-2 The SUN Working Group Descriptors of Uveitis

CATEGORY	DESCRIPTOR	COMMENT
Onset	Sudden	
	Insidious	
Duration	Limited	<3 months' duration
	Persistent	>3 months' duration
Course	Acute	Episode of sudden onset and limited duration
	Recurrent	Repeated episodes separated by periods of inactivity without treatment >3 months in duration
	Chronic	Persistent uveitis with relapses in <3 months after discontinuing treatment

SUN, Standardization of Uveitis Nomenclature.

TABLE 22-1 The SUN Working Group Classification of Uveitis

TYPE	PRIMARY SITE OF INFLAMMATION	INCLUDES
Anterior uveitis	Anterior chamber	Iritis
		Iridocyclitis
		Anterior cyclitis
Intermediate uveitis	Vitreous	Pars planitis
		Posterior cyclitis
		Hyalitis
Posterior uveitis	Retina or choroid	Focal, multifocal, or diffuse choroiditis
		Chorioretinitis
		Retinochoroiditis
		Retinitis
		Neuroretinitis

SUN, Standardization of Uveitis Nomenclature.

TABLE 22-3 Characteristics of Children with Chronic Uveitis and Arthritis

CHARACTERISTIC	OVERALL AVERAGE
Female-to-male ratio	4.4:1
Mean age at onset of arthritis (years)	4
Arthritis subtype (% with uveitis)	
Oligoarthritis	30
Polyarthritis (RF negative)	15
Psoriatic arthritis	10
Polyarthritis (RF positive)	<1
Systemic arthritis	<1
Enthesitis-related arthritis	<1
Serology (%)	
RF positive	<1
Antinuclear antibody positive	80

Acute uveitis ~7%.
Data summarized from published studies.

products are vital participants in the process, and that the innate immune system plays a role.[31] Involvement of the immune response and perturbation of inflammatory cytokines are documented in animal and human studies, although there is limited direct evidence from studies of uveitis in JIA. Ooi and colleagues[32] have reviewed the evidence that interleukin (IL)-1β, IL-2, IL-6, interferon-γ, and tumor necrosis factor (TNF)-α are present in ocular fluids and tissues of adults with ankylosing spondylitis, and that higher levels of these cytokines are associated with more severe uveitis. Levels of TNF-α were especially elevated in the aqueous of patients with ankylosing spondylitis–associated uveitis. The clinical responsiveness of uveitis to the administration of some, but not all, anti–TNF-α agents provides strong support for the premise that TNF-α is at least in part responsible for the inflammation. Serum levels of IL-6 and IL-8 are higher when uveitis is active in adults with posterior uveitis, anterior uveitis, or panuveitis.[33] IL-6 influences the maturation of Th17 CD4+ T cells, which participate in autoimmune diseases. In a murine model, primarily of posterior uveitis or retinitis, Yoshimura and colleagues[34] demonstrated that absence of both IL-6 and IL-23 prevented the production

of Th17 cells and reduced the ocular inflammation. Keino and colleagues[35] demonstrated that the oral administration of an inhibitor of IL-12/IL-23 prevented autoimmune uveoretinitis in animals by reducing production of IL-17–producing cells. Other animal studies have shown that anti-Th17 can block the development of uveitis in uveitis-susceptible mice, but that administration of the cytokine itself into uveitis-susceptible rats has a mitigating effect on disease development.[36] Anti-IL-17 treatment of human uveitis (principally posterior disease) has not demonstrated any significant effect, however.[37] Despite the implication of IL-17 in uveitis, some models involve either Th1[38] or Th2[39] cells exclusively. Animal models may not be entirely relevant to understanding human disease, however. In addition, in the most widely studied T cell–dependent mouse model of uveitis, experimental autoimmune uveitis (EAU) is predominantly a chorioretinitis whose pathogenesis might differ significantly from anterior uveitis. Sijssens and colleagues have demonstrated age-related differences in aqueous humor cytokines in patients, including some with JIA.[40]

Parikh and colleagues[41] have suggested, on the basis of the characteristics of the cellular infiltrate seen in histological studies of enucleated eyes, that the pathogenesis probably involved B lymphocytes as well. In addition to the high frequency of ANAs of undetermined specificity, autoantibodies to ocular antigens have been described in children with arthritis and uveitis. There have been unconfirmed reports that children with uveitis and JIA have a higher frequency of immunity to soluble retinal antigen (S antigen)[42,43] than do children with arthritis alone. It is not clear whether immunity to these ocular antigens is pathogenic or merely reflects the inflammatory process.

The basis of the association between inflammatory joint disease and inflammatory ocular disease is unexplained, but it is likely that a shared genetic predisposition plays a part.

Genetic Background

Genetic susceptibility to uveitis in JIA is complex. Although there is limited evidence for the familial occurrence of this disorder, a few case reports have documented the occurrence of oligoarthritis and chronic anterior uveitis in siblings.[44-46]

A number of sometimes contradictory studies have reported an array of HLA alleles associated with chronic anterior uveitis in JIA. The strongest and most consistent associations appear to be with genes in the class II region. Studies from the United States[47,48] have documented a strong association with DRB1*1104 (formerly called DR5), and associations with DQA1*0501 and DQB1*0301, which are in linkage disequilibrium with DRB1*1104. The association of uveitis in JIA with DRB1*11 noted in American children was confirmed in one Italian study[49] but not in another.[50] An association with DRB1*13 has been reported in British[51] and Greek children.[52] An increased prevalence of HLA DR9 (DRB1*09) (odds ratio [OR] 2.33) was also noted in one study.[50]

Acute anterior uveitis is associated with the class I gene HLA-B27.[53,54] Other associations between class I genes and chronic uveitis are less convincing. Single studies have alleged associations with HLA-A19 (OR 2.87), HLA-B22 (OR 4.52),[50] and A2*06,[55] but these studies have not yet been confirmed.

Genetic polymorphisms of non-HLA genes have been less well studied. TNF gene polymorphisms (−238 GA and −308 GA) have been linked with HLA B*27–associated uveitis.[56] In patients with acute anterior uveitis, an association was found with another single nucleotide polymorphism (SNP) (857T) in the TNF gene.[57] The TNF locus is located in the HLA/major histocompatibility complex (MHC), and large studies are needed to determine whether TNF associations reflect linkage disequilibrium with class I or class II loci.

Clinical Manifestations
Insidious Onset, Chronic Uveitis

Insidious onset, chronic uveitis is characteristic of oligoarticular JIA (persistent or extended), and most children with psoriatic arthritis or RF-negative polyarthritis develop uveitis (see Table 22-3). The onset of chronic uveitis is usually insidious and often entirely asymptomatic, although up to half of the children have some symptoms attributable to the uveitis (pain, redness, headache, photophobia, change in vision) later in the course of their disease (Table 22-4). Uveitis is detected in less than 10% of patients before the onset of arthritis,[28] usually in the course of a routine ophthalmic examination. In almost half of all patients with uveitis, it occurs just before arthritis is diagnosed, at the time of diagnosis, or shortly thereafter.[17,28,47] A Finnish study of children with JIA and uveitis documented the appearance of uveitis within the first 3 months after onset of arthritis in 49%; 90% developed uveitis within the first 4 years after onset of arthritis.[58] The risk is never entirely absent, however[17,59] (Fig. 22-2). The disease is bilateral in 70% to 80% of children.[2,3,17,25] Patients with unilateral disease are unlikely

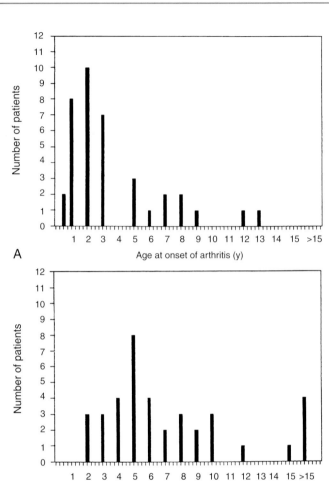

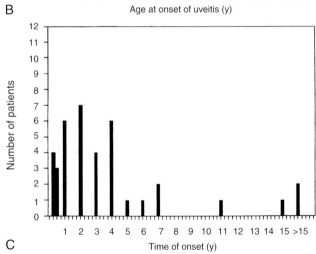

FIGURE 22-2 Graphs showing the temporal relationships between arthritis and uveitis in children with juvenile idiopathic arthritis. **A,** The distribution of age at onset of arthritis in a series of 38 children who developed uveitis. **B,** The distribution of age at onset of uveitis in the same children. Note that in four patients, uveitis began after their 15th birthday: at 15½, 18, 31, and 39 years of age. **C,** Interval between onset of arthritis and diagnosis of uveitis in these patients. Note that for one patient the interval was 29 years, and for another, 34 years.

to develop bilateral involvement after the first year of disease; however, there are exceptions, and unilateral uveitis may persist for many years in a few children before the other eye is involved.

The early detection of chronic uveitis requires slit-lamp biomicroscopy, which should be performed at the time of diagnosis in every child with JIA and repeated at prescribed intervals during the first few years of the disease. The recommended frequency of ophthalmological examinations is influenced by the level of risk of uveitis (Table 22-5).[60] It is recommended that slit-lamp examinations be performed every 3 months for the first 2 years in children in the high-risk group (early

age at onset, oligoarthritis or polyarthritis, ANA positivity) and every 4 to 6 months thereafter for a period of 7 years at a minimum. In children with ANA-negative disease, slit-lamp examinations should be done initially at 4- to 6-month intervals. Children with psoriatic arthritis are also at considerable risk for the development of uveitis and should be followed at the same frequencies as children with oligoarticular or polyarticular JIA. In children with systemic onset JIA, examinations once a year are probably sufficient. Subsequent to the publication of these guidelines, there have been suggestions for their modification.[28,61] Heiligenhaus et al. proposed guidelines that conformed to the ILAR classification of JIA[28] (Table 22-6). Any child who has had uveitis should be considered to be at high risk, even if it has remitted, and continued surveillance is essential.

The diagnostic signs of anterior uveitis on slit-lamp examination are the presence of inflammatory cells and increased protein concentration ("flare") in the aqueous humor of the anterior chamber of the eye (Fig. 22-3). Deposition of inflammatory cells on the inner surface of the cornea (keratic precipitates) may be detected at presentation or develop later.

TABLE 22-4 Ocular Signs and Symptoms in Children with Chronic Uveitis and Arthritis

CHARACTERISTIC	PERCENT AFFECTED (RANGE)
Bilateral uveitis	25-89
Symptoms	
Ocular pain and or redness	0-25
Change in vision	0-30
Photophobia	0-8
Headache	0-6
None	51-97

Data summarized from published studies.

TABLE 22-5 American Academy of Pediatrics Guidelines for the Ophthalmological Screening of Children with JIA

		SCREENING SCHEDULE	
JIA ONSET TYPE	ANA	ONSET <7 YEARS*	ONSET >7 YEARS†
Oligoarthritis	Positive	Every 3-4 months‡	Every 4-6 months
Oligoarthritis	Negative	Every 4-6 months	Every 4-6 months
Polyarthritis	Positive	Every 3-4 months‡	Every 4-6 months
Polyarthritis	Negative	Every 4-6 months	Every 4-6 months
Systemic	Negative or positive	Every 12 months	Every 12 months
High risk: Screen every 3 months			
Moderate risk: Screen every 4-6 months			
Low risk: Screen every 12 months			

*All patients are considered to be at low risk 7 years after onset of arthritis; they should have yearly ophthalmological examinations indefinitely.
†All patients are considered to be at low risk 4 years after onset of arthritis; they should have yearly ophthalmological examinations indefinitely.
‡All high-risk patients are considered to be at medium risk 4 years after onset of arthritis.
Adapted from [No authors listed], American Academy of Pediatrics Section on Rheumatology and Section on Ophthalmology: Guidelines for ophthalmologic examinations in children with juvenile rheumatoid arthritis. Pediatrics 93 (1993) 295–296.

TABLE 22-6 Recommendations for Screening Based on the ILAR Classification of JIA

JIA SUBGROUP	ANA	AGE AT ONSET OF JIA	DURATION OF JIA	SCREENING
Oligoarthritis	+	<7 years	<5 years	3 months
RF-negative polyarthritis				
Psoriatic arthritis				
Undifferentiated arthritis				
	+	<7 years	>4 years	6 months
	+	<7 years	>7 years	12 months
	+	>6 years	<3 years	6 months
	+	>6 years	>2 years	12 months
	—	<7 years	<5 years	6 months
	—	<7 years	>4 years	12 months
	—	>6 years	NA	12 months
Enthesitis-related arthritis	NA	NA		12 months
RF-positive polyarthritis	NA	NA		12 months
Systemic arthritis	NA	NA		12 months
Patients in any category with uveitis	NA	NA		According to uveitis course

Adapted from Heiligenhaus et al.[28]

Complications of chronic anterior uveitis are frequent and increase with increasing duration of active disease.[3] In recent series, the frequency of complications is somewhat lower than in earlier reports, presumably due to earlier treatment. Posterior synechiae, inflammatory adhesions between the iris and anterior surface of the lens, result in an irregular or poorly reactive pupil (Table 22-7; Fig. 22-4). This abnormality may be the first obvious clue to the presence of uveitis on ophthalmoscopic examination, but it is often a sign of disease of considerable duration or severity. Synechiae that are circumferential prevent the free flow of aqueous humor between the posterior and anterior chambers, resulting in bulging of the iris (iris bombé) and increased intraocular pressure.

Band keratopathy is caused by deposition of calcium in the corneal epithelium and tends to be a late occurrence (Fig. 22-5). Initially, crescentic gray-to-brown depositions are seen at the corneal limbus. With time, the band progresses centrally at the equator of the eye and impairs light entry through the pupil. Cataracts result either from the inflammatory disease or the use of corticosteroid. Glaucoma and hypotony are serious complications, as is phthisis bulbi, a rare occurrence late in the disease course.[13,62,63] Cystoid macular edema, which affects central vision, is reported in some series[13,64] (Fig. 22-6). Wide variation in the reported frequency of these complications is a reflection of the differences in duration of active disease as well as the time to initiation of therapy and the intensity of therapy. These complications are still occasionally encountered in some children with chronic uveitis in spite of vigorous and carefully monitored ophthalmic treatment, although their frequency may be diminishing. Even in recent series, however, cataracts occurred in up to 64% of children, glaucoma in up to 25%, and band keratopathy in up to 59%.[49] Nonetheless, visual acuity was normal or good in almost 66% of these children. Rare ocular diseases associated with childhood rheumatic diseases include papillitis, scleritis, episcleritis, and keratoconjunctivitis sicca. Complication frequencies reported from several studies are summarized in Table 22-7.

Keenan and colleagues[65] suggest that granulomatous uveitis may be more common than has been thought. Using a definition of granulomatous uveitis as the presence of Busacca or angle nodules, mutton-fat keratic precipitates (KPs), or hyalinized ghost KPs, they observed granulomatous uveitis in 28% of 71 children with JIA. Granulomatous uveitis may be more common in black patients (67% of those patients with granulomatous disease in the series) than white patients (25%). Many of these patients had only ghost KP as evidence of disease; this may account for the higher incidence of granulomatous uveitis than in other studies of juvenile arthritis.

Pars planitis is a form of uveitis characterized by inflammatory cells accumulating over the inferior pars plana, the portion of the eye just posterior to the ciliary body. Patients with this form of uveitis usually complain of visual floaters. The disease is generally bilateral with an insidious onset. This disease commonly begins in childhood or

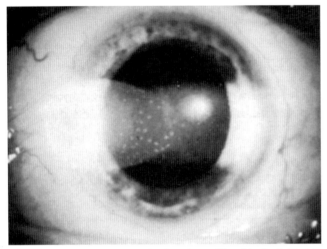

FIGURE 22-3 A slit-lamp examination shows "flare" in the fluid of the anterior chamber (caused by increased protein content) and keratic precipitates on the posterior surface of the cornea, representing small collections of inflammatory cells. (Courtesy of Dr. H.J. Kaplan)

TABLE 22-7 **Frequency of Complications of Chronic Uveitis in Reported Cases**	
COMPLICATION	REPORTED RANGE (%)
Synechiae	37-75
Band keratopathy	11-56
Cataract	6-75
Glaucoma	8-25
Hypotony	5-10
Phthisis bulbi	0-14
Cystoid macular edema	3-6

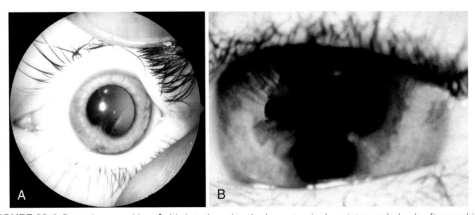

FIGURE 22-4 Posterior synechiae. **A.** Iris is tethered to the lens at a single point revealed only after mydriatics were given in this 4-year-old girl with oligoarthritis. **B.** The eye of a 7-year-old boy shows an irregular pupil that resulted from multiple adhesions of the iris to the anterior surface of the lens.

TABLE 22-8 Terms Used by Ophthalmologists to Describe Abnormalities in Uveitis

TERM	DEFINITION
Anterior uveitis	Ocular inflammation that is predominantly anterior to the lens. Subsets of anterior uveitis include iritis and iridocyclitis; the latter term is preferred if the ciliary body is involved.
Intermediate uveitis	Ocular inflammation in which the predominant manifestation is leukocytes in the vitreous humor.
Panuveitis	Ocular inflammation involving the anterior chamber, the vitreous humor, and the retina and/or choroid.
Mutton-fat precipitates	Large concretions of leukocytes attached to the endothelial surface of the cornea.
Granulomatous uveitis	Uveitis usually characterized by large concretions of cells on the corneal endothelium (granulomatous keratic precipitates) or iris nodules. Although these findings are more common in a granulomatous disease such as sarcoidosis or tuberculosis, the histology of these lesions is not a granuloma.
Nodules	Cellular nodules in a patient with uveitis including Koeppe's nodule at the pupillary margin and Busacca's nodules in the iris stroma.
Pars planitis	A subset of intermediate uveitis in which the inflammation is predominantly over the pars plana, an anatomic region just posterior to the ciliary body.
Cystoid macular edema	Collection of fluid in the macula, a common cause of vision loss in patients with uveitis.
Vitritis	Inflammation in the vitreous humor.
Cyclitic membrane	Fibrotic tissue that forms posterior to the lens capsule and impedes the visual axis.
Cataract	Opacification of the lens as occurs from aging, chronic oral or topical corticosteroid use, or chronic inflammation.
Glaucoma	Optic nerve injury usually resulting from a chronic elevation of intraocular pressure.
Hypotony	Excessively low intraocular pressure.
Posterior synechiae	Adhesions between the iris and the anterior lens capsule.
Anterior synechiae	Adhesions between the iris and the cornea.
Iris bombé	Circumferential posterior synechiae resulting in impaired flow of aqueous humor and a marked elevation of intraocular pressure.
Keratic precipitates	Concretions of cells that deposit on the corneal endothelium during uveitis.
Band keratopathy	Deposition of calcium in the corneal epithelium as can occur from chronic anterior uveitis in JIA.
Phthisis	The irreversible end stage of chronic inflammation or infection.
Snowbanking	The cellular exudate over the pars plana, a characteristic of pars planitis.

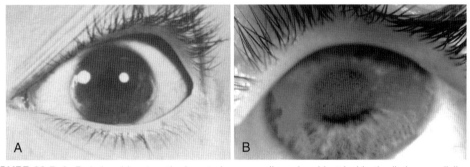

FIGURE 22-5 **A,** Early band keratopathy is noted as a semilunar band just inside the limbus medially and laterally. It does not extend across the pupil. **B,** The semiopaque band extends across the midplane of the cornea in this example of more advanced band keratopathy.

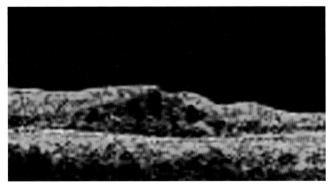

FIGURE 22-6 Cystoid macular edema. Optical coherence tomography (OCT) images the retina and its layers by reflectance. The normal macula is concave. The convex appearance of the macula in this example is due to cystoid edema.

adolescence and may last for decades. Visual acuity is often only moderately impaired by pars planitis, but macular edema is an especially common complication. Pars planitis is a relatively common cause of uveitis in childhood, but it is not characteristic of JIA. Terms used to describe uveitis and its complications are listed in Table 22-8.

Sudden-Onset (Acute) Uveitis

Sudden-onset (acute) uveitis differs in several ways from the more common insidious-onset chronic uveitis and is strongly associated with HLA-B27 and enthesitis-related arthritis (ERA). In a large series reported by Saurenmann and colleagues,[11] 7.8% of children with ERA had uveitis. It is much more common in boys (as is ERA), is more often unilateral, and is characterized by a painful, red, photophobic eye. Until the patient is evaluated by an ophthalmologist, the symptoms are often mistakenly attributed to a foreign body, infection, or an allergy. Slit-lamp examination reveals the presence of cells and flare in the anterior chamber. Because of the symptomatic nature of this type of anterior uveitis, the process is usually identified and appropriately treated soon after onset; as a result, long-term sequelae are uncommon and visual prognosis is excellent. The reasons for the differences in clinical appearance between sudden-onset acute uveitis and insidious-onset chronic uveitis are unknown.

Differential Diagnosis

Anterior uveitis without evidence of joint or systemic involvement probably accounts for most children with anterior uveitis.[2,3] Such children should be evaluated for the presence of occult inflammatory joint disease (including leg length inequality, and muscle wasting), and monitored for the possible development of arthritis or other systemic disease over time. Some experts think that a subset of these children have a *forme fruste* of JIA.

Uveitis and arthritis occur together with high frequency in a number of diseases other than JIA. Inflammation of the anterior uveal tract may complicate the arthropathy of inflammatory bowel disease and reactive arthritis. Uveitis also occurs in chronic infantile neurological cutaneous and articular syndrome (CINCA), sarcoidosis, Blau syndrome, Behçet disease, and Kawasaki disease. Uveitis that occurs in these disorders is discussed in the respective chapters. Uveitis rarely occurs in systemic lupus erythematosus, polyarteritis nodosa, or Henoch–Schönlein purpura. Rheumatoid arthritis in adults is not associated with uveitis unless it induces scleritis with secondary uveal involvement. Syndromes associated with uveitis are listed in Box 22-1.

Uveitis in Other Diseases
Tubulointerstitial Nephritis and Uveitis

Tubulointerstitial nephritis and uveitis (TINU) is the second most common type of childhood uveitis in Japan[66]; in an American series[67]

BOX 22-1   Diseases Most Often Associated with Anterior Uveitis in Children

Rheumatic Diseases
Juvenile Idiopathic Arthritis
Oligoarthritis
Psoriatic arthritis
Polyarthritis (rheumatoid factor negative)
Enthesitis-related arthritis (acute uveitis)

Reactive Arthritis, Urethritis, Conjunctivitis Syndrome
Vasculitis
Kawasaki disease
Behçet disease
Henoch–Schönlein purpura, rheumatic fever (very rare)
Granulomatosis with polyangiitis (very rare)

Infection
Cat scratch disease
Herpes simplex, Epstein–Barr and other viral diseases
Human immunodeficiency virus (HIV) syndrome

Other
Tubular interstitial nephritis and uveitis (TINU)
Masquerade syndromes
Pars planitis
Crohn's disease
Sarcoidosis, Blau syndrome

---

nearly one third of patients under the age of 20 years with sudden-onset bilateral anterior uveitis had TINU. This diagnosis is frequently missed, and its prevalence may be underestimated.[68] TINU usually manifests as a bilateral, sudden-onset, anterior uveitis with eye redness and photophobia before or after the presentation of renal disease.[69] The child with TINU is usually systemically ill with fever, arthralgias, fatigue, and abdominal pain. The renal disease, manifested by sterile pyuria, may be transient. There may be elevation of liver enzyme levels, an elevated erythrocyte sedimentation rate, and mild anemia. Association with HLA DRB1*0102 and HLA DQA*01 is quite strong.[70] Treatment with moderate doses of corticosteroids for 8 to 12 weeks is usually effective treatment for all aspects of this syndrome, although some children go on to develop chronic uveitis.[69] The cause of TINU is unknown.

Infectious Causes of Uveitis

Uveitis was identified in seven South African boys who had human immunodeficiency virus–associated arthritis.[71] Intermediate uveitis was present in four children, and nongranulomatous anterior uveitis was present in three patients. The range of complications was similar to that seen in children with JIA.

Infection with *Bartonella henselae*, the most commonly identified cause of cat-scratch fever, may result in arthritis[72,73] and a neuroretinitis characterized by exudates in the retina (macular star).[74] Cells in the vitreous humor indicate the presence of uveitis. Diagnosis is confirmed serologically. Treatment with antibiotics is usually effective. Lyme disease is associated with a variety of ocular manifestations, including, rarely, anterior and intermediate uveitis[75] (see Chapter 42). Epstein–Barr viral infection is another rare cause of anterior uveitis. Infection with *Toxoplasma gondii* is relatively common as an identifiable cause of a panuveitis.[76] *Toxocara canis* infection should also be considered in children with uveitis.[77] Both *toxoplasma* and *toxocara* usually cause a focal chorioretinitis that narrows the differential diagnosis. Tuberculosis may cause granulomatous uveitis affecting both the anterior and posterior uvea.

Other Syndromes Associated with Uveitis

Vogt–Koyanagi–Harada syndrome is a rare autoimmune disease possibly induced by immunity to the enzyme tyrosinase, leading to vitiligo, aseptic meningitis, encephalitis, uveitis, and hearing loss, as well as changes in the retinal pigment epithelium.[78] Poliosis (patchy loss of pigment of eyelashes, eyebrows, or hair) is a characteristic finding. The disease is usually responsive to corticosteroid given over a period of months; rarely, methotrexate or biologics may be necessary. Some authorities recommend using pulse intravenous methylprednisolone for this disease when it presents in childhood.

So-called masquerade syndromes, caused by juvenile xanthogranuloma or infiltration of the uveal tract with retinoblastoma or leukemic cells, may mimic the presence of uveitis.[79] Children with leukemia frequently have bone pain and occasionally frank joint effusions (see Chapter 50), suggesting the possible diagnosis of JIA and adding to the risk of misinterpretation of uveitis. Uveitis has been described in adults experiencing graft-versus-host disease after stem-cell transplantation for malignancies.[80,81]

PATHOLOGY

Reports of the histopathology of uveitis in JIA are few. Descriptions of the pathology in patients with extremely severe, long-standing disease that led to blindness do not necessarily illuminate the pathogenic process. Such studies describe an intense immunoinflammatory response in the iris, ciliary body, and pars plana, as well as increased iris vascularity.[82] Evidence of B lymphocyte involvement is suggested by the presence of scanty lymphocyte and plasma-cell infiltrates[41,83-85]; increased immunoglobulin (Ig) levels in the aqueous humor[85-87]; and high IgG concentration, activated complement, and C1q binding in the vitreous.[88] Kaplan and associates[89] found that 90% of vitreous lymphocytes in one adult with uveitis and "juvenile" rheumatoid arthritis (RA) were B lymphocytes. Evidence of T-cell infiltrations is limited.[85] Given the strong MHC class II associations, it seems likely T cells play a role, whether in the eye or in local lymph nodes. The keratic precipitates on the endothelial surface of the cornea consist of mononuclear phagocytes, with plasma cells and lymphocytes.[90]

LABORATORY EXAMINATION

The most characteristic laboratory abnormality found in children with arthritis and insidious chronic uveitis is the presence of ANA, usually in low titer (<1 : 640).[2,3] The specificities of these antibodies are usually unknown, although reactivity to histones has been reported to occur more commonly in children with JIA and uveitis than those with JIA alone.[91] ANAs and RFs are uncommon in children with sudden-onset uveitis, as they are in the JIA subtype (ERA) with which this type of uveitis is usually seen. In children with acute anterior uveitis, HLA-B27 is often present. Abnormalities of the acute phase response reflect the extent and activity of arthritis, rather than uveitis.

MANAGEMENT

Investigations

In the child with uveitis in whom no rheumatic disease such as JIA is immediately evident, consideration should be given to other possible systemic disorders before coming to the conclusion that the child has isolated idiopathic uveitis. An approach to investigation is outlined in Box 22-2.

BOX 22-2 Suggested Investigations for the Child with Uveitis

Investigations for all patients should include the following:
  ANA
  Urinalysis
  HLA-B27 (only if uveitis is acute and symptomatic)
  Consider Lyme serology, Bartonella serology, toxocara serology, toxoplasmosis serology only in appropriate historical and clinical context
  Urine beta 2 microglobulin, serum blood urea nitrogen and creatinine, erythrocyte sedimentation rate and complete blood count for bilateral, sudden-onset anterior uveitis
Investigations for patients with granulomatous uveitis should also include the following:
  Mantoux skin test or Quantiferon blood test
  Chest x-ray if suspicion of tuberculosis
  Note: tests such as angiotensin converting enzyme (ACE) inhibitor, serum calcium, etc., are considered too nonspecific to be of value in excluding sarcoid
Investigations for patients with posterior uveitis should also include the following:
  Toxoplasmosis serology (if ophthalmologist regards the chorioretinal lesion as characteristic)
  Cytomegalovirus serology and *polymerase* chain reaction on aqueous fluid
    HIV serology

Medical Management of Chronic Uveitis Associated with JIA

The treatment of chronic uveitis should be supervised by an ophthalmologist who is experienced in management of children with this disease.[92] The goal of therapy is to achieve normal vision by completely controlling inflammation in the eye so that no cells (or only occasional cells) are demonstrable in the anterior chamber on slit-lamp examination. The initial approach consists of glucocorticoid eye drops (such as dexamethasone or methylprednisolone), with or without a mydriatic agent to dilate the pupil and help prevent the development of posterior synechiae. A short-acting mydriatic drug is preferred, given, if possible, once a day in the evening so that pupillary dilatation does not interfere with schoolwork and reading. Some data suggest that oral nonsteroidal antiinflammatory drugs (NSAIDs) may be of some benefit.[93,94] Although this effect is not a major one, it should be considered when NSAID treatment of arthritis is altered.

In unresponsive disease, glucocorticoid drops may be given as often as hourly during waking hours, with glucocorticoid ointment placed in the conjunctival sac at bedtime. Such frequent eye drop instillation may be very difficult, particularly in the school-age child. The approach to management of uveitis that does not respond completely to the use of topical corticosteroids is changing rapidly. Systemic corticosteroids (prednisone, 1 to 2 mg/kg/d orally, or methylprednisolone, 30 mg/kg intravenously on 1 to 3 consecutive days) are occasionally used to achieve rapid control of inflammation prior to surgery or to help manage hypotony. In a few instances, sub-Tenon injections of glucocorticoid may be required. Although the results of slit-lamp examination may quickly return to normal soon after treatment is initiated, relapses are common. Long-term systemic administration of corticosteroids may lead to the development of cataracts, increased intraocular pressure, and even Cushing syndrome, and should be avoided if possible. For these reasons, systemic corticosteroids are currently used less frequently, and limited response to topical corticosteroids usually requires initiation of second-line therapy, most commonly methotrexate. Foeldvari and Wierk[95] retrospectively reviewed the treatment of 38 children with uveitis (31 associated with oligoarticular JIA and 7 with psoriatic JIA). Twenty-five patients were treated with methotrexate. Remission (no active uveitis without topical or systemic corticosteroids) occurred in 21 of 25 patients. Heiligenhaus and colleagues[96] reported that methotrexate allowed control of uveitis with (n = 21) or without (n = 4) topical corticosteroids in 25 of 35 patients. Both of these studies concluded that methotrexate was very effective in managing uveitis in children with JIA, but that topical corticosteroids were often required in addition. It is not entirely clear how rigorous the definition of remission was in these studies. Charuvanij and colleagues[97] reviewed the medication history in 43 children with JIA and anterior uveitis. Only 16% achieved satisfactory control with topical corticosteroids alone. The addition of methotrexate controlled the uveitis in three quarters of the children, but six required the addition of infliximab, with disease control in four patients.

Tappeiner et al.[98] reported a retrospective study of 82 children with JIA and uveitis (137 affected eyes); all were on corticosteroids, 55% were on methotrexate, and 18% were on azathioprine. The authors concluded that cyclosporine had a limited role in treating uveitis. Remission (1 cell or less in the anterior chamber) occurred in 6 of 25 patients receiving cyclosporine as monotherapy. When cyclosporine was used together with methotrexate, uveitis became inactive in approximately half of patients, with reduction in requirements for topical or systemic corticosteroids in many. However, over the 2.9-year follow-up period, 45% developed new complications of uveitis.

Goebel et al.[99] reported the benefit of azathioprine (1.4 to 3.2 mg/kg/d) in 41 children with JIA who had chronic active uveitis in spite of topical corticosteroids and, in 29%, methotrexate or cyclosporine. Azathioprine as monotherapy resulted in remission in 16 of 26 patients with a mean follow-up of 2.2 years. The addition of azathioprine to methotrexate or cyclosporine also achieved disease control in 60% to 70% of patients.

Mycophenolate mofetil (MMF) has recently received attention as an effective agent in patients resistant to other therapy.[100,101] Doycheva and colleagues[100] noted a considerable steroid sparing effect, improvement in inflammation, and reduction in relapse rate in 17 children with uveitis (only one with JIA) treated with MMF (600 mg/m²/day) during the average of 3 years of follow-up. However, additional immunosuppression was required in some patients. Sobrin and colleagues[101] reported that MMF was effective in treating uveitis in children but was less effective in those with JIA.

The anti–TNF-α agents—etanercept, infliximab, and adalimumab—have advanced the therapy of methotrexate-resistant uveitis, including that associated with JIA. Reiff[102] reported the effectiveness of etanercept in an uncontrolled study of seven children with active uveitis and chronic arthritis who had not responded satisfactorily to corticosteroids and methotrexate or cyclosporine. Follow-up of these patients indicated that at least four had a sustained response.[103] Smith and co-workers[104] conducted a randomized, blinded, placebo-controlled trial in 12 children with juvenile RA (JRA) and uveitis in whom the methotrexate response was insufficient; they found no difference between etanercept and placebo at 6 months. Saurenmann and colleagues[105] reported results of treatment with etanercept (n = 6) or infliximab (n = 8) in 12 patients with JIA and concluded that infliximab was superior to etanercept in both clinical response and frequency of uveitis complications. Tynjala and colleagues[106] reported similar results. In most studies, the response was partial, with approximately one third of patients achieving complete remission of uveitis. Simonini et al.[107] reported complete remission in eight children with JIA and uveitis who received infliximab but noted that the beneficial effect waned over time. Similar results were noted by Tugal-Tutkun et al.[108] There are also reports of new onset or worsening of uveitis during treatment with anti-TNF agents, particularly etanercept.[109]

In an interventional prospective case series, Magli and colleagues[110] gave adalimumab to 21 children with JIA and chronic uveitis who were resistant to treatment with corticosteroids, methotrexate, or infliximab, and noted resolution of anterior chamber inflammation in 76% of the children and significant reduction in the flare rate. Concomitant medications (methotrexate, topical corticosteroids) were reduced or discontinued in many children. Beister and colleagues reported comparable results in a similar patient group.[111] Zannin et al.[112] compared the efficacy of infliximab and adalimumab after 1 year of treatment in 91 children with oligoarticular JIA and uveitis who were resistant to methotrexate (10 to 15 mg/m²/wk) or cyclosporine (4 to 5 mg/kg/day), or were corticosteroid dependent at 6 months of therapy. The authors concluded that adalimumab and infliximab were both effective but that a higher remission rate was seen in the adalimumab group (67%) compared with the infliximab group (43%) (P < .025). Case reports record the benefit of the TNF inhibitor, golimumab,[113] tocilizumab (anti-IL6),[114] abatacept (anti-CTLA4),[115] and rituximab (anti-CD20).[116] Refractory uveitis has also been treated with intravenous immunoglobulin.[117] We think that there is no longer a role for chlorambucil in the management of uveitis in children with JIA. Current clinical trials can be viewed online at www.ClinicalTrials.gov.

A consensus recommendation for treatment of refractory uveitis with JIA has been recently published[118] (Box 22-3). These guidelines provide a step-by-step outline for the time-limited administration of

---

> **BOX 22-3   Suggested Guidelines for the Treatment of Uveitis in Juvenile Idiopathic Arthritis**
>
> **Initial Therapy**
> Topical corticosteroids with or without mydriatics
>   Continue for up to 3 months provided inflammation is controlled, before gradually tapering frequency of eye drops
>   If disease activity increases or does not respond add second line agent
>
> **Second-Line Therapy**
> Add methotrexate (0.35 to 0.65 mg/kg) by mouth or by subcutaneous injection once a week for up to 3 months. If inflammation is controlled, continue using methotrexate and taper topical corticosteroids. Monitor methotrexate toxicity (liver enzymes, albumin, complete blood count every 2 months). If disease control is unsatisfactory or disease worsens, add third-line therapy.
>
> **Third-Line Therapy**
> Add anti–TNF-α agent—preferably intravenous infliximab (4 to 10 mg/kg every 6 to 8 weeks) or adalimumab (20 to 40 mg subcutaneously every 1 to 2 weeks). If rapid control of inflammation is not achieved, consider substituting mycophenolate mofetil or cyclosporine; local corticosteroid injections.

methotrexate or azathioprine, followed by infliximab, adalimumab, or cyclosporine, in intractable disease. At the present time, there are no studies indicating the optimal duration of biological therapy after remission of uveitis is achieved. Experience indicates, however, that relapses following cessation of biologics or methotrexate are quite common. The longer methotrexate therapy was continued after remission of uveitis was achieved, the lower the risk of posttreatment flare.[119]

Surgical Management

Band keratopathy has been treated with topical chelation and by lasers. Cataracts seldom interfere significantly with vision in childhood, but they may require surgical removal. The management of complicated uveitis and glaucoma remains unsatisfactory, but the results of lensectomy or vitrectomy for complicated cataracts are improved.[96] It is recommended that cataract surgery be performed only in the absence of vitreous opacities, hypotony, or cyclitic membrane formation and that the anterior chamber be free of inflammatory cells for a minimum of 3 months prior to surgery. Perioperative glucocorticoids are recommended. The timing of cataract extraction challenges the judgment of the ophthalmologist as they weigh the danger of an operation on an inflamed eye against the risk of amblyopia. An unresolved controversy is whether to replace the lens with an intraocular lens or require that the child use a contact lens or a thick corrective lens. Operative complications are minimized with microsurgery and phacoemulsification.

DISEASE COURSE AND PROGNOSIS

The course of chronic anterior uveitis in patients with JIA is variable; it may last for months to a decade or longer, and may persist into adulthood, although new approaches to therapy suggest that the course may be much shorter if it is treated aggressively. In some children, the course is intermittent; in others it is persistent. In a retrospective review of 62 patients with JIA and uveitis, Hoeve et al.[120] noted a biphasic disease course, with highest disease activity early in the disease course and during adolescence, as measured by anterior chamber cell count. The activity of the uveitis does not appear to parallel that of the arthritis,[121] and it may occur for the first time after the arthritis is in remission.

Visual loss may occur because of complications of the uveitis or as a result of amblyopia related to suppression of visual images from a cataract in a young child. In early studies, the frequency of blindness (visual acuity less than 20/400) in both eyes was as high as 15% to 30%. In more recent reports, visual outcome is much improved. As reported by Sabri and colleagues[62] in 2008, in a large series of patients who had been followed for a mean of 6.3 years, visual acuity of 20/40 or better was present in 91% of affected eyes; 3.4% had visual impairment, and 5.7% were blind. It seems likely that earlier identification of the disease, more effective medical therapy, and improved surgical management are responsible for this improvement in outcome in the past decade. Avoidance of long-term systemic or topical corticosteroids has probably contributed to the reduction in the frequency of cataract and glaucoma.

The prognosis for uveitis is worse in children in whom the onset of uveitis occurs before diagnosis of arthritis or shortly thereafter.[26] It is also worse in those with an initial severe inflammatory response, chronicity of inflammation, or ANA negativity.[26] Boys were found to have a prognosis for sight loss that was significantly worse than that for girls.[122] The effects of uveitis may have lasting impact on the child's quality of life.[123]

Uveitis persists into adulthood in a small number of patients.[124-126] Each of these studies represents findings in a highly selected group of patients in whom uveitis has persisted or has resulted in significant visual impairment. In a long-term follow-up study of 123 patients with onset of JIA between 1976 and 1995,[124] active uveitis was defined as the presence of three or more cells in the anterior chamber or the requirement for topical corticosteroids was diagnosed in 25 patients. At the time of clinic reevaluation (a mean of 16 years after diagnosis), uveitis was still active in 8 of the 19 patients with insidious-onset, chronic, anterior uveitis. Oligoarthritis tended to become extended and to be active in those with active uveitis. Acute, symptomatic, anterior uveitis was seen in six patients between the ages of 14.5 and 22 years, all of whom were HLA-B27 positive. Visual outcome was good. These observations are similar to those reported by Skarin and colleagues.[13]

There have been significant advances in the diagnosis and management of uveitis in JIA, but there is a need for evaluation of the early institution of second-line therapies, and for prospective controlled trials of biologics.

REFERENCES

1. D.A. Jabs, R.B. Nussenblatt, J.T. Rosenbaum, Standardization of uveitis nomenclature for reporting clinical data: results of the first international workshop, Am. J. Ophthalmol. 140 (2005) 509–516.
2. G.N. Holland, C.S. Denove, F. Yu, Chronic anterior uveitis in children: clinical characteristics and complications, Am. J. Ophthalmol. 47 (2009) 667–678.
3. J.A. Smith, F. Mackensen, H.N. Sen, et al., Epidemiology and course of disease in childhood uveitis, Ophthalmology 116 (2009) 1544–1551.
8. R.E. Petty, T.R. Southwood, P. Manners, et al., International League of Associations for Rheumatology classification of juvenile idiopathic arthritis: second revision, Edmonton, J. Rheumatol. 31 (2004) (2001) 390–392.
10. S.T. Angeles-Han, C.F. Pelajo, L.B. Vogler, et al., Risk markers of JIA-associated uveitis in the childhood arthritis and rheumatology research alliance (CAARA) registry, J. Rheumatol. 40 (2013) 2088–2096.
11. R.K. Saurenmann, A.V. Levin, B.M. Feldman, et al., Prevalence, risk factors and outcome of uveitis in juvenile idiopathic arthritis: a long-term followup study, Arthritis Rheum. 56 (2007) 647–657.
13. A. Skarin, R. Elborgh, E. Edlund, et al., Long-term follow-up of patients with uveitis associated with juvenile idiopathic arthritis: a cohort study. Ocular. Immunol, Inflammation 17 (2009) 104–108.
14. H.-H. Yu, P.-C. Chen, L.-C. Wang, et al., Juvenile idiopathic arthritis-associated uveitis: a nationwide population-based study in Taiwan, PLoS ONE 8 (8) (2013) e70625. doi:10.1371/journal.pone.0070625.
15. A. Heiligenhaus, C. Heinz, C. Edelsten, et al., Review for disease of the year: epidemiology of juvenile idiopathic arthritis and its associated uveitis: The probable risk factors, Ocul. Immunol. Inflamm. 21 (2013) 180–191.
16. A.T. Vitale, E. Graham, J.H. Boer, Juvenile idiopathic arthritis-associated uveitis: clinical features and complications, risk factors for severe course and visual outcome, Ocul. Immunol. Inflamm. 21 (2013) 478–485.
27. R.K. Sauermann, A.V. Levin, B.M. Feldman, et al., Risk factors for development of uveitis differ between girls and boys with juvenile idiopathic arthritis, Arthritis Rheum. 62 (2010) 1824–1828.
28. A. Heiligenhaus, M. Niewerth, G. Ganser, et al., Prevalence and complications of uveitis in juvenile idiopathic arthritis in a population-based nation-wide study in Germany suggested modification of current screening guidelines, Rheumatology 46 (2007) 1015–1019.
29. I. Asproudis, T. Felekis, E. Tsanou, et al., Juvenile idiopathic arthritis-associated uveitis: data from a region in western Greece, Clin. Ophthalmol. 4 (2010) 343–347.
31. F. Willerman, J.T. Rosenbaum, B. Bodaghi, et al., Interplay between adaptive and innate immunity in the development of non-infectious uveitis, Prog. Retin. Eye Res. 31 (2012) 182–194.
34. T. Yoshimura, K.-H. Sonoda, N. Ohguro, et al., Involvement of Th17 cells and the effect of anti-IL-6 therapy on autoimmune uveitis, Rheumatology (Oxford) 48 (2009) 347–354.
37. A.D. Dick, I. Tugal-Tutkun, S. Foster, et al., Secunkinumab in the treatment of non-infectious uveitis: results of three randomized controlled clinical trials, Ophthalmology 120 (2013) 177–187.
38. D. Luger, D. Caspi, New perspectives on effector mechanisms in uveitis, Semin. Immunol. 30 (2008) 135–143.
40. K.M. Sijssens, G.T. Rijkers, A. Rothova, et al., Distinct cytokine patterns in the aqueous humor of children, adolescents and adults with uveitis. Ocular Immunol, Inflammation 16 (2008) 211–216.
46. K. Julian, C. Terrada, P. Lehoang, P. Quartier, Uveitis related to juvenile idiopathic arthritis: familial cases and possible genetic implications in the pathogenesis, Ocul. Immunol. Inflamm. 18 (2010) 172–177.
54. T.M. Martin, J.T. Rosenbaum, An update on the genetics of HLA-B27 associated acute anterior uveitis, Ocul. Immunol. Inflamm. 19 (2011) 108–114.
55. M. Yanagimachi, T. Miyamae, T. Naruto, et al., Association of HLA-A*02:06 and HLA DRB1*0405 with clinical subtypes of juvenile idiopathic arthritis, J. Hum. Genet. 56 (2011) 196–199.
60. [No authors listed], American Academy of Pediatrics Section on Rheumatology and Section on Ophthalmology: Guidelines for ophthalmologic examinations in children with juvenile rheumatoid arthritis, Pediatrics 93 (1993) 295–296.
61. K. Reininga, K. Los, N.M. Wulffraat, The evaluation of uveitis in juvenile idiopathic arthritis (JIA) patients: are current screening guidelines adequate?, Clin. Exp. Rheumatol. 26 (2008) 367–372.
62. K. Sabri, R.K. Sauernmann, E.D. Silverman, A.V. Levin, Course, complications and outcome of juvenile arthritis-related uveitis, J. AAPOS 12 (2008) 539–545.
63. J.E. Thorne, F. Woreta, S.R. Kedhar, et al., Juvenile idiopathic arthritis-associated uveitis: incidence of ocular complications and visual acuity loss, Am. J. Ophthalmol. 43 (2007) 840–846.
67. F. Mackensen, J.R. Smith, J.T. Rosenbaum, Enhanced recognition, treatment, and prognosis of tubulointerstitial nephritis and uveitis syndrome, Ophthalmology 114 (2007) 995–999.
71. J.G. Zaborowski, D. Parbhoo, K. Chinniah, et al., Uveitis in children with human immunodeficiency virus-associated arthritis, J. AAPOS 12 (2008) 608–610.
75. H.-I. Huppertz, D. Münchmeier, W. Lieb, Ocular manifestations in children and adolescents with Lyme arthritis, Br. J. Ophthalmol. 83 (1999) 1149–1152.

77. S.J. Lim, S.E. Lee, S.H. Kim, et al., Prevalence of toxoplasma gondii and toxocara canis among patients with uveitis, Ocul. Immunol. Inflamm. 22 (2014) 360–366.

92. Q.D. Nguyen, C.S. Foster, Saving the vision of children with juvenile rheumatoid arthritis-associated uveitis, JAMA 280 (1998) 1133–1134.

95. I. Foeldvari, A. Wierk, Methotrexate is an effective treatment for chronic uveitis associated with juvenile idiopathic arthritis, J. Rheumatol. 32 (2005) 362–365.

98. C. Tappeiner, M. Roesel, C. Heinz, et al., Limited value of cyclosporine A for the treatment of patients with uveitis associated with juvenile idiopathic arthritis, Eye 23 (2009) 1192–1198.

99. J.C. Goebel, M. Roese, C. Heinz, et al., Azathioprine as a treatment option for uveitis in patients with juvenile idiopathic arthritis, Br. J. Ophthalmol. 95 (2011) 209–213.

100. D. Doycheva, C. Deuter, N. Stubiger, et al., Mycophenolate mofetil in the treatment of uveitis in children, Br. J. Ophthalmol. 91 (2007) 180–184.

101. L. Sobrin, W. Christen, C.S. Foster, Mycophenolate mofetil after methotrexate failure of intolerance in the treatment of scleritis and uveitis, Ophthalmology 115 (2008) 1416–1421.

102. A. Reiff, S. Takei, S. Sadeghi, et al., Etanercept therapy in children with treatment-resistant uveitis, Arthritis Rheum. 44 (2001) 1411–1415.

103. A. Reiff, Long-term outcome of etanercept therapy in children with treatment-refractory uveitis, Arthritis Rheum. 48 (2003) 2079–2080.

104. J.A. Smith, D.J. Thompson, S.M. Whitcup, et al., A randomized, placebo controlled, double-masked clinical trial of etanercept for the treatment of uveitis associated with juvenile idiopathic arthritis, Arthritis Rheum. 53 (2005) 18–23.

105. R.K. Sauernmann, A.V. Levin, J.B. Rose, et al., Tumor necrosis α inhibitors in the treatment of childhood uveitis, Rheumatology (Oxford) 45 (2005) 982–989.

106. P. Tynjala, P. Lindahl, V. Honkanen, et al., Infliximab and etanercept in the treatment of chronic uveitis associated with refractory juvenile idiopathic arthritis, Ann. Rheum. Dis. 66 (2006) 548–550.

107. G. Simonini, M.E. Zannin, R. Caputo, et al., Loss of efficacy during long-term treatment for sight-threatening childhood uveitis, Rheumatology (Oxford) 47 (2008) 1510–1514.

109. L.L. Lim, F.W. Fraunfelder, J.T. Rosenbaum, Do tumor necrosis factor inhibitors cause uveitis?, Arthritis Rheum. 56 (2007) 3248–3252.

110. A. Magli, R. Forte, P. Navarro, et al., Adalimumab for juvenile idiopathic arthritis-associated uveitis, Graefes Arch. Clin. Exp. Ophthalmol. 251 (2013) 1601–1606.

112. M.E. Zannin, C. Birolo, V.M. Gerloni, et al., Safety and efficacy of infliximab and adalimumab for refractory uveitis in juvenile idiopathic arthritis: 1-year followup data from the Italian registry, J. Rheumatol. 40 (2013) 74–79.

113. M. William, S. Faez, G.N. Papaliodis, A.-M. Lobo, Golimumab for the treatment of refractory juvenile idiopathic arthritis-associated uveitis, J Ophthalmic Inflamm Infect 2 (2012) 231–233.

114. C. Tappeiner, Is tocilizumab an effective option for treatment of refractory uveitis associated with juvenile idiopathic arthritis?, J. Rheumatol. 39 (2012) 1294–1295.

115. F. Zulian, M. Balzarin, F. Falcini, et al., Abatacept fore severe anti-tumor necrosis factor-refractory juvenile idiopathic arthritis-related uveitis, Arthritis Care Res. 62 (2010) 621–625.

116. A. Heiligenhaus, E. Miserocchi, C. Heinz, et al., Treatment of severe uveitis associated with juvenile idiopathic arthritis with anti CD-20 monoclonal antibody (rituximab), Rheumatology (Oxford) 50 (2011) 1390–1394.

118. A. Heiligenhaus, H. Michels, C. Schumacher, et al., Evidence-based interdisciplinary guidelines for anti-inflammatory treatment of uveitis associated with juvenile idiopathic arthritis, Rheumatol. Int. 32 (2012) 1121–1133.

119. V. Kalinina Ayuso, E.L. van de Winkel, A. Rothova, J.H. de Boer, Relapse rate of uveitis post-methotrexate treatment in juvenile idiopathic arthritis, Am. J. Ophthalmol. 151 (2011) 217–222.

120. M. Hoeve, V.K. Ayuso, N.E. Schalij-Delfos, et al., The clinical course of juvenile idiopathic arthritis-associated uveitis in childhood and puberty, Br. J. Ophthalmol. 96 (2012) 852–856.

122. V. Kalinina Ayuso, H.A. Ten Cate, P. van der Does, et al., Male gender and poor visual outcome in uveitis associated with juvenile idiopathic arthritis, Am. J. Ophthalmol. 149 (2010) 994–999.

123. S.T. Angeles-Han, K.W. Griffin, T.J.A. Lehman, et al., The importance of visual function in the quality of life of children with uveitis, J. AAPOS 14 (2010) 163–168.

The entire reference list is available online at www.expertconsult.com.

CHAPTER 23

Systemic Lupus Erythematosus

Marisa Klein-Gitelman, Jerome Charles Lane

Systemic lupus erythematosus (SLE) is the prototypic autoimmune disease. It is characterized by multiple autoantibodies associated with a multisystem illness. Antibodies most commonly associated with SLE are antinuclear antibodies (ANAs) and anti-double stranded (native) DNA (anti-dsDNA). The presentation, disease course, and outcome of SLE are unpredictable. Patients often experience disease flares and, more rarely, remissions. Pediatric lupus patients typically have more severe disease,[1] and, if untreated, the 5-year mortality rate reaches 95%. Treatment requires the clinician to balance the immunosuppression necessary to reduce organ damage and autoimmune dysfunction with the morbidity from such therapies.

HISTORICAL REVIEW

The word *lupus* was originally attributed to Rogerius, a monk in the thirteenth century, who labeled a disease of facial ulcerations seen in his patients that reminded him of wolves. Cazenave, a French dermatologist, added *erythematosus* to *lupus* in his descriptions of the rash. Kaposi, a Hungarian dermatologist who became a faculty member in the department of dermatology at the University of Vienna under Dr. von Hebra, was the first dermatologist in the late 1800s to describe the acute and chronic skin lesions seen in lupus erythematosus. At the end of the nineteenth century, Osler at Johns Hopkins connected the renal failure of young women to the rash and was the first to describe systemic nature of lupus as well as its flares and remissions. The early twentieth century was associated with many medical advances. Libman and Sacks described the cardiac manifestations of the disease while Baehr, Klemperer, and Schifrin described internal organ involvement through pathological evaluations. The mid-twentieth century was marked by the discovery of the lupus erythematosus cell by Hargraves, Richmond, and Morton. This was followed by Friou's discovery of the ANA by indirect immunofluorescence and Kunkel and Tan's identification of anti-dsDNA in the serum and organs of affected patients. These discoveries gave the clinician the ability to identify patients with SLE earlier, particularly in those with atypical signs of disease. Furthermore, the presence of pathological autoantibodies led to the concept of lupus as an inflammatory immune complex disease, associated with complement activation, B-cell hyperactivity, and altered cell-mediated immunity. Our current understanding of disease pathophysiology also includes changes in innate immunity, dendritic cells, and neutrophils.

CLASSIFICATION CRITERIA

The American Rheumatism Association, now known as the American College of Rheumatology (ACR), developed a classification system in 1971. This system was modified in 1982 and 1997 (Table 23-1).[2,3] The Systemic Lupus International Collaborating Clinics (SLICC) reviewed the classification system and published a new set of criteria in 2012 (Table 23-2).[4]

The SLICC criteria include 11 clinical and 6 immunologic items. Classification criteria require four items with at least one clinical and one immunologic item, or biopsy-proven nephritis compatible with lupus in the presence of an ANA or anti-dsDNA. Studies of specificity and sensitivity of the SLICC classification criteria in pediatric lupus were recently published.[5] In this study, the ACR criteria had 76.6% sensitivity and 93.4% specificity while the SLICC criteria had 98.7% sensitivity and 85.3% specificity. Thus the SLICC criteria were more sensitive and less specific. Further study of larger populations is needed to confirm these findings. Although the classification criteria are excellent guides, diagnosis of childhood lupus is not dependent on meeting criteria, and the clinician should use clinical judgment to determine the care of individual patients. However, the ACR criteria appear to be very useful in pediatric SLE (pSLE).

EPIDEMIOLOGY

Incidence and Prevalence

The incidence and prevalence of pSLE is variable depending on factors such as access to care, referral patterns, ethnic diversity, and the ability to ascertain cases for calculation. Pineles et al. summarized available data in 2011.[6] There were nine studies that described incidence of lupus from 0.36 to 2.5 per 100,000 individuals. The studies included data from North America, Europe, and Asia. Eight of the studies had an incidence of 0.36 to 0.73 per 100,000 individuals, while the remaining study, from Atlanta, Georgia, had a higher incidence of 2.5 per 100,000 persons, with a rate of 3.6 per 100,000 for African Americans, and a rate of 0.5 per 100,000 for Caucasians. Five studies describe prevalence rate from 1.89 to 25.7 per 100,000 persons in studies from Spanish to Hawaiian populations. Differences are likely the result of how the data were collected, and ethnic diversity.[7-11]

TABLE 23-1   The 1982 Revised Criteria for Classification of Systemic Lupus Erythematosus With 1997 Revision

CRITERION	DEFINITION
Malar rash	Fixed erythema, flat or raised, over the malar eminences, tending to spare the nasolabial folds
Discoid rash	Erythematosus raised patches with adherent keratotic scaling and follicular plugging; atrophic scarring may occur in older lesions
Photosensitivity	Skin rash as a result of unusual reaction to sunlight, by patient history or physician observation
Oral ulcers	Oral or nasopharyngeal ulceration, usually painless, observed by physician
Arthritis	Nonerosive arthritis involving two or more peripheral joints, characterized by tenderness, swelling, or effusion
Serositis	Pleuritis—convincing history of pleuritic pain or rubbing heard by a physician or evidence of pleural effusion or pericarditis—documented by ECG or rub or evidence of pericardial effusion
Renal disorder	Persistent proteinuria greater than 0.5 g/day (or >3+ if quantitation nor performed) or cellular casts (may be red cell, hemoglobin, granular, tubular, or mixed)
Neurological disorder	Seizures in the absence of offending drugs or known metabolic derangements (e.g., uremia, ketoacidosis, or electrolyte imbalance) or psychosis in the absence of offending drugs or known metabolic derangements (e.g., uremia, ketoacidosis, or electrolyte imbalance)
Hematological disorder	Hemolytic anemia with reticulocytosis or leukopenia less than $4000/mm^3$ total on two or more occasions, or lymphopenia less than $1500/mm^3$ on two or more occasions, or thrombocytopenia less than $100,000/mm^3$ in the absence of offending drugs
Immunological disorder	(a) Positive anti-DNA antibody to native DNA in abnormal titer, or (b) Presence of anti-Sm nuclear antigen, or (c) Positive finding of APLs based on (1) an abnormal serum level of IgG or IgM anticardiolipin antibodies, (2) a positive test result for lupus anticoagulant using a standard method, or (3) a false-positive serological test and confirmed by *Treponema pallidum* immobilization or fluorescent treponemal antibody absorption test
Antinuclear antibody	An abnormal titer of antinuclear antibody by immunofluorescence or an equivalent assay at any point in time and in the absence of drugs known to be associated with drug-induced lupus syndrome

ECG, Electrocardiogram; *IgG,* immunoglobulin G; *IgM,* immunoglobulin M.
The proposed classification is based on 11 criteria. For the purpose of identifying patients in clinical studies, a person is defined as having SLE if any 4 or more of the 11 criteria are present, serially or simultaneously, during any interval of observation.
Data from E.M. Tan, A.S. Cohen, J.F. Fries, et al., The 1982 revised criteria for the classification of systemic lupus erythematosus, Arthritis Rheum. 25 (1982) 1271–1277; M.C. Hochberg, Updating the American College of Rheumatology revised criteria for the classification of systemic lupus erythematosus, Arthritis Rheum. 40 (1997) 1725.

Age at Onset

Pediatric lupus has been estimated to account for 10% to 20% of all cases of SLE. The average age of onset is 12 years, with rare cases occurring at 5 years of age or younger. Diagnosis of pSLE occurs at a younger age in non-Caucasian populations.

Gender

The gender distribution of pSLE is 4.5-5:1 (female-to-male) as opposed to 9-10:1 (female-to-male) in the adult population. The lower ratio has been attributed to differences in hormone status between children and adults; however, not all series that compare gender differences by age or pubertal status support this concept.[12-21]

Ethnicity

Although SLE is found worldwide, several studies on incidence and prevalence demonstrate higher rates of lupus in non-Caucasian populations. In the United States, a majority of pSLE occurs in the African-American population. Several studies have reported increased incidence in aboriginal, Latino, Asian, and Afro-Caribbean populations.[12,22-35]

ETIOLOGY AND PATHOGENESIS

Immunological Abnormalities

SLE is a complex disease of immune dysregulation, with alterations in both innate and adaptive immunity. Initial observations about the immune mechanisms of lupus come from studies of spontaneous and induced immune dysregulation in mice leading to lupuslike syndromes.[36-41] Human studies were initially more difficult; however,

advances in technology have led to many seminal observations. The identification of monogenic causes of lupus, such as complement deficiencies, genetic overproduction of interferon-α (INF-α), and apoptosis defects, has led to important insights in lupus pathophysiology.[42]

Apoptosis and Innate Immunity

The current hypotheses associated with the generation of lupus and loss of tolerance start with a host defense response gone awry. SLE is characterized by abnormal regulation of type I interferons (INF-α), which stimulate production of innate cells and the inflammatory response.[43-48] Apoptosis or cell death requires rapid clearance of intracellular debris. However, in lupus defective or abnormally regulated apoptotic clearance allows presentation of intracellular materials, including autoantigens, RNA, and DNA.[49-57] Defects in complement, complement receptors, immunoglobulin receptors, Bcl2, Fas/Fas ligand, and programmed cell death 1 (PCD1) all can contribute to different rates of clearance of apoptotic materials.[58-64] Phagocytic immune cells respond to specific RNA and DNA motifs that have been endocytosed through Toll-like receptor (TLR) activation of TLR7 and 9. TLR signaling leads to persistent overproduction of proinflammatory cytokines including type I INFs.[65-70]

Complement plays a dual and seemingly paradoxical role in the pathogenesis of lupus nephritis (LN). Hereditary complement deficiencies, such as homozygous C1, C2, or C4 deficiencies, have a high incidence of LN as a result of impaired clearance of apoptotic cells and immune complexes (ICs). Anti-C1q antibodies have been identified that interfere with interaction among C1q, immunoglobulin G (IgG), and C-reactive protein (CRP), likely resulting in a functional C1q

TABLE 23-2   Clinical and Immunologic Criteria Used in the SLICC Classification System*

Clinical Criteria

1. Acute cutaneous lupus, including:
   - Lupus malar rash (do not count if malar discoid)
   - Bullous lupus
   - Toxic epidermal necrolysis variant of SLE
   - Maculopapular lupus rash
   - Photosensitive lupus rash
     In the absence of dermatomyositis
   - OR subacute cutaneous lupus (nonindurated psoriasiform and/or annular polycyclic lesions that resolve without scarring, although occasionally with postinflammatory dyspigmentation or telangiectasias)
2. Chronic cutaneous lupus, including:
   - Classic discoid rash
   - Localized (above the neck)
   - Generalized (above and below the neck)
   - Hypertrophic (verrucous) lupus
   - Lupus panniculitis (profundus)
   - Mucosal lupus
   - Lupus erythematosus tumidus
   - Chilblains lupus
   - Discoid lupus/lichen planus overlap
3. Oral ulcers
   - Palate
   - Buccal
   - Tongue
   - OR nasal ulcers
     In the absence of other causes, such as vasculitis, Behçet disease, infection (herpesvirus), inflammatory bowel disease, reactive arthritis and acidic foods
4. Nonscarring alopecia (diffuse thinning or hair fragility with visible broken hairs)
   In the absence of other causes such as alopecia areata, drugs, iron deficiency, and androgenic alopecia
5. Synovitis involving two or more joints, characterized by swelling or effusion
   - OR tenderness in two or more joints and at least 30 minutes of morning stiffness

6. Serositis
   - Typical pleurisy for more than 1 day
   - OR pleural effusions
   - OR pleural rub
   - Typical pericardial pain (pain with recumbency improved by sitting forward) for more than 1 day
   - OR pericardial effusion
   - OR pericardial rub
   - OR pericarditis by electrocardiography
     In the absence of other causes, such as infection, uremia, and Dressler syndrome
7. Renal
   - Urine protein-to-creatinine ratio (or 24-hour urine protein) representing 500 mg protein/24 hours
   - OR red blood cell casts
8. Neurological
   - Seizures
   - Psychosis
   - Mononeuritis multiplex
     In the absence of other known causes, such as primary vasculitis
   - Myelitis
   - Peripheral or cranial neuropathy
     In the absence of other known causes such as primary vasculitis, infection, and diabetes mellitus
   - Acute confusional state
     In the absence of other causes, including toxic/metabolic, uremia, drugs
9. Hemolytic anemia
10. Leukopenia ($<4,000/mm^3$ at least once)
    In the absence of other known causes such as Felty syndrome, drugs, and portal hypertension
    - OR
    - Lymphopenia ($<1,000/mm^3$ at least once)
      In the absence of other known causes such as corticosteroids, drugs, and infection
11. Thrombocytopenia ($<100,000/mm^3$) at least once
    In the absence of other known causes such as drugs, portal hypertension, and thrombotic thrombocytopenic purpura

*Criteria are cumulative and need not be present concurrently.
ANA, antinuclear antibody; *anti-dsDNA*, anti-double stranded DNA; *ELISA*, enzyme-linked immunosorbent assay; *SLE*, systemic lupus erythematosus; *SLICC*, Systemic Lupus International Collaborating Clinics.
Ref. 4

deficiency and impaired clearance of apoptotic cells and ICs.[71] Therefore, certain complement components might be protective against SLE and LN by clearing apoptotic fragments and preventing the accumulation of chromatin. In contrast, complement activation also plays a role in glomerular tissue damage.[72-74]

Neutrophil Function

More recently, the role of neutrophils in perpetuating chronic inflammation has been explored. In lupus patients, neutrophils become apoptotic in the presence of autoantibodies, particularly antiribonuclear protein (RNP) antibodies, and release neutrophil extracellular traps (NETs). NETs are rich in DNA, LL37 (the cleaved antimicrobial 37-residue, COOH-terminal peptide of hCAP18 [human cationic antimicrobial protein with a molecular size of 18 kD]), and HMGB1 (high-mobility group protein B1). The latter proteins are associated with activation of plasmacytoid dendritic cells (pDCs) by mammalian

DNA; pDCs have been demonstrated to produce high levels of interferon and are associated with active lupus.[75,76] NETs can activate the inflammasome, leading to upregulation of interleukin (IL)-1β and IL-18. Caspase 1 is a central molecule in the inflammasome. A recent murine model demonstrated an essential role of caspase 1 in the induction of murine lupus and its associated vascular damage.[77]

Adaptive Immunity

Lupus patients have been shown to have abnormalities in B cells, T cells, and antigen-presenting cells.[45,78-88] The hallmark of lupus is the production of autoantibodies and hypergammaglobulinemia. Several different mechanisms can account for this, including antigen stimulation, polyclonal B-cell proliferation, T-cell dysregulation, or intrinsic B-cell defects. The result is antibody-mediated disease by direct cellular injury, seen as cytopenias, as well as IC disease due to an immune system that has an ineffective or overwhelmed clearance mechanism, as seen in lupus nephritis and vasculitis. IC formation leads to activation of complement, leading to inflammation and tissue damage. Other autoantibodies such as anti-dsDNA are thought to arise from somatic mutation induced by environmental stimuli, or from autoantigen materials such as nucleosomes or chromatin. T-cell dysregulation is marked by T-cell cytopenia, particularly of natural killer (NK) cells and regulatory T cells, leading to cytokine profiles that support B-cell activation.[89] Furthermore, there is overexpression of CD40–CD40 ligand leading to B-cell activation.

Over the past decade, the central role of dendritic cells (DCs) in the pathophysiology of lupus has been recognized. In addition to activating complement, ICs activate pDCs, leading to production INF-α. FcγRIIa on the pDC cell membrane delivers ICs to lysosomal TLRs (TLR7, for RNA containing ICs, and TLR9 for DNA containing ICs).[90] TLR-induced production of INF-α leads to a variety of important inflammatory processes, including differentiation of monocytes into DCs and activation of immature myeloid DCs (mDCs), which subsequently activate autoreactive T and B cells, leading to increased autoantibody production. Activated mDCs also cause CD8+ T cells to differentiate into cytotoxic T cells, thereby furthering tissue damage, generation of nucleosomes, formation of ICs, complement activation, activation of DCs, INF-α production, T- and B-cell activation, and autoantibody production.[72] Activated DCs present nuclear antigens (nucleosomes) to lymphocytes, resulting in expansion of autoreactive T-cell clones (cytotoxic T cells and T-helper cells [Th] such as Th17) and autoreactive B cell clones that can differentiate into plasma cells, leading to production of more antinuclear antibody. Nuclear particles also can directly activate B cells via the B cell receptor without the presence of antigen-presenting cells.[91]

Genetics

The first indication that genetic susceptibility played a role in the etiology of SLE came from family and twin studies. Ten percent of first-degree relatives of patients with SLE also have the disease, compared with 1% in control families.[92-94] There is a twentyfold increased risk of siblings having SLE compared with the general population.[92,95] Among twins, 24% of monozygous compared with 2% of dizygous twins are concordant for SLE.[96] One in 10 family members of patients with SLE have another connective tissue disease.[93,94,97-99]

Single gene mutations associated with SLE are rare but give important clues regarding the genetic mechanisms underlying SLE. SLE has been reported in more than 90% of cases of homozygous C1q deficiency.[100] Approximately 33% of patients with homozygous C2 deficiency develop SLE, and there is a higher association of C2 deficiency and anti-Ro antibodies.[101] C4 allele deficiencies are also associated with increased risk of SLE.[102]

Early studies in SLE susceptibility using candidate gene association and linkage analysis implicated a region on chromosome 6 (6p11-21) containing the human leukocyte antigen (HLA) region in susceptibility to SLE.[103] The HLA (or major histocompatibility complex [MHC]) region contains genes from MHC class I (HLA-A, HLA-B, and HLA-C), class II (HLA-DR, HLA-DQ, and HLA-DP), and class III (components of the complement system, cytokines such as tumor necrosis factor-α [TNF-α] and heat shock proteins). This region is characterized by a high degree of linkage disequilibrium, in which long stretches of genes are inherited together as a set (haplotype), making it difficult to identify individual alleles associated with risk of SLE.[104] Haplotypes including HLA-DRB1 and HLA-DQB1 alleles are associated with increased risk of SLE in Caucasian populations. HLA-DR2 and HLA-DR3 increase the risk of SLE in Caucasians by twofold or threefold.[105] DR2 haplotypes also have been associated with anti-Sm antibody, and DR3 haplotypes with anti-Ro antibodies. DR2 and DR7 are associated with SLE in African Americans.[106]

TABLE 23-3	Pathway-Assocaited SLE Candidate Genes (not Including HLA)	
PATHWAY	**GENES**
DNA degradation, apoptosis, and clearance of cellular debris	FCGR2B, ACP5, TREX1, DNASE1, DNASE1L3, ATG5
TLR and type I IFN signaling	TLR7, IRF5, IRF7/PHRF1, IRF8, IRAK1, IFIH1, TYK2, PRDM1, STAT4, TREX1, ACP5
NF-κB signaling	IRAK1, TNFAIP3, TNIP1, UBE2L3, SLC15A4, PRKCB
Immune complex processing and phagocytosis	C1Q, C1R/C1S, C2, C4A/B, FCGR2A/B, FCGR3A/B
B-cell function and signaling	FCGR2B, BLK, LYN, BANK1, PRDM1, ETS1, IKZF1, AFF1, RASGRP3, IL10, IL21, NCF2, PRKCB, HLA-DR2 and DR3, MSH5, IRF8
T-cell function and signaling	PTPN22, TNFSF4, CD44, ETS1, IL10, IL21, TYK2, STAT4, PRDM1, AFF1, IKZF1, HLA-DR2 and DR3
Neutrophil and monocyte function and signaling	ITGAM, ICAMs, FCGR2B, FCGR3A/B, IL10, IRF8

IFN, Interferon; *NF-κB,* nuclear factor κB; *SLE,* systemic lupus erythematosus; *TLR,* toll-like receptor.
From: O.J. Rullo, B.P. Tsao, Recent insights into the genetic basis of systemic lupus erythematosus, Ann. Rheum. Dis. 72 (2013) ii56–ii61.

Prior to 2008, the above approaches identified nine genes linked to an increased risk for SLE. Since 2008, the advent of genome-wide association studies (GWAS) and further candidate gene studies have expanded to list of genes linked to SLE to more than 40. Most of these genes can be grouped into common physiological pathways. These include the following: (1) HLA regulation; (2) DNA degradation, apoptosis, and clearance of cellular debris; (3) defective clearance of immune complexes containing nuclear antigens; (4) TLR and type I IFN pathway activation; (5) nuclear factor-κB (NF-κB) signaling; (6) B-cell function and signaling; (7) T-cell signaling and function; and (8) monocyte and neutrophil signaling and function (see Table 23-3).[107]

In addition to individual genes, it is clear that SLE is a complex disease influenced by the interactive effects of multiple genes. Recent studies have shown that epistasis, or gene–gene interaction, plays an important role in SLE susceptibility. Additionally, epigenetic factors, such as cytosine methylation, histone modifications, and microRNA profile may play a role in the development of SLE, as evidenced by globally decreased DNA methylation in patients with lupus.[108-118]

Hormones

Lupus primarily occurs in female patients between menarche and menopause. Thus, the presence of estrogens and low levels of androgens play a role in disease risk. Past studies of children with lupus have reported high levels of follicle-stimulating hormone, luteinizing hormone, and prolactin, and low levels of androgens.[119] Estrogen has a variety of immune effects, including modulation of the innate and adaptive immune responses; altering the number of immunoglobulin-secreting cells; effects on antigen presentation by DCs and macrophages; and modulation of the Th1 and Th2 responses.[120] Of note, there is an increased risk of lupus in patients with Klinefelter syndrome.[121] Individuals with Klinefelter syndrome have mild disease, unlike the normal adult male population, in which there is a higher risk of nephritis and renal failure.[122] The influence of two X chromosomes versus direct hormone effects is unclear.

Determinants of gene function

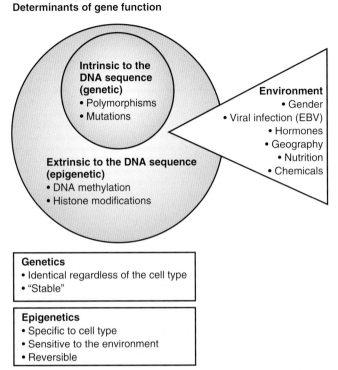

Genetics
- Identical regardless of the cell type
- "Stable"

Epigenetics
- Specific to cell type
- Sensitive to the environment
- Reversible

FIGURE 23-1 Determinants of gene function. Genetic and epigenetic components determine gene function in health and disease. DNA sequence changes (including polymorphisms and mutations) can be considered intrinsic to the DNA sequence, whereas DNA methylation and histone modification, that is, the major epigenetic modifications, are extrinsic to the DNA sequence. Epigenetic modifications are far more sensitive to environmental stimuli than the sequence of DNA. *EBV*, Epstein–Barr virus. (From E. Ballestar, Epigenetic alterations in autoimmune rheumatic diseases, Nat. Rev. Rhematol. 7 (2011) 263–271.)

Environmental Factors

Since monozygous twins do not have a 100% concordance rate for SLE, it is clear that factors in addition to genetics play a role in the disease. It is thought that SLE susceptibility is determined by a complex interaction of environment, genetic predisposition, and differential gene expression through epigenetic modifications (see Fig. 23-1).[123] Some of the environmental factors implicated in SLE include ultraviolet radiation, viral infections, drugs, hormones, and chemicals.

Ultraviolet Radiation

Ultraviolet radiation (UV), in particular UVB, is a well-known trigger of cutaneous as well as systemic lupus. UVB produces a variety of inflammatory responses: It directly induces keratinocytes to release chemokines and cytokines, which recruit memory T cells and pDCs into the skin, and also induces apoptosis and necrosis of keratinocytes, leading to accumulation of nucleic acids and activation of pDCs through TLRs, as previously described (Fig. 23-2).[124] Additionally, UVB can decrease DNA methylation in peripheral blood mononuclear cells, especially in patients with active lupus, which might alter gene expression and play a role in the pathogenesis of SLE.[125]

Viral Infection

Viral infections have been implicated in autoimmunity and SLE. Viruses, such as Epstein–Barr virus (EBV) and cytomegalovirus (CMV), can induce autoimmunity through a variety of mechanisms, including molecular mimicry, activation of T cells by superantigens,

and expansion of previously activated T cells at a site of inflammation (bystander activation).[126]

A higher prevalence of EBV infection has been described in SLE patients compared to the general population.[127-131] This increased incidence of EBV has been described in pSLE as well.[132,133] EBV naturally resides in the B cells of infected hosts and can activate and immortalize B cells, thereby interfering with normal regulation of antibody production. EBV nuclear antigen 1 (EBNA-1) and EBNA-2 cross-react with, or "mimic," lupus autoantigens such as Ro, SmB/SmB$_0$, and SmD. EBV, therefore, might induce SLE through expression of EBNA-1 and EBNA-2, which induce autoimmunity by triggering antibody formation to lupus autoantigens. In normal hosts with EBV infection, these antibodies are limited and effectively cleared. However, in SLE-susceptible individuals who have abnormal immune response to EBV infection, these cross-reactive antibodies persist and become pathogenic.[134]

CMV, like EBV, is another member of the herpesvirus family and has been associated with triggering and exacerbating SLE.[135-137] Higher rates of infection and seropositivity have been found in SLE patients compared to controls.[138,139] CMV can induce antiphospholipid antibodies (APLs) and autoantibodies to erythrocytes, nuclear components, and smooth muscle. CMV early RNA can induce anti-Ro/SSA activity. CMV lower matrix phosphoprotein (pp65) antigen triggers autoimmunity in murine models and SLE patients, and induces autoantibodies to nuclear components.[138] Although parvovirus B19 infection can appear to mimic the clinical features of SLE, there is conflicting evidence regarding the association of parvovirus and SLE.[5,140-147]

Case reports indicate a possible association of vaccination with SLE, especially after hepatitis B and influenza vaccination. Vaccination can result in a transient rise in autoantibody titers. However, vaccination appears to be safe in patients with quiescent disease, and the benefits regarding reduction in infections outweigh the possible risks of vaccination, especially regarding childhood diseases with possible high morbidity and mortality.[148,149]

Drug-Induced Lupus

More than 80 medications have been associated with the drug-induced lupus (DLE). These drugs fall into 10 categories, including antiarrhythmics, hypertension medications, antipsychotics, antibiotics, anticonvulsants, thyroid medications, antiinflammatory medications, diuretics, statins, and biologics (see Table 23-4). Drugs most commonly associated with DLE include hydralazine, procainamide, isoniazid, methyldopa, quinidine, minocycline, and chlorpromazine.[150] In children, antiepileptic medications are most commonly implicated.

Patients with DLE tend to have milder disease manifestations than idiopathic SLE, though severe and even fatal cases of DLE have been described. DLE usually occurs after several months of treatment and might be associated with higher and cumulative medication doses.[150] DLE typically presents with constitutional symptoms, such as arthralgia, myalgia, arthritis, fever, malaise, anorexia, and weight loss. Skin manifestations have been reported in approximately 5% to 40% of patients. Other features of DLE have included pleural or pericardial disease, and hepatosplenomegaly. Major organ involvement is rare, though cases of nephritis have been reported after treatment with hydralazine, sulfasalazine, propylthiouracil, and anti–TNF-α therapy.[151-154]

Complement levels in DLE usually are normal, though low levels have been reported with C-penicillamine and quinidine. Antihistone antibodies are elevated in more than 90% of cases, but may be negative, especially in DLE associated with minocycline, propylthiouracil, and statins. Since antihistone antibodies may occur, though less commonly, in idiopathic SLE, the presence of these antibodies may be suggestive, but not diagnostic, of DLE. Anti-double-stranded DNA antibodies are

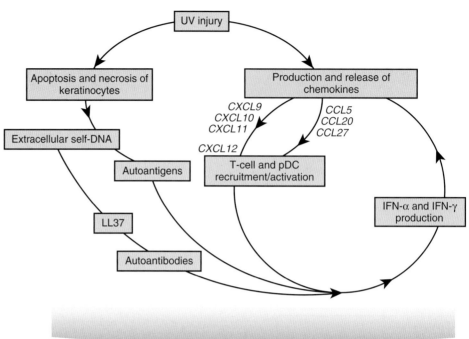

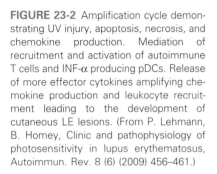

FIGURE 23-2 Amplification cycle demonstrating UV injury, apoptosis, necrosis, and chemokine production. Mediation of recruitment and activation of autoimmune T cells and INF-α producing pDCs. Release of more effector cytokines amplifying chemokine production and leukocyte recruitment leading to the development of cutaneous LE lesions. (From P. Lehmann, B. Homey, Clinic and pathophysiology of photosensitivity in lupus erythematosus, Autoimmun. Rev. 8 (6) (2009) 456–461.)

UV-induced cutaneous LE phenotype

less common in DLE but may be elevated in cases associated with minocycline, propylthiouracil, and quinidine.[151]

DLE is not the result of a typical drug hypersensitivity reaction. Proposed pathogenic mechanisms of DLE include activation of B and T cells, interference with T-cell maturation, cytokine effects, DNA methylation, and formation of reactive metabolites.[150,151,155] DLE usually resolves within weeks to months after discontinuation of the drug that caused the DLE. Lack of reversibility might indicate that the drug unmasked underlying idiopathic SLE. Rarely, corticosteroids or other immunosuppressive therapies might be needed in DLE. Autoantibody titers decline gradually and can persist for months to years after resolution of clinical symptoms. Reexposure to the causative drug typically causes return of DLE manifestations within 1 to 2 days, and with each exposure the time before the onset of symptoms may decrease, and the severity of symptoms may increase.[151]

OTHER ENVIRONMENTAL EXPOSURES

A variety of other environmental, chemical, hormonal, and occupational exposures have been associated with SLE with varying degrees of evidence. These include smoking, pesticides, solvents, silica, heavy metals, and hair dyes. The chemicals in cigarette smoke, including tars, nicotine, carbon monoxide, and polycyclic aromatic hydrocarbons, have multiple effects on the immune system, including tissue hypoxia and damage, toxin-induced cellular necrosis, release of intracellular antigens, and augmentation of autoreactive B cells.[150] Silica inhalation can induce processes of inflammation, fibrosis, and autoimmunity. Silica has been shown to reduce regulatory T cells (Treg) and increase CD4+ T cells, as well as cause apoptosis in macrophages. Lung inflammation and tissue damage might lead to generation of autoantibodies as well.[126,156]

A variety of environmental estrogens and estrogen-like compounds, including oral contraceptives and hormone therapy, insecticides such as DDT, plastics, and phthalates, have been associated with lupus. The

evidence regarding exogenous estrogens is mixed, and further investigation is required.[150]

CLINCIAL DISEASE

Lupus in childhood presents most frequently in the teenage years and accounts for 15% to 20% of the lupus population, depending in the ethnicity of the population studied. The time from symptoms to diagnosis is variable (1 month to 5 years). Recognition and early diagnosis, along with improving therapies, have led to improvements in diagnosis and outcomes.

CLINICAL PRESENTATION

Childhood onset lupus can present with subtle persisting or intermittent symptoms; however, most pediatric patients have more severe disease than their adult counterparts,[1,157] with more organ involvement and more laboratory abnormalities (see Table 23-5). Most lupus patients have vague constitutional symptoms of fever, weight loss, fatigue, and loss of appetite. Generalized signs of immune activation are seen, such as lymphadenopathy and hepatosplenomegaly. SLE may start in a single organ system but will ultimately manifest itself as a multiorgan disease (see Table 23-6). It is important to recognize that the classification criteria that aid in diagnosis are not required to treat severe single organ manifestations.

Kidney Involvement

Involvement of the kidneys is a significant cause of morbidity and mortality in both adult and pediatric patients with SLE. As many as 20% to 75% of children with SLE will develop nephritis, with 18% to 50% progressing to end-stage kidney disease (ESKD).[172-175] In general, the prevalence of LN is higher in children (50% to 67%) than in adults (34% to 48%) with SLE.[176] Eighty percent to 90% of childhood LN develops within the first year of diagnosis. In 10% to 20% of patients,

TABLE 23-4 Drugs Associated With the Development of SLE Drug-induced Lupus

AGENT	RISK
Antiarrhythmics	
Procainamide	High
Quinidine	Moderate
Disopyramide	Very low
Propafenone	Very low
Antihypertensives	
Hydralazine	High
Methyldopa	Low
Captopril	Low
Acebutolol	Low
Enalapril	Very low
Clonidine	Very low
Atenolol	Very low
Labetalol	Very low
Pindolol	Very low
Minoxidil	Very low
Prazosin	Very low
Antipsychotics	
Chlorpromazine	Low
Phenelzine	Very low
Chlorprothixene	Very low
Lithium carbonate	Very low
Antibiotics	
Isoniazid	Low
Minocycline	Low
Nitrofurantoin	Very low
Anticonvulsants	
Carbamazepine	Low
Phenytoin	Very Low
Trimethadione	Very low
Primidone	Very low
Ethosuximide	Very low
Antithyroidals	
Propylthiouracil	Low
Antiinflammatories	
d-Penicillamine	Low
Sulfasalazine	Low
Phenylbutazone	Very low
Diuretics	
Chlorthalidone	Very low
Hydrochlorothiazide	Very low
Miscellaneous	
Anti-tumor necrosis-α	Very low
Lovastatin and other statins	Very low
Levodopa	Very low
Aminoglutethimide	Very low
Interferon α and other cytokines	Very low
Timolol eye drops	Very low

Adapted from R.L. Rubin, Drug-induced lupus, Toxicol. 209 (2005) 135–147.

TABLE 23-5 Frequencies of Clinical Features of Children and Adolescents: Within One Year of Diagnosis and Any Time During Their Disease

CLINICAL FEATURES*	WITHIN FIRST YEAR OF DIAGNOSIS	ANY TIME
Constitutional and Generalized Symptoms		
Fever	35-90%	37-100%
Lymphadenopathy	11-45%	13-45%
Hepatosplenomegaly	16-42%	19-43%
Weight loss	20-30%	21-32%
Organ involvement		
Musculoskeletal		
Arthritis	60-88%	60-90%
Myositis	<5%	<5%
Any skin involvement	60-80%	60-90%
Malar rash	22-68%	30-80%
Discoid rash	<5%	<5%
Photosensitivity	12-45%	17-58%
Mucosal ulceration	25-32%	30-40%
Alopecia	10-30%	15-35%
Other rashes	40-52%	42-55%
Nephritis	20-80%	48-100%
Neuropsychiatric disease	5-30%[†]	15-95%[‡]
Psychosis	5-12%	8-18%
Seizures	5-15%	5-47%
Headache	5-22%	10-95%
Cognitive dysfunction	6-15%	12-55%
Acute confusional state	5-15%	8-35%
Peripheral nerve involvement	<5%	<5%
Cardiovascular disease	5-30%	25-60%
Pericarditis	12-20%	20-30%
Myocarditis	<5%	<5%
Pulmonary disease	18-40%	18-81%
Pleuritis	12-20%	20-30%
Pulmonary hemorrhage	<5%	<5%
pneumonitis	<5%	<5%
Gastrointestinal disease	14-30%	24-40%
Peritonitis (sterile)	10-15%	12-18%
Abnormal liver function	20-40%	25-45%
Pancreatitis	<5%	<5%

*Not all reports commented on all features or incidence in first year.
[†]Had highest prevalence of CNS disease but did not describe incidence in first year.[171]
[‡]Headache reported in 95% of patients.[171]
Data from Refs. 1, 16-21, 23, 24, 158-170.

the nephritis usually occurs between year 1 and year 2 after diagnosis, but late development beyond 5 years can occur.[24,177,178]

PATHOGENESIS OF LN

Extrarenal mechanisms of SLE have been covered in detail elsewhere in this chapter but will be covered in the following section where they pertain to and overlap with intrarenal pathogenic mechanisms. Murine models of LN suggest the LN is initiated by the renal formation of ICs, leading to activation of complement and Fcγ receptors. Indeed, the histological hallmark of LN—the "full-house" pattern of IgG, IgM, IgA,

TABLE 23-6 Common Clinical Manifestations by Organ Involvement

Constitutional	Fever, malaise, weight loss, anorexia
Cutaneous	Butterfly rash, photosensitivity, mucosal ulcerations, periungual erythema, alopecia
Musculoskeletal	Polyarthralgia/arthritis, morning stiffness, tenosynovitis, myositis
Renal	Glomerulonephritis, nephrotic syndrome, hypertension
Neurological	Acute confusional state, seizures, psychosis, cognitive deficits chorea, cerebrovascular accident, pseudotumor cerebri
Cardiac	Pericarditis and effusion, chest pain, Libman–Sacks endocarditis
Pulmonary	Pleuritis, abnormal pulmonary function tests, pneumonitis, pulmonary hemorrhage, infection
Gastrointestinal	Ascites, abdominal pain, peritonitis, colitis, abnormal liver function tests
Reticuloendothelial	Hepatomegaly, splenomegaly, diffuse lymphadenopathy, Kikuchi lymphadenitis
Vascular	Raynaud phenomenon, thrombosis, livedo reticularis
Ocular	Exudates, papilledema, retinopathy

C3, C1q, and κ and λ light chain deposits in the kidney—supports the role of ICs and complement activation in the pathogenesis of LN.[179] Circulating ICs are not deposited in the kidney passively, as previously thought. Instead, ICs form directly in the glomeruli by the binding of autoantibodies to the components of chromatin, likely derived from the nuclear debris of apoptotic renal cells.[73,179-181] As in extrarenal SLE, decreased clearance of apoptotic debris leads to accumulation of chromatin in apoptotic nucleosomes within the kidney. It is also possible that circulating chromatin fragments might reach the kidney, eventually leading to the formation of ICs.[182] IC formation within the kidney leads to activation of complement, leading to inflammation and tissue damage. Intrarenal ICs activate pDCs, leading to various immune responses discussed previously.

Nucleic acids and anti-DNA antibodies can directly activate glomerular endothelial cells and mesangial cells to produce proinflammatory cytokines, INF-α and INF-β. Activation of TLRs, Fcγ, and complement receptors also activate renal cells to produce proinflammatory cytokines and chemokines, as well as induce luminal expression of selectins and adhesion molecules in the renal vasculature. Chemokines recruit macrophages and T cells into the glomeruli and renal interstitium, where they cause inflammation and tissue injury. T and B cells form lymphoid aggregates in the renal tubulointerstitium, in some cases forming germinal centers around follicular DCs. These germinal centers might play a role in persistence of renal inflammation and local generation of autoantibodies.[72,183-185]

Once deposited in the mesangial matrix, ICs appear to downregulate the production of DNase I, the major renal nuclease, through incompletely understood mechanisms that might involve transcriptional interference. Decreased DNase I activity impairs clearance of apoptotic cells and leads to further and large-scale exposure of chromatin fragments (see Figs. 23-3 to 23-7).[182,186]

In a study in which immunoglobulin was eluted from the kidneys of LN patients at autopsy, only 0.3% to 41% of the antibodies reacted to known antigens such as dsDNA, chromatin, Sm, SSA, SSB, and histones. Antibodies generated by isolated memory B cells from LN patients also show only 15% to 26% reactivity to known antigens.

Thus, a large portion of glomerular ICs react to unknown antigens other than dsDNA, and the development of LN is not necessarily associated with autoantibodies of any singular specificity.[187,188]

Once LN has been established, tissue damage can progress to chronic and irreversible stages through processes similar in many different forms of kidney disease. Focal necrosis of glomerular capillaries leads to migration of parietal epithelial cells into the glomerular tuft and production of extracellular matrix, contributing to the process of glomerulosclerosis.[189] Breaks in the glomerular basement membrane (GBM) allow leakage of plasma filtrate into Bowman space. Mitogenic components of plasma induce proliferation of parietal epithelial cells in Bowman space and formation of cellular crescents that fill the urinary space. These parietal cells eventually produce matrix, and the cellular crescents evolve into fibrocellular and fibrous crescents with glomerulosclerosis characteristic of end-stage (class VI) LN.[179,190,191]

CLASSIFICATION OF LUPUS GLOMERULONEPHRITIS

Classification of LN follows the 2003 criteria of the International Society of Nephrology/Renal Pathology Society (ISN/RPS) (Table 23-7). The ISN/RPS 2003 scheme supplanted the old World Health Organization (WHO) classifications and includes assessment of acute and chronic disease. Kidney biopsy tissue is examined by light microscopy to assess general features, cellular findings, glomerular and tubular lesions, and extent of fibrosis; immunofluorescent microscopy to determine the nature and extent of immune deposits; and electron microscopy to determine ultrastructural features and location of immune deposits within the basement membrane. As mentioned previously, LN is defined by the presence of "full-house" immune deposits, predominantly IgG, C3, and, in most cases, C1q, with variable IgA and IgM deposits. Lack of this "full-house" deposition calls into question the diagnosis of LN.[192]

An activity score (AI, range 0-24) and chronicity score (CI, range 0-12) can be used to quantify the degree of acute and chronic changes in a kidney biopsy[193,194] (see Table 23-8), though some studies have questioned the reproducibility and prognostic significance of these scores. Since the degree of active lesions versus chronic lesions can play a role in treatment decisions, the ISN/RPS classification advises, but does not require, the inclusion of AI and CI in assessment of LN.[195]

CLINICAL PRESENTATION

Although correlations often can be made between clinical presentation and histological findings in LN, the presentation of the various classes of LN can overlap, and sometimes patients with the same clinical and laboratory manifestations can have different histological patterns of glomerular involvement. Additionally, severe LN can be "silent" or show minimal clinical and laboratory findings more characteristic of milder forms of the disease.[195-205] Patients with proliferative nephritis often have acute nephritic syndrome, defined by hematuria (microscopic or occasionally macroscopic), usually accompanied by hypertension and a variable degrees of proteinuria. Proteinuria in acute nephritic syndrome can range from mild to nephrotic. Membranous (class V) disease often presents with nephrotic syndrome, defined by nephrotic range proteinuria, hyperlipidemia, hypoalbuminemia, and edema. Isolated asymptomatic hematuria and/or nonnephrotic proteinuria generally is seen in class II LN, but it is sometime seen in other classes, especially if a kidney biopsy is performed after at least several months of immunosuppressive treatment. Depending on the severity

Text continued on p. 296

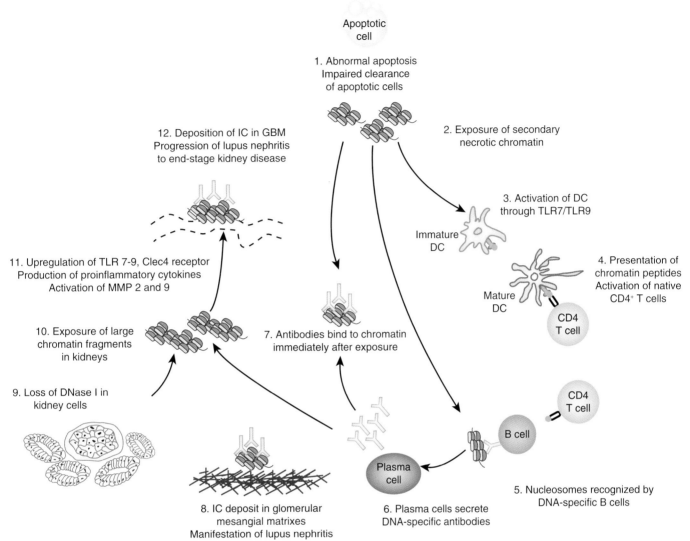

FIGURE 23-3 The role of extracellular chromatin fragments and anti-dsDNA antibodies in progressive lupus nephritis. Retention of chromatin is assumed to start with reduced clearance of apoptotic cells (*1*). Secondary to this, chromatin may be exposed in tissues (*2*) and is assumed to activate dendritic cells (*3*). These cells present chromatin-derived peptides in the context of MHC class II molecules to peptide-specific CD4+ T cells (*4*). When primed, the peptide-specific T cells recirculate and bind the same chromatin-derived peptides presented in the context of MHC class II by chromatin-specific B cells (here recognizing dsDNA in chromatin; *5*). As a consequence of cognate interaction of dsDNA-specific B cells and peptide-specific CD4+ T cells, the B cells transform into plasma cells that secrete IgG anti-dsDNA antibodies (*6*), which bind chromatin fragments (*7*). Immune complexes that consist of IgG antibodies and chromatin fragments bind in the glomerular mesangial matrix and initiate mesangial lupus nephritis (*8*). This early inflammation is followed by silencing of renal DNase I in tubular and glomerular cells (*9*) and accumulation of undigested chromatin fragments (*10*). These fragments promote upregulation of TLRs, proinflammatory cytokines and matrix metalloproteases (*11*). Finally, IgG autoantibodies recognize and bind the chromatin fragments, and these immune complexes deposit in the glomerular basement membranes (GBMs) and aggravate renal inflammation (*12*). In this sense, chromatin fragments and antichromatin (here anti-dsDNA) antibodies are the partners that impose the classic murine and human lupus nephritis. Thus, antichromatin antibodies are pathogenic only in the context of exposed chromatin structures. (From N. Seredkina, J. Van Der Vlag, J. Berden, et al., Lupus nephritis: enigmas, conflicting models and an emerging concept, Mol. Med. 19 (2013) 161–169.)

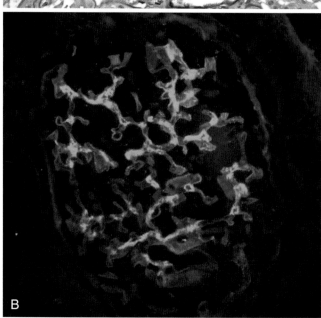

FIGURE 23-4 Mesangial (class II) lupus nephritis. Representative photomicrographs of mesangial (class II) lupus nephritis. **A,** Mesangial proliferation (arrow) but open glomerular capillaries and otherwise normal appearance, Periodic acid-Schiff stain. **B,** Immunofluorescent staining showing a mesangial pattern of IgG deposition. (Photomicrographs provided by Dr. S.M. Meehan, Department of Pathology, University of Chicago.)

FIGURE 23-5 Proliferative lupus nephritis. Representative photomicrographs of proliferative lupus nephritis. Biopsy from a patient with class IV(G)-A lupus nephritis illustrating: **A,** Global (almost the entire glomerulus) endocapillary proliferation and exudation (arrows), Periodic acid–Schiff stain. **B,** Cellular crescents from epithelial proliferation (arrows) and wire loops (arrowhead) from coalescent subendothelial immune deposits, Periodic acid-Schiff stain. **C,** Electron micrograph showing numerous subendothelial (arrows) and mesangial electron dense deposits. **D,** Immunofluorescent staining showing deposition of IgG in glomerular capillary walls and mesangium. (Photomicrographs provided by Dr. S.M. Meehan, Department of Pathology, University of Chicago.)

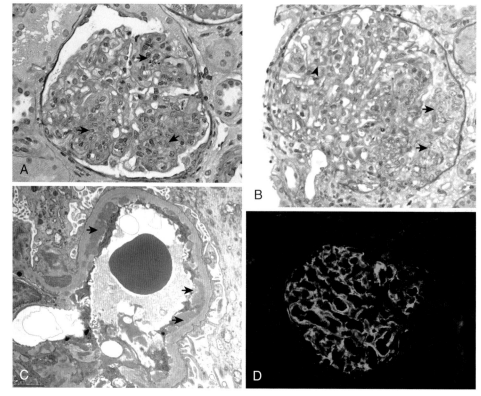

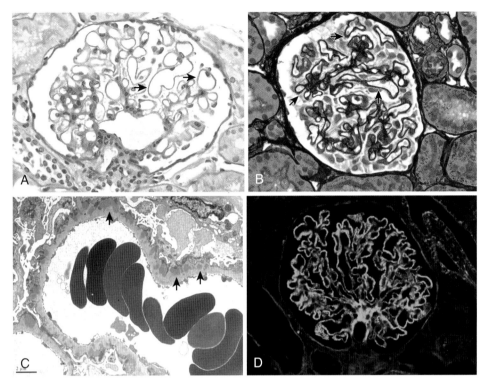

FIGURE 23-6 Membranous (class V) lupus nephritis. Representative photomicrographs of membranous lupus nephritis. **A,** Periodic acid–Schiff stain with thickened basement membranes and "spikes," which appear as fine hairs radiating from the capillary loops (*arrows*) and arise from basement membrane deposition between subepithelial immune deposits. **B,** Jones methenamine silver staining demonstrating spikes (*arrows*). **C,** Electron micrograph with subepithelial and intramembranous deposits (*arrows*). **D,** Immunofluorescent staining showing fine granular staining for IgG in glomerular capillary walls. (Photomicrographs provided by Dr. S.M. Meehan, Department of Pathology, University of Chicago.)

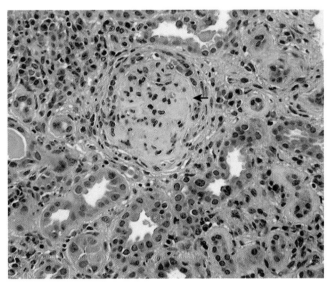

FIGURE 23-7 End-stage (class VI) lupus nephritis. Representative photomicrographs of end-stage (class VI) lupus nephritis illustrating global glomerulosclerosis (*arrow*), with interstitial fibrosis, tubular atrophy, and mononuclear inflammation with numerous plasma cells (hematoxylin-eosin stain). (Photomicrograph provided by Dr. S.M. Meehan, Department of Pathology, University of Chicago.)

TABLE 23-7   International Society of Nephrology/Renal Pathology Society (ISN/RPS) 2003 Classification of Lupus Nephritis

Class I	**Minimal mesangial lupus nephritis**
	Normal glomeruli by light microscopy, but mesangial immune deposits by immunofluorescence
Class II	**Mesangial proliferative lupus nephritis**
	Purely mesangial hypercellularity of any degree or mesangial matrix expansion by light microscopy, with mesangial immune deposits
	A few isolated subepithelial or subendothelial deposits may be visible by immunofluorescence or electron microscopy, but not by light microscopy
Class III	**Focal lupus nephritis**
Class III (A)	Active or inactive focal, segmental or global endocapillary or extracapillary glomerulonephritis involving <50% of all glomeruli, typically
Class III (A/C)	with focal subendothelial immune deposits, with or without mesangial alterations
Class III (C)	Active lesions: focal proliferative lupus nephritis
	Active and chronic lesions: focal proliferative and sclerosing lupus nephritis
	Chronic inactive lesions with glomerular scars: focal sclerosing lupus nephritis
Class IV	**Diffuse lupus nephritis**
Class IV-S (A)	Active or inactive diffuse, segmental or global endocapillary or extracapillary glomerulonephritis involving ≥50% of all glomeruli,
Class IV-G (A)	typically with diffuse subendothelial immune deposits, with or without mesangial alterations; this class is divided into diffuse
Class IV-S (A/C)	segmental (IV-S) lupus nephritis when ≥50% of the involved glomeruli have segmental lesions, and diffuse global (IV-G) lupus
Class IV-G (A/C)	nephritis when ≥50% of the involved glomeruli have global lesions; *segmental* is defined as a glomerular lesion that involves
Class IV-S (C)	less than half of the glomerular tuft; this class includes cases with diffuse wire loop deposits but with little or no glomerular
Class IV-G (C)	proliferation
	Active lesions: diffuse segmental proliferative lupus nephritis
	Active lesions: diffuse global proliferative lupus nephritis
	Active and chronic lesions: diffuse segmental proliferative and sclerosing lupus nephritis
	Active and chronic lesions: diffuse global proliferative and sclerosing lupus nephritis
	Chronic inactive lesions with scars: diffuse segmental sclerosing lupus nephritis
	Chronic inactive lesions with scars: diffuse global sclerosing lupus nephritis
Class V	**Membranous lupus nephritis**
	Global or segmental subepithelial immune deposits or their morphologic sequelae by light microscopy and by immunofluorescence or electron microscopy, with or without mesangial alterations
	Class V lupus nephritis may occur in combination with class III or IV, in which case both will be diagnosed
	Class V lupus nephritis may show advanced sclerosis
Class VI	**Advanced sclerotic lupus nephritis**
	≥90% of glomeruli globally sclerosed without residual activity

Adapted from Ref. 192. : J.J. Weening, V.D. D'Agati, M.M. Schwartz, et al., The classification of glomerulonephritis in systemic lupus erythematosus revisited, J. Am. Soc. Nephrol. 15 (2) (2004) 241–250.

TABLE 23-8   National Institute of Health Version of Activity and Chronicity Indices

ACTIVITY INDEX	CHRONICITY INDEX
Glomerular Abnormalities	
1. Cellular proliferation	1. Glomerular sclerosis
2. Fibrinoid necrosis, karyorrhexis	2. Fibrous crescents
3. Cellular crescents	
4. Hyaline thrombi, wire loops	
5. Leukocyte infiltration	
Tubulointerstitial Abnormalities	
1. Mononuclear cell infiltration	1. Interstitial fibrosis
	2. Tubular atrophy

Each variable is scored from 0 to 3+. Fibrinoid necrosis and cellular crescents are weighted by a factor of 2. The maximum score of the activity index is 24 and that of the chronicity index is 12.
From: B. Mittala, H. Rennke, A.K. Singh, et al., The role of kidney biopsy in the management of lupus nephritis, Curr. Opin. Nephrol. Hypertens. 14 (2005) 1–8.

and duration of disease, patients may also develop chronic kidney disease (CKD), defined by persistent elevation of serum creatinine or reduced glomerular filtration rate (GFR). Advancing degrees of CKD can be accompanied by sequelae such as hypertension, anemia, azotemia, or metabolic bone disease.

When gross hematuria is present in a patient with SLE, it should raise suspicion for other causes such as renal vein thrombosis (as a complication of nephrotic syndrome or APLs), thrombotic microangiopathy, or a clotting factor deficiency (such as prothrombin deficiency).[206,207]

Proteinuria in children is defined by a spot urine protein/creatinine (Up/c) of greater than 0.2 mg/mg creatinine or by a 24-hour urine collection containing protein greater than 4 mg/m²/hour. Nephrotic range proteinuria in children is defined by a Up/c of greater than 2 to 3 mg/mg creatinine or by a 24-hour urine collection containing protein greater than 40 mg/m²/hour. Given the cumbersome nature of 24-hour urine collection, and the possible unreliability in young or incontinent children, Up/c determination is a convenient and reliable method for evaluating and following LN in children and shows good correlation with 24-hour urine collection.[208] First morning urine collection is necessary to eliminate false readings due to the possible contribution of orthostatic proteinuria.

INDICATIONS FOR KIDNEY BIOPSY

The early diagnosis of LN is critical in minimizing the risk of disease progression and ESKD.[209-211] However, there are no evidence-based guidelines regarding when to perform a kidney biopsy in children with SLE. It is generally agreed that evidence of the clinical syndromes mentioned in the previous section are indications for biopsy in the initial evaluation of children with suspected LN. Therefore, clear indications for biopsy include nephrotic syndrome, acute nephritic syndrome, and persistent elevation in creatinine. More controversial are indications for biopsy in mild, asymptomatic hematuria and/or proteinuria.

Given the consequences of missing and undertreating LN, and given the possibility of clinically "silent" LN with minimal laboratory findings and severe histology, it is the authors' practice to have a low threshold for biopsy. We have generally recommended biopsy with any urinary abnormalities such as urine casts, persistent proteinuria (Up/c greater than 0.2 mg/mg) and/or persistent microhematuria (≥5 red blood cell count per high power field [RBC/hpf]) in addition to the more clinically overt presentations such as nephrotic syndrome, acute nephritis, and/or CKD or elevated creatinine levels mentioned above. Additionally, we have recommended kidney biopsy when urine testing has not been performed prior to initiation of treatment. A kidney biopsy generally is not indicated in the new patient with SLE; with no prior steroid or other immunosuppressive therapy; a normal serum creatinine; and a normal urinalysis without hematuria, proteinuria, or casts.

There are few studies that provide evidence regarding when to repeat a kidney biopsy in LN. In general, a repeat biopsy should be considered for persistent or increasing proteinuria, worsening kidney function, or development of active urine sediment (such as hematuria and/or casts) when previously normal (for example, in nonproliferative LN).[195,211] A repeat biopsy also should be considered with flare of renal disease, as defined by increase in proteinuria and/or increase in urine sediment.[212] In general, a repeat biopsy can help to assess the individual's response to treatment and guide subsequent treatment. For example, persistence of active lesions might warrant a change or intensification of immunosuppression, whereas a high degree of chronic, irreversible changes might portend inevitable decline of kidney function and suggest a less aggressive approach.[195] A repeat biopsy might also be useful in determining if and when a patient can be weaned from immunosuppression therapy after LN has gone into remission, though the optimal duration of treatment for LN has yet to be defined.

TREATMENT OF LUPUS NEPHRITIS

Since untreated proliferative (class III and IV) LN is associated with a high rate of mortality and ESKD, drug trials have primarily focused on treatment of proliferative LN. Early drug trials by the National Institutes of Health (NIH) in the 1970s and 1980s established cyclophosphamide (CYC) as the treatment of choice for class III and IV LN. These trials demonstrated that the addition of intravenous CYC to corticosteroids produced better outcomes than treatment with steroids alone.[213-218] The Euro-Lupus Nephritis Trial (ELNT) subsequently demonstrated that low-dose intravenous CYC compared favorably with the higher-dose, longer-duration NIH regimen.[219,220]

Over the past decade, a series of landmark trials in adults have demonstrated that mycophenolate mofetil (MMF) has equivalent or better results than CYC, with lower rates of adverse effects for the 6-month induction phase and long-term maintenance.[221,222] The MAINTAIN Nephritis Trial demonstrated that MMF and azathioprine (AZA) were similar in efficacy for long-term maintenance in rates of relapse, disease activity, and kidney function, with lower rates of anemia and leukopenia in the MMF group.[223] The largest randomized, controlled drug trial in LN to date, the Aspreva Lupus Management Study Group (ALMS) study, recently reported that MMF and CYC had similar rates or remission and that for long-term maintenance of remission, MMF was superior to AZA. African Americans and Hispanics responded better to CYC than they did to MMF.[224,225] A recent and comprehensive Cochrane meta-analysis concurred that MMF was as effective as CYC for inducing remission, with decreased risk of ovarian failure, and that for maintenance therapy the rate of relapse was lower for MMF than AZA.[226]

Regarding biological therapies, the Lupus Nephritis Assessment with Rituximab (LUNAR) trial demonstrated no benefit in renal outcomes with the addition of rituximab (RTX), a monoclonal antibody to CD-20 that depletes circulating B cells, to steroids and MMF. However, a recent review of 26 reports and 300 patients treated with RTX demonstrated combined complete and partial remission in 87% (class III), 76% (class IV), and 67% (class V) LN. Further study is needed to determine the efficacy and optimal use of RTX.[227]

Belimumab, a human monoclonal antibody that prevents activation of B cells by blocking B lymphocyte stimulator (BLyS), was recently approved for treatment of nonrenal SLE. Though belimumab trials (BLISS-52, BLISS-76) excluded patients with severe LN, a post hoc analysis of patients with mild to moderate LN demonstrated greater renal improvement with belimumab added to standard treatment.[228,229] Abatacept is a fusion protein of CTLA-4-Ig that blocks CD80 and CD86 on antigen-presenting cells from interacting with CD28 on T cells, thereby preventing T-cell activation. Recent clinical trials have failed to show a benefit of abatacept over placebo when added to background immunosuppression.[230] However, when the data are reanalyzed with less stringent criteria more in keeping with the LUNAR and ALMS studies, higher rates of renal response are seen for abatacept compared with placebo. The ACCESS study (Abatacept and Cyclophosphamide Combination Therapy for Lupus Nephritis) is in the process of further examining the efficacy of abatacept.[231]

Treatment of mixed membranous and proliferative LN (class III/V or IV/V) generally follows the recommended treatments for proliferative disease. Few studies have examined treatment of pure class V disease, since there is a lower risk of ESKD (20% at 10 years). Class V LN with low-grade proteinuria and well-preserved kidney function might only require treatment with angiotensin-converting enzyme inhibitors (ACEIs) to lower proteinuria and preserve renal function. However, immunosuppressive treatment has been recommended for pure class V disease with nephrotic-range proteinuria and/or decreased kidney function, though there are few randomized controlled trials defining optimal treatment for this condition.[232] Various small studies have combined corticosteroids with another agent, such as MMF, tacrolimus (TAC), cyclosporine A (CSA), AZA, or intravenous CYC, with beneficial results.[224,225,233-239]

There are few pediatric trials, mostly small observational studies, that examine the various adult treatment regimens mentioned above in the context of pediatric LN. These studies have demonstrated beneficial effects in treatment of pediatric LN with different combinations of steroids and MMF, CYC, TAC, and CSA.[240-249] However, there have been no large-scale randomized, controlled trials in pediatric LN; treatment primarily has been determined from the adult studies presented above. An important step in the standardization of treatment and future study of pediatric LN was taken with the publication by the Childhood Arthritis Rheumatology Research Alliance (CARRA) in 2012 of consensus guidelines for induction therapy of proliferative pediatric LN. These guidelines are presented in Fig. 23-8.[212] The CARRA guidelines recommend either MMF or CYC for the initial 6-month induction period, combined with one of three corticosteroid strategies: primarily oral, primarily intravenous (IV), and mixed oral/ IV based on practitioner preference. Methylprednisolone pulses (30 mg/kg/dose up to 1000 mg/dose) may be given at the time of induction for all three potential steroid protocols.

At the present time, given the lack of adequate studies or consensus-based guidelines, maintenance therapy for pediatric proliferative LN should be based on the adult studies above, which favor MMF or AZA for long-term maintenance. For pediatric patients with pure class V disease, treatment can be adapted from the ACR adult guidelines consisting of steroids and MMF or AZA, with change of treatment to intravenous pulse steroids and CYC for disease unresponsive to MMF or AZA.[250]

Hydroxychloroquine reduces rates of flare in SLE and incidence of renal disease, and improves renal outcomes in adult studies; it should be considered for use in pediatric LN.[251-256] Similarly, adult studies have

---

SELECTION OF IMMUNOSUPPRESSIVE AGENT (pick 1 of these 2)
Cyclophosphamide IV q 4 weeks for 6 months
-OR-
Mycophenolate mofetil 600 mg/m2/dose PO BID (max 3000 mg/d) for 6 months
(may substitute mycophenolate sodium 400 mg/m2/dose PO BID [max 1080 mg BID] for 6 months)

SELECTION OF STEROID REGIMEN (pick 1 of these 3)

Primarily ORAL*			OR	*PRIMARILY IV*				OR	*MIXED ORAL/IV*			
Week (wk)	Daily dose >30 kg (mg)	Daily dose ≤30 kg		Week	# Steroid pulses†	Daily dose >30 kg (mg)	Daily dose ≤30 kg (mg)		Week	# Steroid pulses†	Daily dose >30 kg (mg)	Daily dose ≤30 kg (mg/kg/day)
1–4	60–80	2 mg/kg/day		1	3/week	20	10		1	3/week	60	1.5
5–6	60	2 mg/kg/day		2	1–3/week	20	10		2	1/month (month)	60	1.5
7–10	50	↓ by 5–10 mg		3	1–3/week	20	10		3		50	1.2
11–12	40	↓ by 5 mg		4	1–3/week	20	10		4		40	1
13–14	40	↓ by 5 mg		5–7	1–3/week	20	10		5–8	1/month	35	0.9
15–18	30	↓ by 5 mg		8–11	1/month	20	10		9–12	1/month	30	0.8
19–22	25	↓ by 2.5–5 mg		12–18	1/month	15	7.5		13–16	1/month	25	0.7
23–24	20	↓ by 2.5–5 mg		19–24	1/month	10	5		17–20	1/month	20	0.6
*Optional 3-day pulse in week 1 is permitted									21–24	1/month	15	0.5
†Pulse methylprednisolone: 30 mg/kg/dose, maximum: 1000 mg/dose												

FIGURE 23-8 Consensus treatment plans for proliferative juvenile systemic lupus erythematosus–associated lupus nephritis. *BID,* Twice daily; *IV,* Intravenous; *PO,* oral; *q,* every. (From R. Mina, E. von Scheven, S.P. Ardoin etal., Consensus treatment plans for induction therapy of newly diagnosed proliferative lupus nephritis in juvenile systemic lupus erythematosus, Arthritis Care Res. 64 (3) (2012) 375–383.)

demonstrated the benefit of addition of ACEIs has in reducing proteinuria and preserving kidney function, independent from the effect on hypertension.[171,257-261]

OUTCOMES AND PROGNOSIS IN LUPUS NEPHRITIS

Various definitions of complete and partial response and of renal flares have been proposed by the ACR, the European League Against Rheumatism (EULAR) and CARRA (eTable 23-9). Due to the scarcity of studies in pediatric LN, it is difficult to define rates of response to treatment. Outcomes in pediatric LN have improved since the 1980s, presumably from the adaptation of adult innovations in treatment. A retrospective study reported improvement in 5-year pediatric patient survival from 83% to 91%, and renal survival from 52% to 88% over the past three decades. Predictors of poor renal outcome include African Americans, low GFR (less than 60 mL/min/1.73 m^2), and nephrotic-range proteinuria at presentation.[262] Other factors associated with increased risk of ESKD in adult studies include treatment resistance; lack of response in the first 6 months of induction therapy; renal flares; hypertension; delay in diagnosis of LN; higher chronicity score on biopsy; and greater degree of chronic tubulointerstitial disease.[72]

Once a patient approaches ESKD, options include transplantation or renal replacement therapy (peritoneal dialysis or hemodialysis). There is evidence that preemptive transplantation, prior to the need for dialysis, improves graft and patient survival, as well as extrarenal SLE activity.[161] Indeed, in both children and adults with LN, there is an increased risk of death (more than twofold in children) on dialysis compared with patients with non–LN-related ESKD.[263] However, many transplant centers require SLE to be in remission for 6 to 12 months prior to transplantation.[175] Recurrence of SLE after transplantation occurs in approximately 2% to 30% of patients. Recurrence is generally mild and is not associated with decreased patient survival but is associated with a greater rate of graft loss.[72]

Mortality in African-American children with ESKD is double the rate in Caucasian children.[173] In both pediatric and adult LN patients, the leading causes of death, before and after ESKD, are infection and cardiovascular complications.[72]

OTHER RENAL MANIFESTATIONS OF SLE

Other renal manifestations of SLE include tubulointerstitial nephritis and a variety of renal vascular lesions.

Tubulointerstitial (TI) changes, such as tubular epithelial cell alterations, tubular atrophy, interstitial inflammatory infiltrate, and interstitial fibrosis, are commonly found in a wide variety of kidney diseases and often follow primary glomerular disease. TI changes are found in approximately two thirds of all cases of LN and strongly correlate with progression of renal disease.[264-266] Predominant tubulointerstitial nephritis (TIN) without glomerular disease can occur in rare cases in SLE. Patients with predominant TIN generally present with abnormal renal function and normal or mild urinary laboratory findings. Histopathology is characterized by a mononuclear inflammatory interstitial infiltrate and varying degrees of interstitial fibrosis and tubular atrophy.

A variety of renal vascular lesions (RVLs) also are seen in SLE. *Thrombotic microangiopathy* (TMA) is characterized in the acute phase by vessel lumen narrowing or occlusion by accumulation of eosinophilic and fuchsinophilic material with staining properties of fibrin; endothelial cell swelling and denudation; presence of fragmented

erythrocytes; and absence of immune deposits (eFig. 23-9). The chronic phase is characterized by "onion skin" intimal fibroplasia. TMA has been reported in 8% to 17% of LN biopsies.[267-269] TMA often presents clinically as hemolytic uremic syndrome (HUS), thrombotic thrombocytopenic purpura (TTP) and/or antiphospholipid syndrome (APS). *Noninflammatory, necrotizing lupus vasculopathy* (LVO) is characterized by necrotizing vessel wall changes, abundant intramural immune deposits, and luminal narrowing or occlusion with the absence of inflammatory cells. LVO has been reported in 3% to 9% of kidney biopsies for LN.[267-269] *Lupus vasculitis* (LV) is a rare finding characterized by prominent inflammatory cells (neutrophils and mononuclear cells) that infiltrate in the walls of small- and medium-sized arteries with fibrinoid necrosis; it resembles polyarteritis nodosa. *Vascular immune complex deposits* (VIDs) can be found in otherwise normal-appearing renal vessels on light microscopy, with the presence of IC deposits in the vessel walls on immunofluorescent and electron microscopy. VIDs may correlate with more active glomerular LN and might portend a worse renal outcome.[269] In general, patients with RVLs have higher rates of active proliferative nephritis, hypertension, and renal insufficiency. They have poorer survival than patients without RVLs and often progress to ESKD.[267] With the exception of TMA, optimal treatment for RVLs has yet to be defined and usually consists of aggressive immunosuppression with or without plasmapheresis. Of the RVLs, TMA has the worst outcomes regarding patient and renal survival.[267,269]

Mucocutaneous Involvement

The typical rashes of SLE are helpful in the diagnosis of both cutaneous and systemic lupus. Most patients have or develop lupus rashes over the course of disease (up to 85%). Three rashes and mucosal changes were included in the initial classification criteria (Table 23-1), while the SLICC criteria were more inclusive (Table 23-2). The archetypical malar or butterfly rash is classified as a maculopapular rash that includes the nose and cheeks but spares the nasolabial folds (Fig. 23-10). The rash is variable in intensity from a mild blush appearance to an intense erythema with a follicular or scaled appearance (Fig. 23-11). It is also variable in distribution from a more diffuse lesion to multiple satellite lesions including the forehead and chin. This particular rash most often resolves without scarring. Lupus rashes are often, but not necessarily, photosensitive and may be sensitive to fluorescent light as well (Fig. 23-12).[270] The lupus patient may have photosensitive rashes on the limbs and chest as well as the face. The rash may be annular or diffuse. Sun exposure can cause not only a skin flare but a systemic flare as well. It is important to recognize the similarity between the malar rash of lupus and the heliotrope rash of juvenile dermatomyositis. Both rashes are photosensitive; however, the facial rash of dermatomyositis tends to be less thickened, include periorbital skin more frequently, and is associated with dilated vessels and a more significant vasculopathy. Lupus and myositis patients have other distinguishing rashes that are helpful in determining a diagnosis. The other important illness in the differential diagnosis is parvoviral infection. This rash does not usually cross the nasal bridge, and parvovirus patients may have hematologic changes and low total complement. There are other rare syndromes that may cause a photosensitive rash in the malar area, but generally they have different distinguishing features (Table 23-10).

The other distinctive lupus rash is the discoid lesion. This rash is seen more frequently in the adult population both as isolated skin disease or part of systemic lupus. Discoid lesions tend to occur around the eyes and ears of patients but can be distributed over the face, scalp, and body as a generalized rash (Fig. 23-13, A-C). The rash tends to be

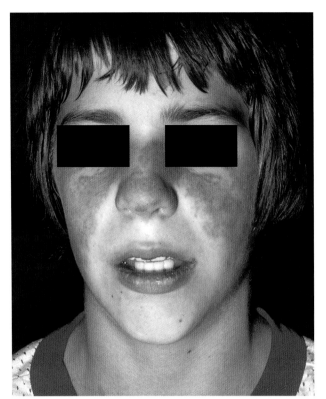

FIGURE 23-10 Malar erythema of acute systemic lupus erythematosus. The classic butterfly rash has erupted over both cheeks and spread over the bridge of the nose. It may be punctate and follicular or an erythematous blush. The rash does not leave a scar.

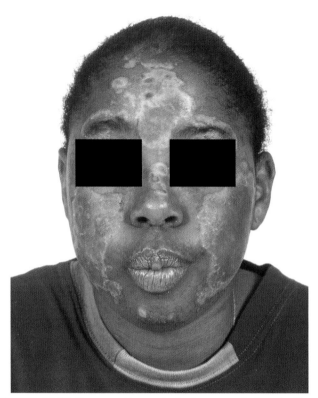

FIGURE 23-12 Photosensitive rash. Rash appeared after significant sun exposure.

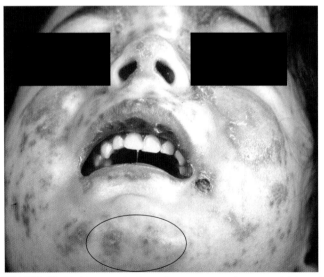

FIGURE 23-11 Malar rash. Butterfly rash extending over bridge of nose. There is sparing below the lip–chin involvement.

TABLE 23-10 Skin Manifestations That May Be Confused with SLE
Parvovirus[271,272]
Erythropoietic protoporphyria[273,274]
Bloom syndrome[275,276]
Cockayne syndrome[277,278]
Rothmund–Thomson syndrome[279,280]
Syndrome of telangiectasia and membranoproliferative glomerulonephritis[281]
Prolidase deficiency[282,283]

Pediatric patients may also present with isolated skin disease due to tumid lupus or subcutaneous lupus. Tumid lupus is a lesion that has induration and erythema but no scale or follicular plugging. Lesions are typically found on the face and trunk and heal without scarring. Subcutaneous lupus (SCLE) is evident most frequently as an annular lesion associated with anti-Ro/SSA and anti-La/SSB antibodies (Fig. 23-14, A-D). As seen in the illustrations of this rash, some patients have postinflammatory hyperpigmentation that can lead to chronic scarring. This is more often seen in patients with darker pigmentation.[16,289,290] Isolated SCLE is also more common in adult SLE than in pSLE.

Bullous lupus erythematosus is a rare complication of lupus. It is important to recognize this diagnosis because of the potential severity of the lesions. It can cause diffuse skin disruption similar to that of a burn patient, as well as cause lesions in the mucosal areas (including the oropharynx) that can compromise an individual's airway.

Another common cutaneous phenomenon in SLE is Raynaud phenomenon. True classic triphasic changes or two-phase changes with

hyperpigmented; however, some patients may develop hypopigmentation as well. The lesion is notable for a thick adherent scale and follicular involvement, leading to hair loss at the area of the lesion. The lesions can become confluent and disfiguring and can lead to chronic alopecia in those who have scalp involvement due to atrophic changes and scarring.[284-288]

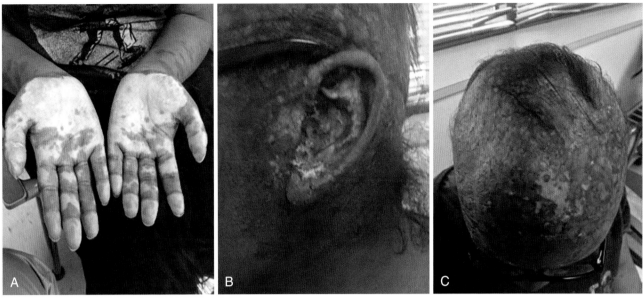

FIGURE 23-13 Discoid rash. Diffuse discoid rash over **(A)** hands; **(B)** ear; **(C)** scalp.

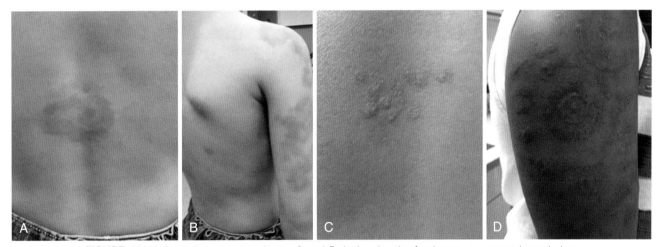

FIGURE 23-14 Subacute cutaneous lupus. **A** and **B,** Isolated rash of subacute cutaneous lupus is less commonly seen in pediatric patients in association with SLE. **C** and **D,** Patients with more pigment may develop postinflammatory hyperpigmentation.

hyperemia are seen frequently. This can be complicated by cold injury or, in rare instances, pernio.[291-293] Patients often respond to typical interventions: keeping the body core warm with layers of insulating clothing, including sock and glove liners, and mittens.

Childhood lupus patients may have cutaneous manifestations of vasculopathy and vasculitis. Subungual erythema is often seen with nonspecific nailfold abnormalities seen by nailfold capillaroscopy, including dilated vessels and loss of capillary loops similar to that seen in dermatomyositis.[294] Livedo reticularis can also be seen and can be associated with the presence of APLs. Patients will also have erythema, palpable purpura (Figs. 23-15 and 23-16), and ulcers or urticaria associated with LV or APS. Poorly controlled cutaneous vasculitis lesions can be associated with complement defects.[295-299] Patients with lupus can present with petechiae and purpura due to thrombocytopenia. The lesions may be similar to that seen in Henoch–Schönlein purpura and acute lymphocytic leukemia.

Alopecia associated with discoid lupus is rare and causes scarring. Alopecia without scarring, however, is a common finding in systemic lupus. It tends to occur at the frontotemporal line but can be more diffuse (Fig. 23-17). It is a frequent symptom at disease onset and can also herald disease flares.

MUCOSAL INVOLVEMENT

The mucosal surfaces of the oropharynx are frequently altered in systemic lupus. True nasal ulcers are seen rarely and ulcers of the tongue and hard palate are uncommon. Nasal septal perforation can occur. The lesions are typically painless although some patients do report discomfort. Hard palate erythema is quite common, supporting the diagnosis of lupus (Fig. 23-18). Again, this finding is shared by patients with juvenile dermatomyositis, although the erythema is typically mild in the latter diagnosis. Hyperemia of the oral and nasal mucosa is

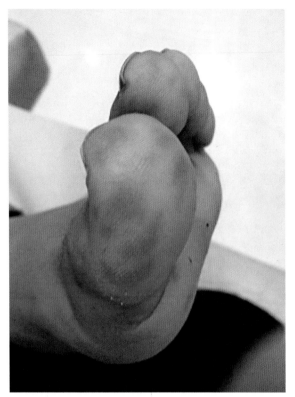

FIGURE 23-15 Vasculitis seen as punctate erythema of the toes of a child with systemic lupus erythematosus.

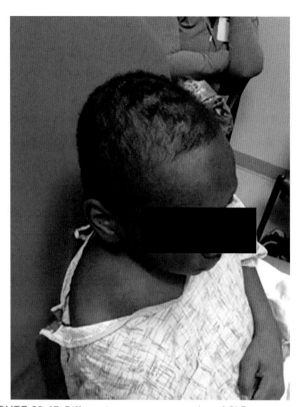

FIGURE 23-17 Diffuse alopecia at presentation of SLE.

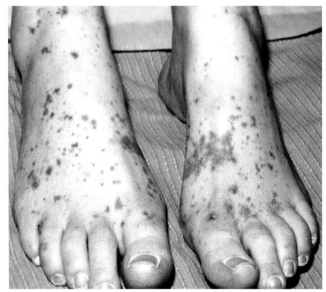

FIGURE 23-16 Vasculitic purpura in a teenage girl with an acute exacerbation of systemic lupus erythematosus.

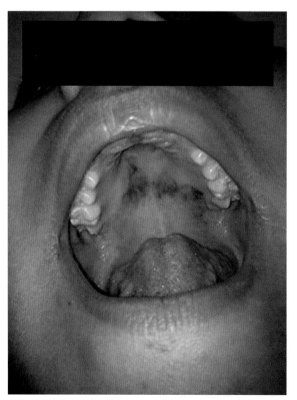

FIGURE 23-18 Mucocutaneous ulcerations of acute SLE. A shallow, painless, erythematous ulceration with an irregular margin is seen on the hard palate.

common but nonspecific. Oral mucosal lesions tend to occur on the hard palate, although involvement of the buccal mucosa may occur. Hard palate lesions range from hyperemia, to petechial rashes, to true ulceration. The ulcers are usually painless unless they come in contact with an irritant.

SKIN PATHOLOGY

Acute lupus skin lesions are notable for disruption of the dermal–epidermal junction with infiltration of T lymphocytes and around the blood vessels. Fibrinoid degeneration of the connective tissues is notable. Chronic cutaneous lesions have a thickening of the keratinic layer, epidermal atrophy, follicular plugging, and fibrosis of the elastic tissues. The presence of ICs by fluorescent staining at the dermal–epidermal junction in normal-appearing skin as well as lesional skin is typical in lupus skin disease.

TREATMENT

Lupus patients require counseling regarding their skin care. Sun avoidance at peak sun hours and sun protection are the cornerstones of care. The use of broad-spectrum (UVA and UVB) 30 SPF or more sunscreens 30 minutes prior to sun exposure allows the chemicals to bind to the skin. Patients may choose to use a physical barrier sunscreen or apply it over a chemical sunscreen (titanium dioxide or zinc oxide). Wide-brimmed hats, dark colors, long sleeves, and tightly woven clothes are helpful. Sunscreen additives can be washed into clothes as well, or clothes with sunscreen additives included can be purchased. Treatment of rashes may require the use of topical or oral steroids (for severe skin lesions). Facial skin is very sensitive and thin and requires the use of mild steroids such as alclometasone. Tacrolimus can also be used to treat lesions topically. Hydroxychloroquine is the standard oral medication used to treat topical lesions and nonscarring alopecia. Some patients will require use of second-line therapies such as dapsone or AZA (Table 23-11).

Musculoskeletal Disease

Pediatric lupus patients often have arthralgia and myalgia that resolves with diagnosis and treatment. True arthritis of the small joints of the hands is frequent, and may also include other peripheral joints. A smaller group of lupus patients have arthritis as a prominent feature with typical joint swelling, range loss, tenderness, and pain on motion (see Tables 23-5 and 23-6). Patients with persisting arthritis require arthritis-specific therapies. Lupus polyarthritis is rarely associated with erosive injury. Tenosynovitis of the hands leading to deformity is a well-described entity.[300-307] Patients may have what appears to be a polyarticular arthritis with some minor constitutional symptoms with or without rheumatoid factors; this may develop into a diagnosis of lupus over time.[308-310] Pediatric lupus patients may also have or develop an inflammatory myositis. Muscle enzyme elevation can be substantial and is responsive to appropriate therapy.

Although musculoskeletal symptoms are typical and common in lupus patients, it is important to also consider other causes of musculoskeletal complaints. Steroid myopathy can present at any time after corticosteroid therapy is started and is more severe when fluorinated steroids are used or the patient is bedridden (myopathy).[311,312] Creatine phosphokinase (CPK) elevations can also be drug induced (statins, hydroxychloroquine). A newly swollen or painful joint, particularly if it is a single joint, can represent infection of the joint, osteonecrosis, or infarction of bone. Patients may have complex regional pain syndromes or pain amplification syndromes when they first show signs of disease or after treatment.

TABLE 23-11	Treatment of Cutaneous SLE	
TREATMENT	**DOSAGE**
Antimalarials	
Hydroxychloroquine	4-7 mg/kg/day (maximum 400 mg/day)
Chloroquine	250 mg/day
Topical (in order of suggested use)	
Corticosteroids	1.0% hydrocortisone or 0.1% betnonvate
Vitamin D analogs (e.g., calcipotriene)	
Calcineurin inhibitors (e.g., pimecrolimus or tacrolimus)	
Immunosuppressive Agents	
Systemic corticosteroids	Usually <0.5 mg/kg/day orally
Methotrexate	Up to 15 mg/m² /week either orally or subcutaneously (maximum 25 mg/weak)
Azathioprine	3 mg/kg/day (maximum 150 mg/day) orally
Mycophenolate mofetil	1 g/m² /day divided twice a day orally
Calcineurin inhibitors	
Cyclosporine	Up to 5 mg/kg/day divided twice a day (measure levels); use lowest effective dose
Tacrolimus	0.10 to 0.20 mg/kg/day maximum 10 mg/day orally divided twice a day (measure levels); use lowest effective dose
Intravenous immunoglobulin	1-2 g/kg/dose (maximum 70 g)

Neuropsychiatric Disease

The prevalence of neuropsychiatric SLE (NP-SLE) in lupus is widely variable (20% to 95%) based on a number of pediatric studies that have defined NP-SLE differently. These studies have had different patient populations and have small sample sizes, all which introduced a number of statistical biases into the data (see Table 23-5).[16,159,313-317] The ACR[1] published a guideline for describing NP-SLE in adults that included 19 specific diagnoses (see eTable 23-12).[318,319] Pediatric rheumatologists have adapted this guideline to pediatric patients and studies. It is notable that NP-SLE is more frequent in the pediatric population[1] and typically presents at disease onset; however, patients may develop NP-SLE at any point in their disease course.[314] The approach to treatment of NP-SLE requires a team approach, which may include neurologists, psychologists and psychiatrists. NP-SLE manifestations are given significant weight in disease activity scores due to the severity of disease manifestations and poor outcomes. Table 23-13 reviews the frequency of the individual NP manifestations in pSLE.

NP Disease Manifestations

Headaches. Headache occurs frequently in lupus patients and is the most common NP-SLE manifestation. Headache is a common medical issue. An NP-SLE headache is differentiated by its definition as a severe, unrelenting headache that requires narcotic analgesia.[318] Pediatric patients are rarely treated with narcotics but often have new, worsening, or migrainous headaches (43% in one study). It is critical for the clinician to evaluate new-onset headache or worsening headache as a symptom of another NP-SLE diagnosis. New or worsening headaches may represent vascular events, infection, or increased

TABLE 23-13 Frequency of NP Manifestations in pSLE

CENTRAL NERVOUS SYSTEM*

Headache (any)	4-55% (95%)
Recurrent	10-50%
Migraine	3-10%
Benign intracranial hypertension	2-4%
Cognitive dysfunction	
Acute confusional state	3-9%
Mood disorder	5-9%
Depression	5-9%
Manic	0-3%
Mixed features	0-1%
Seizure disorder (any)	4-20%
Single episode	4-20%
Epilepsy	0-2%
Anxiety disorder	1-10%
Cerebrovascular disease (any)	4-14%
Transient ischemic attack	0-2%
Cerebral infarction (stroke)	2-9%
Venous thrombosis (sinus vein)	1-4%
Vasculitis	1-2%
Hemorrhage	1-3%
"Chronic multifocal disease"	1-2%
Psychosis	3-24%
Movement disorder (any)	0-6%
Chorea	0-5%
Parkinsonian	Case reports
Demyelinating syndrome	2-3%
Aseptic meningitis—may be idiopathic (acute or chronic) or secondary to drugs[†]	0-2%
Myelopathy	1-2%
Peripheral nervous system	3-5%
Acute inflammatory demyelinating polyradiculoneuropathy (Guillain–Barré syndrome and its variants)	Case reports only
Chronic inflammatory demyelinating polyradiculoneuropathy	Case reports only
Autonomic disorder	Case reports only[‡]
Mononeuropathy, single/multiplex	1-2%
Myasthenia gravis	Case reports only
Neuropathy, cranial	1-4%
Plexopathy	No reported pediatric cases
Polyneuropathy	0-2%

*Many patients have more than one manifestation.
[†]Drugs associated with aseptic meningitis: NSAIDs (ibuprofen, tolmetin, sulindac, naproxen, diclofenac) lamotrigine, trimethoprim-sulfamethoxazole, influenza vaccination, azathioprine).
[‡]One report suggested a 42% rate of subclinical autonomic nervous system involvement.
Sources: Refs. 159, 160, 314, 315, 317, 320-327.

intracranial pressure. A careful neurological examination is required, and imaging may be needed.

Psychosis. The diagnosis of psychosis has been made in 3% to 24% of patients with NP-SLE (Table 23-13). In a recent study of NP-SLE symptoms in a pediatric cohort, 12% had psychiatric features and 9% had psychosis.[328] These patients had visual and auditory hallucinations but rarely tactile hallucinations. Preserved insight appeared to be lost if symptoms were prolonged.[314,320,329] Pediatric patients with psychosis often experience cognitive abnormalities, including problems with memory and attention as well as headaches and other NP-SLE symptoms. Brain imaging is usually normal or has nonspecific abnormalities. There are no specific laboratory studies associated with psychosis, although antiribosomal P antibodies can be found. This finding is not specific or necessary for diagnostic purposes. Twenty percent of pediatric patients with psychosis may have a flare, and the time to remission can be greater than a year. Most patients receive medical therapy for their psychosis along with immunosuppression. Cyclophosphamide has been reported to be the most effective immunosuppressive therapy.[330] Of note, patients with lupus psychosis improve with corticosteroid therapy, while patients with steroid-induced psychosis develop symptoms on therapy, and the symptoms tend to be different.[331,332]

Cognitive dysfunction and acute confusional state. Cognitive impairment in childhood lupus varies from covert subtle abnormalities found only at testing to overt cognitive impairment, including confusion, memory loss, and even coma. Issues with school performance are common and need to be studied as the problems may stem from cognitive impairment, depression, adjustment to a new illness, or impairment caused by medications. There are no specific lab abnormalities or imaging studies that are associated with cognitive difficulties; however, it is appropriate to consider imaging as part of an evaluation of new onset cognitive dysfunction. Formal neuropsychological testing is burdensome, costly, and requires extensive time. A pediatric specific battery of tests requiring $2\frac{1}{2}$ hours was developed and recently published. It includes tests of general intelligence and academic skills, psychomotor speed, verbal working memory, attention, processing speed, verbal and visual memory, executive function, and behavior.[333] Currently, an automated 30-minute test adopted from the military called the Pediatric Automated Neuropsychological Assessment Metrics is being validated for use in the clinical setting.[334] The pathophysiological mechanism for injury is not clear. However, recent studies have demonstrated differences in functional network activity within the brain and changes in brain volume correlated with neurocognitive dysfunction.[335,336]

Mood disorders. A recent study of mood disorders in a pSLE population found 19% of subjects had symptoms of depression, and 21% had symptoms of anxiety. It is not clear if these symptoms are disease specific or a response to having a chronic illness and side effects of therapy.[158,314,321] It is important to understand that this population is particularly vulnerable, and symptom check lists reflect current mood states that often fluctuate in teenagers regardless of the presence of chronic illness or disease pathophysiology.[337]

Cerebrovascular disease. Vascular disease in lupus is most often a vasculopathy of small vessels. It is critical to note that small-vessel disease will not be apparent on vascular imaging. It is possible to infer disease from cerebral blood flow studies; however, tissue is necessary for a specific diagnosis. Medium-vessel vasculitis, which often presents with headache, seizure, or neurological deficits, can be diagnosed by formal angiography.[338,339] Vasculitis is often associated with markers of inflammation and active lupus serology. Patients may develop strokes and cerebral vein thrombosis. Magnetic resonance imaging (MRI) studies are typically adequate to make these diagnoses. Patients with thrombotic phenomena (Fig. 23-19) require anticoagulation and typically have lupus anticoagulants and APLs.[207,340,341]

Seizures. Pediatric lupus patients have seizures associated with cerebrovascular disease and hypertension. Seizures are prominent in the presentation of posterior reversible encephalopathy syndrome (PRES) with kidney disease and hypertension, and are less commonly seen in association with APS than in the adult population.[160,342-345] Seizures are more commonly generalized rather than focal and are

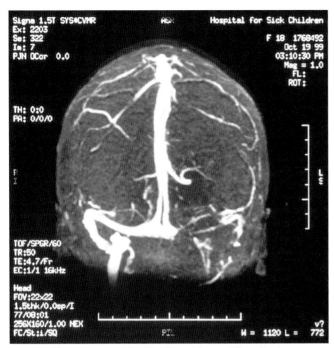

Transverse and Sagittal Sinus Venous Thrombosis

FIGURE 23-19 MRI venogram of cerebral vein thrombosis. Patients reporting severe, unremitting headache should be investigated for a cerebral vein thrombosis. MR venogram demonstrates occlusion of the transverse sinus.

often associated with headaches and cognitive changes. New-onset seizures require a thorough evaluation to consider metabolic and infectious etiologies.

Movement disorders. Basal ganglia injury leading to chorea is a rare complication associated with the presence of APLs in pediatric lupus patients. The overlapping humoral autoimmunity leading to chorea in lupus and rheumatic fever can cause confusion in the differential diagnosis if typical lupus features are not prominent.[346] Lupus patients have also had dystonias and Parkinsonian movement disorders.

Peripheral nervous system. The involvement of the peripheral nervous system in pediatric systemic lupus is very rare. Patients have shown indications of transverse myelitis, which is often associated with APLs.[317,347,348] Patients may also show symptoms of Guillain–Barré or optic neuritis, both of which require urgent treatment. Cranial, peripheral, and autonomic neuropathies are exceedingly rare.

Central nervous system pathology. There are no typical pathological findings of lupus on examination of the brain. The finding of microscopic vasculopathy possibly related to microinfarcts or APS is common.[349] There is brain volume loss, which may be partially related to chronic steroid use or to chronic inflammation.[336] Other lesions are typical of specific events such as hemorrhagic or thrombotic stroke or vasculitis.

NP Disease Investigations

Examinations of patients with psychosis and significant neurocognitive dysfunction are frequently normal, but it is important to exclude other non-SLE causes of NP signs and symptoms such as infection, primary psychiatric disease, metabolic derangements including acute renal failure, endocrinopathies, toxic substances, and trauma. Studies have shown a variety of cerebrospinal fluid (CSF) abnormalities, including elevated cytokine and chemokine levels (eTable 23-14).

Measurement of these important mediators of inflammation may help us to understand the pathophysiology of NP-SLE, but they currently have no clinical utility.[350-352] The presence of antiribosomal P antibodies was initially heralded as a sensitive and specific test for depression and psychosis in SLE. However, antiribosomal P antibodies are frequently present in patients without central nervous system (CNS) disease, and although they appear to have good sensitivity for the presence of depression and psychosis the lack of specificity makes the clinical utility of measuring antiribosomal P antibodies low. The results of investigations into the clinical utility of some "CNS-specific" autoantibodies are shown in eTable 23-15.

Neuroimaging studies are best used to demonstrate arterial or venous occlusion and are important investigations for stroke or seizures and to demonstrate cerebral vein thrombosis (see eTable 23-14, online). NP-SLE–related CNS perfusion defects may be assessed by single-photon emission computed tomography (SPECT) or positron emission tomography (PET) scans. However, they are best used to help differentiate SLE psychosis and non-SLE psychosis.[353-400]

TREATMENT

Once the diagnosis has been established and non-SLE causes excluded, treatment with high-dose steroids and cyclophosphamide (500 mg/m² for 2 to 6 doses) is initiated. Maintenance therapy with AZA or MMF can be considered. In one small study, more than 50% of patients who started treatment with AZA had to be switched to CYC for lack of response.[330] There are no prospective studies in either adult or pediatric lupus populations. Thrombotic phenomena require anticoagulation. Headaches often respond to typical headache prophylaxis if they are constant or persistent. Other manifestations such as mood disorders require symptomatic management.

Antiphospholipid Antibody Syndrome

APS can present as a primary disease or as a secondary disease found most frequently in the setting of lupus but also found in a number of autoimmune diseases including overlap syndromes, vasculitis, and arthritis.[401] Please refer to Chapter 24 for details. *Catastrophic antiphospholipid syndrome* (CAPS) refers to an acute event when thrombosis is found in three different organs over the period of a week, with biopsy evidence of microthrombi and the presence of APLs or lupus anticoagulant in a titer higher than 40 U/L. The international CAPS registry found that presentation of CAPS was the first APS event for 86.6% of the pediatric registrants. About 31% of the patients had a diagnosis of lupus. CAPS requires emergent therapy with high-dose steroids, plasmapheresis, and intravenous immunoglobulin (IVIG). For more severe or unresponsive cases, rituximab has had some efficacy. Hydroxychloroquine may be useful over time to protect the function of Annexin A5. Future therapies may include anticomplement therapies.[402-404]

Cardiovascular Disease

The prevalence of heart disease in children with SLE is approximately 32% to 42%.[405] Variable associations in children and adults have been made between heart disease in SLE and autoantibodies such as anti-Ro/SSA, anti-La/SSB antibodies, anti-Sm, anti-RNP, and APLs. However, there is a clear association between maternal IgG anti-Ro/SSA and congenital heart block in neonatal lupus.[406-409]

Pericarditis

Pericarditis is the most common cardiac manifestation of SLE in adults and children. In children, the incidence of pericarditis is approximately 5% to 38%, with an incidence of cardiac tamponade in 2.5% to 6% of cases.[407,408,410,411] In children and adults, symptoms of pericarditis include fever, tachycardia, and decreased heart sounds. Patients may have substernal or precordial chest pain that is usually positional and aggravated by lying down, and sometimes associated with dyspnea. A pericardial rub can be present but is rare. Chest X-ray can demonstrate an enlarged cardiac silhouette when a large effusion is present. Electrocardiography (ECG) typically demonstrates elevated ST segments and peaked T waves. Pericarditis is usually diagnosed by echocardiography. Effusions are usually small and hemodynamically insignificant.[406,408,410]

On histological examination, the pericardium is thickened by proliferating fibroblasts, edema, and mononuclear inflammatory infiltrate. Immunofluorescence microscopy shows deposition of immunoglobulin, C1q, and C3, supporting ICs in the pathophysiology of pericarditis.[411] Treatment in mild disease consists of nonsteroidal anti-inflammatory medications and/or corticosteroids. In more severe or recurrent cases, intravenous methylprednisolone with or without additional immunosuppressive medications might be required. Pericardiocentesis, pericardial window, or pericardial stripping are rarely needed.[406,408,410]

Myocarditis

The incidence of myocarditis in pSLE is approximately 2% to 19%.[161,407,412] In addition to myocarditis, other causes of myocardial dysfunction in SLE should be considered, including infection, ischemia due to coronary artery disease, hypertension, kidney failure, valvular disease, and toxicity from drugs such as CYC and antimalarials.[410]

Clinical findings in adults and children with lupus myocarditis include fever, dyspnea, palpitations, nonexertional chest pain, jugular venous distension, resting tachycardia out of proportion to fever, gallop or murmur, cardiomegaly, and peripheral edema. Pericarditis and/or endocarditis as well as skeletal myositis may also be present. Typical laboratory findings include elevations in the erythrocyte sedimentation rate (ESR), CRP, cardiac fraction of the creatine kinase myocardial band (CK-MB), and cardiac troponins, though normal CK-MB and troponins do not rule out the disease. Chest X-ray may show enlarged cardiac silhouette and pulmonary edema. ECG may show nonspecific ST and T wave changes, conduction abnormalities, premature complexes, and supraventricular and ventricular tachycardia. Global or focal hypokinesis or reduced left ventricular ejection fraction in the absence of other causes on echocardiography supports the diagnosis. Echocardiography may be useful in following response to treatment. Cardiac MRI and gallium scan may also be helpful in diagnosing myocarditis. Endomyocardial biopsy is the definitive method for diagnosis; however, it is a high-risk procedure with a significant false negative rate. Tissue examination demonstrates interstitial plasma cell and lymphocytic infiltrates and patch fibrosis. As in pericarditis, immunofluorescent microscopy demonstrates immune complex and complement deposition, supporting the possibility that myocarditis is an IC-mediated disease.[406,408,409,411,413,414]

There are not enough studies in the literature to make conclusions regarding optimal treatment of lupus myocarditis. First-line treatment usually consists of high-dose oral and/or intravenous steroids. The use of additional immunosuppressant medications such as CYC, mycophenolate, AZA, IVIG, plasmapheresis, and rituximab have been reported. Treatment also consists of supportive care for arrhythmias and heart failure.[409,413-415]

Endocarditis

The incidence of lupus-related endocarditis in pSLE is unknown, but the disease appears to be rare in children.[416] The most common valvular findings in SLE are left-sided valve thickening and regurgitation. The typical endocarditis associated with SLE is Libman–Sacks

endocarditis (LSE), consisting of sterile, small, verrucous valve lesions, typically on the mitral valve but also found other valves, chordae tendineae, and endocardium. LSE is associated with longer disease duration, higher lupus activity, and APLs. LSE can be found in both primary APS and APS secondary to SLE.[411]

Generally, LSE is asymptomatic. Stroke and thromboembolism can occur in 13% of adult patients,[410] though children appear to be at much lower risk.[417] LSE is usually diagnosed by transthoracic echocardiography (TTE) or transesophageal echocardiography (TEE), though TTE usually is sufficient in children.[418] In asymptomatic LSE, treatment is generally for the underlying disease (SLE and APS). Valvular abnormalities may resolve over time. Valve replacement may be necessary for valvular dysfunction. There is little direct evidence that corticosteroid treatment prevents valvular damage, though the decline in the prevalence of LSE in autopsy studies in the steroid-era suggests that corticosteroids may have a beneficial effect.[410,411,417]

OTHER CARDIAC MANIFESTATIONS OF SLE

The risk of *coronary artery disease* (CAD) is four to eight times higher in SLE patients than in control groups, with the increased risk extending to younger patients. Young women with SLE are 50 times more likely to have an *acute myocardial infarction* (MI).[410,411,417] CAD and MI have been reported in teenage patients and young adults below the age of 35 as well. MI often is not recognized in young patients, even in the presence of angina symptoms, and symptoms may be mistaken for more common complications of SLE such as pericarditis.[419] Even after controlling for traditional cardiovascular risk factors such as hypertension, dyslipidemia, and smoking, individuals with SLE have a threefold higher incidence of coronary artery plaques, as well as a higher incidence of carotid intima-media thickening and plaques.[420] Early cardiovascular changes are also seen in children with SLE who, like adults, have increased carotid–femoral pulse wave velocity and augmentation index (measures of arterial stiffness), increased carotid intima-media thickness (CIMT) and increased left ventricular mass index.[421,422] Mechanisms of CAD in SLE include atherosclerosis, coronary arteritis, thrombosis with or without APLs, embolization of valvular material, vasospasm, and hypertension. The accelerated rate of atherosclerosis in SLE may be linked to inflammation and endothelial dysfunction, as well as atherogenic risk factors such as hypertension and dyslipidemia. Coronary vasculitis also can occur and can be difficult to distinguish from atherosclerotic disease.[410,411] The recent Atherosclerosis Prevention in Pediatric Lupus Erythematosus (APPLE) trial demonstrated that atorvastatin is safe to use in pSLE and lowers total cholesterol, LDL, triglycerides, and CRP, though treatment had no significant effect on the progression of CIMT, the primary outcome of the study. The APPLE study could not recommend routine use of statins in children with SLE at this time, though routine monitoring of cardiovascular risk factors, such as dyslipidemia, hypertension, obesity, smoking, and low physical activity, is recommended.[423]

Pleuropulmonary Disease

Pleuropulmonary involvement in SLE occurs in approximately 5% to 67% of pediatric patients.[424,425] Even in the absence of symptoms and radiological findings, approximately 35% to 84% of children with SLE have abnormal pulmonary function tests (PFTs). In children and adults, the most common PFT findings are restrictive lung disease and/or impaired diffusion.[425-427] A wide variety of pulmonary manifestations occur, from asymptomatic to life-threatening, as described in eTable 23-16.[428-434] Of note, pulmonary alveolar hemorrhage (PAH) is a relatively rare but potentially catastrophic event (mortality rate 50%). PAH patients rarely have hemoptysis but may have fever, cough, and

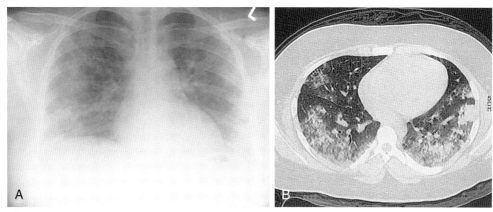

FIGURE 23-20 Radiograph **(A)** and thin-section computed tomogram **(B)** of the chest of a 14-year-old girl with acute onset of pulmonary hemorrhage and thrombocytopenia. There is evidence of widespread airspace and interstitial disease. The abnormalities completely resolved after therapy with high-dose prednisone.

dyspnea. The clinician should consider PAH as well as gastrointestinal (GI) blood loss in the new lupus patient or patient with newly acquired anemia regardless of Coombs status. Computed tomography (CT) scan reveals pulmonary nodules and ground glass changes (Fig. 23-20) in patients who may have patchy infiltrates or normal-appearing chest radiographs. Bronchoscopy demonstrates blood- and hemosiderin-laden macrophages. Patients should receive aggressive management with high-dose IV corticosteroids and secondary immunosuppressants. Plasmapheresis may be helpful in acutely deteriorating patients.[429,430,432-434]

PULMONARY INFECTION

Adult and pediatric patients with SLE are at high risk for lung infection as a result of immunosuppression secondary to disease activity and treatment. Underlying parenchymal disease, atelectasis, lung edema, and respiratory muscle weakness further the risk of infection. Patients with new pulmonary infiltrates and/or respiratory symptoms should be presumed to have a respiratory infection and treated empirically until infection is ruled out. Infection may be caused by common as well as opportunistic organisms. Bacterial organisms include Gram-negative bacilli, Gram-positive cocci, *Chlamydia pneumoniae* and *Mycoplasma pneumoniae*. Vaccination may reduce the rate of pneumococcal infection. Opportunistic infections include aspergillosis, cryptococcosis, *Pneumocystis jiroveci*, cytomegalovirus, and Nocardia. Patients with SLE also have a higher susceptibility to pulmonary and extrapulmonary tuberculosis (TB). Screening for TB should be performed before steroid treatment of SLE begins. Bronchoscopy and bronchoalveolar lavage (BAL) should be considered when infection is suspected.[430,432,434]

Hematological Involvement

Hematological manifestations occur in a range of approximately one third to three quarters of children with SLE.[435-439] A variety of hematological abnormalities occur in childhood SLE (see Table 23-17). *Anemia of chronic disease* is common in adults and children with SLE. This anemia is usually normochromic and normocytic, accompanied by low reticulocyte count, elevated ferritin, and low iron. In response to inflammatory cytokines, the liver releases hepcidin, which inhibits iron release from macrophages and absorption of iron from the intestine, thereby inhibiting erythropoiesis. Most patients do not require treatment; however, severe or symptomatic cases can be treated by injections of darbepoetin alfa or epoetin alfa, though inflammation

may need to be treated with corticosteroids before an adequate response is seen.[440]

Coombs-positive, *autoimmune hemolytic anemia* (AHA) occurs in approximately 10% of pSLE patients, though 30% to 40% may have a positive direct Coombs test without overt hemolysis.[436] AHA is predominantly caused by warm agglutinins, IgG antibodies that react with red cell surface antigens at 37°C, which leads to splenic destruction of red cells and anemia.[440,441] The first line of treatment for AHA is corticosteroids: oral for mild to moderate disease and intravenous for more severe or refractory anemia. In cases unresponsive to steroids, IVIG, plasmapheresis, rituximab, AZA, MMF, and CYC have been used successfully.[437,440-443]

In the patient with SLE and anemia, other causes of anemia besides lupus need to be considered. Iron deficiency is common in SLE, and GI or menstrual losses of blood should be investigated. Kidney disease is an important cause of anemia, due to impaired kidney function and reduced erythropoietin production. Aplastic anemia, due to SLE and/or medications, and lupus-related pure red cell aplasia are rare causes of anemia.[440]

Leukopenia is seen in 46% to 64% of children with SLE.[439] Both lymphopenia and neutropenia can be found, although lymphopenia is more common and usually does not require specific therapy. When the lymphopenia is profound (reduction in the number of lymphocytes to an absolute count persistently <500), an underlying infection with the herpes family of viruses or macrophage activation syndrome (MAS) should be sought.[436] Leukopenia usually occurs during active SLE and subsides, and disease activity abates; therefore, when markers of SLE disease activity are normal, other causes of leukopenia—such as drug toxicity—should be investigated. Additional causes of leukopenia are to antineutrophil antibodies, drugs, and infections. Although the role of leukopenia in the risk of infection in SLE is not clear,[444] a number of recent studies link neutropenia and lymphopenia to increased infection risk.[445-449] SLE-associated leukopenia is usually treated with corticosteroids. Neutropenia also can be treated with granulocyte colony-stimulating factor (GCSF), though there is a risk of SLE flare with GCSF.[437,440]

Thrombocytopenia is present in 7% to 30% of pSLE patients and may be the initial presentation in up to 15% of pediatric cases.[176,436,437] Two types of autoantibodies play a major role in the pathogenesis of lupus-related immune thrombocytopenia: anti-GPIIb/IIIa and anti-thrombopoietin receptor (TPOR) antibodies.[440] Immune thrombocytopenic purpura (ITP) can precede the development of SLE by as much as 10 years.[437] Corticosteroids are the first line of treatment for

TABLE 23-17	Major Cytopenias of SLE			
CYTOPENIA	TYPE	FREQUENCY	KEY LABORATORY FEATURES	MANAGEMENT
Anemia	AHA	Common	↑Retic, ↑LDH, ↓haptoglobin, +DAT	Cs, danazol, rituximab, IVIG, MMF, splenectomy, CYC
	ACD	Most common	NL MCV & MCH	EPO
	IDA	Common	↓MCV, ↓MCH	Iron supplementation
	Megaloblastic	Not rare	↑MCV, ↓B_{12} & FA levels	Folate and B_{12} supplementation
	Aplastic	Very rare		Cs, danazol, CYC, CSA, Plasmapheresis
	PRCA	Rare		Cs, danazol, CYC, CSA, TPE, MMF, IVIG
Leukopenia	Lymphopenia	Very common	<1500/μL	Cs, CSA, MMF, CYC, rituximab
	Neutropenia	Uncommon	<1000/μL	GCSF
Thrombocytopenia	Immune	Common	<150,000/μL	Cs, MMF, CSA, IVIG, splenectomy, danazol, AZA, IL-11, rituximab, TPE
	Drug induced	Common	History	
	Infection	Not rare	Microbiology	
	TMA	Not rare	Schistocytes	
	APS	Not rare	APA	
	DIC	Rare		
	Marrow dysplasia	Rare		

ACD, Anemia of chronic diseases; *AIHA,* autoimmune hemolytic anemia; *APA,* antiphospholipid antibody; *APS,* antiphospholipid antibody syndrome, *AZA,* azathioprine; *Cs,* corticosteroids; *CSA,* cyclosporine A; *CYC,* cyclophosphamide; *DAT,* direct antiglobulin test (Coombs' test); *DIC,* disseminated intravascular coagulopathy; *EPO,* erythropoietin; *FA,* folic acid; *IL-11,* interleukin-11; *IVIg,* intravenous immunoglobulin; *LDH,* lactate dehydrogenase; *MCH,* mean corpuscular hemoglobin, *MCV,* mean corpuscular volume; *μl,* microliter; *MMF,* mycophenolate mofetil; *NL,* normal; *PRCA:* pure red cell aplasia; *Retic,* reticulocyte count; *rhG-CSF,* recombinant human granulocyte-colony stimulating factor; *TTP,* thrombotic thrombocytopenic purpura.
Adapted from K. Newman, M.B. Owlia, I. El-Hemaidi, M. Akhtari, Management of immune cytopenias in patients with systemic lupus erythematosus—Old and new, Autoimmun. Rev. 12 (7) (2013) 784–791.

lupus-related thrombocytopenia, though response can be transient, and relapse is common after the tapering off of treatment. IVIG can rapidly improve platelet count, but results can also be transient; repeated and prolonged administration may be necessary. Successful treatment also has been reported with rituximab, AZA, cyclosporine, MMF, and CYC.[440] The role of splenectomy in the management of thrombocytopenia is unclear. Splenectomy may improve platelet count in cases refractory to medical management but at the cost of increased infection risk.[440] *Evans syndrome* is defined by the simultaneous occurrence of AHA and immune[440] thrombocytopenia and can be associated with SLE, lymphoma, and immunodeficiency; treatment is similar to lupus-related immune thrombocytopenia.[450] Thrombocytopenia also can be caused or exacerbated by drugs commonly used in lupus patients, such as AZA, CYC, methotrexate, nonsteroidal antiinflammatory drugs (NSAIDs), statins, ACE inhibitors, proton pump inhibitors, and antibiotics.[451]

Thrombotic microangiopathies (TMAs) are a group of disorders characterized by microangiopathic hemolytic anemia (fragmented red cells, schistocytes, in peripheral blood) and thrombocytopenia. Histologically, TMAs are characterized by arteriolar thrombi, with intimal swelling and fibrinoid necrosis of the vessel wall. *TTP* and *HUS,* both forms of TMAs, have been reported in SLE. HUS is defined by a combination of microangiopathic hemolytic anemia, thrombocytopenia, and acute kidney injury. TTP is defined by microangiopathic hemolytic anemia, thrombocytopenia, fever, acute kidney injury, and neurological abnormalities. Approximately 1% to 4% of SLE patients develop HUS or TTP during the course of their disease. The diagnosis of a TMA may be missed, since symptoms of HUS and TTP overlap with those of SLE. However, schistocytes are not a feature of SLE in the absence of TMAs, and a positive direct Coombs test does not rule out the possibility of TMAs.[452]

Possible pathophysiological mechanisms in SLE-related TTP/HUS include direct endothelial damage, possibly due to antiendothelial antibodies, which leads to reduced prostacyclin, increased platelet activation, von Willebrand factor (vWF) abnormalities, and resultant TMA. APLs are present in some patients with TMA, though it is unclear what role they play in its pathogenesis, and features of TMAs and APL syndrome can overlap.[452] Lupus-related TMA has a high mortality rate, and recognition and prompt treatment is critical. Treatment of TMA consists of corticosteroids and plasma exchange via plasmapheresis. CYC and rituximab have also been used in combination with steroids and plasmapheresis. Lupus-related TMA has a higher mortality and is more resistant to treatment than the idiopathic disease.[437,440,452,453]

MAS is a rare and potentially life-threatening condition that can be associated with SLE (please see Chapter 49 for details). It is notable that the presentation of MAS is very similar to the presentation of lupus itself. The presence of high ferritin in combination with high soluble IL-2 receptors and NK cell dysfunction help the clinician distinguish the two entities.

Coagulation abnormalities are common in SLE. The lupus anticoagulant (LAC) is positive in approximately 20% of patients with pSLE. Patients with the LAC do not bleed but rather develop thromboembolic events (TEs) and, in particular, venous rather than arterial occlusions. The most common areas for TEs are the legs, cerebral veins, and pulmonary vasculature. Patients with the LAC have approximately a 25- to 30-times greater risk of thrombosis than do patients without the LAC. Patients with an arterial thrombosis tend to have a true vasculitis in addition to the LAC.[207] When patients with the LAC have abnormal bleeding, a second coagulation abnormality should be considered such as an acquired prothrombin deficiency (seen in about 5% of pSLE patients with the LAC) or less commonly acquired factor VIII and IX or von Willebrand deficiencies. Elevated homocysteine levels or acquired protein S, protein C, or anti–thrombin III deficiency may also increase risk of thrombosis, while congenital thrombophilia defects do not seem to be increased in SLE patients.[207,454-463]

Vasculitis

Vasculitis is a common manifestation of SLE. Specific organ-related vasculitis, such as vasculitis of the CNS, intestines, lung, and heart, are discussed under their respective clinical sections in this chapter. LV primarily affects the small arteries and venules in the skin. Medium-sized vessel involvement is less common, and large-vessel disease is rare. Although LV most often appears with skin manifestations, a wide variety of organs can be involved, as mentioned above, with potentially life-threatening consequences.[464,465]

The most common form of cutaneous LV is a leukocytoclastic vasculitis (LCV), presenting with erythematous or violaceous punctate, nonblanching lesions on the fingertips and palms. Skin biopsy in LCV demonstrates perivascular inflammatory infiltrate composed mostly of neutrophils, as well as nuclear dust; swollen endothelial cells; fibrinoid degeneration of the vessel walls; and abundant extravasated erythrocytes.[466] Cryoglobulinemia, unusual in children, can present with lower-extremity purpura; hepatitis C should be ruled out in these cases. Urticarial vasculitis also can be a manifestation of small-vessel LV.[465]

Patients with LV generally have higher disease activity scores, lymphopenia, hypocomplementemia, a high ESR, and anemia. APLs and livedo reticularis also are associated with LV. It is important to distinguish between the thrombosis of APS and the vasculitis lesions of SLE-related vasculitis because the former requires anticoagulation while the latter requires immunosuppression.[465]

Gastrointestinal and Hepatic Manifestations

GI manifestations occur in approximately 20% of children with SLE. Abdominal pain, diarrhea, and/or vomiting are the most common presenting symptoms. The causes of abdominal pain in SLE patients are diverse, including lupus-related and non–lupus-related etiologies, as well as infections and medication side effects (Table 23-18).[467] Adults primarily have non-lupus GI pathology, such as hepatitis, cholecystitis, ulcers, and diverticulitis, whereas children more often have

TABLE 23-18 Leading Causes of Acute Abdominal Pain in SLE Patients

NON-SLE RELATED	SLE RELATED
Appendicitis	Lupus enteritis
Lithiasic cholecystitis	Pancreatitis
Peptic ulcer	Pseudo-obstruction
Acute pancreatitis	Acalculous cholecystitis
Retroperitoneal hematoma	Mesenteric thrombosis
Ovarian pathology	Hepatic thrombosis
Diverticulitis	Medication (NSAIDs, MMF, steroids, HCQ)
Adhesions, intestinal occlusion	Colon perforation (vasculitis)
Infectious enteritis	
Pyelonephritis	
CMV colitis	

HCQ, Hydroxychloroquine; *MMF,* mycophenolate mofetil; *NSAIDs,* nonsteroidal antiinflammatory drugs; *SLE,* systemic lupus erythematosus.
From P. Janssens, L. Arnaud, L. Galicier, et al., Lupus enteritis: from clinical findings to therapeutic management, Orphanet J. Rare Dis. 8 (2013) 67.

lupus-related causes such as lupus mesenteric vasculitis, ascites/peritonitis, and pancreatitis.[467,468]

Acute lupus peritonitis presents with abdominal pain and ascites, usually during acute general SLE activity. It is important to distinguish between primary acute lupus peritonitis and peritonitis/ascites secondary to other causes, such as nephrotic syndrome, pancreatitis, and intestinal infarction or perforation due to vasculitis or thrombosis. In addition, other causes for ascites should be evaluated, such as congestive heart failure, constrictive pericarditis, and protein-losing enteropathy. Examination of peritoneal fluid can be useful to rule out infection. In lupus peritonitis, ascitic fluid is exudative, culture negative, and may have lupus erythematosus (LE) cells, low C3 and C4, and elevated anti-dsDNA antibodies.

Acute pancreatitis is an uncommon but potentially life-threatening SLE manifestation, occurring in about 5% to 6% of childhood cases of SLE. The most frequent symptoms in both adults in children are abdominal pain, nausea, vomiting, and fever. Causes of acute pancreatitis other than lupus that should be excluded are obstruction of the pancreatic duct, hypertriglyceridemia, hypercalcemia, alcohol, medications, and infections (such as CMV). Diagnosis is based on clinical symptoms and elevation of serum amylase and lipase. Pancreatitis generally is associated with higher lupus activity at the time of onset. Possible pathological mechanisms involved in lupus-related pancreatitis include vascular ischemia and damage (from vasculitis, intimal thickening, IC deposition, microthrombi, and APLs, and vascular occlusion), antipancreas autoantibodies, vascular ischemia, as well as pancreatic inflammation due to lymphocyte infiltration and complement activation, viral infection, and drug toxicity. In general, the mortality rate of pancreatitis in children is approximately 2% to 21% and may be higher in lupus-related pancreatitis. In rare instances, pseudocyst formation and pancreatic insufficiency may be sequelae. Although corticosteroids and AZA have been implicated in causing acute pancreatitis, in fact, patients with lupus-related peritonitis respond well to corticosteroid treatment, and steroid treatment has been shown to be associated with better survival in lupus-related pancreatitis.[469-474]

Lupus mesenteric vasculitis (LMV), a leukocytoclastic vasculitis of mesenteric vessel walls, also known as *lupus enteritis,* usually presents with abdominal pain, sometimes associated with impaired intestinal motility and signs of peritonitis.[475] Corticosteroids can mask signs of intestinal perforation in patients who already take steroids. The clinician should have a low threshold when determining when to obtain a CT scan, which will demonstrate multiple segments of focal or diffuse bowel-wall thickening, dilation, abnormal bowel-wall enhancement (target sign), engorgement of mesenteric vessels with increased number of visible vessels (comb's sign), increased attenuation of mesenteric fat, and ascites. These findings, however, also can be seen in pancreatitis, mechanical bowel obstruction, peritonitis, or inflammatory bowel disease, from which LMV must be distinguished.[476]

Lupus-related protein-losing enteropathy (PLE) is a rare GI manifestation that presents with peripheral edema, ascites, diarrhea, and hypoalbuminemia. Infection should be excluded before diagnosing PLE, as should nephrotic syndrome, which also can cause ascites, edema, and hypoalbuminemia. SLE has been associated with celiac disease, which can cause diarrhea, weight loss, and iron-deficiency anemia. Symptoms may not improve with gluten restriction but instead may improve with steroid treatment.[477]

Intestinal pseudoobstruction (IPO) is another rare manifestation of SLE. Richer reported that IPO comprises 2.5% of GI manifestations in children.[467] IPO usually presents with abdominal pain, vomiting, constipation, and a distended and tender abdomen with hypoactive or absent bowel sounds. The small bowel is affected more frequently.

Abdominal radiography demonstrates dilated, fluid-filled bowel loops, thickened bowel wall, and multiple air-fluid levels. Other causes of obstruction must be ruled out before a diagnosis of IPO is made. Interestingly, IPO often has been reported with accompanying interstitial cystitis.

Liver manifestations, generally mild elevations in liver transaminases, have been reported in approximately 25% of children with SLE.[478] Elevated liver enzymes correlate with disease activity and improve with corticosteroid treatment. It is important to distinguish primary lupus-related hepatic disease from infection and drug toxicity. Budd–Chiari syndrome, acute hepatic vein thrombosis associated with APS, is important to diagnose because it requires rapid anticoagulation to preserve liver function. *Lupoid hepatitis,* a chronic, active form of lupus-associated hepatitis, can be difficult to distinguish from non-lupus autoimmune hepatitis (AIH) but generally has a more benign course than the latter disease and does not require steroid treatment.

Endocrine Involvement

The most common endocrine abnormality in systemic lupus is hypothyroidism associated with a high frequency of antithyroid antibodies (close to 40%).[479] Patients should have thyroid studies at disease onset, annually, or if they develop any signs or symptoms of hypothyroidism. The presentation is typical of Hashimoto's thyroiditis, whereas Graves disease is rarely seen. The parathyroid glands by contrast are rarely involved. Rare reports of lupus presenting with Addison disease can be found as well as type I diabetes, psoriasis, and vitiligo.

Endocrinopathies secondary to lupus and its treatment also occur. Patients may develop type II diabetes from corticosteroids or, in the high-risk patient, in association with weight gain from corticosteroid use. Adrenal gland failure due to prolonged corticosteroid use or APS-related infarction can occur. Growth delay or failure, along with delayed puberty, is associated with chronic corticosteroid use, particularly in prepubertal or peripubertal patients.[480] Finally, ovarian or testicular dysfunction, including sterility, may occur secondary to chemotherapeutic agents used to treat disease.

Sjögren Syndrome

See Chapter 30 regarding secondary Sjögren syndrome.

Ocular Disease

Few studies have described the incidence of ocular involvement in pSLE. The most common ocular finding associated with pSLE is cotton-wool spots (cytoid bodies), indicative of retinal vasculitis (Fig. 23-21; Table 23-19). Cotton-wool spots tend to have a paraarteriolar location in the posterior pole of the retina. The lesions represent edema and degeneration of ganglion cells secondary to the arteriolitis and immune complex deposition. Occlusion of the central retinal vein, usually associated with APLs or CNS vasculitis, and severe diffuse retinal vasculitis may occur. Both of these entities are frequently associated with visual loss.[481-483] Both episcleritis and scleritis may be seen. Keratoconjunctivitis sicca is seen in patients with secondary Sjögren syndrome.

Lymphatic Tissues and Cancer Risk

At lupus onset or with flares, patients often have increased lymphatic tissue found on examination as splenomegaly and lymphadenopathy. Occasionally, lymphadenopathy is very impressive, suggesting the presentation of malignancy or Kikuchi disease (histiocytic necrotizing lymphadenitis).[484] These patients are often biopsied if there are no physical findings or lab abnormalities that suggest multisystem disease (lupus). It is important to recognize that there is an increased incidence of malignancy in patients with lupus. Recently, Bernasky et al. reported

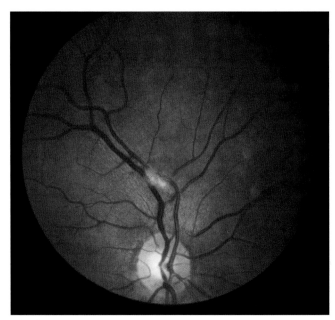

FIGURE 23-21 An oval white cotton-wool spot (CWS) in the posterior retinal pole. A CWS is invariably in a paraarteriolar position and often partially obliterates the adjacent arteriole. CWSs arise from segmental vasculitis within and adjacent to these vessels. The surrounding retina generally shows an edematous sheen. In SLE, usually only a few CWSs are present. Identical lesions may rarely be seen in other connective tissue diseases. In hypertension, diabetes, or septicemia, numerous CWSs may be present.

TABLE 23-19   Ocular Manifestations
External eye disease: discoid rash over eyelids
Lacrimal system: keratoconjunctivitis sicca
Orbital disease: periorbital edema, orbital masses, myositis, panniculitis, ischemia/infarction
Anterior segment: corneal-dry eyes, erosions, punctuate epithelial loss, ulcerative keratitis, conjunctival inflammation (rare), uveitis (rare)
Episcleritis
Scleritis: either anterior or posterior segment
Retinopathy: cotton-wool spots, perivascular hard exudates, retinal hemorrhages and vascular tortuosity, vasoocclusive retinopathy (or "retinal vasculitis"), retinal infections
Choroidal: unifocal or multifocal retinal detachments and choroidal effusions or ischemia infections
Optic nerve disease: optic neuritis and ischemic optic neuropathy (anterior or posterior)
Ocular motor abnormalities: diplopia, internuclear ophthalmoplegia, nystagmus and Miller Fisher syndrome
Drug-induced

Adapted from Ref. 59.

increased rates of cancer in a series of 1020 subjects. Despite the increased risk, the malignancies were rare events and often occurred 10 to 19 years after lupus diagnosis and transition to adult care.[485]

GENERAL ASSESSMENT

Systemic lupus is a disease that is very challenging with regard to diagnosis and to determining the best treatment both at onset and throughout the illness. This is due, in part, to the multisystem nature of the disease in combination with serological abnormalities and the difficulty of determining significant disease activity and disease improvement. This challenge has resulted in a number of disease activity scores. The most commonly used scores are the Systemic Lupus Erythematosus Disease Activity Index or SLEDAI[486-490]; the Safety of Estrogen in Lupus Erythematosus National Assessment Trial (SELENA–SLEDAI), which includes a physician global assessment score[491]; or the British Isles Lupus Assessment Group (BILAG) Activity Index.[492,493] The SLEDAI scores have specific definitions of organ or lab abnormalities that are added to reach a score. The BILAG identifies involvement by system, as well as a grading system of disease severity. Other scoring systems that have been devised include the Lupus Activity Index, the Systemic Lupus Activity Measure (SLAM),[489,494] the European Lupus Activity Measure (ECLAM),[495-497] and the Responder Index for Lupus Erythematosus (RIFLE). All of these indexes have been studied and found to have validity. The ACR response criteria for SLE clinical trials and measures of overall disease activity are also used.[498] Pediatric-specific comparisons demonstrated equal specificity and sensitivity between the SLAM, SLEDAI, and BILAG in the evaluation of clinical change in childhood-onset SLE.[499-503] Disease activity scores are included with other measures such as physician and patient assessment of well-being to create specific measures of disease flare and remission that may be used in interventional trials and patient care.

Another important component of disease activity is a measure of damage. The SLICC Damage Index for SLE provides a measure of accumulated organ damage due to the disease and its treatment. This scoring system has been validated for children in a study that also noted that ongoing disease activity, steroid use, presence of APLs, and thrombocytopenia were associated with pediatric damage, whereas use of immunosuppressive agents reduced that risk.[503] Of note, the SLICC Damage Index does not address growth failure, gonadal failure, onset of diabetes secondary to treatment among other damaging consequences of lupus and its treatment, since these effects are often, but not always, reversible, and therefore, their inclusion in damage indexes creates controversy.[13,504]

Pediatric measures of Health-Related Quality of Life (HRQOL) have been applied and studied in the pediatric lupus population.[505] Children with lupus had significantly lower quality of life compared to healthy controls as measured by the Childhood Health Assessment questionnaire, the rheumatology module, and the core module of the Pediatric Quality of Life Inventory (Peds QL). Interestingly, lower HRQOL was related to flare of some, but not all, disease activity measures. Other useful measures for childhood lupus include the Peds QL Multidimensional Fatigue Scale and the Simple Measure of the Impact of Lupus Erythematosus in Youngsters (SMILEY).[505-511]

GENERAL LABORATORY EVALUATION

Indicators of Inflammation

Acute phase indexes are elevated in proportion to disease activity. ESR is increased,[512,513] though CRP often is normal in pSLE, except in cases of accompanying infection, serositis, or arthritis.[514-522] Serum ferritin is elevated, though not to the degree seen in MAS.[523-527]

Autoantibodies

Antinuclear antibodies are present in more than 99% of children with SLE.[3] However, ANAs also are associated with other rheumatic diseases, infections, malignancies, drug exposures, and first-degree relatives of patients with autoimmune disease.[528] Additionally, as many as 33% of healthy children without SLE may be positive for ANAs.[529]

Anti-dsDNA antibodies have a high specificity for SLE. Several laboratory assays are available to measure anti-dsDNA antibodies. Both the radioimmunoassay, utilizing radiolabeled dsDNA, and the enzyme-linked immunosorbent assay (ELISA) are sensitive but less specific because of higher rates of false positivity. A more specific, though less sensitive, test utilizes fluorescence microscopy and the protozoan *Crithidia luciliae*, which has a kinetoplast comprising only dsDNA. The *Crithidia* assay is generally preferred for diagnostic purposes, whereas the radioimmunoassay or ELISA can be used for monitoring.[530] The sensitivity of anti-dsDNA for predicting SLE flares is approximately 50%. Combining anti-dsDNA with anti-C1q antibodies may improve the ability to predict SLE flares.[531-533]

Antibodies to extractable nuclear antigens include anti-Sm, anti-Ro/SSA, anti-La/SSB, and antiribonucleoprotein (anti-RNP). The Sm antigen is composed of five small uridine-rich RNAs (U1, U2, U4, U5, U6), and anti-Sm antibody is highly specific for SLE. The Ro/SSA antigen is complexed to Y RNAs and has been most strongly associated with neonatal SLE and subacute cutaneous lupus. Anti-Ro/SSA is present in about 25% of SLE patients, and approximately 15% of the general population may test positive for anti-Ro/SSA. The La/SSB antigen also is complexed to Y RNAs. Anti-La/SSB antibody also has been associated with neonatal lupus and almost always occurs in combination with anti-Ro/SSA (though anti-Ro/SSA can be found without anti-La/SS-B).

Antihistone antibodies can be associated with drug-induced lupus, and antiribosomal P antibodies can be associated with neuropsychiatric lupus, though neither antibody is specific to those manifestations. Anti-dsDNA antibodies generally are present in LN. A more complete list of autoantibodies, frequencies, and associated disease manifestations is shown in Table 23-20.

Complement

Complement testing is one of the most important laboratory tests in the diagnosis of SLE and measurement of disease activity. Total hemolytic complement assay (THC, CH_{50}), as well as individual complement levels of C3 and C4, can be followed. A significant portion of lupus patients have a C4 null allele and cannot achieve C4 levels above half of the normal range. Undetectable levels of an individual complement component may indicate a homozygous genetic deficiency. During the course of disease, normal C3 and C4 levels have good negative predictive value in following disease activity (i.e., normal levels are reassuring of quiescent disease), especially in LN. Testing for other specific complement components, such as C2 and C1q, should be considered when genetic complement deficiency is suspected. Anti-C1q antibody may also provide a good marker of LN activity and correlate with the severity of nephritis and proteinuria.[533,537,538]

Other tests

The evaluation of a new lupus patient is not complete without evaluation of a complete blood count (CBC), electrolytes, liver function tests, and urine studies. Patients should be screened for thyroid function, antithyroid antibodies, LAC, and APLs. A baseline echocardiogram; PFT, including the diffusing capacity of lungs for carbon dioxide ($DLCO_2$); and bone density are recommended. If there is any concern about NP function, brain imaging and cognitive testing should also be considered. See eTable 23-21 for suggested lab evaluations upon initial workup and confirmation of SLE.

TREATMENT

The major aims of treatment are to contain disease activity using the least toxic therapies, with the goal of avoiding damage from lupus and

TABLE 23-20 **Autoantibodies in pSLE**

PARTICLE RECOGNIZED	SPECIFICITY OF PARTICLE	COMMON NAME FOR ANTIBODY	SPECIFIC PROTEIN	FREQUENCY AT PRESENTATION[†]	FREQUENCY AT ANY TIME	DISEASE ASSOCIATIONS
Nucleosome (chromatin)	Epitopes on nucleosome (chromatin)	Anti-ds-DNA	Native, ds-DNA	65-95%	84-100%	Highly specific for SLE Active glomerulonephritis
	Histone protein complexes	Antihistone	Histone proteins H1, H2A, H2B, H3, H4	No large studies in pSLE	~90% 30-40%	Drug-induced LE SLE
Ro RNP	Proteins complexed to small cytoplasmic RNAs known as hY-RNAs	Anti-Ro	52- and 60-kD proteins	27-33%	38-54%	Neonatal LE Secondary SS Subacute cutaneous LE Cardiac (one study only)
		Anti-La	48-kD protein	13-19%	16-32%	Neonatal LE Secondary SS Subacute cutaneous LE Cardiac (one study only)
Small nuclear (Sn) RNP	Proteins complexed to Uridine-rich RNAs (U1, U2, U4, U5 SnRNP)	Anti-Sm	B/B/,* D1,[†] D2,[†] D3,[†] E, F, G proteins	32-34%	23-48%	Specific SLE
	Proteins associated with U1 RNP	U1RNP	70-kD, A, C proteins	27-35%	31-62%	SLEMCTD
Rheumatoid factors	Gamma globulins	RF	IgM antibodies	11%	15-35%	SLE-JIA, SS
Ribosomal P proteins	Phosphorylated ribosomal proteins	Anti-P	P0 (38 kD), P1 (19 kD) and P2 (17 kD) proteins[‡]	No large studies in pSLE	21-42%	SLE-hepatitis, renal and psychosis
Chromosomal protein	Nonhistone basic chromosomal protein	Anti–SCI-70	Topoisomerase 1 (70-kD protein)	No large studies in pSLE	15%	More common in progressive systemic sclerosis

*Very few studies reported autoantibodies at presentation.
[†]Major antigens.
[‡]Most antibodies bind to all three.
ds-DNA, Double-stranded DNA; IgM, immunoglobulin M; JIA, juvenile idiopathic arthritis; LE, lupus erythematosus; MCTD, mixed-connective tissue disease; pSLE, pediatric systemic lupus erythematosus; RNP, ribonuclear protein; SLE, systemic lupus erythematosus; SS, Sjögren syndrome.
Sources: See Refs. 1, 17, 21, 24, 162, 163, 166, 170, 381, 407, 534-536.

from the chosen therapies used to manage the disease. Perhaps the most important aspect of treatment is patient education and counseling that utilizes a team approach for support. After diagnosis, outcomes rely on rapid responses to change in disease activity and adherence to medical therapies; thus, engaging the patient and family is critical to successful outcomes. General care also includes appropriate management of infections and vaccinations, including an annual influenza vaccine as well as pneumococcal vaccine. Routine inactivated vaccines should be administered as required. Patients need to understand the importance of sleep, stress management, and exercise as part of daily routines. Nutritional counseling is critical particularly if the patient requires corticosteroids, has renal insufficiency, or dyslipidemias. Lastly, all lupus patients require education about sun protection, which includes the use of sunscreens at least 30 minutes prior to going outside, avoidance of the midday sun, and the use of protective clothing and sun protective additives that can be included in the wash cycle.

Pharmacological Therapy

Pharmacological interventions should be designed for each individual patient based on the type and severity of disease manifestations. See Table 23-22 for a list of commonly used medications in SLE, side effects, and precautions.

Nonsteroidal Antiinflammatory Drugs

NSAID therapy and antimalarial therapies are used to treat musculoskeletal complaints in lupus patients. Patients with arthralgias and myalgias often respond to treatment; however, patients with polyarthritis or myositis are likely to require immunosuppression. Complications from NSAIDs include GI irritation or ulcer, hypersensitivity

TABLE 23-22 Medications Commonly Used in Pediatric SLE (Excluding Corticosteroids)				
MEDICATION	**MAJOR INDICATIONS**	**USUAL DOSE**	**MAJOR SIDE EFFECTS**	**PRECAUTIONS**
Hydroxychloroquine	Most patients	4-7 mg/kg/day, maximum 400 mg	Ophthalmological	Reduce dose in renal insufficiency
			Cardiac muscle	Ophthalmological exam every 6 months
Nonsteroidal antiinflammatory drugs (NSAIDs)	Systemic features Musculoskeletal	Varies by drug	Gastrointestinal Aseptic meningitis	Give with caution with decreased renal function
Methotrexate	Steroid sparing	Up to 15 mg/m^2/week orally or subcutaneously, maximum 25 mg	Hepatitis Bone marrow suppression	Monitor CBC and LFTs Alter dose in renal insufficiency
Azathioprine	Proliferative nephritis Steroid sparing	3 mg/kg/day maximum 150 mg	Bone marrow suppression Hepatitis infection	Monitor CBC and LFTs
Cyclophosphamide	NP disease	1 g/m^2/month intravenously	Bone marrow suppression	Alter dose with renal insufficiency
	Proliferative nephritis		Infection Infertility Malignancy	Give PCP prophylaxis Give mesna Monitor CBC and urine
Mycophenolate mofetil	Proliferative and membranous lupus nephritis	1 g/m^2/day (can measure levels)	Bone marrow suppression	Monitor CBC and LFTs
	NP disease		Hepatitis infection	May need to alter dose with renal insufficiency
	Steroid sparing when other drugs fail			

CBC, Complete blood count; *LFT,* liver function test; *NP,* neuropsychiatric; *PCP, Pneumocystis jiroveci* pneumonia.

reactions, and, rarely, aseptic meningitis.[539] Patients with renal insufficiency should avoid this class of medication. Low-dose aspirin is often prescribed for children with moderate to high positive APLs, although there is no specific evidence that this reduces clotting events in APL-positive patients.

Hydroxychloroquine/Chloroquine

Hydroxychloroquine has been used in the treatment of lupus for more than 50 years. It has been found to improve musculoskeletal symptoms, rash, and alopecia.[540-545] It improves dyslipidemia often associated with corticosteroid use.[546-549] It appears to maintain disease remission and reduce the risk of vascular events, possibly by restoring the function of annexin A5, which is altered by APLs.[550] The usual dosage of hydroxychloroquine is 4 to 7 mg/kg/day. Chloroquine can be substituted if hydroxychloroquine is not tolerated. The general low toxicity of hydroxychloroquine makes it an attractive maintenance therapy; however, retinal toxicity after 5 years of therapy becomes a concern, and patients require monitoring. New recommendations include a baseline examination and annual examinations after 5 years unless there is a specific increased risk. Newer evaluation tools including multifocal electroretinogram (mfERG), spectral domain optical coherence tomography (SD-OCT), and fundus autofluorescence (FAF) allow for more objective measures of toxicity.[551]

Glucocorticoids

Glucocorticoids are the backbone of medication of management for most children with lupus. Often at diagnosis, but sometimes during the course of the disease, children will receive oral or IV therapy or both. There are several corticosteroids that can be given orally or intravenously. Preference is based on training and experience. There is no evidence that supports one type of glucocorticoid over another. The management of corticosteroid therapy is widely variable among

pediatric rheumatology practices. This has been reported in a comparison of four North American rheumatology practices[552] and is also reflected in the recently reported consensus treatment plans for class III and IV LN.[212]

Most pediatric rheumatologists would agree that initial therapy for severe disease requires IV methylprednisolone 30 mg/kg/day up to a maximum of 1000 mg for 1 to 5 consecutive days. There is good evidence that this drug changes the INF signature of the disease[553] and begins management of severe kidney, brain, or hematological disease. Some practitioners prefer equivalent potency of dexamethasone for neurological disease. Daily oral prednisone at a dosage of 0.5 to 2 mg/kg/day divided into two or three doses depending on organ involvement and disease severity may be initiated at the start of moderate disease or follow initial pulsing. Once the patient is stabilized over a period of 3 to 4 weeks, the dose is consolidated and then tapered by 5% to 10% every 1 to 2 weeks. The taper of medication is mindful of clinical and laboratory parameters, as any signs or symptoms of flare require a significant increase in steroid dose. Many practitioners do not alter initial steroid therapy until complement is almost normal (understanding that many lupus patients have a C4 null allele and will not be able to correct C4), anti-dsDNA levels have improved, and significant cytopenias have resolved. Some disease manifestations require the addition of other immunosuppressant therapies at disease presentation. If the patient does not require immediate use of these therapies, the clinician may need to initiate therapy for the patient who does not respond well to steroids or has unacceptable steroid toxicity.

Cyclophosphamide

CYC is primarily used for severe SLE, especially kidney, CNS disease, and other severe organ involvement, as discussed in earlier sections of this chapter (see "Treatment of Lupus Nephritis").

The risk of amenorrhea and infertility with CYC treatment remain a concern. Age at initiation of treatment and cumulative dose are the most important predictors of ovarian failure. CYC treatment before onset of puberty has little risk of amenorrhea. However, because of active proliferation of Sertoli and Leydig cells in the testes even before puberty, prepubertal boys are not as protected as girls from the effects of CYC, and azoospermia has been reported in boys treated with CYC. Gonadotropin-releasing hormone (GnRH) treatment, in the form of depot leuprolide acetate, may provide ovarian protection by suppressing ovulation. Studies of GnRH have been encouraging but not conclusive, and consensus is lacking so far regarding general recommendations for use of GnRH. Another option for postpubertal women is ovarian stimulation followed by oocyte extraction and preservation. As with oral contraceptive pills, ovarian stimulation may increase the risk of SLE flare. For postpubertal men, sperm banking is an option to provide fertility in the event of CYC-induced azoospermia.[554-558]

AZATHIOPRINE AND MYCOPHENOLATE MOFETIL

As mentioned previously (see the section "Treatment of Lupus Nephritis"), attention has shifted away from CYC, especially in the treatment of LN, and toward AZA and MMF. Although AZA has a higher rate of cytopenias, it has the advantage of lower cost, relative safety during pregnancy, and once-daily administration.[559] Genotyping of thiopurine methyltransferase (TPMT), an enzyme that metabolizes AZA and can have reduced or absent activity in some individuals, may help to identify those at risk for AZA toxicity.[560] MMF can result in GI side effects (often mild and temporary), cytopenias, and teratogenicity. The potential risks of MMF during pregnancy led to the U.S. Food and Drug Administration (FDA) to institute a risk evaluation and mitigation strategies (REMS) system in 2012.[561]

Methotrexate

Methotrexate (MTX) is most commonly used in mild to moderate SLE. MTX is effective in the management of SLE with skin and mucocutaneous involvement.[562-566] Methotrexate also can be used as a steroid-sparing agent.[562,563,567,568] MTX also improves complement levels, decreases anti-dsDNA antibody, and improves SLEDAI score.[569] However, there is limited and conflicting information on the use of MTX in pSLE.[570,571]

CYCLOSPORINE AND TACROLIMUS

Small studies have demonstrated a beneficial effect of CSA on proteinuria in LN.[233,244,572] The utility of CSA is limited by its need for careful monitoring of drug levels and its potential toxicities, including hypertension, renal impairment, effects on lipid profile, tremor, hirsutism, and gum hyperplasia.[559] Tacrolimus (TAC), another calcineurin inhibitor, offers a better side-effect profile than CSA, though careful drug monitoring is still required. Similarly, a number of small trials have shown efficacy of TAC in LN.[234,238,239,247,573-578] At this time, and based on limited evidence, CSA and TAC seem to be most useful in treating patients with LN who are resistant to steroids or other drugs.[232,579,580] Regarding nonrenal SLE, a recent multicenter, randomized, controlled trial by BILAG concluded that low-dose CSA was as effective as AZA as a steroid-sparing agent in patients with severe SLE with a similar rate of adverse drug effects.[581] In small studies, TAC has been used effectively in nonrenal systemic lupus and cutaneous lupus.[582-586]

Biological Therapies
Intravenous Immunoglobulin

There are no data to support the use of IVIG in the treatment of systemic lupus. It may temporarily help in the treatment of cytopenias; however, it does not appear to alter the course of the disease.

Plasmapheresis

Plasmapheresis is implemented for acute and life-threatening disease manifestations that may respond to elimination of autoantibodies and ICs such as pulmonary hemorrhage and acute hemolytic anemia, or thrombocytopenia that is unresponsive to corticosteroids. There are no data to support plasmapheresis as a long-term therapy.

Monoclonal Antibodies

Anti-CD20 (rituximab) has been reported to be of benefit in multiple open-label studies of hundreds of patients with all types of SLE. These series suggest that it is particularly effective in patients with treatment-resistant SLE-associated cytopenias.[442,587-591] Randomized, controlled trials failed to show a benefit over placebo.[592,593] However, two recent series of pediatric patients treated with a combination of rituximab and CYC have demonstrated benefit.[594,595] There are several other anti–B-cell therapies available. Anti-CD22 is in phase III trials currently.

BLyS is a cytokine of the TNF superfamily produced by myeloid cells and are required for B-cell maturation, survival, and immunoglobulin production. Belimumab, a monoclonal antibody against soluble BLys, has demonstrated modest efficacy and has been approved for use in adults. There is a double-blind placebo-controlled trial ongoing for children at this time.[596,597] There are four other monoclonal antibodies in this category undergoing evaluation at this time.

Other therapies include anti-IFN-α therapy. Sifalimumab and rontalizumab are undergoing clinical trials. Inhibitors of TLRs 7/8/9 are in the pipeline. Anti-TNF therapies have failed. Newer therapies including nonselective and selective proteasome inhibitors of plasma cells and FcγRIIB receptor therapies are being developed. Use of T-cell inhibitors such as abatacept failed a clinical trial for treatment of LN because of an increased rate of zoster infections but has been useful anecdotally for the treatment of lupus arthritis.[230]

TRANSPLANTATION

Autologous bone marrow transplantation (ABMT) has been tried in the treatment of severe lupus. In 2011, international evaluation of ABMT in more than 200 adult patients with refractory disease demonstrated a 50% to 70% remission rate at 5 years, but a significant early mortality rate needs to be addressed by improved patient selection, improved induction, maintenance, and long-term follow-up of patients.[598] There have been reports of the successful use of allogenic bone marrow transplantation and allogenic bone marrow mesenchymal stem cells in adult SLE patients.[599-601] The pediatric experience is limited to case reports.

MORBIDITY AND MORTALITY

Pediatric lupus patients continue to improve their life expectancy (from 40% to 50% of normal in the 1960s to 90% to 95% currently). As a result, they have accrued a number of morbidities. The causes of death in the pediatric population are unchanged and are most often due to infection, renal failure, and cardiopulmonary disease. A list of morbidities seen in patients with pSLE is shown in Table 23-23. Patients typically have significant morbidity due to steroid therapy, including skin changes, weight changes, cataracts and glaucoma,

TABLE 23-23 Morbidities Associated with pSLE

SYSTEM	MORBIDITY
Renal	Hypertension, dialysis, transplantation
Central nervous system	Organic brain syndrome, seizures, psychosis, neurocognitive disorder
Cardiovascular	Atherosclerosis, myocardial infarction, cardiomyopathy, valvular disease
Immune	Recurrent infection, functional asplenia, malignancy
Musculoskeletal	Osteoporosis, compression fractures, avascular necrosis
Ocular	Cataracts, glaucoma, retinal detachment, blindness
Endocrine	Diabetes, obesity, growth failure, infertility, fetal wastage

TABLE 23-24 Risk Factors for Atherosclerosis in pSLE

Traditional Risk Factors
Dyslipidemia
Hypertension
Family history of premature atherosclerosis
Smoking
Obesity
Diabetes mellitus
Physical inactivity

Nontraditional Risk Factors
Chronic inflammation
Multiple elevated inflammatory markers found
Other lipid abnormalities
Apoproteins
Free fatty acid
Lipoprotein(a)
Oxidized LDL
Proinflammatory HDL
Elevated homocysteine
Endothelial injury
Anti–endothelial cell antibodies
Vasculitis
Autoantibodies
Anti-annexin
Antiphospholipid
Decreased mannose-binding lectin
Prothrombotic state
Abnormal adipokine levels
Abnormal nitric oxide metabolism
Elevated levels of cytokines
Abnormal CD40–CD40 ligand interaction
Corticosteroids
Renal disease

changes in growth, and increased risk of diabetes and hypertension. Pediatric lupus patients have an increased risk of cardiovascular disease (Table 23-24). This is partially due to dyslipidemia often related to steroids; however, persistent inflammation secondary to poorly controlled or persistent disease can also be associated with poor cardiovascular outcomes in the adult population.[602,603] Evaluation of the effect of atorvastatin over a 3-year period on pediatric cardiovascular health and dyslipidemia did not demonstrate benefit but did demonstrate progression of atherosclerosis in the pediatric lupus population. Further study to determine whether specific groups of patients may experience benefits from atorvastatin was undertaken.[423] Preliminary studies have shown abnormalities of myocardial perfusion and early signs of atherosclerosis, including abnormal pulse wave velocity, vascular reactivity, and increased CIMT.[604-609]

Osteoporosis

Chronic inflammatory diseases alter bone mineral metabolism, resulting in osteoporosis. Low bone mineral density (BMD), seen in up to 20% of patients with pSLE, is likely the result of both chronic inflammation and steroid use. In one study, 16% of newly diagnosed pediatric lupus patients were found to have osteoporosis on imaging. Other risks for osteoporosis in this population include disease duration; disease severity; chronic steroid therapy; sun avoidance, which reduces vitamin D production; poor intake of high calcium foods; persistent inflammation; renal disease; and decreased activity due to fatigue and musculoskeletal disease. It is critical to address this issue as individuals complete their peak bone mass in their early 20s. If an appropriate density is not achieved, patients are at higher risk for complications of osteoporosis at midlife when hormones change. Patients should be monitored for appropriate intake of calcium and vitamin D as well as appropriate physical activity. Vitamin D levels should be monitored, and vitamin D supplementation to improve levels to vitamin D sufficiency should be considered. Bone density should be monitored, and consideration of treatment of osteoporosis should be reserved for patients with BMD in the osteoporotic range who experience fragility fractures.[610,611]

The other musculoskeletal morbidity is osteonecrosis, which often occurs at weight-bearing bones, including vertebrae and the long bones of the lower limbs. It occasionally occurs very early in the treatment of lupus but is often associated with steroid use over long periods. It is unclear why some patients are more prone to osteonecrosis. The finding of radiographic changes occurs less frequently than MRI changes, which are more sensitive to edema.[612,613] Treatments include bed rest and core decompression; these modalities have shown modest success. Grafting of vascularized bone has been somewhat helpful.[614,615] Joint replacement is sometimes necessary when there is limited ability to ambulate due to pain or dysfunction.

Drug-induced myopathy is another morbidity associated with lupus. It is usually related to therapy with hydroxychloroquine, statins, or steroids. Drug-induced myopathy is reversible when the causative agent is discontinued.

SUMMARY

Childhood-onset systemic lupus is a challenge for the diagnostician and for the clinician treating the patient. It is one of the diseases that has many faces at presentation, and patients may initially seek advice from specialists of the initial target organ involvement. Through better understanding and education, patients receive earlier diagnoses. It is then up to the treating physician to balance disease activity, treatment options considering medication toxicities, and patient and family lifestyle in order to find the best outcomes. One of the most important goals for the clinician is to have the patient and family embrace the diagnosis as a lifelong challenge, to prepare them through education and experience to take ownership and manage their disease so that these young patients can successfully transition their care and improve their outcomes.

REFERENCES

1. L.B. Tucker, A.G. Uribe, M. Fernández, et al., Adolescent onset of lupus results in more aggressive disease and worse outcomes: results of a nested matched case-control study within LUMINA, a multiethnic US cohort (LUMINA LVII), Lupus 17 (2008) 314–322.

4. M. Petri, A.M. Orbai, G.S. Alarcon, et al., Derivation and validation of the Systemic Lupus International Collaborating Clinics classification criteria for systemic lupus erythematosus, Arthritis Rheum. 64 (2012) 2677–2686.

5. E. Sag, A. Tartaglione, E.D. Batu, et al., Performance of the new SLICC classification criteria in childhood systemic lupus erythematosus: a multicentre study, Clin. Exp. Rheumatol. 32 (2014) 440–444.

6. D. Pineles, A. Valente, B. Warren, et al., Worldwide incidence and prevalence of pediatric onset systemic lupus erythematosus, Lupus 20 (2011) 1187–1192.

21. L.R. Gómez, O.U. Uribe, O.O. Uribe, et al., Childhood systemic lupus erythematosus in Latin America. The GLADEL experience in 230 children, Lupus 17 (2008) 596–604.

24. L.T. Hiraki, S.M. Benseler, P.N. Tyrrell, et al., Clinical and laboratory characteristics and long-term outcome of pediatric systemic lupus erythematosus: a longitudinal study, J. Pediatr. 152 (2008) 550–556.

42. A. Belot, R. Cimaz, Monogenic forms of systemic lupus erythematosus: new insights into SLE pathogenesis, Pediatr. Rheumatol. Online J. 10 (2012) 21.

43. T.B. Niewold, Interferon alpha as a primary pathogenic factor in human lupus, J. Interferon Cytokine Res. 31 (2011) 887–892.

46. E.C. Baechler, F.M. Batliwalla, G. Karypis, et al., Interferon-inducible gene expression signature in peripheral blood cells of patients with severe lupus, Proc. Natl. Acad. Sci. U.S.A. 100 (2003) 2610–2615.

49. L. Casciola-Rosen, A. Rosen, Ultraviolet light-induced keratinocyte apoptosis: a potential mechanism for the induction of skin lesions and autoantibody production in LE, Lupus 6 (1997) 175–180.

75. S. Caielli, J. Banchereau, V. Pascual, Neutrophils come of age in chronic inflammation, Curr. Opin. Immunol. 24 (2012) 671–677.

76. G.S. Garcia-Romo, S. Caielli, B. Vega, et al., Netting neutrophils are major inducers of type I IFN production in pediatric systemic lupus erythematosus, Sci. Transl. Med. 3 (2011) 73ra20.

108. D.M. Absher, X. Li, L.L. Waite, et al., Genome-wide DNA methylation analysis of systemic lupus erythematosus reveals persistent hypomethylation of interferon genes and compositional changes to CD4+ T-cell populations, PLoS Genet. 9 (2013) e1003678.

111. T. Hughes, A. Adler, J.A. Kelly, et al., Evidence for gene-gene epistatic interactions among susceptibility loci for systemic lupus erythematosus, Arthritis Rheum. 64 (2012) 485–492.

113. Q. Lu, The critical importance of epigenetics in autoimmunity, J. Autoimmun. 41 (2013) 1–5.

148. M. Abu-Shakra, Safety of vaccination of patients with systemic lupus erythematosus, Lupus 18 (2009) 1205–1208.

151. A.T. Borchers, C.L. Keen, M.E. Gershwin, Drug-induced lupus, Ann. N. Y. Acad. Sci. 1108 (2007) 166–182.

158. S.M. Benseler, E.D. Silverman, Neuropsychiatric involvement in pediatric systemic lupus erythematosus, Lupus 16 (2007) 564–571.

161. F. Caeiro, F.M. Michielson, R. Bernstein, et al., Systemic lupus erythematosus in childhood, Ann. Rheum. Dis. 40 (1981) 325–331.

195. G. Giannico, A.B. Fogo, Lupus nephritis: is the kidney biopsy currently necessary in the management of lupus nephritis?, Clin. J. Am. Soc. Nephrol. 8 (2013) 138–145.

198. J. Font, A. Torras, R. Cervera, et al., Silent renal disease in systemic lupus erythematosus, Clin. Nephrol. 27 (1987) 283–288.

207. D.M. Levy, M.P. Massicotte, E. Harvey, et al., Thromboembolism in paediatric lupus patients, Lupus 12 (2003) 741–746.

208. R.J. Hogg, R.J. Portman, D. Milliner, et al., Evaluation and management of proteinuria and nephrotic syndrome in children: recommendations from a pediatric nephrology panel established at the National Kidney Foundation conference on proteinuria, albuminuria, risk, assessment, detection, and elimination (PARADE), Pediatrics 105 (2000) 1242–1249.

210. C. Fiehn, Y. Hajjar, K. Mueller, et al., Improved clinical outcome of lupus nephritis during the past decade: importance of early diagnosis and treatment, Ann. Rheum. Dis. 62 (2003) 435–439.

211. G. Moroni, S. Pasquali, S. Quaglini, et al., Clinical and prognostic value of serial renal biopsies in lupus nephritis, Am. J. Kidney Dis. 34 (1999) 530–539.

214. J.E. Balow, H.A. Austin 3rd, L.R. Muenz, et al., Effect of treatment on the evolution of renal abnormalities in lupus nephritis, N. Engl. J. Med. 311 (1984) 491–495.

236. C.C. Mok, K.Y. Ying, C.W. Yim, et al., Very long-term outcome of pure lupus membranous nephropathy treated with glucocorticoid and azathioprine, Lupus 18 (2009) 1091–1095.

239. K.C. Tse, M.F. Lam, S.C. Tang, et al., A pilot study on tacrolimus treatment in membranous or quiescent lupus nephritis with proteinuria resistant to angiotensin inhibition or blockade, Lupus 16 (2007) 46–51.

240. A.A. Al Salloum, Cyclophosphamide therapy for lupus nephritis: poor renal survival in Arab children, Pediatr. Nephrol. 18 (2003) 357–361.

249. D.C. Yan, C.C. Chou, M.J. Tsai, et al., Intravenous cyclophosphamide pulse therapy on children with severe active lupus nephritis, Zhonghua Min Guo Xiao Er Ke Yi Xue Hui Za Zhi. 36 (1995) 203–209.

296. M. Kallel-Sellami, L. Baili-Klila, Y. Zerzeri, et al., Hereditary complement deficiency and lupus: report of four Tunisian cases, Ann. N. Y. Acad. Sci. 1108 (2007) 197–202.

302. R.M. van Vugt, R.H. Derksen, L. Kater, J.W. Bijlsma, Deforming arthropathy or lupus and rhupus hands in systemic lupus erythematosus, Ann. Rheum. Dis. 57 (1998) 540–544.

314. M.I. Steinlin, S.I. Blaser, D.L. Gilday, et al., Neurologic manifestations of pediatric systemic lupus erythematosus, Pediatr. Neurol. 13 (1995) 191–197.

336. D.R. Gitelman, M.S. Klein-Gitelman, J. Ying, et al., Brain morphometric changes associated with childhood-onset systemic lupus erythematosus and neurocognitive deficit, Arthritis Rheum. 65 (2013) 2190–2200.

359. A. How, P.B. Dent, S.K. Liao, J.A. Denburg, Antineuronal antibodies in neuropsychiatric systemic lupus erythematosus, Arthritis Rheum. 28 (1985) 789–795.

370. E. Kinnunen, P. Järvinen, L. Ketonen, R. Sepponen, Co-twin control study on cerebral manifestations of systemic lupus erythematosus, Acta Neurol. Scand. 88 (1993) 422–426.

375. R. Omdal, K. Brokstad, K. Waterloo, et al., Neuropsychiatric disturbances in SLE are associated with antibodies against NMDA receptors, Eur. J. Neurol. 12 (2005) 392–398.

412. S. Lacks, P. White, Morbidity associated with childhood systemic lupus erythematosus, J. Rheumatol. 17 (1990) 941–945.

417. J. Sharma, Z. Lasic, A. Bornstein, et al., Libman-Sacks endocarditis as the first manifestation of systemic lupus erythematosus in an adolescent, with a review of the literature, Cardiol. Young 23 (2013) 1–6.

431. T. Mochizuki, S. Aotsuka, T. Satoh, Clinical and laboratory features of lupus patients with complicating pulmonary disease, Respir. Med. 93 (1999) 95–101.

442. S. Kumar, S.M. Benseler, M. Kirby-Allen, E.D. Silverman, B-cell depletion for autoimmune thrombocytopenia and autoimmune hemolytic anemia in pediatric systemic lupus erythematosus, Pediatrics 123 (2009) e159–e163.

463. J.M. Von Feldt, L.V. Scalzi, A.J. Cucchiara, et al., Homocysteine levels and disease duration independently correlate with coronary artery calcification in patients with systemic lupus erythematosus, Arthritis Rheum. 54 (2006) 2220–2227.

480. M. Rygg, A. Pistorio, A. Ravelli, et al., A longitudinal PRINTO study on growth and puberty in juvenile systemic lupus erythematosus, Ann. Rheum. Dis. 71 (2012) 511–517.

481. A. Au, J. O'Day, Review of severe vaso-occlusive retinopathy in systemic lupus erythematosus and the antiphospholipid syndrome: associations, visual outcomes, complications and treatment, Clin. Experiment. Ophthalmol. 32 (2004) 87–100.

482. R.W. Read, L.P. Chong, N.A. Rao, Occlusive retinal vasculitis associated with systemic lupus erythematosus, Arch. Ophthalmol. 118 (2000) 588–589.

489. P.R. Fortin, M. Abrahamowicz, C. Neville, et al., Impact of disease activity and cumulative damage on the health of lupus patients, Lupus 7 (1998) 101–107.

524. M.K. Lim, C.K. Lee, Y.S. Ju, et al., Serum ferritin as a serologic marker of activity in systemic lupus erythematosus, Rheumatol. Int. 20 (2001) 89–93.

527. S. Vilaiyuk, N. Sirachainan, S. Wanitkun, et al., Recurrent macrophage activation syndrome as the primary manifestation in systemic lupus erythematosus and the benefit of serial ferritin measurements: a case-based review, Clin. Rheumatol. 32 (2013) 899–904.

531. L.M. Campos, M.H. Kiss, M.A. Scheinberg, et al., Antinucleosome antibodies in patients with juvenile systemic lupus erythematosus, Lupus 15 (2006) 496–500.

532. A. Matrat, C. Veysseyre-Balter, P. Trolliet, et al., Simultaneous detection of anti-C1q and anti-double stranded DNA autoantibodies in lupus nephritis: predictive value for renal flares, Lupus 20 (2011) 28–34.

533. L. Watson, M.W. Beresford, Urine biomarkers in juvenile-onset SLE nephritis, Pediatr. Nephrol. 28 (2013) 363–374.

548. P. Rahman, M.B. Urowitz, D.D. Gladman, et al., Contribution of traditional risk factors to coronary artery disease in patients with systemic lupus erythematosus, J. Rheumatol. 26 (1999) 2363–2368.

595. T.J. Lehman, C. Singh, A. Ramanathan, et al., Prolonged improvement of childhood onset systemic lupus erythematosus following systematic administration of rituximab and cyclophosphamide, Pediatr Rheumatol Online J. 12 (2014) 3.

The entire reference list is available online at www.expertconsult .com.

Antiphospholipid Syndrome

Tadej Avčin, Kathleen M. O'Neil

The antiphospholipid syndrome (APS) is an autoimmune multisystem disease characterized by thromboembolic events, pregnancy morbidity, hematological, dermatological, neurological, and other manifestations in the presence of elevated titers of antiphospholipid antibodies (aPLs). APS may occur as an isolated clinical entity (primary APS) or in association with other diseases, mainly systemic lupus erythematosus (SLE). It occasionally occurs with other autoimmune conditions, infections, and malignancies.

DEFINITION AND CLASSIFICATION

Preliminary classification criteria for APS were developed by consensus in 1998.[1] It was proposed that the term *APS* should designate patients who suffered from vascular thrombosis or recurrent fetal losses associated with the presence of aPLs, namely the lupus anticoagulant (LA) or the anticardiolipin antibodies (aCLs) of immunoglobulin G (IgG) and/or IgM isotype in medium or high titers detected on two or more occasions at least 6 weeks apart.[1] The classification criteria for *definite APS* were revised in 2006 and include the presence of antibodies against β_2 glycoprotein I (anti-β_2GPIs) of IgG and/or IgM isotype as part of the updated laboratory criteria and require aPLs to be positive on more than one occasion at least 12 weeks apart[2] (Table 24-1). The revised 2006 criteria were evaluated only in studies in adult populations and require further validation; however, it is generally assumed that they limit the risk of misclassification of patients with transient aPLs and provide a more selective and risk-stratified framework for evaluating patients with persistently positive aPLs.[3-5]

APS in children has been largely reported in patients with vascular thromboses and less frequently in association with isolated neurological or hematological manifestations.[6-8] Pregnancy morbidity, which represents one of the two clinical criteria for definite APS in adults, is not applicable to the pediatric population, and it is possible that current consensus criteria may fail to recognize a subgroup of pediatric patients who do not have vascular thrombosis but demonstrate typical nonthrombotic clinical features and fulfill the laboratory criteria for APS.[9] A classification of *probable APS* has been given to patients with aPLs who have clinical features associated with APS that do not meet the APS criteria, such as heart valve disease, livedo reticularis, thrombocytopenia, nephropathy, and neurological manifestations.[2]

The term *seronegative APS* was proposed for patients with clinical manifestations highly suggestive of APS, but with persistently negative results in the commonly used assays to detect aCLs, anti-β_2GPIs, and LA.[10,11] Some of these patients may have so-called noncriteria aPLs including antibodies to phosphatidylethanolamine, phospholipid-binding plasma proteins (prothrombin, protein C, protein S, annexin V, and domains of β_2GPI), phospholipid–protein complexes (vimentin/cardiolipin complex), and anionic phospholipids other than cardiolipin (phosphatidylserine, phosphatidylinositol, and phosphatidic acid). The clinical relevance of noncriteria aPLs is still controversial; however, it is possible that some of the new aPL assays will be added as a laboratory diagnostic marker in future revisions of classification criteria for APS.[10-12]

Catastrophic antiphospholipid syndrome (CAPS) is another subset of APS that is characterized by acute microvascular occlusive disease with subsequent multiorgan failure and a high mortality rate. Preliminary classification criteria for CAPS were established in 2002[13] (Table 24-2). This syndrome is defined as clinical involvement of at least three organ systems and/or tissues over a very short period of time (less than a week) with histopathological evidence of small-vessel occlusion and laboratory confirmation of the presence of aPLs.[13,14] Diagnostic algorithms for CAPS were updated in 2010 to emphasize possible overlap with other thrombotic microangiopathies.[15]

EPIDEMIOLOGY

APS is considered to be the most common acquired prothrombotic state of autoimmune etiology, with an estimated incidence around 5 per 100,000 persons per year and the prevalence of 40 to 50 cases per 100,000 persons.[16-19] The cumulative retrospective analysis indicates that approximately one third of patients with aPLs have a history of thrombosis.[18,20,21]

There are no reliable data on the incidence or prevalence of APS in the pediatric population because there are no validated criteria, and the diagnosis rests on the application of adult guidelines and clinical judgment. In a large cohort study of 1000 consecutive patients with APS from 13 European countries, 85% of patients were diagnosed between ages 15 and 50 years. Those with disease onset before 15 years of age accounted for 2.8% of patients with APS.[22] Although the incidence of thrombosis in children is significantly lower than in adults, the proportion of thrombosis that is attributable to aPLs in children appears to be higher than in the adult population, which has other common prothrombotic risk factors such as atherosclerosis, cigarette smoking, hypertension, and use of oral contraceptives.[23] The prevalence of aPLs in unselected children with thrombosis was reported between 12% and 25%.[24,25] Meta-analysis of 16 observational studies investigating the association of aPLs and first onset of thromboembolism in children showed persistent aPL positivity in 1% to 22% of arterial and 2% to 12% of venous thrombotic events.[26]

The demographic characteristics of 121 pediatric patients with aPL-related thrombosis, included in an international registry of APS, revealed a mean age at disease onset of 10.7 years (range, 1.0 to 17.9 years).[27] There was a moderate female predominance in pediatric APS studies with a female-to-male ratio ranging from 1.2:1 to 3:1,[27-29] whereas in adult APS studies the female-to-male ratio is over 5:1.[22,30,31]

TABLE 24-1 Revised Classification Criteria for Antiphospholipid Syndrome[2]

Clinical criteria	1. Vascular thrombosis One or more clinical episodes of arterial, venous, or small-vessel thrombosis, in any tissue or organ. Thrombosis must be confirmed by objective validated criteria (i.e., unequivocal findings of appropriate imaging studies or histopathology). For histopathological confirmation, thrombosis should be present without significant evidence of inflammation in the vessel wall. 2. Pregnancy morbidity (a) One or more unexplained deaths of a morphologically normal fetus at or beyond the 10th week of gestation, with normal fetal morphology documented by ultrasound or by direct examination of the fetus. (b) One or more premature births of a morphologically normal neonate before the 34th week of gestation because of (i) eclampsia or severe preeclampsia defined according to standard definitions, or (ii) recognized features of placental insufficiency (c) Three or more unexplained consecutive spontaneous abortions before the 10th week of gestation, with maternal anatomic or hormonal abnormalities, and paternal and maternal chromosomal causes excluded.
Laboratory criteria	1. Lupus anticoagulant (LA) present in plasma, on two or more occasions at least 12 weeks apart, detected according to the guidelines of the International Society on Thrombosis and Hemostasis. 2. Anticardiolipin antibody of IgG and/or IgM isotype in serum or plasma, present in medium or high titer (i.e., >40 GPL or MPL, or greater than the 99th percentile), on two or more occasions, at least 12 weeks apart, measured by a standardized ELISA. 3. Anti-β_2 glycoprotein-I antibody of IgG and/or IgM isotype in serum or plasma (in titer greater than the 99th percentile), present on two or more occasions, at least 12 weeks apart, measured by a standardized ELISA.

Note: APS is present if at least one of the clinical criteria and one of the laboratory criteria are met.

TABLE 24-2 Preliminary Criteria for the Classification of Catastrophic Antiphospholipid Syndrome

1. Evidence of involvement of three or more organs, systems, and/or tissues
2. Development of manifestations simultaneously or in less than a week
3. Confirmation by histopathology of small-vessel occlusion in at least one organ or tissue
4. Laboratory confirmation of the presence of antiphospholipid antibodies

Definite Catastrophic APS
- All four criteria

Probable Catastrophic APS
- All four criteria, except for only two organs, systems. and/or tissues involvement
- All four criteria, except for the absence of laboratory confirmation at least 6 weeks apart due to the early death of a patient never tested for aPL before the CAPS
- Points 1, 2, and 4
- Points 1, 3, and 4, and the development of a third event in more than a week but less than a month, despite anticoagulation

Modified from R.A. Asherson, R. Cervera, P.G. de Groot, et al., Catastrophic antiphospholipid syndrome: international consensus statement on classification criteria and treatment guidelines, Lupus 12 (2003) 530–534.

have primary APS and later during follow-up develop overt SLE.[27,28,32] During the 6.1-year mean follow-up period, 21% of children who were initially diagnosed with primary APS progressed to have either clear-cut SLE or lupuslike disease.[27] Comparisons between pediatric patients with primary APS and those with APS associated with underlying autoimmune disease suggest that children with primary APS are significantly younger and have a higher frequency of arterial thrombotic events, especially cerebrovascular ischemic events. In contrast, children with APS associated with underlying autoimmune disease have a higher frequency of venous thrombotic events associated with hematological and skin manifestations.[27]

Autoimmune Diseases

From the pediatric APS registry data, it is estimated that 50% to 60% of all APS cases in pediatric populations are associated with underlying autoimmune disease.[27,29] There are only limited data addressing how autoimmune disease can modify the clinical expression of APS, and sometimes the clinical distinction between primary APS and APS associated with autoimmune disease can be difficult to make. This is especially true in SLE, which has many overlapping features with APS, including thrombocytopenia, hemolytic anemia, seizures, and proteinuria.[33]

SLE and lupuslike disease account for the majority (80% to 90%) of pediatric APS cases associated with underlying autoimmune disease.[27,29] SLE is the autoimmune disease in which aPLs can be found most often, with the reported aPL frequencies ranging from 19% to 87% for aCL, 27% to 48% for anti-β_2GPI, and 10% to 62% for LA, respectively.[34-50] A meta-analysis of the published studies that investigated the prevalence and clinical significance of aPLs in childhood-onset SLE showed a global prevalence of 44% for aCLs, 40% for anti-β_2GPIs, and 22% for LA.[51]

Patients with juvenile idiopathic arthritis (JIA) very rarely develop aPL-related thrombotic events in spite of the high percentage of positive aPLs.[52,53] Anticardiolipin antibodies were reported in 7% to 53%

This difference may reflect, in part, a sampling bias, because the adult APS studies included patients with thrombosis as well as women with pregnancy morbidity. Very little is known about the geographic and racial distribution of pediatric APS.

Primary Antiphospholipid Syndrome

Primary isolated APS without other underlying disease accounts for 40% to 50% of pediatric patients with APS.[27,29] This percentage may be somewhat overestimated because a number of children initially of JIA patients, but anti-β₂GPIs and LA, felt to be more specific for thrombosis risk than aCL, were detected in less than 5% of patients.[38,42,43,54-57] The aPL profile observed in JIA appears to have limited pathogenic potential and may explain the low incidence of thromboembolism in this disease.[43,57]

Isolated cases of APS were reported in a variety of other pediatric autoimmune diseases including Henoch–Schönlein purpura,[58,59] Behçet disease,[60] polyarteritis nodosa,[61] immune thrombocytopenic purpura,[29,62] hemolytic uremic syndrome,[63,64] and rheumatic fever.[65] The risk of aPL-associated thrombotic events seems to be particularly high in systemic vasculitides, which are generally regarded as hypercoagulable disorders. Patients with immune thrombocytopenic purpura associated with aPLs are at risk for developing both bleeding and thrombotic complications.[66-68]

Infections

Many viral and bacterial infections in childhood can induce *de novo* production of aPL in previously negative patients.[69-73] Infection-induced aPLs tend to be transient, present in low titer, and are generally not associated with clinical manifestations of APS.[72-74] The majority of postinfectious aPLs differ immunochemically from those seen in patients with autoimmune diseases and do not require the presence of cofactor plasma proteins such as β₂GPI for binding.[75-77] Because common viral and bacterial infections occur so frequently in children, a high percentage of incidental aPL positivity might be expected in a pediatric population.[78] The association between infections and aPLs is supported also by some indirect evidence, such as seasonal distribution of aPLs.[79]

The distinction between nonpathogenic "postinfectious aPLs" and thrombogenic "autoimmune aPLs" is not absolute, and it was demonstrated that several infections may induce production of heterogeneous aPLs, including pathogenic antibodies against β₂GPI and prothrombin, resembling those found in autoimmune diseases.[73,74,77,80,81] Preceding or concomitant infections were found in approximately 10% of children with primary APS or APS associated with autoimmune disease[27] and as high as 60% in children with CAPS.[82] Pediatric APS was most frequently reported in association with varicella-zoster virus,[83-85] parvovirus B19,[86] human immunodeficiency virus (HIV),[87] streptococcal and staphylococcal infections, Gram-negative bacteria,[88] and *Mycoplasma pneumonia*.[89-92] The main causes for infectious induction of APS could be molecular mimicry between infectious agents and β₂GPI in certain predisposed subjects or unmasking of cryptic antigenic determinants of naturally occurring anti-β₂GPIs.[77,93]

Malignancies

There have been isolated case reports of the association of aPLs with thrombotic events in children with various malignancies, including solid tumors and lymphoproliferative and hematological malignancies.[94-96] Malignancy is an important risk factor for the development of childhood thrombosis and the presence of aPLs may enhance the thrombophilic state of patients with neoplasms.[95,97] However, aPLs were found as one of the acquired prothrombotic risk factors in less than 3% of thrombotic children with malignancy.[95] Published data suggest that APS associated with malignancies accounts for less than 1% of all children with APS.[27] It appears that aPL-related thrombotic events associated with malignancies are more common in elderly patients, particularly in association with solid tumors.[96-98]

Healthy Children

Low levels of aPLs can be found in up to 25% of apparently healthy children, which is higher than the rate seen in the normal adult population.[78,99-102] Such naturally occurring aPLs are usually transient, present in low titer, and could be the result of previous infections or vaccinations.[69-71,103,104] In apparently healthy children, the estimated frequency of aCLs ranges from 3% to 28%, and of anti-β₂GPIs from 3% to 7%.[78,102] LA has also been described in apparently healthy children, usually as an incidental finding of prolonged activated partial thromboplastin time (aPTT) in preoperative coagulation screening.[99,100] The risk of future thrombosis is exceedingly low in otherwise healthy children who were incidentally found to have positive aPLs.[99]

Increasing evidence suggests that alternative responses of the developing immune system to nutritional antigens can result in production of specific nonpathogenic anti-β₂GPIs during childhood.[78,105,106] It was shown that dietary bovine β₂GPI from milk or meat products may act as an oral immunization agent and induce transitory production of IgG anti-β₂GPIs in up to 55% of healthy infants whose intestinal mucosa is more permeable to large molecules than that of adolescents and healthy adults.[105,106] During the prospective follow-up of infants born to mothers with APS or aPL-positive autoimmune disease, it was observed that aCL titers in the newborns' sera progressively decrease; at 6 and 12 months of age, all infants were negative for aCLs.[106,107] In contrast, anti-β₂GPIs were found at 12 months of age in up to 64% of infants born to aPL-positive mothers and in 33% of infants born to mothers with aPL-negative autoimmune disease, further implying postnatal *de novo* synthesis of anti-β₂GPIs in infants.[106] Current evidence suggests that postnatally produced anti-β₂GPIs found in infants have low thrombosis risk, display unusual epitope specificity directed against domain V of β₂GPI, and are clearly different from pathogenic anti-β₂GPIs found in patients with APS, which preferentially target domain I.[105,108] For clinical practice it seems prudent to consider the detection of aCLs, but not anti-β₂GPIs, to evaluate the disappearance of transplacentally acquired maternal aPLs.

ETIOLOGY AND PATHOGENESIS

Although aPLs are found in healthy children, it is clear these antibodies can be associated with thrombosis (see the section "Clinical Manifestations"); pregnancy morbidity; hematological, skin and neurological conditions; and they can produce signs and symptoms of microangiopathy. Production of aPLs appears to be triggered by infections of all sorts, and in some instances, it can be familial or hereditary.[109] The presence of any one of several prothrombotic risk factors, including underlying autoimmune disease such as childhood-onset SLE, dramatically increases the risk of thromboembolic disease when the child has aPL. This "two hit-theory" implies that although aPL may inhibit repair of endothelial and platelet surface defects, thereby promoting thrombosis, a perturbation of these membranes is in some way required as well. Animal models have contributed significantly to our understanding of the pathogenesis of APS in humans, as discussed in the sections that follow. Still, it is difficult to ascertain which autoantibodies and in what setting aPLs will cause thromboembolic disease in an individual child.

Pathophysiology

aPLs cause disease through a variety of effects on endothelial cells, platelets, monocytes, and neutrophils. These antibodies promote complement activation, inhibit physiological anticoagulants such as activated protein C, antithrombin, and the annexin A5 anticoagulant shield, and can impair fibrinolysis. Furthermore, aPLs increase the procoagulant function of cells such as platelets, endothelial cells, and leukocytes.[110] Recent evidence implicates oxidative stress, including decreases in paraoxonase activity[111]; effects on endothelial nitric oxide synthase[111]; increased lipid peroxidation in plasma[112]; and direct antibody-mediated cross-linking and activation of apolipoprotein E receptor 2 in the pathogenesis of thrombosis as well.[112]

As recently reviewed,[23] aPLs have broad-ranging biological effects that not only perturb the interaction between cells and the plasma that bathes them, but also disrupt the orderly function of biological membranes. There is increasing evidence that aPLs promote atherosclerosis,[113] cardiac valve disease,[114] and directly contribute to trophoblast[115,116] and neuronal dysfunction.[117-120]

Characteristics of aPLs That Influence Pathogenicity

In humans, thrombotic disease related to aPLs is more likely to occur in individuals with abnormal functional assays such as LA, or prolonged phospholipid-dependent clotting assays; very high titers of aPLs confer higher risk of thrombotic disease than do lower antibody titers.[121] IgG and IgM antibodies are generally associated with hypercoagulable complications.[122] However, IgA antibodies to cardiolipin can be found as the only isotype of aPLs in Afro-Caribbean adults with thrombophilia.[122] Furthermore, sera from patients with IgA aCLs can produce thrombosis in mice.[123] IgA aCL in adults with SLE or other related autoimmune diseases is associated with thrombocytopenia.[124] Likewise, in a large multiethnic cohort, IgA anti-β_2GPI, even as the only detectible aPL, was associated with at least one APS-related clinical syndrome in the majority of patients.[125]

Antibodies to specific membrane phospholipids such as phosphatidylcholine, phosphatidylethanolamine, and phosphatidylserine are less reliable indicators of risk of thrombotic disease than protein or protein-phospholipid–directed antibodies. A study of 230 adults with SLE examined six tests for aPLs, including LAs, aCLs, anti-β_2GPIs, solid-phase antiprothrombin, antiphosphatidylethanolamine and antiphosphatidylserine/prothrombin (aPS/PT) (23 possible combinations of test results).[126] Antibodies to domain I of β_2GPI are more closely associated with thrombosis and with abnormalities of functional coagulation tests in children.[127,128] The combination of abnormal results for LA in combination with both the anti-β_2GPI and aPS/PT antibody ("triple positive") was most closely associated with APS (odds ratio [OR] 23.2) than any combination of two positive tests (OR 3.1-7.3). In children as in adults, aPLs that are persistent for at least 12 weeks are more likely to be associated with thrombosis than transient autoantibodies, hence the international consensus definition requiring detection at least 12 weeks apart.[2,23]

Most authors recommend screening with functional tests such as the lupus-sensitive aPTT or dilute Russell viper venom test (dRVVT), then performing a mixing test to ensure that the prolonged clotting test is not due to deficiency of one or more clotting factor, and then confirming with a different phospholipid-dependent assay (kaolin clotting time, hexagonal phospholipid clotting test, etc.). To better assess the risk for thrombosis or obstetric risk in aPL-positive patients and those with a variety of autoimmune diseases, a score was developed by Otomo et al. that utilizes the combined strength of several assays to predict risk.[129] Pathogenic autoantibodies to annexin A2,[130] galectins,[131] and a variety other antigens have been described in association with APS in adults; their diagnostic and prognostic utility has yet to be confirmed, especially in children.

Platelet Effects

Anti-β_2GPI binds to the platelet von Willebrand factor (vWF) receptor, glycoprotein Ib alpha, and the apolipoprotein E receptor 2 (ApoE2R), promoting platelet adherence to endothelium.[132] In vivo platelet activation in patients with APS has been demonstrated by the finding of high levels of urinary thromboxane metabolites; in vitro aPLs induce release of thromboxane from platelets.[133] aPL-induced platelet aggregation in vitro requires partial preactivation of the platelets with thrombin, collagen, or ADP; aPL then completes that activation via p38 mitogen-activated protein (MAP)-kinase phosphorylation, leading to release of thromboxane and activation of phospholipase A2.[134] For anti-β_2GPI to induce this effect, expression of the platelet ApoE2R and the platelet glycoprotein Ib alpha subunit is required. Anti-β_2GPI from sera of APS patients augments the expression of platelet P-selectin in response to thrombin receptor-activating peptide 6, and antibody derived from patients during the catastrophic phase of APS shows greater enhancement than that from quiescent stage donors.[135] The same study showed APS subjects have higher plasma soluble P-selectin, CD40 ligand, monocyte chemoattractant protein 1, and soluble vascular cell adhesion molecule 1. In addition, platelet factor 4, released by activated platelets, promotes dimerization of β_2GPI on the platelet surface.[136] The interaction of aPLs with platelets is illustrated in simplified format in Fig. 24-1. These platelet-activating effects of aPLs are blocked in vitro with hydroxychloroquine,[137] suggesting an important mechanism for the effect of this drug in APS. The hydroxychloroquine effect can be seen in images of artificial membrane bilayers treated with β_2GPI and then with monoclonal anti-β_2GPI. This disrupts the membrane, making globular outcroppings that are dissipated following the addition of hydroxychloroquine[138] (Fig. 24-2).

Endothelial Cells in Antiphospholipid Syndrome

ALPs increase the adhesiveness of endothelial cells to leukocytes and platelets by increasing expression of intracellular adhesion molecule (ICAM)-1, vascular adhesion molecule (VCAM)-1, and E-selectin.[139] Mice genetically deficient in these adhesion molecules have impaired aPL-induced thrombus formation, thereby confirming the importance of this effect in the pathology of APS. Endothelial cells treated with aPLs increase production of interleukin (IL)-6 and reactive oxygen species, promoting an endothelial inflammatory phenotype.[140] Tissue factor, an important initiator of coagulation via the extrinsic pathway, is highly expressed by endothelium of vessels from patients with APS.[141] Anti-β_2GPIs activate p38-MAP kinase on endothelium as well as platelets, increasing expression of tissue factor by endothelium exposed to aPLs. This tissue factor overexpression contributes to the prothrombotic effects of aPLs. Activation of nuclear factor (NF)-κB is an essential step in the endothelial effects of aPLs, and MG132, an inhibitor of NF-κB, blocks the tissue factor upregulation induced by aPLs.[142] Pretreatment with fluvastatin blocks the aPL endothelial cell effects on tissue factor and adhesion molecule expression.[143] β_2GPI blocks vWF-dependent platelet aggregation, and aPLs interfere with this inhibition of platelet aggregation.[144] Plasma concentrations of von Willebrand protein are high in patients with primary APS,[145] further promoting platelet aggregation and the prothrombotic effects of aPLs. IgG from subjects with APS can also stimulate endothelial release of microparticles, which themselves can promote thrombosis.[146]

β_2GPI–aPL complexes bind tightly to endothelial cells, and that binding is mediated by annexin A2.[147,148] Antibodies to annexin A2 produce the same activation of endothelial cells as do anti-β_2GPIs, with the same kinetics. This effect is only present with cross-linking antibodies and not present with F(ab') monomers, suggesting that perturbation of annexin A2 in the membrane mediates the anti-β_2GPI–induced endothelial activation through effects on annexin A2.[149] β_2GPI promotes the activation of plasminogen by tissue plasminogen activator; this suggests that β_2GPI may be an endogenous regulator of fibrinolysis.[150] Consequently, impairment of β_2GPI-augmented fibrinolysis by anti-β_2GPI may contribute to thrombosis in patients with APS.

aPLs activate endothelial cells via the Toll-like receptor 4 (TLR4),[151] activating the adapter protein MyD88 and downstream effects; TLR4 knockout mice are resistant to aPL-induced thrombosis. In mouse fibroblasts a similar role for TLR2 has been demonstrated.[152] This

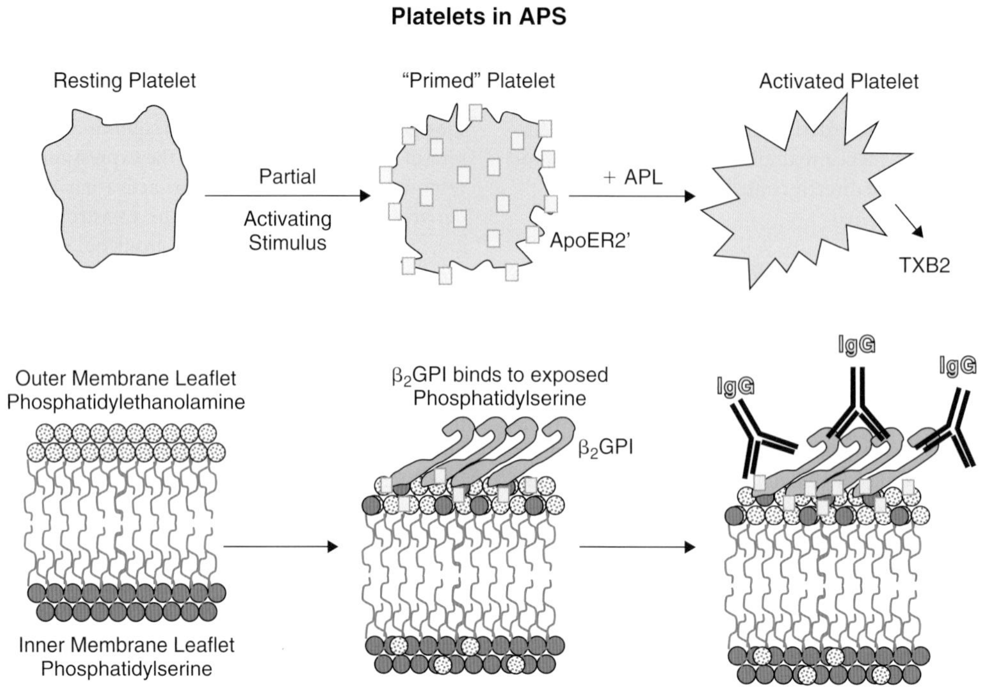

Platelets in APS

FIGURE 24-1 Effects of antiphospholipid antibodies on platelets. Top images: Following a partial activating stimulus such as LPS or cytokine exposure, platelets increase expression of the apolipoprotein E2 receptor (ApoE2R) (yellow squares), and bind β_2GPIs and aPLs, leading to platelet aggregation and release of thromboxane B2. The bottom images show fine detail at the level of the platelet membrane. In the resting state, the neutral phospholipid, phosphatidylethanolamine, is maintained in the extracellular leaflet, and the negatively charged phosphatidylserine (PS) is on the intracellular membrane leaflet. With preactivation, this is perturbed, and PS is expressed on the platelet surface, exposing sites that can bind β_2GPI. This now produces binding sites for aPLs, and total activation of the platelet.

involvement of the innate immune system may be a critical link in comprehending the pathogenesis of this complex disease. The interaction of aPLs with endothelial cells is illustrated in Fig. 24-3.

Leukocyte Activation by Antiphospholipid Antibodies

aPLs affect monocytes in ways similar to how they affect platelets. They upregulate tissue factor expression and adhesion molecule expression, the production of IL-1, IL-6 and IL-8 via phosphorylation of p38 MAPK, and the activation of NF-κB and MEK/ERK kinases.[153] Recently, involvement of both NF-κB and c-Jun/activator protein 1 (AP1) pathways were demonstrated in this effect.[154] Monocyte effects of aPLs are likely important in preactivating endothelial cells to a prothrombotic phenotype. Neutrophils are required for fetal loss related to aPLs, as neutrophil depletion in mice prevents the intrauterine growth retardation and fetal demise related to passive aPL antibody administration. Neutrophil accumulation in decidual tissues is mediated by complement activation products, particularly C5a.[155] Tissue factor expression on neutrophils is increased by aPLs, and blockade of tissue factor by monoclonal antibody treatment prevents fetal injury.[156]

The Effect of aPLs on Placental Trophoblasts

In addition to promoting inflammation and coagulation at the level of endothelial cells and leukocytes within vessels, there is mounting evidence that aPLs have direct toxic effects on the functions of a variety of other cells. Most prominent among these are the effects on placental trophoblasts. This has best been demonstrated in a murine model of APS, where serum IgG antibody and monoclonal human aPL can induce fetal loss in pregnant mice.[157] In particular, aPL can bind

directly to the trophoblast in the developing embryo. Following binding, these antibodies inhibit the normal invasion of the trophoblast into the decidual tissues, which results in defective placentation.[158] Trophoblast production of chorionic gonadotropin and placental lactogen is impaired following aPL treatment.[158] Because trophoblasts express anionic phospholipids on the surfaces during differentiation, they bind β_2GPI in vivo, making them a target for aPLs.[159] Matrix metalloproteinases, required for placental invasion, are underexpressed in APS, and heparin increases trophoblast invasiveness by increasing matrix metalloproteinases expression.[160]

Complement Activation in the APS

Antigen–antibody complexes made of aPLs and the membrane phospholipids to which they are directed, like most immune complexes, can activate complement via the classical pathway. Complement activation generates a variety of biologically active cleavage fragments that have serine protease activity, anaphylatoxic effects, and promote neutrophil adhesion to activated endothelium and influx into tissues. In an animal model of aPL-induced fetal loss, complement activation appears to be necessary for fetal demise and resorption,[155,161,162] and aPL-induced thrombus formation.[161] This complement effect makes intuitive sense, as both complement and the thrombosis systems are cascades of interacting serine proteases. Serine protease inhibitors (serpins), several of which are common to both pathways, regulate both coagulation and thrombosis. Studies utilizing intravital microscopy following immunological "priming" with lipopolysaccharide then intraarterial injection of aPLs in rats demonstrated complement activation in the aPL-treated thrombotic vessels. In contrast, thrombus

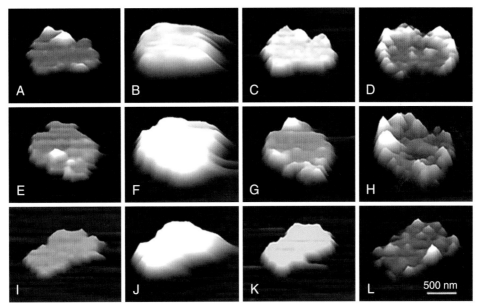

FIGURE 24-2 Atomic force microscopy height images (three-dimensional view with 50-degree pitch) showing the effect of hydroxychloroquine (HCQ) on three separate aPL mAb/β$_2$GPI complexes. Panels **A, E, I:** Addition of β$_2$GPI to buffer covering phospholipid bilayers resulted in the formation of distinct structures raised above the bilayers. Panels **B, F, J:** Subsequent addition of aPL mAb to the phospholipid-bound β$_2$GPI shown in panels **A, E,** and **I** resulted in large aggregates of increased height (indicated by white color) composed of aPL mAb/β$_2$GPI complexes over the lipid bilayers. Panels **C, G, K:** At 12 min after the addition of HCQ to the supernatant fluid covering the bilayer, the immune complexes, shown in panels **B, F,** and **J** were significantly eroded. Panels **D, H, L:** The immune complexes, shown in panels **B, F,** and **J** showed further disintegration 30 min after the addition of HCQ. The color shades represent height variations in the images, with the darker colors (rust) indicating lower heights and the lighter colors (white), the higher profiles. (From D.J. Taatjes, A.S. Quinn, J.H. Rand, B.P. Jena. Atomic force microscopy: High resolution dynamic imaging of cellular and molecular structure in health and disease, J. Cell. Physiol. 228 (2013) 1949–1955.)

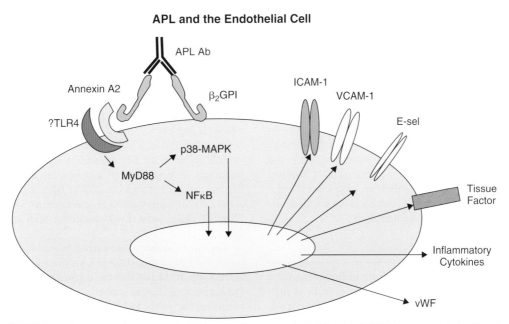

FIGURE 24-3 Effects of antiphospholipid antibodies on endothelial cells. β$_2$GPI binds to endothelial cell membranes via annexin A2, which does not contain a transmembrane domain. aPLs bind to the β$_2$GPI, and through a signaling pathway involving MyD88, p38-MAPK, and NF-κB activation (presumably mediated by TLR4), the endothelial cell becomes activated, increasing expression of the adhesion molecules ICAM-1, VCAM-1, E-selectin (E-sel), and the coagulation protein tissue factor. In addition, inflammatory cytokines and the von Willebrand factor (vWF, the factor VIII–associated antigen) are produced for local activity at the cell surface and are exported into the plasma.

TABLE 24-3   **Mechanisms of Action of Antiphospholipid Antibodies**

Platelet Activation
- Aggregation
- Thromboxane release

Monocyte Activation
- Inflammatory cytokine production
- Increased monocyte tissue factor expression

Endothelial Activation
- Tissue factor expression and secretion
- Increased vWF expression
- Expression of adhesion molecules

Impaired Function of Activated Protein C
Decreased Binding of C4 to C4BP
- Increased C4BP binding of protein S

Promote Clot Formation
Impair Thrombolysis

vWF, von Willebrand factor.

did not form as efficiently in complement-deficient C6-/- animals. In addition, an anti-C5 antibody that blocks C5 activation, C5a release, and C5b-9 assembly also had diminished thrombus formation.[163] Thus complement plays a crucial role in promoting the placental inflammation that leads to fetal demise in APS, and in promoting thrombus formation.

aPLs can have antifibrinolytic effects and have been shown to inhibit the activities of thrombin, activated protein C, plasminogen, and plasmin.[150] Anti-β_2GPIs inhibit the anticoagulant activity of activated protein C.[164] Some APS patients have demonstrable antibody to protein S and/or protein C. There is *in vivo* evidence that this inhibition of thrombolysis contributes to the pathogenicity of aPL.[165,166] In fact, measuring inhibition of activated protein C activity may be more sensitive for pathogenic aPL than currently employed assays.[167]

In summary (see Table 24-3), aPLs have a variety of procoagulant effects, including the activation of platelets to aggregate and release thromboxane, activation of monocytes (inflammatory cytokine production and increased tissue factor expression), and activation of endothelium (increased tissue factor expression and secretion, increased vWF, and expression of adhesion molecules). They also impede downregulation of thrombosis via impairment of activated protein C. Furthermore, through aPL actions on complement, endothelium and neutrophils are activated to promote tissue accumulation of neutrophils, thus promoting local inflammation.

GENETIC BACKGROUND

That APS may be familial in a minority of patients has been recognized for decades.[168-170] The findings of a high incidence of aCLs in first-degree relatives of people with APS or with SLE suggest that the capacity to develop antibodies to charged phospholipids, at the least, may be influenced by genetics, probably with important environmental influences. Allelic variations in β_2GPI protein associated with APS have been identified.[171] Inheritance in familial APS may be autosomal recessive, or dominant/codominant.[169]

In interpreting the studies of familial APS, it is important to remember several factors: although primary and secondary APS share a number of features, it is not clear that their genetic basis is similar. Reports of aPL rates in pediatric family members of patients with APS must be interpreted in light an evidence of higher antibody positivity rates in healthy children than in adults.

There are several reports of an association with aPLs and familial Sneddon syndrome, a syndrome of livedo reticularis with hypertension and cerebrovascular disease, which is inherited as an autosomal-dominant trait.[172,173] The role of aPLs in this disease is as yet uncertain.

Most reports of familial APS are anecdotal and do not provide information on the genetic transmission of the disease. The number of reports and small series published provide evidence that familial occurrence and possibly genetic influence are important, at least in a subset of human APS. Other issues that cloud reports of familial APS are variations in whether, and how completely, patients were evaluated for other prothrombotic traits such as inherited heterozygous deficiency of protein C or protein S, or resistance to activated protein C from such genetic disorders as factor V Leiden and methylenetetrahydrofolate reductase (MTHFR) deficiencies. Any of these defects can coexist with aPLs and increase the likelihood of thrombosis in the presence of aPLs. The number of patients reported with aPLs who have genetic defects predisposing to pathological thrombosis raises the possibility that disordered coagulation itself might indeed predispose to the formation of aPLs. This question has not been directly addressed.

It is not known how often APS is familial. Estimates based on family history usually do not include complete laboratory evaluation of family members for APS, or for concomitant thrombophilia disorders. Consequently, such studies likely overestimate the rate of "affected" relatives. Prospective studies of families utilizing current definitions of APS and standardized testing technology are not yet available.

Genetic Studies

A variety of human leukocyte antigen (HLA)-DR and HLA-DQ antigens have been associated with aPLs and both primary and secondary APS (summarized in eTable 24-4). Many of these associations lose significance when corrected for the number of variables tested, however.[174] These studies are generally small series, and most do not include appropriate ethnic controls. Arnett and colleagues studied major histocompatibility complex (MHC) genotypes in 20 patients with LAs, of whom 8 had primary APS and 12 had other rheumatic diseases (7 with significant thrombotic complications).[175] The strongest association with LAs was seen for DQB1*0301 (DQw7), and all who were negative for this allele had DQB1*0302 (DQw8). These two antigens share an identical 7-amino acid sequence in the third hypervariable region of the DQ molecule, suggesting this epitope might be important in mediating an immune response to phospholipid.[175] Recently, a large genotype analysis of HLA associations with vascular disease and aPL positivity in Swedish patients with SLE showed DRB 1*04/*13 alleles were closely associated with aPLs and thrombotic disease.[176]

The large number of associations reported between various measures of aPLs and related thrombotic disease and alleles in the human MHC support the fact that these genes may play a significant role in facilitating formation of antibody to phospholipid antigens, but other factors are likely to be important in producing familial APS. As of now, single gene associations with APS are not confirmed and remain an area of investigation.

CLINICAL MANIFESTATIONS

Children with aPLs may present with any combination of vascular occlusive events or with a variety of nonthrombotic clinical manifestations. Most of the clinical features that occur in adults with aPLs have also been described in children. However, the clinical expression of aPLs in children is modified by several characteristics such as the immaturity of the immune and other organ systems, the absence of common prothrombotic risk factors often present in adults, the lack of pregnancy morbidity, and the presence of routine immunizations and frequent exposure to common viral and bacterial infections.[6-8] Data from large registries of pediatric patients with APS have provided information on the spectrum of thrombotic and nonthrombotic clinical manifestations.[27,29] At the time of the initial thrombotic event in children with definite APS, the estimated frequencies of associated nonthrombotic manifestations were 38% to 53% for hematological manifestations, 6% to 18% for dermatological manifestations, and 16% to 22% for nonthrombotic neurological manifestations.[27,29]

A high percentage of children with persistent aPLs apparently do not present with overt thrombotic events. Studies in children with aPLs demonstrated that thromboses occurred only in 16% to 36% of patients,[21,177] whereas the nonthrombotic aPL-related clinical manifestations alone were observed in more than 40% of patients.[177]

Thrombosis

The classical clinical picture of APS in pediatric populations is characterized by venous, arterial, or small-vessel thrombosis. Vascular occlusion in APS may involve arteries and veins at any level of the vascular tree and in all organ systems, giving rise to a wide variety of clinical presentations (summarized in Table 24-5).[8,27] Meta-analyses investigating the association of aPLs and thromboembolism in children revealed that the presence of persistent aPLs shows a significant association with a first thrombotic event during childhood with an overall summary OR of 5.9.[26] The association of aPLs appears slightly stronger for arterial thrombosis (OR 6.6) than for venous thrombosis

(OR 4.9).[26] Thrombosis is more likely to occur with the existence of additional hereditary and acquired prothrombotic risk factors.[178,179] It is now well established that APS may develop as an initial manifestation of childhood-onset SLE, and all children presenting with aPL-related thrombosis require thorough assessment for evidence of underlying systemic disease.[27,45,180-182]

Venous thrombosis is the most common vascular occlusive event seen, occurring in up to 60% of pediatric APS patients.[27-29] The most frequently reported site of venous thrombotic events is deep vein thrombosis in the lower extremities, followed by cerebral sinus vein thrombosis, portal vein thrombosis, deep vein thrombosis in the upper extremities, and superficial vein thrombosis.[27-29] Venous thrombotic events are particularly common in APS associated with childhood-onset SLE. In a Canadian retrospective cohort study in childhood-onset SLE, 13 of the 149 patients (9%) had one or more thromboembolic events, and all 13 patients with thromboembolic events were LA positive.[45] In total, venous thrombosis occurred in 76% of episodes (cerebral venous thrombosis in nine, deep vein thrombosis in four, pulmonary embolism in two, and retinal vein occlusion in one) and arterial thrombosis in 24% (arterial stroke in three, retinal artery occlusion in one, and splenic infarct in one). The overall incidence of thromboembolic events in childhood-onset SLE patients with positive LAs was 54% (13 of 24 patients) and with positive aCLs, 22% (12 of 54 patients).[45] LAs were found to be the strongest predictor of thrombosis risk in another study in 58 children with SLE, and positivity for multiple aPL subtypes indicates stronger associations with thromboembolic events than for individual aCL, anti-β_2GPI, or antiprothrombin antibodies.[47] Overall, it has been estimated that childhood-onset SLE patients with persistent LA positivity have a twenty-eight-fold increased risk of thrombotic events compared with patients who are negative for LA.[41]

Arterial thrombosis occurs in approximately 30% of pediatric APS patients. The most frequently reported site of arterial thrombotic event is ischemic stroke, followed by peripheral arterial thrombosis.[27-29] Arterial thrombotic events are significantly more common in primary APS patients than in APS associated with underlying autoimmune disease.[27] Several studies have demonstrated that the prevalence of aPL-related cerebral ischemia is particularly high in pediatric and young adult patients, ranging from 15% to 75%.[183-190] In an Israeli study evaluating the importance of various thrombophilia markers in 58 pediatric patients with stroke, positive aPLs were found in 15% of patients, and only factor V Leiden and aPLs were found to be significant risk factors for ischemic stroke in children.[187] aPLs are also an independent risk factor for recurrent ischemic stroke in children, but this effect has not been confirmed for IgG aCLs.[191] Sneddon syndrome is associated with aPLs in approximately 50% of all patients.[192-195]

Small-vessel thrombosis occurs in less than 10% of pediatric APS patients and may present as an aggressive microvascular occlusive disease (CAPS) or localized small-vessel thrombosis.[27] Localized small-vessel thrombosis has been described primarily in children with isolated thrombosis of digital vessels or renal thrombotic microangiopathy. Peripheral vascular disease leading to digital gangrene is a well-recognized complication of APS, particularly in patients with SLE, and it may be difficult to distinguish this from vasculitis, cryoglobulinemia, or disseminated intravascular coagulation.[196,197] In a group of 32 Mexican children with APS, digital ischemia was reported as the most frequent thrombotic event present in 44% of patients at the onset of APS.[29]

Hematological Manifestations

The most common hematological manifestations associated with APS in children are thrombocytopenia, autoimmune hemolytic anemia,

TABLE 24-5 Venous and Arterial Thrombosis Manifestations of Pediatric Antiphospholipid Syndrome

VESSEL INVOLVED	CLINICAL MANIFESTATIONS
Venous Sites	
Limbs	Deep vein thrombosis
Skin	Livedo reticularis, chronic leg ulcers, superficial thrombophlebitis
Large veins	Superior or inferior vena cava thrombosis
Lungs	Pulmonary thromboembolism, pulmonary hypertension
Brain	Cerebral venous sinus thrombosis
Eyes	Retinal vein thrombosis
Liver	Budd–Chiari syndrome, enzyme elevations
Adrenal glands	Hypoadrenalism, Addison disease
Arterial Sites	
Limbs	Ischemia, gangrene
Brain	Stroke, transient ischemic attack, acute ischemic encephalopathy
Eyes	Retinal artery thrombosis
Kidney	Renal artery thrombosis, renal thrombotic microangiopathy
Heart	Myocardial infarction
Liver	Hepatic infarction
Gut	Mesenteric artery thrombosis
Bone	Infarction

and leucopenia. Thrombocytopenia was observed in 20% to 25% of children with APS, often in association with Coombs-positive hemolytic anemia (Evans syndrome).[27,29] Thrombocytopenia associated with APS is usually mild or moderate, with platelet counts greater than 50 × 10⁹/L. Treatment is usually not required except in cases with a platelet count less than 30 × 10⁹/L and symptomatic with bleeding. The pathogenesis of aPL-related thrombocytopenia is probably heterogeneous, including direct binding of aPL to platelet phospholipids, immune-mediated and platelet activation.[198] Occasionally, thrombocytopenia may be severe, causing major bleeding.[199] Thrombotic events are unusual with severe thrombocytopenia but may occur if the platelet counts increase during the disease course. Leucopenia or lymphopenia were reported in 8% of children with APS.[27]

A high percentage (greater than 25%) of patients with isolated immune thrombocytopenic purpura also have aPLs, particularly in the pediatric population.[200,201] In a case control study of 42 children with immune thrombocytopenic purpura, IgG aCLs were found in 78%, and anti-β_2GPIs were found in all chronic cases, whereas patients with acute immune thrombocytopenic purpura demonstrated IgG aCLs in just 27% and anti-β_2GPIs in 13%, respectively.[201] During a 4-year follow-up period, 17% of children who were initially diagnosed with immune thrombocytopenic purpura developed overt SLE, and closer follow-up has been suggested for these children.[201] Several studies have reported an increased risk of thrombosis in aPL-positive patients who present with isolated hematological manifestations.[32,62,66,202-205] Some patients with aPL-related hematological manifestations, however, continue to have thrombocytopenia or hemolytic anemia as isolated clinical manifestations and do not develop thrombosis or SLE during follow up.[204]

The acquired LA-hypoprothrombinemia syndrome is a rare complication consisting of a severe bleeding diathesis associated with the presence of LA. It has been described in both primary APS and APS associated with SLE, and is often preceded by a viral infection.[206-211] This complication has been attributed to the presence of antiprothrombin antibodies that cause rapid depletion of plasma prothrombin and consequent hemorrhagic diathesis.

Dermatological Manifestations

A wide variety of dermatological manifestations have been reported in patients with APS, ranging from minor signs to life-threatening conditions such as widespread cutaneous necrosis.[22,212-215] The most common dermatological manifestations present in children included in the pediatric APS registry were livedo reticularis (6%), Raynaud phenomenon (6%), and skin ulcers (3%)[27] (Fig. 24-4).

In a single-center series of 200 consecutive pediatric and adult patients with APS, skin manifestations were observed in 49% of the patients and were the presenting symptom in 30%.[216] The most frequent manifestation was livedo reticularis (25%), followed by digital necrosis (7%), subungual splinter hemorrhages (5%), superficial venous thrombosis (5%), postphlebitic skin ulcers (4%), circumscribed cutaneous necrosis (3%), thrombocytopenic purpura (3%), and other changes (7%). Livedo reticularis, and especially the coarser livedo racemosa variant, is considered a major clinical feature of APS, strongly associated with arterial and microangiopathic subtypes of APS[215-217] (Fig. 24-5). The mechanism of livedo reticularis is not well understood and may include both patchy thrombosis and/or the interaction of aPLs with endothelium and induction of vasoconstriction.[215] The association of aPLs with Raynaud phenomenon was noted also in a retrospective study of 123 children, in which at least one aPL subtype was positive in up to 36% of patients with primary and 30% of patients with secondary Raynaud phenomenon.[218]

Neurological Manifestations

Typical neurological manifestations of APS are ischemic stroke and cerebral sinus vein thrombosis, both caused by thrombotic occlusion of cerebral vessels.[27,187,219-221] Several other neurological manifestations have been associated with the presence of aPLs, including various movement disorders, epilepsy, migraine, cognitive defects, psychiatric diseases, transverse myelitis, multiple sclerosis–like disorders, sensorineural hearing loss, and Guillain–Barré syndrome.[221-225] These manifestations are not fully explained by the thrombogenic effects of aPLs and may result from both thrombotic and nonthrombotic immune-mediated mechanisms such as direct interaction between aPLs and neuronal tissue or immune complex deposition in the cerebral blood vessels wall.[226-229]

The most common nonstroke neurological manifestations observed in children with APS were migraine headache (7%), chorea (4%), and seizures (3%).[27] Chorea has been strongly linked to the presence of aPLs as an isolated clinical finding or in children with SLE.[222,230-236] A large retrospective cohort study of 137 children with SLE demonstrated an association between LA and chorea over the disease course, but not between aPLs and other neuropsychiatric manifestations.[48] A significant association was found between aPLs and childhood seizure disorder in two prospective studies,[237,238] but not all studies have found such a link.[239] The association between

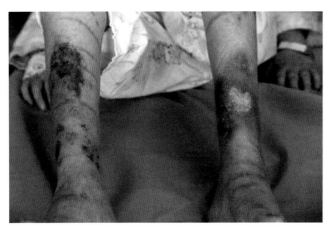

FIGURE 24-4 Chronic leg ulcers in a patient with childhood-onset systemic lupus erythematosus and antiphospholipid antibodies.

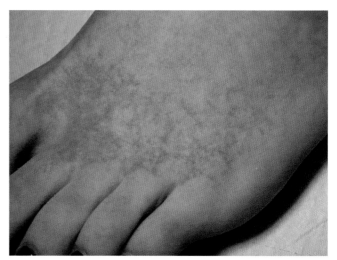

FIGURE 24-5 Livedo reticularis in a patient with childhood-onset systemic lupus erythematosus and antiphospholipid antibodies.

epilepsy and aPLs is clouded also by the role of anticonvulsant drugs that could trigger autoantibody production.[240] There has been controversy concerning a possible association of aPLs and migraines, which has not been confirmed in a prospective study in an unselected group of children with migraines.[241] Prospective studies of adult patients with SLE demonstrated an association between persistent aPLs and cognitive impairments, especially in areas of attention, psychomotor speed, and executive functioning.[242,243] Neurocognitive defects were frequently observed also in childhood-onset SLE patients, but there is no clear evidence suggesting association with aPLs.[49,244-247] In general, APS may constitute a potentially treatable cause of a variety of neurological diseases, and it is recommended to routinely measure aPLs in children with otherwise unexplained neurological disorders.

Other Manifestations

Cardiac manifestations are frequent in adult patients with APS but have not been extensively investigated in childhood. The most prominent cardiac manifestations include valvular disease, occlusive coronary artery disease, cardiomyopathy, and intracardiac thrombosis.[22,248] Nonbacterial (Libman–Sacks) vegetations were disclosed by echocardiographic studies in 11% of adult patients with APS,[22] but were only rarely observed in patients with pediatric APS.[29,249] Several cases of pediatric patients with aPL-related myocardial infarction have been reported, often in association with underlying SLE or congenital heart disease.[32,250-253] Multiple small vascular occlusions are responsible for APS cardiomyopathy, especially in CAPS, in which it is one of the most common causes of death.[254,255]

Pulmonary embolism and infarction constitute the most frequent pulmonary manifestation of APS.[45,182,256-258] aPLs were reported in 30% to 40% of children with pulmonary embolism who were referred for hematology evaluation.[256,258] Rarely, recurrent pulmonary embolism may lead to pulmonary hypertension.[196,259,260]

The kidney is a major target organ of pediatric APS with manifestations that include renal vascular occlusion, thrombotic glomerular microangiopathy, and hypertension.[46,261-265] The term *antiphospholipid syndrome-associated nephropathy* (APSN) was proposed to describe thrombotic microangiopathy involving both arterioles and glomerular capillaries that cause hypertension, acute renal failure, proteinuria, and poor renal function with a tendency to develop end-stage renal disease.[2,266-268] This entity was reported in 16% of Thai patients with childhood-onset SLE who underwent renal biopsy and was significantly more frequent in adult SLE patients (41%).[268] aPLs are also associated with hepatic, digestive, and adrenal manifestations resulting from occlusive vascular disease of intraabdominal vessels.[269-272]

Osteoarticular manifestations such as avascular necrosis of bone, nontraumatic fractures, and bone marrow necrosis are rarely seen in APS patients.[273,274] Adult patients with primary APS and no prior glucocorticoid treatment appear to have an increased risk of avascular necrosis.[275] aPLs were reported as one of the most common prothrombotic alterations in patients with multifocal osteonecrosis, which is present in 20% of cases.[276] Perthes disease has been linked with aPLs in two pediatric studies,[274,277] but the association does not appear to be strong.

Catastrophic Antiphospholipid Syndrome

CAPS is a rare, potentially life-threatening variant of APS, characterized by multiple small-vessel occlusions that can lead to multiorgan failure.[15] Large-vessel occlusions may also occur in CAPS, but they do not dominate the clinical picture. The most commonly affected organ systems include the kidney, lung, central nervous system (CNS), heart, and skin.[278]

In a large cohort of 446 cases collected in the CAPS international registry, 45 patients (10%) developed catastrophic events before 18 years of age, and 87% of pediatric patients had CAPS as initial presentation without any previous history of thrombosis.[82] Primary APS occurred in 69% of pediatric cases with CAPS, and 31% of patients suffered from underlying childhood-onset SLE or lupuslike disease. The most frequently affected organs in pediatric patients with CAPS were kidneys and lung (both 63%), followed by heart (57%), peripheral vessel thrombosis (52%), brain (48%), liver (40%), skin (37%), and gastrointestinal tract (17%). Thrombocytopenia was observed in more than 70% of patients and was one of the hallmarks of pediatric CAPS. Precipitating factors were identified in more than 75% of cases, most frequently infections (61%), malignancy (17%), surgery (6%) and SLE flares (4%).[82]

CAPS has been described also in several pediatric case reports, but overall this aggressive disease represents less than 5% of pediatric APS patients.[27,86,94,279-286] It is not known why this disorder behaves in such an aggressive fashion in some patients. Frequently, patients with CAPS have other non-aPL risk factors that contribute to the acute microvascular thrombosis such as infection with or without sepsis; disseminated, intravascular coagulation; surgery; and underlying autoimmune or malignant disease. The reported mortality rate in pediatric patients with CAPS is significantly higher than in classic APS and ranges between 26% and 33%.[27,82]

Microangiopathic Antiphospholipid-Associated Syndrome

aPLs have also been associated with a variety of microangiopathic syndromes that cannot be attributed simply to the microvascular thrombotic process. The term *microangiopathic antiphospholipid-associated syndrome* was introduced to refer to patients with aPLs and clinical features of thrombotic microangiopathy with hemolytic anemia, severe thrombocytopenia, and the presence of schistocytes.[287,288] The clinical presentations of 46 adult patients with thrombotic microangiopathic hemolytic anemia associated with aPLs included hemolytic uremic syndrome (HUS) (25%), CAPS (23%), acute renal failure (15%), malignant hypertension (13%), thrombotic thrombocytopenic purpura (TTP) (13%), and other clinical presentations (11%).[289]

Two pediatric series reported a high frequency of aCLs in children with diarrhea-associated HUS, but without a clear role in the pathogenesis of microangiopathy.[290,291] Microangiopathic antiphospholipid-associated syndrome was reported in a 4-year-old child who presented with atypical HUS and later developed rapidly progressive thrombotic microangiopathy associated with the transient presence of aPLs, decreased serum factor H, and positive anti–ADAMTS13 antibodies (Fig. 24-6).[63] A study of eight children initially diagnosed with acquired TTP and reduced ADAMTS13 activity showed that SLE was concurrently or subsequently diagnosed in seven of eight patients during 42 months follow-up; all six patients tested for aPLs eventually developed positive aPLs, suggesting a potential association.[292]

In general, published data demonstrate that clinical conditions with thrombotic microangiopathic hemolytic anemia are characterized by major endothelial dysfunction; the pathogenic role of aPLs remains controversial. It is assumed that the majority of these conditions do not form part of APS (with the exception of CAPS), but aPLs can be produced as an immune response to the exposure of phospholipids that occur with endothelial injury. Apparently aPLs represent only one of the pathogenic factors in these conditions, and various infectious causes, inherited defects in complement genes (e.g., complement factors H, I, B, and membrane cofactor protein), acquired autoantibodies against complement regulatory proteins, deficiency of vWF-cleaving protease (ADAMTS13), and inherited prothrombotic disorders must be taken into consideration, particularly in the pediatric population.[287,293,294]

Perinatal Complications Associated with aPLs

The presence of maternal aPLs during pregnancy is associated with a number of serious obstetric and fetal complications, including preeclampsia, uteroplacental insufficiency, intrauterine growth restriction, fetal distress, premature birth, and fetal loss.[295-297] With recent therapeutic approaches including low-dose aspirin alone or together with either unfractionated heparin or low molecular weight heparin (LMWH) throughout pregnancy, the percentage of pregnancies in women with aPLs that end in live births ranges from 75% to 80%.[297-301] The prematurity rate in babies born to mothers with APS

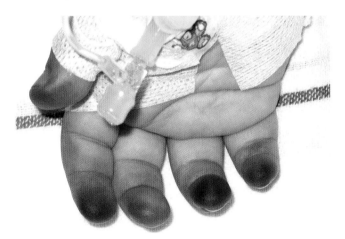

FIGURE 24-6 Necrotic changes on the fingertips in a child with microangiopathic antiphospholipid-associated syndrome. (From A. Meglič, S. Grosek, M. Benedik-Dolnicar, et al. Atypical haemolytic uremic syndrome complicated by microangiopathic antiphospholipid-associated syndrome, Lupus 17 (2008) 842–845.)

is 10% to 15%, and the incidence of growth restriction is 15% to 20%.[297,302-306]

Perinatal thrombosis and other aPL-related clinical manifestations are rare complications of transplacental passage of aPLs in neonates.[306] It is well established that maternal aCLs and anti-β_2GPIs can cross the placenta and be detected in cord blood.[106,107,307,308] The estimated rate of transplacental passage of maternal aPLs is 30% to 50%, significantly lower than that observed for antinuclear antibodies (approximately 80%).[106,306,309] Several cohort studies examining the outcome of infants born to mothers with APS have consistently shown that, except for prematurity and its potential associated complications, these neonates rarely had other clinical manifestations.[302-304,306] A recent report from the European multicenter registry of 134 children born to mothers with APS showed that only 2 neonates (1%) developed thrombocytopenia, but there were no cases of neonatal thrombosis.[306]

In contrast to the encouraging results from the cohort studies, there are a growing number of isolated case reports of perinatal thrombotic events associated with transplacentally transferred aPLs. Analysis of 16 infants with thrombosis born to mothers with aPLs revealed arterial thrombotic events in 80%, and ischemic stroke occurred in approximately half of the cases[310-316] (Fig. 24-7). Moreover, in an Israeli study of 47 infants with perinatal arterial ischemic stroke, aPLs were detected in more than 20% of patients and were identified as a potential risk factor for stroke, together with factor V Leiden.[317] Thromboses in neonatal APS were also reported in other vessels, including the aorta, peripheral arteries, mesenteric arteries, cerebral sinus veins, renal veins, and subclavian veins.[318-330] More than 60% of infants with aPL-related thrombosis had at least one additional thrombophilic risk factor identified, most commonly arterial or venous catheters, sepsis, asphyxia, and/or congenital thrombophilia.[310] In general, transplacentally transferred aPLs alone seem to be insufficient for induction of fetal or neonatal thrombosis, and other inherited and acquired thrombophilic risk factors should be systematically evaluated in case of perinatal thrombotic event in a child born to mother with aPLs.[317,331]

Evidence of neurodevelopmental abnormalities has been described in the prospective long-term studies of children born to mothers with

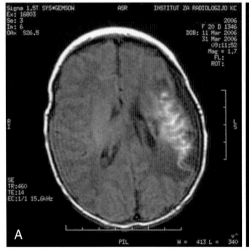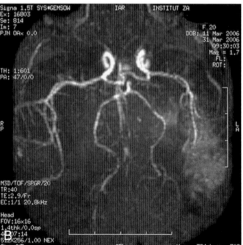

FIGURE 24-7 Magnetic resonance imaging of the head showing ischemic changes in the left hemisphere **(A)** and magnetic resonance angiography showing occlusion of the left middle cerebral artery **(B)** in a neonate with IgG anticardiolipin antibodies and heterozygous methylenetetrahydrofolate reductase C677T and prothrombin G20210A gene mutations. (From D. Paro-Panjan, L, Kitanovski, T. Avčin. Neonatal antiphospholipid syndrome associated with heterozygous methylentetrahydrofolate reductase C677T and prothrombin G20210A gene mutations, Rheumatology 46 (2007) 720–721.)

APS. An Italian study systematically evaluated neuropsychological development in 17 children born to mothers with APS and reported normal cognitive capacity, but with presence of learning difficulties such as dyslexia and dyscalculia in 4 children (24%) upon beginning school.[332] In a recent French study, autism spectrum disorders were observed in 3 of 36 children(8%) born to mothers with primary APS, but in no child born to a mother with SLE.[333] Among the group of 134 children included in the European registry of children born to mothers with APS, 4 children (3%) displayed behavioral abnormalities between 3 months and 3 years of age including autism, hyperactivity disorder, language delay, and learning disabilities.[306] The mechanism of neurodevelopmental abnormalities in children born to mothers with APS is not clear and could be related to prematurity or *in utero* exposure to aPLs, just as prolonged exposure to aPLs induced behavioral and cognitive deficits in an experimental mice model.[226,334,335] Regular psychomotor and cognitive assessments are recommended for long-term follow-up of these high-risk children.

PATHOLOGY

Histopathological changes in APS may be grouped under several categories, including thrombotic, microangiopathic, ischemic, or coincidental with underlying disease–related pathology.[336,337]

Classic vasoocclusive lesions in APS are thrombotic, recent, or organized, and can either be systemic or involve single organs.[336] Thrombotic lesions are characterized by predominant noninflammatory occlusive or mural thrombosis and its consequences. Acute thrombotic lesions may be seen as occlusive thrombi with or without features of thrombolysis and limited reactive changes. Microvascular thrombi can undergo rapid dissolution and disappear. Otherwise, thrombus organization starts early by proliferation of neighboring endothelial cells and is later dominated by intraluminal proliferation of myofibroblasts and recanalization. Occlusive vascular thrombosis causes secondary acute and chronic ischemic changes. True vasculitis may occur as a coincidental finding that is causally not related to APS but to the coexisting underlying disease, most commonly SLE.[336,338]

Microangiopathic lesions are characterized predominantly by endothelial cell injury–subendothelial plasma insudation often associated with thrombotic necrotizing lesions and its chronic consequences. Endothelial cells of the small blood vessels that are activated and injured by aPLs play a major role in the initiation and development of acute microangiopathic lesions. The acute phase is characterized by endothelial cell swelling, detachment, and necrosis, as well as prominent insudation into the subendothelium of blood constituents through a leaky endothelium, which may be seen by immunofluorescence microscopy as intensely positive staining for IgM with a lumpy pattern along the small-vessel walls. Chronic microangiopathic glomerular lesions are characterized by a double-contoured basement membrane in the thickened glomerular capillary walls without thrombosis and no association with inflammatory cell proliferation and exudation. In addition, chronic microangiopathic vascular lesions with obliterating fibrous intimal hyperplasia of arterioles and interlobular arteries may become evident.[268,337,339,340]

DIAGNOSIS AND DIFFERENTIAL DIAGNOSIS

Children with APS will be treated by a wide range of clinical specialists, including pediatric rheumatologists, hematologists, neurologists, and others. A multidisciplinary approach to investigation and management is often appropriate. Testing for aPLs is usually not a first-line investigation and should be limited to those children with an indication as listed in Table 24-6.[8,51,121,341]

TABLE 24-6 Indications for Testing for Antiphospholipid Antibodies
1. Every child presenting with thrombosis
• Venous, arterial, or small vessel
2. Children with clinical features associated with aPLs
• Hematological: unexplained thrombocytopenia, hemolytic anemia
• Dermatological: livedo reticularis, Raynaud phenomenon, digital necrosis, skin ulcers
• Neurological: chorea, refractory epilepsy, migraine, transverse myelitis, psychosis
• Cardiac: Libman–Sacks endocarditis
• Renal: hematuria and hypertension due to thrombotic microangiopathy
3. Children with severe acquired bleeding diathesis, particularly in a child with previous infection, to exclude LA-hypoprothrombinemia syndrome
4. Every child with childhood-onset SLE at the time of diagnosis, and then at least once yearly
5. Children with unexplained prolonged activated partial thromboplastin time (aPTT) in the course of routine laboratory testing (e.g., preoperative coagulation screening)

Given the spectrum of clinical manifestations, the differential diagnosis of APS is very broad and depends on target organ involvement. Characteristically, pathological thrombosis in children requires the presence of multiple risk factors to produce abnormal clotting[342-344]; therefore, clinical assessment of all children who have an aPL-related thrombotic event should include a search for additional congenital and acquired prothrombotic risk factors, and a thorough evaluation for evidence of underlying SLE or other systemic disease.

The main congenital prothrombotic states to be considered include factor V Leiden, prothrombin G20210A mutation, and deficiencies of antithrombin, protein C, and protein S.[342,344] Factor V Leiden is the most common hereditary risk factor for venous thrombosis, and up to 5% of the Caucasian population carry this polymorphism.[345] The G20210A mutation of the prothrombin gene is a common polymorphism associated with venous thrombosis, and its prevalence in Caucasians is 2% to 4%.[178,346] Congenital deficiencies of antithrombin, protein C, and protein S are very uncommon, but acquired deficiency of protein S has been reported in children with APS, particularly in association with varicella infection.[347-349] The evaluation for congenital prothrombotic disorders in children should also include testing of total cholesterol, triglycerides, lipoprotein(a), coagulation factor VIII, and fasting homocysteine concentration.[342,344,350] It is noteworthy that the levels of antithrombin, protein C, and protein S may be transiently decreased because of consumption in the setting of acute thrombosis, whereas factor VIII and lipoprotein(a) can be elevated in inflammatory conditions. The most common acquired factors that may contribute to the risk of thrombosis are infection, malignancy, congenital heart disease, nephrotic syndrome, systemic vasculitis, central venous lines, surgery, and immobilization.

The differential diagnosis of nonthrombotic aPL-related clinical manifestations encompasses a variety of hematological, dermatological, neurological, and other diseases. The differentiation of isolated aPL-related thrombocytopenia from classic idiopathic thrombocytopenic purpura is important and indicates the need for closer follow-up regarding the increased risk of future thrombosis or progression to SLE.[32,201] Neurological manifestations of aPLs should be distinguished from idiopathic neurological conditions, neuropsychiatric involvement in systemic autoimmune diseases, Sydenham chorea, multiple sclerosis, infections, intoxications, and other causes.[351,352]

CAPS should be distinguished from severe SLE vasculitis, sepsis, HUS, TTP, heparin-induced thrombocytopenia, macrophage activation syndrome, and disseminated intravascular coagulation.[8,15,353]

LABORATORY EXAMINATION

Antiphospholipid antibodies is an umbrella term used to describe a heterogeneous group of autoantibodies directed against negatively charged phospholipids or plasma phospholipid-binding proteins. In clinical practice, the most relevant aPLs for identifying patients at risk for immune-mediated thrombosis are aCLs, anti-β_2GPIs, and LA. In a cohort of 121 children included in the pediatric APS registry, the presence of aCL was detected in 81% of cases, anti-β_2GPI in 67%, and LA in 72%.[27]

Persistent positivity of aPLs is of major importance for diagnosing APS, and all abnormal aPL values should be verified on at least two occasions at least 12 weeks apart, preferably at a time when the child has not had a recent infection.[2]

aPLs can be detected by a variety of laboratory tests. The most sensitive test for aPLs is the aCL test, which uses enzyme-linked immunosorbent assay to determine antibody binding to solid plates coated either with cardiolipin or other phospholipids. The specificity of aCLs for APS increases with titer and is higher for the IgG isotype than for the IgM isotype. There have been numerous efforts to standardize the aCL test, but precise reproducible measurement of aCL levels is difficult; for clinical practice the use of semiquantitative measurements (low, medium, and high) is recommended.[354,355] Anticardiolipin antibodies must be persistently present in medium or high titer to meet the definition of APS. The observation that many aCLs are directed at an epitope on β_2GPI led to the development of anti-β_2GPI immunoassays, which have improved specificities over the aCL test. Anti-β_2GPIs have been reported to be associated primarily with thrombosis in patients with APS, particularly in patients with underlying SLE.[77,356] The issue of the standardization of the anti-β_2GPI immunoassay has also been the subject of considerable debate; however, despite these efforts, a considerable degree of interlaboratory variation has been reported.[357,358] Furthermore, recent evidence suggests that IgG antibodies directed against domain I of β_2GPI are more strongly associated with thrombosis than those detected using the standard anti-β_2GPI assay.[77,359] Inadequate data exist as to the clinical utility of other aPL assays for antibodies to prothrombin, phosphatidylethanolamine, anionic phospholipids other than cardiolipin (phosphatidylserine, phosphatidylinositol, and phosphatidic acid), IgA isotype of aCL and anti-β_2GPI, and the annexin A5 resistance test.[2,125]

The LA test is a functional assay measuring the ability of patient plasma containing aPLs to prolong *in vitro* phospholipid-dependent clotting reactions such as the aPTT and the RVVT. *In vivo*, however, the presence of LA is paradoxically associated with thrombotic events rather than with bleeding. LA are a mixture of different antibodies with various target antigens and also include aCL and anti-β_2GPI, among others. According to the updated guidelines of the Scientific Standardization Committee of the International Society of Thrombosis and Haemostasis, the presence of LA should be confirmed with mixing tests with normal plasma and demonstration of the phospholipid-dependent nature of the inhibitor.[360] LA is less frequently positive in APS and is thus regarded as a less sensitive but more specific test for detection of aPLs. The LA assay has been shown to correlate much better with the occurrence of thromboembolic events than the aCL or the anti-β_2GPI assay and is considered to be the most important acquired risk factor for thrombosis.[47,121,361]

Several assays may be required to confirm aPLs in some patients because they may be negative according to one test but positive according to another. Reliance on just one type of assay may lead to false negative aPL assessments. In general, only one third of pediatric APS patients are concurrently positive for three aPL subtypes (aCL, anti-β_2GPI, and LA), whereas other patients are negative for at least one of the aPL subtypes.[27] A full panel of current aPL tests, including aCL, anti-β_2GPI, and LA, should be performed, and if possible, newer assays such as antiprothrombin, anti-β_2GPI domain I, and annexin A5 resistance should be tested.[355] Determination of complete aPL profile is also important for stratification of thrombosis risk and identification of high-risk patients with multiple (particularly triple) aPL positivity.[362]

Measurement of the activation products of coagulation and fibrinolysis, such as D-dimer, prothrombin fragment 1 and 2, soluble fibrin, and thrombin-antithrombin complexes provides additional information on the hypercoagulability state in patients with inherited and acquired prothrombotic disorders such as APS.[363] D-dimer was most extensively studied, and there is substantial evidence that it is a sensitive but nonspecific indicator of deep-vein thrombosis. Because of its high negative predictive value, it is particularly useful for the exclusion of deep-vein thrombosis and pulmonary embolism.[364,365] Persistently elevated concentrations of D-dimer above 500 ng/mL and of coagulation factor VIII above 150 IU are associated with an increased risk of recurrent thromboembolism in children and adults.[366,367]

RADIOLOGICAL EXAMINATION

Thrombosis in patients with APS must be confirmed by objective validated criteria. The ability to detect thrombosis in target organs in infants and children was markedly improved by the development of noninvasive imaging techniques using color-flow and pulsed Doppler ultrasound, echocardiography, computed tomography plus angiography (CT/CTA), and magnetic resonance imaging with or without angiography (MRI/MRA). The diagnosis of deep-vein thrombosis in the lower or upper extremity is usually established by compression and Doppler ultrasound, which can be easily performed in children (Fig. 24-8). Echocardiography, CTA, or MRA can be used for thrombus imaging in the superior vena cava and proximal subclavian veins. MRA, CT pulmonary angiogram, or ventilation-perfusion scans are recommended for diagnosing suspected pulmonary embolism in children.[368] Except during interventional procedures, venography and angiography are rarely used in children because of technical difficulties

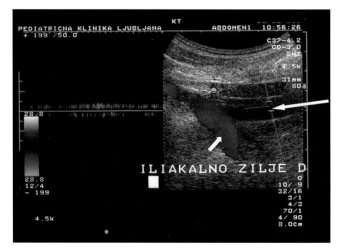

FIGURE 24-8 Color flow Doppler image showing occlusive thrombus in the right external iliac vein (*long arrow*) and normal blood flow in the internal iliac vein (*short arrow*).

(peripheral venous access or arterial catheterization), the requirement for iodinated contrast, and the possibility of extending thrombus.

Brain MRI and positron emission tomography are utilized to assess structural brain lesions such as ischemic infarcts or hemorrhage but are poorly correlated with diffuse or global neurological dysfunction. Cerebral ischemia in APS most often affects the territory of the middle cerebral artery. Cortical MRI findings of middle cerebral artery occlusion are similar to those in large-vessel strokes that result from other etiologies. Diagnosis of cerebral sinus vein thrombosis is confirmed by MRI with venographic sequencing. Neuroimaging findings are often subtle or unremarkable in patients with small-vessel involvement. Newer neuroimaging modalities that assess microstructural white matter damage (i.e., diffusion-weighted imaging and diffusion tensor imaging) along with quantitative perfusion imaging may allow for identification of early CNS damage in APS patients.[221,369,370] Magnetization transfer imaging (MTI) is a quantitative MRI technique that is sensitive to macroscopic as well as microscopic brain tissue changes. In SLE patients with neuropsychiatric manifestations and positive aCL, MTI demonstrated brain damage in the absence of abnormalities on conventional MRI, suggesting that MTI may prove useful in detecting widespread microscopic damage associated with aPLs.[229,371]

TREATMENT

The main goal of therapy in patients with aPLs is prevention of thrombosis in aPL carriers without previous thrombosis (primary thromboprophylaxis), and patients with APS who have already had a thrombotic event (secondary thromboprophylaxis). The treatment of pediatric patients with APS is particularly challenging because of the clinical complexity of the syndrome, different pathogenic potential of aPL subtypes, and a lack of randomized controlled trials in children.[8,51,372-374] Management strategies for children with APS are based on a few pediatric observational cohort studies[27,28,32,45,82] and modified recommendations for adult patients with APS.[375-379] Several differences specific to children must be considered when using the adult recommendations: in particular, the different concentrations of plasma procoagulant and anticoagulant proteins, difficulty of maintaining the appropriate international normalization ratio (INR) levels in infants and children on warfarin anticoagulants, drug side effects in growing children, variable metabolism of oral anticoagulants during infections, a higher risk of hemorrhage during play and sports activities, inconsistent dietary habits, and poor compliance, especially in teenagers.[368,373,374] The optimal management of children with aPLs, whether or not they have had a previous thrombosis, should include the avoidance of additional risk factors for thrombosis such as smoking, hypertension, obesity, and hyperlipidemia. Moreover, the use of oral contraceptives that contain estrogen is contraindicated in adolescent girls with aPLs.

Primary Thromboprophylaxis

Given the severity of thrombotic complications associated with aPLs, the ideal therapeutic approach would be to avoid progression from asymptomatic aPL carrier to patient with definite APS. Primary thromboprophylaxis concerns asymptomatic children—in whom aPLs were incidentally found during laboratory testing performed for other reasons (e.g., LA discovered during routine preoperative coagulation screening)—and children with SLE found to have aPLs in routine serological screening.

The annual thrombosis risk in asymptomatic adult carriers of aPL is estimated to be between 0% and 5%, and is higher in patients with the presence of LA, particularly if combined with aCLs and anti-β_2GPIs (triple positivity).[362,380-382] A randomized controlled trial showed no benefit of low-dose aspirin (81 mg/day) for primary thrombosis

prophylaxis in asymptomatic aPL-positive adults, but the study had important limitations, including the small sample size and the short follow-up period.[383] In contrast, retrospective observational studies suggest a protective effect of low-dose aspirin in asymptomatic aPL carriers.[384,385] A Italian collaborative study evaluated the efficacy of prophylactic treatments including low-dose aspirin, long-term warfarin, or low-dose aspirin/heparin given during high-risk periods (pregnancy/puerperium, immobilization, and surgery) in order to prevent a first thrombotic event in aPL carriers.[386] This study showed that long-term prophylaxis with aspirin does not have a protective role when considered alone; however, in combined long-term and high-risk periods, prophylaxis was found to be an independent, protective factor against thrombosis.[386]

Future thrombotic events are very rare, if not exceptional, in apparently healthy children who were incidentally found to be positive for aPLs,[99] and there is considerable controversy as to whether prophylactic treatment is indicated in this group of children. Because of the increased risk of bleeding during play and sports, which might outweigh the possible but unproven benefit of low-dose aspirin, it is generally recommended that asymptomatic children with aPLs do not need long-term prophylactic treatment. In clinical practice, the final decision on the use of specific prophylactic therapy should be individualized and based on the aPL profile (multiple aPLs, high levels, and persistence) and the presence of additional inherited or acquired prothrombotic risk factors. Prophylaxis with LMWH administered subcutaneously should certainly be considered during high-risk situations, such as prolonged immobilization or surgery.[376] Table 24-7 shows a summary of recommendations for primary thromboprophylaxis in children.

The coexistence of an underlying autoimmune disease, particularly SLE, represents a prothrombotic condition in itself and significantly increases the thrombosis risk, primarily because of chronic systemic inflammation and nephrotic syndrome that depletes endogenous anticoagulants. The highest thrombosis rates in pediatric and adult patients with aPLs were reported in patients with SLE, who have an approximately 50% chance of suffering a thrombotic event within 10 years.[45,387] A systematic review reported moderate levels of evidence that antimalarial drugs prevent thrombosis in SLE,[388] which is further supported by case-control studies.[389] A protective effect of hydroxychloroquine against thrombosis was also observed in SLE patients with aPLs.[390] Hydroxychloroquine has modest anticoagulant properties and decreases endothelial and leukocyte expression of tissue factor.[137] In addition to thrombosis prevention, hydroxychloroquine decreases

---

TABLE 24-7 Recommendations for Primary Thromboprophylaxis in Children With Antiphospholipid Antibodies

Primary thromboprophylaxis in children with aPLs

Asymptomatic individuals with aPLs
- No therapy
- Strict control of cardiovascular risk factors

High-risk situations (surgery, long-lasting immobilization)
- Thromboprophylaxis with low molecular weight heparin

Persistent multiple aPL-positive individuals
- Consider low-dose aspirin (3-5 mg/kg/day)

Patients with childhood-onset systemic lupus erythematosus
- Hydroxychloroquine and consider low-dose aspirin

aPLs, Antiphospholipid antibodies.

damage accrual and increases long-term survival, and is therefore recommended as baseline therapy in all SLE patients[388] (Table 24-7).

Further protection for SLE patients with aPLs may be provided by thromboprophylaxis with low-dose aspirin.[391,392] A decision analysis demonstrated that in patients with SLE the benefit of primary prophylaxis with aspirin outweighs the risk of bleeding, and that aspirin should be given to all patients with SLE to prevent both arterial and venous thrombotic events, especially in patients with aPLs.[393] In this sense, low-dose aspirin (3 to 5 mg/kg/day) has been recommended as thromboprophylaxis in all SLE patients with persistently positive aPLs.[376] No studies evaluated whether the combination of hydroxychloroquine plus low-dose aspirin increases the efficacy of primary thromboprophylaxis in patients with SLE. A recent randomized trial showed that the addition of prophylactic low-intensity oral anticoagulant therapy together with low-dose aspirin does not provide further advantage in comparison with low-dose aspirin alone in aPL-positive SLE patients.[394]

Antithrombotic Therapy and Prevention of Recurrent Thrombosis

The main treatment for APS patients with thrombosis is antithrombotic treatment rather than immunosuppression. Treatment of the acute thrombotic event in children with APS is no different from that of thrombosis arising from other causes and should be organized in consultation with a pediatric hematologist.[374] Most children receive anticoagulation therapy with unfractionated heparin as a loading bolus injection followed by continuous infusion. Because LA prolongs the aPTT and alters the relationship of aPTT-to-heparin concentration, it is recommended to use anti-factor Xa activity assay for heparin monitoring. LMWH is increasingly being used as initial therapy for acute thrombosis in children because it is administered subcutaneously, has a more predictable dose response, and a reduced requirement for monitoring. The target therapeutic anti-Xa activity for children treated with LMWH ranges between 0.5 and 1.0 U/mL.[368,395] Systemic or local thrombolytic therapy represents a key treatment choice in select circumstances of high-risk clots and should be seriously considered in children who are treated within 2 weeks of symptomatic onset. Successful outcome with the use of thrombolytic therapy has been reported in difficult pediatric APS patients.[257,272,396]

Children treated with unfractionated heparin or LMWH as an initial agent are often subsequently transitioned to warfarin for long-term oral anticoagulation. Among children included in the pediatric APS registry, all patients with venous thrombosis received long-term oral anticoagulation therapy, but only 40% of patients with arterial thrombosis received anticoagulation with or without concomitant antiaggregation therapy (low-dose aspirin 3 to 5 mg/kg/day).[27] During the mean follow-up period of 6.1 years, 19% of pediatric patients with initial venous thrombosis and 21% of patients with initial arterial thrombosis developed recurrent thrombotic events.[27] Two previous studies in children with APS also reported a high thrombosis recurrence rate (29%),[28,32] which is significantly higher than recurrence rates reported in adult APS patients during a similar follow-up period (3% to 16%).[397-401] The thrombosis recurrence rate in children with APS appears comparable to the subgroup of high-risk adult APS patients with triple aPL positivity who had a 26% incidence of recurrent thromboembolic events during 5 years of follow-up.[402] Of note, 73% of recurrent thrombotic events in children evolved after cessation of anticoagulation therapy, which represents a situation with the highest risk for thrombosis.[28] Because of the ability of heparin to block complement activation, and in view of the important role of complement in APS pathophysiology, some physicians recommend long-term use of LMWH in children at very high risk of recurrent thrombosis.

Based on two randomized controlled trials in adult APS patients,[397,398] there is general agreement that patients with first venous thromboembolism should receive standard oral anticoagulation at a target INR of 2.0 to 3.0.[375,376] Higher intensity anticoagulation has not been demonstrated to decrease the rate of recurrences for first venous thromboembolism.[397,398] Treatment of APS patients with arterial thrombosis remains more controversial.[376] A systematic review based on observational studies has shown that adult patients with arterial or recurrent thrombosis were at an increased risk for recurrences, even when treated with oral anticoagulation at a target INR of 2.0 to 3.0.[379] Therefore, lifelong anticoagulation at a target INR above 3.0 was advised for patients arterial or recurrent events.[376] This recommendation has been challenged by another systematic review suggesting that patients with first ischemic stroke should receive either aspirin (325 mg/day) or moderate-intensity warfarin with an INR between 1.4 and 2.8.[375] The second recommendation was based on the results of a large randomized trial in patients with ischemic stroke; however, most patients included in this trial had only low levels of aCLs and did not meet classification criteria for APS because repeat testing for aPLs was not performed.[403]

In the absence of controlled trials, the optimal intensity and duration of anticoagulation therapy in pediatric APS patients with thrombosis are still controversial. Given the higher recurrence rate of thrombosis, it seems reasonable to consider anticoagulation in all pediatric patients with definite APS, at least at a target INR suggested for the adult population. In a large retrospective study in pediatric SLE, none of the LA-positive patients who were maintained in the target INR range of 2.0 to 3.0 developed a second thrombotic event.[45] One of the problems of the high-intensity anticoagulation may be a higher risk of bleeding, which should be assessed individually for each patient. Among adult patients with APS, the systematic review showed that repeated thromboses were more frequent and associated with a much higher mortality than hemorrhagic complications in patients taking warfarin.[379] Decisions on how long treatment should be continued must be individualized. As a general rule anticoagulation should be continued until the child becomes aPL negative. Table 24-8 shows a summary of recommendations for secondary thromboprophylaxis in children.

An improved understanding of the pathogenic mechanisms by which aPLs induce thrombosis has suggested some innovative treatments such as an oral direct thrombin inhibitor (dabigatran); anti-factor Xa inhibitors (rivaroxaban, apixaban, edoxaban); antiplatelet drugs other than aspirin (clopidogrel, dipyridamole); hydroxychloroquine: statins (fluvastatin, rosuvastatin); B-cell inhibition (rituximab, belimumab); complement inhibition (eculizumab); peptide therapy (β_2GPI domain I inhibition); and vitamin D.[404] Rituximab, an anti-CD20 chimeric monoclonal antibody that selectively induces depletion of circulating B cells, has been successfully used in APS patients with recurrent thrombosis, severe thrombocytopenia, hemolytic anemia, skin ulcers or necrosis, and aPL nephropathy.[405-407] A smaller open-label trial of rituximab use in 19 adult patients with manifestations of APS that did not meet the criteria showed good safety profile and effectiveness in controlling thrombocytopenia, skin ulcers, and cognitive dysfunction.[408] A few pediatric case reports suggest that rituximab can also offer a therapeutic alternative in severe or resistant pediatric APS patients.[409,410]

Catastrophic Antiphospholipid Syndrome

If CAPS is suspected, immediate aggressive treatment is required. Therapy must be multifaceted and include elimination of possible precipitating factors, treatment of the ongoing thrombotic events, and suppression of the excessive cytokine storm.[411,412] An analysis of 250

TABLE 24-8 Recommendations for Secondary Thromboprophylaxis in Children with Antiphospholipid Antibodies and History of Thrombosis

Secondary thromboprophylaxis in children with aPLs and thrombosis

Children with definite APS and first venous thromboembolism
- Long-term anticoagulation to a target INR 2.0-3.0

Children with definite APS and arterial thrombosis
- Long-term anticoagulation to a target INR 3.0-4.0 or combined anticoagulation and antiaggregation therapy

Children with definite APS and recurrent thrombosis despite oral anticoagulation with a target INR 2.0-3.0
- Long-term anticoagulation to a target INR 3.0-4.0 or alternative therapies such as extended therapeutic dose of low molecular weight heparin

Children with venous thromboembolism with single positive or low level aPLs
- Per usual recommendations for deep vein thrombosis treatment

Children with arterial thrombosis with single positive or low level aPLs
- Per usual recommendations for arterial thrombosis treatment

aPLs, Antiphospholipid antibodies.
Adapted from G. Ruiz-Irastorza, M. Crowther, W. Branch, M.A. Khamashta. Antiphospholipid syndrome, Lancet 376 (2010) 1498–509.[377]

TABLE 24-9 Recommendations for Treatment of Catastrophic Antiphospholipid Syndrome in Children

Clinical suspicion of catastrophic antiphospholipid syndrome
- Fulfilling at least two classification criteria

Treatment of precipitating factors
- Antibiotics if suspected infection
- Excision of necrotic tissues

Effective anticoagulation with intravenous heparin followed by oral anticoagulants
- Long-term anticoagulation to a target INR approximately 3.0

High doses of corticosteroids
- Administered for a minimum of 3 days but may have to be continued for longer depending on the patient's response

Intravenous immunoglobulins
- Recommended dose 0.4 g/day/kg body weight for 4-5 days
- Specifically indicated in patients with severe thrombocytopenia

Plasma exchange with fresh frozen plasma
- Specifically indicated in patients with thrombotic microangiopathy and presence of schistocytes

Cyclophosphamide
- Specifically indicated in patients with CAPS in the presence of cSLE flare

Rituximab
- Specifically indicated in patients with nonresponsive severe thrombocytopenia or autoimmune hemolytic anemia

APS, Antiphospholipid syndrome; *CAPS,* catastrophic antiphospholipid syndrome; *cSLE,* Childhood-onset systemic lupus erythematosus.
Adapted from R. Cervera. Catastrophic antiphospholipid syndrome (CAPS): update from the "CAPS Registry", Lupus 19 (2010) 412–418.[412]

patients included in the CAPS registry showed that the highest recovery rate was achieved by the combination therapy of anticoagulants, corticosteroids, and plasma exchange (78%), followed by the combination of anticoagulants, corticosteroids, plasma exchange, and/or intravenous immunoglobulin (IVIG).[413] Accordingly, the use of a combined treatment of anticoagulants, corticosteroids, and plasma exchange has been recommended as first-line therapy for patients with CAPS.[411,412] This combined treatment regimen was also associated with the highest survival rate in a recent series of pediatric CAPS patients.[82] IVIG has multiple therapeutic actions and may improve outcome in CAPS patients, but rapid infusion of high doses of IVIG may increase the risk of thrombosis. When IVIG and plasma exchange are used simultaneously in the same patient, IVIG is administered after the last day of the plasma exchange to prevent the removal of IVIG by plasma exchange. Concomitant treatment with cyclophosphamide did not demonstrate additional benefit in patients with primary CAPS but improved survival in those with SLE-associated CAPS.[414] Rituximab has been also successfully used in several CAPS patients and may have a role particularly in those with refractory disease.[284,415] Treatment of known precipitating factors in CAPS patients should include prompt use of antibiotics (if infection is suspected) and excision of necrotic tissues. Recommendations for treatment of CAPS are summarized in Table 24-9.

Treatment in patients with microangiopathic antiphospholipid-associated syndrome should be directed toward the underlying condition (i.e., plasma exchange, complement inhibition with eculizumab in atypical HUS) and not to the presence of aPLs, unless there are complicating large-vessel occlusions as in the case of CAPS.[287]

Perinatal Complications Associated with Antiphospholipid Antibodies

There are no uniform guidelines for the therapeutic approach in perinatal thrombosis associated with transplacentally transferred aPLs.[310]

Infants with stroke usually received only symptomatic treatment for the seizures, with or without antiaggregation therapy, and infants with venous or disseminated thrombotic events received additional anticoagulation, thrombolytic therapy, and/or exchange transfusion. Children born to mothers with APS exhibit a higher percentage of neurodevelopmental abnormalities, and the inclusion of regular neuropsychological assessments during their long-term follow-up is recommended.[306,332,333]

COURSE OF THE DISEASE AND PROGNOSIS

An understanding of the course and prognosis of pediatric APS awaits prospective studies in large cohorts. Data from observational studies suggest that the risk of recurrent thrombosis in children with APS during the mean follow-up period of around 6 years is 20% to 30%.[27,28,32] In general, the risk of future thrombosis is very low in asymptomatic children who are incidentally found to have positive aPLs. However, it is high among those in whom thrombosis has already occurred and extremely high in patients with CAPS. A high titer of aPLs, and in particular the presence of LA combined with aCLs and anti-β_2GPIs (triple positivity), increases the risk of thrombosis, as do the concomitant presence of inherited prothrombotic disorders and/or other acquired thrombotic risk factors.[28,362,368,416] The time interval between recurrent thrombotic events varies considerably from weeks to months or even years.

APS is a serious and potentially life-threatening disease. In the cohort of 121 children included in the pediatric APS registry, the estimated mortality rate was 7%. In total, seven patients with APS associated with underlying SLE and two patients with primary APS died during the mean follow-up time of 6.1 years.[27] The most common cause of death was a thrombotic event (seven patients), followed by SLE complications (one patient) and hemophagocytic syndrome associated with splenic infarction (one patient).[27] The mortality rate of 26% was observed at the time of the catastrophic event among 46 pediatric patients included in the European CAPS registry.[82]

Approximately 20% of children who initially develop the features of primary APS may progress over time to develop SLE or a lupuslike disease.[27,32] This percentage is almost three times higher than reported in adult patients with primary APS (7%),[417] and it emphasizes the importance of careful follow-up of all children with primary APS to be alert for the subsequent appearance of manifestations of SLE. The presence of an underlying autoimmune disease influences the occurrence of clinical manifestations of APS. Hematological and skin manifestations have lower prevalence in patients with primary APS, whereas arterial occlusions are less frequent in APS secondary to SLE.[27]

Some pediatric studies noted a positive correlation of aCL titers with SLE disease activity indices.[34,37,39,48] The influence of SLE treatment on aPL titers may reflect the effect of therapy on SLE disease activity; however, there are some pediatric SLE patients who have persistently positive aPLs even when their disease is inactive, and these patients may develop thrombotic events even during SLE remission. Fluctuations of LA are less commonly seen than fluctuations in the level of aCLs in SLE patients; this may also contribute to the more consistent relation of LA with thrombosis compared with aCL.[418] In general, titers of aCL, anti-β_2GPI, and LA should be monitored at least once yearly in every child with SLE.

The presence of aPLs may have a negative impact on the clinical outcome of both childhood-onset and adult-onset SLE.[419-421] Several studies of adult patients with SLE have reported that the presence of APS was an important predictor of irreversible organ damage and death in SLE.[422,423] A retrospective study of 56 children with childhood-onset SLE showed that the risk of irreversible organ damage (as scored by the Systemic Lupus International Collaborating Clinics/ACR Damage Index) in aPL-positive patients was three times higher than in aPL-negative patients.[421] Thus, the presence of aPL in childhood-onset SLE patients could represent not only a risk factor for thrombosis but also a poor prognostic factor overall.

REFERENCES

2. S. Miyakis, M.D. Lockshin, T. Atsumi, et al., International consensus statement on an update of the classification criteria for definite antiphospholipid syndrome (APS), J. Thromb. Haemost. 4 (2006) 295–306.

11. R. Nayfe, I. Uthman, J. Aoun, et al., Seronegative antiphospholipid syndrome, Rheumatology (Oxford) 52 (2013) 1358–1367.

15. D. Erkan, G. Espinosa, R. Cervera, Catastrophic antiphospholipid syndrome: updated diagnostic algorithms, Autoimmun. Rev. 10 (2010) 74–79.

22. R. Cervera, J. Piette, J. Font, et al., Antiphospholipid syndrome clinical and immunologic manifestations and patterns of disease expression in a cohort of 1,000 patients, Arthritis Rheum. 46 (2002) 1019–1027.

23. B. Giannakopoulos, S. Krilis, The pathogenesis of the antiphospholipid syndrome, N. Engl. J. Med. 368 (2013) 1033–1044.

26. G. Kenet, S. Aronis, Y. Berkun, et al., Impact of persistent antiphospholipid antibodies on risk of incident symptomatic thromboembolism in children: a systematic review and meta-analysis, Semin. Thromb. Hemost. 37 (2011) 802–809.

27. T. Avcin, R. Cimaz, E.D. Silverman, et al., Pediatric antiphospholipid syndrome: clinical and immunologic features of 121 patients in an international registry, Pediatrics 122 (2008) e1100–e1107.

28. Y. Berkun, S. Padeh, J. Barash, et al., Antiphospholipid syndrome and recurrent thrombosis in children, Arthritis Rheum. 55 (2006) 850–855.

29. A. Zamora-Ustaran, R.O. Escarcega-Alarcón, M. Garcia-Carrasco, et al., Antiphospholipid syndrome in Mexican children, Isr. Med. Assoc. J. 14 (2012) 286–289.

32. M. Gattorno, F. Falcini, A. Ravelli, et al., Outcome of primary antiphospholipid syndrome in childhood, Lupus 12 (2003) 449–453.

45. D. Levy, M. Massicotte, E. Harvey, et al., Thromboembolism in paediatric lupus patients, Lupus 12 (2003) 741–746.

47. C. Male, D. Foulon, H. Hoogendoorn, et al., Predictive value of persistent versus transient antiphospholipid antibody subtypes for the risk of thrombotic events in pediatric patients with systemic lupus erythematosus, Blood 106 (2005) 4152–4158.

48. T. Avcin, S.M. Benseler, P.N. Tyrrell, et al., A followup study of antiphospholipid antibodies and associated neuropsychiatric manifestations in 137 children with systemic lupus erythematosus, Arthritis Rheum. 59 (2008) 206–213.

74. Y. Shoenfeld, M. Blank, R. Cervera, et al., Infectious origin of the antiphospholipid syndrome, Ann. Rheum. Dis. 65 (2006) 2–6.

77. P.G. De Groot, R.T. Urbanus, The significance of autoantibodies against β_2-glycoprotein I, Blood 120 (2012) 266–274.

82. H. Berman, I. Rodríguez-Pintó, R. Cervera, et al., Pediatric catastrophic antiphospholipid syndrome: descriptive analysis of 45 patients from the "CAPS Registry", Autoimmun. Rev. 13 (2014) 157–162.

99. C. Male, K. Lechner, S. Eichinger, et al., Clinical significance of lupus anticoagulants in children, J. Pediatr. 134 (1999) 199–205.

108. L. Andreoli, C. Nalli, M. Motta, et al., Anti-β_2-glycoprotein I IgG antibodies from 1-year-old healthy children born to mothers with systemic autoimmune diseases preferentially target domain 4/5: might it be the reason for their "innocent" profile? Ann. Rheum. Dis. 70 (2011) 380–383.

113. Y. Motoki, J. Nojima, M. Yanagihara, et al., Anti-phospholipid antibodies contribute to arteriosclerosis in patients with systemic lupus erythematosus through induction of tissue factor expression and cytokine production from peripheral blood mononuclear cells, Thromb. Res. 130 (2012) 667–673.

121. E.S. Sen, M.W. Beresford, T. Avčin, A.V. Ramanan, How to use … lupus anticoagulants, Arch. Dis. Child. Educ. Pract. Ed. 98 (2013) 52–57.

122. J.F. Molina, S. Gutierrez-Ureña, J. Molina, et al., Variability of anticardiolipin antibody isotype distribution in 3 geographic populations of patients with systemic lupus erythematosus, J. Rheumatol. 24 (1997) 291–296.

125. M.L. Bertolaccini, O. Amengual, T. Atsumi, et al., 'Non-criteria' aPL tests: report of a task force and preconference workshop at the 13th International Congress on Antiphospholipid Antibodies, Galveston, TX, USA, April 2010, Lupus 20 (2011) 191–205.

126. S. Sciascia, V. Murru, G. Sanna, et al., Clinical accuracy for diagnosis of antiphospholipid syndrome in systemic lupus erythematosus: evaluation of 23 possible combinations of antiphospholipid antibody specificities, J. Thromb. Haemost. 10 (2012) 2512–2518.

127. A. Banzato, N. Pozzi, R. Frasson, et al., Antibodies to Domain I of β(2) Glycoprotein I are in close relation to patients risk categories in Antiphospholipid Syndrome (APS), Thromb. Res. 128 (2011) 583–586.

128. D.M. Wahezi, N.T. Ilowite, X.X. Wu, et al., Annexin A5 anticoagulant activity in children with systemic lupus erythematosus and the association with antibodies to domain I of β2-glycoprotein I, Lupus 22 (2013) 702–711.

135. A. Bontadi, A. Ruffatti, E. Falcinelli, et al., Platelet and endothelial activation in catastrophic and quiescent antiphospholipid syndrome, Thromb. Haemost. 109 (2013) 901–908.

137. R.G. Espinola, S.S. Pierangeli, A.E. Gharavi, E.N. Harris, Hydroxychloroquine reverses platelet activation induced by human IgG antiphospholipid antibodies, Thromb. Haemost. 87 (2002) 518–522.

138. D.J. Taatjes, A.S. Quinn, J.H. Rand, B.P. Jena, Atomic force microscopy: high resolution dynamic imaging of cellular and molecular structure in health and disease, J. Cell. Physiol. 228 (2013) 1949–1955.

139. S.S. Pierangeli, R.G. Espinola, X. Liu, E.N. Harris, Thrombogenic effects of antiphospholipid antibodies are mediated by intercellular cell

adhesion molecule-1, vascular cell adhesion molecule-1, and P-selectin, Circ. Res. 88 (2001) 245–250.

141. M. Adams, Novel considerations in the pathogenesis of the antiphospholipid syndrome: involvement of the tissue factor pathway of blood coagulation, Semin. Thromb. Hemost. 34 (2008) 251–255.

146. C. Pericleous, L.A. Clarke, P.A. Brogan, et al., Endothelial microparticle release is stimulated in vitro by purified IgG from patients with the antiphospholipid syndrome, Thromb. Haemost. 109 (2013) 72–78.

151. P.L. Meroni, E. Raschi, C. Testoni, et al., Innate immunity in the antiphospholipid syndrome: role of toll-like receptors in endothelial cell activation by antiphospholipid antibodies, Autoimmun. Rev. 3 (2004) 510–515.

154. L. Xia, H. Zhou, L. Hu, et al., Both NF-κB and c-Jun/AP-1 involved in anti-β2GPI/β2GPI-induced tissue factor expression in monocytes, Thromb. Haemost. 109 (2013) 643–651.

156. P. Redecha, R. Tilley, M. Tencati, et al., Tissue factor: a link between C5a and neutrophil activation in antiphospholipid antibody induced fetal injury, Blood 110 (2007) 2423–2431.

159. N. Di Simone, P.L. Meroni, N. de Papa, et al., Antiphospholipid antibodies affect trophoblast gonadotropin secretion and invasiveness by binding directly and through adhered beta2-glycoprotein I, Arthritis Rheum. 43 (2000) 140–150.

163. F. Fischetti, P. Durigutto, V. Pellis, et al., Thrombus formation induced by antibodies to beta2-glycoprotein I is complement dependent and requires a priming factor, Blood 106 (2005) 2340–2346.

171. A.-J. Chamorro, M. Marcos, J.A. Mirón-Canelo, et al., Val247Leu β2-glycoprotein-I allelic variant is associated with antiphospholipid syndrome: systematic review and meta-analysis, Autoimmun. Rev. 11 (2012) 705–712.

179. G. Kenet, L.K. Lütkhoff, M. Albisetti, et al., Impact of thrombophilia on risk of arterial ischemic stroke or cerebral sinovenous thrombosis in neonates and children: a systematic review and meta-analysis of observational studies, Circulation 121 (2010) 1838–1847.

221. E. Muscal, R.L. Brey, Antiphospholipid syndrome and the brain in pediatric and adult patients, Lupus 19 (2010) 406–411.

278. R. Cervera, S. Bucciarelli, M.A. Plasín, et al., Catastrophic antiphospholipid syndrome (CAPS): descriptive analysis of a series of 280 patients from the "CAPS Registry", J. Autoimmun. 32 (2009) 240–245.

306. A. Mekinian, E. Lachassinne, P. Nicaise-Roland, et al., European registry of babies born to mothers with antiphospholipid syndrome, Ann. Rheum. Dis. 72 (2013) 217–222.

310. M.-C. Boffa, E. Lachassinne, Infant perinatal thrombosis and antiphospholipid antibodies: a review, Lupus 16 (2007) 634–641.

360. V. Pengo, A. Tripodi, G. Reber, et al., Update of the guidelines for lupus anticoagulant detection. Subcommittee on Lupus Anticoagulant/Antiphospholipid Antibody of the Scientific and Standardisation Committee of the International Society on Thrombosis and Haemostasis, J. Thromb. Haemost. 7 (2009) 1737–1740.

362. V. Pengo, A. Ruffatti, C. Legnani, et al., Incidence of a first thromboembolic event in asymptomatic carriers of high-risk antiphospholipid antibody profile: a multicenter prospective study, Blood 118 (2011) 4714–4718.

376. G. Ruiz-Irastorza, M.J. Cuadrado, I. Ruiz-Arruza, et al., Evidence-based recommendations for the prevention and long-term management of thrombosis in antiphospholipid antibody-positive patients: report of a task force at the 13th International Congress on antiphospholipid antibodies, Lupus 20 (2011) 206–218.

377. G. Ruiz-Irastorza, M. Crowther, W. Branch, M.A. Khamashta, Antiphospholipid syndrome, Lancet 376 (2010) 1498–1509.

401. R. Cervera, R. Serrano, G.J. Pons-Estel, et al., Morbidity and mortality in the antiphospholipid syndrome during a 10-year period: a multicentre prospective study of 1000 patients, Ann. Rheum. Dis. (2014) doi:10.1136/annrheumdis-2013-204838; [Epub ahead of print].

404. D. Erkan, C.L. Aguiar, D. Andrade, et al., 14th International Congress on Antiphospholipid Antibodies Task Force Report on Antiphospholipid Syndrome Treatment Trends, Autoimmun. Rev. 13 (2014) 685–696.

424. B. de Laat, K. Mertens, P.G. de Groot, Mechanisms of disease: antiphospholipid antibodies-from clinical association to pathologic mechanism, Nat. Clin. Pract. Rheumatol. 4 (2008) 192–199.

425. S. Sciascia, G. Sanna, V. Murru, et al., GAPSS: the Global Anti-Phospholipid Syndrome Score, Rheumatology (Oxford) 52 (2013) 1397–1403.

Entire reference list is available online at www.expertconsult.com.

Neonatal Lupus Erythematosus

Earl Silverman, Jill Buyon, Edgar Jaeggi

ETIOLOGY AND PATHOGENESIS

Neonatal lupus erythematosus (NLE) is a disease of the developing fetus and neonate defined by characteristic clinical features in the presence of specific maternal autoantibodies. It is considered a model of passively acquired autoimmunity. The transplacental passage of these autoantibodies is necessary but not sufficient to cause the disease. The autoantibodies associated with NLE are directed against a group of small cytoplasmic and nuclear ribonucleoproteins (RNPs): Ro/SSA and La/SSSB. Rarely, cutaneous NLE is associated with isolated anti-U1RNP antibodies. The most common clinical manifestations of NLE are cardiac, dermatologic, and hepatic. The term *neonatal lupus erythematosus* is misleading as the affected child does not have systemic lupus erythematosus (SLE), and the mother is frequently healthy, without any symptoms of an autoimmune disease. We will first review the autoantigens and autoantibodies associated with NLE and the genetics of NLE. We will then examine the specific clinical features and proposed pathogenesis of these features.

Autoantigens

Target Antigens of the Ro/La (RoRNP) System

The major candidate autoantigens in NLE are the Ro and La proteins, which are present in all cells. The first Ro protein identified was a 60-kD polypeptide (Ro60). Isolation and cloning of Ro60 identified a zinc finger and an RNA-binding protein consensus motif.[1,2] Crystallographic studies demonstrated a ring-shaped protein with two overlapping RNA binding sites that may serve different functions depending on the cellular location of Ro60.[3] One important function of Ro60 is to protect cells from damage from ultraviolet irradiation.[4] In the nucleus, Ro60 likely plays a role in RNA quality control.[4-6] Ro binds to a class of noncoding RNAs (YRNAs) on the outer surface of the ring. The binding to YRNAs allows for the translocation of Ro60 from the nucleus.[7] This translocation occurs via the zipcode-binding protein ZBP1 and other proteins.[8,9] During apoptosis YRNAs are required for translocation of Ro60 to the cell surface that may be pivotal to the formation of immune complexes on apoptotic cells and a Toll-like receptor–dependent proinflammatory cascade.[10] Murine studies have suggested that Ro60 may protect against the development of autoantibodies by sequestering defective ribonucleoproteins.[6]

The second RoRNP protein recognized was the 48-kD La protein. Although it may, at least transiently, be associated with Ro60,[11] La does not share antigenic determinants with either Ro60 or Ro52.[12,13] La is composed of at least two structural domains, each of which contains a distinct antigenic binding site.[14] La is mainly found in the nucleus, and its nuclear localization is dependent on the C-terminus but not the N-terminus (RNP-consensus motif).[15] Similar to Ro60, it can appear on the cell surface during cell stress or apoptosis, and therefore be a direct target for autoantibodies.[16] La facilitates maturation and termination of RNA polymerase III transcripts including transfer RNA (tRNA), and directly binds multiple different RNAs and precursors to small nucleolar RNAs (SnRNAs) involved in ribosome biogenesis.[17,18] La is required for embryogenesis and normal development.[19,20]

The other recognized target of the autoimmune response is a 52-kD polypeptide, Ro52. Although two isoforms of Ro52 (52α and 52β) have been recognized, postnatally the 52α is the predominate form (now called Trim21). The 52β is derived from the splicing of exon 4 encoding aa168-245 that includes the leucine zipper. This results in a smaller protein with a predicted molecular weight of 45,000 and lacking a leucine zipper.[21] The 52β transcript is the predominant transcript in the early second trimester when maternal antibodies begin to gain access to the fetus. However, by 18 weeks' gestation, 52α becomes the predominant or sole transcript.[22] This evidence is consistent with a role for 52β in the development of congenital heart block (CHB), but further proof is required. The remainder of the discussion will be about 52α/Trim21. The full-length protein 52α/Trim21 has three distinct domains: an N-terminal region rich in cysteine/histidine motifs that contains two distinct zinc fingers known as RING finger and B-box; a central region containing two coiled stations of 52α, one being a leucine zipper with potential for intramolecular dimerization, and the other a C-terminal ret finger protein (rpf)-like domain.[23-25] Ro52 is an E3 ubiquitin ligase that catalyzes the ubiquitination of several proteins, including Ro52 itself.[26-28] Other important functions of Trim21/Ro52 include regulation of proinflammatory cytokine production[29]; the production of type 1 interferon and cytokine production via its ubiquitination of interferon regulatory factors (IRFs) including IRF3, IRF5, IRF7, and IRF8 (reviewed[30]); and regulation of the innate response to intracellular double-stranded DNA.[31]

Calcium Channels

Calcium (Ca++) channels are important in maintaining cardiac rhythm, and antibodies against these ion channels have been hypothesized to be important in CHB. Specifically L-type channels, α_{1c} and α_{1D} subunits, and T-type calcium channels, α_{1G} subunit, have been shown to be present in both adult and fetal conducting tissue. (See the section "Calcium Channels.")

Autoantibodies

The search for the pathogenic antibody specificities that lead to CHB has been attempted by many researchers. The following paragraphs review the history of these efforts. Unfortunately there are important limitations in interpreting many reports; these limitations include small numbers of patients and the failure to use only sera obtained during the pregnancy when comparing autoantibodies from mothers of affected and unaffected children. The problem with this latter approach is that the autoantibody repertoire can change over time.

Anti-Ro60 Antibodies

The first antibodies to be recognized to be associated with the development of NLE were antibodies directed against Ro60 and La48.[32-34] However, it soon became apparent that not all children born to mothers with anti-Ro60 antibodies developed NLE and that although a sensitive marker for the development of NLE, the presence of anti-Ro60 antibodies had poor specificity to identify at-risk pregnancies. Furthermore, the presence of these antibodies alone could not differentiate fetuses or infants at risk to different manifestations of NLE (such as cutaneous NLE [C-NLE]).[35-37] In order to increase the specificity of anti-Ro antibodies as a biomarker for NLE, investigators used different immunologic methods to determine the autoantibody repertoire.

Initial studies used the relatively insensitive method of immunodiffusion assay, which was rapidly usurped with the advent of enzyme-linked immunoassays (ELISAs), using either affinity-purified or recombinant proteins, or an RNA immunoprecipitation assay. The latter assay is quite sensitive and can distinguish anti-Ro60 from anti-Ro52 antibodies. However, it is not commercially available and is only mentioned because it was used as a research tool in studies that helped determine the importance of the anti-Ro52 antibody response in the development of CHB.[38] It is important to note which assay is used when analyzing results, as the type of protein used may give different results. For technical reasons all ELISAs for Ro52 use recombinant proteins, whereas assays for anti-La48 or anti-Ro60 antibodies may use either affinity-purified or recombinant proteins. Assays for anti-Ro antibodies that use affinity-purified proteins cannot identify anti-Ro52 antibodies.

The easiest and cheapest assay to screen pregnant women for the risks of delivering a child with NLE is the anti-Ro ELISA. This assay has excellent sensitivity at greater than 99% to identify all fetuses with CHB, but it has poor specificity. Therefore other autoantibodies have been examined to increase the specificity without decreasing the sensitivity. A prospective study of 146 mothers at risk to deliver a child with cardiac NLE showed that the titer of anti-Ro antibodies was important in determining the risk of developing cardiac NLE.[39] Specifically, none of the mothers with low-titer anti-Ro60 antibodies (less than 50 IU; commercially available ELISA with maximum of 100 IU) delivered a child with NLE, whereas the pregnancies of 5% of mothers with anti-Ro60 antibody titers of 50 IU or more were complicated by fetal cardiac NLE. Based on these data, it was suggested that mothers with low levels of anti-Ro antibodies were at a very low risk for delivering a child with cardiac NLE and therefore may require less intensive screening. Subsequently, a validation cohort confirmed these findings.

Anti-La Antibodies

One of the earliest studies suggested that the presence of both anti-Ro60 and anti-La48 antibodies was sensitive and more specific than the presence of anti-Ro60 antibodies alone for the risk of delivering a child with CHB.[40] Following this observation, a study showed that antibodies directed against a small La polypeptide, named DD, were found only in the sera of mothers of children with NLE and not in sera from mothers of unaffected children.[37] Although this finding was specific for NLE, it had only a 30% sensitivity because many mothers without anti-DD antibodies delivered children with NLE, and anti-DD antibodies were present in only 30% of children with NLE. Subsequent larger studies showed that anti-La48 antibodies were present in up to 50% of sera of mothers of children with CHB and that they had a lower sensitivity than either anti-Ro60 or anti-Ro52 antibodies for the risk

of delivering a child with CHB.[39,41] Therefore testing for the presence of anti-La48 antibodies alone is not a good screening tool to determine at risk pregnancies.

Anti-RO52 Antibodies

Antibodies to Ro52 are found in 70% to 80% of mothers of children with CHB and although less sensitive than anti-Ro60 antibodies, they are more specific for the development of CHB.[38,42,43] Epitope mapping of the anti-Ro52 antibody response revealed an immunodominant region, spanning aa169-291, a region containing the leucine zipper (aa220-232)[44] that was recognized by the majority of the sera from mothers of children with CHB.[43] Examination of the fine specificity of the response to this region showed that the dominant antibody response in mothers of children with CHB was directed against a polypeptide consisting of aa200-239 (p200), whereas a reduced risk of CHB was found when the dominant response was directed against aa176-196 (p176) and aa197-232 (p197). These intriguing data led to replication studies to address the sensitivities and specificities of these antibodies in CHB. The first study showed that although the majority of the maternal sera with anti-Ro52 antibodies had anti-p200 antibodies, the presence of anti-p200 antibodies did not differentiate mothers of children with CHB, C-NLE, or healthy children.[45] Specifically, anti-p200 antibodies were found in 77% of mothers of children with CHB, 80% of mothers of children with C-NLE, and 95% of mothers of unaffected children. The largest study, which was international in scope, found that the mean anti-p200 antibody level in sera from mothers of children with CHB or second-degree heart block (HB) was significantly higher than the mean level in mothers who had children with normal heart rates.[46] Closer examination of one of the cohorts (pregnancies) showed the sera from mothers of children first-, second-, and third-degree HB (detected by fetal echocardiogram during pregnancy) had higher mean anti-p200 antibody levels than the mean anti-p200 antibody level seen in mothers of children without any degree of heart block. However, the first-degree HB resolved by birth.

The most recent study to address this issue used either maternal sera during the pregnancy or cord blood. It was again shown that the frequencies of anti-p200, anti-Ro52, anti-Ro60, and anti-La48 antibodies were not different between affected and unaffected neonates. However, in confirmation of a previous study,[39] mean anti-Ro52 and anti-Ro60 titers were higher in pregnancies with a child with CHB and unaffected siblings of a child with CHB, as compared to those associated with well neonates who never had a sibling with CHB. Maternal anti-p200 antibodies, taken during the pregnancy, were more frequent in mothers who delivered a child with CHB (88%) as compared to mothers who had delivered an unaffected infant (67%). However, the frequency, at 88%, did not differ as compared to that of anti-p200 antibodies in mothers who had previously delivered a child with CHB but had an unaffected child during the study (97%). Overall, anti-p200 antibodies were more specific but less sensitive than anti-Ro60 or anti-Ro52 antibodies for the risk of delivering a child with CHB as compared to delivering an unaffected child.

Translational studies showed that anti-p200 antibodies and anti-Ro52 antibodies both bound the surface of nonpermeabilized apoptotic, but not healthy, human fetal cardiocytes, suggesting that they may be pathogenic in CHB.[47] In vivo rodent models and in vitro culturing systems suggested that anti-p200 antibodies bind neonatal rodent cardiocytes and altered calcium homeostasis.[48]

Anti-L-Type and Anti-T-Type Calcium Channel Antibodies

Anti-Ro/La antibodies were shown to react with, and alter the function of, α_{1c} and α_{1D} subunits of the L-type calcium channel and T-type calcium channels.[49-51] The major target of the anti-T-type Ca^{++}

channel antibodies was an epitope present on an extracellular loop of the channel.[52]

Anti–5-Serotoninergic 5-Hydroxytryptamine A receptor (5-HT₄R) Antibodies

The search for new cardiac targets led investigators[53] to examine whether anti-Ro52 antibodies cross-react with 5-HT$_4$R, which is present in human atrium, including the fetus, and may be important in atrial arrhythmias and fetal cardiac development.[54,55] It was found that two peptides in the C terminus of Ro52—aa365-382 and aa380-396—shared some similarity with the 5-HT$_4$R. Furthermore, the Ro52 365-382 peptide, recognized by sera from patients with SLE, cross-reacted with peptide aa165-185, derived from the second extracellular loop of the 5-HT$_4$R.[53] However, when sera from mothers of children with CHB were examined for the presence of anti-5-HT$_4$R antibodies, they were found only in a minority of the sera, suggesting that these antibodies are not necessary for the development of the CHB in the majority of patients.[56,57]

Anticalreticulin Antibodies

Calreticulin, a calcium-binding protein that is important in cardiac development, was initially thought to be part a Ro protein. However, later studies showed that calreticulin is not a part of the RoRNP although antibodies directed against calreticulin are present in the sera from patients with autoimmune diseases.[58-65] Elevated anticalreticulin antibody levels have been reported in mothers of children with NLE compared with levels in healthy subjects but not when compared with healthy pregnant women.[66] Currently, it is felt that anticalreticulin antibodies are not important in NLE.

Other Autoantibodies

Other antigens present on the fetal heart or placenta have been suggested to be important in the development of, or protection from, atrioventricular (AV) block. Specifically, anti-La, anti-calreticulin, and anti–ERV-3 antibodies can bind to the placenta or placental trophoblast or both. A subset of anti-La antibodies cross-react with laminin (present in the placenta).[67-73] Binding of these autoantibodies to placental tissue may alter the autoantibody repertoire in the fetal circulation and therefore affect binding to fetal tissue. Laminin, calreticulin, or ERV-3 may be targets for maternal autoantibodies, and direct binding to these fetal cardiac proteins may initiate or potentiate inflammation in the fetal heart.[68-70,73] Anti-laminin autoantibodies bind to fetal but not adult heart and cardiac tissue, and ERV-3 and laminin are maximally expressed between 11 and 17 weeks' gestation.[68-70,73]

Two other autoantibodies examined in NLE and CHB were anti-p57 recombinant protein and anti–α-fodrin antibodies. Anti-p57 antibodies were present in one third of sera of mothers of children with NLE, but were almost always associated with anti-Ro antibodies and did not add to sensitivity and specificity testing.[74] Anti–α-fodrin antibodies, present in sera from patients with Sjögren syndrome (SS),[75-77] were demonstrated to be present in the sera of mothers of children with NLE; however, measurement of these antibodies has not been pursued as they do not add to the sensitivity or specificity of autoantibody testing over routine anti-Ro and anti-La antibody testing.[78]

GENETIC BACKGROUND

Maternal Genetics

As early as 1980 it was recognized that human leukocyte antigen (HLA)-DR and HLA-DQ genes were important in the production of anti-Ro/La antibodies.[79,80] DR3 was shown be associated with anti-Ro52 and anti-La48, but not anti-Ro60 antibodies.[81,82] This association

was present in most ethnic backgrounds and differed between patients with primary SS and SLE.[83-89] Further assessment showed that high-titer anti-Ro52 antibodies were associated with the DQw1/DQw2 heterozygote state.[90,91] It is likely that extended haplotypes are more important than single loci in determining production of anti-Ro/La antibodies. In patients of most ethnic backgrounds, high levels of anti-Ro60 and anti-La48 antibodies were associated with all, or at least most, of the DRB1*0301, DQA1*0501, and DQB1*0201 extended haplotypes. If the extended haplotype was not present, then the DQA1*0501 allele was frequently found.[80,90,92] Glutamine at position 34 of DQA1 and leucine at position 26 of DQB1 were shown to be associated with anti-Ro60/La antibodies, although the extended haplotype (in linkage disequilibrium) still had the strongest correlation.[80,93] The genetic control of this response is further complicated by the demonstration that response to individual peptides may be under different genetic control distinct from that found for the response to the whole protein.[94]

In mothers of children with NLE, the HLA profile more closely resembled that present in patients with primary SS than with SLE.[95-98] In Japanese mothers, the production of anti-Ro/La antibodies was associated with the extended haplotypes DRB1*1101-DQA1*0501-DQB1*0301 and DRB1*08032-DQA1*0103-DQB1*0601, as well as the individual alleles DRB1*1101, DRB1*08032, and DQB1*0301.[97] All of the anti-Ro/La antibody–positive mothers had DRB1 alleles that shared the same amino acid residues at positions 14-31 and 71 of DRB1 and were either homozygous or heterozygous at DQ6 and DQ3 alleles that shared the same amino acid residues at positions 27-36 and 71-77 of the hypervariable regions of DQB1.[96] Individual manifestations of NLE may also be influenced by maternal HLA, as DRB1*1101-DQA1*0501-DQB1*0301 (DR5 haplotype) and individual class II alleles making up this haplotype, including DQA1 alleles with glutamine at position 34 of the first domain, were significantly associated with C-NLE but not CHB. DQB1*0602 (carried on DR2 haplotypes) was associated with CHB but not C-NLE.[95,97] Studies in other racial or ethnic backgrounds also have supported a role for maternal HLA-DRB and DQ alleles in the predisposition to deliver a child with NLE, although the alleles differed between ethnicities.[98-101] A few studies have suggested that maternal major HLA class I haplotypes may predispose the delivery of child with CHB.[98,100,102] A review of HLA-DRB1, HLA-DQA1, and HLA-DQB1 loci in Japanese and Caucasian children with CHB showed that these alleles were frequently identical to those in their mothers.[103] However, the specific alleles differed between ethnicities.

In the current genome-wide association study (GWAS) era, a GWAS of children of European ancestry showed that the majority of loci with the most significant associations with cardiac NLE were within the HLA region. However, no individual locus previously implicated in autoimmune diseases achieved genome-wide significance.[104] The finding of the association of cardiac NLE and fetal genes in the HLA region was confirmed in a second study (also of European heritage).[105] Using a family-based approach, these latter authors showed that HLA-DRB1*04 and HLA-Cw*05 variants were transmitted significantly more often to affected individuals, and HLA-DRB1*13 and HLA-Cw*06 variants were transmitted significantly less often to affected children.[105]

GENETICS OF CHILDREN WITH NLE

Despite the strong association of maternal HLA antigens, the association of HLA genes in the offspring is weaker.[99,106-109] Two small studies demonstrated that children with NLE tended to have the same DRB, DQA, and DQB genes as their mothers.[95,108] One report suggested that

DR3 (DRB1*03) in the fetus might protect against *in utero* death,[108] whereas another suggested that DR2 may be protective (associated with maternal DR2-DRB1*02).[101] A large cohort of children with NLE demonstrated that DQB and DRB genes were important in NLE.[110]

Multiple genes outside the major histocompatibility complex (MHC) locus that alter the immune response can influence the onset, susceptibility, and progression of autoimmune diseases.[111-114] The same is likely true in NLE, particularly with regard to amplifying the pathological cascade to scar (e.g., amplification of apoptosis, uptake of opsonized cardiocytes, and ultimately fibrosis). Support for the importance of non-MHC genes in the offspring is suggested by the observation that children with NLE were more likely to have a tumor necrosis factor-α (TNF-α) polymorphism associated with high TNF-α production.[110,115] A tumor growth factor-β (TGF-β) gene polymorphism associated with increased TGF-β production was higher in children with CHB than controls although it did not differ between children with CHB and C-NLE.[115]

A multiethnic cohort showed significantly higher case fatality rates in non-whites affected by CHB compared with whites, and whites were at a lower risk of fetal hydrops and endocardial fibroelastosis (EFE).[116] It is not clear whether the difference in outcomes is the result of maternal or fetal genetics, environment or socioeconomic factors. Further studies are required to confirm these findings and to help determine the factors leading to these observations.

OTHER GENETIC CONTRIBUTIONS

An observation in 1992 suggested that fathers of children with NLE were more likely to carry C4 null alleles than the controls.[117] The only reported study to show a paternal contribution to NLE demonstrated that there may be an increased paternal (but not maternal) HLA-DRB1*04 transmission to offspring with CHB than to unaffected siblings.[105] An interesting observation was enriched transmission of the maternal risk alleles of TNF-α and C6orf10 (Refs. 104, 110, 115) from grandmothers of children with NLE to the mothers of the children with NLE[118]; the significance is unknown.

All of the genetic studies suggest that maternal, paternal, and fetal HLA genes, and fetal non-HLA genes may be important factors that influence the development of NLE. However, all studies are of relatively small size and cannot explain the observation that monozygotic twins are frequently discordant for NLE. In addition, there is a lack of validation cohorts.

CLINICAL FEATURES

Cardiac NLE

The most clinically significant manifestations of NLE are cardiac, specifically CHB. In most cases, the CHB is isolated, but it may be associated with other cardiac lesions, including ventricular septal defect or patent ductus arteriosus. The first reported case of CHB associated with maternal autoimmune disease (i.e., Mikulicz syndrome or SS) was published in 1901.[119] However, it was not until the 1950s that it was generally recognized that autoantibodies in the mother were associated with NLE. It was another 20 to 30 years until the association with anti-Ro and anti-La antibodies was reported.[34,35,38,40,120] Children with cardiac NLE can have first-, second-, or third-degree HB. The HB may be isolated or associated with myocarditis and/or EFE. Myocarditis and EFE associated with NLE can be seen in the absence of conduction abnormalities.

It has been estimated that CHB occurs in approximately 1 in 14,000 live births,[121,122] of which at least 90% of the fetal and neonatal cases, with otherwise structurally normal hearts (isolated CHB), are related to the transplacental passage of maternal autoantibodies. These estimates are based on live births and likely underestimate the true incidence of congenital CHB, as they were performed at a time when fetal echocardiography was not available and more severe fetal cardiac NLE commonly resulted in intrauterine death.[38,40,122-128] Most cases of CHB occur in fetuses of mothers without a diagnosed autoimmune disease. The initial demonstration of autoantibodies in these mothers is during pregnancy or after delivery of a child with NLE. It remains a matter of debate and ongoing research why only some and not all anti-Ro antibody–exposed fetuses acquire cardiac NLE. In prospectively examined pregnancies of mothers with anti-Ro antibodies and a known autoimmune disease, the reported incidence of fetal CHB was approximately 1% to 2%, which increased to approximately 15% for those with a previously affected child with CHB.[129-132] Recent research suggests that the fetal exposure to high-titer anti-Ro antibodies, rather than the presence of these antibodies, is a requirement for the development of fetal cardiac NLE.[39]

Etiology and Pathology of Cardiac NLE

The characteristic pathology of CHB is an absence or a degeneration of the AV node with replacement by fibrosis, calcification, or fatty tissue (Fig. 25-1).[120,133-135] The latter lesion is present in more than 80% of cases of CHB and is associated with maternal anti-Ro/La antibodies, whereas the absence of the AV node without scarring is likely a congenital dysplasia of the conducting system and not associated with maternal autoantibodies.[135,136] We will focus on autoantibody-associated CHB.

In most autopsy cases of CHB there is not only evidence of degeneration of the AV node with replacement by fibrosis and calcification, but also an inflammatory cell infiltrate. Studies have shown a generalized myocardial inflammation with evidence of deposition immunoglobulin G (IgG), complement, and fibrin deposition on the fetal myocardium.[120,137-139] As the fetus is unable to produce IgG, the demonstration of IgG on fetal myocardium implicates maternally derived autoantibodies as an important factor in the fetal pathology. One group was able to elute anti-Ro52 antibodies from the fetal heart, but not unaffected tissue of a fetus that died of CHB, which further implicated maternally derived autoantibodies in the pathogenesis of NLE.[140] Lastly, maternal cells have been found in fetal hearts with CHB.[141] Therefore the transplacental passage of IgG, and possibly maternal lymphocytes, is critical in initiating inflammation leading to CHB. However, it is likely that the fetal immune response to the maternally derived IgG present on the myocardium is important.

The inflammatory infiltrate can be extensive and frequently involves the more distal conducting system and other areas of the heart, including extensive scarring of the atrium and ventricles, and EFE.[137-139] EFE, in association with an inflammatory infiltrate and maternal autoantibodies, has been found without CHB, suggesting that the primary target may be the myocardium and not the specialized conducting tissue.[142,143] Immunohistological evaluation of hearts from fetuses that died with CHB has revealed increased apoptosis, macrophages in zones of fibrosis that colocalize with IgG and apoptotic cells, expression of TNF-α and TGF-β messenger RNA (mRNA) in these cells, and extensive collagen deposition in the conducting system.[115] All of these findings are consistent with an inflammatory response initiated by maternal IgG and expanded by the fetal immune response.

The maternal component is the autoantibody that, by binding to its cognate antigen, initiates the first step to injury. It is logical to hypothesize that the target is a cardiac protein containing either a cross-reactive epitope recognized by anti-Ro/La antibodies or an epitope within the Ro protein itself. Ro itself is intracellular, and therefore either the antibody must be internalized before binding or Ro

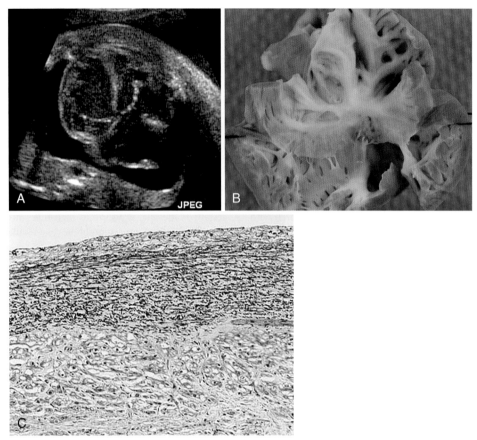

FIGURE 25-1 A, Echocardiographic images of a fetus who presented at 33 weeks with CHB, hydrops fetalis, and a fetal heart rate of 51 beats per minute. The baby was delivered at 35 weeks after the mother went into labor. Care was withdrawn as there was evidence of abnormal brain function. There is some brightness of the papillary muscles but otherwise the myocardium appeared healthy. **B,** Heart at postmortem of the right ventricle at 35 weeks' gestation of the fetus from **A.** There was extensive endocardial fibroelastosis involving both right (shown) and left (not shown) ventricles. **C,** Histological examination of the same heart as in **B.** There is extensive histological evidence of endocardial fibroelastosis with disruption of the normal myocardium.

must be present on, or translocated to, the cell surface. However, a direct pathological consequence to cells by inhibiting function would predict an even higher recurrence rate of CHB in subsequent pregnancies than that observed unless the repertoire changes over time. What is accepted is that without this maternal component, CHB would not ensue, and even the presence of high-titer anti-Ro antibodies is not sufficient.[39] Attempts to generate a robust reproducible animal model exploiting the potential pathogenicity of the antibody as an isolated factor have not met with success. Therefore the exact nature of the maternal component remains unresolved.

A role for the fetal immune response is based on the clinical observations that the rate of recurrence of CHB is 15% to 17% in pregnancies that occur after the birth of a child with CHB[131,144] and that most studies of twins (and triplets) born to a mother with anti-Ro antibodies are discordant for NLE/CHB.[145-149] Histological examination of the fetal heart has shown that in addition to IgG, there is evidence of IgM deposition (unable to cross the placenta) and a T-cell infiltrate.[137,142] These autopsy observations support a role for a fetal component, and therefore differences in fetal response to the maternally derived IgG may be part of the explanation for discordant twins and the low recurrence rate.

Recent studies have demonstrated areas of apoptosis of cardiac myocytes.[142,150] Physiological clearance of apoptotic cardiocytes by resident cardiocytes may be inhibited by maternal autoantibodies, resulting in accumulation of apoptotic cells, inflammation via the production of proinflammatory cytokines, and then scarring.[115,151,152] Many of the cardiocytes had a myofibroblast-like phenotype suggesting that these cells were activated and involved in inducing (or perpetuating) the damage.[150] It is difficult to directly implicate the pathogenic effect of autoantibodies in CHB as not only is the injury an infrequent event but the extent of injury varies among fetuses. Accordingly, CHB is likely to represent the sum of several maternal and fetal components.

These *in vivo* observations are supported by *in vitro* studies. The link between maternal autoantibodies and tissue injury is supported by the demonstration that apoptosis of fetal cardiocytes leads to expression of Ro/La on the cell surface.[153] It was then shown that cardiac cells can phagocytose autologous apoptotic cardiocytes, and anti-Ro antibodies inhibit the ability of these cells to perform this clearance function.[151] Therefore the potential perturbation of the normal remodeling of the developing heart by the presence of anti-Ro antibodies would allow for the uptake of these apoptotic cells by professional phagocytes (including macrophages). *In vitro* studies have shown that macrophages, when coincubated with apoptotic cardiocytes bound by Ro/La antibodies, can secrete proinflammatory and fibrosing cytokines, which could then lead to cardiac damage rather than remodeling.[115,151] Murine studies showed that anti-Ro/La antibodies inhibited the clearance of apoptotic cardiocytes, allowing them to accumulate and thereby leading to an inflammatory reaction and scarring.[152] Studies using human fetal myocytes have shown that the complex of autoantibodies with apoptotic cardiomyocytes leads to transdifferentiation of these cells to a myofibroblast phenotype and the production of the profibrotic cytokine, TGF-β.[154]

The above-mentioned studies have demonstrated that intracellular Ro60, Ro52, and La48 can be translocated to the cell surface and become a target for autoantibodies. An alternative hypothesis has suggested that molecules constitutively present on the surface of cardiac tissue may be the target, and by binding to these antigens the autoantibodies perturb cardiac function. Cardiac calcium channels are present on the cell surface, and based on their importance in conduction, are obvious potential candidate targets. An overview of studies of *in vitro* and *in vivo* data of the targets of maternal autoantibodies in the pathogenesis of NLE is in the "Animal Models" section.

It is logical to assume that there are both fetal and maternal factors that are important in the development of NLE and CHB. In fact, there is increasing evidence of a genetic contribution to the risk, disease pattern, and outcome of NLE (as previous). Lastly, the fact that identical twins are more often discordant than concordant for CHB suggests an environmental factor present *in utero* might be a third factor. Environmental factors would be expected to amplify the injury in susceptible fetuses exposed to the transplacental passage of potentially pathogenic maternal antibodies.

Clinical Approach to CHB, Surveillance of At-Risk Pregnancy, and Treatment of HB

Outcome of cardiac NLE. Risk factors identified to be significantly associated with perinatal death include fetal hydrops; ventricular rates of fewer than 50 to 55 beats per minute; impaired cardiac function/carditis/EFE/cardiomyopathy; and an earlier gestational age at CHB diagnosis.[116,127,155-157] Most children with CHB require a permanent pacemaker during childhood and thus will carry lifelong risks for pacemaker-related morbidity and mortality.[116,128,156,157] In addition, approximately 5% to 10% of children with CHB and normal cardiac function at birth will develop a dilated cardiomyopathy and/or EFE and cardiac death during childhood.[129,158-160] Of note, the experience of five U.S. and Canadian centers demonstrated that the perinatal use of intravenous immunoglobulin (IVIG) and dexamethasone was associated with improved survival of patients affected by EFE and a lower rate of late-onset cardiomyopathy as compared with untreated patients.[161]

Management of cardiac NLE. While there is agreement that immune-mediated complications represent a spectrum of potentially life-threatening cardiac anomalies there is no consensus on the optimal perinatal management of cardiac NLE, at least in part as a result of the absence of evidence from randomized clinical trials.

Pregnancy management options range from no prenatal therapy; therapy targeting the most severely affected fetuses, e.g., with fetal hydrops and/or EFE; to the routine use of antiinflammatory therapy in fetuses with CHB. The rationale for therapy is based on the evidence that CHB carries a significant mortality risk as the fetus needs to overcome the sudden drop in ventricular rate, the loss of normal atrial systolic contribution to ventricular filling, and maternal antibody-triggered myocardial inflammation and/or fibrosis. Although the standard, echocardiography tends to underappreciate the true extent and severity of the cardiac pathology.[139] The reason to treat a fetus with CHB is not to reestablish normal AV conduction but to improve outcome by mitigating cardiac inflammation and damage, and by increasing fetal cardiac output. The fluorinated

steroids dexamethasone and betamethasone, unlike prednisone, are only minimally metabolized by the placenta and pass to the fetus, making them useful in treating fetal inflammation. Dexamethasone is often preferred as it is a single oral daily dose. Repeated transplacental steroid administration has been shown to improve or resolve incomplete fetal AV block, myocardial dysfunction, and pericardial effusions.[162-166]

Concerns with the use of steroids to the fetus are related to neurological development,[167,168] growth retardation, and oligohydramnios.[169] These concerns are based mainly on animal studies. In humans, neuroimaging showed that multiple administration of dexamethasone before birth was associated with decreased cortical involution and brain surface area although the clinical significance was not reported.[170,171] However, follow-up studies showed that by early to mid-childhood fetal exposure to fluorinated steroids had no effect on growth,[172,173] or neurological or psychological development.[174-177] Oligohydramnios resolves with either a reduction in the steroid or temporarily holding the medication. It was shown that roughly a quarter of children with CHB who were treated prenatally with dexamethasone were born with mild growth restriction, but there was catch-up postnatal growth.[178] It is important to note that children with CHB, irrespective of prenatal therapy, had low weight until about 2 to 3 years of age and reached reference standards only at age 9 to 11 years of age.[179,180] A study on neurodevelopment that reviewed that 16% of siblings with (n = 60) and without (n = 54) CHB born to anti-Ro antibody–positive mothers had impaired neurodevelopment at age 13 years.[179] No negative effects on intelligence or neurodevelopment were found in two studies that examined cohorts of preschool- and/or school-age children with CHB who had been prenatally exposed to maternal anti-Ro antibodies with and without prolonged dexamethasone treatment.[181,182]

Potential maternal glucocorticoid side effects include an increased susceptibility to infections, mood changes, weight gain, fluid retention, arterial hypertension, glucose intolerance, insomnia, hirsutism, striae, impaired wound healing, stomach irritation, headache, and, rarely, psychosis. A review of adverse effects associated with the use of antenatal steroids included oligohydramnios in 12% of pregnancies, maternal hypertension in 5%, insulin-dependent diabetes in 2%, and insomnia or mood changes in 7%.[178] However, there was no control group of untreated CHB pregnancies.

The currently used dose of dexamethasone to treat cardiac NLE results in a daily fetal dexamethasone exposure that does not exceed 0.05 mg/kg (maximal 8 mg/day maternal dosage and a cord-to-maternal drug ratio of 30%). This treatment may be maintained over many weeks with tapering at the time of delivery. Significantly higher steroid dosages over a shorter period of time were used in animal studies, for prenatal human pulmonary maturation, and for the treatment of respiratory distress syndrome in premature newborns.

β_1-Adrenergic stimulation with the bronchodilators salbutamol and terbutaline may be used to increase the fetal cardiac output by a change in heart rate and a decrease in systemic vascular resistance.[183,184] The indications of chronic transplacental fetal β-adrenergic therapy are a fetal heart rate fewer than 50 beats per minute and/or significantly reduced cardiac contractility.[169] When given orally to the mother, salbutamol (10 mg every 8 hours to a maximum dosage of 40 mg/day) or terbutaline (2.5 to 7.5 mg every 4 to 6 hours to a maximum dosage of 30 mg/day) typically increased the ventricular rate by 5 to 10 beats per minute.[169,185] Side effects include tremor, palpitations, and sweating, which usually improve or resolve with continuation of therapy. More serious maternal adverse events or intolerable symptoms that required a change in drug treatment have not been reported with oral β-adrenergic stimulation. Nevertheless, β-agonists should be used cautiously in mothers with diabetes, hypertension, hyperthyroidism, and a history of seizures or tachyarrhythmias.

The last modality of therapy advocated by some investigators is the repeated use of IVIG as an adjunct to transplacental steroid treatment, particularly if there is evidence of myocardial inflammation and fibrosis. The prognosis for fetuses and infants with diffuse EFE is poor, with death or need for cardiac transplant in 85% of infants.[137,142,159] In a retrospective review from four centers of 20 fetuses with EFE, perinatal use of both IVIG and dexamethasone was associated with an overall survival rate of 80%, all with normal systolic function.[161] It is not clear whether it was the combination of both therapies or either one individually that was associated with this outcome as IVIG alone was not tried, whereas dexamethasone alone has been associated with improved fetal outcome. It has been proposed that IVIG blocks either the transplacental passage of maternal autoantibody and/or the binding of these autoantibodies to the fetal heart.[186] This would result in decreased macrophages or T cells with decreased cytokine production and complement activation, leading to a reduction in myocardial damage. Immunomodulatory treatment with IVIG is usually well tolerated, but both the mother and fetus carry potential risks associated with the exposure to blood products. The benefit of the use of IVIG is not proven.

The guidelines used in Toronto include the routine initiation of oral dexamethasone therapy at the time of diagnosis of CHB (after confirmation of the presence of maternal anti-Ro antibodies) and maintained for the duration of the pregnancy. If the average fetal heart rate declines below 50 to 55 beats per minute or if the cardiac function is reduced, a β-adrenergic agent is added. Pregnancies are monitored weekly by a team that includes obstetrics, fetal cardiology, and rheumatology. Delivery, usually by cesarean section, is arranged between 37 and 38 weeks' gestation with transfer to the intensive care unit for neonatal care. A study from two Canadian centers using these guidelines showed significant improvement in outcomes of fetal CHB as compared to pregnancies followed in these centers prior to the routine use (beginning in 1997) of the guidelines.[169] Prior to 1997, pregnancies with isolated CHB were typically followed by serial echocardiography without transplacental fetal therapy. Live birth and 1-year survival of fetuses diagnosed between 1990 and 1997 were 80% and 47%, respectively, and improved to 95% for both between 1997 and 2003. Immune-mediated conditions that caused postnatal death or required cardiac transplantation were only observed in fetal survivors of untreated pregnancies. These findings suggest that prolonged administration of dexamethasone rendered a fetus with isolated CHB less likely to develop myocarditis, cardiomyopathy, and/or hydrops fetalis, thus improving overall outcome.

The treatment guidelines used in Toronto were adjusted in recent years to minimize the risk of oligohydramnios.[178] Dexamethasone is started at 8 mg/day then reduced to 4 mg/day after 2 weeks, and then to 2 mg/day at 28 to 30 weeks' gestation in uncomplicated cases. Maternal IVIG (70 g every 2 to 3 weeks) is added if significant EFE is detected. The experience of five U.S. and Canadian centers, including Toronto, that used the contemporary routine prenatal treatment approach demonstrated survival rates to birth and to 10 years of age were 98% and 91%, respectively, for 88 prenatally treated CHB cases. Only 1.1% developed a late-onset dilated cardiomyopathy as compared to historic rates of 10% to 15%. These survival rates compare favorably to the lower survival rates in studies that used no prenatal treatment strategies or targeted ones.[116,157,187]

However, many centers do not advocate the use of any maternal therapy, fluorinated steroids, and/or IVIG for fetuses with CHB. The rationale for nontreatment includes (a) a significant proportion of fetuses with uncomplicated isolated CHB will survive without

antiinflammatory treatment; (b) the potential risks to the fetus and mother, as described above; and (c) the lack of prospective randomized studies that indicate the beneficial effect of treatment.

Prevention of CHB. Most cases of cardiac NLE are diagnosed *in utero* in pregnant women without a history of an autoimmune disease. Unfortunately, at this point, the AV node is usually already irreversibly damaged and replaced by fibrotic scar tissue; antiinflammatory treatment may not restore the fetal AV conduction. However, CHB may be preventable if the disease process is either abolished with preventive therapy (primary prevention) or is detected and treated at an early stage of AV nodal disease (secondary prevention). Strategies used for primary prevention CHB have included prophylactic therapy with plasmapheresis, corticosteroids, and/or IVIG.[188-192] Most researchers do not advocate primary prevention.

Two large, controlled trials of anti-Ro antibody–positive mothers who had previously delivered a child with NLE failed to show a benefit of primary prevention with IVIG.[193,194] In both studies mothers received IVIG at a dosage of 400 mg/kg/dose every 3 weeks from 12 to 24 weeks' gestation. In one study 3 of 15 fetuses developed CHB as compared to 1 of 7 mothers who refused IVIG,[194] whereas in the other study 3 of 19 fetuses developed CHB (all mothers received IVIG).[193] IVIG was well tolerated, but there was no benefit as compared to the predicted 15% to 17% rate of CHB (historic controls). Primary prevention with fluorinated steroids has not been prospectively examined in large numbers of patients.

Most recently interest has focused on the potential beneficial effects of maternal use of antimalarials in decreasing the risk of delivering a child with CHB. The rationale for examining the use of these medications is based on the demonstration that (1) Ro60 can bind to single-stranded RNA (ssRNA), leading to Ro60-associated ssRNA complexes that can activate signaling through Toll-like receptor 7 (TLR7), and activation of TLR7 can lead to fibrosis[195]; and (2) that one of the mechanisms of action of hydroxychloroquine (HCQ) is to inhibit activation of intracellular TLRs, including TLR7.[196] The hypothesis therefore was that Ro60-associated ssRNA complexes lead to abnormal TLR signaling and that maternal use of antimalarial medications, drugs that are known to cross the placenta, would decrease or prevent this signaling and therefore decrease the risk of scarring and CHB. A case-control multicenter study showed that 14% of mothers of fetuses with cardiac involvement used HCQ throughout the pregnancy as compared to 37% of mothers of fetuses without cardiac involvement, thereby giving an odds ratio of 0.46 (95% confidence interval [CI] 0.18-1.18; $P = 0.10$) that HCQ was protective.[197] A second international study examining infants born to mothers with a history of delivering a child with CHB, showed that maternal use of HCQ throughout pregnancy may protect subsequent pregnancies from the development of CHB (odds ratio 0.23; 95% CI 0.06-0.92; $P = 0.037$).[198] The most recent study using Bayesian analysis was a single-center inception cohort study that showed that the probability that antimalarial use was associated with a decreased of the development of CHB was greater than 99%.

Secondary CHB prevention refers to treatment early during the process prior to CHB. It requires that antibody-mediated CHB is the result of progression from first- and/or second-degree AV block to complete AV block rather than the sudden appearance of CHB directly from normal sinus rhythm. In addition, when the abnormality is detected, it must be reversible with treatment. The current evidence suggests that when incomplete HB is detected, treatment with steroids may prevent progression or lead to reversal. However, the diagnosis of incomplete AV block is rare, with fewer than 50 reported cases in the medical literature.[166,199-203] Importantly, progression from first- to third-degree AV block has not been documented in the literature, including in patients who were entered in studies with weekly fetal echocardiograms and within days of a fetal echocardiogram with normal rhythm and no evidence of inflammation.[202] The reason for these observations may be that CHB may develop too fast (within 1 day), progression is not staged, early stages are overlooked, or early treatment of the few suspected cases with first-degree AV block has prevented progression. If the earliest manifestation of evolving AV nodal disease is clinically silent prolongation in AV conduction (first-degree HB), one would predict that a fetal electrocardiogram (ECG), fetal magnetocardiogram (MCG), or fetal echocardiography would be able to demonstrate a first-degree block prior to the emergence of sustained fetal bradycardia. With this concept in mind, many centers have been offering serial echocardiographic assessment of the fetal AV conduction during the period of highest risk of HB (weeks 18 to 24 of gestation) as a strategy to prevent CHB.

Although likely the most sensitive tools to detect early conduction abnormalities, for various reasons, fetal ECG and fetal MCG are available only in very few centers and are predominantly used as research tools.[200,204-208] Alternatively, M-mode, pulse-wave, and tissue Doppler echocardiographic techniques have been used to study the chronology of atrial and ventricular electrical events indirectly by their respective mechanical consequences.[206,209-212] In particular, pulsed Doppler techniques have been found clinically useful to measure mechanical AV time intervals. It is, however, important to realize that reference values differ among modalities, and AV times physiologically prolong with gestational age.[206,213] There have been four large prospective clinical studies that examined the feasibility and utility of serial fetal echocardiographic assessment of antibody-exposed fetuses to detect early, potentially treatable AV conduction disease.[199,202,203,214] While studies demonstrated the feasibility of Doppler-derived AV time measurements, there remains significant controversy about the optimal fetal cardiac surveillance strategy, the clinical relevance of AV prolongation as predictor of emerging CHB, and the indications for *in utero* treatment. An important observation was that most serially followed fetuses had completely normal AV time intervals prior to the detection of CHB, although other findings suggestive of cardiac NLE (tricuspid regurgitation, atrial echodensity, pericardial effusion) were present in some of the fetuses.[199,202,214] These observations suggest that CHB likely results from a rapidly evolving inflammatory process that may not necessarily manifest as a brief episode of incomplete AV block.

Currently there is significant controversy regarding the clinical relevance of AV prolongation, as defined by greater than 2 to 3 standard deviations for gestational age-matched controls, because in most studies this was a relatively frequent observation. In the earliest study, AV intervals were studied in 24 anti-Ro/La antibody–positive women between 18 and 24 weeks' gestation in comparison with 284 pregnant women as controls. The authors found 8 of 24, or 33%, of the autoantibody-associated pregnancies were complicated by statistical prolongation of the AV times.[199] It is important to note, however, that the AV prolongation was transient in all but two of eight pregnancies: one fetus progressed from a borderline prolonged AV interval (140 ms) to CHB within 6 days; the other fetus had second-degree block that reversed to first degree after dexamethasone therapy. The three more recent prospective studies reported AV prolongation with a greater than 2 z-scores in 9% and greater than 3 z-scores in 2% of serially assessed antibody-exposed fetuses.[202,203,214] AV prolongation up to 6 z-scores resolved in all cases regardless of maternal steroid use.[202,203,214] However, to date, in the few cases with first-degree AV block with AV prolongation greater than 90 ms (6 z-scores), all persisted despite steroids.[39,200,215]

In summary, in pregnancies exposed to anti-Ro antibodies, the fetal echocardiographic Doppler finding of the mechanical heart rate (HR) interval prolongation may serve as a surrogate marker of subclinical disease. The two critical issues raised are (1) the clinical significance of a prolonged AV interval and (2) the biological implication with regard to tissue injury. An isolated prolongation of the AV interval may be transient (related to vagal tone or medication use) or reversible injury, or it may be permanent or progress to more marked delay as a result of physical injury to the specialized electrical pathway (e.g., because of inflammation or scarring). It may be that AV prolongation represents a variant of normal, and only in retrospect does it have clinical significance if it progresses to more advanced block. Given the identification of cases with new CHB and severe cardiomyopathy within 1 week of a normal echocardiogram, with the most frequent detection time being between 20 and 24 weeks' gestation, it would seem appropriate to perform weekly or even shorter monitoring intervals between 18 and 24 weeks. The goal of this monitoring would be to identify a biomarker of reversible injury, such as AV interval prolongation, and myocardial echodensity. The task of identifying a biomarker of reversibility is particularly important as dexamethasone and betamethasone may have both maternal and fetal risks. Based on available evidence, the Toronto group currently limits the use of preventive transplacental treatment to those fetuses that either present with AV intervals that have greater than 6 z-scores, with second-degree AV block in association with persistent AV prolongation, or with additional signs of suggestive of cardiac inflammation and tissue damage, such as EFE, effusions, and sudden onset of valvular regurgitation. The potential drawback of this less aggressive approach is that if subtle prolongation of the AV interval does represent tissue injury, untreated CHB might evolve too rapidly in some fetuses and will go unnoticed by weekly screening.

Risk of delivery of a child with CHB. While it is clear that children with NLE are born to mother with anti-Ro/La antibodies, it is important to estimate the risk of delivering a child with NLE from mothers with a rheumatic disease and from mothers who have previously delivered a child with NLE. Large series of pregnancies in women with SLE who had anti-Ro/La antibodies have suggested that the risk of delivering a child with NLE varied between 1% and 10%.[216-218] The most recent, and larger, prospective studies have suggested that the risk of delivering a child with NLE in mothers with anti-Ro and/or anti-La antibodies was 1% to 2%.[39,130,131,219] Large, prospective studies suggest that the risk of delivery of a child with CHB following the delivery of a child with CHB or C-NLE is approximately 15% to 17%.[39,193,194]

Cutaneous Neonatal Lupus Erythematosus

The rash of C-NLE was first reported in 1954 in a child born to a mother with an autoimmune disease.[220] It was not until 1981 that the association of C-NLE and maternal anti-Ro antibodies was described.[221] Similar to mothers of children with CHB, mothers of children with C-NLE are usually clinically healthy despite the presence of circulating anti-Ro/La antibodies. It is likely that a rash is present in 15% to 25% of children with NLE,[222] although it is difficult to determine the true percentage because the rash can be easily missed and spontaneously resolves. There is a female predominance with a female-to-male ratio of 2 : 1 to 3 : 1.[223] The reason for the increased female incidence may be related to the fact that estrogens enhance surface expression of Ro and La proteins on keratinocytes. It should be noted, however, that in the Research Registry for Neonatal Lupus (RRNL) the female predominance was not as pronounced—55% were female and 45% were male.[224]

The photosensitive nature of the cutaneous lesions has led investigators to examine the effect of ultraviolet irradiation on keratinocyte

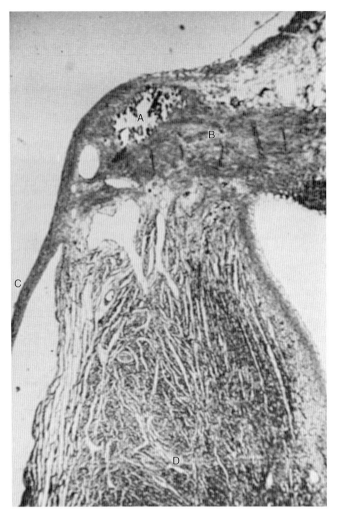

FIGURE 25-2 Section of ventricular septum from the fetus of a mother with systemic lupus erythematosus. The baby died at birth from nonimmune hydrops secondary to complete congenital heart block. (Courtesy Dr. J. Dimmick.)

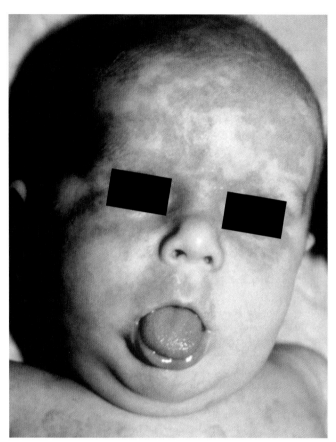

FIGURE 25-3 Neonatal lupus syndrome. This erythematous rash appeared a day after birth, accompanied by thrombocytopenia and leukopenia. (Courtesy Dr. D.C. Rada and T. Kestenbaum.)

surface expression of Ro/La proteins. Clinically, the rash more closely resembles the lesions of subacute cutaneous lupus erythematosus (SCLE) than the malar rash of SLE (Figs. 25-2, 25-3, and 25-4). Most patients with SCLE have anti-Ro60, anti-Ro52, and/or anti-La antibodies; the same antibodies are associated with NLE.[225,226] The rash of C-NLE is less frequently malar, and the lesions are not indurated[227,228]; follicular plugging or dermal atrophy, typical of discoid lupus erythematosus, is rare.[229] The rash may mimic Langerhans cell histiocytosis, resemble capillary malformations, present as targetoid lesions or bullous lesions.[230-233] The face and scalp are the most commonly involved areas, but the rash may occur at any site, including the palms and soles (Fig. 25-5).[228,234-236] Commonly, it develops around the eyes in a raccoonlike distribution (Fig. 25-6). The rash tends to consist of discrete, round, or elliptical plaques with a fine scale that has central clearing, and it tends to be papulosquamous (similar annular erythema).[235] An infant may have one or both of these rashes. In North America, papulosquamous lesions are most common, whereas in Japan, annular erythema is more common.[223,234,235] Bullous lesions may be seen, especially on the soles of the feet.[231] The rash may resemble cutis marmorata telangiectatica congenita, capillary malformation, bullous impetigo, primary herpes simplex infection, and erythema multiforme.[233,236-240]

The rash may be present at birth but more commonly develops within the first few weeks of life.[235] The most common age of appearance is 6 weeks, but it may not be recognized until as late as 12 weeks. New lesions may appear for several months, but they rarely develop beyond 6 months, consistent with the disappearance of maternal antibodies from the infant's circulation. The mean duration of the rash is 17 weeks. The lesions may be induced or exacerbated by sun exposure, but as the rash may be present at birth[241] and may occur on the soles of the feet and diaper area,[236,242] it is evident that sun exposure is not absolutely required for development of the rash. A rash that appears after phototherapy for neonatal jaundice has been reported, but it is uncommon.

The lesions of C-NLE are transient and usually resolve without scarring, although some mild atrophy may result. Cutaneous telangiectasias, beginning at 6 to 12 months, occur in approximately 10% of affected infants.[243-246] The telangiectasias may occur in areas that were not initially involved and therefore are not just the result of healing of the rash. The most common area for telangiectasias is the temple near the hairline, an area not usually affected by the acute lesion (Fig. 25-7). Telangiectasias tend to be bilateral. This lesion may be the presenting feature of C-NLE, although it is not clear in these instances whether the initial rash was missed or the telangiectasias had occurred *de novo*. There have been reports of telangiectasias with atrophy persisting into adolescence.[246,247]

Most mothers of infants with C-NLE are anti-Ro antibody positive, often in combination with anti-La antibodies. The percentage of mothers with elevated anti-Ro antibody levels depends on the assay used. A few cases of C-NLE have been reported in association with

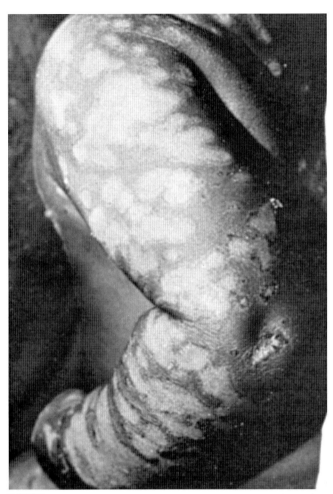

FIGURE 25-4 The rash on this baby is more discoid than the rash on the baby in Fig. 25-3. (Courtesy Dr. D. Kredich.)

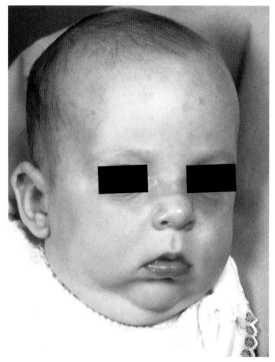

FIGURE 25-6 Rash in raccoon distribution: 4-month-old girl with the erythematous rash across the bridge of her nose, lower eyelids, and superior forehead. Her mother had high titers of anti-Ro antibody.

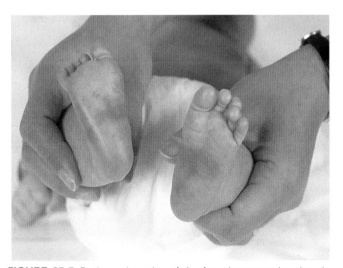

FIGURE 25-5 Rash on the soles of the feet demonstrating that the rash does not only occur in sun-exposed areas.

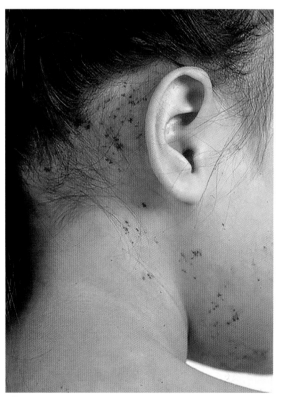

FIGURE 25-7 Three-year-old child with extensive telangiectasias behind her ear, on her chin, and in the temporal region. These lesions began at age 11 months, and she did not have the initial rash in any of these areas.

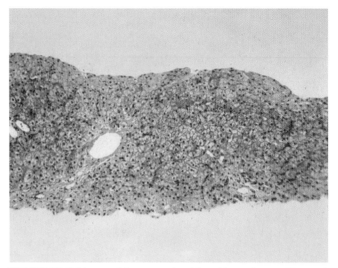

FIGURE 25-8 Mason-trichrome stain of liver biopsy from a 12-month-old child with persistently elevated liver enzymes. There is evidence of a mild inflammatory cell infiltrate and mild fibrosis around the portal tract (shown in green).

TABLE 25-1   Differential Diagnosis of the Rash of Cutaneous NLE

POLYCYCLIC LESION	ANNULAR ERYTHEMA
Urticaria	Erythema annulare centrifugum
Erythema marginatum	Familial annular erythema
Tinea corporis	Infantile epidermodysplastic erythema
Seborrheic dermatitis	Infection with *Pityrosporum*
Ichthyosiform genodermatosis	Annular erythema of infancy
	Erythema gyratum atrophicans

NLE, Neonatal lupus erythematosus.

antibodies to U1RNP in the absence of anti-Ro/La antibodies.[248-251] One infant with C-NLE had anti-U1RNP but not anti-Ro or anti-La antibodies when tested by ELISA but identified by immunoblot.[252]

Biopsies of the lesions of C-NLE demonstrate the typical histopathology of SCLE, which includes epidermal basal cell damage, a mild mononuclear cell dermal infiltrate, vacuolation of the basal layer, and epidermal colloid bodies. IgG, IgM, and complement are deposited usually at the dermoepidermal junction.[253-258] There have been rare reports of neutrophilic as well as lymphocytic infiltrates, as well as nuclear dust and extravasated red blood cells.[232]

Differential Diagnosis

The differential diagnosis of isolated C-NLE includes the other causes of annular and polycyclic lesions (Box 25-1; Table 25-1).

Treatment

The usual approach to management of C-NLE is reassurance and observation as the natural history of the skin lesions is spontaneous resolution without scarring; therefore aggressive treatment is not

indicated. However, topical application of a glucocorticoid cream may hasten the resolution of the lesions and be used for cosmetic reasons, although it is possible, but not proven, that steroid use increases the risk of developing telangiectasias. Some physicians have advocated the use of topical calcineurin inhibitors, but as in the instances of topical steroid use, there is no evidence that they alter the natural history or risk of telangiectasias. Telangiectasias can be treated with pulse dye laser therapy, although they may also spontaneously improve.[246]

Liver Disease

Hepatic dysfunction in NLE is characterized by abnormal levels of liver enzymes and hepatomegaly that were initially ascribed to congestive heart failure, intrauterine fetal hydrops, disseminated intravascular coagulation, or total parenteral nutrition. A large, unselected series demonstrated that liver involvement occurred in approximately 25% of all infants with NLE.[222] Liver disease can present as an isolated disorder or in association with other manifestations of NLE.[222,223,234,236,259] Usually, patients have mild hepatomegaly, with or without splenomegaly, and cholestasis with mildly to moderately elevated transaminase. Although a liver biopsy is usually not clinically indicated, histological abnormalities are similar to idiopathic neonatal giant cell hepatitis with mild bile duct obstruction, occasional giant cell transformation, and mild portal fibrosis (Fig. 25-8).[260-263] It is possible in this regard that idiopathic neonatal hepatitis may be another manifestation of NLE. Liver biopsies should be reserved for infants with clinical evidence of severe dysfunction or with persistent, moderate-to-severe dysfunction.

Liver function abnormalities usually resolve, although deaths secondary to hepatic failure before age 6 months have been reported.[259,264,265] There have not been any instances of late liver failure or cirrhosis.

Hematological Disease

Hematological manifestations occur in 25% to 30% of children with NLE. It has been reported that thrombocytopenia was the most common hematological manifestation, whereas anemia and neutropenia were less frequently present. However, we have found that the incidence and hematological manifestations present are dependent on the timing of the testing. Thrombocytopenia tends to occur within the first week of life, whereas neutropenia usually occurs between 2 and 6 weeks of age. Although uncommon, thrombocytopenia, anemia, neutropenia, and pancytopenia have been reported as isolated manifestations of NLE (NLE should be in the differential diagnosis of neonatal cytopenias). Antiplatelet antibodies are rare, suggesting that other factors may be responsible for the neonatal thrombocytopenia. The thrombocytopenia may be secondary to anti-Ro and/or anti-La antibodies as the Ro60 protein is present on platelets, and thrombocytopenia in SLE is associated with these autoantibodies in the absence of antiplatelet antibodies.[266-268] The neutropenia of NLE is likely secondary to binding of anti-Ro60 antibodies to a cross-reactive protein on the neutrophil membrane surface.[269,270]

There have been isolated reports of aplastic anemia and neonatal thrombosis associated with the transplacental passage of maternal autoantibodies.[271-274] The thrombocytopenia and other hematological manifestations tend to resolve over several weeks and, unless there is bleeding, do not require treatment. However, if the condition is severe or life-threatening, high-dose glucocorticoids or intravenous immunoglobulin may be necessary.

Neurological Involvement

Multiple neurological manifestations have been described. In 1994 two female siblings with C-NLE were reported to have communicating hydrocephalus.[275] Ventricular peritoneal (VP) shunting was performed. A prospective study of 10 children with other clinical features of NLE found one case of macrocephaly.[276] A prospective study of 87 consecutive infants born to mothers with anti-Ro/La antibodies found a significantly increased rate of macrocephaly and hydrocephalus (8%).[277] Only 1 of 7 patients with hydrocephalus was treated with a VP shunt. We have subsequently followed a child with significant hydrocephalus (ventricles enlarged by more than 12 standard deviations for age by ultrasound) who had resolution of the hydrocephalus by age 1 without a shunt, suggesting that a VP shunt is not required in these children. We suggest that measuring head circumferences should be part of the follow-up of children of mothers with anti-Ro/La antibodies.

A myelopathy with a gait abnormality and spastic paraparesis has been reported in two cases of infants with C-NLE.[278,279] The neurological disease became apparent in one child at the age of 1 year and in the other at age 16 months. Although it is possible that there was an undiagnosed intracerebral hemorrhage or infarction without clinical disease, there was no obvious cause other than the presence of anti-Ro antibodies. Similarly, seizures and nonspecific white matter lesions have been described that could not be attributable to any other cause than the transplacental passage of maternal autoantibodies.[280]

Three children with CHB found to have evidence of a vasculopathy in the area of the thalamus suggesting involvement of the gangliothalmic arteries by imaging studies.[281] The short-term follow-up revealed no signs of progression or neurological impairment. There has been one case report of an infant born with CHB who developed moyamoya disease at 17 years of age, and one case report of seizures and central nervous system vasculitis at age 2 months associated with maternally transmitted anti-Ro antibodies in the absence of other features of NLE.[282,283] The latter case was reported in two separate articles.[283,284] A single case of a hemorrhagic stroke in a 33-week-old infant with a platelet count of 66,000 and anti-Ro antibodies was reported.[285] The relationship of these cases to NLE and anti-Ro antibodies is not clear.

A study of 10 children with other clinical features of NLE demonstrated abnormal computed tomography (CT) scans and/or ultrasounds in 9. The CT abnormalities included decreased attenuation of the cerebral white matter, basal ganglia calcifications, ventriculomegaly, and macrocephaly. The ultrasound abnormalities included subependymal cysts, increased echogenicity of the white matter, and

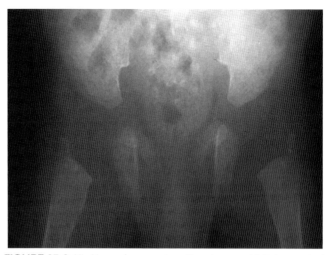

FIGURE 25-9 Hip X-ray of a neonate with cutaneous NLE demonstrating the stippled epiphysis consistent with chondrodysplasia punctata in the proximal femoral epiphysis.

echogenic lenticulostriate vessels. The only clinical abnormality in any of these children was one case of macrocephaly. On follow-up, all were developmentally normal.[276] A second study of 11 infants of mothers with anti-Ro antibodies showed that 64% had nonspecific ultrasound abnormalities consisting of subependymal pseudocysts in the absence of neurological symptoms or any of sign of NLE.[286]

Other Manifestations

There have been numerous reports of different diseases of the newborn associated with the transplacental passage of maternal anti-Ro, anti-La, or other autoantibodies, as well as unusual clinical manifestations in neonates with classic NLE. When there is a single case report, it is not clear whether the illness in the neonate is related to the maternal autoantibodies or is a disease that coincidentally occurs in offspring of mothers with these autoantibodies. Similarly, when unusual features are identified in children with definite NLE, it is not clear whether the other illness is coincidental or the result of autoantibodies.

One interesting associated feature has been the multiple case reports and case series of the association of NLE stippled epiphysis consistent with chondrodysplasia punctata (Fig. 25-9).[287-296] These cases have been associated with anti-Ro/La antibodies and with anti-RNP antibodies. Some of the mothers with the latter have features consistent with mixed connective tissue disease.[293,295] The characteristic epiphyseal changes may be isolated or associated with bone dysplasia.[293]

LONG-TERM RISK OF AUTOIMMUNE DISEASE
Children

It is well known that children born to mothers with SLE have an increased risk of developing SLE as compared to the general population. In 1979 and 1980, the first cases were reported of children with NLE who developed SLE later in life.[297,298] A study from the RRNL showed that 12% (6 of 49) of children with NLE developed an autoimmune disease as compared to none of the 45 unaffected siblings. Only a minority of the children had autoantibodies, and none had anti-Ro antibodies or SLE.[299] A literature review reported 13 cases of autoimmune diseases developing in children with NLE, with SLE and juvenile arthritis being the most commonly reported.[300] A case of a child with NLE who subsequently developed anti-Ro antibody–negative SLE was reported.[301] Although there appears to be an increased risk for children with NLE to develop an autoimmune disease, it is not clear if this risk is truly higher than in unaffected siblings or if this reflects the genetic predisposition of a child born to a mother with an autoimmune disease, as opposed to a direct delayed consequence of having had NLE. However, if there is an increased risk, this increased risk may be secondary to the genetic linkages to the development of NLE as described in previous sections. Parents of these infants should be counseled that the risk of their offspring developing autoimmune diseases is similar to the risk in children of women with SLE.

Mothers

Initially, NLE was the name of the disorder given to infants born with the characteristic skin or cardiac findings in the presence of maternal rheumatic disease, particularly SLE and SS. All mothers of infants with NLE therefore had an autoimmune disease. However, it rapidly became apparent that CHB and C-NLE could be seen in the offspring of mothers with anti-Ro/La antibodies who did not have an autoimmune disease. It was initially assumed that the mothers of children with CHB had a rheumatic disease, although most were healthy at the time of delivery.[129,302-305] A large study showed that mothers of children with C-NLE were more likely to have had an autoimmune disorder at the time of delivery of the child and at long-term follow-up than were mothers of children with CHB.[305]

The long-term outcome of the mothers was addressed in a cohort of 51 mothers who had either minimal symptoms or were asymptomatic at the time of birth of the child with NLE.[306] The majority of these asymptomatic mothers (73%) had either minimal symptoms or remained asymptomatic after a mean of 5.3 years, whereas 12 developed definite or probable SS or SLE, and 2 had an undifferentiated autoimmune syndrome. Similarly, the majority of 37 mothers with minimal symptoms (57%) did not develop new symptoms after a mean of 6 years, whereas 11 developed definite or probable SS or SLE, and 5 an undifferentiated autoimmune syndrome. Mothers with both Ro and La antibodies were nearly twice as likely to develop an autoimmune disease as were mothers with only anti-Ro antibodies. A nationwide survey from Finland reported on 68 mothers who did not have an autoimmune disease at the time of delivery of their child with NLE. After a mean follow-up time of 10 years, the majority of mothers (51%) did not develop a defined autoimmune disease; 30 developed definite or probable SS or SLE, 2 developed autoimmune thyroid disease, and 1 developed rheumatoid arthritis.[307]

EXPERIMENTAL MODELS

Langendorff Experiments

Initial *ex vivo* experiments examined the effect of anti-Ro– and anti-La–containing sera on conduction in isolated rabbit hearts. The perfusion of isolated Langendorff preparations of adult rabbit hearts with either whole sera or affinity-purified IgG from sera containing anti-Ro and anti-La antibodies induced HB and altered the peak slow inward current.[308,309] However, sera from women with SLE or SS without a history of delivering a child with NLE also resulted in HB in the isolated, whole rabbit heart, although the HB occurred only with perfusion with affinity-purified anti–52-kD antibodies. These observations were not unique to anti-Ro antibody–containing sera, because similar alterations of cardiac conduction have been observed with sera from patients with conduction defects associated with Chagas disease.[310]

Perfusion of Langendorff preparations of human fetal hearts with affinity-purified anti–52-kD Ro derived from mothers of children with CHB also resulted in the development of complete AV block. At a whole-cell and single-channel level, perfusion experiments with the human heart demonstrated an inhibition of L-type calcium currents.[311] Similarly, when isolated rat hearts were used, a 2:1 AV block followed by complete inhibition of AV nodal action potential was demonstrated, and calcium channels were inhibited in isolated cellular preparations.[312] These results suggested that rodents may be an appropriate species for monitoring the fetal effects of maternal anti-Ro and anti-La antibodies.

Calcium Channels

As stated above, calcium channels are important in maintaining cardiac rhythm, and therefore anti-calcium channel antibodies maybe important in CHB. Perfusion experiments using whole fetal hearts showed that affinity-purified anti-Ro antibodies (particularly anti-Ro52 antibodies) induced HB and these same antibodies inhibited calcium L-type channels in cultured human fetal cardiomyocyte at a whole-cell and single-channel level.[311] Taken together, these experiments demonstrated that anti-Ro antibodies (particularly anti-Ro52 antibodies) alter calcium L-type channel function. Similarly, when isolated rat hearts were used, a 2:1 AV block followed by complete inhibition of AV nodal action potential was demonstrated, and calcium L-type channels were inhibited in isolated cellular preparations.[312] Subsequent experiments showed that anti-Ro/La antibodies reacted with, and altered the function of, α_{1c} and α_{1D} (Cav1.3) subunits of the L-type calcium channel and also T-type calcium channels.[49-51] There has been a recent resurgence in the interest of the role of calreticulin and the pathogenesis of CHB, as it was shown that calreticulin negatively regulates the cell surface expression of L-type calcium channels.[313]

T-type Ca^{++} channels (in particular the α_{1G} subunit) are also important in Ca^{++} homeostasis, are developmentally regulated, and therefore may be a target for maternal autoantibodies. In 18- to 23-week-old fetal hearts, T-type Ca^{++} channels are present on the cell surface in the area of AV junction. Sera of mothers of children with CHB reacted with an epitope on an extracellular loop of these Ca^{++} channels. These sera also altered T-type current in mouse sinoatrial node cells. Therefore, L-type and/or T-type Ca^{++} may be important antigens in CHB.

The 5-HT₄R, known to be important in activating L-type channel channels, was demonstrated to be present in human fetal atrium and ventricle (extending previous work in mice), and therefore it was an obvious potential target for maternal antibodies leading to CHB.[56,314] However, as discussed previously, there was not an association of anti-5-HT₄R antibodies and the development of CHB; therefore this line of research has been abandoned. Similarly, autoantibodies from mothers of children with CHB have been shown to bind to and modify the response of muscarinic acetylcholine receptor (MAR) activation of neonatal, but not adult, rat atria.[315-317] However, the importance of these antibodies in the pathogenesis of CHB is unclear as there was no correlation with anti-MAR antibodies and anti-Ro or anti-La antibodies in the sera of mothers with children with CHB.

Taken together, it appears that antibodies directed against calcium channels and receptors important in generation of cardiac rhythm, which are present on cardiomyocytes, may play a role in the pathogenesis of CHB.

In Vivo Experiments

Apoptosis has been proposed as a mechanism for the tissue damage.[318] In human fetal cardiac myocytes, apoptosis results in surface translocation of Ro and La antigens.[150] *In vivo* murine experiments have supported this hypothesis because the passive transfer of human IgG containing anti–52-kD Ro, anti–60-kD Ro, and anti-La autoantibodies led to the formation of human IgG–apoptotic cell complexes in organs targeted in NLE (e.g., heart, skin, liver, and bone) but not in thymus, lung, brain, or gut. Experiments with affinity-purified antibodies demonstrated that anti-La, but not anti-Ro, antibodies formed these complexes.[318] It was subsequently demonstrated that the presence of the anti-Ro and anti-La antibodies impaired the clearance of apoptotic cardiomyotcytes.[152] Therefore it is possible that apoptosis, a normal event during cardiac development, may result in the binding of maternal anti-Ro and anti-La antibodies to the apoptotic cells that cause an inflammatory reaction.[319] The neighboring cells may be damaged as bystanders. Initial binding may be by maternal anti–52-kD Ro antibodies or antibodies to isoforms of the La protein, which are maximally expressed early in gestation, with levels decreasing with gestational age until 25 weeks, when adult levels are achieved.[22,320]

Immunization of female BALB/c mice with recombinant Ro/LA proteins generated high-titer antibodies that crossed the placenta during pregnancy and are associated with various degrees of AV conduction abnormalities in the pups. However, conduction abnormalities were seen in only a low percentage of the offspring born to these mice, and advanced conduction abnormalities rarely developed.[321]

Following the establishment of the murine model of CHB by immunizing mice with recombinant Ro or La proteins, and the demonstration that dysregulation of calcium channel conduction may contribute to the pathogenesis of CHB, it was hypothesized that the perturbation of L-type Ca^{++} channels would alter development of CHB in this model.[322] To test this hypothesis, an L-type Ca^{++} channel knockout mouse and a L-type Ca^{++} channel transgenic mouse were developed. Studies using these mice showed that overexpression of the L-type Ca^{++} channel (transgenic mouse) decreased the conduction abnormalities induced by immunization with Ro or La proteins, whereas deletion of the L-type Ca^{++} channel (knockout mouse) exacerbated the conduction abnormalities. The findings of this study support the hypothesis that maternal antibodies can inhibit L-type Ca^{++} channels and perturbation of calcium channels may contribute to the development of CHB.

REFERENCES

1. S.L. Deutscher, J.B. Harley, J.D. Keene, Molecular analysis of the 60-kDa human Ro ribonucleoprotein, Proc. Natl. Acad. Sci. U.S.A. 85 (24) (1988) 9479–9483.
2. E. Ben-Chetrit, B.J. Gandy, E.M. Tan, K.F. Sullivan, Isolation and characterization of a cDNA clone encoding the 60-kD component of the human SS-A/Ro ribonucleoprotein autoantigen, J. Clin. Invest. 83 (4) (1989) 1284–1292.
3. A.J. Stein, G. Fuchs, C. Fu, et al., Structural insights into RNA quality control: the Ro autoantigen binds misfolded RNAs via its central cavity, Cell 121 (4) (2005) 529–539.
4. X. Chen, J.D. Smith, H. Shi, et al., The Ro autoantigen binds misfolded U2 small nuclear RNAs and assists mammalian cell survival after UV irradiation, Curr. Biol. 13 (24) (2003) 2206–2211.
5. C.A. O'Brien, S.L. Wolin, A possible role for the 60-kD Ro autoantigen in a discard pathway for defective 5S rRNA precursors, Genes Dev. 8 (23) (1994) 2891–2903.
6. D. Xue, H. Shi, J.D. Smith, et al., A lupus-like syndrome develops in mice lacking the Ro 60-kDa protein, a major lupus autoantigen, Proc. Natl. Acad. Sci. U.S.A. 100 (13) (2003) 7503–7508.
7. M. Gendron, D. Roberge, G. Boire, Heterogeneity of human Ro ribonucleoproteins (RNPS): nuclear retention of Ro RNPS containing the human hY5 RNA in human and mouse cells, Clin. Exp. Immunol. 125 (1) (2001) 162–168.
8. S. Sim, J. Yao, D.E. Weinberg, et al., The zipcode-binding protein ZBP1 influences the subcellular location of the Ro 60-kDa autoantigen and the noncoding Y3 RNA, RNA 18 (1) (2012) 100–110.

9. M.A. Fouraux, P. Bouvet, S. Verkaart, et al., Nucleolin associates with a subset of the human Ro ribonucleoprotein complexes, J. Mol. Biol. 320 (3) (2002) 475–488.
10. J.H. Reed, S. Sim, S.L. Wolin, et al., Ro60 requires Y3 RNA for cell surface exposure and inflammation associated with cardiac manifestations of neonatal lupus, J. Immunol. 191 (1) (2013) 110–116.
11. G. Boire, J. Craft, Human Ro ribonucleoprotein particles: characterization of native structure and stable association with the La polypeptide, J. Clin. Invest. 85 (4) (1990) 1182–1190.
12. J.C. Chambers, J.D. Keene, Isolation and analysis of cDNA clones expressing human lupus La antigen, Proc. Natl. Acad. Sci. U.S.A. 82 (7) (1985) 2115–2119.
13. J.C. Chambers, D. Kenan, B.J. Martin, J.D. Keene, Genomic structure and amino acid sequence domains of the human La autoantigen, J. Biol. Chem. 263 (34) (1988) 18043–18051.
14. E.K. Chan, K.F. Sullivan, E.M. Tan, Ribonucleoprotein SS-B/La belongs to a protein family with consensus sequences for RNA-binding, Nucleic Acids Res. 17 (6) (1989) 2233–2244.
15. M. Bachmann, D. Grölz, H. Bartsch, et al., Analysis of expression of an alternative La (SS-B) cDNA and localization of the encoded N- and C-terminal peptides, Biochim. Biophys. Acta 1356 (1) (1997) 53–63.
16. M. Bachmann, S. Chang, A. Bernd, W. Mayet, Meyer zum Büschenfelde KH, Müller WE. Translocation of the nuclear autoantigen La to cell surface: assembly and disassembly with the extracellular matrix, Autoimmunity 9 (2) (1991) 99–107.
17. E. Gottlieb, J.A. Steitz, The RNA binding protein La influences both the accuracy and the efficiency of RNA polymerase III transcription in vitro, EMBO J. 8 (3) (1989) 841–850.
18. E. Gottlieb, J.A. Steitz, Function of the mammalian La protein: evidence for its action in transcription termination by RNA polymerase III, EMBO J. 8 (3) (1989) 851–861.
19. S. Gaidamakov, O.A. Maximova, H. Chon, et al., Targeted deletion of the gene encoding the La autoantigen (Sjögren's syndrome antigen B) in B cells or the frontal brain causes extensive tissue loss, Mol. Cell. Biol. 34 (1) (2014) 123–131.
20. J.M. Park, M.J. Kohn, M.W. Bruinsma, et al., The multifunctional RNA-binding protein La is required for mouse development and for the establishment of embryonic stem cells, Mol. Cell. Biol. 26 (4) (2006) 1445–1451.
21. E.K. Chan, F. Di Donato, J.C. Hamel, et al., 52-kD SS-A/Ro: genomic structure and identification of an alternatively spliced transcript encoding a novel leucine zipper-minus autoantigen expressed in fetal and adult heart, J. Exp. Med. 182 (4) (1995) 983–992.
22. J.P. Buyon, C.E. Tseng, F. Di Donato, et al., Cardiac expression of 52beta, an alternative transcript of the congenital heart block-associated 52-kd SS-A/Ro autoantigen, is maximal during fetal development, Arthritis Rheum. 40 (4) (1997) 655–660.
23. E. Ben-Chetrit, E.K. Chan, K.F. Sullivan, E.M. Tan, A 52-kD protein is a novel component of the SS-A/Ro antigenic particle, J. Exp. Med. 167 (5) (1988) 1560–1571.
24. E.K. Chan, J.C. Hamel, J.P. Buyon, E.M. Tan, Molecular definition and sequence motifs of the 52-kD component of human SS-A/Ro autoantigen, J. Clin. Invest. 87 (1) (1991) 68–76.
25. K. Itoh, Y. Itoh, M.B. Frank, Protein heterogeneity in the human Ro/SSA ribonucleoproteins. The 52- and 60-kD Ro/SSA autoantigens are encoded by separate genes, J. Clin. Invest. 87 (1) (1991) 177–186.
26. A. Espinosa, W. Zhou, M. Ek, et al., The Sjogren's syndrome-associated autoantigen Ro52 is an E3 ligase that regulates proliferation and cell death, J. Immunol. 176 (10) (2006) 6277–6285.
27. K. Wada, T. Kamitani, Autoantigen Ro52 is an E3 ubiquitin ligase, Biochem. Biophys. Res. Commun. 339 (1) (2006) 415–421.
28. K. Wada, K. Tanji, T. Kamitani, Function and subcellular location of Ro52beta, Biochem. Biophys. Res. Commun. 340 (3) (2006) 872–878.
29. A. Espinosa, V. Dardalhon, S. Brauner, et al., Loss of the lupus autoantigen Ro52/Trim21 induces tissue inflammation and systemic autoimmunity by disregulating the IL-23-Th17 pathway, J. Exp. Med. 206 (8) (2009) 1661–1671.

30. V. Oke, M. Wahren-Herlenius, The immunobiology of Ro52 (TRIM21) in autoimmunity: A critical review, J. Autoimmun. 39 (1–2) (2012) 77–82.

31. Z. Zhang, M. Bao, N. Lu, et al., The E3 ubiquitin ligase TRIM21 negatively regulates the innate immune response to intracellular double-stranded DNA, Nat. Immunol. 14 (2) (2013) 172–178.

32. D.C. Kephart, A.F. Hood, T.T. Provost, Neonatal lupus erythematosus: new serologic findings, J. Invest. Dermatol. 77 (3) (1981) 331–333.

33. B.R. Reed, L.A. Lee, C. Harmon, et al., Autoantibodies to SS-A/Ro in infants with congenital heart block, J. Pediatr. 103 (6) (1983) 889–891.

34. J.S. Scott, P.J. Maddison, P.V. Taylor, et al., Connective-tissue disease, antibodies to ribonucleoprotein, and congenital heart block, N. Engl. J. Med. 309 (4) (1983) 209–212.

35. P.V. Taylor, K.F. Taylor, A. Norman, et al., Prevalence of maternal Ro (SS-A) and La (SS-B) autoantibodies in relation to congenital heart block, Br. J. Rheumatol. 27 (2) (1988) 128–132.

36. J.S. Scott, P.V. Taylor, Congenital AV-block: role of anti-Ro and anti-La antibodies, Springer Semin. Immunopathol. 11 (4) (1989) 397–408.

37. E.D. Silverman, J. Buyon, R.M. Laxer, et al., Autoantibody response to the Ro/La particle may predict outcome in neonatal lupus erythematosus, Clin. Exp. Immunol. 100 (3) (1995) 499–505.

38. J.P. Buyon, E. Ben-Chetrit, S. Karp, et al., Acquired congenital heart block. Pattern of maternal antibody response to biochemically defined antigens of the SSA/Ro-SSB/La system in neonatal lupus, J. Clin. Invest. 84 (2) (1989) 627–634.

39. E. Jaeggi, C. Laskin, R. Hamilton, et al., The importance of the level of maternal anti-Ro/SSA antibodies as a prognostic marker of the development of cardiac neonatal lupus erythematosus a prospective study of 186 antibody-exposed fetuses and infants, J. Am. Coll. Cardiol. 55 (24) (2010) 2778–2784.

40. E. Silverman, M. Mamula, J.A. Hardin, R. Laxer, Importance of the immune response to the Ro/La particle in the development of congenital heart block and neonatal lupus erythematosus, J. Rheumatol. 18 (1) (1991) 120–124.

41. J.H. Reed, R.M. Clancy, K.H. Lee, et al., Umbilical cord blood levels of maternal antibodies reactive with p200 and full-length Ro 52 in the assessment of risk for cardiac manifestations of neonatal lupus, Arthritis Care Res. (Hoboken) 64 (9) (2012) 1373–1381.

42. J.P. Buyon, R.J. Winchester, S.G. Slade, et al., Identification of mothers at risk for congenital heart block and other neonatal lupus syndromes in their children. Comparison of enzyme-linked immunosorbent assay and immunoblot for measurement of anti-SS-A/Ro and anti-SS-B/La antibodies, Arthritis Rheum. 36 (9) (1993) 1263–1273.

43. S. Salomonsson, T. Dörner, E. Theander, et al., A serologic marker for fetal risk of congenital heart block, Arthritis Rheum. 46 (5) (2002) 1233–1241.

44. M.B. Frank, K. Itoh, V. McCubbin, Epitope mapping of the 52-kD Ro/SSA autoantigen, Clin. Exp. Immunol. 95 (3) (1994) 390–396.

45. R.M. Clancy, J.P. Buyon, K. Ikeda, et al., Maternal antibody responses to the 52-kd SSA/RO p200 peptide and the development of fetal conduction defects, Arthritis Rheum. 52 (10) (2005) 3079–3086.

46. L. Strandberg, O. Winqvist, S.E. Sonesson, et al., Antibodies to amino acid 200-239 (p200) of Ro52 as serological markers for the risk of developing congenital heart block, Clin. Exp. Immunol. 154 (1) (2008) 30–37.

47. R.M. Clancy, A.D. Askanase, R.P. Kapur, et al., Transdifferentiation of cardiac fibroblasts, a fetal factor in anti-SSA/Ro-SSB/La antibody-mediated congenital heart block, J. Immunol. 169 (4) (2002) 2156–2163.

48. S. Salomonsson, S.E. Sonesson, L. Ottosson, et al., Ro/SSA autoantibodies directly bind cardiomyocytes, disturb calcium homeostasis, and mediate congenital heart block, J. Exp. Med. 201 (1) (2005) 11–17.

49. Y. Qu, G. Baroudi, Y. Yue, M. Boutjdir, Novel molecular mechanism involving alpha1D (Cav1.3) L-type calcium channel in autoimmune-associated sinus bradycardia, Circulation 111 (23) (2005) 3034–3041.

50. Y. Qu, G.Q. Xiao, L. Chen, M. Boutjdir, Autoantibodies from mothers of children with congenital heart block downregulate cardiac L-type Ca channels, J. Mol. Cell. Cardiol. 33 (6) (2001) 1153–1163.

51. G.Q. Xiao, K. Hu, M. Boutjdir, Direct inhibition of expressed cardiac l- and t-type calcium channels by igg from mothers whose children have congenital heart block, Circulation 103 (11) (2001) 1599–1604.

52. L.S. Strandberg, X. Cui, A. Rath, et al., Congenital heart block maternal sera autoantibodies target an extracellular epitope on the alpha1G T-type calcium channel in human fetal hearts, PLoS ONE 8 (9) (2013) e72668.

53. P. Eftekhari, L. Salle, F. Lezoualc'h, et al., Anti-SSA/Ro52 autoantibodies blocking the cardiac 5-HT4 serotoninergic receptor could explain neonatal lupus congenital heart block, Eur. J. Immunol. 30 (10) (2000) 2782–2790.

54. D.S. Choi, S.J. Ward, N. Messaddeq, et al., 5-HT2B receptor-mediated serotonin morphogenetic functions in mouse cranial neural crest and myocardiac cells, Development 124 (9) (1997) 1745–1755.

55. L. Castro, J. Mialet-Perez, A. Guillemeau, et al., Differential functional effects of two 5-HT4 receptor isoforms in adult cardiomyocytes, J. Mol. Cell. Cardiol. 39 (2) (2005) 335–344.

56. J.P. Buyon, R. Clancy, F. Di Donato, et al., Cardiac 5-HT(4) serotoninergic receptors, 52kD SSA/Ro and autoimmune-associated congenital heart block, J. Autoimmun. 19 (1–2) (2002) 79–86.

57. R. Kamel, P. Eftekhari, R. Clancy, et al., Autoantibodies against the serotoninergic 5-HT4 receptor and congenital heart block: a reassessment, J. Autoimmun. 25 (1) (2005) 72–76.

58. L.A. Rokeach, J.A. Haselby, J.F. Meilof, et al., Characterization of the autoantigen calreticulin, J. Immunol. 147 (9) (1991) 3031–3039.

59. J.G. Routsias, A.G. Tzioufas, M. Sakarellos-Daitsiotis, et al., Calreticulin synthetic peptide analogues: anti-peptide antibodies in autoimmune rheumatic diseases, Clin. Exp. Immunol. 91 (3) (1993) 437–441.

Entire reference list is available online at www.expertconsult.com.

CHAPTER 26

Juvenile Dermatomyositis

Lisa G. Rider, Carol B. Lindsley, Frederick W. Miller

Juvenile dermatomyositis (JDM) is a multisystem disease of uncertain origin that is defined by chronic inflammation of striated muscle and skin. It is characterized early in its course by perivascular inflammation of varying severity in multiple organ systems and later by the development of calcinosis.

Definition and Classification

In childhood, the chronic idiopathic inflammatory myopathies (IIMs) are relatively heterogeneous disorders, although most affected children have the characteristic muscle and skin abnormalities of JDM.[1-6] The five criteria of Bohan and Peter[7,8] in Box 26-1 are applicable to its diagnosis, and although their sensitivity and specificity have not been validated in children, they are probably 50% to 90%.[3-5,9,10] A diagnosis of probable JDM requires the presence of the pathognomonic rash (the heliotrope rash or Gottron papules over the extensor surfaces of the finger joints, elbows, knees, or ankles) and two of the other criteria; definite JDM requires the characteristic rash and three other criteria.[7,8,11] In general, the first two criteria (i.e., proximal muscle weakness and classic rash) are almost always present; criterion 3 (i.e., elevated serum levels of muscle enzymes), criterion 4 (i.e., electromyographic changes), and criterion 5 (i.e., histopathological changes) provide additional laboratory support for the diagnosis. A diagnosis of JDM is not necessarily excluded by failure to meet one or more of these criteria, except the one related to the dermatitis; however, tests such as electromyography (EMG), magnetic resonance imaging (MRI), or muscle biopsy is preferred to confirm the diagnosis. MRI of the thigh muscles, demonstrating symmetric muscle edema on fat-suppressed T2-weighted or short tau inversion recovery (STIR) sequences, is currently preferred to EMG to confirm a diagnosis of JDM; however, MRI is sensitive in detecting muscle inflammation but is not specific to a diagnosis of myositis because muscular dystrophies and other myopathies can also show edema on MRI.[9,12] A muscle biopsy, however, is considered requisite to confirming a diagnosis of polymyositis (PM), in the absence of the characteristic skin rashes.[13] A method for scoring muscle biopsies has been shown to be reliable and to correlate well with muscle strength; it may help to standardize biopsy readings.[14]

JDM has many similarities with inflammatory myopathies in adults but also has a number of differences (Table 26-1).[1,15-18] Several other types of inflammatory myopathies occur in children, albeit less frequently than JDM (reviewed by Rider et al.[19]). For example, PM (i.e., muscle inflammation without cutaneous disease)[1,3,20,21] and myositis associated with other connective tissue diseases (CTMs)[1,22] such as scleroderma (see Chapter 27) and the myositis overlap syndromes (see Chapter 29) occur in approximately 4% to 8% and 6% to 12% of children, respectively.[19] Amyopathic or hypomyopathic

dermatomyositis (DM), in which patients develop skin rashes—either without weakness or with subclinical muscle weakness detected only by additional testing (e.g., elevated serum muscle enzymes or abnormal EMG, muscle biopsy, or MRI)—occurs in approximately 1% of children with myositis.[23-25] DM in association with malignancy is rare in childhood,[26-28] and an evaluation for occult malignancy is undertaken only if the illness is atypical or if there are other suggestions of a malignancy such as depressed peripheral blood cell counts, a palpable mass, prominent adenopathy, or hepatosplenomegaly. Other types of myositis, which occur rarely in children, include focal myositis,[5,29,30] orbital myositis,[31,32] inclusion body myositis (IBM),[26,33] eosinophilic myositis,[34-37] and granulomatous myositis.[38,39] Macrophagic myofasciitis is a recently recognized entity characterized by predominantly macrophagic infiltration with focal myositis in the deltoids or quadriceps muscles at the injection site of a vaccine containing aluminum.[40-42]

EPIDEMIOLOGY

Incidence

Estimates of the incidence of JDM are given in eTable 26-2.[43-49] Symmons and colleagues[44] calculated a rate of 0.19 cases per 100,000 individuals per year for children younger than 16 years in the United Kingdom and Ireland. Mendez and colleagues[47] calculated an average annual incidence of 3.2 cases per million children (95% confidence interval [CI] 2.5 to 4.1) for children 2 to 17 years of age diagnosed between 1995 and 1998 in the United States based on data obtained from a national registry. Based on inception cohorts in Scandinavia, the annual incidence per million children was estimated to be 2.9 cases in Norway[49] and 1.8 cases (95% CI 0 to 2.6) in Denmark.[48] In general, 16% to 20% of patients with DM have onset in childhood.[43,50] There are no direct studies of prevalence.

Age at Onset and Sex Ratio

The data of Medsger and co-workers[43] suggested a bimodal distribution of age at myositis onset with a peak at age 5 to 14 years old, and a second, much larger peak at age 45 to 64 years.[43,53] In data pooled from nine series derived from divergent geographic areas, the female-to-male ratio was 1.7:1 but as high as 2.7:1 among children with onset at 10 years of age or older.[44,45,51,54-56] More recent data from two national registries in the United States and United Kingdom suggest a median age at onset of 7 years, with 25% of children younger than 4 years of age, and a female-to-male ratio of 2.2:1.[5,57] Onset is especially common from ages 4 to 9, with two peak ages for girls at 6 and 13 years; for boys the most common age at onset is 5.5 years (Fig. 26-1).[57] In recently published registry studies, the average age at onset of JDM ranged from 5.7 to 9.0 years, and the female-to-male ratio ranged from 1.5:1 to

2.6:1.[1-3,9,18,48,49,58,59] For juvenile polymyositis (JPM), the median age at onset is 12.1 years, and for juvenile connective tissue myositis (JCTM) the age at onset ranges from 7.6 to 10.2 years.[1,22] The female-to-male ratio ranges from 2:1 to 2.7:1 for JPM and 2:1 to 8:1 for JCTM.[1,20,22,51]

Geographic and Racial Distribution

Dermatomyositis is widely distributed throughout the world.[60] Striking racial differences in incidence have been described in adults in the United States; the incidence of the disease among black women aged 55 to 64 years is 10 times that of white women in the same age group.[43] Such differences are less marked in children, and in the data of Mendez and colleagues in the United States,[47] the average 4-year annual incidence rate was comparable for whites and blacks and somewhat lower for Hispanic patients.

ETIOLOGY AND PATHOGENESIS

Environmental risk factors. JDM is thought to be the result of environmental triggers in genetically susceptible individuals, leading to immune dysfunction and specific tissue pathology. The potential role of environmental factors in myositis etiology is supported by reports of geographic and seasonal clustering of cases.[4,5,44,61-63] Seasonality has been seen in the birth distributions of patients with JDM who are Hispanic, in those with the human leukocyte antigen (HLA) risk factor DRB1*0301 allele, and in those with the p155/140 (TIF-1) autoantibody, all of which suggest that perinatal or early-life exposures may be implicated in these subgroups.[64]

Evidence for the role of infectious agents in disease etiology is largely indirect.[65] In three large cohorts, an antecedent upper respiratory infection or gastrointestinal illness frequently preceded onset of JDM symptoms by 3 to 6 months.[57,63,66] In a case-control study, children with JDM more frequently reported symptoms of an antecedent illness than did healthy children in the control group.[61] Cases of infections with coxsackievirus, influenza, Group A streptococcus, toxoplasmosis, parvovirus, hepatitis B, Epstein–Barr virus, *Borrelia*, and *Leishmania* preceding the onset of JDM have been documented.[26,67,68] Although acute muscle inflammation may result from viral illness, there are no unequivocal data supporting a viral cause for JDM. Serologic evidence of coxsackievirus B infection was first reported in 83% of children with early JDM, compared with 25% of control subjects,[69] but a second case-control study failed to confirm this association, and enteroviral, herpesvirus, and toxoplasma titers were also not elevated.[61] A search for the presence of viral genome in affected muscle from patients with JDM using the polymerase chain reaction yielded negative results.[70] Acute transitory myositis may occur after influenza and parainfluenza infection.[71-75] A case-control study suggested that

---

BOX 26-1   Criteria for a Diagnosis of Juvenile Dermatomyositis and Polymyositis*

1. Symmetric weakness of the proximal musculature
2. Characteristic cutaneous changes consisting of heliotrope discoloration of the eyelids, which may be accompanied by periorbital edema, and/or erythematous papules over the extensor surfaces of joints, including the dorsal aspects of the metacarpophalangeal and proximal interphalangeal joints, elbows, knees, or ankles (i.e., Gottron papules)
3. Elevation of the serum level of one or more of the following skeletal muscle enzymes: creatine kinase, aspartate aminotransferase, lactate dehydrogenase, and aldolase
4. Electromyographic demonstration of the characteristics of myopathy and denervation, including the triad of polyphasic, short, small motor-unit potentials; fibrillations, positive sharp waves, increased insertional irritability; and high-frequency repetitive discharges
5. Muscle biopsy documenting histological evidence of necrosis; fiber size variation, particularly perifascicular atrophy; degeneration and regeneration; and a mononuclear inflammatory infiltrate, most often in a perivascular distribution

*The presence of three of the five findings indicates a probable diagnosis of myositis, and at least four of five findings indicates definite myositis. Dermatomyositis requires cutaneous changes (#2). A diagnosis of dermatomyositis or polymyositis also requires exclusion of all other conditions in the differential diagnosis. Adapted from A. Bohan, J.B. Peter (1975). Polymyositis and dermatomyositis (parts 1 and 2), New Engl. J. Med. 292: 344–347, 403–407.[7,8]

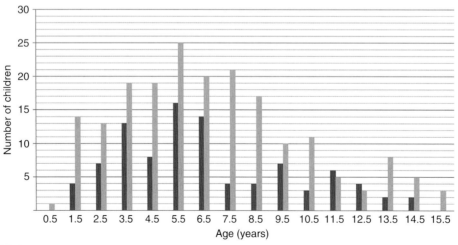

FIGURE 26-1 Age at disease onset of juvenile dermatomyositis (JDM) in 286 children from the JDM National Institute of Arthritis and Musculoskeletal and Skin Diseases Registry. For girls (*light gray bars*), n = 194, mean age ± SD, 6.74 ± 3.54 years; for boys (*dark gray bars*), n = 92, mean age ± SD, 7.33 ± 3.95 years. (Reproduced with permission from L.M. Pachman, R. Lipton, R. Ramsey-Goldman, et al. (2005). History of infection before the onset of juvenile dermatomyositis: results from the National Institute of Arthritis and Musculoskeletal and Skin Diseases Research Registry, Arthritis Rheum. 53: 166–172.)

TABLE 26-1   Similarities and Differences Between Juvenile and Adult Myositis

	JUVENILE MYOSITIS	ADULT MYOSITIS
Classification		
Similarities	Same clinical subgroups	
Differences	JDM is most common, but there are some differences in clinical manifestations or outcomes within a given subgroup in children vs. adults.	DM occurs in approximately 30%; PM, inclusion body myositis, and cancer-associated myositis are also common.
Epidemiology		
Similarities	Female predilection in both.	
Differences	Peak age at onset, 7.6 years.	Peak age at onset, 30-50 years.
Clinical Features		
Similarities	They share many clinical features.	
Differences	Calcinosis, lipodystrophy, and gastrointestinal/cutaneous ulcerations are more frequent.	ILD and myocardial involvement are more frequent. Adult PM and DM patients are weaker than those with JDM and may have more severe disease activity.
Autoantibodies		
Similarities	They share the same autoantibodies and clinical features associated with autoantibody subgroups.	
Differences	Anti-p155/140 (TIF-1) (present in 23% to 30%) and anti-MJ (NXP-2) (present in 20% to 25%) are the most common subgroups in children; antisynthetase autoantibodies are less common (present in up to 5% of juvenile patients).	Antisynthetase autoantibodies are among the most common (present in 20% to 25% of adult patients).
Immunogenetic Risk Factors		
Similarities	They share major immunogenetic risk factors, including MHC region genes HLA-DRB1*0301-DQA1*0501, as well as TNF-α-308A. From genome-wide association studies, they also share risk factor loci common to other autoimmune diseases, including *PLCL1, BLK,* and *CCL21.* Among candidate genes, they share *PTPN22 R620W,* and Gm 3 23 5,13 alleles as risk factors in Caucasians. They share DQA1*01 and motif DQA1 F[25] as protective factors.	
Differences	DQA1*0301 is an additional risk factor for JDM in Caucasians. Gm phenotypes are additional risk factors, and HLA alleles are additional protective factors.	Other cytokine polymorphisms have not yet been studied in adults.
Pathogenesis		
Similarities	They share most elements of pathogenesis with adult DM, including humoral attack on muscle capillaries, upregulation of MHC class I on myofibers, infiltration of plasmacytoid dendritic cells, and type I interferon response.	
Differences	Increased neovascularization of capillaries, increased upregulation of MHC class I on myofibers, increased type I interferon response, especially in JDM and adult DM compared to PM.	PM is mediated primarily by CD8+ T-cell attack on nonnecrotic myofibers and cytotoxic granule release resulting in myofiber destruction.
Responses to Treatment		
Similarities	Prednisone is a mainstay of therapy, with several adjunctive immunosuppressive agents used. Agents used to treat JDM and adult DM are similar, and responses in children are similar to those of adults, but of greater magnitude.	
Differences	Greater magnitude of response to treatment in JDM than in adult DM/PM.	
Outcomes		
Similarities	Survival and outcomes are improving with increased access to immunosuppressive therapies. Many patients, nevertheless, have long-term functional disability and disease damage. Shared predictors of mortality include clinical subgroup (overlap myositis and PM), antisynthetase autoantibodies, ILD, and older age at diagnosis.	
Differences	Lower mortality (≤3%), but comparable standardized mortality ratio as adults (2.4 to 2.6 for JDM); 28% to 41% with functional disability, 37% to 41% with monocyclic course.	Higher mortality (10% to 26%) with 10-year survival 53% to 89%; standardized mortality ratio for DM ranges from 2.4 to 7.6; 35% to 60% with functional disability; 17% to 20% with monocyclic course

DM, Adult dermatomyositis; *HLA,* human leukocyte antigen; *ILD,* interstitial lung disease; *JDM,* juvenile dermatomyositis; *MHC,* major histocompatibility complex; *PM,* polymyositis.

affected juvenile myositis patients had elevated titers of influenza A and parainfluenza virus compared to matched controls.[76] Children with JDM have been reported to express immunoglobulin G (IgG) antibodies against viral non–syncytium-inducing protein, perhaps induced by persistent parvovirus B19 infection.[77] However, a case-control study failed to reveal elevated titers or persistent B19 viral genome in the peripheral blood or muscle of patients with JDM compared with matched healthy control children.[78] Group A streptococcus may be more frequent in JPM patients compared to healthy controls.[79] Relapse with β-hemolytic streptococcal disease may be related to molecular mimicry between the M5 protein and skeletal muscle myosin and immune responses to homologous peptide regions.[80-82]

Toxoplasma gondii was found in muscle in one patient with JDM.[83] Elevated antibody titers to toxoplasma have been reported in some studies,[84,85] but not in a study with appropriate controls.[61] A DM-like disease has been described in a few children with agammaglobulinemia in association with echovirus infection[86-88] and occasionally in patients with selective immunoglobulin A (IgA) deficiency,[89,90] deficiency of the second component of complement (C2),[91] or hyperimmunoglobulin E syndrome,[92,93] in whom an inordinate susceptibility to infection might be anticipated (see Chapter 46).

Less information is available on noninfectious environmental exposures related to the onset of JDM. In a large North American registry of patients with JDM, 38% of patients reported two or more exposures within 6 months prior to diagnosis—generally a combination of infectious and noninfectious exposures, with variation in the exposures in clinical and serologic subgroups of patients.[66] Noninfectious exposures included medications (18%), a number of which were potentially photosensitizing or myopathic; immunizations (11%); stressful life events (11%); unusual sun exposure (7%); and others, including chemicals, animal contact, weight training, and dietary supplement use (less than 5% each).[66] Reports of medication exposures prior to the onset of juvenile myositis include statins, "caine" anesthetics, and growth hormone therapy, with the latter supported by reports of improvement with dechallenge and recurrence upon rechallenge.[26,94] Several other medications have been associated with adult myositis, including D-penicillamine, statins, zidovudine, hydroxyurea, interferons (IFNs), and anti–tumor necrosis factor (TNF) agents.[36,95-98]

In case reports, DM has followed immunizations (e.g., vaccines for hepatitis B, influenza, rubella, diphtheria, or bacillus Calmette–Guérin).[3,26,99-102] Such cases are to be distinguished from macrophagic myofasciitis, a recently described condition thought to result from adjuvants that contain aluminum hydroxide and characterized by muscle weakness at the vaccine injection site (deltoids or quadriceps) accompanied by myalgias, fatigue, arthralgias, an elevated creatine kinase (CK) level, and an elevated erythrocyte sedimentation rate. Children with macrophagic myofasciitis may also have hypotonia, developmental delay, and failure to thrive.[40-42] Muscle biopsy shows infiltration of macrophages and CD8+ T lymphocytes in the epimysium, perimysium, and endomysium, and, on electron microscopy, presence of aluminum hydroxide in the macrophages.[103]

Patients with JDM frequently have photosensitive skin rashes, and some patients anecdotally develop illness after exposure to ultraviolet light. There is increasing evidence of a role for ultraviolet light in the onset of illness from studies of both juvenile and adult myositis. In worldwide population-based studies, the proportion of patients with DM (compared with PM) was most strongly related to global surface ultraviolet light exposure compared with a number of other geoclimatic variables.[104,105] This association, interestingly, also was found for the proportion of patients with anti–Mi-2 autoantibodies, a DM-specific autoantibody.[104] These findings have been confirmed in populations of adult myositis patients in the United States, and the

association with ultraviolet light is stronger in females and in Caucasian patients.[106] In juvenile patients, short-term ultraviolet exposure in the month before illness onset was associated with an increased risk of JDM compared with JPM, particularly in girls and in patients with anti-p155/140 (TIF-1) autoantibodies.[107]

GENETIC BACKGROUND

Familial Autoimmunity and Familial Dermatomyositis

In a large cohort of patients with JDM, approximately 50% reported having at least one other family member with an autoimmune disease, most frequently type I diabetes mellitus or systemic lupus erythematosus (SLE).[108] There are several reports of the rare occurrence of familial JDM.[109-117] In all instances but one, the disease has been typical DM. In one daughter-father pair,[112] the daughter had JDM, and the father had PM with positive lupus erythematosus cell preparations. As reported by Harati and associates,[113] monozygotic twin girls developed JDM within 2 weeks of each other after upper respiratory tract infections. A brother-sister pair was reported.[118] In families with multiplex myositis, there is a higher frequency of homozygosity at the HLA DQA1 locus.[115]

Human Leukocyte Antigen Relationships

HLA-B*08, DRB1*0301, and DQA1*0501 are part of an extended ancestral haplotype in the polymorphic major histocompatibility complex (MHC) class II region that confers risk of myositis in both children and adults in Caucasians, which has been confirmed in several case-control studies (eTable 26-3)[22,119-125] as well as in transmission disequilibrium testing.[126] The MHC region on chromosome 6 is also the region of strongest risk in a large genome-wide association study of JDM and DM in Caucasians.[127] The DQA1*0301 allele is an additional risk factor for JDM, and DRB1 and DQA1 peptide binding motifs confer additional risk.[123] The DQA1*0501/DQB1*0301 locus binds poorly to class II-associated Ii peptide, possibly conferring susceptibility to autoimmunity through access to peptides earlier in antigen processing.[128] HLA-DPB1*0101 also confers independent risk for myositis in both adults and children.[129] The frequency of MHC class II–associated DM molecules (DMA*0103 and DMB*0102) also is higher in Caucasian JDM patients.[130]

Several identified protective alleles have been identified for Caucasian children with myositis, including DQA1*0201, DQA1*0101, and DQA1*0102,[123] which are less frequent in affected patients than in healthy controls and may mechanistically contribute to reduced risk of JDM through binding of self-reactive antigens and elimination of self-reactive T lymphocytes from the thymus. In African Americans, DRB1*0301-DQA1*0501 is a risk factor,[143,144] and in a small series of Hispanic patients, DQA1*0501 was elevated compared to race-matched controls.[143] DRB1*15021 may be the immunogenetic risk factor for JDM in Japanese patients.[145] A number of distinct, stronger HLA associations occur with myositis-specific antibodies.[131,132,146]

Non-HLA Genetic Risk Factors

Several other polymorphic loci have been shown to be risk factors for JDM. From a large study of more than 1000 Caucasian patients with DM or JDM, an examination of non-MHC single-nucleotide polymorphisms (SNPs) previously associated with other autoimmune diseases identified SNPs from three genes that were associated with DM/JDM, including phospholipase C–like 1 (PLCL1), a known risk factor for SLE, B lymphoid tyrosine kinase (BLK), a risk factor for rheumatoid arthritis, and chemokine (C–C motif) ligand 21 (CCL21), also a risk factor for rheumatoid arthritis.[127] Among candidate gene studies, the cytokine genes TNF-α-308A[137,138] and -238A alleles, interleukin

(IL)-1α+4845 GT, IL-1β+3953C,[138] IL-1 receptor antagonist intronic polymorphism VNTR A1,[141] the lymphocyte signaling gene *PTPN22*,[140] and certain serologic polymorphisms of the immunoglobulin heavy chain, called *Gm phenotypes*, are also risk factors for JDM in Caucasian patients (eTable 26-3).[142] A number of these loci are potentially proinflammatory, resulting in the production of more stimulated cytokines,[138] less cytokine receptor antagonist,[141] or higher serum IgG3 levels.[142] In these patients, there is also higher production of TNF-α by peripheral blood mononuclear cells *in vitro* and by regenerating JDM muscle fibers *in vivo*.[147,148]

A polymorphism in the transcription factor IFN regulatory factor 5 appears to be higher in frequency in patients with JDM and may be associated with elevated type I IFN gene expression.[149] Mannose-binding lectin (MBL) polymorphisms, which are more frequent in adult DM, are associated with lower MBL.[150] Of the cytokine and HLA associations, DRB1*0301 is the strongest risk factor.[138] It is not clear whether the TNF-α-308A allele is independent of the HLA-DRB1 locus[138] or due to linkage disequilibrium with the HLA-B locus.[139] The IL-1 loci are less strongly associated than HLA-DRB*0301 or TNF-α-308A.[138]

The TNF-α-308A allele may also be a risk factor for the development of calcinosis and ulcerations[137,138] and has been associated with a prolonged disease course.[137] The IL-1 polymorphism -889CC is a possible additional risk factor for the development of calcinosis[137] as well as photosensitive skin rashes, and IL-1β+3953TT is a possible risk factor for photosensitivity.[138] The HLA-DRB1*0301 allele and other HLA risk factors have not been found to be severity factors for calcinosis, ulcerations, or a chronic course of illness.[123,137,138]

PATHOGENESIS

Most studies suggest that JDM is an autoimmune angiopathy (Fig. 26-2) that results from chronic inflammation in a genetically susceptible individual after interaction with environmental risk factors.[16] Both humoral and cellular components of the innate and adaptive immune systems contribute to the development of JDM and other inflammatory myopathies.[151] Although the earliest events in JDM pathogenesis are not clear, the immune attack on muscle capillary endothelium, infiltration of plasmacytoid dendritic cells with a resulting type I IFN response, and upregulation of MHC class I expression on the surface of myofibers appear to be central events, and limited data suggest that several of these may be early events. Pathogenic aspects of JDM are largely identical to those of adult DM,[133,152,153] except that these central events of pathogenesis, including vasculopathy, type I IFN response, and upregulation of MHC class I, appear to be more prominent in JDM.[154,155] In adults with myositis, there is little evidence for apoptotic muscle,[156] and microchimerism has not been well studied. PM, in contrast, is largely a CD8+ T cell and myeloid dendritic cell–mediated attack on nonnecrotic myofibers, with release of cytotoxic perforin, granulysin, and granzyme B granules that mediate muscle cell death.[157-159] PM does not share a prominent IFN response in the muscle or serum, and infiltrating plasmacytoid dendritic cells are fewer in number and not as mature as in DM.[160,161]

An immune complex–mediated vasculopathy may be an important initiating or perpetuating event.[133,162-166] Complement activation and immune complex deposition have been demonstrated.[165,167] Whitaker and Engel[162] identified immunoglobulin and complement in vessel walls of skeletal muscle in JDM and adult DM, although the frequency and intensity of deposition were more pronounced in children. IgG, IgM, the third component of complement (C3), and the membrane attack complex were deposited alone or in combination in that

study and others.[164] Capillary loss and membrane attack deposition in the muscle appear to occur early, even before other histological changes.[154,166] Angiostatic ELR–CXC chemokines, including IFN-γ-inducible 10-kD protein (IP-10/CXCL10), monokine induced by γ-IFN (MIG/CXCL9), and IFN-γ-inducible T-cell α chemoattractant (I-TAC/CXCL11) are expressed at high levels in biopsy specimens of untreated patients, correlating with the degree of capillary loss and mononuclear cell infiltration.[168] Neovascularization of capillaries might occur later, and this also appears to be of greater intensity in JDM compared to adult DM.[169] Both angiogenic and antiangiogenic genes are expressed in the muscle of JDM and adult DM patients,[169,170] including genes for leukocyte adhesion molecules that participate in both leukocyte trafficking and angiogenesis.[169] Intercellular adhesion molecule 1 (ICAM-1) is selectively upregulated in the capillaries and perimysial large vessels of JDM muscle,[171] compared to adult DM and PM.[172] Elevated plasma levels of factor VIII–related antigen,[173] fibrinopeptide A, C–X–C motif chemokine 10 (CXCL10), and thrombospondin-1 on perimysial vessels[174,175] provide additional evidence of endothelial cell injury that may play a role in susceptibility to vascular thrombosis. Also, in patients with JDM with a short duration of untreated disease, downregulation of microRNA miR-126 is associated with increased vascular cell adhesion molecule 1 (VCAM-1) levels in both muscle and blood, suggesting that VCAM-1 plays an important role early in the development of JDM.[176]

Another central, early event in pathogenesis appears to be the upregulation of MHC class I on the cell surface of muscle fibers, which may also occur prior to and independently of the detection of cellular infiltrates.[155,177-179] Normal muscle cells do not express MHC class I antigens, but in DM, these antigens are strongly expressed.[155,180-182] This response is also evidenced by a transgenic mouse model in which overexpression of MHC class I itself leads to the induction of PM, although the infiltrate is predominantly macrophages.[183] Upregulation of MHC class I on myofibers is associated with the endoplasmic reticular stress response, the unfolded protein response, and activation of the nuclear factor (NF)-κB and ubiquitin proteasome pathway, which can lead to an increase in the ubiquitination of muscle proteins and muscle damage.[184,185]

After the initial vasculopathy and upregulation of MHC class I on myofibers, a perivascular and perimysial infiltration of predominantly plasmacytoid dendritic cells likely results, accompanied by CD4+ T lymphocytes, including T helper (Th)17 cells, B cells, and macrophages.[133,169,175,186,187] The plasmacytoid dendritic cells and T cells undergo local maturation and develop memory responses locally in extranodal lymphoid follicular structures.[186,188] The predominance of activated plasmacytoid dendritic cells in these lesions results in a characteristic type I IFN response with upregulation of many IFN-regulated genes and chemokines.[65,170,189,190] Type I IFN inducible genes and plasmacytoid dendritic cells are also upregulated in the affected skin[191,192] and in peripheral blood, and they correlate with disease activity, perhaps more in the muscle than skin.[187,189,190,193] The type I IFN response may perpetuate these processes, leading to upregulation of MHC class I on myofibers, T-cell survival, and induction of proinflammatory cytokines and chemokines, including MIG/CXCL9, I-TAC/CXCL11, macrophage inflammatory protein (MIP-1), monocyte chemoattractant protein (MCP-1 and MCP-2), IL-4, IL-6, IL-15, IL-17, as well as B-cell survival cytokines (B cell–activating factor [BAFF], ΔBAFF, and a proliferation-inducing ligand [APRIL]), which play roles in recruiting Th1, Th17, and other T and B lymphocytes, as well as macrophages, to sites of inflammation and in angiostasis.[133,151,187,194,195] Production of other proinflammatory cytokines and chemokines, including TNF-α and IL-1α and IL-1β, are also prominently expressed by infiltrating inflammatory cells and by myofibers[147] and endothelial

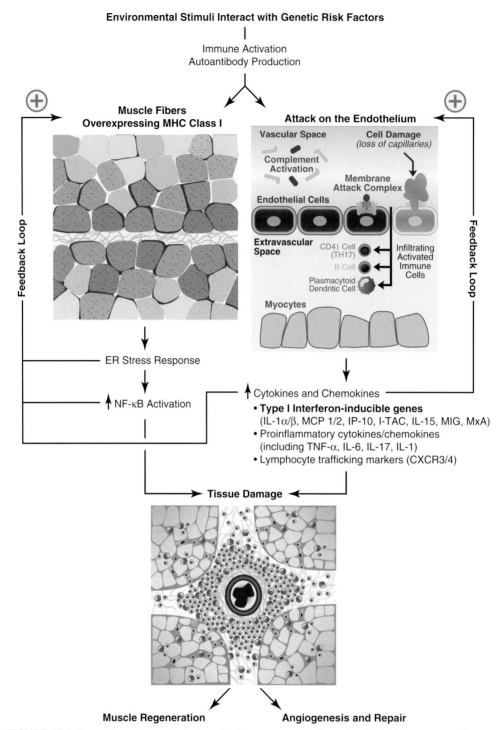

FIGURE 26-2 Key pathogenic events in juvenile dermatomyositis. Note that the initial sequence of events is uncertain and may differ from what is represented in this diagram.

cells (IL-1α).[196] However, transforming growth factor β (TGF-β) has been observed in muscle tissue, which may promote antiinflammatory effects and fibrosis.[196]

Involvement of T cells is apparent through the expression of Th17 cells, a subset of CD4+ T lymphocytes. The involvement of Th17 cells also appears to lead to induction of IL-6 and IL-17, which correlates with the IFN response and with active disease.[187] In a few patients, CD8+ T lymphocytes with unique Vβ repertoires were present in the inflammatory infiltrates of muscle, particularly around blood

vessels, as well as in peripheral blood, suggesting oligoclonal expansion.[197] Cell-mediated immunity to muscle antigens (i.e., activated T cells) may participate in pathogenesis. It is also possible that the aging of T cells could play a role in the pathogenesis of JDM, as indicated by the high frequencies of apoptosis-resistant cytotoxic CD28-null T cells that are seen in the circulation and in muscle tissue of patients with myositis.[198] Muscle biopsies from patients with JDM also demonstrated upregulation of heat shock protein (HSP) 60, as well as induction of T-cell proliferation and production of cytokines in response to HSP60 in the muscle and periphery.[199] Peripheral blood mononuclear cells from patients with JDM also demonstrated increased cytotoxicity to potential self-peptides, including the M5 protein of Group A streptococcus and human myosin.[82] In adults, apoptotic pathways are not active, and TNF-α–related apoptosis-inducing ligand (TRAIL) mediates muscle fiber damage via autophagy.[200] In JDM, however, dysregulation of apoptosis in myofibrils may be operative in pathogenesis, as suggested by the observation of over-expression of B-cell lymphoma 2 (Bcl-2) protein in muscle specimens from children with JDM,[201] as well as the expression of terminal deoxy-nucleotidyl transferase dUTP nick end labeling (TUNEL)-positive myonuclei and caspase 3 within the laminin layer.[202] Hypomethylation of several transcription factors, with resulting upregulation of the Wilms tumor 1 protein, suggests a high capacity for tissue repair in JDM muscle.[203] The finding of activated B cells and plasma cells in lymphoid aggregates and other locations in muscle and skin biopsies of JDM subjects[175,194] has suggested an important role for B-cell factors and autoantibodies in pathogenesis. Although the role of myositis autoantibodies in disease pathogenesis is unclear, hints are emerging. Myositis-specific autoantibodies, which are specific to patients with myositis, are present before the onset of clinical illness, undergo affinity maturation, correlate in titer with disease activity, inhibit the function of their targets *in vitro*, and may subside when disease enters remission.[204-207] Some of the autoantigens associated with myositis-specific autoantibodies are upregulated in regenerating myoblasts[208] and are cleaved by granzyme B, perhaps resulting in their cell surface expression.[209] They may also have a role in initiating or propagating pathogenic events. Sera from patients with anti-histidyl transfer RNA (tRNA) synthetase (Jo-1) and other nucleic acid–directed autoantibodies (Ro/La, U1RNP/Sm), in the presence of RNA and necrotic cellular material, induce production of type I IFN and activation of plasmacytoid dendritic cells in muscle tissue.[210,211] Jo-1-positive sera also upregulate ICAM-1 expression in lung endothelial cells.[212] Histidyl-tRNA synthetase and asparaginyl-tRNA synthetase are chemotactic for CC chemokine receptor 5 (CCR5)- and CCR3-expressing leukocytes; in high concentrations they induce dendritic cell maturation.[213] Ultraviolet light also upregulates the expression of Mi-2 autoantigen in cell cultures.[214]

Maternal cell chimerism is present in more than 70% of peripheral blood T cells and in muscle tissue in 80% to 90% of children with JDM.[215-219] It was identified in 25% of siblings and 15% of controls in those reports. The phenotypes of the microchimeric cells include B cells and plasmacytoid dendritic cells in the muscle.[187] HLA alleles may control the frequency and potential pathogenic mechanisms of this phenomenon. Reed and colleagues[217] found immunologic activity in chimeric cells in 60 of 72 children with JDM, in 11 of 48 unaffected siblings, and in 5 of 29 healthy controls. In all groups, chimerism was associated with the maternal HLA-DQA1*0501 allele. Maternal chimeric cells may be autoreactive against the JDM child's (host's) cells, producing IFN-γ and a memory T-cell response.[217] The maternal HLA genotype influenced the fate of the transferred cells and the activation of chimeric cells.

ANIMAL MODELS

A number of spontaneous, infectious, genetic, and antigen-induced animal models, which each replicate different aspects of human myositis, have been described over the past 4 decades.[220,221] The animal models of myositis that are most similar to human disease in clinical features, pathology, immunology, and therapeutic responses, however, are the DM- and PM-like diseases that spontaneously develop in household dogs.[222-224] A familial form of canine DM in collies and

Shetland sheep dogs is also similar to human disease, including the presence of skin rashes and vasculopathy.[222,223,225-227]

The finding that many infectious[67] and noninfectious[228] agents are temporally associated with human myositis has prompted their investigation in the development of induced animal models. These induced models of myositis have been generated by injecting rodents with muscle antigens, including muscle homogenates, purified muscle antigens, viruses, drugs, and DNA constructs—often with an adjuvant—to boost the immune response. Recent models of experimental autoimmune myositis include immunizing Lewis rats or C57BL6 mice with native C-protein or recombinant skeletal C-protein fragment 2 with complete Freund's adjuvant (CFA) and pertussis toxin[229,230]; injecting myosin or myosin B with CFA and pertussis toxin into C57BL6, SJL/J, or BALB/c mice[231-233]; and immunizing rats with laminin, a muscle structural protein.[234] In the myositis-adjuvant model, mice depleted of regulatory T cells (Tregs) developed more severe myositis, which improved with administration of *in vitro* expanded polyclonal Tregs.[233]

Experimental induction of a PM-like syndrome in neonatal animals has been reported after inoculating mice with picornaviruses, including coxsackievirus[235,236] and encephalomyocarditis virus.[237] Other viral models include injecting influenza B into juvenile BALB/c mice,[238] infecting mice with the alphaviruses Semliki Forest virus[239] and Ross River virus,[240] and encephaloviruses and Mengo viruses,[241] as well as injecting retrovirus into rhesus monkeys.[242] Parasitic models include a mouse model of *Trypanasoma cruzi*[243] and a hamster model of *Leishmania*.[244]

A mouse model of antisynthetase syndrome has been developed by immunizing congenic C57BL/6 or NOD mice with the murine form of histidyl tRNA synthetase (HRS). These mice develop clinical features similar to human disease, with both lung and muscle inflammation.[182] Recent modifications of this model using mice deficient in Toll-like receptor 4 signaling and in DO11.10/Rag2$^{-/-}$ mice expressing an ovalbumin-specific T-cell receptor (TCR) demonstrated that HRS can induce myositis via innate immune mechanisms bypassing both TCR and Toll-like receptor 4 signaling.[245] Furthermore, studies of HRS injected into B6/TLR2$^{-/-}$ and B6/TLR4$^{-/-}$ knockout mice showed that amino acids 60-90 of HRS were required for signaling via multiple MyD88-dependent Toll-like receptor signaling cascades.[246]

Overexpression of MHC class I on the surface of muscle cells in transgenic mice induces muscle inflammation with macrophagic predominance and a clinical syndrome consistent with PM, including the generation of histidyl-tRNA synthetase autoantibodies in some animals.[247] Overexpression of MHC class I in young mice leads to more rapid and severe muscle weakness and pathological changes, paralleled by a more dramatic and rapid upregulation of a number of genes involved in the endoplasmic reticular stress response and downregulation of muscle structural genes.[248] A knockout model of myositis involving deletion of suppressor of cytokine signaling-1 in mice heterozygous for IFN-γ leads to PM and fatal myocarditis.[249] Cytolytic T-lymphocyte-associated antigen and TGF-β knockout mice also develop multifocal inflammation, including involvement of skeletal muscle.[250,251]

PATHOGENESIS OF CALCINOSIS

Studies of the mineral composition of surgically removed calcinosis samples reveal the mineral to be calcium hydroxyapatite or carbonate apatite, with a lesser degree of magnesium also present, which is a mineralization inhibitor. Calcinosis is distinct from bone in its mineral composition and matrix.[252-254] The mineral appears to be deposited in fragments and becomes solid over time.[252,254] Immunohistochemistry reveals a number of small integrin-binding ligand, N-linked glycoprotein (SIBLING) proteins, including osteocalcin, osteopontin, and matrix-Gla protein, that promote and inhibit mineralization within the lesions, and osteoclasts at the periphery of the lesions that are secondarily infiltrating in an attempt to resolve the calcification.[255] Matrix-Gla protein, a calcification inhibitor, is expressed at sites of muscle damage and by infiltrating macrophages in the muscle tissue of patients with JDM. It is also present in adult myositis and childhood muscular dystrophies, whereas only phosphorylated matrix-Gla protein is elevated in biopsies of patients with JDM who developed calcinosis.[256] Liquefied milk of calcium fluid contains macrophages and proinflammatory cytokines, including IL-6, TNF-α, IL-1β, soluble TNF receptors, neopterin, and IL-18, which suggests a role for activated macrophages in the induction of calcinosis.[257,258] Osteopontin and TNF-α receptor knockout mice on a C57BL6 background injected with cardiotoxin in skeletal muscle develop dystrophic calcifications that resemble human calcinosis in mineral composition, although these lesions resolve spontaneously.[259]

CLINICAL MANIFESTATIONS

Classic JDM presents with an insidious progression of malaise, easy fatigue, muscle weakness, fever, and rash that may predate diagnosis by 3 to 6 months (Table 26-4).[1-6,9,18,48,49,260-265] There is, however, great variation in the rapidity of evolution of the clinical manifestations. Onset is usually insidious, with development of progressive muscle weakness and pain; a more acute onset occurs in approximately one third of children. Children with myositis-specific and myositis-associated autoantibodies characteristically present with phenotypically distinct disease.[15,266]

Constitutional Signs and Symptoms

The onset of JDM may be characterized by fever in the range of 38°C to 40°C. An affected child often complains of ease of fatigue, which probably represents muscle weakness. Malaise, anorexia, and weight loss follow. Parents may report that the child had become irritable, with alterations in gross motor function or regression of motor milestones.

Musculoskeletal Disease

Muscle weakness at onset is predominantly proximal, and complaints related to weakness of the limb-girdle musculature of the lower extremities are most common. Weakness of the anterior neck flexors, back, and abdominal muscles leads to inability to hold the head upright or maintain a sitting posture and protrusion of the abdomen. The child may be unable to dress or climb stairs, wash their face or comb their hair, and may stop walking. The affected child may also complain of moderate muscle pain or stiffness.

Physical examination demonstrates symmetric weakness that is maximal in the proximal muscles of the shoulders and hips, in the neck flexors, and in abdominal musculature.[267] The overlying subcutaneous tissue of affected muscles is occasionally edematous and indurated, and the muscles may be tender. Functional muscle examination may demonstrate that the child is unable to arise from a supine position without rolling over, move from sitting to standing, get out of bed without assistance, or is unable to squat or rise from a squatting position without help. Gowers sign is often present. The child with weakness of the pelvic girdle musculature has difficulty climbing or descending stairs. The Trendelenburg sign indicates weakness of the hip abductors. Later in the disease or in children with an especially severe course, the distal muscles of the extremities may become involved and muscle atrophy may develop.[58,268] Occasionally the disease is so severe that the child is unable to rise from bed or move at all. Although not as

TABLE 26-4 Frequency of Manifestations of Juvenile Dermatomyositis, Polymyositis, and Overlap Myositis

| MANIFESTATION | FREQUENCY AT ONSET (%) | | |
	JDM	JPM	OVERLAP MYOSITIS
Progressive proximal muscle weakness	82-100	100	100
Easy fatigue	80-100	85	84
Gottron papules	57-91	0	74-80
Heliotrope rash	66-87	0	40-59
Erythematous rash of malar/facial area	42-100	0-6	20-51
Periungual nailfold capillary changes	35-91	33	67-80
Muscle pain or tenderness	25-83	61-66	55
Weight loss	33-36	52	53
Falling episodes	40	59	29
Arthritis	10-65	0-45	69-80
Fever	16-65	0-41	0-49
Lymphadenopathy	8-75	0-12	20-22
Dysphagia or dysphonia	15-44	39	40
Joint contractures	9-55	17-42	57-60
V- or shawl-sign rashes	19-29	3-6	8-14
Dyspnea on exertion	5-43	17-42	40
Gastrointestinal symptoms	5-37	9-33	6-53
Photosensitive rashes	5-51	0-6	22-40
Raynaud phenomenon	9-28	0-24	41-60
Edema	11-34	15	20
Gingivitis	6-30	9	0-37
Cutaneous ulceration	5-30	3	20-22
Calcinosis	3-34	6	24
Cardiac involvement	2-13	36	19
Interstitial lung disease	5	15	26
Lipodystrophy	4-14	3	0-6
Gastrointestinal bleeding or ulceration	3-4	3	4-10

JDM, Juvenile dermatomyositis; *JPM,* juvenile polymyositis.
Adapted from Refs. 1-6, 9, 18, 20, 48, 260, 265.

clinically dramatic, the distal muscles of the extremities are involved in many patients.[267] Despite considerable muscle weakness, the deep tendon reflexes are usually preserved.

Pharyngeal, hypopharyngeal, and palatal muscles are frequently affected. Difficulty in swallowing may be related to this involvement or to esophageal hypomotility.[269-272] Regurgitation of liquids through the nose may be a sign of impending difficulty. The threat of aspiration is increased in these children. In up to 80% of patients, subtle or even asymptomatic dysfunctional swallowing can be demonstrated by a barium swallow test, which does not necessarily correlate with weakness or other measures of disease activity; thus all children with JDM should undergo evaluation for swallowing dysfunction.[4,271] Dysphonia, weakness of the voice or a gurgling voice quality, and nasal speech are also frequent signs.[273]

Sequential muscle strength examinations, including proximal, axial, and distal muscle groups, by an experienced physician or physical therapist should be recorded using a standard scale.[267,274] The importance of this examination becomes even more critical later during the course of the disease, when serum levels of muscle enzymes may be less dependable indicators of disease activity. Selected muscle groups that should generally be evaluated are the neck flexors; shoulder abductors; elbow flexors and extensors; hip flexors, extensors, adductors, and abductors; and knee flexors and extensors. An abbreviated group of muscles that includes neck flexors, deltoids, biceps, wrist extensors, gluteus maximus and medius, quadriceps, and ankle plantar flexors closely approximates a total set of 24 muscles.[275] Assessment of strength and function can also be documented with the Childhood Myositis Assessment Scale (CMAS); the Childhood Health Assessment Questionnaire (CHAQ); or the Disease Activity Scale (DAS), which includes skin assessment; these assessment tools can demonstrate decreased endurance and physical dysfunction.[276-281] The CMAS, CHAQ, DAS, and other validated myositis assessment tools, including associated training documents, presentations, and videotapes, are available on the International Myositis Assessment and Clinical Studies Group Internet site.[282,283]

Aerobic and anaerobic exercise capacity is reduced in patients with JDM[284-286] and correlates with parameters of disease activity, abnormalities on T1-weighted MRI, and disease duration.[287-290]

Some children with JDM have arthralgia or arthritis that is transient and nondeforming, sometimes accompanied by tenosynovitis or flexor nodules. One report documented the presence of arthritis in 26% to 67% of children with JDM[1-3,48,291,292]; these frequencies are much higher than was previously appreciated. Early development of flexion contractures, particularly at the knees, hips, shoulders, elbows, ankles, and wrists, is common and usually represents the effects of myofascial inflammation rather than synovitis.[1,48,292] The presence of significant, persistent arthritis in a child with myositis and the skin changes of DM also suggest the possibility of an overlapping autoimmune disease.

Mucocutaneous Disease

In more than three fourths of the children diagnosed with JDM, the cutaneous abnormalities are pathognomonic of the disease at presentation; a less characteristic rash occurs in the remainder. Often, dermatitis is the first manifestation of the disorder, although asymptomatic (undiagnosed) muscle weakness frequently occurs in such children. More often, the cutaneous abnormalities become evident in the first few weeks simultaneously with or after the onset of muscle symptoms.[4,5] The two most typical cutaneous manifestations are heliotrope discoloration of the upper eyelids and Gottron papules or sign.[1,293] The classic heliotrope rash occurs over the upper eyelids as a violaceous, reddish-purple suffusion that often is associated with a malar rash resembling that of SLE in its distribution; however, the nasolabial folds are often spared (Fig. 26-3). Edema of the eyelids and face often

accompanies the heliotrope rash and may be extensive. The symmetric changes over the extensor surfaces of joints (i.e., Gottron papules) tend to be associated with shiny, erythematous, scaly plaques (Fig. 26-4). These hypertrophic areas of skin have a bright pink to red appearance. Occasionally, the lesions appear to be pale or atrophic early in the disease course, which may represent ischemia as a result of vasculopathy (Fig. 26-4C). Gottron papules are especially common over the metacarpophalangeal and proximal interphalangeal joints of the hands and less so over the distal interphalangeal joints. The skin overlying the toes is rarely affected. The extensor surfaces of the elbows and knees, and, less frequently, the malleoli, may also be involved.

Abnormalities of the periungual skin and capillary bed are frequent, present in 35% to 90% of patients with JDM. The periungual skin is often intensely erythematous, and careful examination with the naked eye, a ×40 lens of an ophthalmoscope, or a DermLite™ will discern the presence of telangiectasias.[294] Dilatation of isolated loops, thrombosis and hemorrhage (often visible), dropout of surrounding vessels,[291] tortuosity, bushy loop formation, and arborized clusters of giant capillary loops are distinctive and frequent in JDM (eFig. 26-5; Figs. 26-6, and 26-7). There is often associated marked cuticular overgrowth. Similar changes occur in the gingival capillaries.[295,296] Periungual nailfold capillary changes occur in other connective tissue diseases[297,298] but are seldom as dramatic as those seen in JDM. These abnormalities, like the noninflammatory vasculopathy, correlate with skin and muscle disease activity and a longer duration of untreated symptoms. Some studies have also found a relationship between persistently decreased nailfold capillary density and more severe chronic disease course, cutaneous ulceration, or the development of calcinosis.[281,299-301] The acute nailfold abnormalities may abate, and the capillaries may regenerate in patients who experience remission or a unicyclic disease course.[300,301]

Cutaneous involvement varies from the slightest erythematous tinge over the knuckles or eyelids to a generalized pruritic, scaly rash. At onset, edema and induration of skin, periorbital regions, and subcutaneous tissues are common. Less frequently, the extremities and trunk are affected, and severe edema or anasarca indicates severe disease activity.[302-305] Rashes may be photodistributed, including malar, facial erythema, V- and shawl-sign rashes, and linear extensor erythema, or they may involve skin not exposed to sunlight.[293] Scalp dermatitis, which may be misdiagnosed as seborrhea or psoriasis, has been observed in up to 25% of patients.[303] Rashes may also be intradermal or include panniculitis, with inflammation in the subcutaneous tissue, which may also result from an opportunistic infection.[305-307] Photosensitivity occurs in up to 50% of patients.[1,3,308] Sun exposure has been associated with onset of the disease and exacerbations.[106,107]

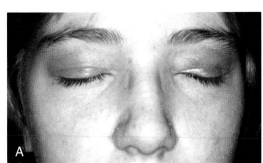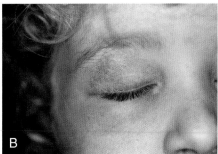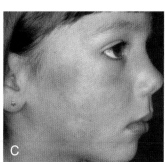

FIGURE 26-3 **A,** Heliotrope discoloration and violaceous suffusion with edema of the upper eyelids in an 11-year-old child with acute dermatomyositis. **B,** Heliotrope rash with erythematous to purplish discoloration on the upper eyelid with telangiectasias. Erythema is also present on the lower lid, temporal region, and ear in a girl with juvenile dermatomyositis. **C,** Erythematous rash in a malar distribution, with perioral sparing.

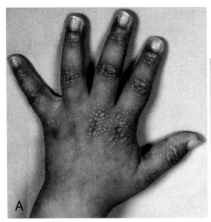
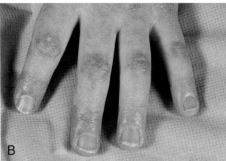
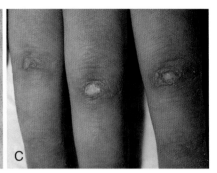

FIGURE 26-4 A, Gottron papules over extensor surfaces of the metacarpophalangeal, proximal, and distal interphalangeal joints. **B,** Erythematous papules over the metacarpophalangeal and proximal and distal interphalangeal joints of the hand of a 6-year-old boy. Also note that some of the papules have areas of central porcelain white infarction with telangiectasia. The periungual capillaries are dilated and tortuous with areas of dropout, and there is cuticular overgrowth on the second and third fingers. **C,** Gottron papules over the proximal interphalangeal joints of the hand of a teenage girl. Note the central porcelain white infarcts, likely the result of vasculopathy.

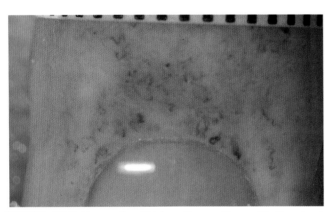

FIGURE 26-6 Abnormal nailfold capillary pattern with the classic changes of dermatomyositis. There is marked capillary dropout, and the remaining capillaries are thickened and tortuous, and show the typical bushy pattern.

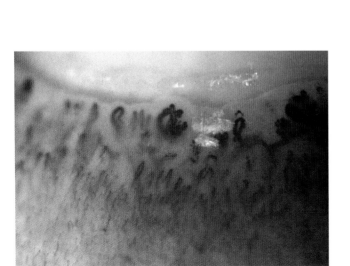

FIGURE 26-7 Advanced changes of the nailfold capillaries, with gross thickening and dropout areas in a child with dermatomyositis. (Courtesy Dr. Jay Kenik.)

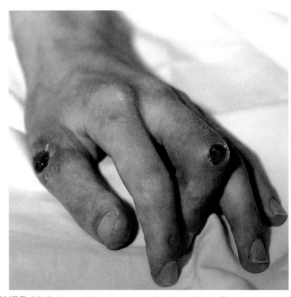

FIGURE 26-8 Vasculitic ulcers on the knuckles of a young boy with severe dermatomyositis. These open ulcerations led to *Staphylococcus aureus* bacteremia and endocarditis.

Gingival and buccal ulcerations develop in 10% to 46% of children, and components of the sicca syndrome may be present.[1,6]

Cutaneous ulceration occurred relatively frequently in the series studied by Crowe and coworkers[309] and in 5% to 30% of patients more recently, possibly more frequently in younger children.[1-3,5,6,9,48,49,260,308,310,311] Vasculitic ulcers at the corners of the eyes, in the axillae, over the elbows or pressure points, and over stretch marks may become a serious problem in management of the disease course (Figs. 26-8). Children with a generalized rash and cutaneous ulcerations may have severe and prolonged disease,[309,312] but this has not been observed in all reports.[265,310,313] Panniculitis has been reported rarely.

Late in the disease course, other cutaneous and subcutaneous changes occur.[293] Thinning and atrophy of the skin and supporting structures may supervene, and alterations in pigmentation become more common.[49,58,268,308,314] Although individual lesions may be hypopigmented, the child may exhibit generalized hyperpigmentation.[6] Poikiloderma, a mixture of atrophy, telangiectasia, and pigmentary changes, is uncommon in children.[49,308,314]

Several tools for assessment of skin disease in JDM have been developed and partially validated,[283] including the Cutaneous Assessment Tool (CAT), which comprehensively assesses skin activity and damage[308,315,316]; the DAS, which includes assessment of skin involvement, particularly the vasculopathic manifestations[278,281]; the Myositis Disease Activity Assessment Tool (MDAAT), in which cutaneous manifestations are assessed along with other systemic disease activity[317]; and the Myositis Damage Index (MDI), to assess damage in skin and other organ systems.[58,268,318] Several tools to assess skin disease in adult DM have also been proposed, including the Cutaneous Dermatomyositis Disease Area and Severity Index (CDASI) and the Dermatomyositis Skin Severity Index (DSSI).[319-321]

Calcinosis

Dystrophic calcification occurs in 12% to 47% of children with JDM.[3,6,9,49,107,308,310,314,322-324] Calcinosis is less frequently present at diagnosis or within 6 months of onset and has been reported in only 3% to 23% of patients,[2-6,49] but it typically occurs after onset of symptomatic myositis.[48] Calcium deposition may occur in subcutaneous plaques or nodules (Box 26-2; Fig. 26-9), as large tumorous deposits in muscle groups (Fig. 26-9 and eFig. 26-10), as calcification within fascial planes, bridging joints, or as an extensive subcutaneous exoskeleton (eFig. 26-11).[312,325,326] Calcinosis affecting the subcutaneous tissues can result in an accompanying cellulitis that may be difficult to distinguish from a true infection, as well as in painful superficial ulceration of the overlying skin. Calcinosis that crosses joint margins may result in flexion contractures, and if those lesions entrap nerves it may result in severe pain.[326,327] Calcinosis deposits may slowly resolve with time, with recurrent extrusion of small flecks or development of liquefied calcium salts that resorb, which appears to be more likely with aggressive antiinflammatory and demineralizing treatments (eFig. 26-11). Rarely, calcinosis is accompanied by hypercalcemia.[328] If deposition in subcutaneous tissues, along fascial planes, and within muscles is extreme, the child may literally be encased within a shell of calcium, known as an *exoskeleton*. This type of calcinosis is unlikely to resolve, and it results in severe disability. Risk factors for calcinosis include delay to diagnosis and the duration of untreated disease, duration of active disease, inadequate therapy, underlying cardiac or pulmonary disease, male gender, older age at illness onset, prolonged persistent disease activity after diagnosis, and the need for corticosteroid-sparing immunosuppressive therapy, which may be an indicator of severe disease activity.[49,58,314,322,323,329] Although the frequency of calcinosis has declined as treatments have improved, it appears to be more frequent in certain regions (e.g., South America more than Europe).[58] Certain myositis autoantibodies, including anti-MJ (NXP-2) and anti-PM-Scl,[22,330] as well as proinflammatory cytokine polymorphisms of TNF-α and IL-1α, are additional risk factors for the development of calcinosis.[137,138] Aggressive treatment to achieve rapid and complete control of inflammation, especially early after onset, may minimize calcinosis.[258,323,327,331,332]

Vasculopathy

Visceral vasculopathy occurs in a minority of children, usually soon after onset of the disorder, but may also occur later in the illness course.[333] It signifies a poor prognosis and sometimes rapidly leads to death.[7,8,309,334] This complication is characterized by diffuse, severe, progressive abdominal pain, pancreatitis, melena, and hematemesis, which represent vasculopathy of the mucosa of the gastrointestinal tract with resulting tissue ischemia or an acute mesenteric infarction.[270,335-339] Free intraperitoneal air radiographically indicates the presence of a perforation of the gastrointestinal tract. Multiple perforations of the duodenum are particularly difficult to recognize and may recur.[335,337-339]

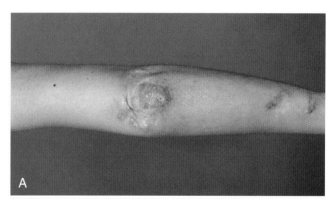

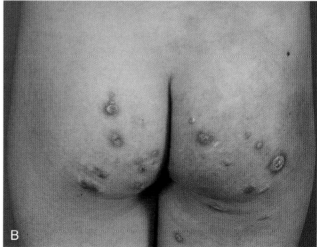

FIGURE 26-9 **A,** Subcutaneous calcification overlying the elbow, resulting in a flexion contracture, and distal forearm in a 10-year-old girl who had juvenile dermatomyositis since the age of 2 years. **B,** Superficial plaques of calcinosis overlying the buttocks in the same child.

BOX 26-2 **Forms of Dystrophic Calcification**	
FORM	**FREQUENCY (%)**
Superficial plaques or nodules, usually on the extremities	33
Deep, large, tumorous deposits, generally in the proximal muscles (i.e., calcinosis circumscripta)	20
Intermuscular fascial plane deposition (i.e., calcinosis universalis)	16
Severe, subcutaneous, reticular exoskeleton-like deposits	10
Mixed forms: superficial plaques or nodules, tumorous deposits, intermuscular fascial plane deposition	22

Adapted from Ref. 314.

Vasculitis of the gallbladder, urinary bladder, uterus, vagina, and testes can also occur.[309,340] Anasarca, cholestasis, pancreatitis, hepatitis, and pneumatosis intestinalis have been reported.[304,305,307,341-343] Widespread vascular disease can involve the central and peripheral nervous systems,[309,344] but severe central nervous system involvement is rare.[345,346] Retinal vessel vasculopathy manifesting as cotton-wool spots has been reported in rare instances.[347]

Cardiopulmonary Disease

The most frequently detected cardiac abnormality is nonspecific sinus tachycardia, but murmurs and cardiomegaly with or without electrocardiographic changes may also be seen.[348] Pericarditis has also been described. Serious cardiac involvement (e.g., acute myocarditis, conduction defects, first-degree heart block) is rare[1,9] but has been associated with death, and onset may be delayed until years after the initial diagnosis.[309,348] Subclinical myocardial involvement may be detected by cardiac MRI.[349,350] Hypertension can occur in 25% to 50% of patients; it may be severe and is sometimes associated with or exacerbated by glucocorticoid therapy.[309,351] However, in long-term outcome studies in which patients received lower doses of glucocorticoids, hypertension is present in less than 15% of patients.[6,49,268,314] Patients with long-term follow-up demonstrated increased systolic cardiac strain, which correlates with myositis damage scores and skin activity at 1 year into the illness.[352] Raynaud phenomenon is unusual but has been diagnosed in 2% to 15% of patients.[6,309,353]

Respiratory muscle weakness results in symptomatic, restrictive pulmonary disease in most children who are moderately to severely affected; dyspnea upon exertion is seen in approximately 25% of patients.[1] However, asymptomatic pulmonary involvement may occur in up to 50% of children, resulting in reduced total lung capacity or diffusion capacity.[354,355] Interstitial pneumonitis is uncommon and is reported in less than 8% of patients.[1,10,49,287] It is associated with anti-Jo-1 and other antisynthease and antimelanoma differentiation–associated gene 5 (MDA5) autoantibodies,[15,356,357] and may be refractory to treatment and a risk factor for increased mortality.[343,358-360] Serum human Krebs Von den Lungen 6 (KL-6) and ferritin levels are elevated in patients with interstitial lung disease, and these may be early markers.[359,361,362] Spontaneous pneumothorax and pneumomediastinum may also rarely occur, presumably due to vasculopathy.[363,364]

Lipodystrophy and Metabolic Abnormalities

Lipodystrophy is a clinically heterogeneous disorder that occurs in acquired and inherited forms.[365] The association of acquired lipodystrophy with JDM may be more common than often appreciated (5% to 50%).[9,47,58,268,314,366-372] This disorder may be generalized; partial, with fat loss from the extremities; or focal, with localized fat loss, particularly overlying sites of calcinosis.[370,373] It is characterized by a slow but progressive loss of subcutaneous and visceral fat, often most noticeable over the upper body and face, that is accompanied most frequently by hypertriglyceridemia, as well as by insulin resistance, acanthosis nigricans, abnormal glucose tolerance, hypertension, and nonalcoholic steatohepatitis, with more severe metabolic sequelae and features related to the degree of fat loss (Fig. 26-12).[369-371,374] Patients with generalized lipodystrophy also frequently have hyperandrogenism, with hypertrichosis, hyperpigmentation, clitoral enlargement, and amenorrhea. Pope et al. reported that JDM is the most common systemic autoimmune disease associated with lipodystrophy, followed by juvenile idiopathic arthritis.[369] Lipodystrophy is most often delayed in presentation until several years after the onset of JDM, and duration of untreated disease may be a risk factor for its development.[58,372] Calcinosis, muscle atrophy, joint contractures, facial rash, greater skin disease activity, and decreased density of periungual nailfold capillaries are the JDM disease

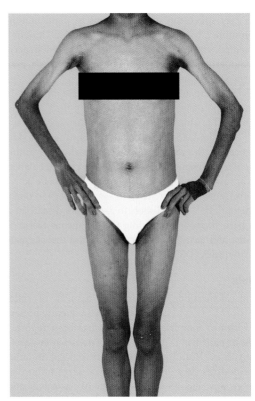

FIGURE 26-12 Generalized lipodystrophy in a teenage girl with long-standing juvenile dermatomyositis. Note loss of body fat from both the extremities and trunk. There is prominent acanthosis nigricans under the axilla and in the neck line. There is generalized hyperpigmentation due to secondary hyperandrogenism. Also note the subcutaneous calcinosis, which is associated with lipodystrophy in juvenile dermatomyositis.

features associated with development of lipodystrophy.[370,372] Panniculitis has been associated with focal lipoatrophy, whereas the anti-p155/140 (TIF-1) autoantibody, a newly described myositis-associated autoantibody, is increased in frequency in patients with generalized lipodystrophy.[370] In addition to the metabolic sequelae, the loss of fat from the lateral thigh, more so than from the medial thigh, which is revealed by MRI, may be an indicator of lipodystrophy.[370] The etiology of acquired lipodystrophy in patients with JDM remains unclear and does not appear to be related to HLA or TNF alleles, lamin mutations, or complement deficiencies.[370]

Metabolic sequelae in the absence of lipodystrophy are also frequent in patients with JDM, especially in patients with chronic disease. Insulin resistance, hyperlipidemia, hypertension, and an increased body mass index in up to 50% of patients, and 25% have the metabolic syndrome, all of which are potential risk factors for the development of early cardiovascular disease.[351,374,375] However, this has not been observed in all JDM cohorts.[352] Patients with a family history of diabetes mellitus may be at increased risk for glucose abnormalities. Glucose abnormalities are correlated with muscle atrophy, as well as with proinflammatory cytokines, rather than prednisone dose,[351] and hyperlipidemia correlates with disease activity and use of cyclosporine.[375] Young adults with long-standing JDM also have evidence of metabolic abnormalities and early cardiovascular disease, with frequent hypertension, increased proinflammatory oxidized high-density lipoprotein, carotid intima-media thickening, and decreased brachial artery reactivity.[376]

Hematologic Manifestations and Osteoporosis

Hematologic manifestations are rare; they have been described primarily in adult DM patients but occasionally in children, and include macrophage activation syndrome, thrombocytopenia, and thrombotic thrombocytopenic purpura.[377-383] Anemia of chronic disease correlates with disease activity.

The majority of patients studied have frank osteopenia or osteoporosis even prior to initiation of corticosteroid therapy, which is worsened by delay to diagnosis as well as long-standing disease activity and may persist years after the patient enters remission.[384-387] Patients have elevated serum levels of receptor activator of NF-κB ligand and decreased osteoprotegerin at the time of diagnosis, resulting in increased osteoclast activity that may result in lower bone mineral density.[387] Vertebral fractures develop in up to 10% of patients treated with 12 months of glucocorticoids, and osteopenia or osteoporosis develops in 6% to 35% of patients in long-term outcome studies.[6,49,58,268,314,388,389] Weight gain associated with steroid use is a risk factor.

PATHOLOGY

The distinctive pathological lesions of JDM involve striated muscles, skin, and the gastrointestinal tract. The severity of clinical disease may or may not correlate with the intensity of the histological findings, which are patchy in distribution in every affected organ and can change over time. Extensive active myopathic changes, including degeneration, vacuolation, sarcoplasmic pallor and necrosis, as well as central nuclei without basophilia, predict a chronic course of illness.[390] Muscle infarction, while not a frequent finding, appears to correlate with a chronic illness course, gastrointestinal ulceration, and mortality.[390,391] Direct immunofluorescence staining of the muscle arteries might also be

associated with a chronic ulcerative course of illness.[390,391] Patients with diffuse infiltrates or lymphocytic aggregates on initial muscle biopsy were responsive to standard therapy with steroids and methotrexate, but those with follicle-like structures, including follicular dendritic cells and high endothelial venules, tended to have severe disease that required treatment with additional agents.[183] A standardized scoring method to examine histopathological features of JDM biopsies—including immunophenotypes of the inflammatory infiltrates, vascular and muscle fiber changes, and connective tissue fibrosis—has good reliability, correlates well with measures of myositis disease activity, and appears to be a promising tool to enable future studies of the relationship of muscle pathology with illness outcomes.[14] The histological characteristics of JDM are contrasted with those in muscular dystrophy and neurogenic atrophy in Table 26-5.

Skeletal Muscle

Muscle fibers characteristically demonstrate group atrophy or necrosis at the periphery of the fascicle (Fig. 26-13).[309] This perifascicular atrophy is often associated with a noninflammatory capillaropathy.[309,392] Nonspecific changes include disruption of the myofibrils and tubular systems, central nuclear migration, and prominent nuclei and basophilia.[85,186] Concomitant degeneration and regeneration of muscle fibers occur and result in moderate variations in fiber size. Areas of focal necrosis are replaced during the healing phase by an interstitial proliferation of connective tissue. An inflammatory exudate is often present. The inflammatory cells, which are often sparse and consist principally of lymphocytes and mononuclear cells, are located predominantly in the perimysium and perivascularly around the septae or in the fascicles (Figs. 26-13 and 26-14). This infiltrate is not in itself diagnostic because the muscular dystrophies may also demonstrate an infiltrate around necrotic fibers. Macrophages, plasma cells, mast cells, and rarely, eosinophils or basophils are also present.

TABLE 26-5   Comparison of Muscle Histopathology in Juvenile Dermatomyositis, Muscular Dystrophy, and Neurogenic Muscle Atrophy

HISTOPATHOLOGY	DERMATOMYOSITIS	MUSCULAR DYSTROPHY	NEUROGENIC ATROPHY
Chronic inflammatory infiltrate			
Endomysial	++	+	−
Perimysial	++	+	−
Perivascular	++	−	−
Fiber degeneration	++	++	−
Fiber regeneration	++	+	−
Perifascicular atrophy	++	−	−
Vasculopathy of blood vessels	++	−	−
Thickened capillaries and capillary loss	++	−	−
Muscle infarction	++	−	−
Endomysial proliferation	++	++	−
MHC class I staining of myocyte	++	±	−
Myofiber necrosis	++	++	−
Phagocytosis of necrotic muscle fibers	+	++	−
Increased perimysial connective tissue	++	+	−
Myofiber size variation	+	++	±
Myofiber hypertrophy	−	++	−
Rounded, hypercontracted myofibers	−	++	−
Muscle fibrosis	±	++	−
Myocytes replaced with fat	±	++	−
Central migration of nuclei	+	++	−
Fiber atrophy	±	+	++
Motor unit atrophy	−	−	++

− Absent; ± possible; + present; ++ characteristic; *MHC,* major histocompatibility complex.

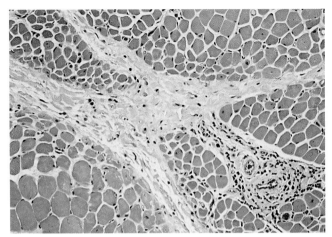

FIGURE 26-13 Muscle biopsy (hematoxylin-eosin stain) with perivascular mononuclear inflammatory infiltrate, arterial wall thickening, endothelial prominence, and perifascicular atrophy. (Reprinted with permission from L.G. Rider, I.N. Targoff, Muscle Diseases, in: R.G. Lahita, N. Chiorazzi, W.H. Reeves (Eds.), Textbook of the Autoimmune Diseases, Lippincott Williams and Wilkins, Philadelphia, 2000, Chapter 22.)

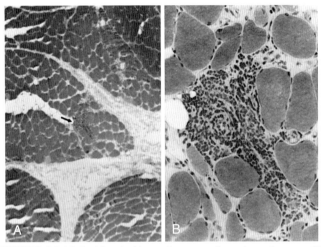

FIGURE 26-14 A, Muscle biopsy (hematoxylin-eosin stain; magnification ×40). Scattered foci (arrow) of perivascular inflammation and resultant perifascicular atrophy. **B,** Enlargement (hematoxylin-eosin stain; magnification ×250) of central area of **(A).** Perivascular mononuclear inflammatory infiltrate, arterial wall thickening, and endothelial prominence.

Immunohistochemistry shows that plasmacytoid dendritic cells are one of the primary infiltrating immunophenotypes.[188] In some cases, lymphoid aggregates and even extranodal lymphoid microstructures are seen in inflamed muscle.[186]

Electron microscopy can confirm focal degeneration of the myofibrils, cytoplasmic masses, disorganization of sarcomeres, disruption of the Z lines and Z-disc streaming, actin-myosin filament disorganization, thickening of the capillary basement membranes, mitochondrial abnormalities, or an increase in vacuole formation. Immunoglobulins are often seen on the sarcolemmal membrane by immunofluorescence microscopy but are of unknown pathogenic significance.[162] Damaged muscle fibers have an increase in calcium content,[393,394] which may explain the uptake of technetium 99m diphosphonate by the muscles in inflammatory myopathy. The regenerative phase probably depends on the mononuclear myoblast that is derived from satellite cells.[395]

Regenerating fibers contain increased aldolase, oxidative enzyme, and alkaline phosphatase activities.[396,397] Studies suggest that sarcolemmal overexpression of MHC class I and class II might be useful to distinguish JDM from other myopathies. MHC class I overexpression along the sarcolemma, which is stronger in JDM than adult myositis, is an early and late event and may remain positive even after initiating corticosteroid therapy.[155,179,398-400] Although overexpression of class I MHC on myofibers has also been seen occasionally in muscular dystrophies, staining appears to be more intense in JDM biopsies.[177,179,401,402]

Blood Vessels

JDM should be considered a systemic inflammatory and noninflammatory vasculopathy rather than simply an inflammation of muscle and skin. Nonnecrotizing vasculitis affects arterioles, capillaries, and venules of the striated muscles, gastrointestinal tract, skin, and subcutaneous tissues. Endothelial vessel wall thickening often develops, as well as thrombotic changes within the vessel, resulting in occlusion and tissue ischemia and infarction.[403] Capillary loss is evident in the muscle, as well as other affected tissues.[154,169] Vasculopathy can lead to infarction, ulceration, and diffuse bleeding, especially in the gastrointestinal tract. The early studies of Banker and Victor[334] identified this type of vasculopathy as an important prognostic factor in survival. Crowe et al.[309] showed that muscle infarction and ulceration of the cutaneous and gastrointestinal tissues were associated with a zonal loss of the capillary bed, areas of focal infarction of muscle, nonnecrotizing lymphocytic vasculitis, and noninflammatory endarteropathy. Conversely, severe vasculopathy was absent from the muscle specimens of children with limited disease.[309] This spectrum of capillary endothelial damage had also been suggested in previous studies.[162,334,404]

Widespread capillaropathy leads to intravascular coagulation, microvascular occlusion and infarction, and associated perifascicular myopathy. These capillary changes, although characteristic, are not specific and have been described in other connective tissue diseases, viral and rickettsial infections, malignancy, and normal wound healing.[404,405] Changes in the capillaries can be identified clinically in the nailfolds (see Figs. 26-6 and 26-7) and in tissues through the use of light and electron microscopy.[309,334,406-409] Endothelial swelling and necrosis, capillary thrombosis and obliteration, and endoplasmic tubuloreticular inclusions (thought to be due to type I IFNs) occur early in the course of disease.[309,334,404,410-412]

Inflammation of small muscular arteries and infarction of muscle results from an immune complex–mediated vasculitis.[309] IgM, IgG, and C3 were deposited in the perimysial veins in 9 of 11 patients studied by Whitaker and Engle.[162] Diffuse linear and occasionally granular vascular wall deposits of IgM, C3d, and fibrin were also observed in the areas of noninflammatory vasculopathy.[309] Deposition of the C5b-9 membrane attack complex on muscle arterioles and capillaries also occurs frequently; for example, it was present in the muscle biopsies of 10 of 12 patients with JDM studied by Kissel et al.[164] Electron microscopy has not confirmed evidence of subendothelial deposition of immunoglobulins within vessel walls, as might be expected in classic immune complex disease, although circulating immune complexes and complement activity are often identified in the blood.[348,413]

Skin

A capillary endothelial change similar to that in muscle is usually observed in involved skin.[309] Histopathological examination of the skin demonstrates perivascular inflammation, vascular changes at the dermal–epidermal junction, telangiectasias, hyperkeratosis in the stratum corneal layer, epidermal atrophy, follicular plugging, and basement membrane thickening.[414,415] The skin histopathological changes are not specific to DM and are also frequently present in

SLE.[415,416] Specialized stains with colloidal iron and periodic acid–Schiff demonstrate increased dermal mucin and basement membrane thickening in most adult DM skin biopsies.[415] Immunofluorescent stains reveal the deposition of C3d, C4d, and the C5b-9 membrane attack complex on blood vessels to a greater degree in DM than in SLE, and immunohistochemistry demonstrates CD123-positive plasmacytoid dendritic cells, primarily in the epidermis in a perivascular distribution, which differs from SLE where they are primarily dermal in location.[192,416-418] Mast cells are also present in higher numbers than normal in lesional skin.[192] Glycosaminoglycans, particularly chondroitin-4-sulfate, is elevated in the dermal matrix of lesional skin.[419,420] In a study of the histopathology of Gottron papules,[415,421] basal layer vasculopathy, periodic acid–Schiff–positive basement membrane thickening, upper dermal mucin deposition, and a diffuse upper dermal mononuclear infiltrate were frequently identified. Epidermal hyperplasia consisting of acanthosis or papillomatosis often occurred, but epidermal atrophy was rare. Lobular panniculitis has also been reported, which may result in focal lipoatrophy or calcification[306,370,422]; it may also be associated with infection with *Staphylococcus* or *Mycobacterium*.[306,423] In the healing phase of the disease, calcium hydroxyapatite or carbonate apatite crystals[252-254] may be deposited or formed in the skin, subcutaneous tissues, and interfascial planes of the muscle.[424]

Gastrointestinal Tract

Ulceration or perforation resulting from vasculopathy can occur in any part of the gastrointestinal tract, including the esophagus.[309,333,334] Serious gastrointestinal disease of this type develops in approximately 10% of children with JDM and may result in bowel perforation.[270,337,338,348] Pneumatosis intestinalis, as well as bowel wall thickening with a stacked coin appearance, has been described.[335,425-427] Constipation, delayed gastric emptying, and prolonged gastrointestinal transit time may occur.[428] Pancreatitis and autoimmune hepatitis are rare.[341,429]

Heart

Cardiac muscle is rarely affected by the primary pathological process,[430,431] but its involvement may be more common than clinically appreciated.[432] A few cases of carditis have been described, with areas of focal myocardial fibrosis and contraction-band necrosis. Interstitial myocarditis and narrowing of the coronary arteries have been reported.[309]

Pulmonary interstitial lung disease is uncommon in children but is a poor prognostic sign. Pathological studies in adults reveal nonspecific interstitial pneumonia to be the most common form of interstitial lung disease.[433,434] Occasionally, bronchiolitis obliterans organizing pneumonia and usual interstitial pneumonia may be seen.[434] Diffuse alveolar damage holds a poor prognosis, with rapid progression, frequent respiratory failure, and even death.[435]

Kidneys

Although microscopic hemoglobinuria related to urine myoglobin may be present, especially at onset, histological renal abnormalities are rare. Thrombotic microangiopathy related to reduced ADAMTS13 (a disintegrin and metalloproteinase with a thrombospondin type 1 motif, member 13) activity has been described.[436]

DIFFERENTIAL DIAGNOSIS

The differential diagnosis includes other forms of IIMs, including JPM, as well as infectious myopathies, noninflammatory myopathies, other systemic diseases that involve weakness, and mimicking rashes such as

---

BOX 26-3   Differential Diagnosis of Juvenile Dermatomyositis

Other forms of idiopathic inflammatory myopathies
  Juvenile polymyositis
  Overlap myositis
  Amyopathic dermatomyositis
  Cancer-associated myositis
  Focal myositis
  Orbital myositis
  Granulomatous myositis
  Eosinophilic myositis
  Macrophagic myofasciitis
  Immune-mediated necrotizing myopathies
Inflammatory myopathies: Infectious myopathies
  Viral (enterovirus, influenza, Coxsackievirus, echovirus, parvovirus, hepatitis B, human T lymphotropic virus I)
  Bacterial and parasitic (*Staphylococcus, Streptococcus, Toxoplasmosis, Trichinosis,* Lyme borreliosis)
Noninflammatory myopathies*
  Muscular dystrophies
  Congenital myopathies
  Myotonic disorders
  Metabolic myopathies—glycogen storage diseases, lipid myopathies
  Periodic paralyses
  Mitochondrial myopathies
  Endocrinopathies
  Trauma
  Toxins
  Drug-induced myopathies
  Disorders of neuromuscular transmission
Systemic rheumatic diseases
  Systemic lupus erythematosus
  Scleroderma
  Juvenile idiopathic arthritis
  Mixed connective tissue disease
  Systemic vasculitis
Autoinflammatory diseases
  Chronic atypical neutrophilic dermatosis with lipodystrophy and elevated temperature (CANDLE)
  Tumor necrosis factor receptor-associated periodic syndrome (TRAPS)
Mimicking rashes
  Psoriasis
  Eczema
  Allergy

*For full listing, see eBox 26-5.

---

psoriasis (Box 26-3). The correct diagnosis is usually straightforward in the presence of the characteristic rash and weak, painful, or tender proximal muscles, but in patients without characteristic rashes, a muscle biopsy is recommended.[13] Early in the disease course, especially in the absence of the characteristic rash, the differential diagnosis can be challenging (Box 26-3). New classification criteria for the inflammatory myopathies are being developed,[437] and a reclassification of inflammatory versus noninflammatory myopathies by identification of specific sets of immune-related genes is still needed.[438]

Other Forms of Idiopathic Inflammatory Myopathies
Juvenile Polymyositis

JPM, defined by the absence of the characteristic skin rashes, is uncommon, with a much lower incidence than JDM and a prevalence of 2%

to 22% among the childhood IIMs.[1,5,6,20,21,44,51] The gender ratio is comparable with JDM, but age at onset is higher, with JPM developing in the preteen or teen years (median 12.1 years).[1] Patients with JPM tend to have a more severe illness onset and higher CK levels. They have more frequent falling episodes as a sign of distal weakness, myalgias, Raynaud phenomenon, weight loss, pulmonary disease, and cardiac abnormalities (Table 26-5).[1] There are no associated cutaneous abnormalities; the nailfold capillary pattern can be abnormal, and calcinosis occurs infrequently.[1,6] Diagnosis can be further hampered by unusual presentation (e.g., anasarca) or delayed appearance of the JDM rash.[439,440] Arthritis, joint contractures, fevers, and dysphagia occur as in JDM.[1,6,21,51] Approximately 50% of patients with JPM have a chronic course of illness, and 30% have used a wheelchair.[1] Muscle biopsy is usually necessary for accurate diagnosis to exclude other myopathies.

Myositis with Other Connective Tissue Diseases (Overlap Myositis)

Children with systemic scleroderma (see Chapter 27), mixed connective tissue disease (see Chapter 29), or occasionally SLE (see Chapter 23) may have skin and muscle abnormalities at onset that suggest a diagnosis of JDM. The differentiation of these diseases is usually not difficult, however, because clinical features unique to each are almost always present. The overlap of JDM or JPM with another systemic connective tissue disease occurs in 3% to 12% of patients, with SLE, juvenile idiopathic arthritis, and scleroderma as the most common overlapping autoimmune conditions. Patients with overlap myositis have more frequent Raynaud phenomenon, interstitial lung disease, arthritis, sclerodactyly, and periungual capillary abnormalities (Table 26-5).[1] Mortality is highest for the overlap myositis subgroup compared to JPM and JDM.[358]

In terms of distinguishing JDM from SLE, the child with JDM may have malar dermatitis that is similar in distribution to the butterfly rash of SLE; however, it often lacks relatively well-defined borders and spares the nasolabial folds. Heliotrope rash and periorbital edema are not characteristic of SLE. Periungual capillary abnormalities are present in many connective tissue diseases, but Gottron papules are present only in children with JDM, whereas linear extensor erythema (erythema between the joints) is present in both JDM and SLE. Systemic features of SLE, such as pericarditis and pleural effusions, are rare in JDM. Hepatosplenomegaly and lymphadenopathy occur in less than 5% of children with JDM. The arthritis of JDM, although not uncommon, is usually mild; that of SLE occurs more frequently and, although nonerosive, may be quite florid at onset and extremely painful.

Although early cutaneous abnormalities of scleroderma and JDM are quite different, the skin changes sometimes tend to become similar during the courses of these diseases. Systemic sclerosis is also a frequent overlapping condition, which shares the HLA-DRB1*03-DQA1*05-DQB1*02 haplotype.[5,6,22] Laboratory evaluation provides supportive or definitive diagnostic information in most instances.

Myositis occurs in systemic scleroderma and mixed connective tissue disease, and, to a limited extent, in SLE and juvenile idiopathic arthritis. The myositis of JDM can be differentiated from that of other connective tissue diseases by its severity, the greater elevation of serum levels of muscle enzymes, and histological examination of muscle obtained by biopsy. In uncomplicated chronic arthritis, acute rheumatic fever, SLE, or scleroderma, muscle biopsy demonstrates focal accumulations of lymphocytes, patchy fiber atrophy, and increased interstitial connective tissue, but no significant vasculopathy.[441-443] Muscle fiber degeneration and atrophy, sarcoplasmic degeneration, and microcyst formation occur in Sjögren syndrome.[444] A necrotizing vasculitis with muscle fiber degeneration and neurogenic atrophy may be identified in polyarteritis.

Dermatomyositis sine myositis or *amyopathic DM* is rare in children, occurring in approximately 1% of patients with juvenile IIM[23,24,445-448]; however, the classic rash of JDM may occur in the absence of clinical muscle involvement or muscle disease may not be initially documented.[25] In the review by Plamondon and Dent,[25] none of 27 patients developed clinical myopathy at a mean follow-up of 32.8 months, although 2 patients developed calcinosis. In another large series, 18 of 68 patients with juvenile-onset clinical amyopathic DM (26%) evolved to classic JDM after a mean follow-up of 3.9 years.[23] Of patients with a normal serum level of CK, 3 of 22 patients tested had an abnormal EMG, 1 of 19 had abnormal muscle biopsy, and 1 of 9 had abnormal MRI, all of which are suggestive of subclinical muscle involvement. Calcinosis developed in 3 of the 68 patients.[23] In contrast to adult amyopathic DM, interstitial lung disease or internal malignancy has not been reported in the cases of juvenile amyopathic DM, and cutaneous ulceration is very rare, suggesting a relatively good prognosis for children.[23,25] Metabolic abnormalities unmasked by exercise as detected by ^{32}P magnetic resonance spectroscopy, in the setting of normal muscle strength, serum levels of muscle enzymes, and standard magnetic resonance imaging, is another sensitive method for detecting muscle abnormalities in patients with amyopathic DM.[449]

Other Inflammatory Myopathies

Cancer-associated myositis has a firm association with adult myositis but is rare in children; hence children are not routinely assessed for occult malignancy.[19,26-28] The associated malignancies include leukemia, lymphoma, and solid-organ tumors, and the DM has atypical or unusual features, with associated adenopathy, hepatosplenomegaly, palpable masses, and atypical rashes. A number of uncommon forms of myositis have been described, especially in adults,[450] including inclusion body myositis[33,451-453] and disease restricted to one muscle group or extremity, such as focal myositis,[29,30,454,455] orbital myositis confined to the extraocular muscles,[31,456] proliferative myositis,[457-459] and granulomatous myositis.[39] IBM tends to respond slowly to immunosuppressive therapy. A DM-like disease has been observed in children with agammaglobulinemia and common variable immune deficiency (see Chapter 46).[86,87,348,460]

Macrophagic myofasciitis, a rare but distinct clinicopathological entity, demonstrates a predominance of macrophagic infiltrates on muscle biopsy, sometimes containing aluminum inclusions, as alum-containing adjuvants in vaccinations may be etiologic.[39,41,461] Children with this condition frequently present with shoulder or thigh weakness, myalgias, fatigue, arthralgias, and high levels of CK. They may also have hypotonia, developmental delay, and failure to thrive.[42]

Some forms of limb-girdle muscular dystrophies, including calpain-3 deficiency (LGMD2A) Becker dystrophy, and gamma-sarcoglycanopathy (LGMD2C) may be present with eosinophilic myositis, which is often accompanied by peripheral eosinophilia.[37,462-464] However, the condition may also be idiopathic or occur after drug exposures, parasitic infection, or be part of an underlying hypereosinophilic syndrome.[35,36,465] Infantile PM results from merosin gene mutations, and this condition has been reclassified as a muscular dystrophy.

Postinfectious Inflammatory Myopathies

Acute, transient myositis may follow certain viral infections, especially influenza A and B[74,75,466] and Coxsackievirus B.[467,468] Coxsackievirus B causes epidemic pleurodynia (i.e., Bornholm disease), which is characterized by fever and sharp pain in the muscles of the chest and abdominal wall. This syndrome is sometimes preceded by a moderate to severe headache, nausea, vomiting, and pharyngitis. The illness is most common in children and adolescents and usually lasts 3 to 5 days (eBox 26-4).

Myositis may occur in up to 6% and 34% of children following influenza A and B infection, respectively, most often in school-age children and more commonly in boys (2 : 1 ratio with girls).[75] After the contagious phase of illness with fever, headache, rhinitis, cough, nausea, and vomiting, muscle symptoms typically begin approximately 3 days (but up to 2 weeks) after the onset of fever and respiratory symptoms. Severe proximal calf pain and tenderness (i.e., myalgia cruris epidemica) is characteristic, which may include tenderness on palpation and difficulty walking. Rhabdomyolysis is uncommon.[74,75] Laboratory studies demonstrate a slightly elevated erythrocyte sedimentation rate, moderate leukopenia with relative lymphocytosis, and concomitant elevation of the serum levels of CK and aspartate aminotransferase (AST). Treatment is supportive, with the illness usually resolving within a few days, but it may last as long as several weeks.

Other infectious causes of myositis include toxoplasmosis; trichinosis; cat scratch fever; staphylococcal and streptococcal bacteremia; clostridial, mycoplasmal, *Borrelia burgdorferi, Salmonella,* or *Serratia* infection; schistosomiasis; trypanosomiasis and other viral infections, including hepatitis and human T-lymphotropic virus.[469-471] Candidiasis and coccidioidomycosis are very uncommon causes. Toxoplasmosis may be associated with a syndrome that resembles DM.[472,473] Trichinosis, caused by ingestion of the larval cyst of the nematode *Trichinella spiralis,* is characterized initially by fever, diarrhea, and abdominal pain, followed in a week by periorbital edema and swelling and tenderness of muscles, especially those of the face, neck, and chest. Peripheral blood eosinophilia is often striking, and biopsy of affected muscles confirms the presence of the larvae and, later, calcified cysts. Treatment includes glucocorticoids to diminish inflammation and agents such as mebendazole or thiabendazole. Other unusual exposures include *Sarcocystis,* malaria, cysticercosis, echinococcosis, and toxocariasis.

Staphylococcal pyomyositis is an abscess in skeletal muscle that occurs after local muscle injury.[469,474] It affects patients of all ages and is more common in boys than in girls. Lesions may be solitary or multiple and are usually located in the thigh, calf, buttock, arm, scapular areas, or chest wall. The abscess is tender and, if not too deep, warm. Patients usually have low-grade fever. Symptoms last for up to a week. This condition is common in Africa, Latin America, and parts of India. Initial blood cultures are often negative.[475] Ultrasonography or gallium-67 citrate scanning may localize the lesion. Severe pustular acne occasionally may be associated with inflammatory disease of muscle and with arthritis.[476]

Rhabdomyolysis may follow an upper respiratory infection, trauma, or extreme muscular exertion.[477] Onset is generally acute and is characterized by profound weakness, myoglobulinuria, very high serum levels of muscle enzymes, and, occasionally, oliguria and renal failure. It may also occur after snakebite; in heat stroke; after certain medications such as lipid-lowering agents and zidovudine; in the familial malignant hyperpyrexia syndrome; and in metabolic and mitochondrial myopathies, particularly disorders of glycogen and lipid metabolism.[478-481]

Neuromuscular Diseases and Myopathies

In the absence of characteristic skin changes, the differential diagnosis includes a wide variety of neuromuscular disorders (eBoxes 26-4, 26-5, 26-6, 26-7, and 26-8).[478,482] Early in the disease or before the development of cutaneous changes, muscular dystrophy or myotonia may be

confused with JDM. In children without the characteristic rashes of JDM, concern about these entities is greater, particularly if chronic inflammation is absent or not prominent on the muscle biopsy and there are prominent myopathic features. Hypotonia in infancy, often associated with projectile vomiting, is a characteristic of the mitochondrial disorders involving the branched chain amino acids. Paroxysmal myoglobinuria or acute rhabdomyolysis occasionally may be encountered, as well as episodic weakness. Certain drugs or toxins, including alcohol, clofibrate, D-penicillamine, glucocorticoids, and hydroxychloroquine, can cause myopathy[481,483,484] (see Chapter 12).

The possibility of *muscular dystrophy* is suggested by a family history of myopathy and an insidious onset of slowly progressive, predominantly proximal muscle weakness, and by absence of the normal progression of achievement of developmental landmarks. Patients with dystrophies often have weakness in muscle groups that are not characteristically weak in the IIMs, including weakness of the scapula, distal muscle groups, or facial or ocular muscles.[486,487] Constitutional signs; muscle tenderness; cutaneous abnormalities, including periungual nailfold capillary changes; arthritis; and a positive antinuclear antibody and myositis autoantibodies are absent. Patients with dystrophies respond less to immunosuppressive therapies.[488] In Duchenne muscular dystrophy, there is a characteristic hypertrophy of the calves, a sign that occurs in other myopathies and occasionally in long-standing JDM or JPM. In other dystrophies, however, there is frequent clinical muscle atrophy.[488] The hereditary nature of Duchenne muscular dystrophy is demonstrated by the presence of markedly elevated levels of serum CK in the patient and the patient's mother. However, approximately one third of these disorders represent new mutations.

Myoadenylate deaminase deficiency (MDD)[489,490] occurs in an autosomal recessive primary form and an acquired disorder associated with rheumatic and neuromuscular diseases. Data suggest that homozygous MDD is relatively common because 2% of muscle biopsies show deficient enzyme activity (less than 2% in the primary form; less than 15% in the secondary form). MDD is due to mutation C34T in the myoadenylate deaminase gene.[491] Muscle fatigue, stiffness, and cramping may be noticed after exercise and may begin in childhood (23%) or adolescence (26%), but these features do not occur in all deficient individuals. Individuals with MDD may demonstrate decreased muscle mass, hypotonia, and weakness. With forearm exercise (ischemic test), there is a failure of the plasma ammonia level to rise along with inosine monophosphate. Electromyographic findings are nonspecific. The muscle tissue in primary MDD is normal histologically except for the absence of adenosine monophosphate deaminase. Activity of this enzyme is normal in other tissues.

Other metabolic myopathies, including lipid and glycogen metabolic pathway defects, may appear with exercise intolerance, muscle cramping, muscle fatigue, decreased endurance (with or without progressive muscle weakness), and myoglobinuria. Weakness may be exacerbated after fasting or food intake and may be episodic.[492-494]

Endocrinopathies, especially hyperthyroidism and hypothyroidism, hyperparathyroidism and hypoparathyroidism, diabetes mellitus, and myopathy associated with idiopathic or iatrogenic Cushing syndrome, should be considered in the differential diagnosis of a myopathy without evidence of cutaneous disease. Myasthenia gravis is rare, and the diagnosis is suggested by a decremental response to repetitive nerve stimulation, involvement of ocular and distal muscles, and improvement of the weakness after administration of cholinergic drugs. Primary neurogenic atrophies, including infantile and juvenile spinal muscular atrophy, are associated with proximal muscle weakness and in rare instances may be confused with inflammatory myopathies.

Miscellaneous Disorders

Fibrodysplasia ossificans progressiva (i.e., myositis ossificans progressiva) is a rare, autosomal dominant inflammatory disorder (usually a new mutation) that results in painful swelling of muscle and fascia (e.g., ligaments, tendons, aponeuroses), followed by fibrosis, calcification, and ossification.[495-499] There is a heterozygous missense mutation, a single nucleotide substitution (c.617G>A; R206H) at codon 206 in the glycine-serine activation domain of activin receptor IA (ACVR1, also known as ALK2), a bone morphogenetic protein type 1 receptor that has been associated with fibrodysplasia ossificans progressiva, although other mutations in ACVR1 and in noggin, a gene located on chromosome 17q22, have also been associated with this disorder.[495,500,501] The patient may present with a spontaneous joint contracture or preosseous soft-tissue lesions. The clinical diagnosis is often elusive until calcification; later, ossification is evident on ultrasound or radiography.[502,503] Biopsy findings of affected sites at an early stage may be misleading and be misinterpreted as malignant sarcoma. The back of the neck and posterior trunk are often the site of the initial tumorlike swellings, followed by the muscles of the limbs. Palmar and plantar fascia may be affected. The great toes are congenitally malformed, usually short and with hallux valgus; the thumbs are sometimes involved. The toe deformity is an early clinical sign to the diagnosis, even before heterotopic ossification occurs.[504] Some patients may also have cranial skeleton abnormalities.[505] After onset in the first year of life the disease is characterized by exacerbations and remissions and slowly progresses to severe debility, restriction of pulmonary capacity, and reduced life expectancy. There is no therapy for prevention or treatment,[506] although bisphosphonates have been advocated.[507] Early diagnosis can prevent misunderstanding and unnecessary procedures and their associated morbidities.

LABORATORY EXAMINATION

Specific Laboratory Diagnostic Studies

The three investigations that are most useful in substantiating a diagnosis of JDM are measurement of serum levels of the muscle enzymes, EMG, and histopathological examination of a muscle specimen obtained by needle or open biopsy (Table 26-6).

Serum Muscle Enzymes

Serum levels of the sarcoplasmic muscle enzymes are important for diagnosis and to monitor the effectiveness of therapy. Considerable individual variation in the pattern of enzyme elevation is observed; it is therefore recommended, at least early in disease, that AST, CK, lactate dehydrogenase (LDH), and aldolase be measured to obtain a baseline evaluation.[12] The degree of elevation in serum concentration ranges from 1.5 to 15 times normal for CK and 1.3 to 5.5 times normal for aldolase, LDH, AST, and alanine aminotransferase (ALT).[1] Serum levels of muscle enzymes are higher in JPM and intermediate in overlap myositis.[1] The CK level does not always correlate with disease activity.[173] A percentage of children (8% to 54%) have normal serum levels of CK during the acute phase of the illness or at the time of diagnosis, particularly with a longer duration of untreated disease. Other enzymes (LDH, aldolase, and transaminase) are normal in 11% to 68% of patients.[1,3,5,10,48,329] Some patients have a persistent elevation of serum muscle enzyme levels late in the course, either associated with ongoing muscle inflammation or in some cases without any other clinical indication of muscle inflammation.[4] In the latter instance, evaluation of serum CK levels in family members may suggest an unrelated or unsuspected genetic abnormality. LDH and ALT levels are elevated in many children with JDM, and LDH appears to correlate best with measures of disease activity.[509] Although relatively less specific, these enzymes often mirror global disease activity. Elevated ALT and LDH activities may also reflect liver disease associated with lipodystrophy and insulin resistance, although gamma glutamyl transferase is often helpful to discriminate these enzyme activities as muscle versus liver in origin.[370,510] Serum levels of all muscle enzymes usually decrease 3 to 4 weeks before improvement in muscle strength and rise 5 to 6 weeks before clinical relapse.[511] As a general rule, changes in CK levels occur first, often falling to the normal range within several weeks of instituting therapy; aldolase or LDH levels are the last to respond. Guzman and colleagues[173] reported that flares of disease are best predicted by a combination of AST and LDH, and that CK functions poorly as a predictor of the exacerbation of myositis.

Creatine Kinase

CK catalyzes the transfer of a phosphoryl group from creatine phosphate to adenosine diphosphate to regenerate adenosine triphosphate in the mitochondria of muscle, brain, and heart. The adenosine triphosphate available to muscle is sufficient to sustain contractile activity for only a fraction of a second. In skeletal muscle, CK constitutes up to 20% of the soluble sarcoplasmic protein, and total CK activity is 225 to 12,000 units per gram of muscle. CK is a dimeric molecule with two subunits: M (muscle) and B (brain). Both consist of 360 amino acids with a molecular mass of 41 kD. Three isoenzymes exist: (1) MM (CK-3) is found in muscle and myocardium; (2) BB (CK-1) is found in the brain; and (3) MB (CK-2) is found in myocardium but also in regenerating muscle, which is often elevated in patients with IIM.[512] There may be a persistent elevation of the MB band in muscle inflammation as a result of muscle regeneration.[511-514] The adult pattern of isozymes is achieved by 4 years of age.

Serum CK concentration is elevated in many cases of muscle injury, motor neuron diseases, vasculitis, metabolic disorders, endocrinopathies, toxic reactions, and infections. Very high levels are most commonly associated with muscular dystrophy and JPM, and somewhat less commonly with JDM. Abnormalities of the junctional sites between the T-tubules and the sarcoplasmic reticulum in muscle cells of children with JDM may be the primary sites of leakage of the enzyme. These abnormal anastomoses are far more extensive in the perifascicular than in the centrofascicular myofibers. Enzyme levels are generally not elevated in diseases in which there is no loss of sarcolemmal integrity (e.g., glucocorticoid myopathy, disuse atrophy); however, muscle enzyme elevation with glucocorticoid myopathy has been reported.[515]

TABLE 26-6	**Specific Diagnostic Studies at Onset of Juvenile Dermatomyositis**
STUDY	**DIAGNOSTIC SUCCESS (%)**
Elevation of serum levels of the muscle enzymes	80-98
Aspartate aminotransferase	48-90
Creatine kinase	54-85
Aldolase	65-84
Lactate dehydrogenase	65-80
Alanine aminotransferase	41-48
Abnormal electromyography	50-95
Abnormal muscle biopsy (inflammation)	76-92

Sources: Refs. 3-5, 9, 48, 508.

Transaminases

AST and ALT are cytosolic and mitochondrial enzymes with a wide tissue distribution. AST has two dimeric isoenzymes: one in the cytosol and the other in the mitochondria. The half-life in human plasma is 47 hours for ALT, 6 hours for mitochondrial AST, and 12 to 17 hours for cytosolic AST. Plasma levels decrease to normal adult ranges by 1 year of age.

Aldolase

Aldolase (1,6-diphosphofructoaldolase) is found in myocardium, liver, cerebral cortex, kidneys, and erythrocytes, but it is present in much higher concentration in skeletal muscle. Aldolase is one of the principal glycolytic enzymes that catalyze the conversion of D-fructose-1,6-diphosphate to dihydroxyacetone phosphate and D-glyceraldehyde-3-phosphate. There are three cytosolic isoenzymes: aldolase A, which predominates in muscle; aldolase B, in the liver; and aldolase C, in the brain. Aldolase A is elevated in active JDM and in some children with chronic disease.

Lactate Dehydrogenase

LDH is abundant in myocardium and skeletal muscle. There are five isoenzymes: I (30%), II (40%), III (20%), IV (6%), and V (4%). In acute adult PM, there is relatively less isoenzyme I and relatively more II, III, IV, and V. In chronic disease, only isoenzymes I and II are disproportionately elevated. In contrast, patients with active muscular dystrophy exhibit an increase in types I and II and a decrease in III, IV, and V, especially in younger patients.

Other Muscle-Derived Markers

Cardiac troponin I may be selectively elevated and aid in distinguishing myocardial from skeletal muscle involvement.[516] The serum level of myoglobin, a normal constituent of cardiac and skeletal muscle with a molecular mass of approximately 17 kD, is elevated in approximately 50% of patients with adult inflammatory myopathies and JPM, but it is probably less frequently elevated in patients with JDM.[513] This elevation does not always correlate with higher serum CK levels. Antibodies to myoglobin are present in 70% of patients and may interfere with its quantitation.[517] Although myoglobin is much more nephrotoxic than hemoglobin, myoglobinuria in cases of JDM seldom reaches levels that are associated with renal damage. Urinalysis is usually normal, although some children have hemoglobinuria associated with urine myoglobin at disease onset.[511,518]

Other Biomarkers

As enzymes often normalize with long-standing disease,[329] and inflammation in the skin, joints, and other systemic organs may not result in an increase in serum muscle enzyme levels, examination of other laboratory biomarkers of active disease is also important in the care of patients with JDM. Nonspecific indicators of inflammation, such as elevation of erythrocyte sedimentation rate, tend to correlate with the degree of clinical inflammation and are helpful to differentiate inflammatory myopathies such as JDM from noninflammatory disorders of muscle such as muscular dystrophy or myotonia; in contrast, C-reactive protein level is normal.[10,511,513,518] Serum acute phase reactants, such as alpha-1 acid glycoprotein, serum albumin, serum amyloid A, ferritin, and cystatin C, also correlate with active disease, particularly outside of the muscles.[514] Leukocytosis and anemia are uncommon at onset, except in the child with associated gastrointestinal bleeding. Patients may have lymphopenia.[513,519] IgG and IgM levels are elevated in 15% to 20% of patients.[513,518] IgE levels have been reported to be elevated in children with calcinosis, recurrent staphylococcal infections, and neutrophil chemotactic defects, suggestive of hyper IgE syndrome.[93,520]

Low levels of C3 or C4 are present in more than one third of patients with JDM.[5]

Serum levels of factor VIII–related antigen (i.e., von Willebrand factor) reflect endothelial damage and are often elevated in children with JDM.[126,173,260,520,521] Fibrinogen and fibrin degradation products are also often elevated.[10] Although abnormal factor VIII–related antigen levels occur in most children with active disease,[522] particularly with active skin disease,[281,513] they were not of value in one study in predicting a flare.[173]

Flow cytometry of peripheral blood lymphocytes demonstrates increases in CD19+ B lymphocytes and in the CD4 (T-helper) to CD8 (T-suppressor) ratio and decreases in CD3− CD16+/CD56+ natural killer cells in newly diagnosed, untreated patients with JDM compared to healthy controls.[523-525] Changes in CD19+ B lymphocytes, activated T lymphocytes (CD3+CD69+), myeloid dendritic cells (HLA-DR-CD11c+), and plasmacytoid dendritic cells (HLA-DR-CD123+) also correlate with change in disease activity, including muscle or extramuscular activity.[151,526]

Neopterin is a derivative of pyrimidine metabolism, and its serum concentration has been considered a marker of IFN-activated monocytes and macrophages. Levels of neopterin are elevated in individuals with inflammation, infections, or malignant diseases. Determination of its concentration has been proposed as a useful laboratory marker of immune activation and disease activity.[522,527] Levels of quinolinic acid, available on a research basis, may be another marker of activity that correlates with macrophage function.[260,527]

Markers in the IFN pathway, important in disease pathogenesis, appear to be promising as biomarkers of disease activity. Serum IFN-α levels correlate with serum levels of muscle enzymes in untreated JDM patients and correlate inversely with disease activity at 36 months.[528] Serum levels of type I IFN-regulated proteins, including I-TAC, IP-10, monocyte chemoattractant protein 1 (MCP-1), MCP-2, and IFN-β, as well as the cytokines IL-6, IL-8, and TNF-α correlate with disease activity and change in activity, including global activity, muscle, skin, and other organs, in patients with JDM and those with adult DM.[187,189,190,529,530] The proinflammatory myeloid-related protein 8/14 correlates with physician global activity and muscle strength and endurance as measured by the CMAS.[195]

Autoantibodies

Antinuclear antibodies have been reported with variable frequency of 41% to 72% of patients with JDM.[1,3-5] Particularly important are antibodies directed against one of a number of extractable nuclear antigens; up to 75% of patients have reactions to one of them (Table 26-7).[211,531,532] Rheumatoid factors are usually absent in patients with JDM. Fifteen percent of patients with JDM have been reported to also have antithyroid and type 1 diabetes autoantibodies, whereas celiac disease and autoimmune hepatitis autoantibodies are less frequent (2% to 5%), and clinical autoimmune diseases associated with these autoantibodies are infrequently seen.[1,429]

Traditional *myositis-specific autoantibodies* (MSAs), such as those directed to the aminoacyl tRNA synthetases, signal recognition particle, and Mi-2, are seen almost exclusively in myositis patients, through the use of validated assays such as immunoprecipitation. These autoantibodies, however, have been described in a minority of children with myositis.[15,22,533,541,542] Recently, however, several myositis autoantibodies, including anti-p155/140 (TIF-1) and anti-MJ (NXP-2), have been identified in a large percentage of children with JDM, each present in 20% to 30% of patients.[136,330,534,535] These autoantibodies appear to be specific for myositis, but require confirmation through additional testing methods, such as reverse immunoprecipitation-immunoblotting or immunoprecipitation-immunodepletion, and

TABLE 26-7	Autoantibodies in Patients With Juvenile Idiopathic Inflammatory Myopathies			
AUTOANTIBODY	**AUTOANTIGEN TARGET**	**FREQUENCY* (%)**	**CLINICAL SUBGROUP**	**CLINICAL FEATURES AND ASSOCIATIONS IN JUVENILE IDIOPATHIC INFLAMMATORY MYOPATHIES**
Myositis-Specific Autoantibodies				
Anti-p155/140	Transcriptional intermediary factor 1 (TIF-1)	23-30	JDM, JDM with overlap myositis	Extensive photosensitive skin rashes, including Gottron papules, heliotrope, malar rash, V- and shawl-sign rashes, linear extensor erythema; also with cutaneous ulcerations and generalized lipodystrophy; frequent chronic illness course. Frequently associated with cancer-associated myositis in adult DM patients only, not JDM. More severe cutaneous involvement, generalized lipodystrophy.
Anti-MJ	NXP-2	20-25	Primarily JDM	Frequent muscle cramps, dysphonia, and joint contractures. Some reports of more frequent calcinosis, muscle atrophy, hospitalization, and gastrointestinal ulceration, suggestive of more severe illness.
Anti-aminoacyl-tRNA synthetases			JDM, JPM, and overlap myositis	More frequent in JPM (9%) and overlap myositis with JPM (8% to 13%). Typically associated with moderate to severe weakness and creatine kinase levels, as well as frequent interstitial lung disease, nonerosive small joint arthritis, mechanic's hands, Raynaud phenomenon, similar to adults with these autoantibodies. Associated with high mortality, resulting from the interstitial lung disease.
Anti-Jo-1	Histidyl-tRNA synthetase	2-5		
Anti-PL-12	Alanyl-tRNA synthetase	1-3		
Anti-PL-7	Threonyl-tRNA synthetase	<1		
Anti-EJ	Glycyl-tRNA synthetase	<1		
Anti-OJ	Isoleucyl-tRNA synthetase	<1		
Anti-Mi-2	NuRD helicases: Mi-2α and Mi-2β, histone deacetylases	2-13	JDM	Mild JDM with classic rashes (Gottron papules, heliotrope rash), and malar rash, often high CK levels. Predominantly seen in Hispanic patients. Children, in contrast to adults with this autoantibody, do not have V- or shawl-sign rashes or cuticular overgrowth.
Anti-SRP	Signal recognition particle (6 polypeptides and 7SLRNA)	1	JPM	More frequent in JPM (18%). Primarily African-American girls with JPM with acute onset of severe proximal and distal weakness, frequent falling episodes, cardiac disease, and Raynaud phenomenon. High frequency of wheelchair use and chronic illness course, refractory to multiple therapies.
Anti-CADM-140	MDA-5	Unknown	JDM	Reported in adult DM and amyopathic DM with frequent rapidly progressive interstitial lung disease, cutaneous ulceration, palmar papules, and high mortality. Case reports, primarily from Japan, in JDM or amyopathic JDM with ILD, high mortality.
Anti-SAE	Small ubiquitin-like modifier activating enzyme	0.2	JDM	Cutaneous manifestations of DM that predate muscle symptoms, absence of constitutional manifestations and interstitial lung disease.
Myositis-Associated Autoantibodies				
Anti-U1-RNP	U1 small nuclear ribonucleoprotein (snRNP)	5-10	JDM, JPM, and overlap myositis	More frequent in JPM (12%) and overlap myositis (20% to 27%). Associated with arthritis, Raynaud phenomenon, and sclerodactyly.

TABLE 26-7 Autoantibodies in Patients With Juvenile Idiopathic Inflammatory Myopathies—cont'd

AUTOANTIBODY	AUTOANTIGEN TARGET	FREQUENCY* (%)	CLINICAL SUBGROUP	CLINICAL FEATURES AND ASSOCIATIONS IN JUVENILE IDIOPATHIC INFLAMMATORY MYOPATHIES
Anti-Ro	52- or 60-kD ribonucleoproteins (hYRNA)	2-6	JDM, JPM, and overlap myositis	More frequent in overlap myositis (12%). Little is known about associated clinical features. May be seen in association with anti-Jo-1 autoantibodies.
Anti-PM-Scl	Exosome protein: 100- and 75-kD	1-4	JDM, JPM, and overlap myositis	More frequent in JPM (6%) and overlap myositis (10% to 25%). In adults, this autoantibody is associated with Raynaud phenomenon, arthritis, interstitial lung disease, and esophageal dysmotility; most frequent in Caucasian patients.
Anti-Ku	DNA binding complex: 70- and 80-kD heterodimers	0.2	JDM, JPM, and overlap myositis	More frequent in overlap myositis (2%). Based on adults with this autoantibody, it is associated with arthralgia, Raynaud phenomenon, myalgias, dysphagia, and interstitial lung disease.
Other MAAs: Anti-U2-, U3-, or U5-RNP, anti-La, anti-Sm, anti-Th	Miscellaneous	<1	JDM, JPM, and overlap myositis	More frequently present in overlap myositis (1% to 10%). Little known, primarily associated with overlap myositis.
Myositis autoantibody negative		28-57	JDM, JPM, and overlap myositis	Heterogeneous with likely several unrecognized autoantibody groups within. Relatively mild.

*Based on data from Refs. 1, 15, 16, 22, 330, 533-540. Modified from Ref. 19.

their antigens appear to be conformationally dependent. *Myositis-associated autoantibodies* (MAAs) occur in approximately 18% of patients with JDM, more often in association with myositis overlap syndromes.[1] With the availability of more extensive testing for the newly identified autoantibodies, the percentage of children with JDM who are negative for myositis autoantibodies is currently estimated to be approximately 30%.[1] The inclusion of myositis autoantibodies has been proposed for the classification of juvenile and adult DM or PM, as well as potentially to aid in their diagnosis.[94,263,543] The titers of these autoantibodies fluctuate with the level of disease activity,[207] and they may become negative when disease enters remission.[204] Testing for MSAs and MAAs using immunoprecipitation is a reliable method available only in a few commercial and research laboratories.

Myositis-Specific Autoantibodies

MSAs are autoantibodies targeted to cytosolic RNAs or proteins involved in protein synthesis, with autoantibodies in DM often directed against nuclear transcription factors and autoantibodies in PM often directed against cellular protein translational machinery; their precise role in disease pathogenesis is not understood. Usually, only one MSA is present in the serum of a patient, and it often can be detected before onset of the phenotype. Patients with a specific MSA are relatively homogeneous in clinical manifestations, response to therapy, and prognosis.[16,544]

Anti-p155/140 autoantibodies immunoprecipitate a 155-kD band along with a fainter 140-kD band and have been present in 23% to 30% of patients with JDM studied to date.[1,15,136,534] It has also been seen in similar frequencies in adult DM, overlap myositis that is associated with DM in adults and children, and in up to 85% of adult DM patients with associated malignancies.[136,545-549] This autoantibody has been detected in the serum of one patient with SLE but not in patients with

PM, muscular dystrophies, or other autoimmune diseases, including rheumatoid arthritis or scleroderma.[136,545-547] The clinical associations with this autoantibody include a high frequency of photosensitive skin rashes, including malar rash, V- and shawl-sign rashes, and erythroderma; cuticular overgrowth; and periungual capillary changes, as well as a higher frequency of cutaneous ulcerations and edema.[15,19,136,534] It is also seen in high frequency in patients with generalized lipodystrophy who have JDM.[370] Patients with anti-p155/140 autoantibodies have lower CK levels, and more often their illness is chronic.[15] The HLA allele associated with this autoantibody is DQA1*0301.[136] The antigenic target has preliminarily been identified as transcriptional intermediary factor-1 (TIF-1).[550] Further studies of the specific isoform are needed.[549]

Anti-MJ, also known as anti-p140, is found in 20% to 25% of patients with juvenile IIM, predominantly in patients with JDM, but also in a few patients with JPM and overlap myositis.[1,15,330,535] Patients with anti-MJ autoantibodies have more frequent muscle cramps, atrophy, and contractures, and a lower frequency of truncal rashes. They may have more frequent calcinosis and associated gastrointestinal bleeding or ulceration and are more frequently hospitalized.[15,330,535] The anti-MJ autoantigen has been preliminarily identified to be nuclear matrix protein NXP-2, a transcription factor and regulator of RNA metabolism.[330,551]

Antisynthetase autoantibodies usually occur in patients with an acute onset in the spring season and rapid progression of disease, but they have been identified in others with slow progression and in asymptomatic adults.[252] The antisynthetases are associated with an increased frequency of the alleles associated with the ancestral haplotype HLA-B*08-DRB1*0301-DQA1*0501-DQB1*0201.[22,129,132,146,553] Anti-Jo-1 is the most common antisynthetase autoantibody. It occurs in approximately 20% of adults and has been described in 2% to 4%

of children with myositis.[15,16,22,142] It is specific for histidyl-tRNA synthetase, a cytoplasmic enzyme that catalyzes the esterification of histidine to its cognate tRNA. Patients who are anti-Jo-1 positive demonstrate a subset of multisystemic features that have been called the antisynthetase syndrome. Patients with this autoantibody have an illness characterized by fever, arthritis, Raynaud phenomenon, and myositis that is often severe.[15,536] Interstitial pulmonary fibrosis, present in approximately 66% of the children and 90% of adults with antisynthetase autoantibodies, may become the dominant feature of the disease course.[537,554] Although the polyarthritis is often mild, it can result in erosions and subluxations. A hyperkeratotic nonpruritic fissuring rash of the palms and lateral aspects of the fingers (i.e., mechanic's hands) is another feature of this syndrome. Non-Jo-1 antisynthetases, including anti-alanyl (PL-12) and anti-threonyl (PL-7) tRNA synthetases, have also been reported in children with myositis,[533] and the timing of the development of myositis and lung disease appears to vary among different antisynthetase autoantibodies.[555] Several other non-Jo-1 antisynthetases, including glycyl, isoleucyl, asparaginyl,[556] phenylalanyl, and tyrosyl tRNA synthetases, have been identified to date only in adults (reviewed by Betteridge et al.[544]). Patients with antisynthetase autoantibodies have the highest mortality, which is associated with interstitial lung disease.[358]

Mi-2 is a 218-kD nuclear helicase that is involved in transcriptional activation, and the autoantibody is often associated with HLA-DRB1*0701 and HLA-DQA1*0201.[144] Anti-Mi-2 has been identified in 2% to 13% of children with JDM and JDM with overlap myositis, particularly in Hispanic individuals.[19] In adults, it is strongly associated with a distinct pattern of rash[22,533,557] and perhaps a more benign course.[558] The areas of most intense involvement often are the V of the neck, the anterior chest area, and the shawl area with involvement of the upper back and shoulders, as well as cuticular overgrowth. Most children have not displayed this characteristic dermatitis, although they have malar erythema and Gottron papules.[15] The disease is responsive to glucocorticoid therapy.

Another subset of patients, approximately 1% of juvenile myositis patients, all exclusively with JPM, has autoantibodies to the signal recognition particle.[15,22,533,538,557,559] Onset of disease is often severe and acute, with severe myositis of the proximal and distal muscles and frequent falling episodes and very high CK levels. These patients have a higher frequency of cardiac disease and Raynaud phenomenon and may respond poorly to glucocorticoid and other therapies.[15,538,557,560] They are uniformly hospitalized, utilize wheelchairs, and their illness is chronic.[15] Muscle biopsy shows an immune-mediated necrotizing myopathy.[96,533,560] Signal recognition particle is a cytoplasmic ribonuclear protein complex that directs the passage of newly synthesized protein from the ribosome to the endoplasmic reticulum. Immunofluorescent tests therefore may demonstrate cytoplasmic staining. HLA-HLA-B*5001 and DQA1*0104 are associated with this autoantibody.[144]

Several autoantibodies have been described in patients with adult myositis, with more limited information in JDM. CADM-140 has been associated with amyopathic DM and rapidly progressive interstitial lung disease with mediastinal emphysema or pneumothorax, frequent skin ulcerations, and vasculopathic palmar papules, and high mortality due to respiratory failure.[539,540,561-564] The autoantibody has been reported in Japanese children, and like many of the adults, they have rapidly progressive interstitial lung disease and high mortality.[356,357] The autoantigenic target has been identified as the cytoplasmic protein MDA5.[565]

Anti–small ubiquitin-like modifier activating enzyme is seen in up to 8% of patients with adult DM, including patients with interstitial pneumonia and cancer, but not in other forms of adult myositis and

rarely in JDM.[1,566] Patients frequently present with skin problems first but progress to muscle weakness and a high frequency of dysphagia.[567] Autoantibodies to 3-hydroxy-3-methyl-glutaryl CoA reductase is associated with an immune-mediated necrotizing myopathy that resembles PM and is more frequent in patients who have taken statins.[96] It has not been described yet in juvenile IIM. Autoantibodies to the DNA mismatch repair enzymes, PMS1 and PMS2, also may be myositis specific and have been identified in 7% of adult myositis patients.[568]

Myositis-Associated Autoantibodies

The MAAs occur in 20% to 70% of children with myositis and consist of several distinct entities.[1,22,142,211] Anti-PM-Scl is suggested by a nucleolar pattern on antinuclear antibody testing.[569-571] It occurs in the overlap syndrome of inflammatory myopathy and systemic scleroderma (i.e., scleromyositis). Clinical features include myositis, arthritis, interstitial lung disease, digital sclerosis, and Raynaud phenomenon.[570,571] The course of the disease is often benign and prolonged, but it has a good prognosis. This autoantibody is associated with HLA-DRB1*0301-DQA1*0501-DQB1*0201.[22] The anti-U1RNP autoantibody is characteristic of overlap myositis with mixed connective tissue disease (see Chapter 29). It is suggested by the presence of a high-titered antinuclear antibody speckled pattern. There is a subgroup of patients (1% to 7%) who have autoantibodies to U3RNP.[128,572] Anti-SSA/Ro antibody often occurs in association with anti-Jo-1.[573] The anti-Ku antibody has not often been described in patients from North America[574] but was reported in approximately 50% of patients from Japan who had an overlap syndrome. In adults it is associated with myalgias, arthralgia, Raynaud phenomenon, dysphagia, and, less commonly, interstitial lung disease. Patients respond well to glucocorticoids alone, except those with lung disease.[575] It has been reported in approximately 1% of children with overlap syndromes.[22] The antigen is a protein kinase that is involved in the phosphorylation of a number of transcription factors.

Electromyography

EMG occasionally is useful to confirm the diagnosis of JDM, to evaluate its distribution and severity, and to select the best site for a muscle biopsy.[576,577] The electromyogram should be evaluated on one side of the body only so that the muscle biopsy, if necessary, can be obtained on the opposite extremity without an artifact created by a needle puncture. Needle EMG is most useful in evaluating myopathies, and a minimal examination of one proximal and one distal muscle from one upper extremity and from one lower extremity as well as the thoracic paraspinal lines is recommended, with additional muscle groups selected based on the pattern of weakness and diagnostic considerations.[576] EMG can be troublesome in the young child, and mild sedation is often necessary. An electromyogram is not mandatory and need not be done unless the diagnosis is in doubt. Currently, EMG is performed in 8% to 55% of children diagnosed with juvenile IIM or JDM.[3,5,12,48]

The characteristic electromyographic changes of myopathy and denervation (Box 26-9) are associated with membrane instability (e.g., increased insertional activity, fibrillations, and positive sharp waves)

BOX 26-9 Electromyography in Inflammatory Muscle Disease

Myopathic motor units (decreased amplitude, short duration, polyphasic)
Denervation potentials (positive sharp waves), spontaneous fibrillations, and insertional activity
High-frequency repetitive discharges

and random fiber destruction (e.g., decreased amplitude and duration of action potentials). The electrical changes in denervation probably result from segmental myonecrosis of the endplate, although the terminal axons may also be affected. Reinnervation may occur after the acute phase of the disease. Nerve conduction velocities and latencies are normal in JDM, unless severe muscle atrophy is present with a decrease in the number of muscle fibers in a motor unit and with electrical irritability of the sarcolemmal membrane or terminal axonal fibers. Corticosteroid usage decreases the extent of detected abnormalities.[578]

The value of EMG in identifying continuing inflammatory activity of muscle during the course of JDM has not been adequately documented. Quantitative EMG may be more informative in this regard.[579-582] In following the course of the disease, increasing muscle strength correlates with less spontaneous activity and a decreasing proportion of high-frequency components. During the initial period of treatment, however, a temporary increase in high-frequency signals is expected.

Muscle Biopsy

A muscle biopsy is primarily indicated in the initial assessment of a child if the diagnosis is in any way uncertain, including in patients without the characteristic skin rashes of JDM. Currently, muscle biopsies are performed in 60% to 75% of children with myositis at the time of diagnosis, although this estimate may be inflated from referral bias.[3,12] A biopsy may be used to evaluate the disease activity, especially late in its course, or if histopathological support for instituting long-term glucocorticoid therapy or immunosuppressive drugs is deemed necessary.[583] A biopsy is also indicated in a child who has failed to respond therapeutically, to rule out disorders such as drug-induced myopathies, dystrophies, metabolic and mitochondrial myopathies, and IBM, particularly if a biopsy was not performed at the onset of illness.[21,452,478,481-483,584,585] A muscle biopsy also provides valuable prognostic information, as discussed above in the section on pathology, with extensive myopathic changes, muscle infarction, or lymphocytic infiltrates with follicle-like structures including follicular dendritic cells and high endothelial venules possibly indicative of a chronic illness course.[186,309,334,390,391]

The muscle to be biopsied, usually the deltoid or quadriceps, should be clinically involved as demonstrated by muscle strength testing on physical examination, EMG, or MRI, but ideally it should not be atrophied. MRI can be used to select an area of muscle that is likely to be affected by the disease and thereby increase the probability of obtaining informative tissue.[586,587] If EMG has been obtained within the previous 6 weeks, the biopsy should be performed on the opposite side of the body.

Care should be taken to prepare the tissue in accordance with the instructions of the pathologist. A generous specimen (12 mm long, 4 mm wide, 2 mm thick) on open muscle biopsy should be obtained in a muscle clamp because muscle involvement is often spotty. The specimen is placed in a transport container and taken immediately to the pathology laboratory. One sample is frozen in isopentane for immunofluorescent and enzyme studies. Another on a separate pediatric clamp is fixed in glutaraldehyde for electron microscopy. The remaining tissue should be stored frozen for additional stains or research studies for situations that are diagnostically unclear. Histopathological results are more likely to be negative or nondiagnostic if the muscle specimen is inadequate in size or is obtained from an inappropriate muscle, obtained after the initiation of glucocorticoid or other immunosuppressive therapy, or taken late in the disease course when the pathological changes may no longer be specific. Occasionally, there is no evidence of inflammatory change even though characteristic abnormalities, such as perifascicular atrophy, are present. In such

cases, or if the biopsy is performed after the initiation of immunosuppressive therapy, a stain for MHC class I to examine for overexpression on the sarcolemma can assist in confirming a diagnosis of inflammatory myopathy.[155,179,398-400] Although an open biopsy is most often performed, needle biopsy is preferred in some centers.[588] Needle biopsy with a spring-activated, 14-gauge needle may offer a convenient and cost-effective alternative to a surgical procedure.[589] With this procedure, three or four cores can be obtained using only surface anesthesia on the patient. However, additional frozen tissue for various histochemical stains and unplanned studies is often limited with this approach. The percutaneous conchotome muscle biopsy technique is less invasive than the open biopsy and provides a sample that is adequate for diagnostic evaluation, with more material than a needle biopsy.[590] The middle deltoid and vastus lateralis are the safest areas to biopsy by this technique from the standpoint of avoiding vascular or neurological damage.

RADIOLOGICAL EXAMINATION

Radiographs in early JDM demonstrate increased soft tissue density caused by edema of the muscle and subcutaneous tissues, and somewhat later, atrophy of muscle. In chronic disease, areas of calcification in soft tissues can be documented by plain radiographs (see eFig. 26-11). Osteoporosis of long bones and of the vertebral bodies is seen in high frequency and is often extensive (eFig. 26-15).[385] Ultrasound studies of muscle demonstrate increased echogenicity in the muscle; less frequently, muscle atrophy; and increased vascularity on power Doppler, which is more evident by microbubble ultrasound (eFig. 26-16).[591-595] Radionuclide scanning can detect early abnormal changes in blood flow in diseased muscles.[596-599] This technique has limited clinical application, however, and has been superseded by MRI, which is more sensitive for localization of inflamed muscle.

MRI dramatically documents the extent and focal nature of the muscle abnormalities (Fig. 26-17).[591,600-604] The STIR image or T2-weighted image with fat suppression demonstrates muscle edema and inflammatory changes by a hyperintense signal[605-607] and inflammation in skin, subcutaneous tissue, and fascia.[607,608] The T1-weighted image demonstrates fibrosis, atrophy, and fatty infiltration, which are characteristic of disease damage. MRI may be helpful in selecting a site for muscle biopsy to reduce the false-negative rate of a blind biopsy.[609] It is also helpful at selected therapeutic junctures to evaluate the extent and severity of active disease compared to muscle atrophy and fatty infiltration.[610] In long-term follow-up, approximately 50% of patients with JDM have evidence of muscle damage on MRI, which is predicted by a high degree of disease activity at 1 year after diagnosis.[125] The presence of subcutaneous edema on an initial MRI examination appears to be a risk factor for a chronic illness course.[611] An increased signal on STIR or T2-weighted MRI of the muscles is seen with inflammation, edema, muscle necrosis and regeneration, rhabdomyolysis, blood, or other proteinaceous material and is not specific for IIMs.[612,613] Active myositis in general is best documented by STIR or fat-suppressed T2-weighted images, even in the absence of serum muscle enzyme elevations or clinical muscle weakness. Although edema is generally enhanced after administration of gadolinium as a contrast agent, it is generally unnecessary, as the lesions are adequately visualized without it, and some contrast agents carry a risk of nephrogenic systemic fibrosis.[614] Quantitation of T2-weighted images with T2 mapping[615-617] and diffusion-weighted MRI—which suggests decreased capillary perfusion in the muscles of adult myositis patients[618]—are currently used research tools. Whole-body MRI is becoming available and may help to reveal the patterns and extent of muscle involvement, including frequent involvement of the calves and

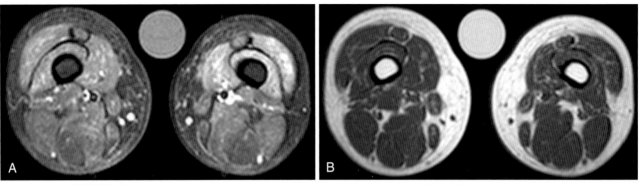

FIGURE 26-17 Cross-sectional magnetic resonance images of the thighs of a child with chronic, severe dermatomyositis. **A,** Short tau inversion recovery depicts widespread mild to moderate muscle hyperintensity, suggesting edema or increased water content, most prominent in the quadriceps, and greater on the left. There is lesser involvement of the hamstrings, with relative sparing of the semitendinosus muscles. **B,** T1 imaging demonstrates mild quadriceps and sartorius muscle atrophy, with fatty infiltration, which is greater on the left.

forearms, in addition to proximal and axial muscle groups and bony abnormalities such as multifocal osteonecrosis.[619-623] Reversal of these changes occurs in response to treatment, but improvement in MRI may lag behind other indicators.[590,601,608,624]

However, exercise-induced changes may mimic active disease.[606] Investigations have suggested that the course of disease in children with JDM can be monitored with ^{32}P-magnetic resonance spectroscopy as an indicator of biochemical defects in energy metabolism.[449,605] Noninvasive ^{32}P-magnetic resonance spectroscopy of thigh muscles in children with JDM was studied to characterize metabolic abnormalities during rest, exercise, and recovery.[625] Adenosine triphosphatase and phosphocreatine levels were low, as were other measures of mitochondrial oxidative phosphorylation, and they correlated with clinical weakness and fatigue. Low levels of free magnesium and magnesium–adenosine triphosphatase were also concordant and in part alleviated by immunosuppressive therapy.[626] Intramyocellular acidification, measured by protocol magnetic resonance spectroscopy, is decreased after exercise in adult patients with DM or PM compared with healthy controls and patients with mitochondrial myopathies.[627] Magnetic resonance elastography demonstrated decreased muscle stiffness in patients with IIM compared to healthy individuals.[628] The use of ^{18}F-fluorodeoxyglucose positron emission tomography or computed tomography may aid in selecting an appropriate muscle biopsy site based on localization of muscle inflammation and aid in discriminating myositis from noninflammatory myopathies or malignancies in adults.[629,630]

Dual energy X-ray absorptiometry has enabled a more accurate assessment of osteopenia and osteoporosis in children with JDM and other chronic rheumatic diseases (see Chapter 9).[385,631] Z scores for these children should be compared with bone mineral density data obtained from healthy, geographically similar children (male and female) in control groups, with normal values adjusted for height, age, and ethnicity.[632] Alternative evaluation has been proposed by comparisons with data obtained from quantitative calcaneal ultrasound.[633]

TREATMENT

In the presteroid era, approximately one third of children with JDM died, one third recovered, and one third were disabled to a moderate or severe extent.[634-636] The introduction of glucocorticoids revolutionized the treatment and prognosis for these children.[109,353,485,508,635,637-647] Currently there is general agreement that glucocorticoids are always

---

BOX 26-10 Medical Treatment of Juvenile Dermatomyositis

Primary Therapy*
Prednisone 1-2 mg/kg/day by mouth
Intravenous methylprednisolone 10-30 mg/kg/pulse
Methotrexate 1 mg/kg/week, or 15 mg/m² by subcutaneous injection
Intravenous immunoglobulin (IVIg) 2 g/kg/month
Cyclosporine 2.5-7.5 mg/kg/day by mouth, divided twice a day
Adjunctive therapies
   Hydroxychloroquine 3-6 mg/kg/day by mouth, divided twice a day
   Physical therapy
   Photoprotective measures
   Topical therapies for skin rashes (topical corticosteroids, tacrolimus, pimecrolimus)
   Calcium and vitamin D for bone protection

Therapies for Refractory Disease
Mycophenolate mofetil 20-40 mg/kg/day by mouth, divided twice a day
Azathioprine 1-3 mg/kg/day
Cyclophosphamide 500-1250 mg/m²/month by intravenous pulse
Rituximab 575 mg/m² or 750 mg/m² (max 1 gm) weekly for 2 weeks
Anti-TNF-α agents (infliximab 3-6 mg/kg/dose; etanercept 0.4 mg/kg [maximum 25 mg] by subcutaneous injection twice weekly)
Combinations of the above

*Agents as primary therapies are those most often used in the initial treatment of juvenile dermatomyositis, whereas other therapies are most often used in the treatment of refractory patients, patients with severe illness features, or patients with unacceptable medication toxicities. The order in which therapies or combinations of therapies are used is not implied by the listing in this table.
Modified from Ref. 19.

required as part of the therapy of JDM, but the specifics of management, including the use of intravenous pulse therapy, vary considerably from physician to physician and patient to patient.[648] A number of additional immunosuppressive and immunomodulatory drugs and biological therapies have also been studied that provide ancillary therapies that are used in conjunction with corticosteroids to spare the amount of steroid given or to provide additional therapy in treatment-refractory individuals (Box 26-10).[649,650] The goals of therapy include the elimination of active disease that results from inflammation, vasculopathy, and myogenic factors (as described in the pathogenesis section), and the prevention of damage to reduce morbidity while minimizing the side effects of medication.[19] Aggressive therapy is also considered to be essential in preventing the development of calcinosis, as well as muscle damage and damage in other organs.[58,275,331] The team approach and general supportive care, including active assisted or passive range-of-motion exercises early in the disease combined with individualized physical therapy, are widely used.[651]

The response of the child to the treatment program is judged on the basis of systemic signs and symptoms such as fatigue, muscle tenderness, and pain (if present); repeated graded muscle examinations by the same observer; skin rashes and other extramuscular manifestations; periungual capillary changes[265,300]; sequential serum levels of selected muscle enzymes, acute phase reactants, and other laboratory examinations if indicated (e.g., factor VIII–related antigen)[173,522]; and occasionally other studies, such as MRI of muscle and ultrasonography.[605] Core set measures of disease activity, including physician and parent global activity assessments, muscle strength and function, extramuscular activity, and enzymes, have been developed and validated by collaborative study groups.[275-277,279,281-283,605,652-656] Other outcomes, including patient-reported outcomes of quality of life and a global index such as the DAS, are also included in some core sets.[281,656] Approximately 20% improvement in most measures—15% improvement in strength and 30% improvement in enzymes—are considered clinically important changes.[509] Indexes that combine clinically important change in measures of disease activity are being validated,[276,657] and criteria for major response and clinically inactive disease are being defined.[658,659] Assessment of disease damage related to cumulative changes from previously active disease and other comorbidities can now be assessed by the MDI.[268,318,660] Collaborative research groups, including the International Myositis Assessment and Clinical Studies Group (IMACS), the Paediatric Rheumatology International Trials Organisation (PRINTO), and the Childhood Arthritis and Rheumatology Research Alliance (CARRA), have been instrumental in developing validated standardized outcomes, standards for the conduct of clinical trials, and consensus treatment guidelines in the care of patients with JDM.[13,283,384,661] These advances have resulted in the development of novel and evidence-based therapies for JDM.

General Supportive Care

The approach to management should be based on the knowledge that the disease remains chronic in the majority of patients. It may remit in 2 to 3 years, especially if it is monophasic, but in a recent study of 84 patients, the median time to remission was 4.7 years.[265] There is no evidence that any therapy is curative; rather, treatment is aimed at suppression of the immunoinflammatory response, maximal preservation of muscle function and joint range of motion, prevention of complications, maintenance of general health, and normal growth and development.

In severe disease, attention must be directed at the adequacy of ventilatory effort and swallowing, and occasionally at monitoring for abdominal perforation or myocarditis with severe arrhythmias or congestive heart failure. Occasionally, weakness is so profound that respiratory assistance, nasogastric feeding, and frequent oral suctioning are required, especially if the patient is bedbound or nonambulatory. Each patient should be monitored carefully for ability to swallow, adequacy of airway, and depth of breathing. Hypoxia may supervene insidiously. In the older child, vital capacity measurements can be a valuable objective measure of response to therapy. Although respiratory problems occur in approximately one third of severely affected children, ventilatory assistance is seldom required. Profound involvement of the

thoracic and respiratory muscles occurs in a few children and leads rapidly to increasing dyspnea at rest, agitation, respiratory insufficiency, aspiration, or death.

Skin care is especially important in children who develop fissures in the axillae and groin or ulcers of the skin over pressure points. Emollients, wound care topical therapies, and padding of pressure areas may help prevent breakdown and ulceration.[662] These ulcerations become sites for secondary infections and abscesses, complications that are abetted by the administration of the glucocorticoid drugs. During the course of the disease, the dermatitis may become markedly photosensitive, and sunblock protective against both ultraviolet (UV-A and UV-B) wavelengths with high sun-protection factor (SPF) numbers (30 and above) are necessary.[663,664] The rash may or may not respond to the use of low-potency topical glucocorticoid or tacrolimus/pimecrolimus creams, and these are often helpful for disease confined to the skin or for more severe rashes, including scalp involvement.[665,666] Long-term use of corticosteroid creams is generally not recommended because of the resulting secondary atrophic effects. Agents to treat pruritus, including antihistamines and emollients, may also be helpful adjuncts in treating skin disease.[667,668] Hydroxychloroquine, which inhibits Toll-like receptor activation, has anecdotally been helpful as an adjunctive agent. It improves cutaneous disease activity and prevents disease damage in patients with SLE.[669] Agents used to treat myositis systemically are also often helpful in treating the skin manifestations of the disease.[667,668]

Frequent counseling and education of the patient and parents are necessary to help allay anxiety and permit understanding of the necessarily slow pace of treatment and recovery.[670,671] The introduction of juvenile and adult myositis patient support groups can assist with education and psychosocial supports (e.g., Cure JM Foundation [www.curejm.org], The Myositis Association [www.myositis.org], and the Myositis UK [www.myositis.org.uk]). Systemic complications, particularly abdominal pain or gastrointestinal bleeding, require urgent surgical consultation and may be life-threatening, especially early in the disease. Attention to nutritional status and intake of potassium and limitation of total caloric and sodium intake may help minimize the side effects of the glucocorticoid drugs.

Glucocorticoid Drugs

Early and adequate treatment with glucocorticoids has been the single most important factor in improved prognosis during the past 50 years. Acute disease is treated with suppressive doses of the synthetic glucocorticoids (Box 26-10).[109,508,635] Prednisone is preferred to other analogues, such as dexamethasone or triamcinolone, because these steroids may have a more potent myopathic effect (see Chapter 12). The drug is given at a dosage of approximately 2 mg/kg/day for the first month of the disease and then, if indicated by the clinical response and a decline in the serum levels of the muscle enzymes, reduced by approximately 10% to 20%.[384,648,672] For patients with more mild disease, some pediatric rheumatologists prefer a lower starting dose, and for patients with moderate to severe disease, some prefer to administer prednisone initially in two divided doses for the first month of therapy.[384,648] For many pediatric rheumatologists, factors that contribute to using an initial dose of oral prednisone at the higher end of the range include length of delay to diagnosis, severity of illness at diagnosis, extramuscular manifestations (presence of dysphagia, gastrointestinal involvement, interstitial lung disease, cutaneous ulcerations), and periungual nailfold capillary dropout that may reflect gastrointestinal vasculopathy and contribute to decreased absorption of oral prednisone.[673] Thereafter, the drug is tapered as permitted by careful monitoring of improvement in muscle weakness, skin rashes, and other symptoms and by assay of serum levels of the muscle enzymes. Alternate-day glucocorticoid therapy is generally not recommended, as disease control is often inadequate. It is axiomatic that satisfactory clinical control is not attained until all of the serum enzymes have returned to normal or near-normal levels and have remained there during continued tapering of the steroids and a gradual increase in the physical activity of the child. It is necessary to maintain some children on very-low-dose glucocorticoids even many years after "clinical control" of myositis. It is difficult to be certain when glucocorticoids can be discontinued without risking an exacerbation of the disease, and this partly appears to be dependent on initiation of adequate therapy at the time of diagnosis,[323] as well as a gradual reduction in corticosteroid dose that is commensurate with the patient's clinical improvement. A shorter course of prednisone therapy has been advocated, with adjunctive use of corticosteroid-sparing agents.[672]

The clinical response of the child to glucocorticoids is not entirely predictable. The fever should abate within a few days, and many patients report improvement in fatigue and malaise within a few days to weeks of initiating therapy. The serum levels of muscle enzymes should appreciably decrease in the first 1 to 2 weeks of therapy. There may be no significant improvement in muscle strength for 1 to 2 months. Improvement in the dermatitis is unpredictable. Of note, the course of the rash does not necessarily parallel that of the muscle disease, and both aspects of illness must be fully treated. An extensive rash at onset or a generalized progression of the dermatitis is, however, a poor prognostic sign, as is persistence of Gottron papules and periungual nailfold capillary abnormalities.[265,300,508]

Children who require high-dose steroids for long periods develop severe osteopenia and osteoporosis, often with vertebral compression fractures.[631] It has not been determined conclusively whether supplementation with dietary calcium and vitamin D can prevent this complication. The efficacy and long-term safety of bisphosphonates are being evaluated, and therefore this therapy is only recommended for patients with recurrent fractures, painful spinal compression fractures, or reduced bone density.[674,675] Cushing syndrome and growth retardation result in any child placed on suppressive doses of corticosteroids for a period of months. The dosage of the glucocorticoid drug and duration of its use should therefore be kept as low as possible, commensurate with the clinical and laboratory responses to therapy. Steroid myopathy, which is common in mild form but rarely severe, might be misinterpreted as an exacerbation of the basic disease process (Box 26-11) (see Chapter 12). The manifestations of this syndrome are insidious onset of hip flexor weakness and atrophy, with normal assays of the serum muscle enzymes and minimal myopathic changes on EMG.[515] MRI may show atrophy of the proximal thigh muscles on T1-weighted axial images but no muscle edema on STIR or fat-suppressed T2-weighted images.

Intravenous pulse glucocorticoid therapy has been proposed to gain rapid control of muscle inflammation while minimizing the exposure of the child to long-term, high-dose daily steroids.[26,648,676-681] An

---

BOX 26-11 Characteristics of Steroid-Induced Myopathy

Insidious onset
Hip flexor weakness and atrophy
Normal serum concentrations of muscle enzymes
Minimal myopathic changes on electromyography
Thigh muscle atrophy without increased muscle edema on magnetic resonance imaging
Type II fiber atrophy on muscle biopsy

---

initial publication by Laxer and associates[679] indicated a satisfactory response in six children; subsequently, two additional patients were treated. Both were boys who had mild early disease; a single intravenous pulse of methylprednisolone (30 mg/kg) led to a decrease in the enzyme levels and improved muscle strength over 2 months. There may be a subgroup of children with JDM for whom this initial approach to management will be successful, thereby abrogating the need for long-term daily glucocorticoid treatment. The majority of pediatric rheumatologists include intravenous pulse methylprednisolone as part of the initial therapy of patients with moderate to severe illness, particularly in North and South America.[648,658] Pachman[54] advanced the concept that early use of intravenous pulse therapy reduces future disability and the extent of calcinosis. The bioavailability of pulse methylprednisolone may be better than that of oral prednisone, particularly in patients with vasculopathy who have reduced periungual nailfold capillary density.[673] As with any form of therapy, this approach to glucocorticoid administration is not always effective and might not impact long-term outcome.[682,683] Pulse therapy can be combined advantageously with methotrexate as part of the initial therapeutic regimen, resulting in less calcinosis, increased frequency of remission, and reduced likelihood of flare later in the illness course, as shown by uncontrolled studies.[323,331,648] Intravenous pulse therapy might also be beneficial for acute or life-threatening manifestations, such as severe weakness, myocarditis, severe dysphagia, interstitial lung disease, or pneumatosis intestinalis.

Hydroxychloroquine

Hydroxychloroquine has been recommended as a steroid-sparing agent and as a drug that is effective in treating the dermatitis of JDM.[684] Olson and Lindsley[685] reported significant improvement of the rash after 3 months and improvement of muscle weakness after 6 months of treatment in a dosage of 2 to 5 mg/kg/day in nine children. Anecdotal experience suggests that the addition of hydroxychloroquine to a glucocorticoid regimen is warranted but has modest efficacy. As such, it tends to be included as part of the therapy of patients with mild to moderate disease.[2,384,648] It is alleged that patients with DM may be prone to non–life-threatening cutaneous reactions from the antimalarial agents.[686]

Immunosuppressive Therapy

Primary indications for the use of immunosuppressive drugs include moderate to severe disease, as well as glucocorticoid resistance or dependence. Consensus from North American pediatric rheumatologists is to introduce methotrexate alone or in combination with intravenous immunoglobulin (IVIG) at the start of therapy in patients with moderate or severe disease activity.[384] A recent large, randomized, controlled trial in Europe concluded that prednisone in combination with methotrexate or cyclosporine leads to a shorter time to inactive disease compared to prednisone alone, with less toxicity in the group that received methotrexate.[687] In steroid-resistant disease, there is inadequate improvement in muscle strength and persistence of elevated serum levels of muscle enzymes in response to a closely monitored glucocorticoid program (prednisone, 1 to 2 mg/kg/day for at least 3 to 4 months). Steroid dependence occurs later in the course of the disease and is characterized by failure of the clinical manifestations of disease to remain suppressed during a gradual reduction of the glucocorticoid dose to an acceptable level, recurrence of progressive muscle weakness despite continuing therapy, or unacceptable steroid toxicity.

Several immunosuppressive drugs have been used as second-line agents in resistant disease, including methotrexate,[681,688-693] IVIG (discussed in the section on IVIG), and cyclosporine.[55,648,658,694-701] Mycophenolate mofetil,[702-704] azathioprine,[692,705] tacrolimus,[706,707] and cyclophosphamide[309,708,709] have been used most often as third-line agents. The efficacy of these drugs is difficult to evaluate because there has been only a single controlled trial.[687] Of the immunosuppressive drugs, weekly oral or subcutaneous methotrexate is the preferred agent among pediatric rheumatologists in North and South America,[2,648] typically at a dosage of 1 mg/kg/week or 15 mg/m² weekly.[384] Careful monitoring of the dose and potential toxicity relative to age, height, and weight is mandatory. Benefit is usually evident within 2 to 3 months. A report of 12 patients with JDM suggested a favorable improvement in all patients over a period of 3 to 78 weeks after initiating therapy, without major toxicity or hepatic disease.[690] Recent reports suggest that early introduction of methotrexate (often subcutaneously) may be associated with reduced corticosteroid toxicity, better growth velocity, and overall reduction in duration and cumulative dose of corticosteroids.[323,331,691] Many North American pediatric rheumatologists now use methotrexate as part of the initial therapy of JDM, regardless of illness severity,[384] and methotrexate is recommended as part of initial therapy for all patients with moderate or more severe disease activity.[384]

There have been several case reports and series of successful cyclosporine therapy.[26,696-701] Some investigators have suggested that this drug should be considered as first-line therapy in the treatment of inflammatory muscle disease,[710] and it is often the preferred second medication for patients receiving treatment in Europe, particularly for illness flares.[658] Except for renal impairment, cyclosporine has less long-term toxicity than the traditional immunosuppressive drugs, and for this reason its use should perhaps be considered earlier, rather than later, in the child who is nonresponsive to steroids or steroid dependent, or who has evidence of interstitial lung disease.[711,712] The efficacy of cyclosporine in the treatment of steroid-resistant or steroid-dependent disease has been reported by Heckmatt and associates.[698] In that study, 14 children who had failed to respond fully to glucocorticoids and immunosuppressive agents were given a dosage of 2.5 to 7.5 mg/kg/day (younger children require a higher dose because drug clearance is age dependent). The investigators reported considerable benefit, with reduced prednisolone requirements in all, including discontinuation of glucocorticoid in six patients. Two of three nonambulatory patients were able to walk after treatment, and six with limited ambulation subsequently regained good independent ambulation. Muscle strength improved but remained significantly reduced. The only notable side effects were hypertension and reversible decreases in renal function.[713] A PRINTO randomized controlled study compared prednisone alone versus prednisone combined with methotrexate versus prednisone in combination with cyclosporine as initial therapy for JDM.[687] The time to inactive disease was shorter in the groups that received combination therapy (prednisone in combination with methotrexate or cyclosporine) compared to prednisone alone, whereas the frequency of adverse events was highest in the group that received cyclosporine compared to methotrexate plus prednisone or prednisone alone.

Intravenous Immunoglobulin

A number of studies and anecdotal reports describe the efficacy of IVIG.[714-717] Initial use of IVIG was inspired by a randomized, double-blind, placebo-controlled trial in adult DM and other controlled studies in adult myositis.[718-720] In these reports, IVIG was of significant benefit, particularly if used early in the disease course and especially with respect to the skin changes. Clinical experience in children has been summarized in several reviews on JDM therapy.[19,26,266] Lang and coworkers[714] reported results of administration of IVIG to five children who were steroid resistant or steroid dependent. All patients exhibited improved muscle strength and diminished rash over the 9-month period with infusions every 4 weeks of 1 g/kg/day on each of 2 consecutive days. A follow-up report in a retrospective review of 18 patients confirmed reduction in disease activity and ability to reduce corticosteroid dose in the majority.[721] Lam et al.[722] retrospectively examined their experience with monthly IVIG infusions in 30 patients with JDM who failed initial therapy with prednisone, intravenous pulse methylprednisolone, and methotrexate, compared to 48 patients who did not go on to receive IVIG. The group receiving IVIG, particularly a steroid-resistant subgroup, achieved lower disease activity 1 month to 4 years after treatment with IVIG, based on analyses that used bias-reduction methods. Although IVIG infusions were generally tolerated well, and most patients remained on IVIG for more than 2 years, IVIG preparations containing a high level of IgA were more frequently associated with fever, lethargy, malaise, nausea, and vomiting.[723] IVIG may also be used in the initial treatment of patients with JDM who have moderately severe disease,[384] as well as in patients with severe weakness or dysphagia, ulcerative disease, or calcinosis.[26] CARRA has developed consensus protocols that include combinations of prednisone and methotrexate with or without IVIG as part of the initial treatment of JDM.[384]

Other Immunosuppressive Drug Therapies

Open-label reports in JDM and adult myositis support the use of mycophenolate mofetil for patients with severe or recalcitrant disease, resulting in improvement in strength, skin rashes, muscle enzymes, and an ability to reduce corticosteroid dose in the majority of patients.[702,703] Fifty treatment-refractory patients with JDM in a retrospective open-label study had improved skin and muscle Disease Activity Scores with mycophenolate mofetil treatment and were able to reduce their corticosteroid dose, which was confirmed in a second case series of eight patients receiving 800 to 1350 mg/m².[704,724] The most common adverse events included minor infections (upper respiratory, otitis media, and sinusitis), with no increase in the frequency of infections after initiation of mycophenolate mofetil.[704] The majority of patients with adult idiopathic inflammatory myositis and several patients with treatment-refractory JDM received tacrolimus in an open-label manner; they demonstrated improvement, which supports its use in treatment-refractory patients.[706,707,725,726] Tacrolimus also appears to be beneficial for the treatment of interstitial lung disease, particularly in patients with antisynthetase and anti-SRP autoantibodies.[712,727,728]

There is little published experience with azathioprine[50,687] or cyclophosphamide. Crowe and colleagues[309] first recommended cyclophosphamide in children with chronic ulcerative illness that was unresponsive to glucocorticoids. An open-label study of intravenous monthly pulse cyclophosphamide in patients with severe or treatment-refractory JDM demonstrated significant improvements in 10 of 12 patients after 6 months, which has been confirmed in a larger open-label series of 56 patients.[709,729] Many of these patients had severe weakness, dysphagia, skin or gastrointestinal ulcerations, central nervous system disease, or calcinosis, all or some of which improved after the initiation of therapy. This therapy may also be beneficial in patients with interstitial lung disease.[730] Intravenous cyclophosphamide therapy, however, is not always successful, particularly in adult patients with chronic, stably active disease.[731]

Combinations of drugs as initial therapy for JDM, including prednisone, methotrexate, and intravenous pulse methylprednisolone, followed by cyclosporine and IVIG, may increase the frequency of remission and decrease the frequency of calcinosis.[323] An experimental protocol in adults that consisted of comparing combination oral methotrexate and azathioprine to high-dose intravenous methotrexate (500 mg/m²) suggested that the combination regimen was superior to methotrexate alone.[732] Case reports in adult patients support other combinations, including cyclosporine or azathioprine with cyclophosphamide,[733,734] as well as cyclosporine or cyclophosphamide with IVIG.[735,736]

Biological Agents and Stem-Cell Transplantation

All seven patients with refractory adult DM who received rituximab (four weekly infusions of 100 mg/m² or 375 mg/m²) responded, beginning 4 to 12 weeks concurrent with the depletion of peripheral blood B lymphocytes, with a maximal response at 12 to 36 weeks, and a response duration of 24 weeks to more than 52 weeks.[737] Marked clinical responses were generally observed following administration of rituximab therapy in patients with refractory, often severe, JDM, but no improvement in calcinosis was noted.[738-740] In one study of refractory adult DM, little improvement in skin disease activity was noted.[741] An overall response rate of approximately 70% was found in the open-label studies, with a mean duration of response of 12 months.[742] A large randomized clinical trial has been completed in which 48 treatment-refractory patients with JDM, along with 152 patients with adult DM and PM, were randomized to receive rituximab (575 mg/m² or 750 mg/m² per dose for 2 weekly infusions) or placebo at weeks 0 and 1 followed by placebo at weeks 8 and 9. Although 83% of patients responded to rituximab and significantly decreased their corticosteroid dosage, there was no difference in the time to clinical response, the primary study end point.[743] The median time to response was 12 weeks in patients with JDM and 20 weeks overall, with the clinical and antibody subgroups of JDM, antisynthetase, anti–Mi-2, and other myositis autoantibodies, as well as less disease damage, predicting a shorter time to improvement.[559,744,745]

The TNF-α inhibitors, including chimeric monoclonal antibodies to TNF-α and recombinant soluble human TNF-α receptor (p75)–Fc fusion protein, have been used with promising results in a few patients.[746] In five patients with severe JDM treated with infliximab (3 mg/kg every 8 weeks to 6 mg/kg every 4 weeks), all had improved disease activity after 8 to 30 months, and in some cases calcinosis also improved, with no serious side effects reported.[332] A larger open-label study of 30 patients with refractory JDM treated with infliximab found improvement in muscle strength and physical function, muscle enzyme levels, skin rashes, and physician global disease activity in more than 70% of patients and up to 50% improvement in calcinosis.[747] In one trial of etanercept, minimal improvement in myositis activity measured by the Disease Activity Score was evident in seven of nine treated patients at week 12; one child experienced a severe worsening in skin rashes and one had worsening muscle disease activity.[748] Responses to anti–TNF-α therapy have been mixed in patients with adult DM/PM,[749] with disease progression in some patients.[750] Reports of the development or exacerbation of adult DM after use of etanercept or adalimumab for treatment of arthritis suggest further caution in the use of anti–TNF-α therapies in the treatment of juvenile IIM.[97] In a randomized, placebo-controlled trial of etanercept in adult DM, 11 patients treated with etanercept had a longer time to disease flare and greater ability to lower prednisone dose compared to 5 patients who received placebo.[751]

There is little evidence for the use of other biological therapies to treat JDM. An open-label trial of anakinra in 15 patients with refractory adult DM, PM, and IBM showed clinical response in 7, generally within 3 months, which correlated best with those who had higher baseline extramuscular activity, as well as muscle macrophages, and IL-1α expression.[752] There are no reports of IL-1 blockade in JDM. In an early phase Ib randomized, placebo-controlled, dose-ranging study of the anti–IFN-α monoclonal antibody sifalimumab in adult DM and PM, the type I IFN gene signature and IFN-inducible proteins were suppressed in the peripheral blood and muscle, and patients who

demonstrated a greater improvement in strength demonstrated more inhibition of the IFN gene signature.[753] A single patient with severe refractory JDM had improved strength, function, and skin activity, including cutaneous ulcerations,[754] and a patient with severe adult PM had improved strength, serum muscle enzymes, and prednisone dosage within a few months of abatacept administration.[755] Two adult patients with refractory PM had improved CK levels and muscle edema on MRI after receiving tocilizumab.[756] A single patient with severe refractory JPM entered a sustained clinical remission 6 to 12 months after receiving an immunoablative dose of alemtuzumab.[757] A nonablative regimen of alemtuzumab was examined in an open-label trial of 13 patients with IBM in which strength and daily life functional activities improved relative to their decline prior to the initiation of treatment. Endomysial inflammation, including expression of CD3+ T lymphocytes and stressor molecules in the muscle, was also reduced following alemtuzumab therapy.[758]

Experience with autologous hematopoietic stem-cell transplantation for JDM is limited but has been successful in a few patients with severe, refractory disease; however, these children are at high risk for developing severe viral infections.[759-761] Plasmapheresis has been of benefit in a few children with severe, life-threatening disease refractory to other therapies, including patients with acute life-threatening multisystem organ failure, severe macrophage activation syndrome, or thrombocytopenia purpura.[377,762-766] Studies suggest that there is no therapeutic effect in adults with stable active disease, based on a randomized controlled trial.[767]

Physical and Occupational Therapy

Physical therapy should be initiated at the time of diagnosis. Although skeletal muscles are actively inflamed, the focus of attention should be on preventing loss of range of motion by giving twice- to thrice-daily active assisted or passive range-of-motion exercises to joints, with the use of gentle stretching to regain lost range.[651] Splinting of knees, elbows, or wrists at night or during periods of rest helps to achieve these goals. During the healing phase, the physical therapy program is increased to normalize function as nearly as possible and to minimize development of contractures from muscle weakness or atrophy. Isometric muscle strengthening should be added to the exercise program only after clinical evidence of acute inflammation has subsided. Later, when disease activity is mild, isotonic strengthening and graded aerobic activity are included.[651] Exercise therapy does not appear to worsen myositis disease activity,[768,769] and studies in adults suggest that strength and functional outcomes improve after muscle-strengthening programs.[769] An open-label pilot trial in 10 patients with JDM who had mild, chronic disease demonstrated improvement in muscle strength and function, aerobic conditioning, bone and muscle mass, disease activity, and health-related quality of life after 12 weeks of twice-weekly aerobic and resistance exercise training.[770]

Management of Calcinosis

None of the many approaches to the treatment of calcinosis has been consistently effective, and no randomized controlled trial has been performed to adequately evaluate such therapies. Therapy aimed at altering calcium metabolism or mineralization, including diltiazem, aluminum hydroxide, probenecid, alendronate, pamidronate and diphosphonates, topical or intravenous sodium thiosulfate, minocycline, intravenous ethylenediaminetetraacetic acid, and warfarin has shown varying success.[326,327] There is general agreement that early aggressive therapy with glucocorticoids and other medications results in decreased frequency and severity of calcinosis.[54,323,331] Antiinflammatory approaches may also decrease calcinosis and its associated inflammation after deposition has occurred, with anecdotal reports of success using IVIG, infliximab, thalidomide, cyclophosphamide, abatacept, and intralesional glucocorticoids.[326,327,729,747,754,771] Colchicine may suppress local and systemic signs of inflammation associated with calcinosis.[772,773] Lithotripsy may decrease associated pain in patients with stable calcinosis.[774] Experimental data suggest that TNF blockade may be beneficial because overexpression of the TNF-α-308A allele is associated with a long duration of active disease and pathological calcifications.[137] Surgical excision of calcifications that mechanically interfere with function or have resulted in breakdown of skin may be indicated,[775] although recurrence of calcinosis and infections in such sites are a risk.[520]

The natural history of many of these calcific deposits is that they spontaneously begin to regress after months or years, coincident with inactivity of the muscle disease and increasing mobility of the patient. However, the one fourth of children who develop calcinosis in interfascial planes tend to have persistent lesions.[312] Hypercalcemia and hypercalcuria have been reported during spontaneous resolution of calcinosis.[328,776]

Management of Lipodystrophy

Management of underlying metabolic sequelae, including diabetes, insulin resistance, and hyperlipidemia, are the primary current therapeutic approaches, including use of metformin, pioglitazone, and other thiazolidinediones.[777,778] Recent data have emphasized the role of leptin deficiency in the abnormalities characteristic of generalized lipodystrophy and the potential role of replacement therapy to treat congenital generalized forms of lipodystrophy, with improvement in glycemic control, insulin sensitivity and plasma triglycerides, and hepatic steatosis.[779-781]

COURSE OF THE DISEASE AND PROGNOSIS

The course of JDM can be divided into three categories: (1) monocyclic, if the patient achieves remission without evidence of active disease within 2 years of diagnosis; (2) polycyclic, if the patient had recurrence of active disease after a definite remission; and (3) chronic continuous, if disease activity persists more than 2 years.[313,324] Some reports have simplified this pattern into monocyclic and chronic continuous.[300]

Four Canadian centers evaluated functional outcome in 80 children treated between 1984 and 1995 (46 girls and 19 boys) with a mean follow-up of 7.2 years (range, 3.2 to 13.9 years).[324] A monocyclic course was characteristic of 37% of the children and a chronic continuous or polycyclic course in 63%. Favorable outcomes were predominant: only 8% had moderate to severe disability, 34% had developed calcinosis, and there was one death. However, persistent rash was seen in 40%, 23% had ongoing weakness, and 35% continued to take medications more than 3 years after disease onset.

More recently, other registry studies have reported on disease course and outcomes. In the United States, a large registry study reported 25% of individuals each with a monocyclic and polycyclic illness course, and 50% with chronic continuous disease.[1]

Predictors of disease course based on early illness features have been difficult to identify (Box 26-12).[265,324] Persistence of rash within the first 6 months after diagnosis, including Gottron papules and periungual nailfold capillary changes, may be predictive of a longer time to remission.[265,300] Shorter delay to diagnosis and less skin disease activity predict a monocyclic course of illness.[300] Children with younger age at onset are more likely to experience a monocyclic illness course,[782] but this was not confirmed in a UK registry cohort.[310] Delay in treatment and inadequate treatment are also important risk factors.[783] The anti-p155/140 and anti-SRP autoantibodies are associated with a chronic illness course.[1] Features on muscle biopsy at diagnosis may predict later

illness course, including extensive myopathic changes and central nuclei without basophilia, which predicted a chronic illness course, and severe arteropathic change, positive arterial direct immunofluorescence, foci of severe capillary loss/endomysial fibrosis, and muscle infarcts, which predict a chronic course of illness with ulceration.[390] Subcutaneous edema on MRI at diagnosis may also predict a chronic illness course.[611] Certain proinflammatory cytokine polymorphisms, including the TNF-α-308A allele may be predictive of a chronic course of illness[137] or of ulcerative disease.[138]

Crowe et al.[309] identified a group of children with noninflammatory vasculopathy who had extensive and chronic ulcerative cutaneous disease. These children and a similar group reported earlier by Banker and Victor[334] were characterized by significant systemic complications, including fatal gastrointestinal hemorrhage. Children with severe generalized erythroderma and cutaneous ulcerations often develop extensive calcinosis and significant overall functional impairment.[322] Approximately 5% of children eventually develop a clinical disease that is more typical of systemic vasculitis.[309,334] A small number of children late in the course of disease may assume more of the characteristics of scleroderma with sclerodactyly and cutaneous atrophy, develop an overlap connective tissue disease,[508,784] or have a recurrence of arthritis.

Late progression has been reported with a recurrence of active disease after a prolonged remission[785,786] or persistent low-level activity many years after onset with multiple physical or dermatologic sequelae.[787-789] Of interest in this regard is the risk from pregnancy in women who have had or currently have JDM.[790-792] Depending on the activity of the disease, residual muscle weakness, calcinosis, and disability, pregnancy should be considered high risk for both mother and baby.

In examining long-term sequelae of disease using sensitive measures, such as the MDI (Table 26-8), almost 80% of patients exhibited measurable damage, including cutaneous scar, joint contractures, persistent weakness, muscle dysfunction, and calcinosis, in 23% to 30% of patients after a median of 6.8 years after diagnosis.[268] In a multicenter cross-sectional study of 490 patients with JDM from Europe and Latin America with a mean disease duration of 7.7 years, 41% to 53% had reduced muscle strength, although only 10% had moderate to

TABLE 26-8   Most Frequent Damage Items in Juvenile Dermatomyositis on Long-Term Follow-up, Ranging From 7.7 to 16.8 Years After Diagnosis

FEATURE	%
Any organ/system with damage	60-79
Cutaneous	43-75
Cutaneous scar	30-63
Calcinosis	21-37
Lipodystrophy	10-17
Muscle	30-63
Muscle dysfunction	16-40
Weakness	11-47
Muscle atrophy	11-27
Skeletal	26-48
Joint contractures	18-45
Osteoporosis with fractures	4-10.5
Endocrine	17-27
Growth failure	8-14
Delay in secondary sexual characteristics	4-21
Irregular menses	0-20
Hirsutism	0-10
Pulmonary	8-17
Dysphonia	2-15
Impaired lung function	4-6
Pulmonary fibrosis	1-6
Gastrointestinal	3-17
Dysphagia	2-13
Gastrointestinal infarction	1-2

From Refs. 49, 58, 268, 314.

TABLE 26-9   Prognosis of Juvenile Dermatomyositis

OUTCOME	% OF PATIENTS
Normal to good functional outcome	65-80
Minimal atrophy or contractures	25-30
Calcinosis*	12-47
Wheelchair dependence	5
Death	1-2

*Children with calcinosis were also included in the other categories.

severe impairment; 41% to 60% had persistently active disease; and 69% had measurable damage.[58] Examples of damage present in 10% to 44% of patients included cutaneous scarring, muscle atrophy, calcinosis and joint contractures, muscle dysfunction, persistent weakness, and hirsutism.[58] These findings have been confirmed in other European cohorts.[48,49] A high level of disease activity at 6 to 12 months after diagnosis, longer disease duration, and older age at disease onset are additional predictors of damage, whereas a shorter duration of active disease is associated with less damage.[48,125,314] In the large European and South American cross-sectional study, disease course was monocyclic in 41% of patients, and chronic polycyclic or continuous in 59%.[58] Patients with a chronic illness course were at greater risk for muscle and skin damage and calcinosis.[58] Individuals with JDM may, as adults, be at higher risk of early atherosclerosis, as seen by increased carotid intimal-medial thickness and brightness in young adulthood; patients with calcinosis and more severe disease activity may be at particularly higher risk.[376]

Calcinosis

Historically, 12% to 47% of children with JDM have developed calcinosis (see Tables 26-6 and 26-9).[6,58,120,268,312,322-324,376,508,783,784] Children with extensive calcinosis were often those who had suffered from a severe and unremitting course.[312] In those children, and to a lesser extent in others, calcinosis was responsible for more long-term disability with limitation of movement of involved muscles or contiguous joints than the residual effects of myositis.[324] Calcinosis appears to be lower in frequency and extent in children treated earlier after symptom onset and in those treated with adequate doses of corticosteroids and/

or other immunosuppressive agents as part of the initial therapy.[323,331,783] Dystrophic calcification occurs in 12% to 47% of children with JDM.[3,6,9,49,107,308,310,314,322-324] Risk factors for calcinosis include delay to diagnosis and the duration of untreated disease, duration of active disease, inadequate therapy, underlying cardiac or pulmonary disease, male gender, older age at illness onset, prolonged persistent disease activity after diagnosis, and the need for corticosteroid-sparing immunosuppressive therapy, which may be an indicator of severe disease activity.[49,58,314,322,323,329] Although the frequency of calcinosis has declined as treatments have improved, it appears to be more frequent in certain regions than in others (e.g., South America as opposed to Europe).[58] Certain myositis autoantibodies, including anti-MJ (NXP-2) and anti-PM-Scl,[22,330] as well as proinflammatory cytokine polymorphisms of TNF-α and IL-1α, are additional risk factors for the development of calcinosis.[137,138] Aggressive treatment to achieve rapid and complete control of inflammation, especially early after onset, may minimize calcinosis.[258,323,327,331,332] Trauma may play a role in the generation of calcific deposits because they also tend to occur in surgical incisions and over pressure points. A study by Moore and coworkers[520] concluded that calcinosis was associated with preceding staphylococcal infection and high levels of IgE and IgE antistaphylococcal antibodies. Granulocyte chemotaxis to staphylococci was depressed.

Functional Disability

In children with a typical monocyclic disease course, functional outcome is usually excellent, although minor flexion contractures and residual skin changes may persist (see Table 26-9). In others in whom the disease remains active beyond 3 years, there may be low levels of myositis and dermatitis disease activity with deposition of calcium salts and progressive loss of function. Factors that adversely influence outcome are listed in Box 26-12. Early and adequate steroid treatment has the greatest impact on a favorable outcome.[508,635] Functional outcome appears best in children who have been diagnosed shortly after onset and treated vigorously, perhaps with initial steroid-pulse administration.[323,331,679,783] Most survivors are able to function independently as adults, although some have flexion contractures and residual atrophy of skin or muscle.[324,788]

In a multicenter study, 72% of patients had no or minimal disability an average of 7 years after onset.[324] In the large cross-sectional multicenter study from Europe and Latin America, 41% of patients had measurable functional disability with a mean follow-up of 7.7 years, although only 6% had severe impairment.[58]

Psychosocial Outcome

A study by Miller and associates[793] suggested that a number of children who enter adulthood continue to have psychological problems and learning disabilities based on unrecognized cerebral abnormalities that occurred at disease onset. Another review of late outcome in JDM indicated that the educational achievements and employment status of

18 patients were better than those of the general adult population or a comparable group who had had chronic arthritis.[794] More recently a Norwegian case-control study of adults with JDM who were assessed a median of 22 years after disease onset showed reduced health-related quality of life in general health measured by the Short Form-36. There was strong correlation between the physical component scores and the Health Assessment Questionnaire but none with the mental health component.[795] Huber et al. reported that 3 of 80 patients experienced school delay of 1 year due to illness, but the population otherwise experienced no educational impairment or difficulty working.[324] In measuring health-related quality of life, the cross-sectional European/Latin American study by Ravelli et al. found that 14% of individuals had mild psychosocial impairment, whereas 4% had substantial impairment.[58] In a large PRINTO study, Apaz et al. measured Child Health Questionnaire physical and psychosocial summary scores in 272 patients with JDM at baseline and 6 months and compared them with healthy controls.[796] Psychosocial scores as well as physical scores decreased with increasing levels of disease activity. Although below the mean of healthy controls at 6 months, patients with JDM had less impairment in psychosocial well-being than in physical well-being.

Death

Long-term survival for patients with JDM is better than 95%; in the presteroid era, this disease was associated with a mortality rate that approached 40%.[309,508,793,797] Children who survived often had devastating residual problems, such as contractures and muscular atrophy. Fatalities most often occur within 2 years of onset and are often associated with progressive involvement of skin or muscle that is unresponsive to steroids. This observation suggests that the basic nature of the inflammatory disease, its early treatment and response, the presence of widespread vasculitis, and involvement of other organ systems (e.g., gastrointestinal tract, lungs) are major factors that should be assessed in estimating prognosis. Death most often results from respiratory insufficiency or interstitial lung disease, myocarditis, or from acute gastrointestinal ulceration, with intestinal perforation or bleeding.[358] Surgical intervention in the latter group of children may be successful.

From the Canadian inception cohort of 80 children diagnosed between 1984 and 1995 with a median of 7.2 years of follow-up, 1 child died of myocardial infarction.[324] In the U.K. JDM registry, only one death was reported in 151 children with juvenile IIM (0.7%) with a mean follow-up duration of 3.1 years.[5] In the European/Latin American multicenter cross-sectional study, with patients diagnosed between 1980 and 2004, the mortality rate was 3.1%.[58] In a Brazilian registry, mortality was 4.2%, with fatal events in five patients, including respiratory failure and sepsis, myocarditis, and sepsis due to neutropenia as a complication of lymphoblastic leukemia.[3] A Danish national registry of JDM tracked all 57 patients hospitalized with JDM from 1977 to 2007 for a median of 7 years. In this cohort, three patients died 3 to 22 months after disease onset: one from an infection and two from bleeding episodes (epistaxis and gastrointestinal ulceration).[48]

Two specific studies recently addressed mortality in patients with juvenile IIM. The first, a national U.S. registry of pediatric rheumatic diseases included almost 50,000 patients from more than 60 centers who were diagnosed between 1992 and 2001, including 662 patients with JDM. Mortality was determined from examination of the Social Security Death Index records, and overall mortality was found to be higher in those individuals with JDM, with a standardized mortality ratio (SMR) of 2.64, representing five deaths in 662 patients (0.8%), with a mean follow-up of 7.9 years. Risk factors for mortality for the entire population included connective tissue diseases (including JDM), male gender, and older age.[798] Huber examined mortality in a large U.S.

registry population by using the Social Security Death Index and/or medical record review.[358] The SMR for individuals with juvenile IIM overall was 14.4 and 8.3 for those with JDM (representing 8 deaths in 329 patients with JDM with a mean follow-up duration of 1.6 years).[358] Clinical subgroup (overlap myositis > JPM > JDM), severity of illness at onset, age at diagnosis, weight loss, and delay to diagnosis were the most important predictors of mortality in multivariable analyses. Antisynthetase autoantibodies, along with interstitial lung disease and Raynaud phenomenon, were significant predictors in univariable models.[358]

REFERENCES

1. M. Shah, G. Mamyrova, I.N. Targoff, et al., The clinical phenotypes of the juvenile idiopathic inflammatory myopathies, Medicine (Baltimore). 92 (2013) 25–41.

5. L.J. McCann, A.D. Juggins, S.M. Maillard, et al., The Juvenile Dermatomyositis National Registry and Repository (UK and Ireland)–clinical characteristics of children recruited within the first 5 yr, Rheumatology (Oxford) 45 (2006) 1255–1260.

6. A.V. Ramanan, B.M. Feldman, Clinical features and outcomes of juvenile dermatomyositis and other childhood onset myositis syndromes, Rheum. Dis. Clin. North Am. 28 (2002) 833–857.

7. A. Bohan, J.B. Peter, Polymyositis and dermatomyositis (first of two parts), N. Engl. J. Med. 292 (1975) 344–347.

8. A. Bohan, J.B. Peter, Polymyositis and dermatomyositis (second of two parts), N. Engl. J. Med. 292 (1975) 403–407.

15. L.G. Rider, M. Shah, G. Mamyrova, et al., The myositis autoantibody phenotypes of the juvenile idiopathic inflammatory myopathies, Medicine (Baltimore). 92 (2013) 223–243.

17. S.L. Tansley, N.J. McHugh, L.R. Wedderburn, Adult and juvenile dermatomyositis: are the distinct clinical features explained by our current understanding of serological subgroups and pathogenic mechanisms?, Arthritis Res. Ther. 15 (2013) 211.

19. L.G. Rider, J.D. Katz, O.Y. Jones, Developments in the classification and treatment of the juvenile idiopathic inflammatory myopathies, Rheum. Dis. Clin. North Am. 39 (2013) 877–904.

47. E.P. Mendez, R. Lipton, R. Ramsey-Goldman, et al., US incidence of juvenile dermatomyositis, 1995-1998: results from the National Institute of Arthritis and Musculoskeletal and Skin Diseases Registry, Arthritis Rheum. 49 (2003) 300–305.

57. L.M. Pachman, R. Lipton, R. Ramsey-Goldman, et al., History of infection before the onset of juvenile dermatomyositis: results from the National Institute of Arthritis and Musculoskeletal and Skin Diseases Research Registry, Arthritis Rheum. 53 (2005) 166–172.

58. A. Ravelli, L. Trail, C. Ferrari, et al., Long-term outcome and prognostic factors of juvenile dermatomyositis: a multinational, multicenter study of 490 patients, Arthritis Care Res. 62 (2010) 63–72.

65. Z. Tezak, E.P. Hoffman, J.L. Lutz, et al., Gene expression profiling in DQA1*0501+ children with untreated dermatomyositis: a novel model of pathogenesis, J. Immunol. 168 (2002) 4154–4163.

68. A.M. Reed, S.R. Ytterberg, Genetic and environmental risk factors for idiopathic inflammatory myopathies, Rheum. Dis. Clin. North Am. 28 (2002) 891–916.

109. R.J.P. Wedgwood, C.D. Cook, J. Cohen, Dermatomyositis. Report of 26 cases in children with a discussion of endocrine therapy in 13, Pediatrics 12 (1953) 447–466.

123. G. Mamyrova, T.P. O'Hanlon, J.B. Monroe, et al., Immunogenetic risk and protective factors for juvenile dermatomyositis in Caucasians, Arthritis Rheum. 54 (2006) 3979–3987.

127. F.W. Miller, R.G. Cooper, J. Vencovský, et al., Genome-wide association study of dermatomyositis reveals genetic overlap with other autoimmune disorders, Arthritis Rheum. 65 (2013) 3239–3247.

137. L.M. Pachman, M.R. Liotta-Davis, D.K. Hong, et al., TNFalpha-308A allele in juvenile dermatomyositis: association with increased production of tumor necrosis factor alpha, disease duration, and pathologic calcifications, Arthritis Rheum. 43 (2000) 2368–2377.

138. G. Mamyrova, T.P. O'Hanlon, L. Sillers, et al., Cytokine gene polymorphisms as risk and severity factors for juvenile dermatomyositis, Arthritis Rheum. 58 (2008) 3941–3950.

175. S. Khanna, A.M. Reed, Immunopathogenesis of juvenile dermatomyositis, Muscle Nerve 41 (2010) 581–592.

187. H. Bilgic, S.R. Ytterberg, S. Amin, et al., Interleukin-6 and type I interferon-regulated genes and chemokines mark disease activity in dermatomyositis, Arthritis Rheum. 60 (2009) 3436–3446.

188. C.M. López de Padilla, A.N. Vallejo, K.T. McNallan, et al., Plasmacytoid dendritic cells in inflamed muscle of patients with juvenile dermatomyositis, Arthritis Rheum. 56 (2007) 1658–1668.

190. E.C. Baechler, H. Bilgic, A.M. Reed, Type I interferon pathway in adult and juvenile dermatomyositis, Arthritis Res. Ther. 13 (2011) 249.

247. K. Nagaraju, N. Raben, L. Loeffler, et al., Conditional up-regulation of MHC class I in skeletal muscle leads to self-sustaining autoimmune myositis and myositis-specific autoantibodies, Proc. Natl. Acad. Sci. U.S.A. 97 (2000) 9209–9214.

255. A.L. Urganus, Y.D. Zhao, L.M. Pachman, Juvenile dermatomyositis calcifications selectively displayed markers of bone formation, Arthritis Rheum. 61 (2009) 501–508.

263. B.M. Feldman, L.G. Rider, A.M. Reed, L.M. Pachman, Juvenile dermatomyositis and other idiopathic inflammatory myopathies of childhood, Lancet 371 (2008) 2201–2212.

264. L.G. Rider, L.M. Pachman, F.W. Miller, H. Bollar, Myositis and You: A Guide to Juvenile Dermatomyositis for Patients, Families and Healthcare Providers, first ed., The Myositis Association, Washington, DC, 2007.

265. E. Stringer, D. Singh-Grewal, B.M. Feldman, Predicting the course of juvenile dermatomyositis: significance of early clinical and laboratory features, Arthritis Rheum. 58 (2008) 3585–3592.

268. L.G. Rider, P.A. Lachenbruch, J.B. Monroe, et al., Damage extent and predictors in adult and juvenile dermatomyositis and polymyositis as determined with the Myositis Damage Index, Arthritis Rheum. 60 (2009) 3425–3435.

276. N. Ruperto, A. Ravelli, A. Pistorio, et al., The provisional Paediatric Rheumatology International Trials Organisation/American College of Rheumatology/European League Against Rheumatism Disease activity core set for the evaluation of response to therapy in juvenile dermatomyositis: a prospective validation study, Arthritis Rheum. 59 (2008) 4–13.

279. A.M. Huber, B.M. Feldman, R.M. Rennebohm, et al., Validation and clinical significance of the Childhood Myositis Assessment Scale for assessment of muscle function in the juvenile idiopathic inflammatory myopathies, Arthritis Rheum. 50 (2004) 1595–1603.

281. R.L. Smith, J. Sundberg, E. Shamiyah, et al., Skin involvement in juvenile dermatomyositis is associated with loss of end row nailfold capillary loops, J. Rheumatol. 31 (2004) 1644–1649.

282. National Institute of Environmental Health Science, International Myositis Assessment & Clinical Studies Group (IMACS), 2013. <http://www.niehs.nih.gov/research/resources/imacs/>, [serial online].

283. L.G. Rider, V.P. Werth, A.M. Huber, et al., Measures of adult and juvenile dermatomyositis, polymyositis, and inclusion body myositis: physician and Patient/Parent Global Activity, Manual Muscle Testing (MMT), Health Assessment Questionnaire (HAQ)/Childhood Health Assessment Questionnaire (C-HAQ), Childhood Myositis Assessment Scale (CMAS), Myositis Disease Activity Assessment Tool (MDAAT), Disease Activity Score (DAS), Short Form 36 (SF-36), Child Health Questionnaire (CHQ), Physician Global Damage, Myositis Damage Index (MDI), Quantitative Muscle Testing (QMT), Myositis Functional Index-2 (FI-2), Myositis Activities Profile (MAP), Inclusion Body Myositis Functional Rating Scale (IBMFRS), Cutaneous Dermatomyositis Disease Area and Severity Index (CDASI), Cutaneous Assessment Tool (CAT), Dermatomyositis Skin Severity Index (DSSI), Skindex, and Dermatology Life Quality Index (DLQI), Arthritis Care Res. 63 (Suppl. 11) (2011) S118–S157.

293. E.M. Dugan, A.M. Huber, F.W. Miller, L.G. Rider, Photoessay of the cutaneous manifestations of the idiopathic inflammatory myopathies, Dermatol. Online J. 15 (2009) 1.

300. S. Christen-Zaech, R. Seshadri, J. Sundberg, et al., Persistent association of nailfold capillaroscopy changes and skin involvement over thirty-six months with duration of untreated disease in patients with juvenile dermatomyositis, Arthritis Rheum. 58 (2008) 571–576.

309. W.E. Crowe, K.E. Bove, J.E. Levinson, P.K. Hilton, Clinical and pathogenetic implications of histopathology in childhood polydermatomyositis, Arthritis Rheum. 25 (1982) 126–139.

312. S.L. Bowyer, C.E. Blane, D.B. Sullivan, J.T. Cassidy, Childhood dermatomyositis: factors predicting functional outcome and development of dystrophic calcification, J. Pediatr. 103 (1983) 882–888.

313. C.H. Spencer, V. Hanson, B.H. Singsen, et al., Course of treated juvenile dermatomyositis, J. Pediatr. 105 (1984) 399–408.

323. S. Kim, M. El-Hallak, F. Dedeoglu, et al., Complete and sustained remission of juvenile dermatomyositis resulting from aggressive treatment, Arthritis Rheum. 60 (2009) 1825–1830.

324. A.M. Huber, B.A. Lang, C.M. LeBlanc, et al., Medium- and long-term functional outcomes in a multicenter cohort of children with juvenile dermatomyositis, Arthritis Rheum. 43 (2000) 541–549.

326. A. Gutierrez Jr., D.A. Wetter, Calcinosis cutis in autoimmune connective tissue diseases, Dermatol. Ther. 25 (2012) 195–206.

330. H. Gunawardena, L.R. Wedderburn, H. Chinoy, et al., Autoantibodies to a 140-kd protein in juvenile dermatomyositis are associated with calcinosis, Arthritis Rheum. 60 (2009) 1807–1814.

331. R.E. Fisler, M.G. Liang, R.C. Fuhlbrigge, et al., Aggressive management of juvenile dermatomyositis results in improved outcome and decreased incidence of calcinosis, J. Am. Acad. Dermatol. 47 (2002) 505–511.

334. B.Q. Banker, M. Victor, Dermatomyositis (systemic angiopathy) of childhood, Medicine (Baltimore). 45 (1966) 261–289.

358. A.M. Huber, G. Mamyrova, P.A. Lachenbruch, et al., Early illness features associated with mortality in the juvenile idiopathic inflammatory myopathies, Arthritis Care Res. 66 (2014) 732–740.

370. A. Bingham, G. Mamyrova, K.I. Rother, et al., Predictors of acquired lipodystrophy in juvenile-onset dermatomyositis and a gradient of severity, Medicine (Baltimore). 87 (2008) 70–86.

384. A.M. Huber, E.H. Giannini, S.L. Bowyer, et al., Protocols for the initial treatment of moderately severe juvenile dermatomyositis: results of a Children's Arthritis and Rheumatology Research Alliance Consensus Conference, Arthritis Care Res. 62 (2010) 219–225.

390. L. Miles, K.E. Bove, D. Lovell, et al., Predictability of the clinical course of juvenile dermatomyositis based on initial muscle biopsy: a retrospective study of 72 patients, Arthritis Rheum. 57 (2007) 1183–1191.

478. Myopathy & Neuromuscular Junction Disorders, Differential Diagnosis, Washington University, St. Louis, MO, 2013. <http://neuromuscular.wustl.edu/maltbrain.html>.

544. Z.E. Betteridge, H. Gunawardena, N.J. McHugh, Novel autoantibodies and clinical phenotypes in adult and juvenile myositis, Arthritis Res. Ther. 13 (2011) 209.

608. R.J. Hernandez, D.B. Sullivan, T.L. Chenevert, D.R. Keim, MR imaging in children with dermatomyositis: musculoskeletal findings and correlation with clinical and laboratory findings, AJR Am. J. Roentgenol. 161 (1993) 359–366.

634. S. Bitnum, C.W. Daeschner Jr., L.B. Travis, et al., Dermatomyositis, J. Pediatr. 64 (1964) 101–131.

657. L.G. Rider, E.H. Giannini, H.I. Brunner, et al., International consensus on preliminary definitions of improvement in adult and juvenile myositis, Arthritis Rheum. 50 (2004) 2281–2290.

658. R. Hasija, A. Pistorio, A. Ravelli, et al., Therapeutic approaches in the treatment of juvenile dermatomyositis in patients with recent-onset disease and in those experiencing disease flare: an international multicenter PRINTO study, Arthritis Rheum. 63 (2011) 3142–3152.

659. D. Lazarevic, A. Pistorio, E. Palmisani, et al., The PRINTO criteria for clinically inactive disease in juvenile dermatomyositis, Ann. Rheum. Dis. 72 (2013) 686–693.

661. N. Ruperto, A. Pistorio, A. Ravelli, et al., The pediatric rheumatology international trials organization provisional criteria for the evaluation of response to therapy in juvenile dermatomyositis, Arthritis Care Res. 62 (2010) 1533–1541.

673. K.A. Rouster-Stevens, A. Gursahaney, K.L. Ngai, et al., Pharmacokinetic study of oral prednisolone compared with intravenous

methylprednisolone in patients with juvenile dermatomyositis, Arthritis Rheum. 59 (2008) 222–226.

691. A.V. Ramanan, N. Campbell-Webster, S. Ota, et al., The effectiveness of treating juvenile dermatomyositis with methotrexate and aggressively tapered corticosteroids, Arthritis Rheum. 52 (2005) 3570–3578.

718. M.C. Dalakas, I. Illa, J.M. Dambrosia, et al., A controlled trial of high-dose intravenous immune globulin infusions as treatment for dermatomyositis, N. Engl. J. Med. 329 (1993) 1993–2000.

722. C.G. Lam, C. Manlhiot, E.M. Pullenayegum, B.M. Feldman, Efficacy of intravenous Ig therapy in juvenile dermatomyositis, Ann. Rheum. Dis. 70 (2011) 2089–2094.

743. C.V. Oddis, A.M. Reed, R. Aggarwal, et al., Rituximab in the treatment of refractory adult and juvenile dermatomyositis and adult polymyositis: a randomized, placebo-phase trial, Arthritis Rheum. 65 (2013) 314–324.

Entire reference list is available online at www.expertconsult.com.

Systemic Sclerodermas

Francesco Zulian

The word *scleroderma* means "hard skin." However, although hardening of the skin is the most signal characteristic common to all types of the disorder, the diseases grouped under this term often involve different organ systems. A classification of the systemic and localized sclerodermas is summarized in Table 27-1. Systemic sclerosis is subdivided by the extent of the skin disease into *diffuse cutaneous systemic sclerosis* (dSSc) and *limited cutaneous systemic sclerosis* (lSSc), previously designated as the CREST syndrome (calcinosis cutis, Raynaud phenomenon, esophageal dysfunction, sclerodactyly, telangiectasia). The localized forms of the disease, such as morphea or linear scleroderma, often are regarded as more dermatological than rheumatological (see Chapter 28).

HISTORICAL REVIEW

The early literature presents a confusing picture of scleroderma in a child because many cases were more compatible with a diagnosis of scleredema. In 1895, Lewin and Heller[1] reviewed 505 cases of scleroderma, mainly from the European literature. Goodman[2] observed that 88 occurred in children from birth to 19 years of age but that most cases were examples of circumscribed disease. Only 1 of 12 children reported as diffuse scleroderma was compatible with current concepts, with the rest being the "acute form," probably scleredema.[3] Another survey concluded that only 12 children with generalized scleroderma had been reported in the world literature through 1960.[4] In 1961, the Mayo Clinic added 63 additional pediatric cases in summarizing experience with 727 patients.[5] A survey (Padua database) of members of the Pediatric Rheumatology European Society and other pediatric rheumatology centers around the world (67 centers in 28 countries) reviewed 153 children with systemic sclerosis, and other American authors reported a series of 111 childhood-onset SSc patients followed at one center.[6,7]

Pathological studies lagged behind clinical reports, and there were no comprehensive descriptions until 1924, when Kraus[8] described pulmonary and cardiac fibrosis in a patient with scleroderma, and Matsui[9] detailed necropsy findings in five patients with scleroderma and cutaneous histological characteristics in another. In 1969, D'Angelo and colleagues[10] examined 58 autopsy cases of adult SSc and reported the abnormalities found at postmortem as percentages in excess of control subjects: skin, 98%; esophagus, 74%; lungs, 59%; kidneys, 49%; small intestine, 46%; pericardium, 41%; large intestine, 39%; pleura, 29%; and myocardium, 26%. Other organs with less frequent involvement were the adrenal glands, lymph nodes, thyroid, and peripheral arteries. Interestingly, vascular lesions suggestive of severe hypertension were found in the kidneys of patients with no history of hypertension and, similarly, vascular lesions suggestive of severe pulmonary hypertension were found in the lungs of patients with no history of pulmonary hypertension.[10]

DIFFUSE CUTANEOUS SYSTEMIC SCLEROSIS

Diffuse SSc is a chronic, multisystem connective tissue disease characterized by sclerodermatous skin changes and widespread abnormalities of the viscera. Rodnan[11] defined dSSc as a disorder in which "symmetrical fibrous thickening and hardening (sclerosis) of the skin is combined with fibrous and degenerative changes in synovium, digital arteries, and certain internal organs, most notably the esophagus, intestinal tract, heart, lungs, and kidneys."

Systemic sclerosis sine scleroderma has been described in adults as a variant of limited cutaneous involvement and not a separate or distinct disorder.[12,13] Other than the absence of skin thickening, this disease has no significant differences in internal organ involvement, laboratory abnormalities, serum autoantibodies, or survival rate compared with lSSc.

Classification

According to old classification criteria of the American College of Rheumatology for adults,[14] definite dSSc requires the presence either of the major criterion (fibrosis/induration involving the skin proximal to the metacarpophalangeal [MCP] or metatarsophalangeal [MTP] joints) or of two minor criteria (sclerodactyly, digital pitting scars, bibasilar pulmonary fibrosis). Subsequently, the widespread use of nailfold capillary microscopy, the more precise autoimmune serological tests, and the early detection of Raynaud phenomenon in patients who, years later, developed SSc, have raised the need for a more comprehensive classification.

In 2001, Leroy and Medsger proposed a set of criteria[15] to identify patients with vascular abnormalities and serological changes typical of scleroderma but who do not yet fulfill criteria for dSSc or lSSc. Patients who exhibit Raynaud phenomenon and either nailfold capillary abnormalities or an antibody profile characteristic of dSSc or lSSc are classified as having the limited form of scleroderma defined as *early systemic sclerosis*. In 2007, an ad hoc International Committee developed classification criteria for juvenile systemic sclerosis.[16] According to these criteria, an individual who is younger than 16 years of age is classified as having dSSc if the one major (presence of skin sclerosis/induration proximal to MCP or MTP) and at least 2 of the 20 minor criteria listed in Table 27-2 are present. This set of classification criteria

TABLE 27-1   Classification of Systemic and Localized Sclerodermas and Scleroderma-Like Disorders

Systemic Sclerosis
Diffuse
Limited

Overlap Syndromes
Sclerodermatomyositis or with other connective tissue diseases
Mixed connective tissue disease

Localized Scleroderma
Plaque morphea
Generalized morphea
Bullous morphea
Linear morphea
Deep morphea

Graft-Versus-Host Disease
Chemically Induced Scleroderma-Like Disease
Polyvinyl chloride
Bleomycin
Pentazocine
Toxic oil syndrome
Adjuvant disease

Pseudosclerodermas
Phenylketonuria
Syndromes of premature aging
Localized idiopathic fibroses
Scleredema
Diabetic cheiroarthropathy
Porphyria cutanea tarda

TABLE 27-2   Preliminary Classification Criteria for Juvenile Systemic Sclerosis*

MAJOR CRITERION	Sclerosis/induration of the skin proximal to MCP	
MINOR CRITERIA	• Skin	Sclerodactyly
	• Vascular	Raynaud phenomenon
		Nailfold capillary abnormalities
		Digital tip ulcers
	• Gastrointestinal	Dysphagia
		Gastroesophageal reflux
	• Renal	Renal crisis
		New-onset arterial hypertension
	• Cardiac	Arrhythmias
		Heart failure
	• Respiratory	Pulmon fibrosis (HRCT/X-ray)
		DL_{CO}
		Pulmonary hypertension
	• Musculoskeletal	Tendon friction rubs
		Arthritis
		Myositis
	• Neurological	Neuropathy
		Carpal tunnel syndrome
	• Serology	Antinuclear antibodies
		SSc selective autoantibodies (anticentromere, anti-topoisomerase I, anti-fibrillarin, anti-PM-Scl, anti-fibrillin or anti-RNA polymerase I or III)

PRES/ACR/EULAR Ad Hoc Committee on Classification Criteria for JSSc (2007). The Pediatric Rheumatology European Society/American College of Rheumatology/European League Against Rheumatism Provisional Classification Criteria for Juvenile Systemic Sclerosis. Arthritis Rheum 57(2): 203–212.
*A patient, aged less than 16 years, shall be classified as having juvenile systemic sclerosis if the one major and at least two of the 20 minor criteria are present. This set of classification criteria have a sensitivity of 90%, a specificity of 96% and kappa statistic value of 0.86.

has a sensitivity of 90%, a specificity of 96%, and kappa statistic value of 0.86.

Similarly, a new set of classification criteria has been recently proposed for adult patients with SSc (Table 27-3).[17] According to these criteria, the skin thickening of the fingers extending proximal to the MCP joints is sufficient to classify the patient as having SSc. If this criterion is lacking, seven alternative criteria should be considered: (1) skin thickening of the fingers, (2) fingertip lesions, (3) telangiectasia, (4) abnormal nailfold capillaries, (5) interstitial lung disease (ILD or pulmonary arterial hypertension, (6) Raynaud phenomenon, and (7) SSc-related autoantibodies. Each of these items has a different weight in defining SSc and patients with a score of 9 or higher can be classified as having SSc.[17]

Epidemiology

Diffuse SSc has been reported worldwide and in all races.[18-26] It has an estimated annual incidence of 0.45 to 1.9 cases per 100,000 persons in the general population and a prevalence of approximately 24 cases per 100,000.[18,20,25-27] The frequency of this disorder increases with age and is highest in individuals who fall into the 30- to 50-year-old age group. The disease is more frequent in African Americans and in Choctaw Native Americans.[26] African-American women are more likely to develop diffuse disease, be diagnosed at a younger age, and have a poorer survival rate.[25]

Onset in childhood is uncommon. Children younger than 10 years of age account for less than 2% of all cases, and patients between 10 and 20 years of age account for only 1.2% to 9%.[21-24,28-35] It has been estimated that approximately 3% of all patients had onset in childhood.[36] A recent study in the United Kingdom reported an incidence rate of 0.27 cases per 1,000,000 children per year.[37]

There is no racial predilection or peak age at onset determined for children. There are several small series and case reports of children with dSSc totaling just over 115 patients, although there are undoubtedly many unreported cases.[3,4,31,38-54] An additional 153 patients in the Padua database are included.[6] Diffuse SSc occurs with equal frequency in boys and girls younger than 8 years old, whereas girls outnumber boys 3 to 1 when disease onset occurs in children who are older than 8 years. Among adults, the female-to-male ratio in the childbearing years is 3:1 to 5:1, whereas in an older age group (older than 45 years) it is 1.8:1.[55] One hypothesis is that factors such as the hormonal milieu, pregnancy-related events, or reproductive-specific exposures are responsible for these differences in disease susceptibility.

Etiology and Pathogenesis

The cause of dSSc is unknown, despite significant advances in understanding of potential pathogenic mechanisms.[56] The disease can be

TABLE 27-3   The American College of Rheumatology/European League Against Rheumatism Criteria for the Classification of Systemic Sclerosis*

ITEM	SUB-ITEM(S)	WEIGHT/SCORE[†]
Skin thickening of the fingers of both hands extending proximal to the metacarpophalangeal joints (sufficient criterion)	—	9
Skin thickening of the fingers (only count the higher score)	Puffy fingers	2
	Sclerodactyly of the fingers (distal to the metacarpophalangeal joints but proximal to the proximal interphalangeal joints)	4
Fingertip lesions (only count the higher score)	Digital tip ulcers	2
	Fingertip pitting scar	3
Telangiectasia	—	2
Abnormal nailfold capillaries	—	2
Pulmonary arterial hypertension and/or interstitial lung disease (maximum score is 2)	Pulmonary arterial hypertension	2
	Interstitial lung disease	2
Raynaud phenomenon	—	3
SSc-related autoantibodies (anticentromere, anti-topoisomerase I [anti-Sd-70], anti-RNA polymerase III) (maximum score is 3)	Anticentromere	3
	Anti-topoisomerase I	
	Anti-RNA polymerase III	

*These criteria are applicable to any patient considered for inclusion in a systemic sclerosis study. The criteria are not applicable to patients with skin thickening that spares the fingers or to patients who have a scleroderma-like disorder that better explains their manifestations (e.g., nephrogenic sclerosing fibrosis, generalized morphea, eosinophilic fasciitis, scleredema diabeticorum, scleromyxedema, erythromelalgia, porphyria, lichen sclerosis, graft-versus-host disease, diabetic cheiroarthropathy).

[†]The total score is determined by adding the maximum weight (score) in each category. Patients with a total score of ≥9 are classified as having definite systemic sclerosis.

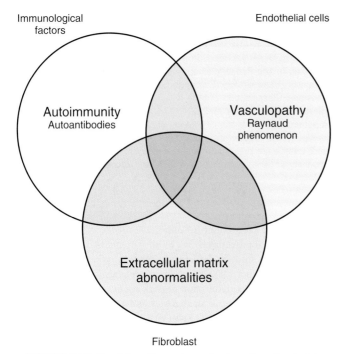

FIGURE 27-1 Possible pathogenic mechanisms in scleroderma.

TABLE 27-4   Cytokines and Growth Factors Involved in the Regulation of the Biologic Behavior of Fibroblasts

BIOLOGIC EFFECT	CYTOKINE OR GROWTH FACTOR
Increased collagen synthesis	TGF-β, PDGF, IL-1, IL-4, IL-6
Decreased collagen synthesis	IFN-β, IFN-γ, TNF-α, β
Fibroblast proliferation	IFN-β, IFN-γ, TGF-β, PDGF, TNF, IL-1, IL-4
Chemoattraction	IFN-γ, TGF-β, PDGF, TNF, IL-4
Glycosaminoglycan synthesis	TGF-β, TNF, IL-1
Fibronectin synthesis	TGF-β, IL-4
Endothelial cell injury	IFN-γ, TNF-α, β, IL-2, NK cell, granzyme A
Reduction of collagen synthesis	TGF-β
Collagenase gene induction	TNF-α

IFN, Interferon; *IL*, interleukin; *NK*, natural killer cell; *PDGF*, platelet-derived growth factor; *TNF*, tumor necrosis factor; *TGF*, transforming growth factor.

represented as a tripartite process in which dysfunction of the *immune system*, *endothelium*, and *fibroblasts* gives rise to a heterogeneous phenotype that is characterized prominently by fibrosis (Fig. 27-1).

Autoimmunity is evident by the elaboration of circulating disease-specific autoantibodies and multiple abnormalities of T-cell function. Raynaud phenomenon, capillary dropout, endothelial injury, and abnormalities in vascular tone are manifestations of endothelial cell dysfunction. Fibroblast dysfunction is represented by fibrosis as the result of increased synthesis and deposition of extracellular matrix proteins. These three areas of abnormal function, although apparently unassociated with each other, are closely linked by several immunological alterations.

Immunological Factors

Many reports suggest that cellular immunity plays a major role in the initiation of scleroderma. These factors include the presence of mononuclear cell (MNC) infiltrates in early lesions, altered function of helper T and natural killer (NK) cells, and release of cytokines, chemokines, and growth factors (Table 27-4). MNC infiltration in various organ systems occurs early and consists of lymphocytes, plasma cells, and fibroblast-histiocytic cells around small blood vessels, eccrine sweat glands, and subcutaneous tissue.[57] Activated T lymphocytes are prominent as evidenced by the expression of surface human leukocyte antigen (HLA) class II molecules.[58]

The early infiltrates of MNCs release a number of cytokines and chemokines that affect endothelial cells and fibroblasts. Several growth factors have also been identified in scleroderma skin, including transforming growth factor-β (TGF-β), connective tissue growth factor (CTGF), and adhesion molecules. TGF-β has pleomorphic cellular actions principally on fibroblasts and endothelial cells.[59] In vitro, it stimulates the synthesis of the extracellular matrix, including types I and III collagen.[60] It also promotes fibrosis indirectly by inhibiting collagenase activity.[61] Fibroblasts from scleroderma skin express in vivo and in vitro increased levels of TGF-β1 and TGF-β2 receptor proteins compared with controls.[62,63] Blockade of TGF-β1 signaling with monoclonal antibodies inhibits upregulation of collagen synthesis in scleroderma fibroblasts.[62] Polymorphisms of the TGF-β1 gene have been reported in Japanese patients.[64] CTGF levels are greatly elevated in the dermis of patients with scleroderma and downregulated by iloprost infusion.[65]

Fibrosis

Although TGF-β1 is known to initiate fibrosis, CTGF may play a greater role in maintaining and promoting fibrosis.[66,67] Once initiated, fibrosis is escalated through multiple feed-forward amplification loops that are generated as a consequence of tissue damage, increased matrix stiffness, hypoxia, oxidative stress, and accumulation of damage-associated molecular patterns (DAMPs), which promote fibroblast activation and differentiation.[68] In the skin, the expanding dermis replaces the subcutaneous adipose layer and obliterates the dermal appendages; blood supply is reduced, leading to progressive tissue hypoxia with induction of local production of vascular endothelial growth factor (VEGF) and other angiogenic factors. Biochemical analysis indicates excessive deposition of the fibrillar collagens (type I and type III); type V and type VII collagens and elastin fibrils; and elevated levels of enzymes that catalyze posttranslational collagen modifications, such as lysyl hydroxylase and lysyl oxidase.

Genetic changes in SSc have been demonstrated. Examination of SSc skin biopsies shows alterations in gene expression as compared with healthy controls[69]; most involved genes are those involved in TGF-β pathway, extracellular matrix proteins, innate immune signaling, lipid metabolism, and hypoxia.[69]

Recent studies have also underlined the role of microRNA (miRNA),[70] short noncoding nucleotides that modulate gene expression at the posttranscriptional level via inhibition of messenger RNA (mRNA) translation or via facilitation of mRNA degradation. In lung fibrosis, changes in expression of some profibrotic and antifibrotic miRNA, regulated by TGF-β, have been shown.[71] The main targets of the regulation are genes involved in matrix repair and remodeling.

Cytokines and Chemokines

Levels of a number of cytokines (e.g., interleukin [IL]-1, IL-2, IL-4, IL-6, IL-8) are increased in the serum.[68-72] Several ILs (e.g., IL-4, IL-6, IL-8) have also been demonstrated in scleroderma skin. Serum levels and spontaneous production of IL-12, a potent inducer of type 1 helper (Th1) T cells, were increased in patients with renal vascular damage.[73] Specific cytokines promote fibrosis; others, such as interferon-γ (IFN-γ), are potent suppressors of collagen synthesis. The effects of some cytokines are mixed. Tumor necrosis factor (TNF) decreases fibroblast production of types I and III collagen while promoting collagenase gene induction.[59] This cytokine also stimulates the

proliferation of some fibroblasts and increases endothelial cell expression of adhesion molecules (i.e., E-selectin, intracellular adhesion molecule-1 [ICAM-1] and vascular cell adhesion molecule-1 [VCAM-1]) and release of endothelin-1. The level of circulating soluble VCAM-1 correlates with impaired left ventricular diastolic function.[74] Serum CD44 (sCD44), another adhesion molecule that regulates the migration of leucocytes, was found to be elevated in scleroderma patients, particularly in those with limited cutaneous disease.[75] As for genetic predispositions, the TNF-863A allele was found to be associated with anticentromere antibody seropositivity.[76]

Chemokines are operative in the recruitment of specific types of leukocytes to involved skin and tissue. Serum levels of MCP-1, which attracts MNCs, and MIP-1, which attracts monocytes and helper T cells, are elevated.[77] A constitutive overexpression of MCP-1 mRNA has been identified in scleroderma skin.[78] Treatment with antibodies to MCP-1 results in reduced chemotactic activity, indicating that this chemokine may be an important agent in the initiation of cutaneous inflammation.[79] Levels of chemokines IL-8 and growth-regulated oncogene-α (GRO-α), which are potent chemoattractants and activators of neutrophils, were found to be elevated in scleroderma; GRO-α correlated particularly with pulmonary involvement.[80] Cell-mediated immunity to laminin, a constituent of basement membrane and to a lesser extent to type IV collagen, has also been demonstrated in patients with dSSc.[81]

Vascular Factors

Endothelial cell injury may be the central pathogenic event and predates fibrotic changes. The endothelial cell may be damaged by protease-dependent mechanisms that are independent of complement and immunoglobulin. Abnormalities of cutaneous mast cell number and type, and abnormalities of mast cell activation as a prefibrotic event have been documented.[82] Damage to the endothelial cell results in increased vascular permeability, which is responsible for the edematous phase of the illness, leading to activation of fibroblasts, increased collagen production, and resultant fibrosis. It also initiates activation of the coagulation pathway, contributing to an accumulation of platelets that release factors leading to proliferation and migration of myointimal cells.

Endothelial Cell Factors

Evidence that the endothelial cell is damaged is provided by studies of the histology of the lesions in dSSc and by demonstration of elevated levels of factor VIII–related antigen,[83] although this has not been a consistent observation.[84] Reduced plasma angiotensin-converting–enzyme activity may be an additional marker of endothelial injury.[85] Endothelial cell apoptosis is accelerated.[86] The microvascular injury leads to arteriolar intimal fibrosis and narrowing of the vascular lumen, which results in ischemic damage.[87] Anti–endothelial cell antibodies are also present[88,89] and lead to endothelial damage, vascular hyperpermeability, and myointimal cell proliferation.

The link between vascular alterations and cellular immunity is represented by adhesion molecules. Three major families have been defined: selectins, integrins, and members of the immunoglobulin gene superfamily. Selectins mediate the initial contact of leukocytes with endothelial cells. Overexpression of E-selectin and P-selectin has been found in sera,[90,91] and in endothelial cells of the skin and minor salivary glands of scleroderma patients.[92] Integrins, a family of heterodimeric transmembrane glycoprotein molecules, serve as a means of communication between extracellular matrix molecules (e.g., collagen, laminin, fibronectin) through the cell membrane to the intracellular compartment. Expression of integrins VLA-2, VLA-4, and LFA-1 is increased on endothelial cells, MNCs, fibroblasts, and dendritic cells in sclerodermatous skin.[92] ICAM-1 and VCAM-1, members of the immunoglobulin gene superfamily on endothelial cells, and LFA-1 and VLA-4, integrin receptors on lymphocytes, play a significant role in the interaction between lymphocytes and endothelial cells or fibroblasts. These molecules are increased on endothelial cells and fibroblasts in sclerodermatous skin[93,94] and facilitate MNC damage to endothelial cells and fibroblasts.

Abnormalities of Collagen

Excessive accumulation of collagen in affected skin led to the hypothesis that there might be abnormalities of collagen type or metabolism.[26,95] There is an increased number of collagen-producing fibroblasts in the skin[96]; however, the ratios of various collagen types are normal.[97] Although reduced, collagenase activity was found in one study,[98] whereas it was normal in another.[99] Abnormalities of glycosylation[100] and hydroxylation[98] of the collagen molecule may prevent normal feedback mechanisms from being effective in controlling synthesis, and permit excessive deposition of collagen. Defects in the regulation of genes controlling fibroblasts apoptosis (i.e., caspase 6, Bcl2, and elastin) have been reported.[101]

Genetic Background

The rare familial occurrence of dSSc has been confirmed in a mother and her 6-year-old son,[45] in a second family with two affected sisters ages 12 and 16 years,[102] and in monozygotic twins.[103]

There is little agreement about the potential associations of histocompatibility antigens with dSSc. Initial studies indicated associations with class I alleles HLA-A9,[104] HLA-B8,[105,106] and HLA-Bw35[107] and class II alleles HLA-DR3,[106] HLA-DR5,[108] and HLA-DRw15.[109] Associations with HLA-DR and HLA-DQ alleles (DQB3.1, DQB1.1, DQB1.2, DQB1.3) have been reviewed by Whiteside and colleagues[110] and Fox and Kang.[111] DRB1*1104 and DRB1*1101 confer odds ratios of 3.5 and 2.3 for the disease in adults.[112]

Prolonged persistence of fetal progenitor cells and microchimerism in T cells has been associated with DQA1*0501.[113,114] Microchimerism, the presence within one individual of a very low level of cells derived from a different individual, was postulated as a possible cause of scleroderma from studies of chronic graft-versus-host disease (GVHD), a chimeric disorder in which donor T cells or NK cells react against HLA molecules of the recipient recognized as "nonself."

Microchimerism occurs in women who had previous pregnancies, individuals who have had blood transfusions, and children with cells from their mother or a twin. Maternal cells can persist in an immunocompetent offspring even in adult life, and fetus-derived hemopoietic cells have persisted in the maternal circulation for many years postpartum.[115] Fetal DNA persists for even longer periods.[116] Although microchimerism can be identified in normal subjects and in other diseases, it has been proposed as an important factor in pathogenesis of autoimmune diseases.[117] In scleroderma, chimeric cells are increased in number and, compared with normal subjects, are more similar to the maternal cells. Quantitative analysis of microchimerism has been reported in sclerodermatous skin.[118] Nelson and co-workers[116] documented high concentrations of male DNA in cells of the vascular compartment of women with scleroderma, many years after having given birth to sons, as compared with women without scleroderma. HLA class II compatibility of the child was more common in dSSc patients than in control subjects. An investigation by Artlett and colleagues[119] also concluded that fetal antimaternal GVH reactions might be involved in pathogenesis. Although this theory of a chronic GVH reaction is attractive, studies offer no data to explain the occurrence of scleroderma in men or women who have never had children.

Clinical Manifestations
Early Signs and Symptoms

Presenting signs and symptoms of dSSc in children are shown in Table 27-5. Onset of the disease is usually insidious, and the course is prolonged, punctuated by periods of inactivity or episodes of severe systemic complications, occasionally ending in remission or more often in chronic disability or death.[120] The onset is often characterized by the development of Raynaud phenomenon; tightening, thinning, and atrophy of the skin of the hands and face; or the appearance of cutaneous telangiectasias about the face, upper trunk, and hands. Because of the subtle nature of this presentation, there is often a diagnostic delay of years. A comprehensive general review of the assessment of patients with systemic sclerosis has been published.[121]

TABLE 27-5 Presenting Signs and Symptoms in Children with Systemic Scleroderma

SIGN	JAFFE ET AL.[3] (N = 5) 1961	GOEL ET AL.[43] (N = 4) 1974	CASSIDY ET AL.[36] (N = 13) 1977	KORNREICH ET AL.[31] (N = 13) 1977	LARRÈGUE ET AL.[49] (N = 3) 1983	SUÁREZ-ALMAZOR ET AL.[51] (N = 4) 1985	LABABIDI ET AL.[52] (N = 5) 1991	MARTINI ET AL.[6] (N = 153) 2006	TOTAL %*
Skin tightening	4	4	15	13	3	4	3	74	82.2
Raynaud phenomenon	5	2	11	5	3	4	3	75	70.4
Soft-tissue contracture	2	1	10	—	2	4	3	—	61.1
Arthralgia	—†	3	9	—	2	1	5	26	28.2
Muscle weakness and pain	—	1	4	—	—	2	2	12	15.2
Subcutaneous calcification	—	—	3	—	—	1	—	9	10.2
Dysphagia	—	—	3	—	—	1	2	10	13.5
Dyspnea	—	—	3	—	—	1	2	10	12.9

*Percentage calculated only on series in which detailed information was provided.
†Dash indicates that information was not provided.

Skin Disease

The onset of cutaneous abnormalities may be especially insidious, but these changes characteristically evolve in a sequence beginning with edema, followed by induration and sclerosis resulting in marked tightening and contractures, eventually resulting in atrophy.

Edema. Tense, nonpitting swelling of the skin and subcutaneous tissues of the digits, hands, arms, and face, or localized areas on the trunk may be the initial manifestation of the disease. Edematous areas may be warm and tender with an erythematous border but are often asymptomatic. Swelling may persist for weeks or months before subsiding or being replaced by sclerosis.

Sclerosis. During the sclerotic phase, the skin develops a waxy texture and becomes tight, hard, and bound to subcutaneous structures. This is particularly noticeable in skin of the dorsal surface of the digits, so-called acrosclerosis (Fig. 27-2), and face (Fig. 27-3); the characteristic immobile, expressionless, unwrinkled appearance of the skin may be the first clue to the diagnosis. The absence of forehead wrinkling and the presence of circumoral furrowing or diminished aperture of the mouth are particularly characteristic. Sclerotic changes usually follow a temporal sequence of development, beginning with bilateral, symmetrical acrosclerosis, followed by involvement of the face, and finally by changes in the skin of the trunk and proximal limbs.

Atrophy. The long-term consequence of edema and sclerosis is atrophy of skin and adnexa. These superficial abnormalities result in a shiny appearance of the skin accompanied by areas of hypopigmentation or hyperpigmentation and often by deposition of calcium salts in the subcutaneous tissues. Cutaneous lesions in all stages of evolution may be observed simultaneously in the same child.

Telangiectasias. Telangiectasias, fine macular dilations of cutaneous or mucous membrane blood vessels, are characteristic (Fig. 27-4). Unlike "spider" angiomata that fill rapidly from central arterioles, telangiectatic vessels fill slowly and lack the characteristic central vessel. The periungual nailfold is often the most obvious early location

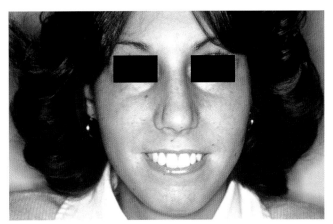

FIGURE 27-3 Shiny skin on the face.

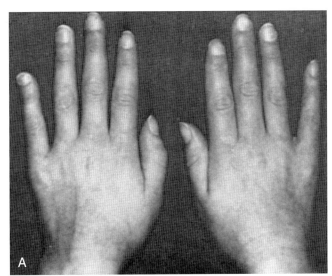
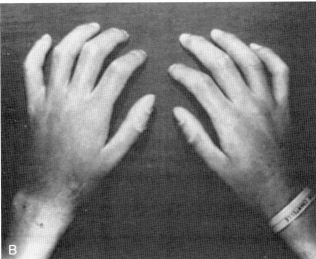

FIGURE 27-2 **A,** The hands of a 9-year-old girl with diffuse cutaneous systemic scleroderma. The skin over the dorsa of the fingers is taut and shiny. **B,** Five years later, the tightening is more evident, and flexion contractures have developed. (Courtesy Dr. K. Oen.)

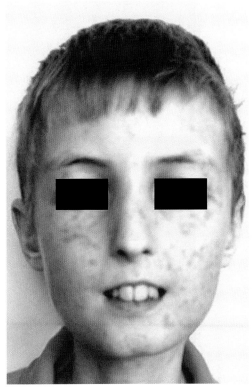

FIGURE 27-4 Telangiectasias.

of abnormal vessels (Fig. 27-5), and examination with an ophthalmoscope, at +40 diopters, demonstrates capillary dropout, tortuous dilated loops, and occasionally distorted capillary architecture (Fig. 27-6).[48,122,123] There is usually redundant cuticular growth; dystrophic changes in the nails have also been reported.[124] Digital pitting, sometimes with ulceration and gangrene, occurs in the pulp of the fingertips as a result of ischemia and is one of the minor diagnostic criteria (Fig. 27-7).

Calcinosis. Subcutaneous calcification, especially over the elbows, MCP joints, and knees, may occur, sometimes with ulceration of surrounding skin. Extensive periarticular calcification (i.e., calcinosis circumscripta) may be a late complication (Fig. 27-8). These lesions, if extensive, lead to a severe reduction in joint mobility. Small, hard, subcutaneous nodules sometimes occur over the extensor surfaces of joints of the fingers and differ histologically from rheumatoid nodules by the absence of fibrinoid necrosis.[125]

Raynaud Phenomenon

Raynaud phenomenon occurs in 90% of children with dSSc and is often the initial symptom of the disorder, preceding other manifestations (in some instances by years).[6,126,127] Raynaud phenomenon represents the first manifestation of the disease in 70% of children with dSSc and in 10%, it is complicated by digital infarcts. During the overall course of the disease, Raynaud phenomenon is also the most frequently reported symptom.[6] Raynaud phenomenon is covered extensively in Chapter 31.

Musculoskeletal Disease

Musculoskeletal symptoms are common and characteristically occur at or near onset. Among the 153 children with dSSc included in the Padua database, 36% had musculoskeletal symptoms during the course of the disease.[6] Morning stiffness and pain of the small joints of the

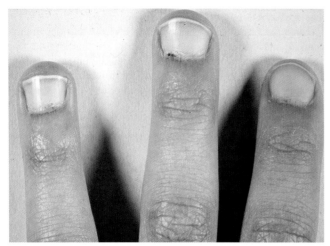

FIGURE 27-5 Changes in the nailfold vessels with visible tortuosity, thickening, and pigmentary extrusion onto the cuticles.

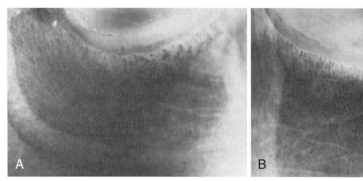

FIGURE 27-6 A, There is a reduction in the number of nailfold capillaries and tortuosity of the remaining vessels in the microvasculature viewed with a microscope (magnification ×100). **B,** Normal vessels. (Courtesy Dr. J. Kenik.)

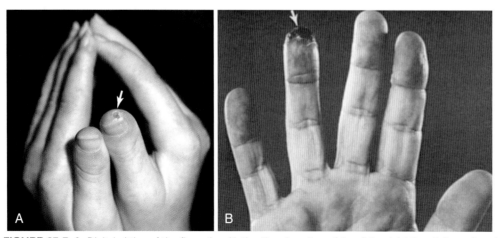

FIGURE 27-7 A, Digital pitting of the fingertips. Notice the ulceration of tip of the right thumb (*arrow*) and shiny, tightly stretched skin over the fingertips bilaterally with pronounced flexion contractures at the metacarpophalangeal joints. **B,** Digital gangrene of the fourth right finger (*arrow*).

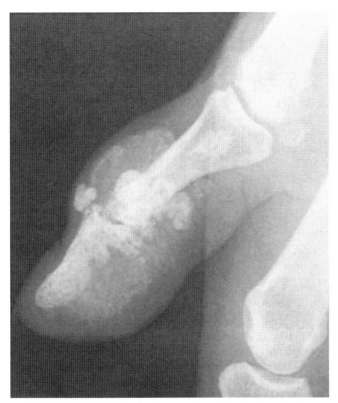

FIGURE 27-8 Calcinosis circumscripta affecting the thumb.

hands, knees, and ankles may also be initial manifestations of the disease. Movement of a thickened tendon through its sheath, which is covered with fibrinous deposits, can often be palpated or detected with a stethoscope as an audible, coarse crepitus.

Joint pain is usually mild and transient. Joint contractures of insidious onset and limitation of motion are most common at the proximal interphalangeal joints and elbows, but other joints can be affected. Objective evidence of articular inflammation is absent or mild in most instances, although small, bland synovial effusions occur. Muscle inflammation characterized by pain and tenderness occurs in up to one fifth of children, and proximal or distal muscle atrophy may be marked.

Gastrointestinal Disease

Gastrointestinal (GI) involvement occurs in approximately 70% to 90% of SSc patients during the course of the disease[128]; however, a recent study[129] has shown that as many as 98.9% of SSc adult patients suffered from GI symptoms. The entire GI tract can be affected, with a prevalence decreasing from 96% for esophageal complications to 10% to 75% for gastric involvement and 10% to 50% for bowel disease[130]; proximal disease usually precedes distal involvement.[6] Lesions of the mouth include mucosal telangiectasias, reduced interincisor distance caused by skin thickening and tightness, parotitis as part of the sicca syndrome, and loosening of the teeth because of changes in the periodontal membrane. The esophagus is involved, often quite early in the disease, and dysphagia may be one of the first signs an individual may exhibit. The most common manifestation is esophageal dysmotility, with asynchronous peristalsis and gastroesophageal reflux disease (GERD), leading to Barrett's esophagus in 7% to 13% of patients.[131] Although many patients are asymptomatic, symptoms (in order of decreasing frequency) include heartburn with postural aggravation, dysphagia, delayed emptying, regurgitation with reflux into the throat, nocturnal aspiration, and cough with swallowing. Esophagitis

with persistent ulceration and stricture along with progressive weight loss because of voluntary restriction of food intake may follow. Dilation of the stomach or duodenum occurs uncommonly. In adults, gastric arteriovenous ectasia ("watermelon stomach") may develop. Small-bowel involvement usually develops in association with esophageal or colonic disease.[10] Abdominal distention and pain with nausea and vomiting result from gut hypotonia that occasionally may be so severe that pseudoobstruction occurs.[132] Pneumatosis intestinalis may develop. Malabsorptive diarrhea and delayed colon transit, when present, reflect long-standing disease.[133] Malabsorption in SSc is primarily due to small bowel bacterial overgrowth and should be treated with rotating oral antibiotics (antibiotic change every 4 weeks) because continuous therapy with one agent may result in the emergence of resistant organisms and an increased relapse rate.

Large-bowel disease, although not uncommon, is usually asymptomatic; however, it may cause severe constipation, bloating, or diarrhea.

Cardiac Disease

Cardiopulmonary disease, although not common at the disease onset, is a leading cause of morbidity.[51,134,135] Pericardial effusions are usually small and asymptomatic, although fever and retrosternal pain may accompany acute disease.[136] Changes in cardiac hemodynamics, reflected by the presence of pedal edema, jugular venous distension, and hepatomegaly, may be present in patients with chronic effusions. Tamponade from pericardial constriction and severe cardiomyopathy are, however, rare, although they can be one of the causes of early death and require prompt and aggressive immunosuppressive treatment.[133]

Cardiac ischemia may result from the equivalent of Raynaud phenomenon of the coronary arteries and is a potential precursor of myocardial fibrosis. Although coronary artery disease is uncommon, electrocardiographic changes and even angina pectoris may occur as a result of disease of the myocardial microvasculature.[137] Systemic and pulmonary hypertension may contribute to myocardial ischemia.

Pulmonary Disease

SSc-associated ILD is diagnosed when radiological evidence of diffuse parenchymal lung disease is detected in a patient with SSc.[17] This complication is frequently asymptomatic, but some studies indicate that in United States up to 90% of adult patients with SSc develop some degree of interstitial lung involvement.[138,139] It usually develops as a complication of SSc, but, occasionally, it can represent the first manifestation of disease.[139]

A minority of patients have a dry, hacking cough or dyspnea on exertion.[140] Occasionally, rales or pleural friction rubs are present. Pulmonary function tests reveal a restrictive pattern with a reduced forced vital capacity (FVC) and a reduced diffusion capacity for carbon monoxide (DL_{CO}). Chest high-resolution computed tomography (HRCT) typically shows a pattern of ground-glass opacities that are bilateral and most prominent in the lower lobes[138,141]; when longstanding, it may be associated with lower lobe traction, bronchiectasis, and fibrotic changes.

The median survival of a patient with SSc who develops an ILD is 5 to 8 years.[142] However, while some patients undergo a rapid pulmonary decline within the first 3 years of disease, others remain stable over time or may spontaneously improve. Some physiological parameters such as advanced age, CT evidence of extensive lung disease, and reduced lung function are predictors of mortality.[143] Chronic gastroesophageal reflux and associated recurrent microaspiration are important contributors to the progression of lung disease. The severity of gastroesophageal reflux is correlated with loss of diffusion capacity and lung volumes, and with the extent of radiographic fibrosis. Pulmonary arterial hypertension, reflecting inherent pulmonary vasculopathy, occurs in up to 20% of patients with SSc-associated ILD, and it has a significant adverse impact on survival.[138,144]

Pulmonary vascular disease results in progressive dyspnea with preserved lung volumes on pulmonary function testing. It can result from pulmonary fibrosis; however, the isolated form of this complication has a much worse prognosis. Pulmonary hypertension (PH) is defined by a mean pulmonary artery pressure of 25 mm Hg or higher at rest, measured during right heart catheterization. Occasionally, it can complicate dSSc associated with anti-fibrillin autoantibodies and is typical also of the lSSc subset of patients.[145] Interstitial pulmonary fibrosis, long recognized as a devastating complication, is being reclassified to reflect differences in histopathology and outcome. It has been postulated that fibrosis also results from pulmonary vascular hyperreactivity similar to Raynaud phenomenon.

Furst and associates[146] demonstrated decreased pulmonary perfusion, as measured by krypton-81m scans, after cold challenge to the hands. Fahey and colleagues[147] noticed a low DL_{CO} in patients with dSSc and Raynaud phenomenon but failed to demonstrate a decrease with cold challenge as found in patients with idiopathic Raynaud disease. Veselý and colleagues[148] measured serum concentrations of KL-6, a high–molecular-weight, mucinlike glycoprotein, expressed on type II pneumonocytes in alveoli and bronchiolar epithelial cells, in patients with juvenile SSc.[148] KL-6 was found significantly higher in SSc patients with ILD as compared with those without ILD or healthy controls. Therefore, KL-6 may represent a useful marker of fibrosis in SSc patients.

Renal Disease

Overt renal disease is one of the most ominous features of dSSc.[149] Although little information is available, it is an impression that children may do better than adults in this regard.[6,51,135] In the Padua database, 5% of the children had renal involvement (as increased urinary protein excretion or raised creatinine level), and one developed renal crisis.[6] Medsger and colleagues indicated that almost 50% of adult patients who developed renal disease did so within the first year after disease onset and that presence of anti-topoisomerase I antibody and rapidly progressing skin involvement are predictors of early and often fatal renal and cardiac involvement.[150]

Scleroderma renal crisis is an infrequent complication of systemic sclerosis. It presents as recent onset, accelerated-phase hypertension and/or rapidly deteriorating renal function, frequently accompanied by microangiopathic hemolysis.[151] Activation of the renin-angiotensin-aldosterone system plays an important role in the pathophysiological process, but the pathogenetic pathway remains poorly understood. There is evidence of a juxtaglomerular apparatus hyperplasia, and blood pressure can usually be controlled with high-dose angiotensin-converting enzyme (ACE) inhibitors.[152] However, elevated plasma renin level does not predict the development of scleroderma renal crisis (SRC).[153,154] Since the introduction of ACE inhibitors, survival has greatly improved, and the 1-year mortality rate decreased from 85% to 24%.[155] However, despite aggressive antihypertensive therapy, 5-year survival with SRC is only 65%.[156,157]

The prevalence of SRC is poorly documented, with disparity among countries.[158] It occurs in about 4% to 6%[159,160] of patients with SSc, predominantly in those with diffuse SSc.[154,159] Clinical signs of SRC are mainly malignant hypertension with hypertensive encephalopathy, congestive heart failure, and arrhythmia; refractory headache and seizures can be the early symptoms. Serum creatinine level can be markedly elevated, and urinalysis often shows mild proteinuria (0.5-2.5 g/L) and microscopic hematuria.[161] Thrombotic microangiopathy occurs in 43% of patients with SRC and is defined by hemolytic anemia and moderate thrombocytopenia.[156] Renal biopsy is not necessary to confirm the diagnosis in typical SRC, but it is mandatory to confirm the diagnosis in case of atypical clinical presentations.[161] Among the risk factors that predict the occurrence of SRC are a duration of SSc of less than 4 years; diffuse and rapidly progressive skin thickening; new-onset anemia; new cardiac events; anti-RNA polymerase III antibodies; and use of corticosteroids, namely prednisone, at dosages greater than 15 to 20 mg/day.[162] Although no study regarding the relationship between the use of high-dose steroids and the development of SRC in pediatric patients has been published, a close monitoring of blood pressure and renal function in patients treated with steroids is recommended, particularly in early diffuse SSc with rapidly progressing skin involvement.

Systemic hypertension occurs in up to one half of adult patients and is usually associated with proteinuria.[163,164] The degree of hypertension ranges from mild or moderate in most patients to malignant hypertension in approximately 25%. This complication often begins during the colder months of the year[163] and may be heralded by the development of microangiopathic hemolytic anemia.[165] Onset is followed rapidly in most patients by death within a few weeks in the absence of intensive intervention. Renal or prerenal azotemia occurs in at least 25% of patients in the presence or absence of hypertension or proteinuria.[164]

Renovascular Raynaud phenomenon, demonstrated by decreased cortical blood flow, may be induced by immersion of the hands in cold water.[163] Even in the absence of angiographic evidence of vascular disease, xenon 133–demonstrated cortical blood flow may be impaired.[163] These reversible changes are mediated by the renin-angiotensin system, and plasma renin levels correlate with the presence of malignant hypertension.[166]

Central Nervous System Disease

The involvement of the central nervous system (CNS) is usually secondary to renal, cardiovascular, or pulmonary involvement, or due to pharmacological treatment. The most frequently reported CNS abnormality is cranial nerve involvement, especially of the sensory branch of the trigeminal nerve.[167-169] However, recent studies based on magnetic resonance imaging (MRI) have described asymptomatic CNS alterations, regardless of severity, complications, or duration of disease.[170,171] Peripheral neuropathies are also uncommon (1.6%).[172] A more subtle abnormality—diminished perception of vibration—probably reflects the damping effect of cutaneous sclerosis on the transmission of the vibrations of a tuning fork.[173] A recent review[174] assessed the frequency of CNS and peripheral nervous system (PNS) disease reported from 1954 to June 2012. The most frequently reported CNS manifestations were psychiatric disease (1490 total events), especially depression (73.2% of total psychiatric events) and anxiety (23.9%); for nonpsychiatric manifestations (177 total reported events), headache (23.73% of total nonpsychiatric events) and seizures (13.6%) were the most frequent, followed by cognitive impairment (8.5%), stroke or transient ischemic attack (TIA) (6.2%), organic brain syndrome (6.21%), and radiculopathy (5.65%). PNS involvement (442 total reported events) was mainly represented by myopathy (50.67% of total PNS involvements), followed by trigeminal neuropathy (16.5%), peripheral sensorimotor polyneuropathy (14.3%), and carpal tunnel syndrome (6.6%). Neuroimaging studies focused on MRI evaluations showed cerebral white matter hyperintensity, including brain stem and cerebellar involvements, in 55.9% of analyzed cases; signs of vasculopathy occurred in 14.3%. CT evaluations reported vasculopathy in 21.6% of the cases, calcification in 21.6% of cases, and paraspinal and intraspinal calcifications in 12.8%.

Sicca Syndrome (Sjögren Syndrome)

Xerostomia (i.e., dry mouth) and *keratoconjunctivitis sicca* (i.e., dry eyes) are common in dSSc (see Chapter 30). Histological evidence of salivary gland involvement was uniformly demonstrable in lip biopsies in a prospective study of Sjögren syndrome in 17 adult patients with dSSc and 8 patients with lSSc[175]; xerostomia and salivary gland enlargement were present in 84%. Scintigraphy of the salivary glands was abnormal in 88%, and sialography was abnormal in 75%. Ocular symptoms of dryness or a foreign-body sensation occurred in 76%. Results of the Schirmer test were abnormal for 40%, and rose bengal staining of the cornea was positive in 55%.

Comparison of SSC in children and adults. As compared with adults, children at diagnosis show a significantly less frequent involvement of all organs, except for the prevalence of arthritis.[6,7,176] Differences with adults become less evident during follow-up with the exception of interstitial lung involvement, gastroesophageal dysmotility, renal involvement, and arterial hypertension, which are significantly more common in adults. Other differences with SSc in adults can be seen in the prevalence of arthritis and muscle inflammation, which are slightly more common in children, whereas Raynaud phenomenon and skin sclerosis are less frequent.[6,176] In children, the limited cutaneous form of SSc, which is most frequent in adults, is rare. However, it has been shown that a substantial number of individuals with childhood-onset SSc have their diagnosis made either during adolescence or as young adults.[7] Indeed, it is possible that the limited cutaneous subset might be underdiagnosed in younger children because of the lack of a full clinical picture.

Pathology

Angiitis is regarded as the initial lesion, with activated lymphocytes infiltrating around small blood vessels. There are increased numbers of T lymphocytes, plasma cells, and macrophages in the deep dermis and subcutaneous tissue and around small blood vessels, nerves, the pilosebaceous apparatus, and sweat glands.[57] Marked hyalinization of blood vessel walls and proliferation of endothelium occur later. Raynaud phenomenon, renal crisis, and pulmonary hypertension are all associated with a distinctive arteriosclerotic fibrotic lesion.[177] Another characteristic finding is an increased number of mast cells in skin and viscera.[178] Hydrophilic glycosaminoglycan in the dermis may account in part for the accumulation of edema.[179]

Later in the course, biopsies document homogenization of collagen fibers with loss of structural detail and an increased density and thickness of collagen deposition (Fig. 27-9, A).[81,179] With electron microscopy, the collagen appears embryonic with narrow fibrils and an immature cross-banding pattern (Fig. 27-9, B).[180] The histological characteristics of the skin in late disease include thinning of the epidermis, and loss of the rete pegs and atrophy of dermal appendages, often with a persistent inflammatory infiltrate of T lymphocytes. The synovial membrane histologically resembles that of rheumatoid arthritis except for the abundance of fibrin and dense fibrosis.[105,181,182]

Biopsy specimens of muscle are abnormal in approximately one half of the patients.[183] The most prominent abnormalities are increased deposition of collagen and fat in interstitial perivascular sites of the perimysium and epimysium, and focal, predominantly lymphocytic, perivascular infiltration. There is a relative loss of type II fibers.[184] Blood vessels are thickened and vessel lumens are narrowed. Immunofluorescence studies have demonstrated no abnormalities.[184]

Histopathological changes in the vasa nervorum, neural dysfunction from fibrosis, and smooth muscle atrophy and fibrosis occur throughout the GI tract but are most prominent in the esophagus, where atrophic muscle is replaced by fibrous tissue. The smooth muscle of the lower two thirds of the esophagus is most commonly affected,

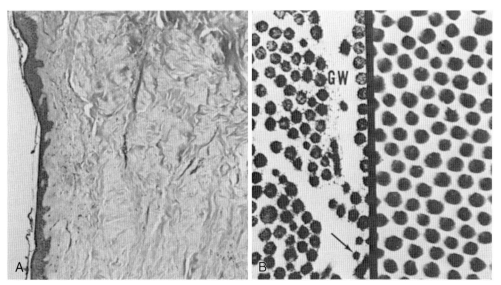

FIGURE 27-9 **A,** The classic histopathological features of the cutaneous disease are visible in this full-thickness section of skin from a patient with diffuse cutaneous systemic scleroderma. The epidermis is thin, and there is atrophy of the dermal appendages. The rete pegs are relatively obliterated (hematoxylin-eosin stain; magnification ×480). **B,** Electron microscopic studies indicate a relative reduction in the fiber size of newly synthesized collagen. Transverse sections of collagen fibers (*left*) are from the skin of a patient. A marked variation in fiber size is apparent when compared with healthy skin (*right*). Many smaller collagen fibers are observed (*arrow*) (normal diameter ×1200). The fine granular and whiskery material (GW) surrounding the sclerodermal collagen probably represents mucopolysaccharides, and their visibility is enhanced by staining with ruthenium red, lead citrate, and uranyl acetate (magnification ×38,610). (Courtesy Dr. C. R. Wynne-Roberts.)

but in some patients, striated muscle of the upper third may also be involved.[185] The lamina propria and Auerbach plexus are infiltrated with mononuclear cells. Arterial walls are thickened.

One half of adult patients in one necropsy series had evidence of myocardial fibrosis that was unrelated to coronary artery disease[186] (Fig. 27-10). Other findings included contraction band necrosis (i.e., myofibrillar degeneration) from transient ischemia in 31% (possibly the equivalent of Raynaud phenomenon of the coronary arteries and a precursor to myocardial fibrosis). Necropsies in adults have demonstrated effusions or fibrous, fibrinous, and adhesive pericarditis in approximately 40%, a frequency similar to that detected by echocardiography.[187] Convincing clinical evidence of pericarditis was present in only 3% to 16% of patients.[186,187]

The main histological abnormality in the lungs is diffuse alveolar, interstitial, and peribronchial fibrosis. The thickened walls lead to a reduction of alveolar space (i.e., compact sclerosis). Rupture of alveolar septae results in small areas of bullous emphysema (i.e., cystic sclerosis) (Fig. 27-11). Extensive bronchiolar hyperplasia, arteriolar endothelial proliferation, fibrous pleuritis, and pleural adhesions are also present. Young and Mark[188] reported that 14 of 30 patients had moderate or marked abnormalities in the pulmonary vasculature at necropsy. They postulated that malignant pulmonary hypertension analogous to malignant renal hypertension was the cause of the rapidly progressive pulmonary failure that culminated in the death of three patients.

The characteristic histopathological change in the renal vasculature is concentric intimal proliferation of the interlobar and arcuate arteries, together with cortical infarcts and fibrinoid necrosis of the media. Vasculitis (other than the changes of malignant hypertension) is uncommon. The glomeruli exhibit a wide spectrum of abnormalities (Fig. 27-12), ranging from acute ischemic necrosis to thickening and sclerosis of the basement membrane. Swelling of the endothelial cells results in vascular narrowing.[189] Deposition of immunoglobulin and

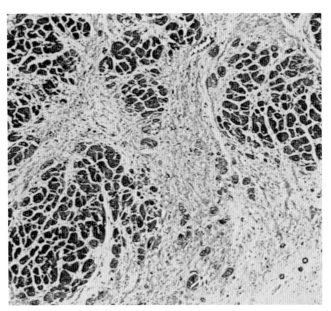

FIGURE 27-10 Fibrosis of the myocardium (hematoxylin-eosin stain; magnification ×480).

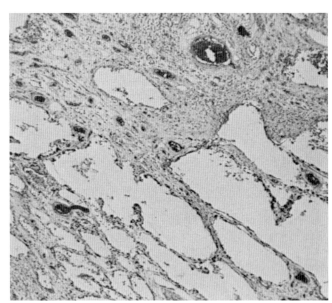

FIGURE 27-11 Biopsy of a lung reveals striking fibrosis and disruption of the alveoli (hematoxylin-eosin stain; magnification ×480).

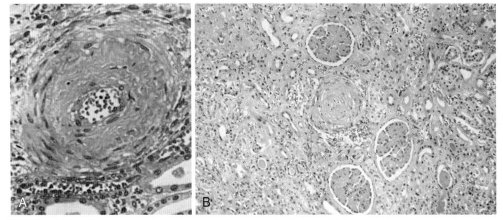

FIGURE 27-12 Necropsy specimen from a patient who died of renal failure and hypertension during the first few months of the disease. **A,** Virtual obliteration of the lumen of an arteriole by subintimal proliferation, thrombus formation, and mucoid hyperplasia of the media. **B,** Glomerulus from the same patient, showing fibrinoid necrosis and effacement of capillary loops without significant inflammatory cell infiltration (hematoxylin-eosin stain; magnification ×480).

complement in the renal vasculature has been reported[189-191] but is generally sparse. On electron microscopy, intimal thickening of the vessels is associated with the presence of myointimal cells resembling those of smooth muscle, but with the capability to produce collagen and elastin.[192]

Laboratory Examination

Anemia, although uncommon, occurs in approximately one fourth of patients and is characteristic of the anemia of chronic disease. Less commonly, it reflects vitamin B_{12} or folate deficiency resulting from chronic malabsorption. Microangiopathic hemolysis[193] or bleeding from mucosal telangiectasias may also occur. Autoimmune hemolytic anemia is rare.[193] Leukocytosis is not prominent but correlates in degree with advanced visceral or muscle disease. Eosinophilia occurs in approximately 15% of patients.[194] Synovial fluid analysis was reported to exhibit increased protein content and high numbers of polymorphonuclear leukocytes that had inclusions similar to those seen in rheumatoid arthritis.[195] Pericardial fluid has the characteristics of an exudate.[196]

High titers of antinuclear antibodies (ANAs) are frequent; the predominant patterns on HEp-2 cell substrate are speckled and nucleolar. ANA seropositivity in two large pediatric series was 81% to 97%, a frequency similar to that reported in adults.[6,7] Anti-topoisomerase I (anti–Scl-70) autoantibodies are present in 28% to 34% of patients, whereas the prevalence of anticentromere antibodies is lower in children (7.1%) than in adults (22.5%).[6]

In contrast, a large study of adults with dSSc indicated that 26% had anti–Scl-70 antibodies and 22% anticentromere antibodies.[197] No patient had reactivity to both antigens, an observation also confirmed by Kikuchi and Inagaki.[198] Antibody to Scl-70 occurred most frequently in patients with peripheral vascular disease, digital pitting, pulmonary interstitial fibrosis, renal involvement, and a high mortality rate.[199,200] Anticentromere antibody occurred almost exclusively in patients with lSSc in association with calcinosis and telangiectasias.

Anti–PM-Scl and anti–U1RNP antibodies correlate with scleroderma in overlap syndromes with musculoskeletal involvement. Anti–RNA-polymerase III antibodies are very unusual, in parallel with the rarity of renal involvement in juvenile SSc.[7] The frequency of occurrence of rheumatoid factor (17% vs 22.9%) and antiphospholipid antibodies (14.8% vs 10.2%) is similar in adults and children with SSc.[6,176]

Serological and genetic markers help to predict particular complications. Patients with anti–Scl-70 autoantibodies or the HLA-DR52a genotype are at increased risk for developing interstitial pulmonary fibrosis, irrespective of their apparent clinical subset.[199] In contrast, anti-RNA polymerase I or III antibodies are associated with renal involvement.[201] Anticentromere antibodies in lSSc are an indicator of risk for isolated pulmonary hypertension and severe GI involvement,[202] and in at least one study in children, they were a marker of Raynaud phenomenon.[203] An association between the presence of antibody to Scl-70 and malignancy has been observed in adults.[204] Antibodies that are specific for a 70-kD mitochondrial antigen have been described in a small proportion of patients.[205] The associations of antibodies to the PM-Scl antigen have been reviewed.[206] Antineutrophil cytoplasmic antibodies have been reported with specificities to bactericidal or permeability protein and cathepsin G.[207]

Cardiac Function

Electrocardiographic abnormalities include first-degree heart block, right and left bundle branch block, premature atrial and ventricular contractions, nonspecific T-wave changes, and evidence of ventricular hypertrophy.[208] The most frequent cardiac arrhythmias in children are of supraventricular origin, whereas ventricular arrhythmias are uncommon.[209]

Thallium-201 radionuclide scans will often document abnormalities of myocardial perfusion, ventricular wall motion, chamber size, and left ventricular ejection fraction.[210] Echocardiographic abnormalities in addition to effusions include thickening of the left ventricular wall in 57% of children with SSc and diminished left ventricular compliance in 42%.[211] Ultrasonic videodensitometric analysis has been introduced as an additional mechanism to evaluate myocardial alterations.[212] Contrast-enhanced cardiac MRI has been recently introduced in adult patients with SSc.[213] In one series, myocardial fibrosis was detected in 43% of the patients.[214] The main finding observed was a late enhancement showing a linear pattern without coronary distribution in 27% of the patients, whereas a patchy nodular enhancement pattern was observed in the remaining 16%. With the application of stress perfusion and late gadolinium enhancement (LGE) it was possible to show early nonsegmental, stress perfusion defects with rest amelioration in both limited and diffuse SSc[215] LGE, unrelated to coronary distribution, is a late event. These findings seem to be correlate with the presence of Raynaud phenomenon and digital ulceration. Unfortunately, no data in pediatric patients are available.

Pulmonary Function

Characteristic findings of involvement of the respiratory tract include a decrease in timed vital capacity and forced expiratory flow, an early decrease in diffusion, and an increase in functional residual volume.[216-218] In one series, 11 of 15 children with dSSc had diminished pulmonary diffusion.[36] The two-dimensional echocardiogram is important in confirming early pulmonary hypertension by documentation of a dilated right ventricle with thickening of the ventricular wall and straightening of the septum. One-dimensional (M-mode) echocardiography is characterized by changes in the midsystolic movement of the pulmonary valve. Right heart catheterization provides definitive confirmation but is often unnecessary.

Steen and colleagues[219] reported that only 38% of 77 adults with dSSc and 28% of 88 with lSSc had normal pulmonary function studies. Restrictive lung disease and isolated reduction of DL_{CO} were the most common abnormalities, occurring in 34 dSSc patients (18%) and 23 (26%) patients with lSSc. The earliest change was a decrease in the forced vital capacity with an forced expiratory volume (FEV_1)/FVC less than 70%. This abnormality was present in 8% of patients with diffuse disease and 16% of those with limited disease. Guttadauria and associates[220] also found a high prevalence of small airways disease (42%), usually in the absence of symptoms, chest radiographic changes, or other abnormalities of pulmonary function.

Renal Function

Renal plasma flow is decreased in most patients, especially in the cortex, although normal glomerular filtration may be preserved by intrarenal shifts in blood flow.[221] Even in patients without clinical evidence of renal disease, plasma renin levels correlate with the degree of histological abnormality of the renal arteries and arterioles.[221] Renal arteriography may document irregular arterial narrowing, tortuosity of the interlobular and arcuate arterioles, cortical hypoperfusion, and other changes of malignant hypertension. Kidney size is small to normal.

Skin Scoring

One of the most used scoring systems for the skin involvement is the modified Rodnan Skin Score (mRSS).[222] According to this score the body surface is divided into 17 regions and the skin thickness is assessed on a 0- to 3-point scale (0, normal; 1, thickened skin; 2, decreased ability; 3, unable to pinch or move skin). The score ranges from 0 to 51. The mRSS, routinely used in adult SSc, is the only instrument available, and it is also used in pediatric patients. However, it has been shown that the mRSS in children correlates with the body mass index and the Tanner stage and should be corrected for these two parameters.[223]

Radiological Examination

Joint complaints are common in SSc, and are generally ascribed to arthralgia rather than true arthritis. However, focal joint-space findings of arthritis, including narrowing, periarticular osteopenia, and erosions, are frequently reported in hand radiographs of SSc patients. Bony erosions usually develop at the distal and proximal interphalangeal joints. Involvement of the first carpometacarpal joint is particularly characteristic of dSSc.[224] The most characteristic radiological findings in the hands are a marked decrease in soft tissue and resorption of the tufts of the distal phalanges (acroosteolysis), particularly in patients with severe Raynaud phenomenon (Fig. 27-13). Resorption of the distal tufts is particularly common in children.[36,225] It may also occur in ribs, clavicles, distal radius and ulna, and other sites. An increase in the thickness of the periodontal membrane results in radiolucent widening between the teeth and the jaw.[226] Periarticular or subcutaneous calcification occurs in 15% to 25% of patients (Fig. 27-8).[36] Asymmetric distribution in the dominant hand and involvement over bony prominences, such as the fingertips, elbows, and knees, suggest that focal injury may play a role.

Radiological studies of the GI tract often demonstrate characteristic abnormalities even in the absence of symptoms. All portions of the GI tract from the esophagus to the anus may be involved. Although barium esophagography and enterography are the traditional methods for imaging the GI tract in SSc, CT or MR imaging of the bowel may be preferable.[227] Cine esophagogram may document decreased or absent peristalsis in the lower part of the esophagus with distal dilation and, frequently, a hiatal hernia with stricture and shortening of the esophagus (Fig. 27-14). Esophageal motility studies by manometry and pH probe monitoring of the distal esophagus for 12 to 24 hours provide more sensitive indicators of diminished lower sphincter tone and the presence of reflux.[228] The most frequent radiographic changes

in the small bowel are dilation of the second and third parts of the duodenum and the proximal jejunum (Fig. 27-15). The stomach is the least common site of GI involvement in SSc, but delayed gastric emptying and gastric antral vascular ectasia (GAVE) may be present.[227] Although gastric dilation can be seen on radiographs or CT in advanced cases, delayed gastric emptying as well as GER are best diagnosed by nuclear medicine scintigraphy that demonstrates abnormal retention of radiolabeled solids.[229] Abnormalities in the colon are characterized by loss of colonic haustrations[230] and the presence of wide-mouthed diverticula or pseudosacculations on the antimesenteric border. Colonic transit is delayed.

The accuracy of conventional radiography for detecting and characterizing lung disease in SSc is significantly limited. HRCT is more sensitive than radiography at detecting early ILD and can better quantify the degree of interstitial fibrosis.[231] SSc-related ILD is the most common pulmonary manifestation of SSc and one of the leading cause of death.[135] On HRCT, two thirds of SSc patients show evidence of

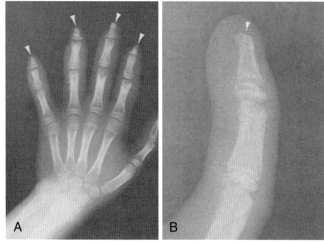

FIGURE 27-13 A, Radiograph of a boy with early resorption of the tufts of the distal phalanges (*arrowheads*). **B,** Magnified view of acroosteolysis of the index finger (*arrowhead*).

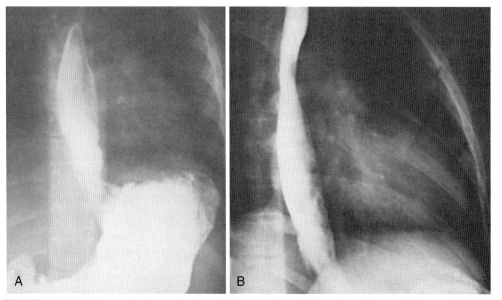

FIGURE 27-14 Barium-contrast examinations of the esophagus illustrate moderate dilation and lack of a normal peristaltic pattern. **A,** Supine anteroposterior view. **B,** Lateral view.

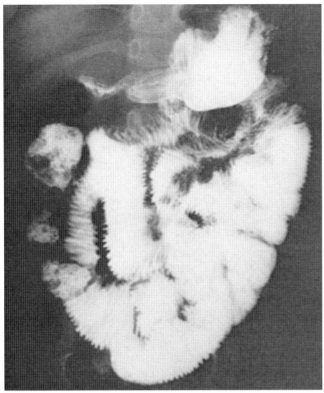

FIGURE 27-15 Upper gastrointestinal barium series with small bowel follow-through in a 3-year-old girl with dilation of the jejunum and closely approximated valvulae conniventes (the "closed accordion" sign) caused by thickening of the ileal mucosa.

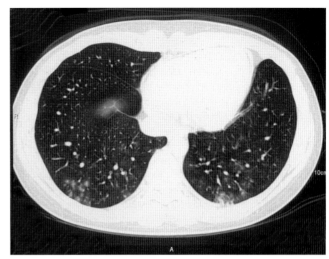

FIGURE 27-16 **A,** Posteroanterior radiograph of the chest illustrates a fine reticular pattern in both lower lobes. **B,** Lateral view of the chest.

SSc-ILD, whereas 30% to 40% of SSc patients have significant pulmonary symptoms.[231] It is now accepted that most SSc-ILD has the imaging and histopathological pattern of nonspecific interstitial pneumonia (NSIP).[232] On HRCT, NSIP demonstrates reticular interstitial markings predominantly involving the posterior basilar aspects of the lower lobes, traction bronchiectasis ground-glass opacities, and "honeycomb" sign.[231,233] In children, the most frequent HRCT findings are (in order) ground-glass opacification, subpleural micronodules, linear opacities, and "honeycombing"[234] (Fig. 27-16).

Assessment of Disease Activity and Severity

Assessment of disease activity or severity is difficult. Regular follow-up and clinical review are the cornerstones of monitoring activity and progression. Serological markers of activity have long been sought, and those that may be useful include soluble adhesion molecules such as sICAM-1, collagen propeptides,[235] products of type I collagen breakdown,[236] and immunological markers such as sIL-2 receptor, neopterin, or vascular activation markers (e.g., E-selectin, thrombomodulin, von Willebrand factor).[237] For organ-based complications such as pulmonary fibrosis, pulmonary hypertension, or renal involvement, objective assessment is easier. Sequential skin scores can be recorded.

Modified health assessment questionnaires have been developed in the United States[238] and Europe.[239,240] They will undoubtedly be of considerable value, particularly because constitutional symptoms and functional impairment are among the most troublesome consequences of this disorder. The European Scleroderma Study Group has developed three different 10-point indexes of disease activity, one for scleroderma as a group, one for dSSc, and one for lSSc.[240] To provide a more global index of severity, a scoring system has been proposed in adults.[241] Recently, a similar severity score, called the Juvenile Systemic

TABLE 27-6 Treatment Approach for Systemic Sclerosis in Children

General supportive measures	• Avoid cold and trauma with appropriate clothing, avoid excessive sun exposure and heat in the hot seasons • General skin care: daily application of lanolin or water-soluble cream as an emollient • Rehabilitation program to preserve maximal function and dynamic splints to treat or prevent contractures • Patient support groups	
Organ-based treatment	Raynaud phenomenon	CCBs, iloprost, sildenafil
	Digital ulcers	CCBs, iloprost, bosentan
	Fibrosing alveolitis	cyclophosphamide, corticosteroids
	Pulmonary arterial hypertension	prostanoids, sildenafil, bosentan
	Gastroesophageal reflux	PPIs, prokinetics
	Midgut disease	Rotating antibiotics
	Musculoskeletal involvement	Low-dose corticosteroids, MTX
	Renal disease	ACE inhibitors
	Skin involvement	MTX, MMF

ACE, Angiotensin-converting enzyme; *CCBs,* calcium channel blockers; *CPM,* cyclophosphamide; *ERAs,* endothelin receptor antagonists; *MMF,* mycophenolate mofetil, *PPIs,* proton pump inhibitors.

Scleroderma Severity Score (J4S), has been proposed to evaluate SSc in children.[242] J4S allows an overall evaluation of the disease status based on general signs and symptoms, such as body mass index and hemoglobin level, plus clinical parameters related with eight organ systems involvement (vascular, cutaneous, osteoarticular, muscular, GI, respiratory, cardiac and renal; see Table 27-6). Innovative features of this score are the use of variables adapted for children and the inclusion of coefficients to appropriately weight the importance of the each organ involvement.

Treatment

Management of SSc in children represents one of the most difficult and frustrating challenges in all of rheumatology because no uniformly effective therapy is available. Disease severity ranges from mild and stable to rapidly progressive and fatal. Management can be divided into two general areas: general supportive measures, and therapy directed at controlling the underlying disease process and complications (e.g., fibrosis, immunological abnormalities, vasculopathy).

General Supportive Measures

Supportive therapy is of utmost importance in managing a chronic, unpredictable, and potentially debilitating or fatal disease. Education of the child and parents should be undertaken early in an attempt to prevent unnecessary psychological uncertainty and trauma. In general, "optimistic veracity" regarding complications, outcome, and treatment is appropriate. Patient support groups may be helpful and important, albeit difficult to assemble for such a rare disease. Patients should be instructed to avoid cold and trauma. Especially in cold climates, the family should keep the child warm by maintaining a satisfactory household temperature and by use of appropriate clothing, including well-insulated mittens (not gloves), boots, and a hat. The child should avoid excessive sun exposure and heat in the summer because of the susceptibility to hyperpigmentation of the skin and a relative inability to dissipate heat through sclerotic skin.

General skin care should include avoidance of drying or irritating substances and daily application of lanolin or water-soluble cream as an emollient. The child should be encouraged to be as physically active as possible within the constraints of the disease. Active range of motion and gentle passive range of motion are essential to preserve maximal function. Dynamic splints may be necessary to treat or prevent contractures. Nonsteroidal antiinflammatory drugs may relieve some of the musculoskeletal symptoms but may be detrimental to renal function.

Therapy of the Disease Process and Complications

Few of the drugs used as disease-modifying agents have undergone placebo-controlled evaluation, and the results from those that have are often disappointing. No drug has been of unequivocal benefit, and even if such data were available, therapeutic gain must be carefully balanced against toxicity and considered in the context of the natural history of the disorder.

The treatment of dSSc is mainly symptomatic and focuses on clinical manifestations, and organ involvement. The European League Against Rheumatism (EULAR) Scleroderma Trials and Research (EUSTAR) group has established a group of evidence-based recommendations to be used in clinical practice.[243] The main aim of these recommendations is to provide guidance to adult and pediatric rheumatologists to correctly approach and choose the treatment for SSc patients. Possible combinations of these approaches to treatment are suggested in Table 27-7.

Digital vasculopathy

Raynaud phenomenon (see also Chapter 31). In addition to avoidance of precipitating circumstances such as cold or emotional stress, specific treatment of Raynaud phenomenon may be necessary. The most commonly used vasodilator agents are the calcium channel blockers (CCBs). Nifedipine is the most widely recommended agent. It has been well tolerated in several controlled trials, has reduced the frequency and severity of Raynaud phenomenon, and has promoted healing of cutaneous ischemic ulcers.[244-248] A meta-analysis, including the results of five randomized clinical trials (RCTs) with intravenous iloprost and one with oral iloprost, indicates that iloprost is effective in reducing the frequency and severity of SSc-related Raynaud

TABLE 27-7 Organ System Involvement During the Course of Systemic Sclerosis in Children				
	NO. WITH INVOLVEMENT/NO. OBSERVED			
ORGAN SYSTEM	**CASSIDY ET AL.[36]**	**%**	**MARTINI ET AL.[6]**	**%**
Skin				
Subcutaneous calcification	4/15	27	28/151	18
Ulcerations	9/15	60	60/150	40
Telangiectases	4/15	27	—	
Pigmentation	3/15	20	—	
Digital arteries (Raynaud phenomenon)	11/15	73	128/152	84
Musculoskeletal System				
Contractures	11/15	73	—	
Resorption of digital tufts	9/11	82	—	
Muscle weakness	6/15	40	37/152	24
Muscle atrophy	6/15	40	—	
Gastrointestinal Tract				
Abnormal esophageal motility	11/15	73	45/150	30
Dilation of duodenum	1/15	7	—	
Colonic sacculations	3/5	60	—	
Lungs				
Abnormal diffusion	11/15	73	40/150	27
Abnormal vital capacity	10/15	67	63/150	42
Heart				
Cardiomegaly	2/15	13	—	
Electrocardiographic abnormalities	4/15	27	15/153	10
Congestive heart failure	2/15	13	11/150	7

phenomenon.[249] Iloprost, given intravenously (0.5 to 2 ng/kg/min for 3 to 5 consecutive days sequentially) significantly reduced the frequency of ischemic attacks and improved the Raynaud phenomenon severity score in comparison with placebo. Oral prostanoids seem to be generally less effective. Iloprost has been reported to be safe and effective in treatment of ischemic digits in children with dSSc and other connective tissue diseases.[250]

In view of costs and feasibility, CCBs should be considered the first-line therapy in the treatment of SSc-related Raynaud phenomenon. Intravenous prostanoids should be used when CCBs fail and there is severe ischemia.

Other agents include drugs that inhibit or suppress the sympathetic nervous system, thereby indirectly promoting vasodilation, and those that act directly on the smooth muscle of the vessel wall, such as reserpine, methyldopa, and ketanserin.[251-256] One drug may be effective in one patient, whereas a different agent is effective in another. It is therefore worth trying several, one at a time, until the desired effect is obtained.

Sildenafil, a selective type 5 phosphodiesterase inhibitor, may be beneficial in treatment of SSc-related vasculopathy by reducing symptoms of Raynaud phenomenon and improving digital ulcer healing.[257] A recent meta-analysis[258] examined six RCTs on the efficacy of PDE-5 inhibitors on Raynaud phenomenon in an adult population. Active molecules used in these trials were sildenafil, modified-release sildenafil, tadalafil, and vardenafil. Overall, the treatments showed a significant but moderate benefit on Raynaud's Condition Score, frequency and duration of Raynaud phenomenon attacks. However, the lack of pediatric data represents the main limitations for their wide recommendation in children.

Digital ulcers. Digital ulcers (DUs) are another severe and disabling complication of dSSc. A recent meta-analysis[259] compared the role of two PDE-5 inhibitors (sildenafil or tadalafil) in the healing and prevention of DUs. Both drugs showed they had beneficial effects on DU healing and DU improvement, although significant adverse events, including headaches, myalgias, nonpainful erections, and allergic reaction were reported.

As for prostacyclin analogs, intravenous or oral iloprost showed no statistically significant difference as compared to placebo in DU healing or improvement. Only intravenous iloprost was shown to prevent new DU formation.[260]

Targeting mediators of immune or vasoactive reactions has been an innovative step in the treatment of connective tissue diseases. Endothelin-1, a potent vasoconstrictor and smooth muscle mitogen, is a possible target in patients with DUs. Bosentan, a dual endothelin receptor antagonist, was evaluated in two placebo-controlled RCTs involving 310 SSc patients in total. Bosentan was given at an oral dose of 62.5 mg twice daily for 4 weeks, then increased to 125 mg twice daily for 12 weeks[261] or 20 weeks.[262] There was no statistically significant difference in DU healing in either trial; however, bosentan was efficacious in DU prevention, with a statistically significant reduction in the mean number of new DUs per patient.

Two major concerns related to the use of bosentan include potential liver toxicity and teratogenicity. Elevated liver aminotransferases have been reported in 11% to 14% of patients treated with bosentan, but these abnormalities were reversible after the drug was discontinued.[263,264] All endothelin receptor antagonists including bosentan are considered to be teratogenic.[265] Accordingly, pregnancy must be excluded before the start of treatment and prevented thereafter by the use of reliable contraceptive measures.[266]

The available evidence concerning CCBs and prostanoids in the prevention of new DUs in SSc patients is far less comprehensive and robust than that of bosentan, but their toxicity pattern is milder, and long-term clinical experience suggests a good safety profile. In view of overall risk-to-benefit considerations, CCBs and intravenous prostanoids should be used as first-line therapy in SSc-related DUs. If the clinical response is unsatisfactory, bosentan should be considered as an adjunct treatment, aiming at the prevention of new DUs rather than for healing them.

Interstitial lung disease. Pulmonary complications are very serious, and there may be no effective long-term therapeutic approach to fibrosing alveolitis or pulmonary hypertension. Alveolitis is predominant early, and later progresses to fibrosis. In general, cyclophosphamide is recommended when there is evidence of active alveolitis or ILD (usually determined by a ground-glass HRCT scan or by the presence of neutrophils in bronchoalveolar lavage). The efficacy and safety of cyclophosphamide in the treatment of SSc-ILD were evaluated in three RCTs.[267-269] In general, cyclophosphamide was not efficacious in increasing the DL$_{CO}$ but showed improvement in the Health Assessment Questionnaire (HAQ) disability index and health-transition domains of the SF36. Although the beneficial effect of cyclophosphamide persisted or increased for some months after therapy was stopped, it were no longer evident after 12 months. Oral

cyclophosphamide was shown to be superior to azathioprine in improving FVC.[269] Although the efficacy of cyclophosphamide was considered moderate, it is currently the only drug with proven efficacy in SSc-ILD and should be considered the drug of choice in progressive SSc-ILD. Toxicity related to cumulative cyclophosphamide doses suggests the use of an intermittent intravenous pulsed regimen.

Mycophenolate mofetil (MMF) is an antiproliferative immunosuppressive agent with a better safety profile than cyclophosphamide. In adults, it is given at a daily oral dose of 2 g.[270] Although to date the evidence is limited to small observational studies only, and no RCT has been conducted, it is the most commonly used immunosuppressor in SSc-ILD maintenance therapy in adults.[271]

Rituximab is a chimeric monoclonal antibody directed against a surface antigen of B cells (CD20). Because elevated levels of B lymphocytes have been described in the lung of patients with SSc-ILD, its use in these patients may be considered.[272] Two small, open-label clinical studies have evaluated the effects of rituximab in SSc-ILD. Treatment consisted of a dose of 1000 mg at baseline and after 15 days. The results showed a stabilization of the pulmonary function test after 6 months.[273,274] Another open-label, randomized, controlled study of 14 SSc-ILD patients showed that the 8 who received rituximab (four weekly infusions with a dosage regimen of 375 mg/m²/week) had a significant improvement of FVC and DL$_{CO}$ in comparison to the 6 who continued the previous treatment (prednisone, cyclophosphamide, mycophenolate, or combination therapies).[275] In a follow-up study, the eight patients who had been treated with rituximab received another two cycles of therapy with an interval of 6 months and showed significant improvement of FVC and DL$_{CO}$ after 2 years.[276] Despite the apparent moderate efficacy and good tolerability profile, to date no RCTs have been conducted on the efficacy of this monoclonal antibody on SSc-ILD, and no pediatric data are available.

MMF has been successfully used for early diffuse scleroderma and lung disease.[277] The apparent safety and tolerability of this drug was confirmed in a retrospective study[278] in which 109 patients with diffuse cutaneous systemic sclerosis who were treated with MMF were compared with 63 control subjects who received other immunosuppressive drugs. A lower frequency of clinically significant pulmonary fibrosis and better 5-year survival from disease onset were reported in the MMF-treated group. MMF seems also to induce improvement of the mRSS, Medsger score, peripheral vascular status, patient's perceived health status, and stabilization of respiratory function.[278-280] MMF has been successfully used in pediatric patients with localized scleroderma[281]; therefore its use in SSc could be reasonable.

Imatinib, a tyrosine kinase inhibitor and a potent inhibitor of TGF-β and PDGF production, has been considered for the treatment of SSc. In 2011, a phase I-IIa open-label pilot trial assessed the safety of high doses of imatinib in 20 patients with SSc-related ILD.[282] Seven discontinued due to adverse events, which included fatigue, facial or lower extremity edema, nausea and vomiting, diarrhea, generalized rash, and new-onset proteinuria. Treatment with imatinib showed a trend toward an improvement of FVC and the mRSS. A randomized, double-blind, placebo-controlled trial on 10 patients with dcSSc[283] showed a poor tolerability and high rates of adverse events in patients on active drug. Two more studies confirmed these unsatisfactory results.[284,285] In conclusion, imatinib failed to show a clear-cut efficacy in SSc. It is poorly tolerated and often associated with adverse events.

One of the most aggressive approaches to therapy is immunoablation followed by reconstitution with hematopoietic stem-cell transplantation (HSCT).[286] Retrospective analyses of independent cohorts of systemic sclerosis patients treated with autologous SCT showed significant improvement of skin thickening, lung function, and quality of life, but with a 6% to 17% increase in treatment-related mortality. Because of this high mortality rate, HSCT must be carefully considered for pediatric patients,[287,288] and unfortunately, it may only be rational therapy early in disease course (3 years or less from the first non-Raynaud sign or symptom) before irreparable damage has resulted (e.g., fibrosis). In patients with SSc-related end-stage respiratory involvement, lung transplantation represents a viable therapeutic option to consider for those with limited extrapulmonary manifestations.[289]

Pulmonary arterial hypertension. One of the most lethal complications of SSc is pulmonary arterial hypertension (PAH), which can occur in the context of established interstitial fibrosis or without it in lSSc.

During the past decade, the targeting mediators of immune or vasoactive reactions has been an innovative step in the treatment of connective tissue diseases. Endothelin-1, a potent vasoconstrictor and smooth muscle mitogen, is a possible target in patients with primary or secondary PAH. Bosentan, an endothelin-1 inhibitor, significantly improved exercise capacity in 6-minute walk test, pulmonary artery pressure (PAP), and cardiac index.[290] The oral formulation and the potential use of these agents for other vascular complications represent important arguments for its potential value in pediatric patients with dSSc.

A subsequent placebo-controlled RCT showed that bosentan significantly improved the 6-minute walk time after 12 and 16 weeks in a heterogeneous population of PAH patients.[291] Indeed, the long-term extension study suggested that bosentan may improve survival in SSc-PAH in comparison with historical controls (1-, 2-, and 3-year survival rates: 82%, 67%, and 64%, respectively, versus 45%, 35%, and 28%).[292]

Sildenafil significantly improves 6-minute walk test results, functional class, and hemodynamics in PAH of different origin.[293] In a subgroup of 84 patients with connective tissue disease–PAH (including 38 SSc-pulmonary arterial hypertension (PAH) patients), sildenafil significantly improved walking distance, functional class, and mean PAP in comparison to placebo.[294]

Skin involvement. In two RCTs involving 29 and 73 SSc patients with early dSSc or lSSc, respectively, methotrexate showed a trend toward improvement of the total skin score.[295,296] In view of these results, methotrexate should be considered as an option in early dSSc that does not require other immunosuppressants for internal organ involvement. Adverse events associated with methotrexate included oral ulcers, liver toxicity, and pancytopenia.[295]

Renal disease. Until recently, the prognosis for renal crisis was uniformly dismal. Immediate and effective lowering of the blood pressure in patients with malignant hypertension is mandatory. Any sudden change in plasma volume should be avoided because marked reductions in renal blood flow may precipitate acute clinical deterioration. The introduction of ACE inhibitors (e.g., captopril or enalapril) brought about a remarkable improvement in the outlook for prevention of vascular damage, effective long-term control of blood pressure, and stabilization of renal function.[155,297-299] Despite the lack of RCTs, ACE inhibitors are indicated for the treatment of SRC.[155,300]

In cases of irreversible renal failure or uncontrollable hypertension, some success has followed the use of hemodialysis with or without bilateral nephrectomy and transplantation.[301] Dialysis may lead to improvement in the cutaneous abnormalities, too.

Musculoskeletal involvement. The treatment of myositis, arthritis, and tenosynovitis includes the use of prednisone, at a dosage of 0.3 to 0.5 mg/kg/day, in children. Because several studies suggest that the use of corticosteroids, particularly in patients with a high skin score and joint contractures, is associated with a higher risk of SRC (43% vs 21% of patients without corticosteroids),[162] patients on steroids should

be carefully monitored for blood pressure and renal function. Attention should be paid especially to patients with early dSSc and high or rapidly progressing skin score.

Gastrointestinal disease. Few studies in children address the most effective management for GI disease. Except for symptomatic approaches, definitive therapy is materially lacking. Treatment of erosive esophagitis often is characterized by considerable delay in healing with the standard approaches of small, more frequent meals, with the last meal taken well before bedtime, and elevation of the head of the bed. Acid reflux and esophageal hypomotility are also complementary factors for the development of pulmonary fibrosis.[302]

Proton pump inhibitors (PPIs) are the drugs of choice for prevention of SSc-related GERD, esophageal ulcers, and strictures. The efficacy of PPIs in the treatment of GERD in the general population is well documented in meta-analyses of RCTs.[303,304] Considering the efficacy of PPIs in the management of GERD in the otherwise healthy population and the high frequency of esophageal involvement in SSc patients, PPIs should be used, even in the early phase, for the prevention of SSc-related upper GI involvement.

Several nonrandomized or uncontrolled studies in adults suggest that prokinetic drugs (octreotide, erythromycin) may improve GI signs and symptoms (dysphagia, early satiety, bloating, pseudoobstruction) in SSc patients.[305-307]

Malabsorption is difficult to manage. Diarrhea and bloating are most often caused by bacterial overgrowth and are treated by rotating antibiotics because continuous therapy with one agent may result in the emergence of resistant organisms. The choice of antibiotic is usually empirical and includes amoxicillin with clavulanate or oral cephalosporins. In refractory cases, metronidazole can be added for 5 to 7 days to treat anaerobic flora. Hyperalimentation may be necessary but has not been demonstrated to be a wise long-term choice.

Course of the Disease and Prognosis

The ultimate prognosis of a child with SSc depends primarily on the extent and nature of visceral involvement. The outcome has been poor but may be improving. Skin tightness and joint contractures inevitably lead to severe disability in some patients (Fig. 27-17).[308] It is a curious but often-repeated observation that the skin may eventually soften years after onset. Progressive GI involvement may lead to severe complications and inanition. Cardiac arrhythmias may result from myocardial fibrosis. Congestive heart failure is often a terminal event. Pulmonary interstitial disease and vascular lesions are probably

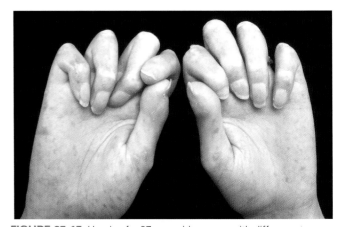

FIGURE 27-17 Hands of a 27-year-old woman with diffuse cutaneous systemic scleroderma that began in childhood. There was essentially no movement possible in these fingers because of joint contractures. Notice the extensive telangiectasias.

universal, even if not clinically evident. Renal failure or acute hypertensive encephalopathy supervenes as a potentially fatal outcome in a few children.

A study investigating clinical and genetic variables at presentation that predict survival showed that absence of anticentromere antibodies, the presence of hypertension, chest radiograph suggestive of pulmonary fibrosis, and low body mass index were significant predictors of mortality in adults with SSc.[309]

Survival rates have not been determined in any large series of children because of the rarity of this disease. The age-specific mortality rate in one epidemiological study for the 0- to 14-year-old age group was 0.04 per million person-years.[310] Recent studies have shown that the prognosis of SSc in children appears to be better than in adults. The survival rates of childhood-onset SSc at 5, 10, 15, and 20 years after diagnosis were 89%, 80% to 87.4%, 74% to 87.4%, and 69% to 82.5%, respectively. These rates are significantly higher than for those in adult-onset disease.[7,135,311]

In general, juvenile SSc may have two possible evolutions: some children have a rapid development of internal organ failure leading to severe disability and eventually to death, whereas most patients experience a slow, insidious course of the disease with lower mortality.[135] The most common causes of death are related to the involvement of cardiac, renal, and pulmonary systems (Table 27-8). Cardiomyopathy is a leading cause of early death and is usually associated with diffuse cutaneous disease and features of polymyositis.[134,135]

In adult series the presence of anti-topoisomerase I and anti-RNA polymerase III antibodies, and the male sex have been associated with poorer survival, whereas in children no clear relationship was found between serological features, age at onset, sex, and mortality.[135,312,313]

As children with SSc live into adulthood, complications associated with pregnancy become a concern.[314,315]

LIMITED CUTANEOUS SYSTEMIC SCLERODERMA

Definition

Limited SSc is the designation for patients previously classified as having the CREST syndrome. Winterbauer[316] first described this syndrome as a variant of systemic scleroderma. Very few instances of lSSc in children have been reported.[6,49-51] Whether it is a relatively mild form of dSSc or an entirely separate, although related, disorder is uncertain.[11,317] The combination of scleroderma and calcinosis was designated as *acrosclerosis* in the older literature, or has been referred to as the *Thibierge–Weissenbach syndrome*.[318]

Epidemiology

Overall, lSSc accounts for approximately one third to one half of the adult patients with scleroderma.[319] Limited disease is more common among women and tends to occur at an earlier age than dSSc. A long interval between the onset of Raynaud phenomenon and diagnostic skin changes is characteristic.

Clinical Manifestations

Calcinosis is usually more severe in patients with lSSc than in dSSc (Fig. 27-18), Raynaud phenomenon is more frequently complicated by digital ulceration and gangrene, and telangiectasias are more widespread.[316] Limited SSC is by no means a mild disease, however, and severe systemic involvement, especially pulmonary fibrosis and hypertension, occurs, although renal disease is less frequent than in dSSc.

Diagnosis

Cutaneous sclerosis is restricted to the distal segments of the digits; telangiectasias, Raynaud phenomenon, and calcinosis are prominent.

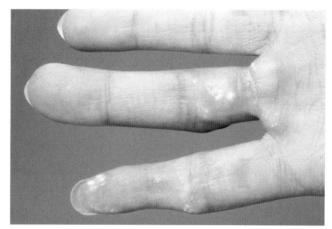

FIGURE 27-18 Striking subcutaneous calcification with extrusion of calcaneous material.

TABLE 27-8	Causes of Death in Children with Systemic Sclerosis			
STUDY	**SEX**	**AGE AT ONSET (YEARS)**	**DISEASE DURATION**	**CAUSE OF DEATH**
Kornreich et al.[31]	M	4	10 years	Cerebral hemorrhage due to thrombocytopenia
	F	6	9 years	Cardiac failure
	M	7	23 months	Renal failure
	F	10	15 months	Cardiac failure
	F	10	22 months	Pulmonary emboli
	F	15	5 months	Cardiac failure
Cassidy et al.[36]	F	12	6 months	Cardiac failure
	F	11	10 years	Cardiac failure
	F	8	9 years	Central nervous system disease, hypertension
Bulkley[186]	M	13	2 years	Pulmonary hypertension
	F	16	1 years	Pulmonary hypertension
Suárez-Almazor et al.[51]	M	10	2 years	Cardiac failure
Martini et al.[135]	5 M, 10 F	5-15	0.5 months to 18 years	Cardiac failure (10)
				Renal failure (2)
				Respiratory failure (2)
				Infection (2)

Isolated proximal scleroderma supports a diagnosis of dSSc rather than limited disease. In other ways, however, these two syndromes closely resemble each other, and clinical separation of these disorders may be entirely artificial.

Immunological Characteristics

Antibody to centromere has been described as the serological hallmark of lSSc, and its discovery historically supported the rationale for clinical differentiation of the CREST syndrome from dSSc.[317,320] This antibody specificity is directed at the kinetochore of components of the mitotic spindle. It is evident, however, that anticentromere antibody is associated with diseases other than lSSc,[321] notably with primary biliary cirrhosis; occasionally with dSSc, Sjögren syndrome, or isolated Raynaud phenomenon; and rarely with rheumatoid arthritis, systemic lupus erythematosus, and other connective tissue diseases. Other ANAs (e.g., anti-ssDNA, anti-RNP) occasionally may be present.[322] Elevated levels of soluble CD31 were reported in patients who had a relatively early age at onset and a lower frequency and severity of pulmonary fibrosis. Because this marker is associated with an antiinflammatory effect by inhibiting transendothelial migration of leukocytes, it could represent a protective factor for the development of cutaneous and pulmonary fibrosis.[323]

Treatment

The management of children with lSSc is not materially different from that for dSSC and modified according to each patient's specific organ involvement and severity (see Table 27-6).

Course of the Disease and Prognosis

It was initially believed that patients with this variant of scleroderma had a more benign course and lower mortality rate than those with dSSc, but this distinction has not been entirely substantiated. The mortality rate for lSSc, although somewhat less than in dSSc, is substantial, with a 10-year survival rate of approximately 75% in adults.[324]

Scleroderma-Like Disorders

Because dSSc usually involves internal organs, muscles, and skin, the differential diagnosis includes many disorders such as juvenile dermatomyositis (see Chapter 26), mixed connective tissue disease, and other undifferentiated connective tissue diseases (see Chapter 29).[325] There are other "scleroderma-like" disorders; a description of them follows.

Chronic Graft-Versus-Host Disease

Chronic GVHD is a complication of allogeneic bone marrow transplantation for the treatment of marrow aplasia, leukemia, or malignant diseases. GVHD results from the interaction between immunocompetent T lymphocytes from the donor and host cells bearing histocompatibility antigens that are recognized as foreign. The graft attempts to "reject" the host because, under the circumstances of the transplantation, the recipient is rendered immunologically incompetent by immunosuppression and x-irradiation. The resulting scleroderma-like disease may follow acute GVHD or occur *de novo* up to 100 days after transplantation. It is characterized by dermatitis, usually beginning with erythema of the face, palms, soles, and other regions that are distal in location, or is sometimes generalized, involving only one side of the body in a harlequin-type syndrome. Hyperpigmentation and hypopigmentation follow. A hidebound skin and extreme tightening of the tendons, subcutaneum, and periarticular structures may severely limit motion. GI disease with severe diarrhea and hepatitis is common. Other SSc features, such as Raynaud phenomenon and respiratory or esophageal involvement, are less frequent in GVHD. The histology in these two conditions is similar but not

identical.[326] D-penicillamine may be beneficial for some patients. Extracorporeal photopheresis after sensitization of host leukocytes by methoxypsoralen, a procedure successfully used for the treatment of T-cell lymphoma, is one of the therapeutic choices.[327] However, modifications of the chemotherapeutic preparation of the graft recipient are actually the best prevention of this complication.[328]

Nephrogenic Systemic Fibrosis

Nephrogenic systemic fibrosis (NSF) is a recently identified fibrosing disorder seen only in patients with kidney failure. It is characterized by thickening and hardening of the skin overlying the extremities and trunk and marked expansion and fibrosis of the dermis in association with CD34-positive fibrocytes.[329] NSF was originally named *nephrogenic fibrosing dermopathy* because of the characteristic skin findings.[330] However, subsequent studies showed that some patients had fibrosis of deeper structures, including muscle, fascia, lungs, and heart.[329]

NSF is characterized by skin involvement in all patients and systemic involvement in some.[329] Among patients with gadolinium exposure (discussed later), the latent period between exposure and disease onset is usually 2 to 4 weeks.[331,332] However, the reported range is as short as 2 days and as long as 18 months.[333] Skin disease in NSF typically manifests as symmetrical, bilateral fibrotic indurated papules, plaques, or subcutaneous nodules that may or may not be erythematous.[329,330] In the majority of cases, the lesions first develop on the feet and hands and then move proximally to involve the thighs, forearms, and, less often, the trunk or buttocks. The head is spared. The lesions are often preceded by edema and may initially be misdiagnosed as cellulitis. The edema usually resolves and the involved skin retains a thickened and firm texture.[329] The lesions may be pruritic and accompanied by sharp pain or a burning sensation. Movement of the joints may be quite limited by the fibrosis. Unlike autoimmune sclerosing conditions, Raynaud phenomenon and livedo reticularis are not present in NSF. Late in the disease course, hyperpigmentation, hairlessness, and epidermal atrophy have been described.[334]

The prevalence of systemic involvement is unknown, but a number of different organ system manifestations have been described. Muscle induration may be seen, but strength is normal or only slightly reduced.[335] Joint contractures are common in advanced disease, but the limitation in motion appears to be due to periarticular skin thickening because there is no evidence of synovitis or arthritis. Computed tomography shows fibrosis of the fascia and muscles in the most severely affected patients. Fibrosis has also been identified in the lungs (reduced DL_{CO}) and diaphragm (respiratory failure),[336-338] myocardium,[336,338,339] pericardium and pleura,[337] and dura mater.[339] Asymptomatic yellow scleral plaques may be seen. Patients with systemic disease may have marked elevations in erythrocyte sedimentation rate and serum C-reactive protein.[340]

The diagnosis of NSF is based upon histopathological examination of a biopsy of an involved site. A deep incisional biopsy should be performed because the typical changes can extend into the subcutaneous fat, fascia, and muscle.[341] On microscopic examination, there is a subtle proliferation of dermal fibroblasts in early lesions and florid proliferation of fibroblasts and dendritic cells in more advanced disease. Inflammatory infiltrates are usually absent. Collagen bundles with surrounding clefts are prominent, and dermal mucin and elastic fibers are variably increased. Electron microscopy confirms these findings, which in some cases resemble a sarcomatous process.

The evaluation of possible NSF should include asking whether the patient has had a recent MRI procedure that might have involved gadolinium administration. Gadolinium is a non–tissue-specific contrast agent that is primarily administered during MRI. In healthy individuals, the gadolinium half-life is very short (1.3 hours for some agents), whereas in patients with impaired renal function it can be prolonged, from 10 hours to several weeks, depending of the estimated glomerular filtration rate.[342,343] The gadolinium accumulation in the body seems to be responsible of this syndrome. Support for the pathogenic role of gadolinium comes from the demonstration of gadolinium deposition in tissue specimens of some patients with NSF.[344-346] In addition, observational clinical studies from the United States and Europe show a link between NSF and exposure to gadodiamide (Omniscan), a form of gadolinium that is the only approved MRI contrast agent in Europe.

In case series from Austria and Denmark, end-stage renal disease patients developed NSF 2 to 4 weeks after their exposure to gadodiamide (Omniscan) for MRI.[331,332] There was no correlation with age, sex, underlying renal disease, drug therapy, dialysis modality, or comorbid conditions. Of note, around one half of the patients had been previously exposed to gadolinium without developing NSF. These initial observations have been confirmed in review of 75 cases of NSF in the United States performed by the U.S. Food and Drug Administration (FDA)[333] and by the International NSF Registry.[347] However, there is some suggestive evidence that the risk may vary with the different gadolinium preparations. According to the most recent recommendations, if a gadolinium preparation must be given in patients with end-stage renal failure, gadoteridol in the lowest possible dose is the preferred agent.[348,349]

The epidemiology of NSF in children is unclear. A recent report[350] identified 23 documented pediatric cases (mean age, 13.6 years; range, 6 to 18 years) with prevalence in males (11 boys, 3 girls, 9 unreported gender). Of these children, 10 were on dialysis, 6 had a chronic kidney disease, and 2 had an acute kidney injury; exposure to contrast agents that contained gadolinium was reported in 74% of the children. The outcome was indicated only for 10 patients, of whom 5 had died and 5 had improved their clinical condition after treatment or kidney transplant.

Chemically Induced Scleroderma-Like Disease

Several chemicals have been implicated in the induction of scleroderma.[351] Polyvinyl chloride, initially used as an anesthetic agent,[352] caused a scleroderma-like disease among workers. It is characterized by Raynaud phenomenon; localized papular skin lesions, especially on the fingers and hands, excluding the face and trunk; and osteolysis of the distal phalanges. Bleomycin, an antineoplastic agent, causes skin changes resembling scleroderma[353] and pulmonary fibrosis.[354] This syndrome is not accompanied by Raynaud phenomenon and may improve on cessation of the drug.[355] Pentazocine, a nonnarcotic analgesic drug, has been reported to cause cutaneous sclerosis with or without ulceration.[356] Predisposing factors may include diabetes mellitus and alcohol abuse.

The toxic-oil syndrome, caused by ingestion of aniline-denatured rapeseed cooking oil, occurred in epidemic proportions in Spain in early 1981.[357,358] It affected approximately 20,000 persons and resulted in at least 350 deaths.[359] A report of 21 children indicated that complications may have been less severe in the younger group and that the female-to-male sex ratio was closer to equal (2.5:1) than in adults (6:1).[360] Onset of the disease was characterized by fever, eosinophilia, dyspnea caused by pulmonary edema, a pruritic rash, and malaise. Sclerodermatous skin lesions, alopecia, conjunctivitis sicca, Raynaud phenomenon, myositis, neuropathy, joint contractures, dysphagia, and liver disease evolved over a period of months.

Adjuvant disease, a systemic scleroderma-like condition, has followed cosmetic surgery involving injection of paraffin or silicone.[361,362] An inflammatory reaction in surrounding tissue occurs when silicone gel leaks from implants used for augmentation mammoplasty. A granulomatous reaction can also be demonstrated in regional lymph nodes. Silicone synovitis is well documented in patients after arthroplasty.[363] A variety of atypical "connective tissue diseases," principally, scleroderma-like conditions with chronic fatigue, myalgia, arthralgia, and arthritis, had been reported in women who had had silicone breast implants. Causality had been based on extrapolation of epidemiological data.[364] Although there was concern about a possible relationship between silicone exposure, primarily in breast implant recipients, and SSc or SSc-like disease, a large epidemiological study and a meta-analysis failed to provide evidence supporting a causative role.[365,366] A recent report has raised new doubts about this possible relationship.[367]

Pseudosclerodermas

The term *pseudoscleroderma* describes a diverse group of disorders that are characterized by scleroderma-like fibrotic changes in the skin in association with other nonrheumatic diseases. This discussion is restricted to disorders of significance in the pediatric population.

Phenylketonuria. A minority of children with phenylketonuria (i.e., phenylalanine hydroxylase deficiency) develop sclerodermatous skin lesions.[368-371] These lesions, which usually appear within the first year of life, are symmetrical, poorly demarcated, and resemble morphea. They occur most frequently on the lower extremities and trunk. The lesions may regress on introduction of a low-phenylalanine diet.[372,373] Although no differences in serum phenylalanine or tryptophan levels were found in children with phenylketonuria who did or did not have sclerodermatous changes, urinary excretion of 5-hydroxyindoleacetic acid, indoleacetic acid, and tryptamine was much higher in affected children.[372] The relationship of these biochemical abnormalities to the pathogenesis of the accompanying skin lesions or to that of scleroderma *per se* is unclear. The experimental use of a low-phenylalanine diet in patients with dSSc produced inconclusive results.[372,373]

Syndromes of premature aging. Two rare autosomal recessive disorders accompanied by dwarfing, premature aging, and early death from atherosclerotic heart disease are associated with sclerodermatous skin changes. In *progeria*, the cutaneous changes usually develop before 1 year of age and are characterized by thickened, bound-down skin on the abdomen, flanks, proximal thighs, and upper buttocks.[374-376] During the second year of life, the skin becomes thinner, subcutaneous vascularization is more evident, and alopecia and nail dystrophy develop. *Werner syndrome* most often presents in adolescence with generalized atrophy of muscle and subcutaneous tissue, graying of the hair, baldness, and scleroderma-like skin changes and ulcers involving the extremities.[375-378] The histological features of this disorder mimic those of scleroderma. Metastatic calcification may also develop.[379]

Localized idiopathic fibroses. Several relatively rare disorders in children result in fibrosis of specific organs or structures.[380-382] Keloids are an obvious example. Retroperitoneal fibrosis usually occurs in the region of the sacral promontory and affects vital structures such as the great vessels and ureters. It is more common in males than in females and occurs in children and adults. The syndrome may be idiopathic or associated with IgG4-related disease[383] Retractile mesenteritis, mediastinal fibrosis, fibrosing pericarditis, fibrosing carditis, and peritoneal fibrosis may represent similar disorders that have been related also to administration of certain drugs, notably methysergide and some antihypertensives and anticonvulsants.[384,385]

Some variants of fibromatosis restricted to childhood are distinctive pathologically.[380,386-388] *Congenital torticollis* or *fibromatosis colli* affects the lower sternomastoid muscle and is present at birth or shortly thereafter. It is associated with other anomalies such as congenital dislocations of the hip. *Fibromatosis hyalinica multiplex* is a morphologically distinctive type of *familial multiple fibromatosis* that affects children but is not present at birth. *Infantile digital fibromatosis* affects predominantly the distal fingers or toes. A distinctive microscopic abnormality is the presence of eosinophilic cytoplasmic inclusions. *Infantile myofibromatosis* is manifested as solitary or multiple nodules limited to superficial soft tissues or associated with internal organ involvement. This disorder probably represents an inborn error of metabolism with possible autosomal dominant transmission. It is characterized microscopically by hyalinization of connective tissues of the skin, oral cavity, joint capsules, and bones. Microscopically, areas that resemble smooth muscle alternate with hemangiopericytoma-like foci with a more typical fibroblastic configuration. Central necrosis and intravascular growth may be present.

Gardner syndrome is a form of fibromatosis associated with multiple colonic polyps and osteomas. The fibrosis has a tendency to involve intraabdominal structures, such as the omentum and mesentery or to occur after an operative procedure. *Dupuytren contracture* is a nodular thickening of the palmar fascia and flexion contractures of the digits. Unassociated with disorders such as diabetes, it is rare in children. *Lipogranulomatosis subcutanea of Rothmann–Makai* produces scleroderma-like changes in the skin of the lower extremities with subcutaneous nodules. Morphea or linear scleroderma may be the initial diagnostic consideration. Systemic involvement is absent. The *stiff-skin syndrome* represents congenital scleroderma-like indentations of fascia, predominantly of the buttocks and thighs.

Scleromyxedema is characterized by papular cutaneous lesions with induration of underlying subcutaneous tissues. The lesions occur predominantly on the hands, forearms, trunk, face, and neck. Histological characteristics include a prominent fibrohistiocytic infiltrate and dense acid mucopolysaccharide deposits in the upper dermis. The disease in adults has been associated with monoclonal gammopathies.

Scleredema

Scleredema, a nonsuppurative disorder that is primarily of historical interest, follows β-hemolytic streptococcal infection and is characterized by edematous induration of the face, neck, shoulders, thorax, and proximal extremities, but not the hands.[389,390] Onset is characteristically insidious, and resolution spontaneously occurs after 6 to 12 months. Cardiac abnormalities suggesting the concurrence of acute rheumatic fever have been reported. Diagnosis is based on documentation of nonpitting, indurated edema or stiffness of the skin in the typical locations. Dysphagia may be present, but Raynaud phenomenon and telangiectasias are not. Histologically, the dermis is thickened; there are multiple fenestrations between swollen collagen bundles, a scant perivascular lymphocytic infiltrate, and minimal deposits of acid mucopolysaccharides within the fenestrations. Immunofluorescent staining is negative. Although some children with scleredema have poorly controlled insulin-dependent diabetes, the disorder is presumably distinct from diabetic cheiroarthropathy.

Diabetic Cheiroarthropathy

Diabetic cheiroarthropathy, a syndrome of juvenile-onset diabetes mellitus, causes short stature and tightening of the skin and soft tissues, leading to contractures of the finger joints in as many as 29% of children (see Chapter 41).[391]

REFERENCES

6. G. Martini, I. Foeldvari, R. Russo, et al., Systemic sclerosis in childhood: clinical and immunological features of 153 patients in an international database, Arthritis Rheum. 54 (12) (2006) 3971–3978.

7. K. Scalapino, T. Arkachaisri, M. Lucas, et al., Childhood onset systemic sclerosis: classification, clinical and serologic features, and survival in comparison with adult onset disease, J. Rheumatol. 33 (2006) 1004–1013.

12. H. Poormoghim, M. Lucas, N. Fertig, et al., Systemic sclerosis sine scleroderma: demographic, clinical, and serologic features and survival in forty-eight patients, Arthritis Rheum. 43 (2000) 444–451.

16. F. Zulian, P. Woo, B.H. Athreya, et al., The PRES/ACR/EULAR Provisional Classification Criteria for Juvenile Systemic Sclerosis, Arthritis Rheum. 57 (2007) 203–212.

17. F. van den Hoogen, D. Khanna, J. Fransen, et al., 2013 classification criteria for systemic sclerosis: an American college of rheumatology/European league against rheumatism collaborative initiative, Ann. Rheum. Dis. 72 (2013) 1747–1755.

26. M.D. Mayes, Scleroderma epidemiology, Rheum. Dis. Clin. North Am. 29 (2003) 239–254.

37. A.L. Herrick, H. Ennis, M. Bhushan, et al., Incidence of childhood linear scleroderma and systemic sclerosis in the UK and Ireland, Arthritis Care Res. 62 (2010) 213–218.

54. R. Vancheeswaran, C.M. Black, J. David, et al., Childhood-onset scleroderma: is it different from adult-onset disease, Arthritis Rheum. 39 (1996) 1041–1049.

56. S.A. Jimenez, C.T. Derk, Following the molecular pathways toward an understanding of the pathogenesis of systemic sclerosis, Ann. Intern. Med. 140 (2004) 37–50.

58. A.D. Roumm, T.L. Whiteside, T.A. Medsger Jr., et al., Lymphocytes in the skin of patients with progressive systemic sclerosis. Quantification, subtyping, and clinical correlations, Arthritis Rheum. 27 (1984) 645–653.

68. S. Bhattacharyya, J. Wei, J. Varga, Understanding fibrosis in sistemi sclerosis: shifting paradigms, emerging opportunities, Nat. Rev. Rheumatol. 8 (1) (2011) 42–54.

70. K.V. Pandit, J. Milosevic, N. Kaminski, MicroRNAs in idiopathic pulmonary fibrosis, Transl. Res. 157 (2011) 191–199.

102. K.M. Burge, H.O. Perry, G.B. Stickler, "Familial" scleroderma, Arch. Dermatol. 99 (1969) 681–687.

103. F. De Keyser, I. Peene, R. Joos, et al., Occurrence of scleroderma in monozygotic twins, J. Rheumatol. 27 (2000) 2267–2269.

119. C.M. Artlett, J.B. Smith, S.A. Jimenez, Identification of fetal DNA and cells in skin lesions from women with systemic sclerosis, N. Engl. J. Med. 338 (1998) 1186–1191.

122. H.R. Maricq, G. Spencer-Green, E.C. LeRoy, Skin capillary abnormalities as indicators of organ involvement in scleroderma (systemic sclerosis), Raynaud's syndrome and dermatomyositis, Am. J. Med. 61 (1976) 862–870.

134. P. Quartier, D. Bonnet, J.C. Fournet, et al., Severe cardiac involvement in children with systemic sclerosis and myositis, J. Rheumatol. 29 (2002) 1767–1773.

135. G. Martini, F. Vittadello, O. Kasapçopur, et al., Factors affecting survival in juvenile systemic sclerosis, Rheumatology (Oxford) 48 (2) (2009) 119–222.

162. V.D. Steen, T.A. Medsger, Case-control study of corticosteroids and other drugs that either precipitate or protect from the development of scleroderma renal crisis, Arthritis Rheum. 41 (1998) 1613–1619.

176. A. Della Rossa, G. Valentini, S. Bombardieri, et al., European multicentre study to define disease activity criteria for systemic sclerosis. I. Clinical and epidemiological features of 290 patients from 19 centres, Ann. Rheum. Dis. 60 (2001) 585–591.

183. T.A. Medsger Jr., G.P. Rodnan, J. Moossy, et al., Skeletal muscle involvement in progressive systemic sclerosis (scleroderma), Arthritis Rheum. 11 (1968) 554–568.

189. D. Lapenas, G.P. Rodnan, T. Cavallo, Immunopathology of the renal vascular lesion of progressive systemic sclerosis (scleroderma), Am. J. Pathol. 91 (1978) 243–258.

190. A.R. McGiven, W.G. De Boer, A.J. Barnett, Renal immune deposits in scleroderma, Pathology 3 (1971) 145–150.

200. A. Perera, N. Fertig, M. Lucas, et al., Clinical subsets, skin thickness progression rate, and serum antibody levels in systemic sclerosis

patients with anti-topoisomerase I antibody, Arthritis Rheum. 56 (8) (2007) 2740–2746.

206. C.V. Oddis, Y. Okano, W.A. Rudert, et al., Serum autoantibody to the nucleolar antigen PM-Scl. Clinical and immunogenetic associations, Arthritis Rheum. 35 (1992) 1211–1217.

209. J. Wozniak, R. Dabrowski, D. Luczak, et al., Evaluation of heart rhythm variability and arrhythmia in children with systemic and localized scleroderma, J. Rheumatol. 36 (1) (2009) 191–196.

213. A.-L. Hachulla, D. Launay, V. Gaxotte, et al., Cardiac magnetic resonance imaging in sistemic sclerosis: a cross-sectional observational study of 52 patients, Ann. Rheum. Dis. 68 (1878) 84–2009.

214. E. Di Cesare, S. Battisti, A. Di Sibio, et al., Early assessment of sub-clinical cardiac involvement in systemic sclerosis (SSc) using delayed enhancement cardiac magnetic resonance (CE-MRI), Eur. J. Radiol. 82 (2013) e268–e273.

216. B.Z. Garty, B.H. Athreya, R. Wilmott, et al., Pulmonary functions in children with progressive systemic sclerosis, Pediatrics 88 (1991) 1161–1167.

218. K.M. Antoniou, A.U. Wells, Scleroderma lung disease: evolving understanding in light of newer studies, Curr. Opin. Rheumatol. 20 (6) (2008) 686–691.

222. G. Valentini, S. D'Angelo, A. Della Rossa, et al., European Scleroderma Study Group to define disease activity criteria for systemic sclerosis. IV. Assessment of skin thickening by modified Rodnan skin score, Ann. Rheum. Dis. 62 (2003) 904–905.

223. I. Foeldvari, A. Wierk, Healthy children have a significantly increased skin score assessed with the modified Rodnan skin score, Rheumatology (Oxford) 45 (2006) 76–78.

234. D.M. Koh, D.M. Hansell, Computed tomography of diffuse interstitial lung disease in children, Clin. Radiol. 55 (2000) 659–667.

242. F. La Torre, G. Martini, R. Russo, et al., A preliminary disease severity score for juvenile systemic sclerosis, Arthritis Rheum. 64 (2012) 4143–4150.

243. O. Kowal-Bielecka, R. Landewé, J. Avouac, et al., EULAR recommendations for the treatment of systemic sclerosis: a report from the EULAR Scleroderma Trials and Research group (EUSTAR), Ann. Rheum. Dis. 68 (5) (2009) 620–628.

249. J. Pope, D. Fenlon, A. Thompson, et al., Iloprost and cisaprost for Raynaud's phenomenon in progressive systemic sclerosis, Cochrane Database Syst. Rev. (2) (2000) CD000953.

250. F. Zulian, F. Corona, V. Gerloni, et al., Safety and efficacy of iloprost for the treatment of ischaemic digits in paediatric connective tissue diseases, Rheumatology (Oxford) 43 (2004) 229–233.

257. R. Fries, K. Shariat, H. von Wilmowsky, M. Böhm, Sildenafil in the treatment of Raynaud's phenomenon resistant to vasodilatory therapy, Circulation 112 (19) (2005) 2980–2985.

263. J.H. Korn, M. Mayes, M. Matucci-Cerinic, et al., Digital ulcers in systemic sclerosis: prevention by treatment with bosentan, an oral endothelin receptor antagonist, Arthritis Rheum. 50 (2004) 3985–3993.

264. J.R. Seibold, M. Matucci-Cerinic, C.P. Denton, et al., Bosentan reduces the number of new digital ulcers in patients with systemic sclerosis, Ann. Rheum. Dis. 65 (2006) 90.

267. D.P. Tashkin, R. Elashoff, P.J. Clements, et al., Cyclophosphamide versus placebo in scleroderma lung disease, N. Engl. J. Med. 354 (2006) 2655–2666.

268. R.K. Hoyles, R.W. Ellis, J. Wellsbury, et al., A multicenter, prospective, randomized, double-blind, placebo-controlled trial of corticosteroids and intravenous cyclophosphamide followed by oral azathioprine for the treatment of pulmonary fibrosis in scleroderma, Arthritis Rheum. 54 (2006) 3962–3970.

277. S.N.C. Liossis, A. Bounas, A.P. Andonopulos, Mycophenolate mofetil as first-line treatment improves clinically evident early scleroderma lung disease, Rheumatology (Oxford) 45 (2006) 1005–1008.

278. S.I. Nihtyanova, G.M. Brough, C.M. Black, C.P. Denton, Mycophenolate Mofetil in diffuse cutaneous systemic sclerosis—a retrospective analysis, Rheumatology 46 (2007) 442–445.

279. T. Chris, E. Grace, M. Shenin, et al., A prospective open-label study of mycophenolate mofetil for the treatment of diffuse systemic sclerosis, Rheumatology 48 (2009) 1595–1599.

282. D. Khanna, R. Saggar, M.D. Mayes, et al., A one-year, phase I/IIa, open-label pilot trial of imatinib mesylate in the treatment of systemic sclerosis-associated active interstitial lung disease, Arthritis Rheum. 63 (11) (2011) 3540–3546.

283. J. Pope, D. McBain, L. Petrlich, et al., Imatinib in active diffuse cutaneous systemic sclerosis: Results of a six-month, randomized, double-blind, placebo-controlled, proof-of-concept pilot study at a single center, Arthritis Rheum. 63 (2011) 3547–3551.

284. R.F. Spiera, J.K. Gordon, J.N. Mersten, et al., Imatinib mesylate (Gleevec) in the treatment of diffuse cutaneous systemic sclerosis: results of a 1-year, phase IIa, single-arm, open-label clinical trial, Ann. Rheum. Dis. 70 (2011) 1003–1009.

290. R.N. Channick, G. Simonneau, O. Sitbon, et al., Effects of the dual endothelin-receptor antagonist bosentan in patients with pulmonary hypertension: a randomised placebo-controlled study, Lancet 358 (2001) 1119–1123.

292. V.V. McLaughlin, Survival in patients with pulmonary arterial hypertension treated with first-line bosentan, Eur. J. Clin. Invest. 36 (Suppl. 3) (2006) 10–15.

296. J.E. Pope, N. Bellamy, J.R. Seibold, et al., A randomized, controlled trial of methotrexate versus placebo in early diffuse scleroderma, Arthritis Rheum. 44 (2001) 1351–1358.

299. J.A. Lopez-Ovejero, S.D. Saal, W.A. D'Angelo, et al., Reversal of vascular and renal crises of scleroderma by oral angiotensin-converting-enzyme blockade, N. Engl. J. Med. 300 (1979) 1417–1419.

300. V.D. Steen, T.A. Medsger Jr., Long-term outcomes of scleroderma renal crisis, Ann. Intern. Med. 133 (2000) 600–603.

309. S. Assassi, D. Del Junco, K. Sutter, et al., Clinical and genetic factors predictive of mortality in early systemic sclerosis, Arthritis Rheum. 61 (10) (2009) 1403–1411.

312. L. Scussel-Lonzetti, F. Joyal, J.P. Raynauld, et al., Predicting mortality in systemic sclerosis. Analysis of a cohort of 309 French Canadian patients with emphasis on features at diagnosis as predictive factors for survival, Medicine (Baltimore) 81 (2002) 154–167.

317. M.J. Fritzler, T.D. Kinsella, The CREST syndrome: a distinct serologic entity with anticentromere antibodies, Am. J. Med. 69 (1980) 520–526.

320. E.M. Tan, G.P. Rodnan, I. Garcia, et al., Diversity of antinuclear antibodies in progressive systemic sclerosis. Anti-centromere antibody and its relationship to CREST syndrome, Arthritis Rheum. 23 (1980) 617–625.

329. A. Galan, S.E. Cowper, R. Bucala, Nephrogenic systemic fibrosis (nephrogenic fibrosing dermopathy), Curr. Opin. Rheumatol. 18 (2006) 614–617.

357. E.M. Kilbourne, J.G. Rigau-Perez, C.W. Heath Jr., et al., Clinical epidemiology of toxic-oil syndrome. Manifestations of a new illness, N. Engl. J. Med. 309 (1983) 1408–1414.

359. J.L. Diaz-Perez, J. Zubizarreta, J. Gardeazabal, et al., Familial eosinophilic fascitis induced by toxic oil, Med. Cutan. Ibero. Lat. Am. 16 (1988) 51–58. [Article in Spanish].

360. M. Izquierdo, I. Mateo, M. Rodrigo, et al., Chronic juvenile toxic epidemic syndrome, Ann. Rheum. Dis. 44 (1985) 98–103.

366. E.C. Janowsky, L.L. Kupper, B.S. Hulka, Meta-analyses of the relation between silicone breast implants and the risk of connective-tissue diseases, N. Engl. J. Med. 342 (11) (2000) 781–790.

368. H.K. Kornreich, K.N. Shaw, R. Koch, et al., Phenylketonuria and scleroderma, J. Pediatr. 73 (1968) 571–575.

375. R. Fleischmajer, J.L. Pollock, Progressive systemic sclerosis: pseudoscleroderma, Clin. Rheum. Dis. 5 (1979) 243.

377. C.J. Epstein, G.M. Martin, A.L. Schultz, et al., Werner's syndrome a review of its symptomatology, natural history, pathologic features, genetics and relationship to the natural aging process, Medicine (Baltimore) 45 (1966) 177–221.

381. V. Falanga, Fibrosing conditions in childhood, Adv. Dermatol. 6 (1991) 145–158.

390. P.Y. Venencie, F.C. Powell, W.P. Su, et al., Scleredema: a review of thirty-three cases, J. Am. Acad. Dermatol. 11 (1984) 128–134.

Entire reference list is available online at www.expertconsult.com.

Localized Scleroderma

Suzanne C. Li, Elena Pope

Scleroderma refers to hard skin that develops because of an excessive accumulation of collagen.[1] In the localized form (localized scleroderma [LS], also called *morphea*), inflammation in the skin and subcutaneous tissues triggers the fibrosis. LS and the systemic form, systemic sclerosis (SSc), are chronic diseases that share some pathophysiological pathways but differ greatly in their clinical features and morbidities. LS is usually unilateral, less extensive, and has a different pattern of extracutaneous involvement. The prognosis is generally much better for LS than SSc but depends upon subtype, response to treatment, and extracutaneous involvement.

HISTORICAL REVIEW

Addison is credited with describing areas of skin hardness that he called *keloids* in 1854.[2] In 1868, Fagge pointed out similarities between Addison's keloids and scleroderma, and described different forms of localized scleroderma, including sclerodermie en coup de sabre, and the atrophy associated with linear forms.[3] Parry–Romberg syndrome was described by Parry in 1825 and Romberg in 1846.[4] Eulenburg provided the name *progressive facial hemiatrophy* for this subtype in 1871.[4] The first reported case of disabling pansclerotic morphea may have been that of Roudinesco and Vallery-Radot in 1923.[5]

DEFINITION AND CLASSIFICATION

LS is an umbrella term encompassing a large spectrum of clinical presentations and severities. The Mayo classification divides LS into five general types: (1) plaque morphea, (2) generalized morphea, (3) bullous morphea, (4) linear morphea, and (5) deep morphea.[6] Because this classification includes some conditions that are not uniformly accepted as LS subtypes (atrophoderma of Pasini and Pierini, eosinophilic fasciitis, bullous morphea, and lichen sclerosus et atrophicus) and omits a category (mixed morphea), which accounts for 15% to 23% of juvenile LS cases,[7-9] a revision of the classification was developed by the Pediatric Rheumatology European Society (PRes).[10] It includes five subtypes: (1) circumscribed morphea, (2) linear scleroderma, (3) generalized morphea, (4) pansclerotic morphea, and (5) the new mixed subtype in which a combination of subtypes is present (Table 28-1). Three forms of the plaque morphea subtype of the Mayo classification (morphea en plaque, guttate morphea, and keloid morphea) are included in the superficial type of circumscribed morphea, and two forms of deep morphea (subcutaneous morphea and morphea profunda) are included in the deep type of

circumscribed morphea of the PRes classification.[6] One of the other deep morphea forms, disabling pansclerotic morphea of children, is put into its own separate category in the PRes classification. Generalized morphea and linear morphea are similar between the two classifications, with the PRes classification dividing the linear scleroderma subtype into two types based on lesion location (trunk/limbs or head). Bullous morphea is not included in the PRes classification, as bullous lesions may represent a reaction related to lymphatic dilatation or trauma rather than indicating a specific subtype.[11]

Circumscribed morphea refers to oval or round lesions that are centrally indurated with a waxy, ivory color and a violaceous rim (Fig. 28-1). There are two depths of involvement. *Superficial circumscribed morphea* is confined to the epidermis and superficial dermis, initially presenting with skin discoloration and minimal skin thickening and resolving with hyperpigmentation and mild skin depression with visible venous pattern. *Deep circumscribed morphea* affects the deeper dermis and subcutaneous tissues, resulting in tight and bound down skin. Circumscribed morphea lesions occur most frequently on the trunk and less often on the extremities. The face is usually spared. Guttate morphea is a rare variant of superficial circumscribed morphea that presents as multiple small (2 to 10 mm), initially erythematous or violaceous, and later yellowish or whitish sclerotic lesions with a shiny or depressed surface.[6,12] These lesions can develop hypopigmentation or hyperpigmentation, and primarily affect the trunk.[6]

Generalized morphea (Fig. 28-1B) consists of four or more individual lesions, typically with a diameter larger than 3 cm, involving at least two out of seven anatomical sites (head-neck, right upper extremity, left upper extremity, right lower extremity, left lower extremity, anterior trunk, posterior trunk). Unilateral generalized morphea usually begins in childhood.[13]

Linear scleroderma is the most common subtype of LS in children and adolescents, and is characterized by one or more longitudinal, bandlike lesions that typically involve upper or lower extremities.[8,14,15] The lesions may not appear contiguous at the outset, but they have a linear configuration and may coalesce later. The distribution of the lesions frequently follows Blaschko's lines, an embryonic pattern that may represent genetic mosaicism.[8,16,17] Linear lesions may start superficially and remain so, or become progressively more indurated, bound down with various degrees of involvement of dermis, subcutaneous tissue, and underlying muscle to bone (Fig. 28-2).

Linear lesions of the face or scalp are called the *en coup de sabre* (ECDS) variety, due to the resemblance to a sword stroke (Fig. 28-3). Extension onto the scalp causes scarring alopecia, which is often irreversible. Progressive hemifacial atrophy, which is also known as *Parry–Romberg syndrome* (PRS), is a form of linear scleroderma of the head

TABLE 28-1   **Classification of Juvenile Localized Scleroderma**

MAIN GROUP	SUBTYPE	DESCRIPTION
(1) Circumscribed morphea	(a) Superficial	Oval or round circumscribed areas of induration, limited to the epidermis and dermis, often with altered pigmentation and violaceous, erythematous halo (lilac ring). They can be single or multiple.
	(b) Deep	Oval or round circumscribed deep induration of the skin, involving subcutaneous tissue, extending to fascia, and may involve underlying muscle. The lesions can be single or multiple.
		Sometimes the primary site of involvement is in the subcutaneous tissue without involvement of the skin.
(2) Linear scleroderma	(a) Trunk/limbs	Linear induration involving dermis, subcutaneous tissue, and sometimes muscle and underlying bone, and affecting the limbs and/or the trunk.
	(b) Head	En coup de sabre (ECDS). Linear induration that affects the face and/or the scalp and sometimes involves muscle and underlying bone.
		Parry–Romberg syndrome (PRS) or progressive hemifacial atrophy (PHA). Loss of tissue on one side of the face that may involve the dermis, subcutaneous tissue, muscle, and bone. The skin is mobile.
(3) Generalized morphea		Induration of the skin starting as individual plaques (four or more and larger than 3 cm) that become confluent and involve at least two out of seven anatomical sites (head-neck, right upper extremity, left upper extremity, right lower extremity, left lower extremity, anterior trunk, posterior trunk)
(4) Pansclerotic morphea		Circumferential involvement of limb(s), affecting the skin, subcutaneous tissue, muscle, and bone. The lesion may also involve other areas of the body without internal organs involvement.
(5) Mixed morphea		Combination of two or more of the previous subtypes. The order of the concomitant subtypes, specified in brackets, will follow their predominant representation in the individual patient (i.e., mixed [linear-circumscribed])

Associated conditions: eosinophilic fasciitis, bullous morphea, lichen sclerosus et atrophicus, and atrophoderma of Pasini and Pierini can be concomitant, or precede or follow each of the localized scleroderma subtypes, but are not included in the classification.
From Laxer and Zulian (Ref. 10).

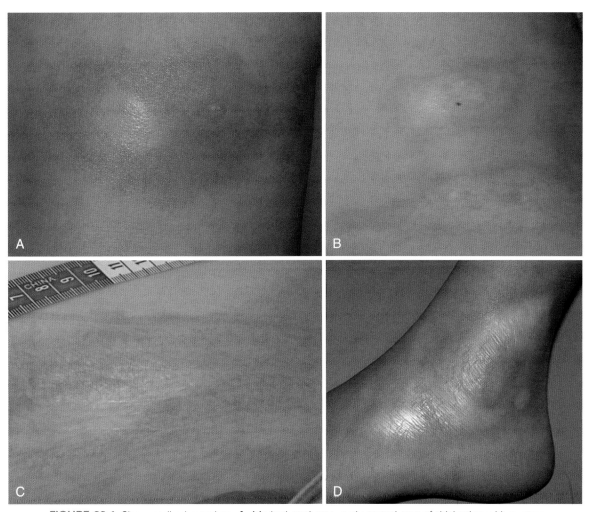

FIGURE 28-1 Circumscribed morphea. **A,** Marked erythema, early central area of thickening with a waxy appearance. **B,** Multiple coexistent plaques displaying activity features: yellow-white discoloration, skin thickening surrounded by a violaceous border, and outer erythema. **C,** Active lesion with central, waxy infiltration surrounded by violaceous border; mild epidermal and superficial dermal atrophy is also noted with visible venous pattern. **D,** Active plaque with marked central thickening/sclerosis surrounded by a thin "lilac" ring.

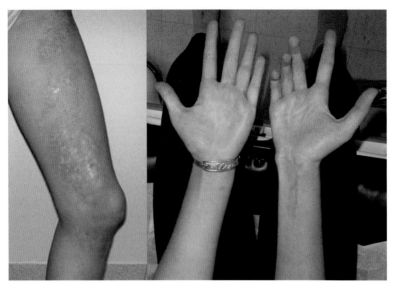

FIGURE 28-2 Linear morphea. **A,** Yellow-white sclerotic plaques coalescent into a linear configuration, crossing over the knee joint. **B,** Linear distribution of a band of subcutaneous atrophy involving the forearm, hand, and third, fourth, and fifth fingers with associated contractures of affected fingers.

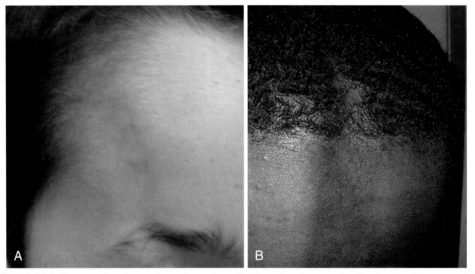

FIGURE 28-3 En coup de sabre variant of morphea. **A,** Linear band across the forehead, with a waxy infiltration toward the eyelid causing dermal and subcutaneous atrophy, and eyebrow and eyelash losses. **B,** Linear band across the forehead with extension onto the scalp with hyperpigmentation, dermal and subcutaneous atrophy, and scarring alopecia.

that may occur with or without ECDS[18,19] (Fig. 28-4). The hallmark of this presentation is varying degrees of atrophy below the forehead, affecting the subcutaneous fat, muscle, and underlying bone structures, with mild or absent epidermal and dermal changes.[10,20] Extensive cases usually cause marked hemifacial atrophy, resulting in severe facial asymmetry and major permanent disfigurement.

Disabling *pansclerotic morphea* of childhood is extremely rare and the most severe subtype of LS because it is widespread, has full-thickness skin involvement, and commonly involves underlying muscle and bone. There is circumferential involvement of all affected anatomic sites, except for the fingertips and toes, which are usually spared.[5] Skin tightness may lead to chronic extensive ulcers with a potential for development of squamous cell carcinoma.[21]

The *mixed subtype* results from a combination of two or more subtypes, such as linear scleroderma and circumscribed morphea, or linear scleroderma and generalized morphea, and can be seen in up to 23% of the cases.[9]

Associated Conditions

Several skin disorders can precede, coexist, or follow LS.[10]

Lichen sclerosus et atrophicus presents as violaceous discoloration progressing to shiny, white, superficial plaques. Typical locations are in the anogenital area and over the wrists and ankles. Sometimes clinical distinction from circumscribed morphea may be difficult. Genital involvement creates an "hourglass" appearance due to the discoloration surrounding the vaginal and perianal area. It is usually

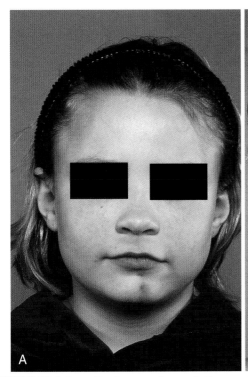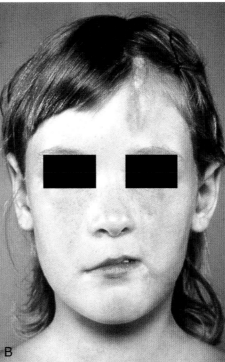

FIGURE 28-4 Parry–Romberg syndrome. **A,** En coup de sabre linear scleroderma of approximately 2 years' duration affects the chin just to the left of midline resulting in a depression and mild asymmetry of the jaw. **B,** En coup de sabre linear scleroderma involves the left face with hyperpigmentation, atrophy of subcutaneous tissues, and early hemifacial atrophy. (Pictures courtesy R. Laxer and F. Zulian).

accompanied by significant pruritus and/or burning sensation due to fissuring. Occasionally hemorrhagic blistering may develop, raising concern about child abuse. There is a high prevalence of lichen sclerosus et atrophicus in patients with circumscribed and generalized morphea.[22]

Atrophoderma of Pasini and Pierini is characterized by asymptomatic hyperpigmented, atrophic patches, with well-demarcated, "cliff-drop" borders (Fig. 28-5, *B*). These lesions, primarily seen on the trunk, lack the typical inflammatory changes of circumscribed morphea and may represent the "burned-out" phase of deep morphea.

Bullous morphea is extremely rare, occurring with most subtypes, including typical circumscribed morphea. The pathogenesis of the bullous lesions is not well understood; local lymphatic obstruction from collagen deposition may play a role.[11,23]

Eosinophilic fasciitis is a rare presentation of primarily fascial involvement with hypergammaglobulinemia, eosinophilia, and high inflammatory markers.[24-27] Eosinophilic fasciitis starts as painful swelling with progressive induration and thickening of the skin creating a typical "peau d'orange" appearance. It tends to involve extremities, and in pediatric patients, often the hands and feet.[28]

EPIDEMIOLOGY

LS is rare, with an estimated incidence of 0.34 to 2.7 cases per 100,000 per year.[16,29] It appears to be more prevalent in the white population (73% to 82%).[8,9,14,29] Pediatric prevalence is estimated at 50 per 100,000. In a current U.S. registry of over 8000 pediatric rheumatology patients (Childhood Arthritis Rheumatology Research Alliance [CARRA] registry), LS is 17 times less common than juvenile idiopathic arthritis and 3 times less common than systemic lupus erythematosus. Most pediatric patients develop the disease in the first decade of life.[30]

The mean age of onset ranges from 6.4 to 10.5 years, and median age from 6.1 to 8.1 years.[8,9,14,17,29,31-33] The female-to-male ratio in children is 1.7-3.7:1, lower than that reported for adults (2.6-7:1).[9,16,31,34] No significant difference in age of onset or sex ratio has been found between subtypes for children.[8,14]

Most pediatric patients have the linear scleroderma subtype (51% to 74%), either alone or as part of the mixed morphea subtype, followed by circumscribed morphea and mixed morphea.[8,9,14,29,32,33] Recent studies report subtype frequencies of 41.8% to 66.7% for linear scleroderma, 15% to 36.8% for circumscribed morphea, 3% to 23% for mixed morphea, and 6.6% to 11% for generalized morphea.[8,9,14,29,32,33] Pansclerotic morphea is extremely rare, with only 5 pansclerotic morphea patients reported in more than 1100 juvenile LS patients.[8,16,31,33]

Adults have a different subtype distribution, with circumscribed morphea the most common presentation (43.9% to 69%), followed by generalized morphea (8% to 23.6%), linear scleroderma (9.8% to 10%), and mixed morphea (3.5% to 11%),[9,16,31] although one study reported a distribution of 13.2% circumscribed morphea, 52.6% generalized morphea, and 21.7% linear scleroderma.[34] Pansclerotic morphea is also extremely rare in adults.[35]

The variable presentations combined with disease rarity result in frequent delays in diagnosis; pediatric studies report a mean time between initial symptom and diagnosis of 11 to 21.6 months,[8,14,36,37] and in over 30% of LS patients in the CARRA registry, a diagnosis was not made for 5 or more years.[38]

ETIOLOGY AND PATHOGENESIS

The etiology and pathogenesis of LS are not completely understood, but they seem to share many similarities with SSc.[39] A recent gene

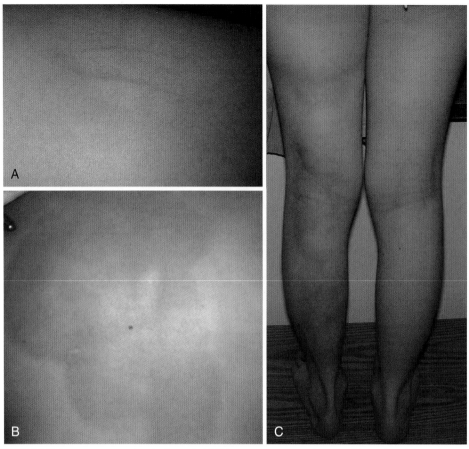

FIGURE 28-5 Late-stage morphea lesions. **A,** Visible venous pattern due to epidermal and dermal atrophy. **B,** Hyperpigmentation and dermal loss with a "cliff-drop" appearance. **C,** Marked areas of dermal and subcutaneous atrophy.

expression profiling study of scleroderma patients found a common inflammatory pattern for LS and diffuse and limited SSc patients, and additional unique patterns for diffuse and limited SSc.[40] A complex interplay of genetic predisposition, autoimmunity, and environmental factors leads to local inflammation and ultimately increased collagen synthesis and deposition in the skin.[41,42] The proposed initiating event is endothelial cell injury resulting in release of cell mediators, upregulation of cell adhesion molecules such as intracellular (ICAM), vascular (VCAM), endothelial leukocyte (E-selectin), and the recruitment of neutrophils. Th-1 and Th-17 immune responses are characteristic for early stages of the disease.[42] The release of interferon (IFN)-γ, interleukin (IL)-2, -6, and -8, and tumor necrosis factor (TNF)-β are thought to be responsible for the increased inflammatory responses. Patients with LS have evidence of upregulation of IL-6 and IL-2R compared with controls.[43,44] On the other hand, high levels of Th-2 cytokines (IL-4, -6, -8, and -13) tend to correlate more with disease damage and fibrosis.[42] Patients with LS have elevated serum levels of B-cell activating factors belonging to the transforming growth factor (TGF) family.[45] Upregulation of TGF-α and TGF-β induces production of platelet-derived growth factor (PDGF); connective tissue growth factor (CTGF); and IL-2, -4, -6, -8, and-13, and soluble receptors (IL-2R and IL-6R), which results in increased mitogenic activity of fibroblasts and production of collagen.[42,46] In one study, the elevated serum levels of TGF correlated with the severity of LS and the presence of antihistone antibodies.[45] Milder cases of LS, such as circumscribed morphea, have levels of TGF-β1 similar to those of healthy controls.[47] The increased production of collagen is further augmented by the decrease in the enzymatic degradation of collagen due to inhibition of matrix metalloproteinases (MMPs).[48]

An autoimmune pathogenesis for LS is supported by the frequent occurrence of autoantibodies, concurrent autoimmune conditions, and family history of autoimmune conditions. A positive antinuclear antibody (ANA) has been found in 26% to 59.4% of juvenile LS patients, with homogeneous, speckled, and nucleolar the most commonly identified patterns.[9,14,31,33,49,50] It is estimated that 5% to 10% of patients with LS have other autoimmune diseases.[9,14,51,52] The frequency of a concurrent autoimmune disease is higher in adults (30%).[9] A 17% to 26% frequency of a concurrent autoimmune disease was reported in juvenile LS patients at median disease durations of 12 to 13 years,[53,54] suggesting that autoimmunity may increase in LS patients over time. However, a cross-sectional study did not find any relationship between age of onset or disease duration and concurrent autoimmunity.[55] A family history of autoimmune conditions is present in 11% to 24% of cases.[8,9,14,51]

The presence of chimeric infiltrating cells in the biopsies of affected skin and similarities to the clinical and histopathological findings of chronic graft-versus-host disease suggest that chimerism may be involved in the pathogenesis of the disease.[56]

An environmental factor, including medication, infection, or trauma may be the initiating event in some cases of LS.[8,49,57] Some medications (bisoprolol, bleomycin, bromocriptine, carbidopa, d-penicillamine, and ergot) have produced scleroderma-like lesions.[58,59] Recent studies report the association of anti–TNF-α medications with onset of LS although these agents have also been used to treat LS.[60,61]

A toxin contained in some lots of L-tryptophan was implicated in a large epidemic of *eosinophilia-myalgia syndrome*, a disease similar to eosinophilic fasciitis and LS.[62,63] Among infectious agents, *Borrelia species* organisms have been extensively studied; at present this etiological link is not supported by the existing evidence, especially outside Europe.[7,48,64]

Typical LS lesions have been reported after local contusion; injection with aluminum-absorbed allergen extracts for allergy desensitization, mepivacaine, pentazocine, vaccinations, vitamin B$_{12}$, or vitamin K$_1$; and radiation treatment.[58,65-69] A preceding history of trauma at the lesion site was reported in 23% to 35.7% of linear scleroderma patients,[49,70] and 11.8% of circumscribed morphea patients.[70] More recent larger juvenile LS studies have reported frequencies of 9% to 12% of a local mechanical event (trauma, insect bite, or vaccination) prior to disease onset[8,14]; there may be a higher frequency of preceding trauma in patients with Parry–Romberg Syndrome.[71-73] Trauma and vigorous exercise may also be inciting events for some cases of eosinophilic fasciitis.[24,74]

Clinical Manifestations

The presentation of LS varies, related to differences in subtype, site of involvement, extracutaneous involvement, and disease duration. Because diagnosis is often delayed, patients commonly show signs of both activity and damage. Most patients have subtle, slowly evolving skin lesions, but some—especially those with pansclerotic morphea—develop rapidly progressive skin and deep tissue involvement. In a few patients, skin lesions only develop after they are diagnosed with arthritis or a neurological problem.[8,75-77] Rarely, LS is evident at birth as areas of faint violaceous discoloration or atrophy without epidermal changes.[78] The skin discoloration can be easily mistaken for a nevus flammeus or port-wine stain,[79] whereas areas of atrophy may raise the possibility of either localized lipoatrophy or early stages of generalized lipodystrophy syndromes.

Early skin lesions, reflecting the initial inflammatory phase, are often erythematous to violaceous plaques with normal skin texture and thickness.[6,7,80] Erythema varies from subtle pink to deep red, with some lesions showing a combined erythematous-violaceous color (Fig. 28-1). Over time, fibrosis becomes more prominent; lesions can develop induration with a central white to yellow, waxy area surrounded by an erythematous or violaceous margin (lilac ring)[6,7] (Fig. 28-1). Later on, damage features predominate. These include postinflammatory hyperpigmentation; atrophy of epidermis (shiny skin with visible venous pattern), dermis (loss of hair follicles and adnexal structures, and cliff-drop atrophy) and subcutaneous tissue (loss of fat) (Fig. 28-5); and progressive skin thickening[7] (Fig. 28-6).

More than 20% of juvenile LS patients have extracutaneous manifestations, including musculoskeletal, neurological, vascular, ocular, and gastrointestinal involvement.[14,52] Extracutaneous manifestations can occur in any subtype, with risk for their development not associated with age of disease onset or disease duration.[9,14,51,52] Subtype and lesion location influence the type of extracutaneous manifestation: growth defects (undergrowth) of extremities, trunk, and face/head are associated with linear scleroderma[10,31]; and neurological, oral, and ocular problems are associated with linear scleroderma of the head.[9,51,52] Joint involvement is associated with linear lesions of extremities, and with pansclerotic, generalized, and deep morphea.[5,9,14,51] Extracutaneous manifestations are usually related to the anatomic site of the skin lesion, but involvement remote from the lesions has been reported in 25% or more of those with arthritis, neurological, or ocular problems.[52] Between 4% and 9% of patients have multiple extracutaneous manifestations, with the risk higher in patients with neurological or ocular involvement.[14,52,75,81]

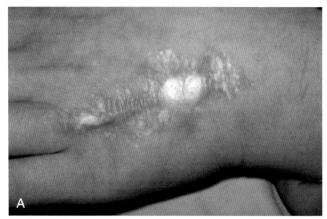

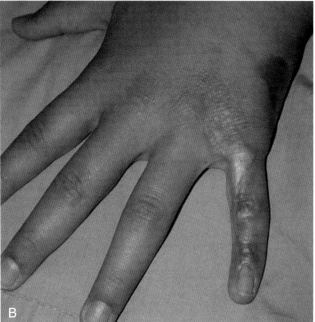

FIGURE 28-6 Inactive morphea. **A,** Band of bound down, sclerotic skin. **B.** Linear morphea causing hyperpigmentation, sclerotic bands, atrophy, and contractures.

Musculoskeletal problems include arthralgia, arthritis, limited range of motion, contractures, and scoliosis.[31] Oligoarticular or polyarticular arthritis has been reported in 12% of childhood-onset LS patients.[52] Muscle atrophy, myositis, muscle spasm, osteomyelitis, and bone and soft tissue growth defects also occur. Musculoskeletal problems are the norm for patients with pansclerotic morphea who are also at risk for soft-tissue calcifications and secondary osteoporosis.[5,82] Growth defects may be subtle until the child has a growth spurt that makes the asymmetry obvious. Defects can be severely disabling or disfiguring; limb length differences of 7 cm have been reported,[83] and patients with PRS can have severe facial hemiatrophy (Fig. 28-4).[71]

Lesions on the head are often associated with neurological, ocular, oral, and bone problems. Neurological problems have been found in 4.4% to 10% of children with LS, with seizures and headache most commonly reported.[14,52,75,84] Seizures include absence, complex partial, generalized tonic clonic, and status epilepticus, and can be refractory to treatment.[75,85] Other neurological problems include cranial nerve palsies, trigeminal and peripheral neuropathy, neuropsychiatric problems, movement disorders, slurred speech, cognitive problems, cavernomas, and central nervous system vasculitis.[32,75,85,86]

Ocular involvement has been found in 2.1% to 6% of children with LS.[9,36,52] The most common ocular complications are fibrotic changes in eyelids, eyelashes, or lacrimal gland and anterior segment inflammation (uveitis, episcleritis).[81] Many other ocular and vision problems have been reported, including hemianopsia, diplopia, ptosis, keratitis, strabismus, acquired glaucoma, enophthalmos, orbital myositis, pupillary mydriasis, and papilledema.[81,85] Because eye involvement can be asymptomatic, patients with facial or head lesions should undergo routine ophthalmological monitoring.

Defects in growth of the lower third of the face, skeletal malocclusion, and paranasal sinus defects occur frequently in children with facial lesions.[87] These children are at risk for delayed permanent tooth eruption, root resorption and underdevelopment, impaired mandibular movement, and masticatory contractions or spasms.[87] Hemiatrophy of the tongue may occur in half of the children with PRS.[71]

Gastrointestinal, pulmonary, cardiac, and renal problems are uncommon in most patients with LS (1% to 2.6%) and rarely life-threatening.[14,31,52,88] The most common gastrointestinal problem is gastroesophageal reflux. More children with LS may have asymptomatic esophageal abnormalities.[74] A few children with LS have dyspnea, chronic cough, or respiratory insufficiency, and they can be found to have a restrictive pattern and/or a decreased diffusion capacity for carbon monoxide on pulmonary function tests[14,31,52] Conduction abnormalities including ventricular premature beats and right bundle branch block have been found in LS.[89,90] A 10-year prospective study found children with LS developed asymptomatic hypertension and diastolic dysfunction at a significantly higher frequency than healthy controls.[89,90] Abnormal pulmonary function tests have been found in more than 25% of patients with pansclerotic morphea, who may also be at risk for more serious cardiac involvement including decreased ejection fraction and cardiomyopathy.[5,21,91]

Eosinophilic fasciitis, unlike LS, usually manifests as acute onset of painful rapidly progressive symmetric involvement of the extremities. Early on, there is edema and erythema, followed by induration and dimpling of the skin giving a peau d'orange appearance, with progressive fibrosis of the subcutaneous tissues causing a bound-down, rock-hard consistency.[28,92-94] Joint contractures and myositis are common in children, and 25% to 44% have polyarthritis.[28,74,93] Up to 29% may have LS lesions of eosinophilic fasciitis.[92]

PATHOLOGY

Histological documentation is helpful but not essential in confirming the clinical diagnosis. The findings are dependent on the stage of the sampled lesion. Ideally, biopsies should be taken from a relatively active border (infiltrative, red and warm lesion). Older sclerotic lesions provide less diagnostic clarity. Early inflammatory stages are characterized by a mixed perivascular and periadnexal infiltrate of predominantly lymphocytes with rare plasma cells and eosinophils in the reticular dermis. There may be dermal edema, swelling and degeneration of collagen fibers, and some thickened collagen bundles.[36,95] Histiocytes may surround individual collagen fibers, creating a "floating" appearance.[96] ECDS variant may present with more prominent vacuolar degeneration at the dermoepidermal junction.[97] Goh et al. described a pattern of perineural lymphoplasmacytic infiltration in alopecia occurring in an ECDS lesion,[98] an interesting potential mechanism explaining linearity and multiple tissues involvement.

In the later stages of the disease, the inflammatory infiltrate is minimal or absent, replaced by excessive deposition of dense collagen, with a shift from type III to type I collagen.[99] The eccrine glands become atrophied and the subcutaneous fat appears "trapped" in the

dermis because of the extension of collagen into the subcutaneous tissues. Blood vessels walls are thickened.

The characteristic histological findings of lichen sclerosus et atrophicus are an atrophic epidermis, edema, and homogenized hyalinized collagen in the papillary dermis. These changes can also be found in LS plaques, typically associated with additional alterations as listed previously.[8,16,100]

Eosinophilic fasciitis is characterized by a significant inflammatory infiltrate (lymphocytes, plasma cells, and eosinophils) at the dermohypodermal junction, dense collagen, and thickening of the fascia. Inflammation and later fibrosis in the hypodermis is robust and also found in the muscle and reticular dermis, and the epidermis can show atrophic changes.[101,102] The sparing of the papillary dermis, marked inflammatory infiltrate, and presence of eosinophils should allow pathological differentiation from classical LS lesions.[103]

The histopathological differentiation between LS and SSc is sometimes difficult, as both biopsies show increased amounts of abnormal collagen and perivascular, interstitial, and periadnexal inflammation.[95] However, in LS the inflammatory infiltrate is more intense and often found at the dermal–subcutaneous junction, a site not involved in SSc inflammation.[95] In addition, because collagen bundles are distributed throughout the dermis in LS but concentrated in the lower reticular dermis in SSc, the papillary dermis shows sclerosis in LS but not in SSc.[95]

DIFFERENTIAL DIAGNOSIS

The manifestations of localized scleroderma are easily overlooked or attributed to other etiologies, particularly in the early stages (Table 28-2).[36,104] Early recognition is important because it allows intervention limiting the ultimate damage. Generalized or pansclerotic morphea may pose more diagnostic dilemmas; differentiation from systemic variants of scleroderma may sometimes be difficult. Children with LS, in contrast to children with SSc, rarely develop Raynaud phenomenon or internal organ involvement (lung, kidney, gastrointestinal). There is also a difference in the pattern of skin involvement: pansclerotic and generalized morphea can affect the entire back, whereas SSc generally spares the central back and more severely affects the fingers and hands.[105] Deep forms of morphea that manifest with contractures of the hands, arthralgias, and sometimes synovitis require further testing to differentiate them from juvenile idiopathic arthritis or other rheumatic diseases, although LS can coexist with these diseases in some patients. As children with LS may also have a positive test for ANA, the absence of erosive joint disease and laboratory findings such as the presence of antihistone antibodies (AHAs), elevated muscle enzymes, and eosinophilia may help to differentiate LS from juvenile idiopathic arthritis.

LABORATORY EXAMINATION

There are no diagnostic or characteristic laboratory findings for LS; it is diagnosed based on clinical findings. A biopsy is sometimes needed to distinguish LS from other conditions. The diagnosis of eosinophilic fasciitis requires documentation of fascia involvement, either on biopsy or magnetic resonance imaging (MRI) findings of hyperintensity and enhancement of fascia.[28]

Patients with eosinophilic fasciitis usually have an elevated erythrocyte sedimentation rate (ESR), C-reactive protein (CRP), eosinophilia, and hypergammaglobulinemia.[74,106,107] Some have elevated muscle enzymes, with aldolase more commonly elevated than creatine kinase (CK).[108] The same abnormalities are infrequently found in children with LS, primarily in those with deeper, more extensive disease,

TABLE 28-2 Differential Diagnosis of Localized Scleroderma

INFLAMMATORY PHASE	INFILTRATIVE (INDURATED) PHASE	INACTIVE ("DAMAGE") PHASE	
		PRIMARILY SKIN	PRIMARILY JOINTS
• Port-wine stain • Lichen sclerosus et atrophicus • Bruising • Annular erythemas (erythema migrans, tinea corporis, erythema marginatum, acrodermatitis chronica atrophicans) • Eosinophilic fasciitis	• Systemic sclerosis • Lipodermatosclerosis • Pretibial myxedema • Panniculitis • Eosinophilic fasciitis • Chronic graft-versus-host disease • Connective tissue/smooth muscle hamartomas (collagenoma, elastoma, smooth muscle, and fibrous hamartoma) • Nephrogenic skin sclerosis • Eosinophilia, myalgia syndrome • Progeria • Scleredema	• Postinflammatory hyperpigmentation • Vitiligo • Lipoatrophy (localized/generalized) • Porphyria cutanea tarda • Bleomycin-induced flagellate hyperpigmentation • Poikiloderma	• Stiff skin syndrome • Progeria • Diabetic cheiroarthropathy • Eosinophilic fasciitis • Winchester syndrome • Metabolic diseases (mucopolysaccharidoses, Niemann–Pick, phenylketonuria)

such as pansclerotic morphea, and in some children with active linear scleroderma or generalized morphea.[5,8,14,21,106] For both eosinophilic fasciitis and LS, abnormal tests tend to normalize as the disease becomes less active.[49,108] In pediatric eosinophilic fasciitis, unlike adult disease, hematological abnormalities are uncommon.[74,93]

Many autoantibodies are found in LS. ANA positivity ranged from 42.3% to 50% in three large juvenile LS cohorts.[8,38] ANA was associated with extracutaneous manifestations in one study, and with more extensive skin involvement in linear scleroderma in another.[50,52] Rheumatoid factor (RF) is found in 15.9% to 26% of LS patients, more frequently in those with arthritis or other extracutaneous manifestations.[8,52,109] In linear scleroderma, antihistone antibodies and anti-single-stranded DNA antibodies (ssDNA ab) have been associated with activity, extensive disease, and joint contractures or functional limitation.[49,50,110] Single-stranded DNA antibodies have also been associated with muscle disease.[111] Antiphospholipid antibodies (anticardiolipin, lupus anticoagulant, anti-phosphatidylserine–prothrombin complex) have been found most commonly in generalized morphea.[8,112,113] Only rarely have patients had thromboembolic events, most commonly with anti-phosphatidylserine–prothrombin complex antibodies.[112] Other antibodies such as antitopoisomerase I antibody and anticentromere antibody, two antibodies commonly associated with SSc, are rare in LS (3.2% and 1.7%, respectively).[8] Neither antibody is associated with presence of extracutaneous manifestations. About 30% of children with eosinophilic fasciitis were found to have ANAs, and 10% had RF.[74,93]

An initial screen of a child with new-onset linear, deep, or more extensive LS could include a complete blood count, ESR, CRP, transaminases, CK, aldolase, ANA, AHA, and ssDNA antibody. Elevations in transaminases, CK, and/or aldolase suggest possible muscle involvement, and these abnormalities, as well as an elevated eosinophil count, ESR, or CRP can be tracked during treatment. If a positive ANA, RF, anti-ss DNA, and/or antihistone antibody is found, more careful monitoring may be advisable as these markers can be associated with more severe or extensive disease.

Disease Monitoring

Several semiquantitative clinical scoring measures have been used to evaluate patient response during treatment. Current measures score both activity (erythema, new or larger lesion, increased skin thickness), and damage (hyperpigmentation, telangiectasias, skin thickness).[114-116] The modified Localized Scleroderma Severity Index (mLoSSI)[115] and Modified Skin Score (MSS)[116] divide the body into multiple anatomic sites for scoring. These measures are easy to use, but they are limited by their subjective assessments, arbitrary scoring weights, and possible limited sensitivity for evaluating activity, because both activity and damage features are combined. Evaluation of additional features, such as lesion warmth, blue or violaceous color, and waxy white to yellow lesions,[117] and use of a weighted clinical activity measure[118] may improve activity assessment.

The Computerized Skin Score (CSS) is a quantitative method that longitudinally evaluates change in lesion size, accounting for changes related to normal growth.[119,120] This method focuses on monitoring one lesion, and is limited by cost and size of tracing film, and sometimes site of involvement.

Several imaging techniques have been used to evaluate LS. Infrared thermography (IT) has high sensitivity for detecting higher surface temperature in active versus inactive lesions, but is limited by low specificity for facial, scalp, and lesions with marked atrophy of the underlying soft tissue.[121] Laser Doppler flowmetry (LDF) and laser Doppler imaging (LDI) assess dermal blood flow and were found to have similar sensitivity and better specificity than IT for identifying active versus inactive lesions.[122,123] Scanning LDI has the advantage over LDF of being able to evaluate a much larger anatomic area and does not require direct skin contact; this latter feature eliminates a major cause for LDF reading variation.[123,124] IT, LDF, and LDI all require patient acclimatization in a temperature-controlled room prior to imaging.

Several adult studies have used high-frequency ultrasound as an outcome measure as it can monitor changes in echogenicity and thickness related to initial edema and later sclerosis.[125-127] Combined histology and sonographic studies have found a range of dermal echogenicity patterns to be associated with active disease.[125,128,129] A pediatric study found hyperechogenicity in the dermis, hypodermis, and muscle to be associated with activity.[130] Increased color Doppler signal (hyperemia) was also associated with activity in pediatric and adult patients,[128,130] similar to the increased dermal blood flow detected by LDF/LDI and increased surface temperature detected by IT. The primary limitation of ultrasound is that it is operator dependent, so training is required to ensure accurate and reliable studies. In addition, because sonographic features vary across sites and between subjects, images of the lesion must be compared to those from a control site, ideally the unaffected contralateral site.[131,132]

Patients with neurological symptoms often have abnormal neuro-imaging studies,[75] and it is recommended that those with craniofacial LS and neurological symptoms have an MRI with gadolinium.[75] The most common computed tomography (CT) abnormalities are cerebral calcifications, skin/skull atrophy, and cortical depression.[75] The most common MRI abnormalities are white matter hyperintensities, abnormal gyral pattern, blurring of gray-white matter, and cerebral atrophy.[75] Brain biopsies have shown inflammation including vasculitis, and gliosis, sclerosis, and abnormal and ectatic blood vessels.[32,75] Imaging abnormalities have also been found in asymptomatic LS patients, and there is evidence that subclinical neurological disease may be present in many.[32,72,133] However, as most patients do not develop overt neurological disease, it is not clear if extensive evaluation of asymptomatic patients is appropriate.[75]

MRI has identified many musculoskeletal abnormalities in LS, including fascial thickening and enhancement, articular synovitis, tenosynovitis, perifascial enhancement, myositis, and enthesitis.[134] Patients with pansclerotic morphea can show bone marrow involvement resembling osteomyelitis.[134,135] MRI use is limited by cost and the need for sedation in young children.

TREATMENT OF LOCALIZED SCLERODERMA

Medical: Topical, Systemic

There are no established guidelines for LS treatment, and many different treatment strategies have been used. Pediatric rheumatologists favor systemic immunosuppressant treatment for patients with moderate to severe disease, which includes most patients except those with circumscribed superficial morphea.[136] Dermatologists favor topical agents and phototherapy but also support the use of systemic immunosuppressants for patients with severe involvement.[48]

Superficial circumscribed morphea commonly causes only minimal permanent skin changes, so therapy primarily consists of topical agents such as topical glucocorticoids, and vitamin D or its analogs.[114] More significant circumscribed morphea lesions may benefit from other immunomodulators such as tacrolimus 0.1% ointment or imiquimod, both of which have been evaluated in trials.[137,138]

There is excellent evidence supporting use of methotrexate (MTX) for moderate to severe disease. Retrospective case series of juvenile LS patients have reported improvement in 74% to 100% of those treated with MTX or a combination of MTX and corticosteroids.[139-143] A 12-month randomized placebo-controlled trial showed that MTX-treated patients (15 mg/m^2/week, maximum 20 mg) achieved better clinical improvement and had a 2.8-fold lower flare rate than placebo-treated patients; all patients had an initial 4-month course of prednisone (1 mg/kg/day, maximum 50 mg per day, for 3 months and then tapered off).[120] Side effects were mild and did not lead to withdrawal of any patient from the trial.

Corticosteroids have primarily been evaluated in conjunction with MTX, as corticosteroid treatment alone has not been found to provide sustained benefit.[144,145] There is no consensus on corticosteroid or MTX regimens, with enormous variation in route of administration, dose, and duration of treatment.[136] CARRA developed standardized treatment regimens based upon best available evidence and current North American treatment practices.[117] The recommended MTX dose is 1 mg/m^2/week (maximum 25 mg) administered subcutaneously. The MTX-based standardized regimens are: (a) MTX alone, (b) MTX plus

oral corticosteroids (2 mg/kg/day, maximum 60 mg, tapered to 1 mg/kg/day by 4 weeks, and then tapered off by 1 year), and (c) MTX plus intravenous corticosteroids (methylprednisolone, 30 mg/kg/dose, maximum 1 gram; administered either 3 consecutive days per month for 3 months, or for 12 weekly doses).[117]

The optimal duration of treatment is not known. Despite mean MTX treatment durations of 27.5 to 36 months,[139,143,145] flares occurred in 15.4% to 44% of patients[141,143,145] at a mean of 4 to 20.4 months off treatment.[140-143,145,146] Possible risk factors for flares include a relapsing course in the first 2 years of treatment, longer follow-up time, and linear subtype.[141,143,145] Mirsky et al. identified an older age at disease onset (mean 9.25 years versus 7.08 years) as another possible risk factor, whereas Weibel et al. found a younger age of onset associated with risk of flare or relapse (mean 3.3 years versus 5.3 years).[141,143] Most children who flare will respond to re-treatment, sometimes with escalation of MTX dose.[141,143,145,147]

Mycophenolate mofetil has been helpful for some patients who are steroid dependent, do not tolerate MTX, or have an inadequate response to MTX; it can be used either alone or in combination with MTX.[148] The CARRA standardized treatment plans recommend dosing according to the U.S. Food and Drug Administration recommendations for pediatric renal disease (600 mg twice a day for patients less than 1.25 m^2; 750 mg twice a day for patients 1.25 m^2 to 1.5 m^2; and 1000 mg twice a day for patients greater than 1.5 m^2).[97] Biological agents are also being considered as a treatment option for more difficult patients.[61,149-151]

Phototherapy, Surgical, and Other Treatment and Care

Phototherapy has been found to have both antifibrotic and immunosuppressive effects, increasing the expression of collagenases (metalloproteinases), decreasing collagen synthesis and proinflammatory cytokines, and causing T-cell apoptosis.[152,153] Many phototherapy regimens have been found to be effective for LS, including narrow band ultraviolet B (UVB) and ultraviolet A1 (UVA1) at low, medium, or high doses, with most studies being open label trials that evaluated changes in skin thickness.[152-155] Several open studies including pediatric patients have reported that psoralen UVA (PUVA) bath photochemotherapy is effective in reducing skin hardness in LS.[156-158] Although UVA1 has greater skin depth penetration than UVB, it only penetrates to the hypodermis and is not recommended for patients with deeper tissue or extracutaneous involvement.[152] The use of phototherapy in children is tempered by concern about potential long-term side effects such as carcinogenesis and skin aging.[153]

For some patients with severe contractures, options such as ablative fractional laser treatment or surgical reconstruction or correction may be helpful.[159,160] Flashlamp pulsed dye laser treatment was reported to improve clinical and histological features of circumscribed morphea lesions that had failed prior treatment. Patients received 7.5 to 8.5 J/cm^2 fluence every 2 weeks for an average of eight sessions.[161]

Patients with significant skin involvement should have physical or occupational therapy directed at counteracting the development of flexion contractures. Moisturizers are recommended to improve xerosis and increase suppleness of the sclerotic areas. Patients with muscle spasm or abnormal movements may benefit from botulinum toxin injection. Botulinum toxin injection into the scalene muscle relieved thoracic outlet syndrome in a patient with linear scleroderma extending from her arm to her trunk, and relieved facial hemidystonia and myokymia in two patients with ECDS.[162-164]

Different surgical strategies have been used to correct atrophy and other deformities associated with ECDS/PRS, including autologous fat injections, Medpor implants, bone paste cranioplasty, and free groin flap, with good outcomes reported.[165,166] Flare of disease following surgery has been reported,[14] and surgery should ideally only be considered when the disease is inactive, and possibly when growth is complete.

Treatment of Pansclerotic Morphea

Treatment of children with pansclerotic morphea is challenging. These patients have deep, extensive, and rapidly progressive disease that often fails to respond to treatment with MTX, corticosteroids, and other immunosuppressive medications including cyclophosphamide.[5,21,167,168] Patients often develop problematic soft-tissue calcifications and ulcerations, secondary osteoporosis, destructive arthritis, and severe flexion contractures that cause profound disability.[5,21] Some pansclerotic morphea patients may benefit from photochemotherapy, combinations of systemic immunosuppressive medications and photochemotherapy, or antithymocyte globulin and cyclosporine.[168-170] For very severe pansclerotic cases, autologous stem-cell transplantation may be considered. Patients with refractory ulcers from pansclerotic morphea or bullous morphea may benefit from N-acetylcysteine, bosentan, or sildenafil.[21,171,172]

Treatment of Eosinophilic Fasciitis

Both oral and intravenous corticosteroids have been used to treat eosinophilic fasciitis; intravenous administration may be more effective.[173] MTX has been found to be helpful for some patients who fail to respond to corticosteroids or who are steroid dependent,[28,147] and a combination initial treatment with MTX or mycophenolate mofetil and corticosteroids may help to reduce cumulative corticosteroid dose and morbidity.[107] Case studies have reported benefit from intravenous immunoglobulin, infliximab, rituximab, cyclosporine, D-penicillamine, phototherapy, dapsone, and allogeneic stem-cell transplant in patients who have responded poorly to other treatments.[174-182]

COURSE OF THE DISEASE AND PROGNOSIS

The prognosis for most children with LS is good in contrast with those with SSc. Those with pansclerotic morphea have the poorest prognosis because they usually fail to respond to standard treatment and develop severe, extensive atrophy; contractures; and skin ulceration.[5,21,183] Deaths are extremely rare, and those deaths are associated with the pansclerotic subtype due to chronic skin ulcer complications (sepsis, squamous cell carcinoma).[5,21,184] Progression to SSc is extremely unlikely (1 of 1134 patients).[9,14,31,52] LS has been reported to coexist with juvenile idiopathic arthritis, systemic lupus erythematosus, and Sjögren's syndrome,[9,51,185] so the rare association of LS with SSc may represent coexistence rather than progression. Up to 6% of adult SSc patients have been found to have circumscribed morphea lesions.[186]

The natural history for many LS patients is a self-limited course, with initial worsening and spread of the lesion(s), followed by resolution of activity features, stabilization of damage features, and softening of lesions occurring in half of the patients with circumscribed morphea by 2.7 years after diagnosis, and by 5 to 5.5 years for the patients with generalized, linear, or deep morphea.[16] Current practice has improved this time course with a recent incidence study reporting improvement in 65% of patients and disease stabilization in another 18% by 1 year.[29]

In some patients, active disease persists for decades. One study found that 35% of linear scleroderma patients had active disease after 10 years, which only declined to 20% at 20 years.[16] Two recent studies of patients with childhood disease onset found that 28% to 88% continued to have active disease as adults, either as continuous activity or as a relapsing and remitting course.[53,54]

Damage occurs frequently. After about 5 years, nearly all linear scleroderma patients were found to have dyspigmentation, cutaneous atrophy, or both.[53] Many patients have functional impairment related to limited joint mobility and limb atrophy. Disability was present in 25% to 44% of patients with linear scleroderma or deep morphea.[16] Functional limitation was present in 28% to 38% of juvenile LS patients in three recent studies, including an ongoing prospective registry.[36,38,53] A study of 27 adult patients with childhood disease onset found that half had permanent damage (75% in those with linear scleroderma).[54] The morbidity of patients who have involvement of the face and head may also be underreported, as about half of 205 surveyed PRS patients reported migraine headache, facial pain, and/or eye or vision problems.[187]

Most adults with eosinophilic fasciitis achieve remission,[173] but many children develop persistent cutaneous fibrosis. Risk factors for persistent fibrosis include extensive disease (three to four extremities and trunk involvement) and younger age (younger than 7 years reported in one study, younger than 12 years in another) at diagnosis.[92,93] In adults, a delay in diagnosis (more than 6 months) was a risk factor for poorer outcome.[173]

Two studies in patients with childhood LS did not find any overall impairment in health-related quality of life (HRQOL),[188,189] but another found that two thirds of patients with linear scleroderma had dissatisfaction with their appearance.[53] Somatic and psychological problems, such as pain, itch, fatigue, or anxiety, occur frequently in adult eosinophilic fasciitis and LS patients, especially those with generalized morphea.[190,191]

Although improvements in treatment have resulted in earlier induction of disease inactivity for most children with LS, many continue to have recurrent or persistent active disease and functional impairment. More work is needed to identify optimal treatment for achieving sustained remission and preventing severe morbidities to improve the long-term outcome for these children.

REFERENCES

5. J. Diaz-Perez, S. Connolly, R. Winkelmann, Disabling pansclerotic morphea of children, Arch. Dermatol. 116 (1980) 169–173.

6. L. Peterson, A. Nelson, W. Su, Classification of morphea (localized scleroderma), Mayo Clin. Proc. 70 (1995) 1068–1076.

7. N. Fett, V. Werth, Update on morphea: part I. Epidemiology, clinical presentation, and pathogenesis, J. Am. Acad. Dermatol. 64 (2011) 217–228.

8. F. Zulian, B. Athreya, R. Laxer, et al., Juvenile localized scleroderma: clinical and epidemiological features in 750 children. An international study, Rheumatology. 45 (2006) 614–620.

9. J. Leitenberger, R. Cayce, R. Haley, et al., Distinct autoimmune syndromes in morphea, Arch. Dermatol. 145 (2009) 545–550.

10. R. Laxer, F. Zulian, Localized scleroderma, Curr. Opin. Rheumatol. 18 (2006) 606–613.

14. S. Christen-Zaech, M. Hakim, F. Afsar, A. Paller, Pediatric morphea (localized scleroderma): review of 136 patients, J. Am. Acad. Dermatol. 59 (2008) 385–396.

15. H. Christianson, C. Dorsey, P. O'Leary, R. Kierland, Localized scleroderma: a clinical study of two hundred thirty-five cases, Arch. Dermatol. 74 (1956) 629–639.

16. L. Peterson, A. Nelson, W. Su, et al., The epidemiology of morphea (localized scleroderma) in Olmstead County 1960 1993, J. Rheumatol. 24 (1997) 73–80.

20. R. Lewkonia, Progressive hemifacial atrophy (Parry-Romberg syndrome) report with review of genetics and nosology, Am. J. Med. Genet. 14 (1983) 385–390.

21. L. Wollina, M. Buslau, B. Heinig, et al., Disabling pansclerotic morphea of childhood poses a high risk of chronic ulceration of the skin and

squamous cell carcinoma, Int. J. Low. Extrem. Wounds 6 (2007) 291–298.

22. A. Kreuter, J. Wischnewski, S. Terras, et al., Coexistence of lichen sclerosus and morphea: a retrospective analysis of 472 patients with localized scleroderma from a German tertiary referral center, J. Am. Acad. Dermatol. 67 (2012) 1157–1162.

24. L. Shulman, Diffuse fasciitis with eosinophilia: a new syndrome? Trans. Assoc. Am. Physicians 88 (1975) 70–86.

26. I. Pinal-Fernandez, A. Selva-O'Callaghan, J. Grau, Diagnosis and classification of eosinophilic fasciitis, Autoimmun. Rev. 13 (2014) 379–382.

29. A. Herrick, H. Ennis, M. Bhushan, et al., Incidence of childhood linear scleroderma and systemic sclerosis in the UK and Ireland, Arthritis. Care. Res. 62 (2010) 213–218.

31. A. Marzano, S. Menni, A. Parodi, et al., Localized scleroderma in adults and children. Clinical and laboratory investigations on 239 cases, Eur. J. Dermatol. 13 (2003) 171–176.

32. Y. Chiu, S. Vora, E.-K. Kwon, M. Maheshwari, A significant proportion of pediatric morphea en coup de sabre and Parry-Romberg syndrome patients have neuroimaging findings, Pediatr. Dermatol. 29 (2012) 738–748.

34. W. Johnson, H. Jacobe, Morphea in adults and children cohort II: patients with morphea experience delay in diagnosis and large variation in treatment, J. Am. Acad. Dermatol. 67 (2012) 881–890.

36. L. Weibel, B. Laguda, D. Atherton, J.I. Harper, Misdiagnosis and delay in referral of children with localized scleroderma, Br. J. Dermatol. 165 (2011) 1308–1313.

39. J. Canady, S. Karrer, M. Fleck, A. Bosserhoff, Fibrosing connective tissue disorders of the skin: molecular similarities and distinctions, J. Dermatol. Sci. 70 (2013) 151–158.

41. I. Badea, M. Taylor, A. Rosenberg, I. Foldvari, Pathogenesis and therapeutic approaches for improved topical treatment in localized scleroderma and systemic sclerosis, Rheumatology (Oxford) 48 (2009) 213–221.

42. K. Kurzinski, K. Torok, Cytokine profiles in localized scleroderma and relationship to clinical features, Cytokine 55 (2011) 157–164.

49. V. Falanga, T. Medsger Jr., M. Reichlin, G. Rodnan, Linear scleroderma. Clinical spectrum, prognosis, and laboratory abnormalities, Ann. Intern. Med. 104 (1986) 849–857.

50. J. Dharamsi, S. Victor, N. Aguwa, et al., Morphea in adults and children cohort III. Nested case-control study-the clinical significance of autoantibodies in morphea, JAMA Dermatol 149 (2013) 1159–1165.

51. M. Pequet, K. Holland, S. Zhao, et al., Risk factors for morphoea disease severity: a retrospective review of 114 paediatric patients, Br. J. Dermatol. 170 (2014) 895–900. doi:10.1111/bjd.12758.

52. F. Zulian, C. Vallongo, P. Woo, et al., Juvenile Scleroderma Working Group of the Pediatric Rheumatology European Society (PRES), Localized scleroderma in childhood is not just a skin disease, Arthritis. Rheum. 52 (2005) 2873–2881.

53. M. Piram, C. McCuaig, C. Saint-Cyr, et al., Short-and long-term outcome of linear morphea in children, Br. J. Dermatol. 169 (2013) 1265–1271.

54. S. Saxton-Daniels, H. Jacobe, An evaluation of long-term outcomes in adults with pediatric-onset morphea, Arch. Dermatol. 146 (2010) 1044–1045.

62. R. Martin, J. Duffy, A. Engel, et al., The clinical spectrum of the eosinophilia-myalgia syndrome associated with L-tryptophan ingestion. Clinical features in 20 patients and aspects of pathophysiology, Ann. Intern. Med. 113 (1990) 124–134.

64. B. Weide, T. Walz, C. Garbe, Is morphoea caused by borrelia burgdorferi? A review, Br. J. Dermatol. 142 (2000) 636–644.

71. A. Somner, T. Gambichler, M. Bacharach-Buhles, et al., Clinical and serological characteristics of progressive facial hemiatrophy: a case series of 12 patients, J. Am. Acad. Dermatol. 54 (2006) 227–233.

72. M. Blaszczyk, L. Królicki, M. Krasu, et al., Progressive facial hemiatrophy: central nervous system involvement and relationship with scleroderma en coup de sabre, J. Rheumatol. 30 (2003) 1997–2004.

75. I. Kister, M. Inglese, R. Laxer, J. Herbert, Neurologic manifestations of localized scleroderma. A case report and literature review, Neurology 71 (2008) 1538–1545.

85. T. Amaral, F. Peres, A. Lapa, et al., Neurologic involvement in scleroderma: a systematic review, Semin. Arthritis Rheum. 43 (2013) 335–347.

92. Y. Endo, A. Tamura, Y. Matsushima, et al., Eosinophilic fasciitis: report of two cases and a systematic review of the literature dealing with clinical variables that predict outcome, Clin. Rheumatol. 26 (2007) 1445–1451.

95. J. Torres, J. Sánchez, Histopathologic differentiation between localized and systemic scleroderma, Am. J. Dermatopathol. 20 (1998) 242–245.

97. T. Taniguchi, Y. Asano, Z. Tamaki, et al., Histological features of localized scleroderma "en coup de sabre": a study of 16 cases, J. Eur. Acad. Dermatol. Venereol. (2013) doi:10.1111/jdv.12280; [Epub ahead of print].

100. F. Succaria, M. Kurban, A. Kibbi, O. Abbas, Clinicopathological study of 81 cases of localized and systemic scleroderma, J. Eur. Acad. Dermatol. Venereol. 27 (2013) e191–e196.

104. J. Nashel, V. Steen, Scleroderma mimics, Curr. Rheumatol. Rep. 14 (2012) 39–46.

109. A. Herrick, H. Ennis, M. Bhushan, et al., Clinical features of childhood localized scleroderma in an incidence cohort, Rheumatology (Oxford) 50 (2011) 1865–1868.

110. T. Arkachaisri, N. Fertig, S. Pino, T. Medsger Jr., Serum autoantibodies and their clinical associations in patients with childhood- and adult-onset linear scleroderma. A Single-Center Study, J. Rheumatol. 35 (2008) 2439–2444.

115. T. Arkachaisri, S. Vilaiyuk, S. Li, et al., The localized scleroderma skin severity index and physician global assessment of disease activity: a work in progress toward development of localized scleroderma outcome measures, J. Rheumatol. 36 (2009) 2819–2829.

117. S. Li, K. Torok, E. Pope, et al., Childhood Arthritis and Rheumatology Research Alliance (CARRA) Localized Scleroderma Workgroup, Development of consensus treatment plans for juvenile localized scleroderma: a roadmap toward comparative effectiveness studies in juvenile localized scleroderma, Arthritis Care Res. 64 (2012) 1175–1185.

120. F. Zulian, G. Martini, C. Vallongo, et al., Methotrexate treatment in juvenile localized scleroderma, Arthritis. Rheum. 63 (2011) 1998–2006.

122. L. Weibel, K. Howell, M. Visentin, et al., Laser doppler flowmetry for assessing localized scleroderma in children, Arthritis. Rheum. 56 (2007) 3489–3495.

123. L. Shaw, J. Shipley, E. Newell, et al., Scanning laser Doppler imaging may predict disease progression of localized scleroderma in children and young adults, Br. J. Dermatol. 169 (2013) 152–155.

125. A. Kreuter, T. Gambichler, F. Breuckmann, et al., Pulsed high-dose corticosteroids combined with low-dose methotrexate in severe localized scleroderma, Arch. Dermatol. 141 (2005) 847–852.

128. X. Wortsman, J. Wortsman, I. Sazunic, L. Carreño, Activity assessment in morphea using color Doppler ultrasound, J. Am. Acad. Dermatol. 65 (2011) 942–948.

129. K. Nezafati, R. Cayce, J. Susa, et al., 14-MHz ultrasonography as an outcome measure in morphea (localized scleroderma), Arch. Dermatol. 147 (2011) 1112–1115.

130. S.C. Li, M.S. Liebling, K.A. Haines, et al., Initial evaluation of an ultrasound measure for assessing the activity of skin lesions in juvenile localized scleroderma, Arthritis. Care. Res. 63 (5) (2011) 735–742.

134. S. Schanz, G. Fierlbeck, A. Ulmer, et al., Localized scleroderma: MR findings and clinical features, Radiology 260 (2011) 817–824.

139. K. Torok, T. Arkachaisri, Methotrexate and corticosteroids in the treatment of localized scleroderma: a standardized prospective longitudinal single-center study, J. Rheumatol. 39 (2012) 286–294.

141. L. Mirsky, A. Chakkittakandiyil, R. Laxer, et al., Relapse after systemic treatment in paediatric morphoea, Br. J. Dermatol. 166 (2011) 443–445.

142. Y. Uziel, B. Feldman, B. Krafchik, et al., Methotrexate and corticosteroid therapy for pediatric localized scleroderma, J. Pediatr. 136 (2000) 91–95.

143. L. Weibel, M. Sampaio, M. Visentin, et al., Evaluation of methotrexate and corticosteroids for the treatment of localized scleroderma (morphoea) in children, Br. J. Dermatol. 155 (2006) 1013–1020.

145. F. Zulian, C. Vallongo, A. Patrizi, et al., A long-term follow-up study of methotrexate in juvenile localized-scleroderma (morphea), J. Am. Acad. Dermatol. 67 (2012) 1151–1156.

148. G. Martini, A. Ramanan, F. Falcini, et al., Successful treatment of severe or methotrexate-resistant juvenile localized scleroderma with mycophenolate mofetil, Rheumatology (Oxford) 48 (2009) 1410–1413.

152. A. Kreuter, UV-A1 phototherapy for sclerotic skin diseases, Arch. Dermatol. 144 (2008) 912–916.

153. N. Fett, V. Werth, Update on morphea. part II. Outcome measures and treatment, J. Am. Acad. Dermatol. 64 (2011) 231–242.

154. B. Zwischenberger, H. Jacobe, A systematic review of morphea treatments and therapeutic algorithm, J. Am. Acad. Dermatol. 65 (2011) 925–941.

155. E. Kroft, N. Berkhof, P.C.M. van de Kerkhof, et al., Ultraviolet A phototherapy for sclerotic skin diseases: a systematic review, J. Am. Acad. Dermatol. 59 (2008) 1017–1030.

The entire reference list is available online at www.expertconsult.com.

Mixed Connective Tissue Disease and Undifferentiated Connective Tissue Disease

Peri H. Pepmueller, Carol B. Lindsley

Connective tissue diseases (CTDs) are inflammatory conditions with characteristic signs and symptoms defining specific disorders. Classification criteria developed by the American College of Rheumatology have provided guidelines for diagnosis in adult patients and have been used to some extent in children. The criteria were developed initially to ensure diagnoses for clinical investigations. Some children, however, simultaneously manifest signs and symptoms characteristic of two or more of the major rheumatic disorders, such as juvenile idiopathic arthritis (JIA), systemic lupus erythematosus (SLE), juvenile dermatomyositis (JDM), cutaneous systemic scleroderma (CSS), and vasculopathy. Children with these disorders are often difficult to categorize under existing classification criteria and are properly referred to as having *overlap syndromes*. The most studied of these conditions is *mixed connective tissue disease* (MCTD), which will be further discussed in this chapter.

MIXED CONNECTIVE TISSUE DISEASE

Definition and Classification

MCTD was initially described by Sharp and colleagues in 1972[1] in 25 adults as a disorder with an excellent initial response to relatively low-dose glucocorticoid therapy and a favorable prognosis. The syndrome included clinical features of rheumatoid arthritis (RA), scleroderma, SLE, and dermatomyositis in conjunction with a high antibody titer to an extractable nuclear antigen (ENA). However, reassessment of the original patients indicated that the inflammatory manifestations (e.g., arthritis, serositis, fever, myositis) tended to become less evident over time, whereas sclerodactyly and esophageal disease, which were less responsive to treatment with glucocorticoids, persisted and began to dominate the clinical picture.[2] Severe renal disease continued to remain an unusual feature. Although the concept of MCTD as a clinical entity separate from the other CTDs has remained controversial, classifications employing more precise serological criteria and human leukocyte antigen (HLA) typing have confirmed the uniqueness of this disorder (Table 29-1).[3-6]

Criteria for MCTD have been evaluated for adults but not for children (Table 29-2).[7-10] These criteria are summarized in the review by Smolen and colleagues.[11] Shen and co-workers[12] studied 50 patients from China during a 2- to 8-year period and indicated that Sharp's criteria[7] were the most reliable for the diagnosis of MCTD. Among 23 patients fulfilling these criteria, only one (4.3%) developed scleroderma. Among 23 patients satisfying the criteria of Kasukawa and colleagues,[8] 7 (30.4%) developed another CTD. Of the 27 who met the criteria of Alarcón-Segovia and colleagues,[9] 12 (44%) fulfilled classification criteria for another major rheumatic disease. The frequencies

of HLA-DR4 and HLA-DR5 were significantly higher among the patients whose disease fulfilled Sharp's criteria.[7] Different conclusions were reached, however, in a comparative study of four diagnostic criteria from France by Amigues and co-workers.[13] These investigators analyzed the criteria developed by Sharp,[7] Kasukawa and colleagues,[8] Alarcón-Segovia and co-workers,[9] and Kahn and associates,[10] respectively, in 45 patients with anti-uridine rich (U1) ribonucleoprotein (RNP) antibodies who were classified as having MCTD. They found that the criteria of Alarcón-Segovia and co-workers[9] had the highest sensitivity (62.5%) and specificity (86.2%), with an overlap of 16% with other major CTDs. These results were comparable with those obtained with the criteria of Kahn and associates.[10]

Epidemiology

MCTD is one of the least common disorders in a pediatric rheumatology clinic. It had a frequency of 0.1% in a Finnish nationwide prospective study[14] and 0.3% in the U.S. Pediatric Rheumatology Database.[15] Data from the British Pediatric Rheumatology Association Disease Registry[16] and the Canadian Pediatric Rheumatology Association Disease Registry[17] showed frequencies of 0.5% and 0.2%, respectively. The median age at onset was approximately 11 years (range: 4 to 16 years). MCTD occurred three times more frequently in girls than in boys.[15] There was one report of this disorder occurring in siblings.[18]

Immunogenetic Background

In studies from several continents, including North and South America, Japan, and Europe, the predominant HLA class II specificity associated with MCTD has been DR4; association with HLA-DR2 is less well established.[5,11,19-25] Individuals with DR4 or DR2 have a region of homology of seven amino acids (numbers 26, 28, 30, 31, 32, 70, and 73) in the highly polymorphic antigen-binding segment of the DRB1 gene *(HLA-DRB1)*.[25,26] These HLA specificities are also linked to antibodies to the uridine-rich small nuclear ribonucleoprotein (U1snRNP) that are characteristic of the disorder. It is notable that major histocompatibility complex (MHC) haplotypes most commonly associated with CSS (DR5) or SLE (DR3) are uncommon.

Etiology and Pathogenesis

MCTD is characterized immunologically by the presence of autoantibodies and T cells reactive with U1-RNP and polypeptides of the spliceosome complex, including their associated uridine-rich (U) small nuclear ribonucleic acids (RNAs). A number of immunological factors have been associated with MCTD and may contribute to disease pathogenesis.[27,28] The 70-kD peptide of the U1-RNP antigen appears to be a dominant autoantigen in MCTD and consists of a 437 residue

TABLE 29-1 Clinical Characteristics of Mixed Connective Tissue Disease

Clinical Signs of at Least Two of the Following Diseases
Juvenile rheumatoid arthritis
Systemic lupus erythematosus
Juvenile dermatomyositis
Systemic scleroderma

Positive Serological Findings
High-titer of antibodies to U1 snRNP and the 70-kD A and C polypeptides
Anti-U1-RNA antibodies

Presence of HLA-DR4

polypeptide, which noncovalently associates with U1-RNA through an RNA binding domain on the polypeptide spanning residues 92-202.[29] There are a variety of potential and proven structural modifications, which occur to the U1 70-kD polypeptide and RNP, any of which might influence antigenicity of the RNP complex.[30,31] The apoptotically modified 70-kD has been shown to be antigenically distinct from intact 70-kD, which may have clinical implications in breaking immune tolerance to the autoantigen.[32-34] One study reported that autoantibodies reactive with apoptotic 70-kD are superior markers to those against intact 70-kD for MCTD.[33]

Various independent observations over the years have led to the conclusion that the innate and adaptive immune systems play a central role in the development of many systemic autoimmune diseases, including MCTD.[35-37] As noted previously, the dominant epitopes

TABLE 29-2 Classification Criteria for Mixed Connective Tissue Disease (MCTD)

SHARP	ALARCÓN-SEGOVIA	KASUKAWA	KAHN
Criteria			
Major			
(a) Severe myositis	(1) **Serological**	(1) **Common Symptoms**	(1) **Serological**
(b) Lung involvement: DLCO <70% and/or pulmonary hypertension and/or proliferative vascular lesions on biopsy	(a) Anti-RNP at hemagglutination titer >1:1600	(a) Raynaud phenomenon	(a) High-titer anti-RNP corresponding to speckled ANA at titer >1:2000
	(2) **Clinical Criteria**	(b) Swollen fingers	
	(b) Swollen hands	(2) **Anti-RNP Ab**	(2) **Clinical**
(c) Raynaud phenomenon or esophageal hypomotility	(c) Synovitis	(3) **Symptoms**	(a) Raynaud phenomenon
	(d) Biologically or histologically proven myositis	*SLE*	(b) Synovitis
(d) Swollen hands or sclerodactyly	(e) Raynaud phenomenon	(a) Polyarthritis	(c) Myositis
	(f) Acrosclerosis with or without proximal systemic sclerosis	(b) Adenopathies	(d) Swollen fingers
(e) Anti-ENA ≥1:10,000 with anti-RNP+ and anti-S−		(c) Malar rash	
		(d) Pericarditis or pleuritis	
		(e) Leukopenia or thrombocytopenia	
Minor			
(a) Alopecia		*SSc*	
(b) Leukopenia <4000		(a) Sclerodactyly	
(c) Anemia		(b) Pulmonary fibrosis or restrictive changes in lung function or reduced DLCO	
(d) Pleuritis			
(e) Pericarditis		(c) Hypomotility or esophageal dilation	
(f) Arthritis		**PM**	
(g) Trigeminal neuralgia		(a) Muscle weakness	
(h) Malar rash		(b) Elevated muscle enzymes	
(i) Thrombocytopenia		(c) Myogenic signs on EMG	
(j) Mild myositis			
(k) History of swollen hands			
Diagnosis			
MCTD Certain	*MCTD*	*MCTD*	*MCTD*
4 major criteria, no anti-Sm, anti-U1-RNP >1:4000	If serological criterion above is met, and at least 3 clinical criteria are identified [if (a), (d), and (e) are present, (b) or (c) are also required]	If presence of at least 1 of the 2 common symptoms, anti-RNP antibodies, *and* the presence of at least 1 sign of at least 2 of the following connective tissue diseases: SLE, SSc, and PM	If serological criteria fulfilled, and Raynaud phenomenon, *and* at least 2 of the 3 following signs are present: synovitis, myositis, and swollen fingers
MCTD Probable			
3 major criteria and no anti-Sm, or 2 major criteria and 1 minor criterion, anti-U1-RNP >1:1000			

Adapted from Reference 13.

recognized in MCTD reside within the RNA binding domains of the peptide. These observations coincided with the discovery of a series of pathogen-associated pattern recognition receptors, including the Toll-like receptors (TLRs), especially those that recognize double-stranded RNA or single-stranded RNA, and normally play a vital role in host defense through their recognition of bacterial and viral cell products. These findings led to a series of studies examining TLRs in autoimmunity. Studies have shown that U1-RNA can activate cells of a TLR3 using U1-RNA and TLR-deficient mutant endometrial cell lines.[38]

Autoantibodies are widely recognized as a hallmark of many of the rheumatic diseases, including MCTD.[39] Two studies have supported a role for anti-RNP antibodies in the pathogenesis of MCTD by providing linkage between the emergence of antibodies and clinical disease.[40,41] B cells can function in several other key immunological pathways beyond antibody production; these include functioning as antigen-presenting cells, secreting pathological cytokines, and mediating tissue injury through a variety of antibody-directed mechanisms.[27]

T cells appear to have a central role in the pathogenesis of MCTD. RNP-reactive CD4[+] T cells have been identified from peripheral blood of MCTD patients. Both anti-RNP and anti-U1-RNA antibodies found in patients' sera have, in most instances, undergone isotope switching to immunoglobulin G (IgG) subtypes. Also, there is dense lymphocyte infiltration, with many T cells found in the sites of tissue injury at autopsy and in biopsy specimens from patients. Findings have also shown that human RNP reactive T cells can provide B-cell help *in vitro* to anti-RNP autoantibody production.[27,39]

Vascular alterations result in some of the most severe clinical manifestations in patients with MCTD. Uncontrolled overexpression of angiogenic and angiostatic factors (vascular endothelial growth factor [VEGF] and endostatin) were found in adult MCTD patients. Levels of VEGF were higher in MCTD patients with pulmonary arterial hypertension (PAH) and myositis, possibly characterizing patients with a more severe course of disease.[42]

A murine model for MCTD has been developed, and it will assist in advancing preclinical and translational research in MCTD.[43]

Clinical Manifestations

MCTD has been recognized with increasing frequency in childhood.[23,44-60] These children present with features of more than one CTD, a speckled antinuclear antibody (ANA) pattern, and high titers of antibody to RNP (see Table 29-1). The condition characteristically evolves over time from a more limited presentation of clinical disease to one with overlapping features of JRA, SLE, CSS, or JDM. Manifestations develop sequentially, but not in any predictable order or over any circumscribed period. The rashes of SLE or JDM are common at onset. Sclerodermatous skin changes are slow to develop but may become the most prominent feature of the disease late in its course. Moderately asymptomatic involvement, such as myositis with minimal weakness, mild atrophy, and minimal to moderate increases in the serum muscle enzyme concentrations, is common. Van der Net et al. showed that proximal muscle strength, as well as aerobic capacity, was significantly impaired in one cohort.[61] Dysphagia and bowel dysmotility also may occur. Manifestations of the sicca syndrome with xerostomia, keratoconjunctivitis sicca, or parotid gland enlargement occur in one third of the children.[62] Although children typically do not complain of shortness of breath (depending on cognitive development or unconsciously self-imposed restriction of activity), they often have pulmonary functional impairments.

Clinical characteristics of children from selected studies are summarized in Table 29-3. Polyarthritis (93%) and Raynaud phenomenon (85%) are the most common manifestations at onset (Fig. 29-1). The

TABLE 29-3 Disease Characteristics of Children with Mixed Connective Tissue Disease

CHARACTERISTIC	NUMBER REPORTED*	NUMBER PRESENT†	PERCENT
Arthritis	72	67	93
Raynaud phenomenon	72	61	85
Sclerodermatous skin	67	33	49
Rash of systemic lupus erythematosus	67	22	33
Rash of dermatomyositis	67	22	33
Fever	61	34	56
Abnormal esophageal motility	56	23	41
Cardiac disease	67	20	30
Pericarditis	67	18	27
Muscle disease	72	44	61
Sicca syndrome	66	24	36
Central nervous system disease	61	14	23
Lung			
Abnormal diffusion	56	24	43
Restrictive disease	56	8	14
Hypertension	56	4	7
Effusion	56	13	23
Radiographic changes only	56	1	2
Splenomegaly	63	18	29
Hepatomegaly	68	19	28
Renal disease	72	19	26
Anti-dsDNA positive	64	13	20
Anti-Sm positive	58	6	10
Anti-RNP positive	72	72	100
Rheumatoid factor positive	57	39	68

*The number of children in whom the characteristic was identified.
†The number in whom the abnormality was present.
Data from 10 reports with a total of 72 children: References 1, 44, 45, 46, 47, 48, 51, 52, 63, 75.

arthritis may be relatively painful; erosive disease is uncommon, but deformity may develop with flexion contractions or swan-neck deformities. The arthritis is often associated with rheumatoid factor (RF) seropositivity, which often presents early, in approximately two thirds of the children. Cutaneous changes include scleroderma-like disease in one half of MCTD patients, the rash of SLE in one third, and the rash of JDM in one third. Nailfold capillary abnormalities are similar to those in CSS.[63-65] Cardiopulmonary disease and esophageal dysmotility occur more frequently than clinical symptoms indicate.[66] Vasculitis can occur and be severe (i.e., transverse myelopathy). Although nephritis occurs in about one fourth of the patients with MCTD, it is less common and is usually less severe than in those with SLE. However, children with MCTD may have more frequent and more severe renal disease, more hematological complications, such as thrombocytopenia, and less pulmonary hypertension than do adults with MCTD.[57,59,67] Trigeminal neuropathy has been reported as a presenting symptom.[68,69]

Pulmonary disease is a major source of morbidity and mortality among adults who have MCTD. In a prospective longitudinal study, 31

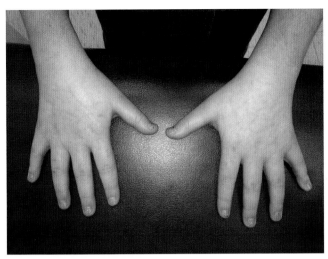

FIGURE 29-1 The hands of a 9-year-old patient with MCTD demonstrating swelling and mild skin rash.

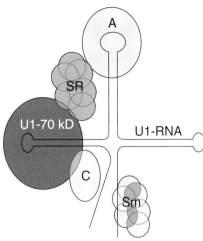

FIGURE 29-2 The U1-RNP. The U1-RNP is composed of an RNA backbone, U1-RNA, three proteins highly specific for the U1-RNP (the U1-A, U1-C, and U1-70 kD proteins), and a series of additional proteins common to multiple U-RNP and RNA splicing macromolecules (Sm and SR). From E.L. Greidinger, R.W. Hoffman, Autoantibodies in the pathogenesis of mixed connective tissue disease, Rheum. Dis. Clin. N. Am. 31 (2005) 437–450.

of 34 adults with high titers of RNP antibody had typical MCTD in which pulmonary disease, often initially asymptomatic, was common.[70] Pulmonary hypertension was the most frequent serious complication. One retrospective study in pediatric patients found restrictive pulmonary disease in up to 35% and abnormal carbon monoxide diffusion (DLCO) in up to 42%.[59] This retrospective data may represent a select patient population. A cross-sectional study focusing on chest manifestations in juvenile-onset MCTD patients identified interstitial lung disease in 25% of the cohort. All but one had mild disease affecting 5% or less of the parenchyma. DLCO was abnormal in 33%. The authors concluded that the prevalence of interstitial lung disease in childhood-onset MCTD was lower than previously thought.[71]

Pathology

Widespread intimal proliferation and medial hypertrophy of vascular walls have been described in four children with MCTD who died.[72] Renal biopsies in eight additional patients confirmed abnormalities of the glomerular basement membrane or vascular sclerosis. These investigators commented that although the histopathology of MCTD resembled that of CSS, the extent of fibrosis was less, and intimal vascular abnormalities in larger vessels such as the aorta, and the coronary, pulmonary, and renal arteries, were more prominent. Another study reported pulmonary hypertension and proliferative vasculopathy in the virtual absence of interstitial fibrosis in patients with MCTD, in contrast to those with CSS.[70]

Histological analysis of esophageal muscular layers was reported from 27 autopsy cases in adults with MCTD. The most striking change observed was atrophy and loss of smooth muscle cells followed by fibrosis. Immunohistochemically, the degenerated muscular tissues of the esophagus were positive for anti-IgG and anti-C3 antibodies, but not for IgM antibodies. The IgG fractions isolated from MCTD patients reacted with smooth muscle from nonconnective tissues disease cases, suggesting that serum antibodies may be involved in tissue damage.[73]

Laboratory Examination

Very high titers of ANAs are usually present initially, often in a speckled pattern on HEp-2 cell substrate. These antibodies react specifically with an RNase-sensitive component of ENA and RNP. Anti-RNP antibodies in high titers have been the serological hallmark of MCTD, but these antibodies may be present in low titers in other diseases, such as

SLE.[11,39,45,74] Further investigations confirmed that the most characteristic specificities of the anti-RNP antibodies in MCTD were directed against a uridine-rich (U1), small nuclear RNP (snRNP) complex (U1 snRNP) of the spliceosome consisting of U1-RNA and the associated 70-kD, A, and C polypeptides (Fig. 29-2).[27,39,75-79] The anti-U1 snRNP profile of patients with MCTD is characterized by a high-titer antibody response, predominantly or solely of IgG antibodies, and specificity for an epitope different from that of SLE sera[11]; a false-positive anti-U1 snRNP antibody response may be observed in cases of SLE.[80] IgM-specific anti-U1 snRNP responses have been shown to distinguish SLE from MCTD patients.[81] Reports indicate that antibodies to U1-RNA are even more closely associated clinically with disease activity during the course of MCTD than are U1-RNP antibodies,[82-84] although assays for U1-RNA antibodies themselves are poorly standardized and of limited availability to clinicians in most areas; this makes this observation primarily one of research relevance.

Substantial advances have been made in employing specific autoantibody activities against the U1 snRNP polypeptides for classification of disease.[11,85] In contrast to patients with CTDs who did not demonstrate these antibody activities, there were significant clinical associations with Raynaud phenomenon, swollen hands, sclerodactyly, telangiectasia, and abnormal esophageal motility among adult patients with high titers of autoantibodies against the U1-70 kD antigen.[24] In the study by DeRooij and colleagues,[23] all five children who had antibodies against the U1-70 kD antigen had clinical disease characterized by arthralgia or arthritis, swollen hands, Raynaud phenomenon, and abnormalities of pulmonary function.

Some MCTD sera, including those from patients without renal disease, also react with B/B′ polypeptides, but probably to one or more epitopes different from those characteristic of the anti-Sm antibody activity found in SLE.[85,86]

In a prospective investigation of 11 children with MCTD,[19] antibodies to U1 snRNP polypeptides were compared sequentially during the course of the disease. All patients had high-titer anti-ENA antibodies determined by hemagglutination (greater than 1:1,000,000) and positive anti-RNP reactivity by immunodiffusion. Antigenic specificity identified by immunoblot analysis and enzyme-linked immunosorbent assay was to the 70-kD polypeptide in 11 patients; A in 10; C in 2; B/B′ in 9; and D in 3. Four children had both IgG and IgM antibodies to the 70-kD protein, five to the A peptide, two to B/B′, and only one to D. One patient developed low-titer anti-Sm antibodies, and three developed low-titer, transient anti-double-stranded DNA (anti-dsDNA) seropositivity. Three had anti-Ro/SS-A antibodies. Anti-ENA titers and 70-kD reactivity decreased in patients during prolonged remission; positive reactions remained in those with continuing active disease and in patients receiving only symptomatic treatment. The predominant HLA antigens were DR2 in six of nine children and DR4 in four of nine; all children were either DR2 or DR4 positive, similar to findings in adults with MCTD.

Hematological abnormalities are seen in childhood MCTD. Anemia in up to 64%[87] and leukopenia in 9% to 58%[11,57,58,79] have been reported. Thrombocytopenia in 40% was emphasized in early series of children with MCTD[45]; however, later series have reported 9% to 21%.[11,59,74,87,88] When it occurs, it can be severe and resistant to conventional therapy.[45,74] Hypocomplementemia has been reported in 10% to 30% of patients.[58,59,60,74] RF is commonly seen, as are elevated muscle enzymes. Hypergammaglobulinemia is noted to be common when it is reported.[81] Some patients have marked elevations of serum Ig levels, especially of IgG.[46-51] Two children with selective IgA deficiency have been reported.[43,74] Vitamin D insufficiency was prevalent in a population of adult MCTD patients.[89] Vitamin D levels in children with MCTD have not been studied.

In a study of adults with MCTD,[90] 48 anti-U1-70 kD antibody–positive patients with MCTD were compared with 59 anti-U1-70 kD antibody–negative patients with classic SLE. Although levels of antiphospholipid antibodies were increased in the patients with MCTD compared with control subjects, levels of these antibodies were even higher in the patients with SLE who had clinical manifestations of the antiphospholipid antibody syndrome in which deep vein thrombosis, pulmonary embolism, recurrent fetal loss, chorea, livedo reticularis, severe thrombocytopenia, and avascular necrosis occurred. In adult patients, the presence of antiphospholipid antibodies and antiendothelial cell antibodies correlated with the development of pulmonary hypertension.[90,91] A study of adult Hungarian individuals with MCTD found that the presence of antiphospholipid antibodies raised the risk of mortality.[92]

Treatment

There is no specific treatment for MCTD. Management should address the predominant problems of the child, such as arthritis, cutaneous disease, or visceral involvement. Many children respond satisfactorily to low-dose glucocorticoids, nonsteroidal antiinflammatory drugs, hydroxychloroquine, or a combination of these medications.[59,74,87] Raynaud phenomenon should be treated with nonpharmacological measures, such as avoidance of cold and emotional stress. Patients should be instructed to keep their entire body warm, not just their hands. Vasodilating agents, most commonly calcium channel blockers, are used in severe cases. Nifedipine is the most extensively studied agent. Patients with severe myositis, renal, or visceral disease generally require high-dose glucocorticoids and sometimes require cytotoxic drugs (cyclophosphamide), especially for life-threatening complications such as pulmonary hypertension.[93] In recent years, several new agents have emerged for the treatment of pulmonary hypertension in adults, including prostacyclin analogs[94-96] and endothelin receptor antagonists.[96,97,98] There is limited experience with the use of these agents in children, but the results are promising.[99] Methotrexate has been advocated,[59,100] and authors have also reported the use of mycophenolate mofetil, etanercept, azathioprine, cyclosporine, and

infliximab in children with MCTD.[59,87] Case studies have described the use of imatinib and immunoadsorption.[101,102] Rituximab has been used, especially in cases of refractory thrombocytopenia.[103] Autologous hemopoietic stem-cell transplantation has been attempted for refractory, life-threatening disease.[104]

Course of the Disease and Prognosis

The long-term outcomes of children with MCTD are varied and unpredictable.[57,58,74,78,87] Deaths have been reported from disease resembling that of SLE accompanied by renal failure. In contrast to SLE, however, morbidity and mortality in MCTD are more often associated with development of pulmonary hypertension (7%)[49,52,74,70,105] or gradually evolving restrictive pulmonary disease (15%) with minimal fibrosis.[45,49,67] Pulmonary dysfunction may be underestimated clinically, because it tends to develop insidiously.[70] Another ominous development is severe thrombocytopenia (20%), which is often resistant to conventional therapy. This complication is more common in children than in adults.[74]

In a retrospective review, Tiddens and colleagues[87] (see Table 29-4) reported 14 children with MCTD who met the criteria of Kasukawa and co-workers,[8] with a mean follow-up of 9.3 years (range: 3.8 to 14.1 years) and a mean age at onset of 10.6 years (range: 5.2 to 15.6 years of age). Features of the disease characteristic of SLE and JDM tended to disappear over time, whereas those of CSS, Raynaud phenomenon, and JRA persisted. At follow-up, thrombocytopenia persisted in three children; four had extensive limitation of range of joint movement, all had abnormal esophageal function, but none had active renal disease. No pulmonary hypertension was documented, although one half of the children had restrictive disease on function studies. Glucocorticoids were judged successful in managing MCTD but were associated with osteonecrosis in three children and growth retardation in one child.

The outcomes of children with MCTD were evaluated in a study in three U.S. Midwestern clinics[74] (Fig. 29-3). There were 21 girls and 6 boys, with a mean age at onset of 13 years (range: 5 to 18 years of age) and a mean duration of disease of 8 years (range: 1 to 18 years). Organ systems predominantly involved at onset and at follow-up at 8 years or more were the joints (24 and 11 patients, respectively); muscles (8 and 9); skin (16 and 8); lungs (10 and 13); heart (7 and 4); gastrointestinal tract (5 and 5); and kidneys (3 and 4). A characteristic onset involved Raynaud phenomenon, arthritis, swollen hands, myositis, and the cutaneous features of JDM or SLE. Cutaneous disease, esophageal dysfunction, myositis, and arthritis were prominent during the entire course of the disease. These clinical features were similar to those of adults with MCTD, with less frequent and less severe pulmonary disease, and only one instance of pulmonary hypertension. Five patients developed severe thrombocytopenia. All patients had positive immunodiffusion results for anti-RNP antibodies. Anti-ENA antibodies were found in titers up to 1:16,000,000 by hemagglutination and were often maintained at high levels for many years; concentrations ultimately declined if the course stabilized or the patient entered remission. Transient, low-titer anti-dsDNA antibodies were present in eight patients. Hypocomplementemia occurred in eight patients, and high titers of RF in seven patients. Twelve patients had good or stable outcomes, and five had prolonged remissions. Seven developed progressive disease, and four died of renal disease, diffuse intravascular coagulation, or cardiopulmonary failure.

Michels[88] reviewed the course of MCTD in 224 children reported until 1996, including 33 patients from the Rheuma-Kinderklinik in Garmisch-Partenkirchen, Germany. Because this review involved a number of studies over many years that were often retrospective and without serological or genetic characterization by current standards,

TABLE 29-4 Clinical Findings of Childhood MCTD at Presentation, Cumulative over Time, and at Most Recent Evaluation

	HOFFMAN ET AL.[19]		MIER ET AL.[59]			TIDDENS ET AL.[87]	
	PRESENTATION (%)	CUMULATIVE (%)	PRESENTATION (%)	CUMULATIVE (%)	MOST RECENT EVALUATION (%)	PRESENT DURING DISEASE COURSE (%)	MOST RECENT EVALUATION (%)
Raynaud phenomenon	9 (82)	9 (82)	81	94	88	13 (93)	12 (86)
Polyarthropathy	11 (100)	11 (100)	91	94	48	10 (71)	7 (50)
Swollen hands	6 (55)	9 (82)	65	68	19	11 (79)	6 (43)
Sclerodactyly	4 (36)	7 (64)	12	26	24	12 (86)	12 (86)
Proximal muscle weakness	4 (36)	6 (55)	34	—	9	7 (70)	7 (50)
Pleuritis/pericarditis	4 (36)a	5 (45)a	—	12/16		3 (21)	0 (0)
Esophageal dysmotility	3 (27)b	6 (55)b	25	21d	33	—	10/10 (100)b
Pulmonary dysfunction	3 (27)c	9 (82)c	22/21e	35/42f	64/58g	9 (64)h	7/2 (53/15)i
Leukopenia/lymphopenia	1 (9)	4 (36)	—	36	—	7 (50)	9 (64)
Thrombocytopenia	1 (9)	2 (18)	—	18	—	3 (21)	1 (7)

aPleural effusion.
bDetermined by barium esophagography, manometry, or both.
cDecreased carbon monoxide (CO) diffusion.
dDocumented objectively.
eRestrictive lung disease, 22; decreased CO diffusion, 21.
fRestrictive lung disease, 35; decreased CO diffusion, 42.
gRestrictive lung disease, 64; decreased CO diffusion, 58.
hRestrictive lung disease.
iRestrictive lung disease, 7/13; decreased CO diffusion, 2/13.

Disease characteristics of MCTD

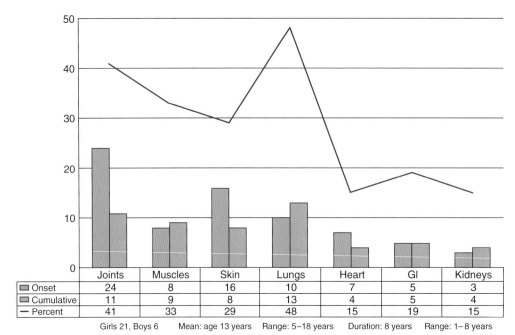

	Joints	Muscles	Skin	Lungs	Heart	GI	Kidneys
▨ Onset	24	8	16	10	7	5	3
▨ Cumulative	11	9	8	13	4	5	4
— Percent	41	33	29	48	15	19	15

Girls 21, Boys 6   Mean: age 13 years   Range: 5–18 years   Duration: 8 years   Range: 1–8 years

FIGURE 29-3 Characteristics of MCTD at disease onset and cumulative for 27 children from three U.S. Midwestern clinics. Data from J.T. Cassidy, R.W. Hoffman, D.W. Wortmann et al., Long-term outcome of children with mixed connective tissue disease (MCTD), J. Rheumatol. 27 (2000) 100.

it predominantly reflects the clinical classifications and historical conclusions of the various centers. Nevertheless, this meta-analysis indicated that most of the children improved over time, and that remissions occurred in 3% to 27% of the series. Raynaud phenomenon and scleroderma-like skin changes were reported in up to 86% of the children. Long-term problems included loss of range of joint motion in 29%, renal disease in up to 47%, pulmonary restrictive disease in up to 57%, and esophageal dysmotility in up to 29%. Cardiovascular disease included cardiomyopathy, pericarditis, and pulmonary hypertension. Central nervous system (CNS) involvement was rare but could be severe: 17 (7.6%) of the 224 patients died of sepsis (7 patients), cerebral disease (3 patients), heart failure (2 patients), pulmonary hypertension (2 patients), renal failure (2 patients), or gastrointestinal bleeding (1 patient). It was concluded that this mortality rate was in a similar range as that for other major systemic CTDs and that otherwise the long-term problems in patients who survived were minor.

Mier and colleagues reviewed several reports of pediatric MCTD[57,60,87,88] and supplemented the data with information collected by the authors from 34 pediatric patients with MCTD from seven pediatric rheumatology centers.[59] Similar to other studies, they noted in their series that manifestations of inflammation, such as muscle weakness, arthritis, and hand swelling, were present more often at disease onset, and they decreased in frequency over time, whereas scleroderma-like manifestations increased in frequency. In the authors' cohort, 3% had achieved remission, 82% exhibited a favorable outcome, and 15% exhibited an unfavorable outcome. Other features of the authors' cohort are shown in Table 29-4. Similar findings were noted in a cohort of 12 Taiwanese patients retrospectively reviewed.[106]

Kotajima and colleagues[57] compared two groups of Japanese patients with MCTD, one with onset when patients were younger than 16 years old and another with onset when patients were 16 years old

or older. Signs typical of SLE, such as facial erythema, photosensitivity, the presence of lupus erythematosus cells, lymphadenopathy, and cellular casts, were more common in the juvenile-onset group. Conversely, scleroderma-like symptoms, such as esophageal dysmotility, sclerodactyly, and pulmonary disease, were more common in the older group. The investigators also found that swelling of the hands occurred less frequently in children. The mortality rate was approximately 2.8% for the juvenile-onset group. Compared with other CTDs, these outcomes were interpreted as relatively favorable.

The long-term outcomes of 47 adults and children with MCTD who met the criteria of Kasukawa and co-workers[8] and were followed for 3 to 29 years, were studied by Burdt and colleagues.[105] In 23% of the patients, the disease began during childhood. All patients had antibodies to the 70-kD polypeptide of U1-RNP; 81% to A; 79% to B/B'; 48% to C; and 14% to D. Anti-U1-RNA was positive in 89% of the patients, and these antibody levels correlated with the activity of the disease. Initially, epitope spreading was observed as a feature of active MCTD, and with time, antibody reactivity was selectively reduced in patients in remission (i.e., epitope contraction). HLA-DR4 and HLA-DR2 were present in 23 (85%) of 27 patients. Inflammatory features of the disease, such as Raynaud phenomenon and esophageal hypomotility, diminished over time, whereas pulmonary hypertension and CNS disease persisted despite treatment. Sclerodactyly was frequent (49%), but diffuse sclerosis occurred in only 19% of patients. Antibodies to centromere, Scl-70, and PM-1/PM-Scl antigens were not detected. Renal disease developed in five patients (11%; World Health Organization class III in two patients, class IV in two, and classes III and V in one). Eleven patients died 3 to 25 years after the onset of MCTD, with pulmonary hypertension the major contributory factor in nine deaths and often associated with the presence of anticardiolipin antibodies. A favorable outcome was documented in 62% of the patients, with 36% in remission leading normal lives without functional disabilities at the time of the study.

UNDIFFERENTIATED CONNECTIVE TISSUE DISEASE AND OVERLAP SYNDROMES

A number of patients have some features of CTD but lack adequate clinical or diagnostic features to fit a recognizable clinical syndrome. The term *undifferentiated connective tissue disease* (UCTD) is often used to designate such patients. The term was first used by Leroy and colleagues in 1980 to describe an early phase of CTDs when the findings were nonspecific and indistinct.[107] Subsequent authors have used the term, although uniform criteria have not been determined. The patient's characteristics may range from the presence of a single clinical or laboratory finding, such as a positive ANA, to the presence of a number of clinical or serological features. Disease initially classified as UCTD may evolve into a clinically recognizable rheumatic disease, or the condition may remain with inadequate features for classification as a well-recognized rheumatic disease. Several reports of adult cohorts have been published.[107-116] Alarcon and colleagues have published a series of studies examining the evolution of UCTD and classification of the rheumatic diseases. Their studies indicate that a moderate percentage of patients will evolve into recognizable disease, although many remain characterized as UCTD.[108-113] Observations by Bombardieri indicated that in their cohort, patients with UCTD did not progress into distinctively recognizable rheumatic diseases.[114-115]

An individual's antibody response to a self-antigen is usually focused on one or two epitopes within the protein, which are termed *dominant*. However, the entire protein or particle (such as a spliceosome) is taken up by the antigen-processing cells and is therefore subject to antigen processing. Depending on the polymorphisms of the individual's HLA molecules, there may be diversification of the antibody response to include some other antigens. This process is called *epitope spreading* and is important in the development of the linked antibody responses observed in patients with autoimmune disease.[117-118] In this way, an immune response may become modified over time; this change has been associated with changes in the clinical picture.[105] This may occur in patients with UCTD or in patients with a well-established CTD.

The term *overlap syndrome* is sometimes confused with the term *undifferentiated connective tissue disease*. The term *overlap syndrome* is typically applied to patients who have two or more distinctly recognizable rheumatic diseases. Although the concept seems uncomplicated, classification remains somewhat controversial; e.g., a patient with features of RA and systemic lupus may represent a distinct clinical entity or may reflect the coexistence of two rheumatic conditions in a patient, which is based on chance rather than a specific entity. There may also be some question (e.g., of an erosive arthritis occurring in systemic lupus) whether it is the coexistence of RA or the fact that erosive arthritis could be a feature of systemic lupus at times. The precise relationship of such coexisting conditions ultimately awaits a more complete understanding of the genetics and pathogenesis of autoimmunity and the CTDs.

One approach to classification of rheumatic diseases is the use of antibodies as disease markers. There are several overlap syndromes, such as MCTD, identifiable by the presence of specific autoantibodies. These conditions are clinically defined by the presence of characteristics of two or more defined rheumatic diseases and the presence of specific autoantibodies. In addition to MCTD, other well-defined overlap syndromes associated with specific autoantibodies include synthetase syndromes associated with antibodies to aminoacyl-transfer RNA synthetases and clinically associated with myositis, arthritis, and pulmonary involvement. Anti-Jo-1 antibody (anti-histidyl-tRNA synthetase) is the most common and best characterized of the antisynthetase antibodies. Patients with PM-Scl autoantibodies have features of polymyositis and limited scleroderma.[119,120] These overlap syndromes have been described in children.[121,122]

REFERENCES

1. G.C. Sharp, W.S. Irvin, E.M. Tan, et al., Mixed connective tissue disease: an apparently distinct rheumatic disease syndrome associated with a specific antibody to an extractable nuclear antigen (ENA), Am. J. Med. 52 (1972) 148–159.
2. S.H. Nimelstein, S. Brody, D. McShane, et al., Mixed connective tissue disease: a subsequent evaluation of the original 25 patients, Medicine (Baltimore) 59 (1980) 239–248.
5. R.W. Hoffman, G.C. Sharp, Is anti-U1-RNP autoantibody positive connective tissue disease genetically distinct? J. Rheumatol. 22 (1995) 586–589.
7. G.C. Sharp, Diagnostic criteria for classification of MCTD, in: R. Kasukawa, G.C. Sharp (Eds.), Mixed Connective Tissue Disease and Anti-Nuclear Antibodies, Excerpta Medica, Amsterdam, 1987, pp. 23–32.
8. R. Kasukawa, T. Tojo, S. Miyawaki, et al., Preliminary diagnostic criteria for classification of mixed connective tissue disease, in: R. Kasukawa, G.C. Sharp (Eds.), Mixed Connective Tissue Disease and Anti-Nuclear Antibodies, Excerpta Medica, Amsterdam, 1987, pp. 41–48.
9. D. Alarcón-Segovia, M. Villarreal, Classification and diagnostic criteria for mixed connective tissue disease, in: R. Kasukawa, G.C. Sharp (Eds.), Mixed Connective Tissue Disease and Anti-Nuclear Antibodies, Excerpta Medica, Amsterdam, 1987, pp. 33–40.
11. J.S. Smolen, G. Steiner, Mixed connective tissue disease: to be or not to be? Arthritis Rheum. 41 (1998) 768–777.
13. J.M. Amigues, A. Cantagrel, M. Abbal, et al., Comparative study of 4 diagnosis criteria sets for mixed connective tissue disease in patients with anti-RNP antibodies. Autoimmunity Group of the Hospitals of Toulouse, J. Rheumatol. 23 (1996) 2055–2062.
15. S. Bowyer, P. Roettcher, Pediatric rheumatology clinic populations in the United States: results of a 3 year survey, pediatric rheumatology database research group, J. Rheumatol. 23 (1996) 1968–1974.
19. R.W. Hoffman, J.T. Cassidy, Y. Takeda, et al., U1-70-kd autoantibody-positive mixed connective tissue disease in children: a longitudinal clinical and serologic analysis, Arthritis Rheum. 36 (1993) 1599–1602.
23. D.J. de Rooij, T. Fiselier, L.B. van de Putte, et al., Juvenile-onset mixed connective tissue disease: clinical, serological and follow-up data, Scand. J. Rheumatol. 18 (1989) 157–160.
24. R.W. Hoffman, L.J. Rettenmaier, Y. Takeda, et al., Human autoantibodies against the 70-kd polypeptide of U1 small nuclear RNP are associated with HLA-DR4 among connective tissue disease patients, Arthritis Rheum. 33 (1990) 666–673.
27. R.W. Hoffman, M.E. Maldonado, Immune pathogenesis of Mixed Connective Tissue Disease: a short analytical review, Clin. Immunol. 128 (2008) 8–17.
28. R.W. Hoffman, E.L. Greidinger, Mixed connective tissue disease, Curr. Op. Rheumatol. 12 (2000) 386–390.
36. A. Marshak-Rothstein, Toll-like receptors in systemic auto-immune disease, Nat. Rev. Immunol. 6 (2006) 823–835.
39. E.L. Greidinger, R.W. Hoffman, Autoantibodies in the pathogenesis of mixed connective tissue disease, Rheum. Dis. Clin. North Am. 31 (2005) 437–450.
40. M.R. Arbuckle, M.T. McClain, M.V. Rubertone, et al., Development of autoantibodies before the clinical onset of systemic lupus erythematosus, N. Engl. J. Med. 349 (2003) 1526–1533.
42. J.H.W. Distler, T. Strapatsas, D. Huscher, et al., Dysbalance of angiogenic and angiostatic mediators in patients with mixed connective tissue disease, Ann. Rheum. Dis. 70 (2011) 1197–1202.
44. D.Y. Sanders, C.C. Huntley, G.C. Sharp, Mixed connective tissue disease in a child, J. Pediatr. 83 (1973) 642–645.
45. B.H. Singsen, H.K. Kornreich, K. Koster-King, et al., Mixed connective tissue disease in children, Arthritis Rheum. 20 (1977) 355–360.
46. A. Fraga, J. Gudino, F. Ramos-Niembro, et al., Mixed connective tissue disease in childhood: relationship to Sjögren's syndrome, Am. J. Dis. Child. 132 (1978) 263–265.

47. M. Rosenthal, Juvenile sharp syndrome (mixed connective tissue disease), Helv. Paediatr. Acta 33 (1978) 251–258.

48. S.A. Peskett, B.M. Ansell, P. Fizzman, et al., Mixed connective tissue disease in children, Rheumatol. Rehabil. 17 (1978) 245–248.

51. W.J. Oetgen, J.A. Boice, O.J. Lawless, Mixed connective tissue disease in children and adolescents, Pediatrics 67 (1981) 333–337.

57. L. Kotajima, S. Aotsuka, M. Sumiya, et al., Clinical features of patients with juvenile onset mixed connective tissue disease: analysis of data collected in a nationwide collaborative study in Japan, J. Rheumatol. 23 (1996) 1088–1094.

58. S. Yokota, T. Imagawa, S. Katakura, et al., Mixed connective tissue disease in childhood: a nationwide retrospective study in Japan, Acta Paediatr. Jpn. 39 (1997) 273–276.

59. R.J. Mier, M. Shishov, G.C. Higgins, et al., Pediatric-onset mixed connective tissue disease, Rheum. Dis. Clin. North Am. 31 (2005) 483–496.

60. S. Yokota, Mixed connective tissue disease in childhood, Acta Paediatr. Jpn. 35 (1993) 472–479.

61. J. van der Net, B. Wissink, A. van Royen, et al., Aerobic capacity and muscle strength in juvenile-onset mixed connective tissue disease (MCTD), Scand. J. Rheumatol. 39 (2010) 387–392.

70. W.D. Sullivan, D.J. Hurst, C.E. Harmon, et al., A prospective evaluation emphasizing pulmonary involvement in patients with mixed connective tissue disease, Medicine (Baltimore) 63 (1984) 92–107.

71. T.M. Aaløkken, V. Lilleby, V. Søyseth, et al., Chest abnormalities in juvenile-onset mixed connective tissue disease: assessment with high-resolution computed tomography and pulmonary function tests, Acta Radiol. 4 (2009) 430–436.

72. B.H. Singsen, V.L. Swanson, B.H. Bernstein, et al., A histologic evaluation of mixed connective tissue disease in childhood, Am. J. Med. 68 (1980) 710–717.

73. M. Uzuki, A. Kamataki, M. Watanabe, et al., Histologic analysis of esophageal muscular layers from 27 autopsy cases with mixed connective tissue disease (MCTD), Pathol. Res. Pract. 207 (2011) 383–390.

74. J.T. Cassidy, R.W. Hoffman, D.W. Wortmann, et al., Long-term outcome of children with mixed connective tissue disease (MCTD), J. Rheumatol. 27 (2000) 100.

76. I. Pettersson, G. Wang, E.I. Smith, et al., The use of immunoblotting and immunoprecipitation of (U) small nuclear ribonucleoproteins in the analysis of sera of patients with mixed connective tissue disease and systemic lupus erythematosus: cross-sectional, longitudinal study, Arthritis Rheum. 29 (1986) 986–996.

85. Y. Takeda, G.S. Wang, R.J. Wang, et al., Enzyme-linked immunosorbent assay using isolated (U) small nuclear ribonucleoprotein polypeptides as antigens to investigate the clinical significance of autoantibodies to these polypeptides, Clin. Immunol. Immunopathol. 50 (1989) 213–230.

86. M. Takano, S.S. Golden, G.C. Sharp, et al., Molecular relationships between two nuclear antigens, ribonucleoprotein and Sm: purification of active antigens and their biochemical characterization, Biochemistry 20 (1981) 5929–5936.

87. H.A. Tiddens, J.J. van der Net, E.R. Graeff-Meeder, et al., Juvenile-onset mixed connective tissue disease: longitudinal follow-up, J. Pediatr. 122 (1993) 191–197.

88. H. Michels, Course of mixed connective tissue disease in children, Ann. Med. 29 (1997) 359–364.

90. G.R. Komatireddy, G.S. Wang, G.C. Sharp, et al., Antiphospholipid antibodies among anti-U1-70 kDa autoantibody positive patients with mixed connective tissue disease, J. Rheumatol. 24 (1997) 319–322.

91. T. Nishimaki, S. Aostsuka, H. Kondo, et al., Immunological analysis of pulmonary hypertension in connective tissue disease, J. Rheumatol. 26 (1999) 2357–2362.

92. A. Hajas, P. Szodoray, B. Nakken, et al., Clinical course, prognosis, and causes of death in mixed connective tissue disease, J. Rheumatol. 40 (2013) 1134–1142.

93. X. Jais, D. Launay, A. Yaici, et al., Immunosuppressive therapy in lupus- and mixed connective tissue disease-associated pulmonary arterial hypertension: a retrospective analysis of twenty-three cases, Arthritis Rheum. 58 (2008) 521–531.

95. R.J. Barst, L.J. Rubin, W.A. Long, et al., A comparison of continuous intravenous epoprostenol (prostacyclin) with conventional therapy for primary pulmonary hypertension: The Primary Pulmonary Hypertension Study Group, N. Engl. J. Med. 334 (1996) 296–302.

96. T.M. Bull, K.A. Fagan, D.B. Badesch, Pulmonary vascular manifestations of mixed connective tissue disease, Rheum. Dis. Clin. North Am. 31 (2005) 451–464.

98. L.J. Rubin, D.B. Badesch, R.J. Barst, et al., Bosentan therapy for pulmonary arterial hypertension, N. Engl. J. Med. 46 (2002) 896–903.

99. S.G. Haworth, A.A. Hislop, Treatment and survival in children with pulmonary arterial hypertension: the UK Pulmonary Hypertension Service for Children 2001–2006, Heart (2009) 312–317.

100. S. Nakata, K. Uematsu, T. Mori, et al., Effective treatment with low-dose methotrexate pulses of a child of mixed connective tissue disease with severe myositis refractory to corticosteroid, Nihon Rinsho Meneki Gakkai Kaishi 20 (1997) 178–183 (Article in Japanese).

103. B. Jovancevic, C. Lindholm, R. Pullerits, Anti B-cell therapy against refractory thrombocytopenia in SLE and MCTD patients: long term follow-up and review of the literature, Lupus 22 (2013) 664–674.

106. Y.Y. Tsai, Y.H. Yang, H.H. Yu, et al., Fifteen-year experience of pediatric-onset mixed connective tissue disease, Clin. Rheumatol. 29 (2010) 53–58.

107. E.C. LeRoy, H.R. Maricq, M.B. Kahaleh, Undifferentiated connective tissue syndromes, Arthritis Rheum. 23 (1980) 341–343.

108. G.S. Alarcon, G.V. Williams, J.Z. Singer, et al., Early undifferentiated connective tissue disease. I. Early clinical manifestation in a large cohort of patients with undifferentiated connective tissue diseases compared with cohorts of well-established connective tissue diseases, J. Rheumatol. 18 (1991) 1332–1339.

111. H.J. Williams, G.S. Alarcon, R. Joks, et al., Early undifferentiated connective tissue disease (CTD). VI. An inception cohort after 10 years: disease remissions and changes in diagnoses in well-established and undifferentiated CTD, J. Rheumatol. 26 (1999) 816–825.

113. J. Calvo-Alen, H.M. Bastian, K.V. Straaton, et al., Identification of patient subsets among those presumptively diagnosed with, referred, and/or followed up for systemic lupus erythematosus at a large tertiary care center, Arthritis Rheum. 38 (1995) 1475–1484.

115. M. Mosca, A. Tavoni, R. Neri, et al., Undifferentiated connective tissue diseases: the clinical and serological profiles of 91 patients followed for at least 1 year, Lupus 7 (1998) 95–100.

117. C.L. Vanderlugt, S.D. Miller, Epitope spreading in immune-mediated diseases: implications for immunotherapy, Nat. Rev. Immunol. 2 (2002) 85–95.

The entire reference list is available online at www.expertconsult.com.

SUGGESTED READINGS

M. Reichlin, P.J. Maddison, I. Targoff, et al., Antibodies to a nuclear/nucleolar antigen in patients with polymyositis overlap syndromes, J. Clin. Immunol. 4 (1984) 40–44.

CHAPTER 30

Sjögren Syndrome

Lori Tucker

The syndrome of chronic inflammation of the exocrine glands, principally the salivary and lacrimal glands, was first described by Henrik Sjögren, a Swedish ophthalmologist, who published in 1933 the first complete description of a disorder he named *keratoconjunctivitis sicca*.[1] He reported that the disorder occurred most often in menopausal women and that arthritis was a prominent feature of the disease, as well as raised erythrocyte sedimentation rate (ESR), anemia, and fever. This disease has been considered to be rare in children and adolescents; however, it has almost certainly been underdiagnosed and is probably more common than previously realized. It is now recognized that this disorder can affect children and adolescents, and that the presentation may be different from that in adults with this condition, which is one factor contributing to the low recognition of the disorder.

DEFINITION AND EPIDEMIOLOGY

Sjögren Syndrome (SS) is defined as a chronic autoimmune disease characterized by inflammation of the exocrine glands. The principal inflammatory targets are the salivary and lacrimal exocrine glands, resulting in dryness of the mucosal surfaces of the mouth and eyes. However, there can be more extensive exocrinopathy involving the skin, respiratory tract, and urogenital tracts. Extraglandular or systemic features can also be part of the disorder. Table 30-1 outlines the principal clinical manifestations of SS.

The reported incidence and prevalence of primary SS in the adult population varies depending on population studied. Estimates range from a prevalence rate of 0.098% to 3.6%, and an incidence rate ranging from 3.9 to 5.3 per 100,000 individuals.[2] A recent population-based epidemiology study done in Olmstead County, Minnesota, USA, using a medical records linkage data system and the American-European Consensus Group classification criteria for identification of cases, reported an annual incidence of 5.1 (95% confidence interval [CI] 4.1-6.1) per 100,000 individuals, increasing with age to 10.7 per 100,000 in people over the age of 75.[3] To date, there have been no studies reporting accurate incidence or prevalence of SS in childhood.

CLASSIFICATION

Sjögren syndrome is described as *primary Sjögren syndrome* (pSS) when there is no association with other autoimmune disease, and as *secondary Sjögren syndrome* (sSS) when there is another autoimmune disease present, most commonly systemic lupus erythematosus (SLE) or rheumatoid arthritis (RA).

Accurately diagnosing pSS is challenging, as many of the cardinal symptoms are common, and there is currently no gold standard diagnostic test. Therefore, since the mid-1960s, a number of classification criteria sets have been proposed.[4] However, none of the proposed classification criteria sets for pSS in adults have gained universal acceptance.[5] The American-European Consensus Group (AECG) criteria, revised in 2002 (shown in Box 30-1), have been validated in adults with SS in whom the criteria has a sensitivity of 89.5% and a specificity of 95.2%.[6] In 2012, a new set of classification criteria was published by Shiboski et al.[7] and called the Sjögren International Collaborative Clinical Alliance criteria (SICCA-ACR) (Box 30-2). These criteria were developed in an attempt to simplify the process of making an accurate diagnosis while also defining a uniform group of patients to participate in clinical trials. The new criteria put less emphasis on subjective oral symptoms and do not include any objective salivary gland testing such as sialography or scintigraphy. A positive labial salivary gland biopsy is required. Patients with a positive antinuclear antibody (ANA) and rheumatoid factor (RF) but without positive anti-SSA or anti-SSB can satisfy the autoantibody criteria. A recent comparison of these two criteria sets was done by Rasmussen and colleagues[8] using a study cohort of 646 adult patients seen at two specialty clinics in the United States. There was a concordance rate of 81% between the two criteria sets, which suggests they are not significantly different. However, there was a subset of patients who fulfilled only one set of criteria but not the other; these differences primarily related to differences in the evaluation and scoring of ocular disease. In this comparison study, the most valuable criteria for confirming the diagnosis of SS regardless of classification system used were presence of anti-Ro/La serology and a positive minor salivary gland biopsy.[8] In a small case series of eight children diagnosed with pSS, reported by Saad-Magalhaes and colleagues, all patients underwent minor salivary gland biopsy, and all samples showed lymphocyte infiltration, although only five of eight had definitive focus scores. However, this paper demonstrates the possible value of this procedure in diagnosing pSS in children and adolescents.[9]

Bowman and Fox reviewed the current state of classification criteria for SS and suggest that moving toward a single valid accepted consensus criteria set would be most important for international standardization, particularly in relation to research.[4]

Bartunkova and colleagues[10] have proposed a set of criteria for the diagnosis of pSS in children, but these have not been validated (Box 30-3). The proposed pediatric criteria include parotid enlargement or recurrent parotitis, and additional laboratory tests not included in the adult classification criteria sets (elevated amylase, evidence of renal tubular acidosis [RTA], leukopenia, elevated ESR, ANAs, RF, and hypergammaglobulinemia). These clinical and laboratory findings seem to occur with increased frequency in pediatric SS. Houghton and colleagues[11] compared the usefulness of the AECG adult criteria and

TABLE 30-1 **Clinical Manifestations of Sjögren Syndrome**

Dry eyes	Xerophthalmia, keratoconjunctivitis sicca
Dry mouth	Xerostomia
Parotid swelling	
Extraglandular manifestations	Fatigue
	Arthritis
	Purpura
	Raynaud phenomenon
Pulmonary involvement	Interstitial pulmonary disease
	Small airways disease
Renal involvement	Nephritis
	Renal tubular acidosis
Neurological involvement	Peripheral neuropathy
	Central nervous system disease—rare

BOX 30-1 **American-European Consensus Group Classification Criteria for Sjögren Syndrome**

Ocular symptoms (positive answer to at least one of the following):
1. Have you had daily, persistent, troublesome dry eyes for more than 3 months?
2. Do you have a recurrent sensation of sand or gravel in the eyes?
3. Do you use tear substitutes more than three times a day?

Oral symptoms (positive answer to at least one of the following):
1. Have you had a daily feeling of dry mouth for more than 3 months?
2. Have you had recurrently or persistently swollen salivary glands as an adult?
3. Do you frequently drink liquids to aid in swallowing dry food?

Ocular signs (objective finding, positive result on at least one of the following):
1. Schirmer test, without anesthesia ($\leq$5 mm in 5 min)
2. Rose Bengal score ($\geq$4)

Histopathology: Focal lymphocytic sialadenitis from a minor salivary gland biopsy, evaluated by an expert histopathologist, with a focus score of $\geq$1 (defined as a number of lymphocytic focuses adjacent to normal mucous acini and containing >50 lymphocytes per 4 mm^2 of glandular tissue)

Salivary gland involvement: Objective evidence of salivary gland involvement defined as a positive result for at least one of the following diagnostic tests:
1. Unstimulated whole salivary flow ($\leq$1.5 mL in 15 min)
2. Parotid sialography showing the presence of diffuse sialectasis, without evidence of obstruction in the major ducts
3. Salivary scintigraphy showing delayed uptake, reduced concentration, and/or delayed excretion of tracer

Autoantibodies: Presence in the serum of antibodies to Ro (SSA) or La (SSB) antigens, or both

For diagnosis of primary SS:
Presence of four of six items, provided either histopathology or serology are positive
Presence of three of four objective items (ocular signs, histopathology, salivary gland involvement, or autoantibodies)

For diagnosis of secondary SS:
In patients with a potentially associated disease, presence of either ocular or oral symptoms, plus any two of ocular signs, histopathology, or salivary gland involvement.

Revised 2002, from Vitali, Bombardieri, Jonsson, et al., Classification criteria for Sjögren syndrome: a revised version of the European criteria proposed by the American-European Consensus Group, Ann. Rheum. Dis. 61 (2002) 554–558.

the proposed pediatric criteria in a group of six patients in British Columbia, and 128 cases found on literature review. The adult criteria were fulfilled by 14% of the local cases and 39% of reported pediatric cases, whereas the proposed pediatric criteria were fulfilled by 71% of the local cases and 76% of the reported pediatric cases. Although the new proposed pediatric criteria improved the diagnostic accuracy considerably, the conclusion of this study was that neither set of criteria was sensitive when compared with the gold standard of pediatric rheumatologist clinical diagnosis.

CLINICAL MANIFESTATIONS

Oral Manifestations

One of the principal clinical findings of SS is dryness of the oral mucosa (xerostomia), which is described in 90% of adults with SS.[12] Poor oral salivary flow can result in difficulty in swallowing dry food, a change in taste, halitosis, and an increase in dental caries. Report of these symptoms may be difficult to elicit from children or young adults.[13] Upon examination of the mouth, one may see dry, "sticky" mucosa, dental caries, or atrophy of the filiform papillae on the dorsum of the tongue.

Parotid enlargement is described in two thirds of adults with pSS, but it may be a more frequent feature in children diagnosed with SS. Review of the reported cases of pediatric SS demonstrates that parotitis is the most common presenting feature, present overall in 50% to 70% of children.[13,14] In many cases, the sole presenting complaint may be recurrent parotitis. Parotitis may be unilateral but frequently becomes bilateral and can be painful or painless. It is most often episodic, but it may be chronic in some patients. Children with recurrent episodes of parotid swelling are generally seen by a pediatrician or pediatric otolaryngologist for diagnosis. The differential diagnosis of recurrent parotid swelling in childhood (Box 30-4) includes infection, juvenile recurrent parotitis,[15] lymphoma, hemangiomas, and other rare inflammatory conditions.[16] Primary SS should be strongly considered in the differential diagnosis of a child with recurrent parotid swelling, and a complete diagnostic evaluation should be performed.[14,17,18] The reason that SS has been considered a "rare" disease in pediatrics is almost certainly the lack of recognition of SS as a potential cause of recurrent parotid swelling in children.

Ocular Manifestations

Patients with SS may experience a decrease in tear production due to inflammation of the lacrimal glands, which leads to damage to the corneal and bulbar epithelium (keratoconjunctivitis sicca). The symptoms of ocular involvement in SS include burning sensations in the eye, a feeling of having a foreign body in the eye, a "sandy" or scratchy feeling under the lids, itchiness, erythema of the eyes, or photosensitivity. Description of these symptoms may be difficult to elicit from children. On examination, one may find pericorneal irritation, dilation of conjunctival vessels, or enlargement of the lacrimal glands.

BOX 30-2 American College of Rheumatology SICCA (Sjögren International Collaborative Clinical Alliance) Classification Criteria

The classification of SS, which applies to individuals with signs and symptoms that may be suggestive of SS, will be met in patients who have at least two of the following three objective features:

1. Positive serum anti-SSA/Ro and/or anti-SSB/La or positive rheumatoid factor and ANA titer ≥1:320
2. Labial salivary gland biopsy exhibiting focal lymphocytic sialadenitis with a focus score ≥1 focus/4 mm^2
3. Keratoconjunctivitis sicca with ocular staining score ≥3 (assuming that the individual is not currently using daily eye drops for glaucoma and has not had corneal surgery or cosmetic eyelid surgery in the previous 5 years)

Prior diagnosis of any of the following conditions would exclude participation in SS studies or therapeutic trials because of overlapping clinical features or interference with criteria tests:

History of head and neck radiation treatment

Hepatitis C infection

Acquired immunodeficiency syndrome

Sarcoidosis

Amyloidosis

Graft-versus-host disease

IgG4-related disease

From Shiboski, Shiboski, Criswell, et al., American College of Rheumatology classification criteria for Sjögren's syndrome: a data-driven, expert consensus approach in the Sjögren's International Collaborative Clinical Alliance cohort, Arthritis Care Res. 64 (4) (2012) 475–487.

BOX 30-3 Proposed Criteria for Juvenile Primary Sjögren Syndrome

I. Clinical symptoms
  1. Oral (dry mouth, recurrent parotitis, or enlargement of parotid glands)
  2. Ocular (recurrent conjunctivitis without obvious allergic or infectious etiology, keratoconjunctivitis sicca)
  3. Other mucosal involvement (recurrent vaginitis)
  4. Systemic (fever of unknown origin, noninflammatory arthralgias, hypokalemic paralysis, abdominal pain)
II. Immunological abnormalities (presence of at least one of the following: anti-SSA, anti-SSB, high-titer ANA, RF)
III. Other laboratory abnormalities or additional investigations
  1. Biochemical (elevated serum amylase)
  2. Hematological (leucopenia, high ESR)
  3. Immunological (polyclonal hyperimmunoglobulinemia)
  4. Nephrological (renal tubular acidosis)
  5. Histological proof of lymphocytic infiltration of salivary glands or other organs
  6. Objective documentation of ocular dryness (Bengal red staining, Schirmer test)
  7. Objective documentation of parotid gland involvement (sialography)
IV. Exclusion of all other autoimmune diseases
Presence of four or more criteria required for diagnosis

From Bartunkova, Sediva, Vencovsky, et al., Primary Sjögren's syndrome in children and adolescents: proposal for diagnostic criteria, Clin. Exp. Rheumatol. 17 (1999) 381–386.

BOX 30-4 Differential Diagnosis of Recurrent Parotitis in Children

Juvenile recurrent parotitis

Diffuse infiltrative lymphocytosis (associated with HIV)

Streptococcal or staphylococcal infection

Hemangioma

Neoplastic (benign or malignant)

Viral infection
  Epstein–Barr
  Cytomegalovirus
  Parvovirus
  Paramyxovirus

Unilateral parotitis:
  Bacterial infection
  Sialolithiasis

Other Glandular Involvement

Less commonly, dryness can affect the upper respiratory tract or oropharynx, resulting in hoarseness, bronchitis, or pneumonitis. The skin may be dry, and there may be loss of exocrine function in other glands, resulting in pancreatic dysfunction and hypochlorhydria.

Extraglandular Manifestations

Extraglandular manifestations of childhood SS may be less common than those in adults. However, general systemic complaints, such as fatigue, low-grade fever, myalgias, and arthralgias are frequent, particularly at the time of parotitis attacks.

Extraglandular manifestations can be considered in two different pathophysiological groups: (1) Peripheral organ involvement due to lymphocytic invasion in the epithelia of organs other than the exocrine glands, e.g., interstitial nephritis or obstructive bronchiolitis; and (2) extraepithelial involvement secondary to immune complex deposition and subsequent inflammation.

The types of extraglandular manifestations that may be seen in SS are shown in Table 30-1, with further details on more common findings described below.

Skin Manifestations

Raynaud phenomenon is reported to be relatively common among individuals with SS, and it may precede sicca complaints by years. Purpura or pernio have been reported in SS, and they may be signs suggesting a poor prognosis.

Arthritis

Adults with SS commonly complain of arthralgia, and inflammatory arthritis is reported in approximately 20% of patients.[19] The presence of arthritis has rarely been commented on in case series of children with SS, and it is difficult to determine how often it occurs.

Pulmonary Involvement

Pulmonary manifestations in patients with pSS are common and may be present in as many as 75% of patients.[20] Dryness of the epithelium of the trachea can result in a dry cough. Small airway obstructive disease and airway hyperactivity may result from lymphocytic infiltration around bronchi and bronchioles.

Interstitial lung disease (ILD) occurs in approximately 8% of adults with pSS and has the appearance of lymphocytic interstitial pneumonitis in many cases.[21,22] Among a population-based retrospective cohort of patients with SS by Nannini et al. from Rochester, Minnesota,[3] there was a cumulative incidence of ILD of 10% at 1 year after diagnosis, increasing to 20% by 5 years after diagnosis. In this study, patients with SS and ILD had a worse survival rate compared to those without ILD (95% CI 0.99-4.74).

Patients with lung disease may present with cough and/or dyspnea, although some are asymptomatic early in their course. Chest x-ray films may be abnormal, showing interstitial changes in 27% (pSS) to 75% (sSS) of asymptomatic patients. A high-resolution computed tomography scan can detect abnormalities not seen on plain radiographs. Abnormalities detected in 65% of asymptomatic patients include interlobular and intralobular thickening and ground glass appearance in lower lung fields. Pulmonary function tests may demonstrate decreased peak flows or diffusing capacity. Less commonly, pulmonary arterial hypertension has been reported.[23] If hilar and/or mediastinal adenopathy or lung nodules are found, an evaluation to rule out lymphoma should be conducted.

Houghton and colleagues reported fraternal twin girls with pSS, one of whom presented with mild dyspnea and was found to have large pulmonary nodules.[24] Biopsy of these nodules substantiated the diagnosis of pSS, with lymphocytic interstitial pneumonitis. Five years after the diagnosis of pSS, clinical worsening prompted reinvestigation, and repeat biopsy demonstrated a mucosa-associated lymphoid tissue (MALT) lymphoma.

Renal Involvement

Renal involvement in patients with SS is not common, but patients may develop interstitial nephritis or glomerulonephritis. Interstitial nephritis, due to activated lymphocytes infiltrating tubular epithelium, can result in distal renal tubular acidosis (RTA), with hyposthenuria. Glomerulonephritis in SS results from immune complex deposition. Goules et al.[25] reported that 4.9% (35 of 715 adult patients with pSS) of patients had clinically evident renal disease, with 49% of these having glomerulonephritis and 37% interstitial nephritis. Patients with interstitial nephritis had a generally benign long-term outcome; however, the presence of glomerulonephritis was associated with higher mortality or progression to lymphoma.

One report reviewed 12 cases of RTA in children with SS.[26] In this small series, RTA was more frequently seen in pSS in childhood than in adults. Clinically significant hypokalemia was seen in the majority, and some patients had proximal or mixed RTA. Other more rare manifestations in patients with SS include proximal tubular acidosis, membranous or membranoproliferative glomerulonephritis, tubulointerstitial nephritis,[27] and interstitial cystitis.

Neurological Involvement

The spectrum of neurological manifestations associated with SS is broad and includes meningitis, myelopathy, cranial neuropathy, sensorimotor polyneuropathy, and mononeuritis multiplex.[28,29] A syndrome of purely sensory neuropathy is said to be relatively unique to SS among the rheumatic diseases and has been reported in childhood.[30] A peripheral neuropathy may precede the appearance of sicca symptoms in many patients. There have been reports of optic neuropathy in pediatric-onset SS.[31] Other central nervous system (CNS) manifestations include hemiparesis, movement disorders, brainstem, motor neuron, and cerebellar syndromes.[32,33] The CNS manifestations reported in SS overlap with those seen in patients with CNS lupus, making the differentiation between these disorders difficult.

Connection between Neonatal Lupus and Sjögren Syndrome

Neonatal lupus syndrome, including congenital heart block, can occur in offspring of women who have anti-Ro and/or anti-La antibodies

during their pregnancy (see Chapter 25). These autoantibodies are those most commonly found in women with SS.[34] Among mothers of infants with neonatal lupus, SS is as common as lupus.[35] Counseling older adolescents with SS and anti-Ro/La antibodies about the risk of neonatal lupus in future pregnancies is advisable; more intensive pregnancy screening should take place for teenagers with SS who become pregnant.

PATHOLOGY

The primary pathological finding in SS is of lymphocytic infiltration of affected tissues. Salivary gland biopsies show focal aggregates of lymphocytes, plasma cells, and macrophages; there may be larger foci with the appearance of germinal centers. This appearance is characteristic of chronic lymphocytic sialadenitis. A minor salivary gland biopsy is said to be specific for the diagnosis of SS if it is obtained through normal-appearing mucosa, has 5 to 10 glands present but separated by surrounding connective tissue with focal lymphocytic infiltration, and with all or most of the glands abnormal.[36] Focus scores are determined by counting the number of lymphocytes in a 4-mm^2 area, and classified on a scale from grade 0 (no histological abnormalities) to grade 4 (more than one lymphoid nodule present); a score of grade 3 or 4 is indicative of SS.[37]

PATHOGENESIS

The proposed model of the pathogenesis of SS is that genetically predisposed individuals are exposed to environmental factors, such as viral infection, which lead to a protracted autoimmune response focused in the epithelial cells of exocrine glands.[38-40] However, the specifics of these pathways are not well understood, and the pathogenic relationship between initial autoimmune disease in exocrine glands and further extraglandular disease is unknown. To date, there have been relatively few gene association studies of large SS patient groups, and no genome-wide association studies. The few genetic association studies done demonstrate a set of genes as potential risk alleles, including STAT 4 and IRF 5, which are also susceptibility genes for systemic lupus erythematosus (SLE).[41] Larger genetic studies are required to identify the more specific genetic associations of this disease.

Autoantibodies

Patients with SS have a variety of autoantibodies, which include RF, with ANA most commonly directed against the extractable nuclear antigens Ro/SSA and La/SSB, and others directed against organ-specific antigens such as thyroid cells or gastric mucosa. At least three pieces of evidence support the possibility that autoantibodies against Ro and La may have a pathogenic role: (1) they are present in the saliva of patients with SS; (2) there is increased messenger RNA for La in conjunctival epithelial cells in SS; and (3) B cells infiltrating salivary glands in SS have intracytoplasmic immunoglobulin directed against Ro and La.[42]

More recently, autoantibodies directed against the cytoskeletal protein β-fodrin and muscarinic receptor M3 have been described,[42] although their pathogenic roles are not yet known.

Potential Viral Triggers of Sjögren Syndrome Autoimmunity

Although both clinical and experimental observations suggest a role for viruses as triggers for SS, no specific infectious agent has been identified. Several retroviruses have been associated with pSS, including human T lymphotropic virus type 1, human retrovirus 5, hepatitis C virus, and Coxsackie virus.[38,43] Viral activation of the innate immune system may play a role in inciting SS, with a maladaptive response leading to autoimmunity.

Immunopathological Mechanism of Disease

The majority of lymphocytes infiltrating the affected glandular tissue are activated CD4+ T cells and activated B cells. The involvement of the innate immune system in the pathogenesis of SS is increasingly an area of study, with a focus on the potential role of interferon (IFN)-α and a possible role for B-cell activating factor (BAFF).[39]

There is increased expression of IFN-regulated genes in the salivary glands of SS patients,[44,45] and plasmacytoid dendritic cells, known to be a major source of IFN-α, are present.[45] In addition, this IFN signature was found in peripheral blood mononuclear cells of SS patients, and correlated with anti-SSA and anti-SSB levels.[46]

In addition to IFN genes, which are markers for innate immunity, an increase in BAFF, one of the cytokines upregulated by IFN-α, has been shown in salivary glands, saliva, and serum of SS patients.[47] BAFF promotes B-cell survival, and BAFF-deficient mice develop a lupuslike disease with infiltrates in the salivary glands and decreased salivary flow.[48] These data suggest a pathogenic role for BAFF in SS; however, the specifics of this role are not currently known.

LABORATORY EXAMINATION

Laboratory testing in SS is important, although not specific. Patients frequently have a very elevated ESR, although this is likely related to significant hypergammaglobulinemia seen in nearly 100% of patients.[11,49,50] The majority of patients with SS also have ANA; RFs are found in 57% to 87.5% of pediatric patients.[11,49,50] Approximately 20% of adults with SS are reported to have cryoglobulins in their serum,[51] an indicator of poor prognosis, which puts them at a higher risk of developing additional organ involvement and with a greater potential for developing lymphoma. Autoantibodies to nuclear antigens Ro/SSA and La/SSB are considered the "hallmark" feature of this disease; however, these autoantibodies are found in only 60% to 90% of patients. The presence of anti-Ro and anti-La has been reported to be associated with a higher prevalence of systemic, hematological, and immunological abnormalities.[52]

RADIOLOGICAL STUDIES

Salivary flow can be measured by sialometry, but this procedure is difficult to do, particularly in younger children; in addition, there are no appropriate age-matched normal values for children. Sialography is a radiocontrast method of examining the anatomical detail of the parotid ductal system. In SS, sialectasis can be demonstrated on sialography. The radiographic features found in sialograms in 21 pediatric patients with either pSS or sSS ranged from punctuate or globular ectasia sialectasis (Fig. 30-1) to considerable narrowing of the ductal system and destroyed parenchyma.[13] The authors of the study suggested that sialography provided highly accurate and sensitive findings in children with suspected SS.

Parotid Scintigraphy and Ultrasound

Salivary gland scintigraphy assesses salivary gland function, using 99Tc-pertechnetate injection, and demonstrates the uptake and distribution of the isotope. In patients with SS, the uptake and secretion of the isotope is delayed or absent. Abnormal parotid scintigraphy is included as one of the criteria the AECG diagnostic criteria for SS, with abnormal results classified into grades 1-4 (1, least severe; 4, most severe) by an accepted system proposed by Schall et al.[53] A prospective study of 405 adult patients with SS who had scintigraphy performed

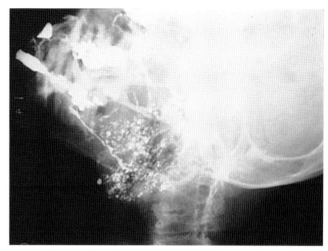

FIGURE 30-1 Typical sialogram in Sjögren syndrome.

at disease diagnosis demonstrated that severe scintigraphic findings early in disease were significantly associated with a higher risk of systemic features, progression to lymphoma, and lower survival rate over a mean 7-year follow-up.[54] However, more recently, some experts have questioned the value of using scintigraphy as a diagnostic requirement in pSS.[55]

Ultrasound can also be used to demonstrate abnormal salivary gland architecture, with the advantage of being noninvasive. A simple scoring system has been proposed by de Vita et al.,[56] which is based on parotid gland homogeneity and presence of hypoechoic lesions, leading to grading on a scale 0 (normal gland) to 4 (multiple hypoechogenic areas greater than 6 mm, or multiple calcifications with echogenic bands); a score of grade 3 or 4 is considered most suggestive of a diagnosis of pSS. A comparative study of salivary gland ultrasound, scintigraphy, and salivary gland biopsy in 107 adult patients demonstrated that ultrasound was highly accurate as a diagnostic test, with 90.8% specificity and 87.1% sensitivity.[57] In this study, the ultrasound score was shown to be of value in differentiating adult patients with pSS who have more systemic involvement, higher disease activity, and risk factors for lymphoma development. Although to date there have been no studies of salivary gland ultrasound in children, this clearly has great potential as a useful and accurate noninvasive diagnostic test.

Schirmer's test is a standardized valid method of testing the amount of tear secretion. A small specially measured strip of filter paper is slipped under the inferior lid of the eye for 5 minutes; the wet length of paper is measured. If the tear secretion is less than 5 mm, a significant decrease in tear secretion is demonstrated. Although this is a simple test, it may be difficult to apply in many children. In these cases, Rose Bengal staining, which dyes the corneal and conjunctival epithelium damaged secondarily to low tear output, may be performed by an ophthalmologist.

Minor Salivary Gland and Parotid Biopsy

Biopsy of the minor salivary glands of the lower lip has been used widely as a diagnostic tool, particularly for adults with a presumptive diagnosis of SS. The AECG diagnostic criteria include the finding of focal sialadenitis from a minor salivary gland biopsy as a major diagnostic parameter.[58] Periductal lymphocytic infiltration or chronic sialadenitis are findings from the minor salivary gland biopsy that indicate a diagnosis of SS. However, in some cases, these biopsies may be nondiagnostic or may not provide adequate glandular tissue for diagnostic confirmation. In one retrospective single center study, Caporali and colleagues studied the usefulness of a minor salivary gland biopsy in 435 adult patients who underwent the procedure as part of the diagnostic evaluation for possible SS.[59] The procedure was safe with no major adverse events, and only 1% of samples had inadequate material for testing. Ninety-three patients (24.5%) had a positive biopsy; in 51 patients, the minor salivary gland biopsy results were essential in making a definitive diagnosis. In a study of 23 children with pSS and sSS, 20 patients had typical pathological findings of SS, which was important information to substantiate the diagnosis, as reported symptoms of xerostomia or xerophthalmia were not reliable, particularly in younger children.[13] These data support the view that in a child or youth with suspected SS, a minor salivary gland biopsy can be a very useful and important procedure to determine a definite diagnosis.

Parotid biopsy is suggested by some as a more definitive diagnostic procedure. McGuirt and colleagues reported six pediatric patients (6 to 12 years old),[50] four of whom underwent parotid biopsy to confirm the diagnosis of SS. In all four, parotid swelling was present, but the minor salivary biopsy was normal. The authors suggest that the parotid biopsy is a minor procedure, which can be a safe method of confirming the diagnosis of SS in the pediatric population.

MANAGEMENT

For the majority of patients with SS, the management of their disease is focused on symptom relief of dry eyes and dry mouth or episodic treatment of parotitis. Compared with many other of the rheumatic conditions, such as SLE, the disease course is more indolent, and it less frequently requires immunosuppressive therapy.

The treatment of dry eyes is generally the application of topical artificial tears as necessary. Avoidance of conditions that may add to dry eyes, such as smoking or medications that may have anticholinergic side effects, may also be helpful.[19] In some patients, topical cyclosporine has been reported to improve tear production and decrease ocular symptoms. For younger children who may not complain of dry eyes, annual ocular screening should be considered to look for keratitis or scarring.

The treatment of dry mouth may be challenging, but luckily this symptom is rare in pediatrics. The use of sugar-free lozenges or chewing gum may help to stimulate salivary flow. Good dental hygiene and more frequent dental check-ups are very important for patients with SS to prevent or detect caries. Pilocarpine hydrochloride may be useful in some individuals to increase salivary secretion.[19]

Hydroxychloroquine is widely prescribed for patients with SS, and it may be helpful in treating constitutional symptoms, arthralgias, or fatigue associated with the disease. One study evaluating the effect of hydroxychloroquine on xerostomia in adults with pSS showed a significant increase in saliva production after 6 months of treatment.[60] There have been conflicting results from other reported studies, with some suggestions of improvement in ocular or oral symptoms in many patients but with few studies demonstrating improvements in laboratory parameters.[61]

Immunosuppressive agents are not uniformly required in patients with SS. However, patients with extraglandular organ manifestations, severe ocular or mucosal symptoms, or disabling constitutional problems may require more aggressive treatment. Corticosteroids do not seem to stop the progression of SS or improve salivary flow, but they have been demonstrated in one randomized trial to result in a decrease in episodes of parotid swelling, and improvement in systemic complaints of fatigue and arthralgia.[62] Based on these results, corticosteroid treatment may be beneficial to treat troublesome recurrent parotid swelling and constitutional symptoms. Although not frequently recommended for patients with SS, methotrexate was shown to result in clinical symptom improvement and decreased parotid gland swelling in one trial in adults with pSS.[63]

More recently, there has been interest in the effects of biological agents in the treatment of SS. There have been several publications describing the use of the anti–tumor necrosis factor agents etanercept and infliximab in the treatment of SS. One trial using etanercept did not show, by specific testing, clinically significant effectiveness for treating oral or ocular symptoms of SS or for improving salivary or lacrimal flow.[64] Infliximab was shown to be effective in reducing global and local disease manifestations in a small open-label pilot study of 16 patients with pSS, with sustained improvement over a 1-year period.[65]

Rituximab, a chimeric monoclonal antibody directed against CD20 molecules present on the surface of mature B cells, began to be used in small series of patients with pSS (reviewed by Isaksen and colleagues[66]). These early reports suggested the lack of objective effect on the sicca phenomenon, but significant improvement in systemic complaints, such as fatigue, arthritis, arthralgia, and cryoglobulin-associated vasculitis. Meijer et al. performed a careful randomized controlled trial of rituximab versus placebo in 30 adult patients with active pSS, 20 of whom received rituximab.[67] Patients who received rituximab demonstrated improved stimulated saliva flow, compared with placebo patients whose stimulated saliva flow declined over the 48-week follow-up period. In this study, rituximab-treated patients did report improvement in their symptoms of dry mouth and eyes, as well as significant improvements in quality of life scores using the SF-36. Gottenberg et al. reported on patients enrolled in the French Society of Rheumatology AutoImmune and Rituximab Registry (AIR) who received rituximab for pSS.[68] The 78 adult patients described were given rituximab primarily for systemic disease manifestations. At mean follow-up of 35 months after registry entry, 60% of patients were reported to have clinical improvement by physician rating 6 months after a course of rituximab. In this patient cohort, rituximab was particularly efficacious for patients with hematological involvement; 63% of patients with articular involvement also improved. However, only 44% of those with nervous system involvement were reported as improved. Additional courses of rituximab were given to 52% of patients; although the mean number of cycles reported was 2, nine patients had 5 to 12 cycles. Interestingly, eight patients were persistent responders 30 months after a single course of rituximab, suggesting that this therapy may be advantageous for a subset of patients.

Adverse events in pSS patients treated with rituximab have been generally transient and mild, usually related to infusions; some patients developed later serum sickness–like reactions.[66,67] Of 12 patients who reported pSS-related lymphoma and were treated with rituximab, 7 went into a full remission, 3 remained stable, and only 2 did not respond, suggesting an important role for this medication in treating this serious complication of pSS.

Belimumab, a monoclonal anti-BAFF antibody, has been tested in patients with pSS in a small open label proof-of-concept study.[69] It has been reported that serum BAFF levels were raised in patients with pSS and in pSS-associated lymphoproliferative disease.[70] Of 31 patients enrolled from two sites in Europe in the Mariette study, 60% achieved improvement in one of the primary endpoints at a 28-week assessment point. Patients treated with belimumab reported improvement in dryness but not fatigue or pain; physician assessment of systemic disease improved significantly, as did biological B-cell markers. The mean EULAR Sjögren Syndrome Disease Activity Index (ESSDAI) score decreased significantly, suggesting a moderate positive impact of the treatment. Overall the treatment was well tolerated, with infections as the majority of adverse events reported. One patient developed severe pneumococcal meningitis. This first study of belimumab in pSS

TABLE 30-2   Disease Activity, Patient Symptoms, and Damage Indices in Sjögren Syndrome

DISEASE ACTIVITY INDICES	YEAR PUBLICATION	COMMENTS
SSDAI (Sjögren Syndrome Disease Activity Index)	2007	Simple, but has floor effect (>60% of patients with score of 0-1)
SCAI (Sjögren Systemic Clinical Activity Index)	2007	Complex for use in routine practice
ESSDAI (EULAR Sjögren Syndrome Disease Activity Index)	2009	Developed by worldwide consensus process, best accuracy in predicting clinical change
PATIENT SYMPTOM INDICES		
SSI (Sicca Symptoms Inventory)	2002	Assessment of oral/ocular/vaginal/skin dryness only
PROFAD (Profile of Fatigue and Discomfort)	2004	Includes assessment of fatigue, arthralgia, Raynaud symptoms
ESSPRI (EULAR Sjögren Syndrome Patient Reported Index)	2010	Assessment of dryness, fatigue, pain
DAMAGE INDICES		
SS Disease Damage Index		Developed by the same group as SSDAI
SSDI (Sjögren Syndrome Damage Index)		Modified version of the SLICC Damage Index for SLE

demonstrates encouraging modest positive outcomes and suggests that larger randomized controlled trials are warranted.

OUTCOME MEASURES

Accurate standardized assessment of disease activity and outcome has become more important for patients with Sjögren syndrome, as new therapies have become available that require testing in randomized controlled trials. Disease domains considered important for assessment include sicca symptoms, measures of tear and saliva production, fatigue, quality of life, and disease activity and damage. Measures of disease activity, patient symptoms, and disease damage have been published and validated to some degree[71] (Table 30-2). The EULAR-developed measures, ESSDAI and ESSPRI (EULAR Sjögren Syndrome Patient Reported Index) appear to have advantages of good accuracy in detecting clinical change and simplicity in use and scoring.[72,73] None of these tools have been used or tested in a pediatric population, and there remains a need to validate the metric properties of these measures to allow their use in clinical trials and daily clinical care of patients.

PROGNOSIS AND OUTCOME

Despite a significantly increased risk for B-cell lymphoma in some patients with SS, the prognosis for most adult patients with SS is very good, with many patients having a stable and benign course of disease. Long-term prognosis of pediatric patients with SS has not been studied. Skopouli and colleagues[51] analyzed outcomes of 261 adult Greek patients with SS and determined that overall mortality in SS was only increased in the presence of particular predictive factors. Factors associated with an adverse outcome included purpura, glomerulonephritis, low C4, or a mixed monoclonal cryoglobulinemia. Patients who developed arthritis, Raynaud phenomenon, interstitial nephritis, or lung or liver involvement had a more favorable outcome. In general, serological profiles of patients did not change over time.

Progression to Lymphoma

It has been well demonstrated that patients with SS are at high risk of developing malignancy; they have a relative risk for development of lymphoma 44 times greater when compared with age-matched peers.[74] Lymphoma develops in approximately 5% of patients with pSS. Although this is well reported in adult patients, lymphoma in pediatric SS patients has not been reported in the literature. This may be because the development of lymphoma may take years to become clinically

apparent, and therefore it is not "revealed" in the pediatric patients. The majority of the lymphomas are non-Hodgkin lymphoma, with the most common being extranodal B-cell lymphomas of the MALT cell type. The salivary glands are the most commonly affected site, but other organs can be involved. Lymphoma development in SS is thought to be driven by a combination of factors, including chronic antigenic stimulus, lymphocyte persistence due to defective apoptosis, and additional oncogenic events involving oncogenes.[74]

Clinical features thought to be predictive of lymphoma development include persistent enlargement of parotid glands, lymphadenopathy, splenomegaly, or palpable purpura.[75] Laboratory features indicating a predisposition to lymphoma include the presence of a mixed monoclonal cryoglobulinemia, low level of C4, or monoclonal bands in the serum or urine.[74] A more recent Italian study, by Quartuccio et al.,[70] examined a large prospective cohort of adult patients with pSS to define biomarkers associated with a higher risk of lymphoma evolution. Of 661 patients with pSS selected for study, 40 of these patients had progressed to lymphoma and were compared with 180 patients with persistent salivary gland swelling, 17 patients with cryoglobulinemic vasculitis, and 424 patients with pSS but none of the other findings. Variables significantly associated with lymphoma were low C4 (relative risk ratio 8.3), positive anti-La autoantibody (relative risk ratio 5.2), leucopenia (relative risk ratio 3.3), and cryoglobulinemia (relative risk ratio 6.8). Absence of these biomarkers was reported to have a negative predictive value of 98% in patients who had persistent parotid swelling. This study provides useful clinical and laboratory findings to guide clinicians' care of patients with SS.

IGG4-RELATED DISEASES

In the past decade there has been recognition of a diverse group of inflammatory diseases characterized by very high serum levels of IgG4 (over 140 mg/dl), marked IgG4-producing plasma cell infiltrate, characteristic "storiform" fibrosis, obliterative phlebitis, and mild to moderate eosinophilia in affected tissues. Originally described in patients with chronic pancreatitis,[76] the group includes diseases that affect many organ systems.[77] Table 30-3 shows the spectrum of diseases now considered to be part of the IgG4-related disease group. Clinically, the presentation includes enlargement of the lacrimal and salivary glands, which might suggest a diagnosis of Sjögren syndrome; marked submandibular lymphadenopathy, which might suggest a malignancy; pancreatitis; hepatobiliary disease and ocular inflammatory disease (retro-orbital pseudotumor); and joint disease.[78,79] Diagnosis of IgG4 disease may be difficult, with the most definitive method of diagnosis

TABLE 30-3 Conditions Once Considered Unrelated That Are Now Recognized as Part of the IgG4-Related Disease Spectrum

CONDITION	AFFECTED ORGAN) OR TISSUE
Enterocolitis	Gut
Eosinophilic angiocentric fibrosis	Orbits, upper respiratory tract
Fibrosing mediastinitis	Mediastinum
Hypertrophic pachymeningitis	Dura mater
Idiopathic hypocomplementemic tubulointerstitial nephritis with extensive tubulointerstitial deposits	Kidney
Inflammatory aortic aneurysm	Aorta
Inflammatory pseudotumor	Orbits, lungs, kidneys, and other organs
Küttner tumor	Submandibular glands
Mikulicz syndrome	Salivary and lacrimal glands
Multifocal fibrosclerosis	Orbits, thyroid gland, retroperitoneum, mediastinum, and other tissues and organs
Periaortitis and periarteritis	Aorta and large blood vessels
Retroperitoneal fibrosis	Retroperitoneum
Riedel's thyroiditis	Thyroid
Sclerosing cholangitis	Liver, biliary tract
Sclerosing mesenteritis	Mesentery
Sclerosing pancreatitis	Pancreas

Data from Mahajan (Ref. 77) and Takahashi (Ref. 79).

being histological examination of affected tissues for the classic fibrosis lesions and staining to look for IgG4+ plasma cells.

IgG4-related disease is rare in adults and has been described most commonly in middle-aged men. It has been even more rarely recognized in children, but it may be underdiagnosed. Reports of this disorder in children include three children with an IgG4-related pseudotumor[80,81]; a youth with autoimmune pancreatitis[82,83]; a 15-year-old boy with pulmonary disease[84]; a 15-year-old boy with mastoiditis, hypertrophic pachymeningitis and ankle joint arthritis[78]; and a boy with sclerosing sialadenitis of the submandibular salivary gland.[85] Recognition of this condition is important because it is usually responsive to treatment with corticosteroids, mycophenolate mofetil,[81,82] or rituximab.[86]

REFERENCES

2. A. Binard, V. Devauchelle-Pensec, B. Fautrel, et al., Epidemiology of Sjögren's syndrome: where are we? Clin. Exp. Rheumatol. 25 (2007) 1–4.
3. C. Nannini, A.J. Jebakumar, C.S. Crowson, et al., Primary Sjögren's syndrome 1976–2005 and associated interstitial lung disease: a population-based study of incidence and mortality, BMJ Open 3 (2013) e003569.
5. M.P. Novljan, B. Rozman, M. Berse, et al., Comparison of the different classification criteria sets for primary Sjögren's syndrome, Scand. J. Rheumatol. 35 (2006) 463–467.
7. S. Shiboski, C.H. Shiboski, L. Criswell, et al., American College of Rheumatology classification criteria for Sjögren's syndrome: a data-driven, expert consensus approach in the SICCA cohort, Arthritis Care Res. (Hoboken) 64 (2012) 475–487.
8. A. Rasmussen, J.A. Ice, K. Grundahl, et al., Comparison of the American-European Consensus Group Sjögren's syndrome classification criteria to newly proposed American College of Rheumatology criteria in a large, carefully characterised sicca cohort, Ann. Rheum. Dis. 73 (2014) 31–38.
9. C. Saad-Magalhaes, P.B. de Souza Medeiros, J.O. Sato, M.A. Custodio Domingues, Clinical presentation and salivary gland histopathology of paediatric primary Sjögren's syndrome, Clin. Exp. Rheumatol. 29 (2011) 590–594.
11. K. Houghton, P. Malleson, D. Cabral, et al., Primary Sjögren's syndrome in children and adolescents: are proposed diagnostic criteria applicable? J. Rheumatol. 32 (2005) 2225–2232.
12. F.N. Skopouli, J. Dafni, J.P. Ioannidis, H.M. Moutsopoulos, Clinical evolution, and morbidity and mortality of primary Sjögren's syndrome, Semin. Arthritis Rheum. 29 (2000) 296–304.
13. M. Stiller, W. Golder, E. Doring, et al., Primary and secondary Sjögren's syndrome in children-a comparative study, Clin. Oral Investig. 4 (2000) 176–182.
14. M. Civilibal, N. Canpolat, A. Yurt, et al., A child with primary Sjögren's syndrome and a review of the literature, Clin. Pediatr. 46 (2007) 738–742.
15. C.M. Leerdam, H.C. Martin, D. Isaacs, Recurrent parotitis of childhood, J. Paediatr. Child Health 41 (2005) 631–634.
19. P.J. Venables, Management of patients presenting with Sjögren's syndrome, Best Pract. Res. Clin. Rheumatol. 20 (2006) 791–807.
20. A.L. Parke, Pulmonary manifestations of primary Sjögren's syndrome, Rheum. Dis. Clin. North Am. 34 (2008) 907–920.
22. V. Dalvi, E.B. Gonzalez, L. Lovett, Lymphocytic interstitial pneumonia in Sjögren's syndrome: a case report and a review of the literature, Clin. Rheumatol. 26 (2007) 1339–1343.
23. D. Launay, E. Hachulla, P.Y. Hatron, et al., Pulmonary arterial hypertension: a rare complication of Sjogren syndrome: report of 9 new cases and review of the literature, Medicine (Baltimore) 86 (2007) 299–315.
24. K. Houghton, D. Cabral, R. Petty, L. Tucker, Primary Sjögren's syndrome in dizygotic adolescent twins: one case with lymphocytic interstitial pneumonia, J. Rheumatol. 32 (2005) 1603–1606.
25. A.V. Goules, I.P. Tatouli, H.M. Moutsopoulos, A.G. Tzioufas, Clinically significant renal involvement in primary Sjögren's syndrome: clinical presentation and outcome, Arthritis Rheum. 65 (2013) 2945–2953.
26. F. Pessler, H. Emery, L. Dai, et al., The spectrum of renal tubular acidosis in paediatric Sjögren syndrome, Rheumatology (Oxford) 45 (2006) 85–91.
27. S. Johnson, S.A. Hulton, M.A. Brundler, et al., End-stage renal failure in adolescence with Sjögren's syndrome autoantibodies, Pediatr. Nephrol. 22 (2007) 1793–1797.
28. B. Segal, A. Carpenter, D. Walk, Involvement of nervous system pathways in primary Sjögren's syndrome, Rheum. Dis. Clin. North Am. 34 (2008) 885–906.
29. S.I. Meligren, L.G. Goransson, R. Omdal, Primary Sjögren's syndrome associated neuropathy, Can. J. Neurol. Sci. 34 (2007) 280–287.
32. J.A. Gottfried, T.H. Finkel, J.V. Hunter, et al., Central nervous system Sjögren's syndrome in a child: case report and review of the literature, J. Child Neurol. 16 (2001) 683–685.
35. A.R. Neiman, L.A. Lee, W.L. Weston, J.P. Buyon, Cutaneous manifestations of neonatal lupus without heart block: characteristics of mothers and children enrolled in a national registry, J. Pediatr. 137 (2000) 674–680.
36. R. Amarasena, S. Bowman, Sjögren's syndrome, Clin. Med. (Northfield Il) 7 (2007) 53–56.
38. N. Delaleu, M.V. Jonsson, S. Appel, R. Jonsson, New concepts in the pathogenesis of Sjögren's syndrome, Rheum. Dis. Clin. North Am. 34 (2008) 833–845.
39. N.P. Nikolov, G.G. Illei, Pathogenesis of Sjögren's syndrome, Curr. Opin. Rheumatol. 21 (2009).
40. G. Nordmark, G.V. Alm, L. Ronnblom, Mechanisms of disease: primary Sjögren's syndrome and the type I interferon system, Nat. Clin. Pract. Rheumatol. 2 (2006) 262–269.
41. R.H. Scofield, Genetics of systemic lupus erythematosus and Sjögren's syndrome, Curr. Opin. Rheumatol. 21 (2009) 448–453.
42. J.G. Routsias, A.G. Tzioufas, Sjögren's syndrome: study of autoantigens and autoantibodies, Clin. Rev. Allergy Immunol. 32 (2007) 238–251.

43. A. Triantafyllopoulou, H.M. Moutsopoulos, Persistent viral infection in primary Sjögren's syndrome: Review and perspectives, Clin. Rev. Allergy Immunol. 32 (2007) 210–214.
44. J.E. Gottenberg, N. Cagnard, C. Lucchesi, et al., Activation of IFN pathways and plasmacytoid dendritic cell recruitment in target organs of primary Sjögren's syndrome, Proc. Natl Acad. Sci. U. S. A. 103 (2006) 2770–2775.
45. T.O. Hjelmervik, K. Petersen, I. Jonassen, et al., Gene expression profiling of minor salivary glands clearly distinguishes primary Sjögren's syndrome patients from healthy control subjects, Arthritis Rheum. 52 (2005) 1534–1544.
46. E.S. Emamian, J.M. Leon, C.J. Lessard, H. Emery, Peripheral blood gene expression profiling in Sjögren's syndrome, Genes Immun. 10 (2009) 285–296.
47. F. Lavie, C. Miceli-Richard, M. Ittah, et al., B-cell activating factor of the tumour necrosis factor family expression in blood monocytes and T cells from patients with primary Sjögren's syndrome, Scand. J. Immunol. 67 (2008) 185–192.
48. M. Ittah, C. Miceli-Richard, J.E. Gottenberg, et al., Viruses induce high expression of BAFF by salivary gland epithelial cells through TLR- and type-I IFN-dependent and -independent pathways, Eur. J. Immunol. 38 (2008) 1058–1064.
49. J. Bartunkova, A. Sediva, J. Vencovsky, V. Tesar, Primary Sjögren's syndrome in children and adolescents: Proposal for diagnostic criteria, Clin. Exp. Rheumatol. 17 (1999) 381–386.
50. W.F. Mcguirt Jr., C. Whang, W. Moreland, The role of parotid biopsy in the diagnosis of pediatric Sjögren's syndrome, Arch. Otolaryngol. Head Neck Surg. 128 (2002) 1279–1281.
52. M. Ramos-Casals, R. Solans, J. Rosas, et al., Primary Sjögren's syndrome in Spain: clinical and immunologic expression in 1010 patients, Medicine (Baltimore) 87 (2008) 210–219.
54. M. Ramos-Casals, P. Brito-Zeron, M. Perez-de-lis, et al., Clinical and prognostic significance of parotid scintigraphy in 405 patients with primary Sjögren syndrome, J. Rheumatol. 37 (2010) 585–591.
57. E. Theander, T. Mandl, Primary Sjögren's syndrome: the diagnostic and prognostic value of salivary gland ultrasonography using a simplified scoring system, Arthritis Care Res (Hoboken) 66 (2014) 1102–1107.
59. P. Caporali, E. Bonacci, O. Epis, et al., Safety and usefulness of minor salivary gland biopsy: retrospective analysis of 502 procedures performed at a single center, Arthritis Rheum. 59 (2008) 714–720.
60. M. Rihl, K. Ulbricht, R.E. Schmidt, T. Witte, Treament of sicca symptoms with hydroxychloroquine in patients with Sjögren's syndrome, Rheumatology (Oxford) 48 (2009) 796–799.
61. S.E. Carsons, Issues relating to clinical trials of oral and biologic disease-modifying agents for Sjögren's syndrome, Rheum. Dis. Clin. North Am. 34 (2008) 1011–1023.
64. V. Sankar, M.T. Brennan, M.R. Kok, et al., Etanercept in Sjögren's syndrome: a twelve-week randomized, double-blind, placebo-controlled pilot clinical trial, Arthritis Rheum. 50 (2004) 2240–2245.
65. S.D. Steinfeld, P. Demols, I. Salmon, et al., Infliximab in patients with primary Sjögren's dyndrome: a pilot study, Arthritis Rheum. 44 (2001) 2371–2375.
66. K. Isaksen, R. Jonsson, R. Omdal, Anti-CD20 treatment in primary Sjögren syndrome, Scand. J. Immunol. 68 (2008) 554–564.
68. J.E. Gottenberg, G. Cinquetti, C. Larroche, et al., Efficacy of rituximab in systemic manifestations of primary Sjogren's syndrome: results in 78 patients of the AutoImmune and Rituximab registry, Ann. Rheum. Dis. 72 (2013) 1026–1031.
69. X. Mariette, R. Seror, L. Quartuccio, et al., Efficacy and safety of belimumab in primary Sjogren's syndrome: results of the BELISS open-label phase II study, Ann. Rheum. Dis. (2013) doi:10.1136/annrheumdis-2013-203991; [Epub ahead of print].
70. L. Quartuccio, M. Isola, C. Baldini, et al., Biomarkers of lymphoma in Sjögren's syndrome and evaluation of the lymphoma risk in prelymphomatous conditions: Results of a multicenter study, J. Autoimmun. 51 (2014) 75–80. doi:10.1016/j.jaut.2013.10.002.
71. R. Seror, H. Bootsma, S.J. Bowman, et al., Outcome measures for primary Sjögren's syndrome, J. Autoimmun. 39 (2012) 97–102.
72. R. Seror, E. Theander, H. Bootsma, et al., Outcome measures for primary Sjögren's syndrome: a comprehensive review, J. Autoimmun. 51C (2014) 51–56.
73. M. Ramos-Casals, P. Brito-Zeron, R. Solans, et al., Systemic involvement in primary Sjögren's syndrome evaluated by the EULAR-SS disease activity index: analysis of 921 Spanish patients (GEAS-SS Registry), Rheumatology (Oxford) 53 (2014) 321–331.
77. V.S. Mahajan, H. Mattoo, V. Deshpande, et al., IgG4 related disease, Ann. Rev. Pathol. Mech. Dis. 9 (2014) 315–347.
78. M. Hufnagel, P. Henneke, A. Schmitt-Graeff, IgG4-related disease, N. Engl. J. Med. 366 (2012) 1643–1644, author reply 1646–1647.
79. H. Takahashi, M. Yamamoto, C. Suzuki, et al., The birthday of a new syndrome: IgG4-related diseases constitute a clinical entity, Autoimmun Rev 9 (2010) 591–594.
81. G.J. Griepentrog, R.W. Vickers, J.W. Karesh, et al., A clinicopathologic case study of two patients with pediatric orbital IgG4-related disease, Orbit 32 (2013) 389–391.
82. M. Mannion, R.Q. Cron, Successful treatment of pediatric IgG4-related systemic disease with mycophenolate mofetil: case report and review of the pediatric autoimmune pancreatitis literature, Pediatr. Rheumatol 9 (2011) 1.
84. M. Pifferi, M. DiCicco, A. Bush, et al., Uncommon presentation of IgG4-related disease in a 15-year-old boy, Chest 144 (2013) 669–671.
86. A. Khosroshahi, D.B. Bloch, V. Deshpande, J.H. Stone, Rituximab therapy leads to rapid decline of serum IgG4 levels and prompt improvement in IgG4-related systemic disease, Arthritis Rheum. 62 (2010) 1755–1762.

The entire reference list is available online at www.expertconsult.com.

Raynaud Phenomenon and Vasomotor Syndromes

Robert Fuhlbrigge

Episodic color changes of the hands and feet in response to cold or stress, known as Raynaud phenomenon (RP), are a frequent complaint among patients presenting to pediatric rheumatology clinics. The first description of vasomotor instability triggered by cold exposure, or "local asphyxia of the extremities," is ascribed to A.G. Maurice Raynaud, a French medical student, whose name is eponymously linked with this disorder.[1] Despite 150 years of clinical observation and basic research, it is only recently that significant inroads been made regarding the biological basis for this condition and establishing evidence-based therapeutic interventions.

CLINICAL PRESENTATION

The clinical presentation of RP is characterized by recurrent episodes of vasospasm following exposure to cold or emotional stress.[2] Episodes of RP typically occur as sudden onset of pallor (ischemia) of the digits, often triggered by changes in the ambient temperature or contact with cold surfaces, followed by blue (cyanosis) and then red (hyperemia) upon rewarming. Attacks commonly begin in a single finger or toe and then spread to other digits, symmetrically involving both hands and/or feet (Fig. 31-1). The areas involved are often sharply demarcated and can be accompanied by sensations of pins and needles, aching, numbness, and/or clumsiness of the hands and feet. The index, middle, and ring fingers are the most frequently involved digits, whereas the thumb is often spared. Patients may also display symptoms of cutaneous vasospasm at other sites, including the ears, nose, face, knees, and nipples, and livedo reticularis involving the distal arms and legs.[3] Vascular spasm within viscera, such as the esophagus or coronary arteries, may accompany peripheral symptoms, particularly in patients with systemic sclerosis (SSc).

The symptoms of RP attacks reflect transient arterial vasospasm that can last from minutes to hours and is typically readily reversed by mechanical warming measures. Upon warming, blood flow is often exaggerated: the skin appears reddened or flushed and the digits may swell or itch. With more severe episodes, tender, red subcutaneous nodules (pernio) and peeling or ulceration of skin overlying the involved areas may result from local tissue ischemia (Fig. 31-2).

The triggers of RP in children are similar to those described in adults, with cold, emotional stress, and exercise as the most commonly reported initiators.[3-5] Although exposure to absolute cold (e.g., air temperature below 0° C) is readily recognized as a stimulus, provocation may also occur upon transition from warmer to relatively cooler temperatures. In this way a seemingly modest cold exposure, such as entering an air-conditioned space or handling cold food, may cause an attack. A general body chill or exposure of the face can also trigger an episode, even if the hands or feet are kept warm. In some patients, RP occurs after nonspecific stimulation of the sympathetic nervous system (e.g., periods of intense emotional stress, startle response).

Primary RP, Raynaud sign, or *idiopathic Raynaud disease* are terms used to describe those patients without a definable cause for their symptoms beyond nonspecific vascular hyperreactivity (Box 31-1).[6] In this setting, RP is considered an exaggeration of the normal vasoconstriction response to cold exposure or stress, the clinical features are generally benign, and the symptoms are reversible with rewarming. Use of the word "disease" in this context may cause undue concern; thus, many clinicians prefer the term *primary RP* for otherwise healthy individuals. *Secondary RP,* or *Raynaud syndrome,* refers to patients in whom an associated disease or known cause of vascular injury drives the frequency and severity of symptoms.[7,8]

EPIDEMIOLOGY

Primary RP is a common disorder that is frequently presented to rheumatologists because of concern for an underlying connective tissue disease. Estimates of the prevalence of RP range from 5% to 20% in women and 4% to 14% in men.[2,6,9] The large variation between studies reflects, in part, the ethnic balance of the populations studied and the climate where the study patients live.[10,11] For obvious reasons, patients living in colder climates are more likely to present for evaluation and at younger ages.[10] A study of children 12 to 15 years old in Manchester, United Kingdom, reported an overall prevalence of 18% in females and 12% in males, with values increasing with age in this population.[12] In general, RP is more common among women, adolescent, and young adult age groups, and family members of individuals with RP.[9,13] Although the large majority of persons with RP do not have, nor will they develop, an associated rheumatological or vascular disorder, it is important to recognize that RP may herald significant rheumatic disease. RP occurs at high frequency (80% to 90%) in children with SSc or mixed connective tissue disease (MCTD) and is often the initial symptom of these disorders, preceding other manifestations of disease in some instances by years.[4] New-onset RP should, therefore, prompt consideration and examination for signs and symptoms of systemic disease and, potentially, further rheumatological evaluation.

ETIOLOGY/PATHOGENESIS

In his thesis published in 1862, Raynaud ascribed the features he saw to "increased irritability of the central parts of the cord presiding over

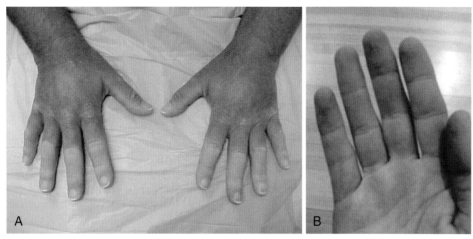

FIGURE 31-1 **A,** Classic presentation of Raynaud phenomenon with symmetrical, sharply demarcated pallor affecting all fingers and sparing the thumbs. **B,** Cyanosis associated with Raynaud phenomena typically follows after pallor and represents deoxygenation of slow flowing blood.

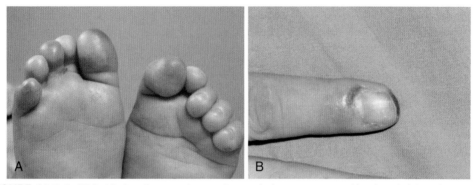

FIGURE 31-2 **A,** Digital ischemia secondary to Raynaud phenomenon resulting in painful erythematous plaques (pernio) on the tips of affected toes (from http://emedicine.medscape.com/article/1087946-media). **B,** Necrosis of the fingertip and the proximal periungual area associated with Raynaud phenomenon (from http://asps.confex.com/asps/2006am/techprogram/paper_10931.htm).

BOX 31-1   Clinical Features of Primary and Secondary Raynaud Phenomenon

Primary Raynaud phenomenon
- Episodic vasospastic attacks precipitated by cold or emotional stress
- Symmetrical involvement of distal extremities
- No evidence of peripheral vascular disease
- Absence of tissue necrosis, digital pitting, or gangrene
- Normal nailfold capillary examination
- Negative antinuclear antibody (ANA) test and normal erythrocyte sedimentation rate (ESR)

Secondary Raynaud phenomenon
- Older age at onset
- Male gender
- Painful, asymmetric attacks with signs of digital ischemia (pernio or ulceration)
- Ischemia proximal to the fingers or toes
- Abnormal nailfold capillary examination with enlarged or distorted capillary loops
- Abnormal laboratory parameters suggesting vascular or autoimmune disease (e.g., elevated ESR or CRP), autoantibodies (ANA, antitopoisomerase, anti-Smith antigen, antiphospholipid), decreased complement levels

---

the vascular innervations."[1,14] Observing that local sympathectomy did not cure RP, Sir Thomas Lewis proposed in 1929 that RP was due to a "local fault," rather than a defect in the central nervous system (CNS).[15] Current data continue to support this view, suggesting that RP primarily represents exaggerated physiological vasomotor responses

to cold temperature (i.e., lowering of blood flow to the skin, thereby reducing the loss of body heat and preserving core body temperature) and/or emotional stress.[2,16-19] In broad terms, blood flow volume is regulated by an interactive system involving central and peripheral neural signals, cellular mediators, circulating hormones, and soluble vasoactive compounds.[20,21] The inherent tone, or basal contractile activity, of vascular smooth muscle varies substantially between different arterial structures, ranging from relatively high in the coronary circulation to low or absent in the pulmonary circulation, and it can increase or decrease dramatically.[20] Numerous mechanisms participate in the regulation of vascular tone, including both the intrinsic characteristics of vascular smooth muscle and endothelial cells, and extrinsic activities of local nerves, adjacent tissues, circulating cells, and soluble factors (Box 31-2).[21]

The pathophysiological mechanisms influencing RP can be segregated into three broad categories of abnormality: vascular, neural, and intravascular.[22] The effects seen in primary RP are, by definition, fully reversible, whereas secondary RP may combine defective function and structural abnormalities, leading to irreversible tissue damage.

Endothelial cells play an active role in regulating vascular tone. Depending on their state of activation, endothelial cells can produce both potent vasodilating agents (e.g., prostacyclin and nitric oxide [NO]) and potent vasoconstricting agents (e.g., endothelins and angiotensin). Endothelial NO production, in particular, has a large effect on vascular tone, regulating vascular smooth muscle contraction, proliferation, and migration. NO also stimulates platelet disaggregation and hinders the adhesion of platelets, lymphocytes, and neutrophils to the endothelial surface, which can have secondary effects on vascular function. SSc-associated RP differs fundamentally from primary RP due to its associated vasculopathy involving fibrous intimal proliferation with associated intravascular thrombi. Endothelin-1 and angiotensin are potent vasoconstrictors with profibrotic activities that have been shown to be overexpressed in the skin of patients with SSc and other forms of secondary RP.[22] These are but a few examples from a long list of agents and functions that may contribute to the pathogenesis of vascular abnormalities in SSc (summarized in Box 31-2 and discussed in greater detail in Chapter 27).[16]

BOX 31-2 Factors Influencing Vascular Reactivity

Arterial smooth muscle cells
  Transmural pressure (autoregulation)
  Oxygen tension/ischemia
  Temperature (decreased temperature selectively increases response to norepinephrine)
Endothelial cell products
  Nitric oxide (vasodilation)
  Prostacyclin (vasodilation)
  Endothelin-1 (vasoconstriction)
Sympathetic nervous system
  Norepinephrine (vasoconstriction)
Neuropeptides
  Substance P (vasodilation)
  Vasoactive intestinal peptide (vasodilation)
  Calcitonin gene-related peptide (vasodilation)
  Neurokinin A (vasodilation)
  Somatostatin (vasoconstriction)
  Neuropeptide Y (vasoconstriction)
Other
  Shear stress
  Platelet products (thromboxane, serotonin)
  Blood viscosity
  Blood cell deformability
  Estrogen

Neurotransmitters from both autonomic and sensory afferent nerves also influence digital vascular tone. Blood vessels can receive innervation from three main classes of neurons: sympathetic vasoconstrictor neurons, sympathetic or parasympathetic vasodilator neurons, and sensory neurons that mediate vasodilation. Although the sympathetic nervous system, via release of norepinephrine, is considered a major mediator of vasoconstriction in the skin, local nerve endings can produce both vasodilating (substance P, vasoactive intestinal peptide, calcitonin gene-related peptide, neurokinin A) and vasoconstricting (somatostatin, neuropeptide Y) neuropeptides in response to local microenvironmental effects.[23] Although many patients report stress as a trigger for RP, suggesting CNS influence on local vasospasm, studies that investigated the differential effects of mental stress in patients with RP have produced mixed results and have failed to clarify the role of the CNS in the pathogenesis of this disorder.[24]

Vascular reactivity is also affected by shear stress, vasoactive substances released by platelets (thromboxane, serotonin), changes in blood viscosity, and changes in the rheological properties of blood (e.g., altered red blood cell deformability), which highlights the complexity of regulatory mechanisms involved.[17,20]

The marked sensitivity to cold in both primary and secondary RP appears to be mediated, at least in part, by an enhanced response to stimulation of alpha adrenergic receptors in the digital and cutaneous vessels of patients with RP.[21,22,25] Alpha adrenergic receptors are increased in small vessels relative to larger vessels in normal subjects, and are particularly numerous in cutaneous arteries and veins relative to other tissue beds.[22] In humans, the administration of "selective" alpha-1 and alpha-2 adrenergic agonists causes a reduction in skin or finger blood flow.[26] Cold exposure has been shown to selectively amplify the vascular smooth muscle constriction response to norepinephrine mediated through alpha adrenergic receptors.[22] Estrogen has also recently been shown to increase expression of alpha-2 adrenergic receptors in vascular smooth muscle and to increase cold sensitivity, which may explain the greater prevalence of RP among postpubertal females.[27-29] Within the alpha-2 adrenergic receptor family, individual subtypes (e.g., alpha-2a, -2b, and -2c) have been shown to display differing sensitivity to cold in both humans and mice.[30,31] Under normal conditions (37°C), alpha-2c adrenoreceptors in cutaneous arteries are stored within the Golgi apparatus. Cooling induces activation of Rho/Rho kinase signaling pathways, prompting translocation of alpha-2c adrenoreceptor from the Golgi complex to the plasma membrane and augmenting sensitivity of contractile proteins to calcium ions.[32] One trigger for Rho/Rho kinase signaling may be a rapid increase of reactive oxygen species (ROS) seen in smooth muscle cells following cold exposure (below 28° C).[33] Ischemia and reperfusion, in turn, induce production of additional ROS by mitochondria, leading to further activation of the Rho/Rho kinase pathway and provoking repeated or persistent cycles of vasospasm. Selective inhibition of alpha-2 adrenergic receptors abolishes cold-induced vasoconstriction of isolated blood vessels *in vitro*,[30] and inhibition of Rho kinase signaling pathways prevents translocation of alpha-2 adrenoreceptors from the Golgi to the cell surface in response to cooling.[32]

Increased contractile protein responses to alpha-2 adrenergic agonists and cooling, and the associated changes in Rho/Rho kinase and protein tyrosine kinase activity, are observed in both primary and secondary RP compared to healthy controls. These findings provide a possible unifying explanation for cold-induced vascular reactivity in primary and secondary RP, identify a family of targets through which mutations may contribute to familial and ethnic clustering, and highlight opportunities for the development of new therapeutic agents.[34,35]

A large number of diseases, disorders, medications, and chemical agents have been associated with secondary RP, presumably reflecting a common end point of vascular injury and the complex mechanisms responsible for control of vessel reactivity (Box 31-3).[2,21,36] As noted previously, changes in the microvascular system are seen in association with intimal fibrosis and endothelial dysfunction in SSc. Endothelial cell dysfunction appears at an early stage and is associated with increased platelet adhesion, decreased storage of von Willebrand factor, and decreased adenosine uptake.[22,37-39] Ischemic reperfusion injury results in increased production of ROS, which further alters vascular tone.[40] However, not all increased vascular reactivity in patients with SSc can be attributed to endothelial injury or fibrosis. These mechanisms may occur with, or even induce, the increase in alpha-2 adrenergic receptor reactivity discussed previously.[41] Other observations in SSc include enhanced endothelial cell proliferation, reduced activity of

NO, increased circulating levels of endothelin-1, and increased expression of endothelin receptors.[16,38,42]

Intravascular or circulating factors have also been implicated in the pathogenesis of RP, in particular in patients with SSc. Abnormal platelet activation, defective fibrinolysis, and oxidant stress have also been reported. Although their actions are not fully understood, intravascular factors may exacerbate the effect of digital vasospasm by reducing basal blood flow in the microvasculature and promoting coagulation.

DIAGNOSIS

History

Patients with primary RP are frequently referred to rheumatologists due to concerns that they might have an underlying rheumatological disorder. A detailed patient history should be collected, including the distribution of affected sites; frequency, severity, and duration of attacks; color pattern; triggers; seasonality; and associated symptoms (i.e., numbness, paresthesia, pain). Patients should also be questioned for any features suggestive of connective tissue disease (CTD) such as unexplained fever, fatigue, rash, morning stiffness, arthralgia, myalgia, dysphagia, peripheral edema, lymphadenopathy, or oral ulcers; about changes in digits, such as nail pitting, ulcers, or poor healing; and about the incidence of infection. Potential associated or precipitating factors should also be assessed, including frostbite, drug or toxin exposure, infection, vibration injury, personal and family history of RP or CTD, migraines, weight loss or eating disorders, and cardiovascular disease.

Clinical Criteria

The complaint of cold hands or feet is very common and must be distinguished from RP, which involves both cool skin and cutaneous color changes. Normal individuals may have cool skin and digital pallor or skin mottling on cold exposure. However, unlike RP, onset is not abrupt, the recovery phase of vascular flow is not delayed, and there is no prolonged or sharp demarcation of color changes in skin. A diagnosis of RP may be made if the patient provides a history of symptoms characteristic of a Raynaud episode; history alone is accepted as diagnostic in general practice, because no simple clinical test consistently triggers an attack. If necessary, or for research studies, digital arteriolar blood flow can be documented by Doppler flow ultrasound.[43] Characteristic changes have also been reported by plethysmography and arteriography, although the latter is not usually necessary or indicated and is performed with some danger of precipitating acute catastrophic arteriolar spasm in patients with severe RP. In practice, digital artery ultrasound is readily available and interrogates the same anatomical structures as angiography, and it is cheaper, faster, and noninvasive. Although measurement of digital blood pressure, digital blood flow, or skin temperature responses to cooling may be predictive in a research setting, attempts to induce and measure attacks in an office setting are not consistent, even in patients with definite RP.[44-47] A simple approach employing the use of standard questionnaires and color photos of typical features has proven useful in clinical trials and epidemiological studies.[48,49]

Specific criteria for the diagnosis of RP were first proposed in 1932.[50] Several modifications designed to improve the differentiation of primary and secondary RP have been proposed and validated (see Box 31-1).[48,51] The diagnosis of RP is fundamentally based on a history of episodic vasospastic attacks precipitated by cold or stress. Characteristic features include sharply demarcated lesions; bilateral symptoms; and white, blue, and/or red color changes, although the spectrum of symptoms observed is broad.[18] Maricq and colleagues have reported that, among adults who were cold sensitive, only 1% had triphasic color changes, and 37% had white or blue color only.[10] In a retrospective review of 123 pediatric patients, Nigrovic and colleagues reported that 24% of children with primary RP and 19% of children with secondary RP reported triphasic color changes, whereas 40% to 50% had only monophasic color changes.[5] An interesting cross-sectional study of patients in the Netherlands indicated that reactive hyperemia at the end of an attack and discoloration of the earlobes and nose were more highly associated with primary RP than with secondary RP.[52]

Significant factors differentiating primary from secondary RP are the absence of evidence for vascular disease by clinical examination (including blood pressure, pulses, and nailfold capillaroscopy) in primary RP, and the presence of abnormal nailfold capillaries and/or laboratory findings suggesting systemic disease in secondary RP. Primary RP attacks typically involve all fingers in a symmetrical pattern and are not commonly associated with significant pain. Asymmetrical finger involvement and severe pain, by contrast, are suggestive of an underlying pathology and should prompt a more vigorous evaluation. Although patients with primary RP are, by definition, generally healthy, comorbid conditions, including hypertension, atherosclerosis, cardiovascular disease, and diabetes mellitus, can increase the frequency or severity of symptoms. Anatomical variants, such as incomplete palmar arterial arch (clinical positive Allen test), can augment the symptoms of vasospasm, leading to earlier and more severe presentations.[53] An issue important in the evaluation of children with RP is the use of stimulants for attention deficit disorder, which may exacerbate vasospasm and vascular dysfunction.[54]

As discussed, the regulation of regional blood flow is complex and susceptible to a variety of insults. Also, the number of disorders associated with RP is extensive (see Box 31-3).[2] As research progresses, the border between idiopathic and "disease"-associated symptoms blurs. Ultimately, primary RP is a diagnosis of exclusion supported by lack of progression over time toward development of an associated disorder. Although extensive special testing is not always necessary, every patient with a diagnosis of RP should be carefully evaluated for features of concurrent or incipient disease. Among these, the rheumatological diagnoses most often associated with secondary RP are SSc, MCTD, and other CTD (e.g., systemic lupus erythematosus [SLE], overlap syndromes, polymyositis, dermatomyositis, Sjögren syndrome, and vasculitis). Other conditions that must be considered include occlusive vascular disease, drug effects, hematological or coagulation abnormalities, and other vasospastic syndromes (see Box 31-3 and later discussion).[2,55]

Nailfold Capillary Microscopy

Nailfold capillary microscopy is a simple, yet powerful diagnostic tool shown to significantly improve the predictive power of clinical evaluation.[51,56-60] The examination can be performed at the bedside using a handheld magnifier (e.g., DermLite) or with a low-power microscope (Fig. 31-3). Enlarged or distorted capillary loops, telangiectasias, and a relative paucity or loss of capillary loops strongly suggest a concurrent or incipient CTD. The presence of these features in a patient with RP should prompt a vigorous search for related findings.

Laboratory Testing

If the history and physical examination, including nailfold capillary microscopy, are not suggestive of a cause for secondary RP, a diagnosis of primary RP may be made, and there is no need for further specialized testing. In particular, blood tests such as the erythrocyte sedimentation rate and antinuclear antibody (ANA) are not necessary and may be misleading. If, however, there is a moderate or higher clinical suspicion of a secondary cause of RP, then special testing as indicated by the clinical assessment is appropriate. Recommended laboratory studies for possible connective tissue disorders include a complete blood count, a general blood chemical analysis with tests for renal and liver function, urinalysis, complement (C3 and C4), and ANA. If the

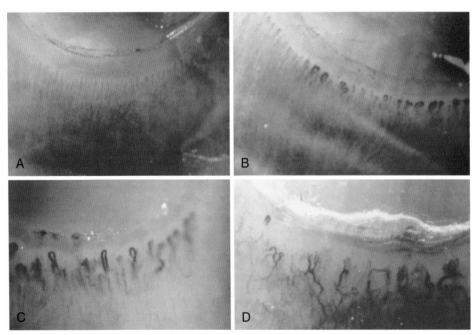

FIGURE 31-3 Nailfold capillaroscopy. **A,** Normal nailfold capillary size and distribution. **B,** Early changes of scleroderma showing dilation, tortuosity, and disorganization. **C,** Active stage scleroderma showing increasingly disorganized architecture, giant capillaries and hemorrhage, decreased number of vessels, and increased frequency of abnormal vessels. **D,** Late-stage scleroderma showing severe dropout and abnormal vessels with arborization. (From www.hakeem-sy.com/main/node/20196.)

ANA is positive, tests for specific autoantibodies may assist with formulating a diagnosis (e.g., anti-double-stranded DNA, anti-SSA [Ro], anti-SSB [La], antiribonucleoprotein, antitopoisomerase [anti-Scl 70], and antiphospholipid antibodies). Anticentromere pattern ANA and anti-Scl 70 antibodies have the highest sensitivity for predicting evolution to SSc and risk for development of digital ischemia.[18,61,62] It is important to recognize that while most pediatric patients with secondary RP will have a positive ANA (85% to 100%), a significant number of pediatric patients with primary RP will have nonspecific elevation of ANA titer without evidence for an associated rheumatic disorder.[4,5,63,64] Conversely, in a cohort of 1039 adult patients monitored prospectively, only 6.3% of patients with negative autoantibody studies developed CTD over more than 10 years of follow-up, whereas nearly 60% of patients with RP and a positive ANA were ultimately diagnosed with a CTD.[65] About 30% of pediatric patients with primary or secondary RP were also found to have antiphospholipid antibodies, although none of the patients had features of systemic antiphospholipid syndrome.[5]

Although anticentromere and antitopoisomerase antibodies are associated with development of SSc,[62] the combination of autoantibodies and nailfold capillary microscopy may be more informative than either finding alone. In a 20-year prospective study of 586 patients with RP who had no known CTD at enrollment, the overall incidence of limited (CREST variant) or diffuse SSc was 13%.[66] In patients with one or more related autoantibodies or abnormal nailfold capillary microscopy, the incidence of SSc was 47%, whereas in those with both an autoantibody and abnormal nailfold capillary microscopy, the incidence of SSc was nearly 80%. Further discussion of the clinical evaluation of systemic rheumatological disorders and the significance of autoantibodies in the prognosis of SSc are included elsewhere in this text (Chapter 27).

Differential Diagnosis

The differential diagnosis for RP includes the extensive list of conditions in Box 31-3. In patients who present with prolonged peripheral vascular obstruction, it is particularly important to distinguish whether they are experiencing a thrombotic event rather than transient vasospasm. Although an exhaustive discussion of these possibilities is beyond the scope of this chapter, the following paragraphs represent disorders commonly considered in the differential diagnosis of non-classic RP.

Acrocyanosis is an uncommon, painless, vasospastic disorder causing persistent coldness and bluish discoloration of the hands (and less commonly of the feet).[42] Patients with acrocyanosis have cold and diffusely cyanotic color changes that can involve the entire hand and foot, extending proximally without a sharp demarcation between affected and unaffected tissue. Mild diaphoresis may be present, creating a clammy feel to the extremities. Mild capillary abnormalities may exist but do not show the avascular regions or giant capillaries found in patients with scleroderma.[67] Both acrocyanosis and RP are more common in individuals with low body weight or who have anorexia nervosa.[68] Evaluation for cyanotic heart disease, celiac disease, eating disorders, or GI malabsorption should be considered.

Perniosis, or chilblains, is a cold-induced condition marked by the appearance of painful, erythematous, papular, or nodular lesions, usually located on the fingers, toes, thighs, and/or buttocks.[69,70] As with RP, pernio may present as an idiopathic process or in association with systemic disease (e.g., SLE). It is distinguished from RP by the lack of blanching and absence of a sharp line of demarcation. Although clinically and histologically distinct from RP, the treatment paradigms are similar and based primarily on nonpharmacological lifestyle modifications. Although definitive data are lacking, many of the agents used

for RP can be considered for pernio if pharmacological intervention is necessary.

Frostbite is relatively common in cold climates and can have prolonged sequelae including tissue loss and persistent cold sensitivity. In a study of 30 individuals who had suffered moderate (second degree) frostbite, Ervasti and colleagues reported subjective symptoms at 4 to 11 years after injury in 63% of the subjects, including hypersensitivity to cold, numbness, and decreased touch sensitivity. Cold air provocation testing revealed an increased tendency for vasospasm in these individuals, including white fingers in 20%.[55]

Carpal tunnel syndrome is relatively rare in children and is more often idiopathic or secondary to metabolic disorders (e.g., lysosomal storage diseases), rather than related to overuse as is seen in adults.[71] Symptoms are more characteristically numbness and reduced manual dexterity, rather than color changes, and are generally not related to cold exposure. Although the wrist-flexion test (Phalen maneuver) and the nerve compression or percussion test (Tinel sign) can be informative, they are often nondiagnostic in pediatric patients, and electrophysiological testing is indicated to confirm a diagnostic suspicion.

Brachial or *lumbosacral plexus neuropathies* are also rare in children, outside of those related to birth injury, but may be present in older adolescents and young adults presenting for evaluation in pediatric clinics.[72] The typical presentation of idiopathic brachial plexus neuritis (Parsonage–Turner syndrome) or lumbosacral plexopathy includes acute onset of shoulder or proximal leg pain, respectively, associated with weakness and muscle wasting in the extremity and without restricted passive range of motion. Numbness and color changes in the extremity are variable, but gradual in onset, fixed in nature, and typically less prominent a complaint than pain and neuromuscular symptoms. Idiopathic plexus neuropathies often follow an upper respiratory infection and may be recurrent. Electromyographic findings are characteristic and diagnostic. Prognosis is generally good, though recovery may be protracted and may require intensive physical therapy to reduce contractures and restore muscle strength.

Erythromelalgia is a relatively rare condition of paroxysmal vasodilation.[73,74] Erythromelalgia can be thought of as the opposite of RP. Symptoms manifest as episodic burning pain accompanied by erythema, warmth, and swelling of the hands and/or feet; symptoms are brought on by heat, exercise, or friction, and affected patients report dramatic relief with application of ice or cold water. Erythromelalgia also presents in both primary and secondary forms. Primary erythromelalgia (also termed *erythermalgia*) appears in childhood and can be familial (autosomal dominant) or sporadic. It affects girls more than boys, and symptoms are most often symmetrical; it is frequently resistant to treatment. Recent studies have attributed a majority of both familial and sporadic cases to gain-of-function mutations of SCN9A, the gene that encodes the voltage-gated sodium channel Na(v)1.7.[73] Loss-of-function mutations in the same gene are associated with congenital insensitivity to pain.[73] Secondary erythromelalgia is more common and typically presents in older children and adults. The majority of cases are associated with essential thrombocytosis and are characteristically responsive to low-dose aspirin therapy.[74] Erythromelalgia can also develop in individuals with small fiber neuropathies of various etiologies, including multiple sclerosis, hypercholesterolemia, mercury and other heavy-metal poisoning, and a variety of autoimmune diseases. These patients are not responsive to aspirin, but the condition typically responds to treatment of the underlying disorder. Management of erythromelalgia includes avoidance of triggers (heat, friction) and application of cold during acute attacks. Although controlled studies are lacking, if aspirin or treatment of associated conditions is unsuccessful, case studies have reported successful use of a range of approaches: pharmacological (e.g., nifedipine, verapamil, propranolol, nitroprusside), nonpharmacological (e.g., biofeedback, hypnosis), and surgical (sympathectomy, amputation, stereotactic destruction of regions of the hypothalamus).

Complex regional pain syndrome (CRPS), or reflex sympathetic dystrophy, will often present with altered temperature and coloration of the involved extremity.[75] Persons with CRPS usually have unilateral distal limb involvement, with the affected area showing differences in temperature (warmer or colder) and color (red, pale, or mottled) compared with the unaffected side. These individuals typically display severe diffuse allodynia; paresthesia, causalgia, or other abnormal sensations; refusal to move the affected region; and unusual positioning of the affected extremity. A detailed discussion of CRPS can be found elsewhere in this text (Chapter 52).

TREATMENT

The primary aim of treatment of patients with RP is to increase blood flow, which can be accomplished by increasing vasodilation or decreasing vasoconstriction. Treatment choices depend on the severity of digital ischemia and the presence of underlying disease.[76] Patients with primary RP do not generally report significant disability, although quality of life may be affected by symptoms and the need for cold avoidance. Spontaneous remission or improvement is also relatively common. In a prospective survey of a middle-aged white population with new-onset RP, remissions occurred in 64% of both women and men over a 7-year period.[9] Thus, a conservative, nonpharmacological approach is often sufficient and most appropriate for these patients. By comparison, individuals with secondary RP are more likely to have more severe attacks and require pharmacological agents to achieve symptomatic control.[2,76,77] Treatment of RP patients with moderate to severe disease is often problematic, because pharmacological side effects are often dose-limiting, responses to vasodilators are idiosyncratic, and there is lack of agreement as to objective measures of improvement. Clinical trials also consistently demonstrate a high rate of improvement (10% to 40%) among placebo-treated patients with either primary or secondary RP. This not only supports the recommendation that general education is an important factor in controlling attacks, but it emphasizes the importance of placebo-controlled trials in evaluating the efficacy of specific therapies.

General Measures

Patients with either primary or secondary RP benefit from education regarding the common triggers of Raynaud attacks and simple interventions to help prevent and terminate episodes (Box 31-4).[2,78] Nonpharmacological therapeutic interventions include avoidance of cold temperatures, stress, and vasoconstrictors; the use of warm/layered clothing; and techniques to terminate an attack, such as massage, windmill motions of the arms, and immersion in warm water. Because sympathetic tone and sensitivity to sympathetic mediators are enhanced in patients with RP, reduction of emotional stress and anxiety are useful treatment goals.[79]

Behavioral Therapy

A variety of behavioral therapies (e.g., biofeedback, autogenic training, classic conditioning) have been employed in patients with RP.[78] Multiple studies have demonstrated that normal subjects can voluntarily control peripheral blood flow and skin temperature using these techniques.[80,81] Studies exploring their use in RP, however, vary greatly in methodological rigor. Many lack no-treatment controls and, in general, they report an effect size similar to that of the placebo-response seen in other trials. In one well-controlled randomized study of patients with primary RP, the authors found no benefit with temperature or

---

BOX 31-4 **General Measures for the Management of the Raynaud Phenomenon**

Avoid cold exposure

Minimize emotional stress

Dress warmly (layered clothing, long sleeves and pants, socks, thermal underwear, and heat-conserving hats)

Keep hands/feet warm and dry (e.g., mittens, boots, electric or chemical hand/foot warmers)

Use warming methods to terminate attacks, e.g., place hands under warm water or in a warm body fold (e.g., axillae), rotate arms in a windmill pattern or swing-arm maneuver (forceful side-to-side swinging motion)

Avoid rapid changes in temperature, e.g., transitions from hot to cool environments, cool breezes, or humid cold air

Avoid smoking and exposure to secondhand smoke

Avoid sympathomimetic drugs and central nervous system stimulants (e.g., decongestants, amphetamines, methylphenidate, and dextroamphetamine)

---

electromyogenic biofeedback, and found that sustained-release nifedipine was superior to either behavioral method.[82] Similarly, a study of biofeedback in 24 scleroderma patients failed to demonstrate either symptomatic improvement or increased finger temperature in response to voluntary control or cold stress.[83] Although controlled trials have not shown dramatic effects, behavioral therapies and education are helpful to reduce stress related triggers and to improve compliance with both pharmacological and nonpharmacological interventions. Although these approaches alone are unlikely to be sufficient to control symptoms in moderate and severe forms of RP, they can provide substantial benefit as an adjunct to medical interventions. Overall, these approaches appear to be safe.

Pharmacological Measures

Pharmacological agents targeting various physiological pathways have been used to treat RP with varying degrees of support from controlled trials (Box 31-5).[2,61,84] Calcium channel blockers (CCBs) are the most commonly prescribed agents, and their efficacy has been well proven in controlled trials with both children and adults.[85] Use of alternative vasodilator agents as first-line therapy for the treatment of RP is not recommended, because CCBs have been shown to be the most consistently effective and are often better tolerated. However, because individual responses may be idiosyncratic, patients who do not tolerate or who fail to respond adequately to CCBs can be treated with other vasoactive agents alone or, more commonly, in combination with a CCB.[2,61,84] A brief summary of major findings is included below, and algorithms for management of primary or mild RP and complex RP with digital ischemia are shown in Figs. 31-4 and 31-5. It should be emphasized that corticosteroids and immunosuppressive agents are not appropriate in the management of primary or SSc-related RP.

For patients with uncomplicated primary RP, medical therapy should only be considered in those who fail vigorous application of nonpharmacological measures. In these cases, a long-acting CCB such as controlled-release nifedipine or amlodipine is the initial treatment of choice. Titrating to lowest effective dose and use of medications only during periods of expected cold exposure (e.g., winter months) can help to minimize medication exposure in patients with minimal risk (primary RP and mild secondary RP).[2,86] Patients with secondary or more severe RP are likely to require more aggressive therapy. In these patients, it is unlikely that medical therapy will completely terminate attacks, and it is not useful to use this as the primary goal or measure of effectiveness of treatment. Instead, the major goals

BOX 31-5   The Pharmacological Treatment of Raynaud Phenomenon

Calcium channel blockers (dihydropyridine)
  Nifedipine, nicardipine, amlodipine, felodipine, nisoldipine, and isradipine
Calcium channel blockers (non-dihydropyridine)
  Diltiazem
Direct vasodilators
  Nitroglycerin, nitroprusside, hydralazine, papaverine, minoxidil, niacin, and nitric oxide (via a generating system)
Indirect vasodilators
  Angiotensin-converting enzymes inhibitor (captopril, enalapril)
  Angiotensin II receptor blockers (losartan)
  Endothelin-1 receptor antagonists (bosentan)
  Phosphodiesterase inhibitors (sildenafil, tadalafil, vardenafil, pentoxifylline)
  Serotonin reuptake inhibitors (fluoxetine)
Sympatholytic agents (alpha-adrenergic receptor antagonists)
  Methyldopa, reserpine, phentolamine, and prazosin
Prostaglandins
  Prostaglandin E1 (PGE1) (alprostadil)
  Prostacyclin (PGI2) (epoprostenol)
Antioxidant agents
  Zinc gluconate
  N-acetylcysteine
Anticoagulation, antithrombotic and thrombolytic agents
  Aspirin
  Dipyridamole
  Heparin
  Tissue plasminogen activator
Other
  Botulinum toxin-A

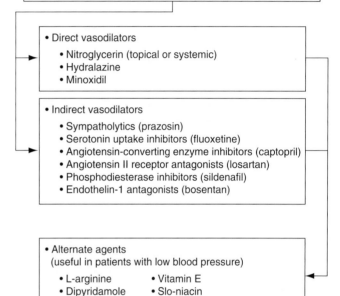

FIGURE 31-4 Treatment algorithm for uncomplicated Raynaud phenomenon.

of treatment in secondary RP are to reduce the frequency and severity of attacks, to prevent new digital ulceration and to promote healing of existing lesions.

Calcium Channel Blockers

CCBs are the most widely used class of drugs in the treatment of RP. In addition to their vasodilating properties, CCBs have other biological effects, including inhibition of platelet activation, that are beneficial in management of RP.[87] Among the different pharmacological classes, the dihydropyridine group (nifedipine, amlodipine, felodipine) is the least cardioselective and appears to be the most efficacious. Variability of reported responses occurs, in part, because patients with secondary RP (particularly those with SSc) are less likely to benefit from nifedipine and other CCBs than those with primary RP, and not all trials clearly segregate these different RP populations. Two meta-analyses of randomized, double-blind, placebo-controlled trials assessing efficacy of CCBs (primarily nifedipine) in primary and secondary (SSc-associated) RP have reported therapeutic benefit, with a significant reduction in the mean number of attacks and the severity of symptoms in both groups.[85,88] Results were more significant for secondary RP than primary RP, as might be expected. Patients with primary RP generally have lower degrees of severity and were treated with lower doses of CCBs, which may have lowered the measured effectiveness in these studies. Therapeutic benefit in practice, therefore, may be even greater than predicted from these results. For the management of nonurgent RP, slow-release or long-acting preparations of nifedipine (30 to

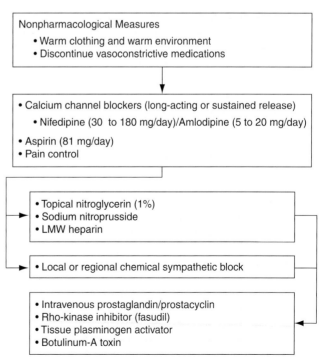

FIGURE 31-5 Treatment algorithm for complex Raynaud phenomenon with digital ischemia.

180 mg daily) or amlodipine (5 to 20 mg daily) are recommended to improve compliance, reduce the incidence of adverse effects, and potentially achieve more sustained vascular improvement. Adverse effects, including headache, light-headedness, and lower extremity edema, require discontinuation or dose modification in approximately 15% of patients and can be minimized by initiating therapy at a low dose with a sustained-release preparation and advancing over several weeks.

Angiotensin Inhibitors

Angiotensin-converting enzyme inhibitors and angiotensin II receptor antagonists have experienced expanded use, particularly in patients with SSc, due to increased awareness of their effects on endothelial function and vascular remodeling, though only limited trials have been completed.[84] A randomized, parallel-group, controlled trial of losartan, an angiotensin II receptor antagonist, significantly reduced the frequency and severity of vasoconstrictive episodes in patients with primary and SSc-related RP, with effects comparable to sustained-release nifedipine.[89] Although these results are promising, further investigation is needed to establish the role of these agents in the treatment of RP.

Serotonin Receptor Inhibitors

Selective serotonin receptor inhibitors such as fluoxetine and ketanserin have engendered strong interest due to their potential effects on both local and CNS-mediated mechanisms regulating vasoconstriction. Although there are anecdotal reports of therapeutic benefit,[84] there have been few well-designed, placebo-controlled trials of the use of SSRIs in RP. Results of these studies have been mixed.

Phosphodiesterase Inhibitors

Phosphodiesterase-5 (PDE-5) inhibitors potentiate the effect of NO by preventing the degradation of cyclic guanosine monophosphate, leading to enhanced vasodilation and increased blood flow. Interest in these agents has grown as a number of case reports and small series have reported their benefit in the treatment of RP.[17,61,84,90] However, several controlled trials of PDE-5 inhibitors have been published in recent years with somewhat conflicting results. A recent systematic review and meta-analysis concluded PDE-5 inhibitors provide moderate, but significant, benefit for treatment of secondary RP, particularly in combination with CCBs.[90] Although these studies are supportive, additional work is needed to assess adequately the role of these agents in primary and secondary RP and in critical digital ischemia.

Endothelin Inhibitors

Endothelin-1 induces vasoconstriction and is thought to play a key role in the pathogenesis of SSc. Bosentan, an oral, nonpeptide endothelin receptor antagonist, has been shown to be effective in the treatment of both idiopathic and SSc-related pulmonary hypertension.[17,61] Two placebo-controlled randomized clinical trials among SSc patients (RAPIDS-1 and RAPIDS-2) have demonstrated the efficacy of bosentan in preventing new digital ulcers although there was no reduction in frequency or intensity of RP attacks, and no improvement in the healing of existing digital ulcers.[91] Endothelin receptor antagonists, including bosentan, are considered teratogenic and should be used only when appropriate measures to prevent pregnancy are in place.[92]

Antioxidants

Increased awareness of the importance of oxidative stress in the pathogenesis of RP has stimulated interest in antioxidant therapy; however, evidence of benefit from controlled studies is lacking. In a pilot study of 22 patients with SSc, treatment with intravenous *N*-acetylcysteine

improved the frequency and severity of RP episodes and reduced the number of unhealed ulcers.[93] A randomized, parallel-group study of 40 patients with primary and secondary RP treated with probucol, a cholesterol-lowering and antioxidant agent, showed only a modest effect on the frequency and severity of Raynaud attacks.[94] Similarly, a double-blind, placebo-controlled study of 33 patients with SSc-associated RP demonstrated no benefit after 20 weeks of treatment with micronutrient antioxidants (selenium, beta-carotene, vitamin C, vitamin E, and methionine) and allopurinol (which blocks superoxide).[95] It is possible that early initiation of antioxidant therapy would be more effective, but the current data do not support a substantial benefit.

Nitric Oxide

Although the specific role NO plays in the pathophysiology of RP remains to be elucidated, there is considerable interest in its therapeutic use. Supplementation of NO has been explored in several ways, including administration of its precursor, L-arginine, and treatment with NO donors, including topical glyceryl trinitrate and parenteral sodium nitroprusside. Small studies of topical glyceryl trinitrate (1%) significantly reduced the number and severity of Raynaud attacks in both primary and secondary RP when compared with placebo.[96,97] Oral L-arginine supplementation for 28 days did not produce any benefits in RP, but intra-arterial L-arginine and sodium nitroprusside both significantly improved the response to an acute cold challenge in patients with SSc.[98-100]

Calcitonin Gene Related Peptide

Calcitonin gene-related peptide (CGRP), a neuropeptide found in sensory nerves, has been shown to be reduced in patients with RP when compared with controls. In one study of patients with severe RP, intravenous CGRP improved hand and digital blood flow, skin temperature, and hand rewarming, compared to saline, and treatment resulted in healing of digital ulcers in four of five patients.[101]

Alpha-Adrenergic Blockade

As highlighted previously, it is increasingly clear that sympathetic adrenergic stimulation, particularly of the alpha-2 adrenergic receptors on the digital arteries, plays an important role in the pathogenesis of RP.[2] Although a variety of sympatholytic drugs have been tried in RP patients, few controlled studies are available to define the role of these agents, and there is some evidence that patients become refractory with prolonged use. In a placebo-controlled trial, the alpha-1 adrenergic receptor antagonist prazosin provided modest improvement in SSc-associated RP, but frequent side effects were noted.[102] Preclinical studies and early trials of more selective alpha-adrenergic blockers, including selective alpha-2c adrenergic receptor antagonists, have stimulated interest in evaluating the digital vascular effects of agents in this drug class.[103,104]

Rho-Kinase Inhibition

Data indicating that Rho-kinases are directly involved in cold-induced vasoconstriction has prompted increasing interest in inhibition of this pathway.[105] Fasudil, a Rho-kinase inhibitor, has been shown to have significant acute vasodilator effects in patients with RP, as well as pulmonary hypertension and other vasospastic conditions.[106-108] Rho-kinase inhibitors represent an innovative and distinct set of therapeutic agents for RP that merit further clinical investigation.

Botulinum Toxin-A

Botulinum toxin-A (Botox®) inhibits acetylcholine signaling, causing flaccid paralysis and inhibition of signaling through C-type pain fibers.

In a case series of 11 patients with vasospasm who failed aggressive medical therapy, all patients treated with perivascular injections of botulinum toxin-A experienced significant pain reduction, and 9 of 11 patients reported digital ulcer healing and decreased severity and frequency of vasospastic episodes.[109]

Prostanoids

Prostanoids can be predicted to have a number of potentially beneficial effects in patients with RP, including vasodilation, inhibition of platelet aggregation, suppression of profibrotic cytokines and connective tissue growth factors, and effects on vascular remodeling. However, limited availability of oral agents and significant side effects of therapy have limited use primarily to treatment of severe refractory RP and ischemic digital ulcers. A variety of studies have examined the efficacy of preparations of prostaglandin E1 (PGE1),[110] prostacyclin (PGI2),[111] and iloprost (a PGI2 analog)[112-115] in SSc-related RP and digital ischemia, and reported mixed results. Intravenous iloprost has been shown to be beneficial in children with RP, but it is not available in the United States. An iloprost formulation for inhalation (Ventavis) is available in the United States with an indication for treatment of pulmonary hypertension, though experience with its use for RP is limited.[116] Intravenous prostacyclin (epoprostenol) has also been reported as beneficial in pediatric patients with severe RP with digital ischemia, although cost and the need for continuous intravenous infusion limit clinical use.[117] New oral and transdermal prostanoid agents are approaching the market, and will presumably be studied for effectiveness in patients with moderate to severe RP.[118]

Antithrombotic Agents

Antithrombotic agents are commonly utilized in patients with RP in whom ulceration and thrombosis have occurred, although published data are largely case-based and limited.[119] Antiplatelet therapy with aspirin (75 or 81 mg/day) may be considered in patients with secondary RP who have a history of ischemic ulcers or other thrombotic events; however, aspirin could theoretically worsen vasospasm via reduction in the production of prostacyclin and other vasodilating prostaglandins. Dipyridamole has been used in a similar fashion for its antiplatelet and vasodilating properties, but this agent does not appear to have a major impact in patients with severe RP.[119] Anticoagulation or thrombolytic therapy can be considered during the acute phase of an ischemic event, but controlled trials are lacking, and these treatments are best limited to acute care of embolic or vascular occlusive disease associated with new thrombosis.[119] A small placebo-controlled study of long-term therapy with low molecular weight heparin showed a reduction in the severity of RP after 4 weeks that was maximal by 20 weeks.[120] Small studies have also suggested that thrombolytic therapy, such as tissue plasminogen activator, may be helpful in patients with RP and scleroderma.[121] However, controlled studies will need to be performed before it is known if this approach will improve acute ischemia in severe RP.

Other Measures
Sympathectomy

Sympathectomy has been used for more than 80 years to treat RP.[2,76] Temporary local (digital or wrist block) or regional (cervical or lumbar) chemical sympathectomy to reverse vasoconstriction can be performed with lidocaine or bupivacaine (without epinephrine). This form of transient sympathectomy may not have a long-lasting benefit, but it is sometimes successful in reversing severe acute vasospasm (e.g., critical digital ischemia) that is slowly or poorly responsive to medical therapy.[86] Localized microsurgical digital sympathectomy has been introduced as an alternative to proximal sympathectomy.[122] Although

case series have reported successful responses and few complications, the role of sympathectomy in management of severe RP has not been defined by controlled studies. Differences in the causes of ischemia, surgical techniques, and outcome measures make interpretation of the reported series difficult. It is also unclear whether the benefits of sympathectomy persist over time; the available data suggest high rates of relapse and variable benefit at 1 year.[86] At present, it appears these procedures should be limited to patients who have failed medical treatment and who have digital ischemia or other severe manifestation of RP.

Vascular Reconstruction

Occlusion of a major artery can occur in patients with secondary RP.[123] In patients with SSc, in particular, arterial occlusion is not rare and occurs most commonly in the ulnar artery. Microsurgical revascularization of the hand and digital arterial reconstruction in this setting may improve digital perfusion and promote healing of digital ulcers.[123]

Management of Critical Digital Ischemia

The keys to success in the setting of critical digital ischemia are early intervention and rapid escalation (Fig. 31-5). Patients with severe digital ischemia, uncontrolled pain, or impending digital autoamputation should be hospitalized and kept warm and quiet. Pain due to severe ischemia may be intense, and adequate pain control may require the use of narcotic analgesics or a regional nerve block. All complex cases should be fully evaluated for reversible processes that may be causing or aggravating the crisis, including correctable macrovascular disease, vasculitis, or hypercoagulable states. Doppler ultrasound can be helpful in distinguishing sources of obstruction and in directing further diagnostic and therapeutic decisions.

Hospitalized patients should receive aggressive vasodilator therapy with either extended release nifedipine or amlodipine (at the highest tolerated dose) and antiplatelet therapy with low-dose aspirin as an initial agent. Antibiotics should be considered if the area of ischemia is necrotic or appears infected. If normal blood flow is not restored within a few hours, then combination therapy, such as the addition of transdermal nitroglycerin or a sympatholytic agent, is suggested. Treatment with heparin for a period of 24 to 72 hours is commonly suggested if digital ischemia progresses during vasodilator therapy, and/or the onset of arterial occlusion is thought to be secondary to acute thrombosis or embolization. However, there have been no trials that have assessed this treatment. Temporary chemical sympathectomy should be considered when oral and/or topical vasodilator therapy does not quickly result in improvement in digital blood flow. If temporary chemical sympathectomy succeeds in reversing vasospasm and relieving critical ischemia, it suggests that the structural arterial disease is not advanced. If ischemia recurs as the effects of chemical sympathectomy wane, despite the ongoing use of vasodilator therapy, surgical sympathectomy or perivascular injection of botulinum toxin-A can be considered. If these measures do not reverse the ischemia, or if the clinical presentation is severe (e.g., multiple ischemic digits, limb-threatening ischemia), an intravenous infusion of a prostaglandin (PGE1) or prostacyclin (PGI2) analog may be beneficial.[110,112-115,124] Intravenous iloprost, in particular, has been reported to be safe and effective in the treatment of ischemic digits in children with SSc and other CTDs.[125] In patients with late-stage ischemia or severe structural arterial disease that cannot vasodilate in response to medical therapy, pain control and surgical amputation may be the only options.

Summary and Future Directions

RP is a common presenting feature among patients seen in pediatric clinics and should be evaluated with an eye toward identification of the causes of secondary RP. Individuals with both primary and secondary RP will benefit from education and nonpharmacological control measures. This is often all that is required for primary RP, whereas patients with secondary RP more often require medical therapy. First-line drug therapy for RP is most commonly a long-acting CCB, given during symptomatic periods or seasons. A variety of alternate agents is available that can be used alone or in combination with CCB therapy for patients who require more aggressive care. Severe or critical digital ischemia requires immediate evaluation to identify reversible vascular and coagulation defects, and aggressive intervention to restore blood flow. Consideration should be given to pain control, vasodilatation, anticoagulation, and chemical or surgical sympathectomy in management of these patients.

The complexity involved in conducting clinical trials of RP and the lack of standard outcome measures remain a challenge to investigators. However, advances in the understanding of the pathogenesis of RP and the development of complementary therapeutics continue to provide improved outcomes for patients, particularly for those with severe disease. The indication that primary RP reflects a genetic variant or fundamental vascular disorder is a target of active investigation. Preliminary results with novel vasoactive agents suggest opportunities exist for development of more effective therapies.

REFERENCES

2. R. Bakst, J.F. Merola, A.G. Franks Jr., M. Sanchez, Raynaud's phenomenon: pathogenesis and management, J. Am. Acad. Dermatol. 59 (2008) 633–653.

3. B.H. Athreya, Vasospastic disorders in children, Semin. Pediatr. Surg. 3 (1994) 70–78.

4. C.M. Duffy, R.M. Laxer, P. Lee, et al., Raynaud syndrome in childhood, J. Pediatr. 114 (1989) 73–78.

5. P.A. Nigrovic, R.C. Fuhlbrigge, R.P. Sundel, Raynaud's phenomenon in children: a retrospective review of 123 patients, Pediatrics 111 (2003) 715–721.

6. F.M. Wigley, Clinical manifestations and diagnosis of the Raynaud phenomenon, in: J. Axford (Ed.), UpToDate, Wolters Kluwer Health, UpToDate, Inc., Waltham, MA, 2009.

8. E.C. LeRoy, T.A. Medsger Jr., Raynaud's phenomenon: a proposal for classification, Clin. Exp. Rheumatol. 10 (1992) 485–488.

9. L.G. Suter, J.M. Murabito, D.T. Felson, L. Fraenkel, The incidence and natural history of Raynaud's phenomenon in the community, Arthritis Rheum. 52 (2005) 1259–1263.

10. H.R. Maricq, P.H. Carpentier, M.C. Weinrich, et al., Geographic variation in the prevalence of Raynaud's phenomenon: a 5 region comparison, J. Rheumatol. 24 (1997) 879–889.

12. G.T. Jones, A.L. Herrick, S.E. Woodham, et al., Occurrence of Raynaud's phenomenon in children ages 12–15 years: prevalence and association with other common symptoms, Arthritis Rheum. 48 (2003) 3518–3521.

16. N.A. Flavahan, S. Flavahan, S. Mitra, M.A. Chotani, The vasculopathy of Raynaud's phenomenon and scleroderma, Rheum. Dis. Clin. North Am. 29 (2003) 275–291.

17. L. Landry, Current medical and surgical management of Raynaud's syndrome, J. Vasc. Surg. 57 (2013) 1710–1716.

18. F.M. Wigley, Clinical practice. Raynaud's Phenomenon, N. Engl. J. Med. 347 (2002) 1001–1008.

19. R. Bakst, J.F. Merola, A.G. Franks, M. Sanchez, Raynaud's phenomenon: pathogenesis and management, J. Am. Acad. Dermatol. 59 (2008) 633–653.

21. F.M. Wigley, Pathogenesis of Raynaud Phenomena, in: J. Axford (Ed.), UpToDate, Wolters Kluwer Health, UpToDate, Inc., Waltham. MA, 2014.

22. A.L. Herrick, The pathogenesis, diagnosis and treatment of Raynaud's phenomenon, Nat. Rev. Rheumatol. 8 (2012) 469–479.

30. M.A. Chotani, S. Flavahan, S. Mitra, et al., Silent alpha(2C)-adrenergic receptors enable cold-induced vasoconstriction in cutaneous arteries, Am. J. Physiol. Heart. Circ. Physiol. 278 (2000) H1075–H1083.

31. M.A. Chotani, S. Mitra, B.Y. Su, et al., Regulation of alpha(2)-adrenoceptors in human vascular smooth muscle cells, Am. J. Physiol. Heart. Circ. Physiol. 286 (2004) H59–H67.

32. S.R. Bailey, A.H. Eid, S. Mitra, et al., Rho kinase mediates cold-induced constriction of cutaneous arteries: role of alpha2C-adrenoceptor translocation, Circ. Res. 94 (2004) 1367–1374.

34. P.B. Furspan, S. Chatterjee, M.D. Mayes, R.R. Freedman, Cooling-induced contraction and protein tyrosine kinase activity of isolated arterioles in secondary Raynaud's phenomenon, Rheumatology (Oxford) 44 (2005) 488–494.

36. J.A. Block, W. Sequeira, Raynaud's phenomenon, Lancet 357 (2001) 2042–2048.

39. M.B. Kahaleh, Raynaud phenomenon and the vascular disease in scleroderma, Curr. Opin. Rheumatol. 16 (2004) 718–722.

40. M. Matucci Cerinic, M.B. Kahaleh, Beauty and the beast. The nitric oxide paradox in systemic sclerosis, Rheumatology (Oxford) 41 (2002) 843–847.

42. J.P. Cooke, J.M. Marshall, Mechanisms of Raynaud's disease, Vasc. Med. 10 (2005) 293–307.

43. W.A. Schmidt, A. Krause, B. Schicke, D. Wernicke, Color Doppler ultrasonography of hand and finger arteries to differentiate primary from secondary forms of Raynaud's phenomenon, J. Rheumatol. 35 (2008) 1591–1598.

47. S.H. Kim, H.O. Kim, Y.G. Jeong, et al., The diagnostic accuracy of power Doppler ultrasonography for differentiating secondary from primary Raynaud's phenomenon in undifferentiated connective tissue disease, Clin. Rheumatol. 27 (2008) 783–786.

48. P. Brennan, A. Silman, C. Black, et al., Validity and reliability of three methods used in the diagnosis of Raynaud's phenomenon. The UK Scleroderma Study Group, Br. J. Rheumatol. 32 (1993) 357–361.

50. E. Allen, G. Brown, Raynaud's disease: A critical review of minimal requisites for diagnosis, Am. J. Med. Sci. 183 (1932) 187.

51. M. Hudson, S. Taillefer, R. Steele, et al., Improving the sensitivity of the American College of Rheumatology classification criteria for systemic sclerosis, Clin. Exp. Rheumatol. 25 (2007) 754–757.

52. H. Wollersheim, T. Thien, The diagnostic value of clinical signs and symptoms in patients with Raynaud's phenomenon. A cross-sectional study, Neth. J. Med. 37 (1990) 171–182.

54. W. Goldman, R. Seltzer, P. Reuman, Association between treatment with central nervous system stimulants and Raynaud's syndrome in children: a retrospective case-control study of rheumatology patients, Arthritis Rheum. 58 (2008) 563–566.

56. F. Ingegnoli, P. Boracchi, R. Gualtierotti, et al., Prognostic model based on nailfold capillaroscopy for identifying Raynaud's phenomenon patients at high risk for the development of a scleroderma spectrum disorder: PRINCE (prognostic index for nailfold capillaroscopic examination), Arthritis Rheum. 58 (2008) 2174–2182.

58. S. Pavlov-Dolijanovic, N. Damjanov, P. Ostojic, et al., The prognostic value of nailfold capillary changes for the development of connective tissue disease in children and adolescents with primary Raynaud phenomenon: a follow-up study of 250 patients, Pediatr. Dermatol. 23 (2006) 437–442.

60. C. Kayser, J.Y. Sekiyama, L.C. Prospero, et al., Nailfold capillaroscopy abnormalities as predictors of mortality in patients with systemic sclerosis, Clin. Exp. Rheumatol. 31 (2 Suppl. 76) (2013) 103–108.

61. J.E. Pope, The diagnosis and treatment of Raynaud's phenomenon: a practical approach, Drugs 67 (2007) 517–525.

63. P. Navon, A. Yarom, E. Davis, Raynaud's features in childhood. Clinical, immunological and capillaroscopic study, J. Mal. Vasc. 17 (1992) 273–276.

64. M. Hirschl, K. Hirschl, M. Lenz, et al., Transition from primary Raynaud's phenomenon to secondary Raynaud's phenomenon identified by diagnosis of an associated disease: results of ten years of prospective surveillance, Arthritis Rheum. 54 (2006) 1974–1981.

65. G.J. Landry, J.M. Edwards, R.B. McLafferty, et al., Long-term outcome of Raynaud's syndrome in a prospectively analyzed patient cohort, J. Vasc. Surg. 23 (1996) 76–85, discussion 85–86.

73. S.D. Dib-Hajj, Y. Yang, S.G. Waxman, Genetics and molecular pathophysiology of Na(v)1.7-related pain syndromes, Adv. Genet. 63 (2008) 85–110.

76. A.L. Herrick, Management of Raynaud's phenomena and digital ischemia, Curr. Rheumatol. Rep. 15 (2013) 303–310.

77. O. Kowal-Bielecka, R. Landewe, J. Avouac, et al., EULAR recommendations for the treatment of systemic sclerosis: a report from the EULAR Scleroderma Trials and Research group (EUSTAR), Ann. Rheum. Dis. 68 (2009) 620–628.

78. F.M. Wigley, Nonpharmacologic therapy for the Raynaud phenomenon, in: J. Axford (Ed.), UpToDate, Wolters Kluwer Health, UpToDate, Inc., Waltham, MA, 2008.

84. P. Sinnathurai, L. Schreiber, Treatment of Raynaud phenomena in systemic sclerosis, Intern. Med. J. 43 (5) (2013) 476–483.

85. A.E. Thompson, J.E. Pope, Calcium channel blockers for primary Raynaud's phenomenon: a meta-analysis, Rheumatology (Oxford) 44 (2005) 145–150.

87. K. Takahara, A. Kuroiwa, T. Matsushima, et al., Effects of nifedipine on platelet function, Am. Heart J. 109 (1985) 4–8.

88. A.E. Thompson, B. Shea, V. Welch, et al., Calcium-channel blockers for Raynaud's phenomenon in systemic sclerosis, Arthritis Rheum. 44 (2001) 1841–1847.

102. J. Pope, D. Fenlon, A. Thompson, et al., Prazosin for Raynaud's phenomenon in progressive systemic sclerosis, Cochrane Database Syst. Rev. (2000) CD000956.

115. F.M. Wigley, J.H. Korn, M.E. Csuka, et al., Oral iloprost treatment in patients with Raynaud's phenomenon secondary to systemic sclerosis: a multicenter, placebo-controlled, double-blind study, Arthritis Rheum. 41 (1998) 670–677.

116. A. Pakozdi, K. Howell, H. Wilson, et al., Inhaled iloprost for the treatment of Raynaud's phenomenon, Clin. Exp. Rheumatol. 26 (2008) 709.

125. F. Zulian, F. Corona, V. Gerloni, et al., Safety and efficacy of iloprost for the treatment of ischemic digits in pediatric connective tissue diseases, Rheumatology 43 (2004) 229–233.

The entire reference list is available online at www.expertconsult.com.

32 | CHAPTER

Vasculitis and Its Classification

Ross E. Petty, David A. Cabral

The term *vasculitis* indicates the presence of inflammation in a blood vessel wall. The inflammatory infiltrate may be one that is predominantly neutrophilic, eosinophilic, or mononuclear. *Perivasculitis* describes inflammation around the blood vessel wall but without mural involvement. *Vasculopathy*, a broader term, indicates an abnormality of blood vessels that may be inflammatory, degenerative, or may result from intimal proliferation.

CLASSIFICATION

The vasculitides are the most difficult of all rheumatic diseases to classify. Traditionally, vasculitis syndromes have been categorized according to features that include clinical phenotype, the predominant size of the involved vessels, or the histopathology of the involved vessel. Within such a framework, in 1990 a committee of the American College of Rheumatology (ACR) provided formal classification criteria for many, but not all, individual types of vasculitis.[1] In 2012, the International Chapel Hill Consensus Conference (CHCC 2012)[2] updated the 1994 consensus recommendations (CHCC 1994)[3] on the names of diseases, preferred abbreviations, and disease definitions (Table 32-1). CHCC 2012 retained the ACR framework for categories of vasculitis based on the size of predominantly affected blood vessels defined as follows. Large-vessel vasculitis (LVV) involves arteries outside organs, including muscles, nerves, kidneys, and skin; medium-vessel vasculitis (MVV) involves the main visceral arteries and their branches; small-vessel vasculitis (SVV) involves intraparenchymal arteries, arterioles, capillaries, and venules. Variable-vessel vasculitis (VVV) involves vessels (arteries, veins, capillaries) of any size and includes Behçet disease and Cogan syndrome. Also added are categories of single organ vasculitis (which includes isolated central nervous system vasculitis), vasculitis associated with systemic disease (such as systemic lupus erythematosus) and vasculitis associated with a probable etiology (such as hepatitis or drug-induced vasculitis). The most notable addition has been the incorporation of the presence or absence of antineutrophil cytoplasmic antibody (ANCA) within the classification framework, and thus small vasculitis is subcategorized into immune complex and ANCA-associated vasculitis. Subcategorization according to histopathology (e.g., granulomatous versus nongranulomatous) has not been retained because of the limited consistency of histopathological findings. The use of eponyms have also been phased out, particularly where

a noneponymous replacement could reflect some pathophysiological specificity. Thus, Wegener granulomatosis, Churg–Strauss syndrome, and Henoch–Schönlein purpura have been replaced, respectively, with the terms *granulomatosis with polyangiitis* (GPA), *eosinophilic granulomatosis with polyangiitis* (EGPA), and IgA vasculitis.

The CHCC 2012 nomenclature and the definitions[2] do not provide diagnostic and classification criteria. Therefore, the 1990 ACR criteria, derived primarily from adult-patient data, remains the most widely used system for classifying patients with vasculitis.[1] These ACR criteria have limited usefulness when applied to children with chronic vasculitis and result in a significant proportion being described as unclassifiable.[4-6] A pediatric adaptation of the ACR criteria, taking into account common pediatric manifestations and the presence of ANCA, was developed by consensus by a group of pediatric experts and reported in 2006[7] (Box 32-1). Proposed criteria for four diseases (GPA, Takayasu arteritis [TAK], polyarteritis nodosa [PAN], and Henoch–Schönlein purpura [HSP]) were subsequently tested and improved upon using a cohort of pediatric patients. The final validated criteria had improved sensitivity when compared with the ACR criteria and were subsequently published in 2010, after having been endorsed by the European League Against Rheumatism, the Pediatric Rheumatology International Trial Organization, and the Pediatric Rheumatology European Society (EULAR/PRINTO/PRES).[8] Unfortunately, these criteria retain some inherent limitations of the ACR criteria that have also been recognized in the adult literature. Specifically, the lack of any criteria for microscopic polyangiitis (MPA) has led to difficulties in discriminating GPA patients from MPA patients (see Chapter 36). This conundrum has led, on the one hand, to the convenient grouping of GPA and MPA in adult clinical trials under the rubric of ANCA-associated vasculitis (AAV). On the other hand, complex algorithms have been proposed or required to differentiate patients with the various types of AAV and PAN for study.[9-11] Because of this and other classification inadequacies, the whole system for classifying vasculitis currently remains under scrutiny.[12] The CHCC 2012 initiative provides a framework for developing and rigorously verifying new criteria. The Diagnostic and Classification of Vasculitis (DCVAS) prospective study is an international initiative launched in 2010[13] aiming to develop both revised classification criteria and a validated set of diagnostic criteria for systemic vasculitis in adult patients. This will have implications for the diagnosis and classification of pediatric patients that will be evaluated in an integrated Pediatric Vasculitis Initiative (PedVas).

TABLE 32-1 2012 Chapel Hill Consensus Conference on Nomenclature of Systemic Vasculitis

Large-vessel vasculitis (LVV)*

Giant cell (temporal) arteritis (GCA)	Granulomatous arteritis of the aorta and its major branches with a predilection for the extracranial branches of the carotid artery. *It often involves the temporal artery. Usually occurs in patients older than 50 years of age and is often associated with polymyalgia rheumatica.†*
Takayasu arteritis (TAK)	Granulomatous inflammation of the aorta and its major branches. *Usually occurs in patients much younger than 50 years of age.*

Medium-vessel vasculitis (MVV)*

Polyarteritis nodosa (PAN)	Necrotizing inflammation of medium-sized or small arteries without glomerulonephritis or vasculitis in arterioles, capillaries, or venules and not associated with ANCAs.
Kawasaki disease (KD)	Arteritis involving large, medium-sized, and small arteries associated with the mucocutaneous lymph node syndrome. *Coronary arteries are often involved. Aorta and veins may be affected. Usually occurs in children.*

Small-vessel vasculitis (SVV)*

ANCA-associated vasculitis (AAV)

Granulomatosis with polyangiitis (GPA)	Granulomatous inflammation involving the respiratory tract associated with necrotizing vasculitis affecting small- to medium-sized vessels. *Necrotizing glomerulonephritis is common.*
Eosinophilic granulomatosis with polyangiitis (EGPA)	Eosinophilic and granulomatous inflammation involving the respiratory tract accompanied by necrotizing vasculitis affecting small- to medium-sized vessels associated with asthma and eosinophilia.
Microscopic polyangiitis (MPA)	Necrotizing vasculitis with few or no immune deposits, affecting small vessels. *Necrotizing arteritis involving small- and medium-sized arteries may be present. Necrotizing glomerulonephritis is common. Pulmonary capillaritis often occurs.*

Immune complex small vessel vasculitis

IgA vasculitis (Henoch–Schönlein) (IgAV)	Vasculitis characterized by immunoglobulin A–dominant immune deposits affecting small vessels. *Typically involves skin, gut, and glomeruli. Arthralgias and arthritis are common.*
Cryoglobulinemic vasculitis (CPV)	Vasculitis with cryoglobulin immune deposits affecting small vessels associated with cryoglobulinemia. *Skin and glomeruli are often involved.*
Antiglomerular basement membrane (anti-GBM) disease	Vasculitis affecting pulmonary and renal capillaries with deposition of antiglomerular basement membrane antibodies.
Hypocomplementemic urticarial vasculitis	Associated with anti-C1q antibodies. *Affects kidney, joints, lungs, and eyes.*
Variable vessel vasculitis (VVV)	Affects arteries and veins with thrombosis, arteritis, and arterial aneurysms. *Oral and/or*
Behçet disease (BD)	*genital aphthous ulcers, and can involve skin, eyes, joints, and central nervous system.*
Cogan syndrome (CS)	Affects small, medium, or large arteries; aortitis, aortic, and mitral valvulitis.
Single organ vasculitis (SOV)	
Cutaneous leukocytoclastic angiitis	Vasculitis. Isolated cutaneous leukocytoclastic angiitis without systemic vasculitis or glomerulonephritis.
Cutaneous arteritis	Cutaneous vasculitis not associated with systemic vasculitis.
Primary central nervous system vasculitis	CNS vasculitis not associated with systemic vasculitis.
Isolated aortitis	Aortitis not associated with systemic vasculitis.
Others	

Vasculitis associated with systemic disease
Lupus vasculitis
Rheumatoid vasculitis
Sarcoid vasculitis
Others

Vasculitis associated with probable etiology
Hepatitis C–associated cryoglobulinemia
Hepatitis B–associated vasculitis
Syphilis-associated vasculitis
Drug-associated immune complex vasculitis
Drug-associated ANCA-associated vasculitis
Cancer-associated vasculitis
Others

Adapted from J.C. Jennette, R.J. Falk, P. Bacon, et al. (Ref. 2).
*Large vessels: aorta and its larger branches directed toward major anatomic regions; medium vessels: renal, hepatic, coronary, and mesenteric arteries; small vessels: venules, capillaries, arterioles, and intraparenchymal distal arteries and arterioles.
†Essential components are in normal type; *italicized type* represents usual, but not essential, components.

BOX 32-1 EULAR/PReS Classification of Childhood Vasculitis

I. Predominantly large-vessel vasculitis
 Takayasu arteritis
II. Predominantly medium-sized vessel vasculitis
 Childhood polyarteritis nodosa
 Cutaneous polyarteritis
 Kawasaki disease
III. Predominantly small-sized vessel vasculitis
 A. Granulomatous
 Wegener granulomatosis
 Churg–Strauss syndrome
 B. Nongranulomatous
 Microscopic polyangiitis
 Henoch–Schönlein purpura
 Isolated cutaneous leukocytoclastic vasculitis
 Hypocomplementemic urticarial vasculitis
IV. Other vasculitides
 Behçet disease
 Vasculitis secondary to infection (including hepatitis B-associated polyarteritis nodosa), malignancies, and drugs (including hypersensitivity vasculitis)
 Vasculitis associated with connective tissue diseases
 Isolated vasculitis of the central nervous system
 Cogan syndrome
 Unclassified

From Ozen et al. (Ref. 7).

BOX 32-2 Features That Suggest a Vasculitis Syndrome

Clinical Features
Fever, weight loss, fatigue of unknown origin
Skin lesions (palpable purpura, fixed urticaria, livedo reticularis, nodules, ulcers)
Neurological lesions (headache, mononeuritis multiplex, focal central nervous system lesions)
Arthralgia or arthritis, myalgia or myositis, serositis
Hypertension, hematuria, renal failure
Pulmonary infiltrates or hemorrhage
Myocardial ischemia, arrhythmias

Laboratory Features
Increased erythrocyte sedimentation rate or C-reactive protein level
Leukocytosis, anemia, thrombocytosis
Eosinophilia
Antineutrophil cytoplasmic antibodies
Elevated factor VIII–related antigen (von Willebrand factor)
Cryoglobulinemia
Circulating immune complexes
Hematuria

In practice, the classification of vasculitis is very much dependent on the clinical presentation. The classification used in this book accommodates the new nomenclature described in CHCC 2012, pediatric specific classification criteria that have been validated,[12] and ACR classification criteria[1] used in the absence of validated pediatric criteria.

EVALUATION OF VASCULITIS

Ideally, accurate disease classification in a given patient at disease onset should also assist in determining the disease course (trajectory), prognosis (predicted outcome), and treatment choices (toxic versus less toxic). In addition, treatment choices (when to stop, start, increase, or decrease therapy) at disease onset and during the disease course are determined after assessing disease activity and severity. Disease severity and activity plus disease damage assessment are used to measure disease outcome and/or effectiveness of a specific treatment. Clinical assessment tools in adults have enabled a more systematic and formal approach to staging levels of disease activity and damage in vasculitis.[14-17] Two adult tools, the Birmingham Vasculitis Activity Score (BVAS) and the Vasculitis Damage Index (VDI),[14-16] are widely used for evaluation of adult AAV and accepted by the Outcome Measures in Rheumatology Clinical Trials (OMERACT) initiative.[18] These tools are not fully applicable to childhood cryoglobulinemic vasculitis (CPV),[19] but a pediatric adaption of the BVAS known as the *pediatric vasculitis activity score* (PVAS)[20] and initiatives to establish a pediatric adaption of the VDI are discussed in Chapter 36.

GENERAL CLINICAL ASPECTS OF VASCULITIS

Childhood vasculitis is a complex and fascinating area of pediatric rheumatology. It is a clinical field often shared with other pediatric subspecialists such as dermatologists, cardiologists, and nephrologists,

which is a reflection of the multisystem nature of these diseases. The type of pathological change, site of involvement, size of vessel, and systemic extent of the vascular injury determine the clinical expression of the disease and its severity. Box 32-2 summarizes features that suggest a vasculitic syndrome. The onset of some vasculitides (e.g., Henoch–Schönlein purpura [HSP], Kawasaki disease [KD]) is usually abrupt, and characteristic features of the disease become apparent in a few days to a week, with diagnosis usually based on syndrome recognition without the need for a biopsy. In many of the vasculitides, however, presentation is more indolent, and various signs and symptoms, which offer persistent evidence of inflammation that develops over weeks to months, are characteristic. In this case, the diagnosis is often difficult and delayed, and it requires a high index of suspicion; a thorough investigation; and repeat clinical examinations of symptomatic and asymptomatic (but potentially affected) organs, such as the heart, lungs, liver, brain, and kidneys. Diagnosis of both acute-onset or indolent disease may require exclusion of the mimics of vasculitis or causes of secondary vasculitis (Box 32-3). There may be some general correlation of clinical features with the predominant size of blood vessels involved. Diseases of large- and medium-sized vessels (TAK, PAN, and KD) occur with ischemic pain or claudication involving heart or gut or limbs; hypertension; or focal central neurological symptoms. For diseases of small vessels (GPA, MPA, HSP) the symptoms may reflect involvement of rich vascular beds of the lungs, kidneys, gastrointestinal tract, and brain, with hemoptysis, hematuria, and gastrointestinal or neurological dysfunction. There are characteristic skin lesions (Box 32-2). Definitive diagnosis frequently requires a biopsy of one or more sites, magnetic resonance angiography, or arteriography. The clinical and pathological characteristics of the vasculitides in childhood are discussed in greater detail in subsequent chapters.

EPIDEMIOLOGY

The incidence and prevalence of vasculitis in children are unknown. In the pediatric population, the most common vasculitides are HSP and KD. All others are very uncommon or rare. There are striking

TABLE 32-2 Relative Frequencies of Vasculitides in Childhood

VASCULITIDES	UNITED STATES* N = 434	%	CANADA† N = 225	%	TURKEY‡ N = 376	%
Kawasaki disease	97	22.4	147	65.3	78	9.0
Henoch–Schönlein purpura	213	49.1	38	16.9	218	81.6
Wegener granulomatosis	6	1.4	5	2.2	1	0.4
Polyarteritis nodosa	14	3.2	4	1.8	60	5.6
Behçet disease	—	—	2	0.9	5	1.9
Takayasu arteritis	8	1.8	2	0.9	14	1.5
Unclassified	96	22.1	27	12.0	—	—

*Data from Bowyer and Roettcher, J. Rheumatol. 23 (1996) 1968–1974 (Ref. 4).
†Data from P.N. Malleson, M.Y. Fung, A.M. Rosenberg, J. Rheumatol. 23 (1996) 1981–1987 (Ref. 5).
‡Data from Ozen et al. (Ref. 21).

BOX 32-3 Causes of Secondary Vasculitis and/or Mimics of Vasculitis

Drugs and Toxic Exposure
Leflunomide, anti-TNFs, antithyroids, cocaine, marijuana

Infections
Bacterial/fungal: subacute endocarditis and bacteremia, particularly meningococcemia
Viral: human immunodeficiency virus (HIV), hepatitis B virus (HBV), cytomegalovirus (CMV), Epstein–Barr virus (EBV), parvo B19, herpes, and herpes zoster/varicella
Other: tuberculosis, syphilis, typhus, and rickettsial pox

Malignancy
Lymphoma, leukemia

Autoimmune/Systemic Inflammatory Disorders
Systemic lupus erythematosus (SLE), dermatomyositis, scleroderma, sarcoidosis, inflammatory bowel disease (IBD)

Noninflammatory Mimics
Thrombocytopenia, antiphospholipid syndrome (APL), embolic conditions, coarctation

geographic differences in relative disease frequency. KD and TAK are most prevalent in Japan. Without a doubt, KD and HSP are the most common disorders in North America and Europe. Comprehensive studies of the frequencies of the vasculitides in other parts of Asia are not available, but it is probable that KD and TAK constitute a larger proportion of vasculitis in that area of the world. PAN and cutaneous polyarteritis may also be more common in Japan and Turkey. In a multicenter survey in Turkey, Ozen and colleagues[21] noted that HSP was much more common than KD; that PAN was possibly increased relative to other vasculitides; and that Wegener granulomatosis, which appears to be more common in Western Europe and North America, is rare in the Turkish population. Isolated vasculitis of the central nervous system has only recently been recognized in childhood,[22] and its classification and relative frequency have yet to be established. Studies in African populations have not been reported.

In national diagnostic registries, the various forms of vasculitis account for 1% to 6% of pediatric rheumatic diseases.[4,5] The proportions of children from three registries that identified specific vasculitides are shown in Table 32-2. The wide differences in frequencies may just as likely reflect referral patterns as determinable geographic differences.

Although childhood vasculitis is uncommon, it is an important component of referrals to pediatric rheumatology clinics, and these children often require disproportionately large amounts of time and expertise. Diagnosis can be difficult, monitoring disease activity is problematic, and the outcome for some of the vasculitides may be serious or fatal.

REFERENCES

Entire reference list is available online at www.expertconsult.com.

33 CHAPTER

Leukocytoclastic Vasculitis: Henoch–Schönlein Purpura and Hypersensitivity Vasculitis

Paul Brogan, Arvind Bagga

Necrotizing vasculitis that affects small blood vessels (especially the postcapillary venules, capillaries, and arterioles) and is often caused by immune complex deposition may show *leukocytoclastic vasculitis* on histology (Fig. 33-1 and Box 33-1).[1,2] The term *leukocytoclasis* refers to the infiltration of polymorphonuclear leukocytes into vessel walls, resulting in necrosis with scattered nuclear debris, and thus is not a diagnosis in itself. This is the predominant inflammatory reaction in Henoch–Schönlein purpura (HSP), hypersensitivity angiitis, and mixed cryoglobulinemia. It is also observed in the antineutrophil cytoplasmic antibody (ANCA)-associated vasculitides and the vasculitis of other connective tissue diseases, such as systemic lupus erythematosus (SLE). Leukocytoclastic vasculitis is sometimes observed as a sequel of drug hypersensitivity, infectious endocarditis, or hematological malignancies. This chapter focuses on HSP and hypersensitivity vasculitis; other causes of leukocytoclastic vasculitis are described elsewhere.

HENOCH–SCHÖNLEIN PURPURA

Definition and Classification

HSP is one of the most common vasculitides of childhood.[3-7] It is characterized by nonthrombocytopenic purpura, arthritis and arthralgia, abdominal pain and gastrointestinal hemorrhage, and glomerulonephritis. A diagnostic triad of purpuric rash, arthritis, and abnormalities of the urinary sediment was proposed by Schönlein in 1837, and Henoch described the association of purpuric rash, abdominal pain with bloody diarrhea, and proteinuria in 1874. The term *anaphylactoid purpura* was applied by Gairdner in 1948.[8] The American College of Rheumatology (ACR) criteria[9] are now superseded by new pediatric criteria.[10] The original ACR criteria were derived by comparing 85 patients with HSP to 722 controls with other vasculitides and had a sensitivity of 87.1% and specificity of 87.7% for the classification of HSP.[9] In 2010 the vasculitis working group of the Pediatric Rheumatology European Society (PRES) proposed new classification criteria for pediatric vasculitides, endorsed by the European League Against Rheumatism (EULAR), which required palpable purpura with lower limb predominance (as mandatory criteria) plus at least one among the following four features: (1) diffuse abdominal pain, (2) biopsy showing typical leukocytoclastic vasculitis or proliferative glomerulonephritis with predominant immunoglobulin A (IgA) deposition, (3) arthritis or arthralgia, and (4) renal involvement (any hematuria and/or proteinuria).[10] In the case of purpura with atypical distribution, a demonstration of IgA deposit in a biopsy is required.[10] The PRES/EULAR criteria have been prospectively validated through international, Web-based prospective data that included 827 patients with HSP and 349 with other vasculitides. The

sensitivity and specificity of the new classification criteria were 100% and 87%, respectively.[10] Table 33-1 summarizes the new criteria, and the sensitivity and specificity of individual clinical features for the classification HSP.

In 2012, a new definition was proposed as part of an overall updating of nomenclature of systemic vasculitides undertaken at an international consensus conference that took place in Chapel Hill.[11] It must be emphasized that definitions of disease are not the same as formal, validated classification criteria, however.[11] Using that nomenclature, HSP is now referred to as *IgA vasculitis (Henoch–Schönlein)* and is defined as vasculitis, with IgA1-dominant immune deposits affecting small vessels (predominantly capillaries, venules, or arterioles); it often involves the skin and the gastrointestinal tract, and frequently causes arthritis. Glomerulonephritis indistinguishable from IgA nephropathy may occur.

Epidemiology

HSP is predominantly a disease of childhood, although a similar syndrome has been reported in adults.[12-15] It occurs most frequently between the ages of 3 and 15 years and is more common in boys than in girls (1.5 : 1).[15,16] The condition is rare in children younger than 2 years old.[17] Prospective data from an international cohort of 827 patients (49% girls) with HSP showed a mean age at onset of 6.9 ± 3 (range, 1 to 16.2) years, and at diagnosis at 7 ± 3 years.[10]

An incidence of 13.5 cases per 100,000 children per year was observed in an unselected childhood population in Belfast, Northern Ireland.[18] An incidence of 9 to 86 per 100,000 children was estimated by Farley and colleagues.[19] In the latter study, incidence was highest among Hispanic children (86 per 100,000) and children in lower socioeconomic groups (69 per 100,000), compared with children in higher socioeconomic or different racial groups (9 to 11 per 100,000). In a study from Britain, although the combined incidence was 20.4 per 100,000, it was 70.3 per 100,000 in the 4- to 6-year-olds age group.[20] Striking seasonal variations have been observed,[19] with most cases occurring in winter, often (30% to 50%) preceded by an upper respiratory tract infection.[21,22]

Etiology and Pathogenesis

Many reports have implicated infection, particularly with β-hemolytic streptococci, as a potential trigger for this disease.[8,23-25] Some investigators have, however, doubted this association.[21,22,26] Other preceding infections, including vaccination,[27,28] viral infection[29-32] (e.g., varicella,[33-35] rubella, rubeola, hepatitis A and B),[36,37] *Mycoplasma pneumoniae*,[38,39] *Bartonella henselae*,[40] and *Helicobacter pylori*[41] have been described.

As the term *anaphylactoid purpura* suggests, allergy has been regarded by some as the basis for development of this disease after insect bites[42] and exposure to drug and dietary allergens.[43] A possible pathogenic role of IgE in HSP has been suggested for some cases of HSP nephritis; it has been suggested that stimulation of IgE-sensitized mast cells by specific antigens in the presence of IgA circulating immune complexes leads to release of vasoactive substances, increased capillary permeability, and perivascular deposition of IgA immune complexes.[44]

The characteristic vascular deposition of IgA strongly suggests, however, that HSP is a predominantly IgA-mediated dysregulated immune response to antigen and may operate through the alternative complement pathway.[45] Although the pathogenic mechanisms of nephritis are still not delineated, studies suggest that galactose-deficient IgA1 is recognized by antiglycan antibodies, leading to the formation of circulating immune complexes and their mesangial deposition, which results in renal injury in HSP.[46] An increase in the levels of poorly galactosylated IgA1 appears insufficient in itself to cause HSP

nephritis or IgA nephropathy, because first-degree relatives may have high serum levels of poorly galactosylated IgA1 but no signs of nephritis.[47,48] Thus it is likely that a "second hit" is required for high levels of poorly galactosylated IgA1 to form immune complexes that result in nephritis.[48] It is suggested that this second hit is the formation of antiglycan IgG or IgA antibodies (perhaps triggered by infection) that then go on to form large circulating immune complexes with the poorly galactosylated IgA1 that are prone to deposition.[48] Currently,

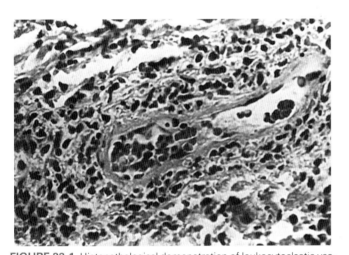

FIGURE 33-1 Histopathological demonstration of leukocytoclastic vasculitis. The characteristic "nuclear dust" is seen as granular, dark-stained material in the vessel wall. Hematoxylin-eosin stain.

BOX 33-1   Conditions Associated with Leukocytoclastic Vasculitis

Henoch–Schönlein purpura
Hypersensitivity angiitis
Hypocomplementemic urticarial vasculitis
Mixed cryoglobulinemia
Cutaneous polyarteritis
ANCA-associated small-vessel vasculitis*
Goodpasture syndrome
Rheumatic disorders
   SLE, juvenile dermatomyositis, MCTD, scleroderma, JIA
Mucha–Habermann disease
Relapsing polychondritis
Köhlmeier–Degos syndrome
Antiphospholipid antibody syndrome
CANDLE syndrome
Malignancy-associated disease
Sweet syndrome
Cronkhite–Canada syndrome
Stevens–Johnson syndrome
Erythema elevatum diutinum

ANCA, Antineutrophil cytoplasmic antibody; *CANDLE*, chronic atypical neutrophilic dermatosis with lipodystrophy and elevated temperature; *JIA*, juvenile idiopathic arthritis; *MCTD*, mixed connective tissue disease; *SLE*, systemic lupus erythematosus.
*Leukocytoclastic vasculitis may occur in cutaneous lesions in some patients with ANCA-associated vasculitis and collagen vascular diseases.

TABLE 33-1   2010 Classification Criteria for Henoch–Schönlein Purpura

CRITERION	DEFINITION	SENSITIVITY	SPECIFICITY
Purpura (mandatory)	Purpura (palpable, in crops) or petechiae, with lower limb predominance,* not related to thrombocytopenia	89%	86%
And at Least 1 Out of 4 of the Following:			
Abdominal pain	Diffuse, acute, colicky pain; may include intussusception and gastrointestinal bleeding	61%	64%
Histopathology	Leukocytoclastic vasculitis with predominant IgA deposits; or proliferative glomerulonephritis with predominant IgA deposits	93%	89%
Arthritis, arthralgias	Arthritis: acute joint swelling or pain with limitation of motion	78%	42%
	Arthralgia: acute joint pain without joint swelling or limitation of motion		
Renal involvement	Proteinuria: >0.3 g/24 hr; spot urine albumin to creatinine ratio >30 mmol/mg; or ≥2+ on dipstick	33%	70%
	Hematuria: red cell casts; urine sediment showing >5 red cells per high-power field or red cell casts		

The sensitivity and specificity of the above classification for HSP is 100% and 87%, respectively.
*If purpura presents with atypical distribution, demonstration of IgA deposit on biopsy is required.
Adapted from: Ozen, et al. EULAR/PRINTO/PRES criteria for Henoch-Schönlein purpura, childhood polyarteritis nodosa, childhood Wegener granulomatosis and childhood Takayasu arteritis: Ankara 2008. Part II: Final classification criteria, Ann. Rheum. Dis. 69 (2010) 798–806.

the genes controlling IgA1 glycosylation are unknown. Other factors that may modulate IgA synthesis and galactosylation include B-cell programming at the time of antigen encounter, Toll-like receptor activation, and local cytokine production.[48] It has been suggested that the genetic mechanisms controlling these processes should be further explored to try to better understand the genetic contribution to the pathogenesis of HSP nephritis and IgA nephropathy.[48] Thus, although there remain many unanswered questions in relation to this pathogenetic model, increased serum levels of poorly galactosylated IgA1 remain the most consistent finding in patients with HSP nephritis and IgA nephropathy, and these almost certainly predispose to the formation of IgA immune complexes with resulting vasculitis.

Disorders of coagulation and its activation are also associated with the development of HSP or an HSP-like vasculitis.[49] It is recognized that disease activity may be linked to a rapid decline of factor XIII, particularly in patients with severe abdominal involvement.[50-52] This may be useful as a prognostic or diagnostic marker because the decline occurs before classic skin rash and thus could allow early diagnosis of HSP, when abdominal symptoms and signs predominate. There is no information regarding the diagnostic specificity of a fall in factor XIII, however. Anecdotal reports of factor XIII replacement to successfully treat severe abdominal symptoms in HSP are described[52]; no high-quality controlled data relating to this treatment are available, however. Factor XIII also declines prior to recurrence of HSP, but it is unknown whether this is a merely a secondary epiphenomenon or a true causative association.

One study concluded that oxidant stress, especially lipid peroxidation, was involved in the origin of renal injury.[53] Vasculitis may develop after antirheumatic therapy, including administration of methotrexate[54] and anti–tumor necrosis factor agents.[55]

Genetic Background

Familial clusters of the disease may occur, with siblings affected simultaneously or sequentially.[19,56,57] Investigations from Spain have presented preliminary data on genetic associations. The frequency of human leukocyte antigen (HLA)-B35 was increased in patients who developed nephritis.[58] The incidence of HLA-DRB1*01 was also increased compared with matched controls, and HLA-DRB1*07 was decreased.[59] A study of unselected children with HSP from Turkey showed that HLA-A2, -A11, and -B35 antigens were associated with a significantly increased risk of HSP, whereas HLA-A1, -B49, and -B50 antigens were associated with decreased risk for the disease.[60] There was no association, however, between HLA class 1 alleles and renal involvement.[60]

Although there were no general associations with the expression of intercellular adhesion molecule 1 in patients compared with controls,

a K/E polymorphism at codon 469 was significantly decreased in those who did not develop severe gastrointestinal manifestations (and possibly in patients without renal sequelae).[61] In studies from Israel and Turkey, mutations in the familial Mediterranean fever (MEFV) gene were frequent in patients with HSP.[62,63] Other genetic polymorphisms have also been implicated and have been reviewed elsewhere.[64]

Several polymorphisms relating to disease susceptibility, severity, and/or risk of renal involvement have been described. Studies of this nature have been hampered by relatively small patient numbers and thus lack the power to be definitive or necessarily applicable to all racial groups. It is, however, increasingly apparent that the genetic contribution is complex and probably polygenic in nature.[64]

Clinical Manifestations

Clinical characteristics of HSP are presented in Table 33-2.[65-69] The onset is often acute, with the principal manifestations appearing sequentially over several days to weeks. Nonspecific constitutional signs, such as a low-grade fever or malaise, are often present.[3]

Cutaneous Involvement

The presence of *palpable purpura* is characteristic.[10] This rash is most prominent on dependent or pressure-bearing surfaces, especially the lower extremities and buttocks, but it may occur in other areas. The cutaneous lesions range from small petechiae to large ecchymoses to rare hemorrhagic bullae; they tend to occur in crops and progress in color from red to purple to brown (Figs. 33-2 and 33-3). Ulceration may occasionally develop in large ecchymotic areas. The rash is often preceded by maculopapular or urticarial lesions. Subcutaneous edema over the dorsa of the hands and feet and around the eyes, forehead, scalp, and scrotum may occur early in the disease, particularly in the very young child.

Gastrointestinal Disease

Gastrointestinal manifestations occur in approximately two thirds of children, usually within a week after onset of the rash and almost always within 30 days; in 14% to 36% of cases, abdominal pain precedes other manifestations.[68,70,71] Edema and submucosal and intramural hemorrhage resulting from vasculitis of the bowel wall occasionally lead to intussusception (usually confined to the small bowel), gangrene, or overt perforation. Less common involvement includes acute pancreatitis,[72] hepatobiliary disease,[73] ulcerative colitis, other forms of enteropathy,[74] and steatorrhea.

In one study, abdominal pain was usually intermittent, colicky, and periumbilical.[68] Rebound tenderness was uncommon. Vomiting occurred in 60%, hematemesis in 7%, and melena in 19% of children, although occult blood was present in the stools of 50% of the patients.

TABLE 33-2	**Clinical Features of Henoch-Schönlein Purpura (Percent Patients)**					
FEATURE	EMERY ET AL.[66] N = 43	ROSENBLUM & WINTER[68] N = 43	BAGGA ET AL.[65] N = 47	SAULSBURY ET AL.[14] N = 100	NONG, ET AL.[67] N = 107	AVERAGE %
Purpura	100*	97	96	100*	95	96
Arthralgia, arthritis	79	65	47	82	47	64
Abdominal pain	63	100*	64	63	72	66
Gastrointestinal bleeding		26	26	33		28
Renal involvement	37		51	40	28	39
Subcutaneous edema	63		21			42
Orchitis			6	4		5

*Criterion used for inclusion in the series.

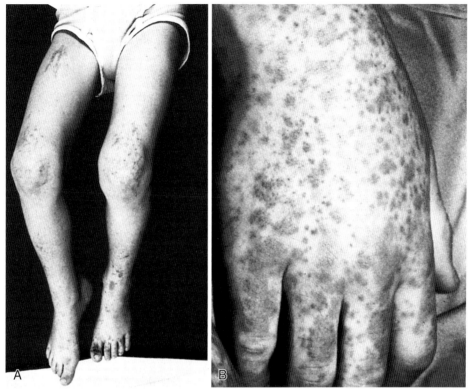

FIGURE 33-2 Henoch–Schönlein purpura. **A,** These purpuric lesions appeared on the lower extremities of a 10-year-old boy who had an acute, self-limited illness characterized by fever, arthritis, melena, and transient hematuria. Notice the periarticular swelling around the ankles and knees. **B,** Purpura on dorsum of the hand of a 14-year-old boy with Henoch–Schönlein purpura.

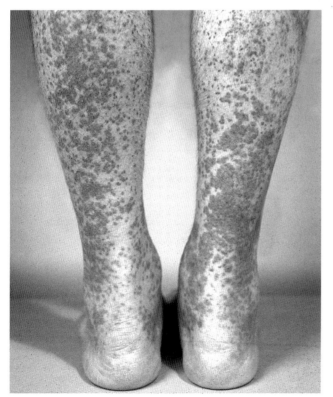

FIGURE 33-3 Palpable purpuric lesions involve the heels and ankles of a patient with Henoch–Schönlein purpura.

Massive gastrointestinal hemorrhage or intussusception occurred in less than 5% of children, but it could develop suddenly without preceding abdominal symptoms.

Renal Disease

Glomerulonephritis affects up to one third of the children, but it is serious and potentially life-threatening in less than 10%.[4,7,10] In the Belfast study of 155,000 unselected children, 55 of 270 patients (20%) had evidence of nephritis at onset.[18] Renal disease, like abdominal pain, seldom precedes the purpura, and, in most instances, serious renal disease develops within 4 to 6 weeks of the onset of the rash. The spectrum of features ranges from microscopic hematuria and mild proteinuria to the less-common nephrotic syndrome, acute nephritic syndrome, hypertension, or renal failure. Age at onset of more than 7 years old, persistent purpuric lesions, severe abdominal symptoms, and decreased factor XIII activity are associated with an increased risk of nephritis.[75-77] The intensity of renal symptoms at onset determines the severity of glomerular lesions.[78]

The initial 3 months are critical in determining the eventual extent of the illness. In a few children, however, nephritis may not occur until much later in the course of disease, sometimes after a number of recurrences of the purpura. Renal involvement characteristically develops early, but end-stage disease may not be obvious for a number of years. In a small number of children, renal abnormalities occur alone, and clinically and immunopathogenically resemble IgA nephropathy in adults.

In a systematic review involving 1133 select patients with HSP, renal manifestations (proteinuria, hematuria) were found in 34.2%. These features developed in 85% of cases within 4 weeks of the diagnosis of

HSP, in 91% within 6 weeks, and in 97% within 6 months.[79] Permanent renal impairment never developed after normal urinalysis, but occurred in 1.6% of those with isolated urinary abnormalities and in 19.5% of those who developed nephritic or nephrotic syndrome. Based on these findings, it is recommended that patients with HSP should be followed up for a minimum of 6 months to detect renal involvement.

Arthritis

Arthralgia or arthritis involving only a few joints occurs in 50% to 80% of children with HSP. Large joints, such as the knees and ankles, are most commonly affected, but other areas, including the wrists, elbows, and small joints of the fingers, may be involved. Characteristic findings include periarticular swelling and tenderness, usually occurring without erythema, warmth, or effusions, but with considerable pain and limitation of motion. The joint disease is transient, although usually not migratory, and resolves within a few days to a week without residual abnormalities. Occasionally, arthritis may precede the appearance of the rash by 1 or 2 days.[66]

Other Manifestations

Other features of HSP include an isolated central nervous system vasculitis, seizures, coma and hemorrhage[80]; Guillain–Barré syndrome[81]; ataxia and central and peripheral neuropathy[82,83]; ocular involvement[68,84]; intramuscular, subconjunctival, or pulmonary hemorrhages[85,86]; interstitial pneumonitis[87]; recurrent epistaxis; parotitis[22]; carditis[4,88,89]; and stenosing ureteritis.[90] Scrotal pain and swelling are frequent, occurring in 13% (range, 2% to 38%)[69,91-93] of boys evaluated for HSP.

Pathology

The pathological lesion of HSP is leukocytoclastic vasculitis (Fig. 33-4), although in routine practice biopsies are not always performed.[10] In the skin, this is demonstrated in the dermal capillaries and postcapillary venules. Deposition of IgA (principally IgA$_1$) in these lesions is characteristic.[14,45,94-96] It is possible to fail to detect IgA deposition in vascular tissue in some cases of HSP, especially if the biopsy was obtained from the middle of a lesion where the presence of proteolytic enzymes can result in negative staining for IgA.[96]

In the kidneys, proliferative glomerulonephritis ranges from focal and segmental lesions to severe crescentic disease (Fig. 33-5).[95,97] Group A streptococcal antigen (i.e., nephritis-associated plasmin receptor) was identified by immunofluorescent microscopy in the mesangium

of 10 of 33 children.[25] Levy and co-workers[22] provided a comprehensive review of the renal pathology. The principal lesion is an endocapillary proliferative glomerulonephritis with an increase in endothelial and mesangial cells. All gradations of severity may be present in the same biopsy. There may be marked interstitial inflammatory disease, but vasculitis *per se* is usually not present. Fluorescence microscopy confirms deposits of Ig, principally IgA,[45,94,98] but it is often accompanied by IgG, fibrin, C3, and properdin in most involved glomeruli. These deposits are invariably in mesangial cells, but peripheral capillary loops also are involved in more severe cases. Dense deposits in the mesangium and occasionally in the subendothelial and paramesangial regions are present on electron microscopy. Thickening and splitting of the basement membrane, caused by the interposition of mesangial cell cytoplasmic material, are notable.

Differential Diagnosis

HSP must be distinguished from immune thrombocytopenic purpura, acute poststreptococcal glomerulonephritis,[2] SLE, septicemia, disseminated intravascular coagulation, hemolytic-uremic syndrome, the papular-purpuric gloves-and-socks syndrome,[99] and other types of vasculitis.[10] FMF can also mimic or occur in association with HSP in areas where FMF is endemic.[100,101]

The more common causes of an acute surgical abdomen with abdominal pain and gastrointestinal tract bleeding must be considered. A tender abdominal mass may indicate intussusception, and abdominal tenderness with an elevated level of serum amylase and/or lipase

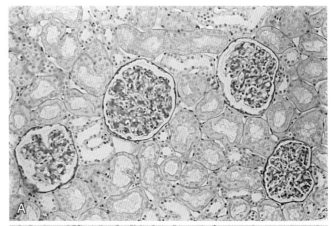

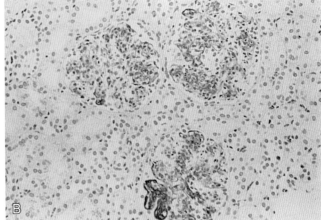

FIGURE 33-5 **A,** Diffuse, mesangial, proliferative nephritis in Henoch–Schönlein purpura. Hematoxylin-eosin stain. **B,** Mesangial and capillary wall deposition of immunoglobulin A (immunoperoxidase stain) in Henoch–Schönlein purpura.

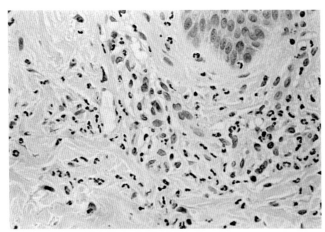

FIGURE 33-4 Leukocytoclastic vasculitis in the skin of a patient with Henoch–Schönlein purpura. Hematoxylin-eosin stain; original magnification ×480.

suggests acute pancreatitis. Punch biopsy of a cutaneous lesion may assist in the diagnosis of difficult cases by demonstrating leukocytoclastic vasculitis characterized by deposition of IgA and C3.[45] A renal biopsy is indicated only in children with persistent or significant renal manifestations. Indications for diagnostic renal biopsy in children with HSP are as follows[102]:

- Acute nephritic or nephrotic syndrome at presentation
- Raised blood level of creatinine; hypertension or oliguria
- Heavy proteinuria (early morning urine protein to creatinine ratio greater than 100 mg/mmol)
- Persistent proteinuria (not declining) after 4 weeks
- Impaired renal function (GFR less than 80 mL/min/1.73 m^2)

Infantile Acute Hemorrhagic Edema

Infantile acute hemorrhagic edema (Finkelstein–Seidlmayer syndrome) affects infants between 4 and 24 months of age with an acute onset of fever, purpura, ecchymoses, and inflammatory edema of the limbs, ears, and face.[103-107] Although spontaneous remission in 1 to 3 weeks and a benign course are characteristic, attacks may recur. Involvement of viscera (kidneys, gastrointestinal tract) is rare. Histopathology shows leukocytoclastic vasculitis with occasional demonstration of perivascular IgA deposition.[108] This disorder in older children overlaps clinically with HSP.

HSP in Adults

HSP is uncommon in adults, with a reported incidence of 0.12 cases per 100,000 persons. Males are affected as commonly as females.[12,13,109-112] In a study of clinical features and outcomes in an unselected population of 46 adults and 116 children with HSP, cutaneous lesions were the principal initial manifestation in both groups.[113] However, adults had a lower frequency of abdominal pain and fever and a higher frequency of joint symptoms and severe renal involvement. Adults often required aggressive therapy with glucocorticoids or cytotoxic agents, or both. Outcome was relatively good in both age groups, with a complete recovery in 94% of children and 89% of adults.

Another study showed that leukocytosis, thrombocytosis, and high levels of serum C-reactive protein were more common in children, whereas elevated serum IgA and cryoglobulin levels were common in adults.[110] HSP in adults may represent a more severe form of the disease with a higher frequency of significant renal involvement and risk of progressive kidney disease, but without the other manifestations of HSP.[110-114]

Laboratory Examination

There are no diagnostic laboratory abnormalities.[9] The platelet count is normal or increased, differentiating this form of purpura from that caused by thrombocytopenia. A moderate leukocytosis up to 20,000 white cells/mm^3 (20×10^9/L) with a shift to left is identified in some children. Normochromic anemia is often related to gastrointestinal blood loss, confirmed by a positive stool guaiac examination in 80% of patients with abdominal complaints. Antinuclear antibody (ANA) and rheumatoid factor (RF) are usually absent.

Although renal disease may occur in the absence of overt urinary findings and minimal abnormalities, such as hematuria, are not necessarily associated with a severe glomerular lesion, these laboratory abnormalities usually demonstrate a direct correlation with the severity of the proliferative changes. Patients occasionally have decreased concentrating ability and creatinine clearance. Proteinuria, severe enough to result in hypoalbuminemia, may occur.[115]

Although levels of C1q, C3, and C4 are usually normal,[116] activation of the alternate complement pathway is demonstrated in half of patients during the acute illness by presence of C3d, low levels of total hemolytic complement, and decreased serum concentrations of properdin and factor B.[116,117] Plasma levels of von Willebrand factor antigen are elevated, indicating endothelial cell damage.[118,119]

Circulating IgA-containing immune complexes[120,121] and cryoglobulins[122] may be present. Serum IgA and IgM concentrations are increased in half of the patients during the acute phase of the disease.[123] An increased number of circulating IgA-producing cells was found in one study in definite HSP cases but not in other forms of leukocytoclastic vasculitis.[124] ANCAs are typically absent.

Radiological Examination

Plain radiographs may demonstrate decreased intestinal motility with dilated loops of bowel in children with abdominal involvement. Ultrasound studies can identify specific gastrointestinal abnormalities in children with abdominal complaints.[70] Magnetic resonance imaging and magnetic resonance angiography of the brain can define the extent of cerebral vasculitis.[125-127] Occasionally, intussusception is identified on a barium study and is relieved by it if performed early in the course.[69,128] Epididymal enlargement, subcutaneous scrotal swelling, hydrocele, or, rarely, testicular torsion can be confirmed if necessary by scrotal ultrasonography.

Treatment

Treatment is supportive with maintenance of good hydration, nutrition, and electrolyte balance; control of pain is accomplished with simple analgesics such as acetaminophen. If necessary, control of hypertension is attempted.[129] Although glucocorticoids dramatically decrease the severity of joint and cutaneous disease, they are not usually indicated for management of these manifestations.[14] Short-term glucocorticoid therapy is effective in relieving the pain of severe orchitis. Prednisone has been advocated in children with severe gastrointestinal disease or hemorrhage.[68,130-132] The severity of disease may occasionally prompt the use of intravenous corticosteroids.[132,133] However, studies do not demonstrate a clear advantage of prednisone over supportive therapy (e.g., nasogastric suction, parenteral nutrition, antibiotics). Pulmonary hemorrhage is an extremely rare and sometimes fatal complication, which requires aggressive immunosuppressive treatment, combining intravenous (IV) methylprednisolone with another immunosuppressive agent such as cyclophosphamide or cyclosporine, and supportive care.[134]

Management of HSP Nephritis

The management of HSP nephritis has recently been reviewed by Zaffanello and Fanos.[135] The authors highlighted that currently prescribed treatments for HSP nephritis are not guided by evidence obtained in robust randomized placebo-controlled trials with outcome markers related to the progression to end-stage renal disease.

Treatment to prevent renal disease. Various treatment strategies to prevent the occurrence of HSP nephritis have been reported with variable effect. The efficacy of corticosteroids to prevent complications, such as abdominal pain is debated.[136] Chartapisak and colleagues systematically reviewed randomized controlled trials (RCTs) for the prevention or treatment of renal involvement in HSP.[137] Meta-analyses of four RCTs, which evaluated prednisone therapy at presentation of HSP, showed that there was no significant difference in the risk of development or persistence of renal involvement at 1, 3, 6, and 12 months with prednisone compared with placebo or no specific treatment. Findings from this review, and a recent large placebo-controlled RCT involving 352 children[138] suggests that prophylactic therapy with corticosteroids does not prevent the onset of HSP nephritis.

That said, there could still be a role for early use of corticosteroids in patients with severe extrarenal symptoms and in those with renal involvement, as suggested by Ronkainen and colleagues.[139] Prednisone (1 mg/kg/day for 2 weeks, with weaning over the next 2 weeks) was effective in reducing the intensity of abdominal pain and joint pain. Prednisone did not prevent the development of renal symptoms but was effective in treating them if present; renal symptoms resolved in 61% of the prednisone patients after treatment, compared with 34% of those receiving placebo.[139]

Treatment of rapidly progressive glomerulonephritis. There are good data indicating that crescents in greater than 50% of glomeruli and nephrotic range proteinuria carry an unfavorable prognosis, thus highlighting the need for an effective intervention. To date, there has been only one RCT that evaluated the benefit of treatment, which showed no difference in outcome using cyclophosphamide versus supportive therapy alone.[140] However, this study did not examine combined therapy with cyclophosphamide and steroids, a regimen used in most other severe small vessel vasculitides. For patients with rapidly progressive glomerulonephritis with crescentic changes on renal biopsy, uncontrolled data suggest that treatment may comprise aggressive therapy with intravenous methylprednisolone,[140-143] cyclophosphamide, and plasma exchange,[135] as for other causes of crescentic nephritis. Warfarin and heparin have been used with disputable effect, as have cyclosporine,[13,144-146] azathioprine,[135] intravenous Ig, and plasma exchange.[147,148] Shenoy and colleagues reported 14 children with severe HSP nephritis were treated successfully with plasma exchange alone.[149] These treatment options, although potentially important in select cases, are not supported by RCTs.

Treatment of HSP nephritis that is not rapidly progressive. Patients for whom HSP nephritis is not rapidly progressive may exhibit the following features: less than 50% crescents on renal biopsy; suboptimal GFR; or heavy proteinuria, which is not necessarily nephrotic in range.[102] There are no robust clinical trials to guide therapy of this type of presentation, although many physicians would advocate corticosteroids. Others advocate the addition of cyclophosphamide to corticosteroids in HSP nephritis when biopsy shows diffuse proliferative lesions or sclerosis, but with less than 50% crescentic change in those who have ongoing heavy proteinuria. A typical regimen would comprise 8 to 12 weeks of oral cyclophosphamide (2 mg/kg/day) with daily prednisolone, converting to alternate day prednisolone and azathioprine for 12 months.[102] The published evidence for the efficacy of this approach is lacking, but it may be a reasonable option for selected patients. In patients with greater than 6 months' duration of proteinuria, an angiotensin converting enzyme inhibitor may be used to limit secondary glomerular injury, although evidence to support this therapy is lacking.[135]

Renal transplantation has been successful in some children with renal failure.[150-152] In pooled data,[150,151] there was a 35% risk of recurrence 5 years after transplantation and an 11% risk of graft loss. A study of the long-term outcome of renal transplantation in adult patients with HSP showed a 15-year patient and graft survival rate of 80% and 64%, respectively.[153] Forty percent of patients, particularly those with necrotizing or crescentic glomerulonephritis of native kidneys, developed recurrent HSP nephritis resulting in graft loss in half.

Course of the Disease and Prognosis

In two thirds of children, HSP runs its entire course within 4 weeks of onset.[129] Younger children have a shorter course and fewer recurrences than do older patients. One third to half of the children have at least one recurrence that commonly consists of a rash and abdominal pain, with each episode usually being similar but briefer and milder than the preceding one.[14] Most exacerbations take place within the initial 6-week period but may occur as late as 2 years after onset. They

may be spontaneous or coincide with repeated respiratory tract infections. The severity of the cutaneous leukocytoclastic vasculitis does not correlate with visceral involvement.[154]

Prognosis is excellent for most children.[155] Significant morbidity or mortality is associated with gastrointestinal tract lesions in the short term and with nephritis in the long term.[156] The development of major indications of renal disease, particularly those with a mixed nephritic-nephrotic syndrome within the first 6 months after onset or the occurrence of numerous exacerbations associated with nephropathy suggests a poor prognosis for renal function.[97,157] Additional poor prognostic factors[157] are decreased factor XIII activity; hypertension; renal failure at onset, and, if a renal biopsy had been performed, an increased number of glomeruli with crescents; macrophage infiltration; and tubulointerstitial disease.

The reported outcome of children with renal disease is highly variable.[158] With minimal lesions, more than 75% recover within 2 years; in contrast, 66% of children with crescentic glomerulonephritis in more than 80% of glomeruli progress to renal failure within the first year. The worst outcome is associated with the presence of the nephrotic or nephritic syndrome at onset.[79,159,160] Almost half of such children have active renal disease or renal insufficiency at follow-up periods of 6 or more years. Thus the extent of the renal disease is an important determinant of long-term outcome.

Overall, less than 5% of children progress to end-stage renal failure. HSP accounts for less than 1% of children with renal failure from all causes. In a follow-up evaluation of 64 children,[161] the renal survival rate at 10 years was 73%, and initial renal insufficiency was the best predictor of the future course of nephritis. Similar results were found in a multicenter study on 443 patients with HS nephritis from Turkey, in which 87% patients had a favorable outcome and 13% an unfavorable one; 1.1% children showed end-stage renal disease at follow-up.[162] All patients who showed end-stage renal disease had nephritic-nephrotic syndrome at presentation and greater than 50% crescents on renal biopsy.[162]

Patients who have had clinical nephritis should be followed closely for at least 5 years.[157-159] In one study, 8 of 12 patients had mesangial IgA deposition at follow-up of 2 to 9 years, despite an apparent clinical remission of their renal disease. Later, 16 of 44 pregnancies in adults were complicated by proteinuria or hypertension, even in the absence of active renal disease.[158] Of 18 patients in the Belfast study who had a nephrotic or nephritic syndrome at onset and who were followed for a mean of 8.3 years, one died and three had persistent urinary abnormalities but no azotemia.[18] The overall mortality rate was less than 1%, and the morbidity rate was 1.1%. This somewhat optimistic outcome is tempered by a study of 16 children from Minnesota, which indicated that the longer a child was followed, the more likely it was that renal disease would become clinically evident.[163]

HYPERSENSITIVITY VASCULITIS

Vascular inflammation in hypersensitivity angiitis occurs more typically in smaller vessels than in those involved in the classic form of polyarteritis nodosa; in this regard, it resembles HSP. Previously, it was the most frequently encountered form of vasculitis after the administration of therapeutic antisera.[164] The Chapel Hill International Consensus Conference did not use the term *hypersensitivity vasculitis*.[165] It was proposed instead that *microscopic polyarteritis* and *cutaneous leukocytoclastic vasculitis* were best equated with the common usage of this designation. The terminology used to describe leukocytoclastic vasculitis resulting from an allergic reaction remains confusing. The ACR criteria define hypersensitivity vasculitis (Table 33-3)[166] as palpable purpura, with or without a maculopapular rash precipitated by

TABLE 33-3   Criteria for the Diagnosis of Hypersensitivity Vasculitis

CRITERION	DEFINITION
Age at onset >16 years	Development of symptoms after age 16 years
Medication at disease onset	Medication that may have been a precipitating factor was taken at the onset of symptoms
Palpable purpura	Slightly elevated purpuric rash over one or more areas; does not blanch with pressure and not related to thrombocytopenia
Maculopapular rash	Flat and raised lesions of various sizes over one or more areas of the skin
Biopsy, including arteriole and venule	Histological changes showing granulocytes in perivascular or extravascular location

For purposes of classification, a patient is said to have hypersensitivity vasculitis if at least three of these criteria are present. The presence of any three or more criteria has a diagnostic sensitivity of 71.0% and specificity of 83.9%. The age criterion is not applicable for children.
From L.H. Calabrese, B.A. Michel, D.A. Bloch, et al. The American College of Rheumatology 1990 criteria for the classification of hypersensitivity vasculitis, Arthritis Rheum. 33 (1990) 1108–1113.

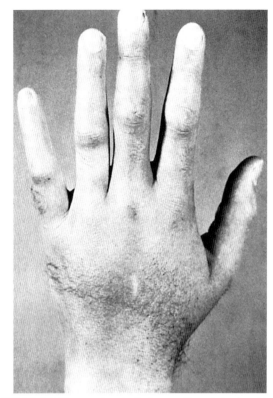

FIGURE 33-6 Diffuse and periarticular swelling of the hand in a boy with acute serum sickness.

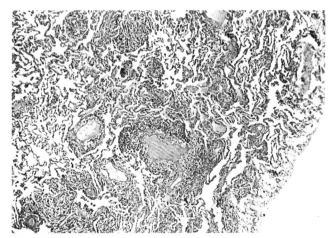

FIGURE 33-7 Hypersensitivity angiitis is demonstrated in a lung biopsy specimen from a young drug addict with a short history of increasing dyspnea on exertion and purpura. This section shows prominent infiltration by inflammatory cells and eosinophils of the alveolar walls and around blood vessels. Hematoxylin-eosin stain.

a medication or other agent, and a biopsied lesion characterized by a neutrophilic perivascular or extravascular infiltration in small vessels (like those affected in HSP). The new pediatric vasculitis classification suggested by Ozen et al. refers to hypersensitivity vasculitis under the subheading "other vasculitis."[167] The revised Chapel Hill 2012 nomenclature suggest that vasculitis associated with a probable etiology should have a prefix specifying the association (e.g., hydralazine-associated vasculitis), emphasizing that a primary cause should always be sought in a patient with vasculitis.[11]

A report of serum sickness–like arthritis in Finland estimated its frequency at 4.7 cases per 100,000 children younger than 16 years, establishing it as one of the most common causes of acute arthritis in childhood.[168] In this study, the arthritis was transient, usually lasting only a few weeks, and most commonly affected the ankles, metacarpophalangeal joints, wrists, and knees (Fig. 33-6). Occasionally, pulmonary, renal, and other vasculature systems were affected (Fig. 33-7).

Leukocytosis usually occurs in cases of hypersensitivity angiitis and is sometimes accompanied by eosinophilia and circulating immune complexes.[168] The erythrocyte sedimentation rate is often normal. IgG antibodies to the putative antigen may be demonstrable. Synovial fluid examination in one report demonstrated 8800 to 59,000 leukocytes/mm^3 (8 to 59 × 10^9/L), of which 38% to 80% were polymorphonuclear leukocytes.[168] Biopsy of a cutaneous lesion confirms that small venules and capillaries are the predominantly involved vessels. Inflammatory lesions are at a similar stage of development in all areas of involvement, and the cellular infiltrate contains large numbers of neutrophils and eosinophils.

Systemic treatment is directed at the relief of symptoms, because the course—although often acute and variable—is self-limited. Removal of the precipitating agent, if identified, is the first step in treatment. In the absence of systemic features, management is usually symptomatic. Antihistamines and nonsteroidal antiinflammatory drugs (NSAIDs) alleviate cutaneous symptoms and arthralgia. Glucocorticoid therapy may be indicated in children with severe cutaneous symptoms or systemic vasculitis.

Historically, serum sickness, a classic example of immune complex-mediated disease in humans, was encountered after the administration of heterologous antiserum to treat or prevent specific infections such as diphtheria and tetanus. Although current indications for use of heterologous antiserum are uncommon, it has been superseded as a cause of serum sickness by myriad drugs, notably cefaclor, penicillin, quinolones, allopurinol, thiazide diuretics, NSAIDs, phenytoins, antithyroid drugs, and, rarely, streptokinase, recombinant human growth hormone, cytokines, and monoclonal antibodies.

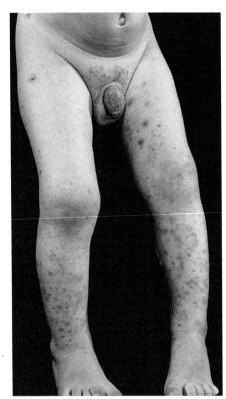

FIGURE 33-8 Skin lesions of a patient with hypersensitivity vasculitis.

The clinical syndrome begins 7 to 14 days after primary exposure to the antigen and is characterized by fever, arthralgia, arthritis (sometimes), myalgia, lymphadenopathy, and a rash. The rash may be purpuric, linear, urticarial, or ecchymotic and distributed predominantly over the lower legs, although the trunk and arms may be involved (Fig. 33-8). Kunnamo and colleagues[168] described a patchy discoloration over the affected joints, with urticaria predominantly on the trunk. With the use of equine antithymocyte globulin in the treatment of bone marrow failure, 30 of 35 patients developed serum sickness characterized by malaise, headache, fever, cutaneous eruptions, arthralgias, arthritis, myalgias, gastrointestinal complaints, and lymph node enlargement, beginning 7 to 9 days after infusion and lasting 10 to 14 days.[164]

A study that compared the clinical features of HSP and hypersensitivity angiitis found that transient arthralgias and oligoarthritis, myalgias, cutaneous nodules, ulcerations, livedo, gangrene, and eosinophilia were more common in patients with hypersensitivity angiitis. Gastrointestinal bleeding, hematuria, and palpable purpura were frequent in those with HSP.[169]

REFERENCES

1. J.T. Lie, Illustrated histopathologic classification criteria for selected vasculitis syndromes. American College of Rheumatology Subcommittee on Classification of Vasculitis, Arthritis Rheum. 33 (1990) 1074–1087.
2. A. Yalcindag, R. Sundel, Vasculitis in childhood, Curr. Opin. Rheumatol. 13 (2001) 422–427.
5. S. Mrusek, M. Kruger, P. Greiner, et al., Henoch-Schönlein purpura, Lancet 363 (2004) 1116.
8. D. Gairdner, The Schönlein-Henoch syndrome (anaphylactoid purpura), Q. J. Med. 17 (1948) 95–122.
9. J.A. Mills, B.A. Michel, D.A. Bloch, et al., The American College of Rheumatology 1990 criteria for the classification of Henoch-Schönlein purpura, Arthritis Rheum. 33 (1990) 1114–1121.
10. S. Ozen, A. Pistorio, S.M. Iusan, et al., EULAR/PRINTO/PRES criteria for Henoch-Schönlein purpura, childhood polyarteritis nodosa, childhood Wegener granulomatosis and childhood Takayasu arteritis: Ankara 2008. Part II: final classification criteria, Ann. Rheum. Dis. 69 (2010) 798–806.
11. J.C. Jennette, R.J. Falk, P.A. Bacon, et al., 2012 Revised International Chapel Hill Consensus Conference Nomenclature of Vasculitides, Arthritis Rheum. 65 (2013) 1–11.
14. F.T. Saulsbury, Henoch-Schönlein purpura in children. Report of 100 patients and review of the literature, Medicine (Baltimore) 78 (1999) 395–409.
16. M.C. Calvino, J. Llorca, C. Garcia-Porrua, et al., Henoch-Schönlein purpura in children from northwestern Spain: a 20-year epidemiologic and clinical study, Medicine (Baltimore) 80 (2001) 279–290.
18. M. Stewart, J.M. Savage, B. Bell, B. McCord, Long term renal prognosis of Henoch-Schönlein purpura in an unselected childhood population, Eur. J. Pediatr. 147 (1988) 113–115.
19. T.A. Farley, S. Gillespie, M. Rasoulpour, et al., Epidemiology of a cluster of Henoch-Schönlein purpura, Am. J. Dis. Child. 143 (1989) 798–803.
20. J.M. Gardner-Medwin, P. Dolezalova, C. Cummins, T.R. Southwood, Incidence of Henoch-Schönlein purpura, Kawasaki disease, and rare vasculitides in children of different ethnic origins, Lancet 360 (2002) 1197–1202.
21. S.R. Atkinson, D.J. Barker, Seasonal distribution of Henoch-Schönlein purpura, Br. J. Prev. Soc. Med. 30 (1976) 22–25.
22. M. Levy, M. Broyer, A. Arsan, et al., Anaphylactoid purpura nephritis in childhood: natural history and immunopathology, Adv. Nephrol. Necker Hosp. 6 (1976) 183–228.
23. M. Al-Sheyyab, A. Batieha, H. el Shanti, A. Daoud, Henoch-Schönlein purpura and streptococcal infection: a prospective case-control study, Ann. Trop. Paediatr. 19 (1999) 253–255.
24. D.M. Allen, L.K. Diamond, D.A. Howell, Anaphylactoid purpura in children (Schönlein-Henoch syndrome): review with a follow-up of the renal complications, AMA J. Dis. Child. 99 (1960) 833–854.
25. M. Masuda, K. Nakanishi, N. Yoshizawa, et al., Group A streptococcal antigen in the glomeruli of children with Henoch-Schönlein nephritis, Am. J. Kidney Dis. 41 (2003) 366–370.
26. H. Matsukura, A. Ohtsuki, T. Fuchizawa, T. Miyawaki, Acute poststreptococcal glomerulonephritis mimicking Henoch-Schönlein purpura, Clin. Nephrol. 59 (2003) 64–65.
45. J. Giangiacomo, C.C. Tsai, Dermal and glomerular deposition of IgA in anaphylactoid purpura, Am. J. Dis. Child. 131 (1977) 981–983.
46. K.K. Lau, H. Suzuki, J. Novak, R.J. Wyatt, Pathogenesis of Henoch-Schönlein purpura nephritis, Pediatr. Nephrol. 25 (2010) 19–26.
47. K. Kiryluk, Z. Moldoveanu, J.T. Sanders, et al., Aberrant glycosylation of IgA1 is inherited in both pediatric IgA nephropathy and Henoch-Schönlein purpura nephritis, Kidney Int. 80 (2011) 79–87.
48. J.K. Boyd, J. Barratt, Inherited IgA glycosylation pattern in IgA nephropathy and HSP nephritis: where do we go next?, Kidney Int. 80 (2011) 8–10.
51. H. Kamitsuji, K. Tani, M. Yasui, et al., Activity of blood coagulation factor XIII as a prognostic indicator in patients with Henoch-Schönlein purpura. Efficacy of factor XIII substitution, Eur. J. Pediatr. 146 (1987) 519–523.
58. M.M. Amoli, W. Thomson, A.H. Hajeer, et al., HLA-B35 association with nephritis in Henoch-Schönlein purpura, J. Rheumatol. 29 (2002) 948–949.
59. M.M. Amoli, W. Thomson, A.H. Hajeer, et al., HLA-DRB1*01 association with Henoch-Schönlein purpura in patients from northwest Spain, J. Rheumatol. 28 (2001) 1266–1270.
60. H. Peru, O. Soylemezoglu, S. Gonen, et al., HLA class 1 associations in Henoch Schönlein purpura: increased and decreased frequencies, Clin. Rheumatol. 27 (2008) 5–10.
61. M.M. Amoli, D.L. Mattey, M.C. Calvino, et al., Polymorphism at codon 469 of the intercellular adhesion molecule-1 locus is associated with

protection against severe gastrointestinal complications in Henoch-Schönlein purpura, J. Rheumatol. 28 (2001) 1014–1018.

62. R. Gershoni-Baruch, Y. Broza, R. Brik, Prevalence and significance of mutations in the familial Mediterranean fever gene in Henoch-Schönlein purpura, J. Pediatr. 143 (2003) 658–661.

63. Z.B. Ozcakar, F. Yalcinkaya, N. Cakar, et al., MEFV mutations modify the clinical presentation of Henoch-Schönlein purpura, J. Rheumatol. 35 (2008) 2427–2429.

64. D. Eleftheriou, P.A. Brogan, The molecular biology and treatment of childhood systemic vasculitis, in: J.W. Homeister, M.S. Willis (Eds.), Molecular and Translational Vascular Medicine, first ed., Springer, New York, 2012, pp. 35–70.

65. A. Bagga, S.K. Kabra, R.N. Srivastava, U.N. Bhuyan, Henoch-Schönlein syndrome in northern Indian children, Indian Pediatr. 28 (1991) 1153–1157.

66. H. Emery, W. Larter, J.G. Schaller, Henoch-Schönlein vasculitis, Arthritis Rheum. 20 (1977) 385–388.

69. F.T. Saulsbury, Henoch-Schönlein purpura, Pediatr. Dermatol. 1 (1984) 195–201.

76. J.I. Shin, J.M. Park, Y.H. Shin, et al., Predictive factors for nephritis, relapse, and significant proteinuria in childhood Henoch-Schönlein purpura, Scand. J. Rheumatol. 35 (2006) 56–60.

77. J.L. de Almeida, L.M. Campos, L.B. Paim, et al., Renal involvement in Henoch-Schönlein purpura: a multivariate analysis of initial prognostic factors, J. Pediatr. (Rio J) 83 (2007) 259–266.

78. F. Assadi, Childhood Henoch-Schönlein nephritis: a multivariate analysis of clinical features and renal morphology at disease onset, Iran. J. Kidney Dis. 3 (2009) 17–21.

79. H. Narchi, Risk of long term renal impairment and duration of follow up recommended for Henoch-Schönlein purpura with normal or minimal urinary findings: a systematic review, Arch. Dis. Child. 90 (2005) 916–920.

100. E. Flatau, D. Kohn, D. Schiller, et al., Schönlein-Henoch syndrome in patients with familial Mediterranean fever, Arthritis Rheum. 25 (1982) 42–47.

101. H. Ozdogan, N. Arisoy, O. Kasapcapur, et al., Vasculitis in familial Mediterranean fever, J. Rheumatol. 24 (1997) 323–327.

102. L. Rees, N.J.A. Webb, P.A. Brogan, Vasculitis, in: L. Rees, N.J.A. Webb, P.A. Brogan (Eds.), Paediatric Nephrology (Oxford Handbook), first ed., Oxford University Press, Oxford, 2007, pp. 310–313.

135. M. Zaffanello, V. Fanos, Treatment-based literature of Henoch-Schönlein purpura nephritis in childhood, Pediatr. Nephrol. 24 (2009) 1901–1911.

136. A.M. Huber, J. King, P. McLaine, et al., A randomized, placebo-controlled trial of prednisone in early Henoch Schönlein Purpura [ISRCTN85109383], BMC Med. 2 (2004) 7.

137. W. Chartapisak, S. Opastiraku, N.S. Willis, et al., Prevention and treatment of renal disease in Henoch-Schönlein purpura: a systematic review, Arch. Dis. Child. 94 (2009) 132–137.

138. J. Dudley, G. Smith, A. Llewelyn-Edwards, et al., Randomised, double-blind, placebo-controlled trial to determine whether steroids reduce the incidence and severity of nephropathy in Henoch-Schönlein Purpura (HSP), Arch. Dis. Child. 98 (2013) 756–763.

139. J. Ronkainen, O. Koskimies, M. la Houhala, et al., Early prednisone therapy in Henoch-Schönlein purpura: a randomized, double-blind, placebo-controlled trial, J. Pediatr. 149 (2006) 241–247.

140. P. Tarshish, J. Bernstein, C.M. Edelmann Jr., Henoch-Schönlein purpura nephritis: course of disease and efficacy of cyclophosphamide, Pediatr. Nephrol. 19 (2004) 51–56.

141. J.T. Flynn, W.E. Smoyer, T.E. Bunchman, et al., Treatment of Henoch-Schönlein Purpura glomerulonephritis in children with high-dose corticosteroids plus oral cyclophosphamide, Am. J. Nephrol. 21 (2001) 128–133.

142. K. Iijima, S. Ito-Kariya, H. Nakamura, N. Yoshikawa, Multiple combined therapy for severe Henoch-Schönlein nephritis in children, Pediatr. Nephrol. 12 (1998) 244–248.

143. P. Niaudet, R. Habib, Methylprednisolone pulse therapy in the treatment of severe forms of Schönlein-Henoch purpura nephritis, Pediatr. Nephrol. 12 (1998) 238–243.

144. D.C. Huang, Y.H. Yang, Y.T. Lin, B.L. Chiang, Cyclosporin A therapy for steroid-dependent Henoch-Schönlein purpura, J. Microbiol. Immunol. Infect. 36 (2003) 61–64.

145. T. Someya, K. Kaneko, S. Fujinaga, et al., Cyclosporine A for heavy proteinuria in a child with Henoch-Schönlein purpura nephritis, Pediatr. Int. 46 (2004) 111–113.

146. J.I. Shin, J.M. Park, Y.H. Shin, et al., Cyclosporin A therapy for severe Henoch-Schönlein nephritis with nephrotic syndrome, Pediatr. Nephrol. 20 (2005) 1093–1097.

147. E. Wright, M.J. Dillon, K. Tullus, Childhood vasculitis and plasma exchange, Eur. J. Pediatr. 166 (2007) 145–151.

148. D. Donghi, U. Schanz, U. Sahrbacher, et al., Life-threatening or organ-impairing Henoch-Schönlein purpura: plasmapheresis may save lives and limit organ damage, Dermatology 219 (2009) 167–170.

152. J.S. Cameron, Recurrent primary disease and de novo nephritis following renal transplantation, Pediatr. Nephrol. 5 (1991) 412–421.

156. J. Ronkainen, M. Nuutinen, O. Koskimies, The adult kidney 24 years after childhood Henoch-Schönlein purpura: a retrospective cohort study, Lancet 360 (2002) 666–670.

159. R. Counahan, M.H. Winterborn, R.H. White, et al., Prognosis of Henoch-Schönlein nephritis in children, Br. Med. J. 2 (1977) 11–14.

165. J.C. Jennette, R.J. Falk, K. Andrassy, et al., Nomenclature of systemic vasculitides. Proposal of an international consensus conference, Arthritis Rheum. 37 (1994) 187–192.

166. L.H. Calabrese, B.A. Michel, D.A. Bloch, et al., The American College of Rheumatology 1990 criteria for the classification of hypersensitivity vasculitis, Arthritis Rheum. 33 (1990) 1108–1113.

167. S. Ozen, N. Ruperto, M.J. Dillon, et al., EULAR/PReS endorsed consensus criteria for the classification of childhood vasculitides, Ann. Rheum. Dis. 65 (2006) 936–941.

Entire reference list is available online at www.expertconsult.com.

34 | CHAPTER

Polyarteritis Nodosa

Despina Eleftheriou, Seza Ozen

INTRODUCTION

Polyarteritis nodosa (PAN) was first described by Kussmaul and Maier in 1866.[1] The original and subsequent descriptions identified the pathological features of necrotizing arteritis with nodules along the walls of medium and small muscular arteries, affecting multiple organ systems throughout the body.[2-5] Despite some overlap with smaller vessel disease, PAN is a distinct entity.[6] Notably, the disease varies in its presentation from a relatively benign cutaneous form that may resolve without treatment to a severe systemic form that can be fatal.[2-5] In this chapter, the systemic and cutaneous forms of PAN will be described under separate headings.

POLYARTERITIS NODOSA (SYSTEMIC)

Definitions and Classification Criteria

In the Chapel Hill Consensus Conference held for the nomenclature and definition of vasculitides, classical PAN was defined as necrotizing inflammation of medium- or small-sized arteries without vasculitis in arterioles, capillaries, or venules.[7] PAN was separated from the distinct group of antineutrophil cytoplasmic antibody (ANCA)-associated microscopic polyangiitis (MPA), which was defined as necrotizing vasculitis with few or no immune deposits affecting small vessels.[7] MPA is predominantly a renal disease and usually presents in childhood as rapidly progressive, crescentic, glomerulonephritis.[7]

The widely accepted classification criteria for PAN have been the American College of Rheumatology (ACR) criteria, which were introduced in the 1990s and based solely on an adult registry.[8] There have been two early attempts to introduce specific pediatric criteria for PAN, one by Ozen and colleagues in 1992 and one by Brogan and colleagues in 2002.[5,9] These criteria were based on the pediatric practice and experience in children with PAN, although neither was tested for specificity, and there were no attempts at validation.[5,9]

In 2006, the first unique childhood criteria for systemic PAN were published with the endorsement of the European League against Rheumatism (EULAR) and the Paediatric Rheumatology European Society (PRES), with the participation of the European Society of Paediatric Nephrology (ESPN) and the ACR.[10] These criteria were established in two steps: initially, opinions were gathered from pediatric rheumatologists and nephrologists worldwide through a Delphi technique.[10] Subsequently, the final criteria were agreed on in a consensus conference with 10 experts, using the nominal group technique.[10] This was followed by a large validation exercise based on international Web-based registry for childhood vasculitides.[11] The 2006 criteria were revised and validated based on this international registry and the consensus of an expert panel.[11] After minor revisions, the final criteria with the highest sensitivity and specificity for childhood PAN were agreed upon; they are summarized in Box 34-1. It should be emphasized that these are classification criteria and not diagnostic criteria, although they are often incorrectly used as such.

Epidemiology

There is currently a lack of data describing the epidemiology of childhood PAN; however, systemic PAN is generally considered the third most common systemic vasculitis encountered in children.[12] In adults, at least in Europe and the United States, an estimated incidence ranges from 2 to 9 per million individuals per year.[12] Childhood PAN seems to be of worldwide distribution, with no sex bias and with the majority of cases presenting in mid-childhood, although with a wide spectrum of ages affected.[4,13-15]

In a multinational survey registering 110 childhood PAN patients (both systemic and cutaneous), the majority of respondents were from the eastern Mediterranean and South America.[4] Because not all countries are represented in this survey, there is a certain bias involved, and future studies are needed to define whether there are true geographic or even ethnic differences. The majority of patients in another large case series of children with PAN in the UK were Caucasian (81%), 15% were Asian, and 2% were Afro-Caribbean.[13]

Etiopathogenesis

The immunopathogenesis leading to vascular injury in PAN is probably heterogeneous. A number of infectious triggers have been implicated, and PAN-like illnesses have additionally been reported in association with cancers and hematological malignancies.[16-20] However, associations between PAN and these infections or other conditions are rare in childhood. Streptococcal infection may be an important trigger, and indirect evidence suggests that bacterial superantigens may play a role in some cases.[19-21] On the other hand, hepatitis B virus has been associated with PAN; however, this association has almost disappeared with recent vaccination protocols in children.[2,4] The hepatitis B virus–associated PAN was an immune complex disease in which antiviral treatment was also required.[2,4] In the revised 2012 Chapel Hill nomenclature, hepatitis B–associated PAN is classified under the "secondary vasculitis" category because there is a clear association with this virus.[7]

In terms of pathogenic mechanisms it seems likely that the immunological processes involved are similar to those in other systemic vasculitides and include cell adhesion molecules, cytokines, growth factors, chemokines, neutrophils, and T and B cells.[22] Of note, immunohistochemical studies performed on biopsied perineural and muscle vessels from homogeneous populations of PAN patients showed that inflammatory infiltrates consist mainly of macrophages and T lymphocytes, particularly of the CD8[+] subset.[23] To date, there is no reliable

BOX 34-1   **Classification Criteria for Childhood Polyarteritis Nodosa**

Evidence of necrotizing vasculitis in medium or small arteries or an angiographic abnormality showing aneurysm, stenosis, or occlusion of a medium- or small-sized artery (histopathology or angiography mandatory), plus one out of five of the following criteria:

1. Skin involvement (livedo reticularis, skin nodules, or infarcts)
2. Myalgia or muscle tenderness
3. Hypertension (systolic/diastolic blood pressure greater than 95th percentile for height)
4. Peripheral neuropathy (sensory peripheral neuropathy or motor mononeuritis multiplex)
5. Renal involvement (proteinuria >0.3 g/24 hours or >30 mmol/mg of urine albumin/creatinine ratio on a spot morning sample; hematuria or red blood cell casts, >5 red blood cells/high-power field, red blood cell casts in the urinary sediment, or equal to 2+ on dipstick; or impaired renal function, measured or calculated glomerular filtration rate [Schwartz formula] <50% normal)

Adapted from S. Ozen, A. Pistorio, S.M. Iusan, et al., EULAR/PRINTO/PRES criteria for Henoch Schönlein purpura, childhood polyarteritis nodosa, childhood Wegener granulomatosis and childhood Takayasu arteritis: Ankara 2008. Part II: Final classification criteria, Ann. Rheum. Dis. 69 (2010) 798–806.

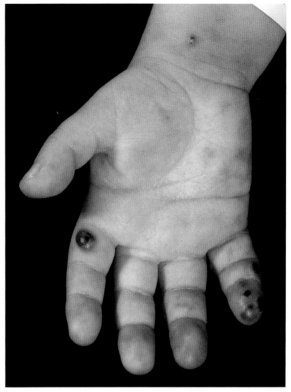

FIGURE 34-1 Lesions on the hand of a 2-year-old girl with polyarteritis nodosa. The biopsy revealed severe necrotizing vasculitis. (Courtesy Dr. P.A. Brogan.)

animal model of the disease. The PAN-like disease in cynomolgus macaques, which is very similar to the human disease, occurs only sporadically.[24] Snyder et al. described a PAN-like illness arising spontaneously in beagle dogs, but to date this animal model has not provided insight to the pathogenesis of PAN in humans.[25]

Genetic predisposing factors may make individuals vulnerable for developing PAN.[2] Recently, an association of childhood PAN with mutations in the familial Mediterranean fever (MEFV) gene has been shown in Turkish children.[26,27] This suggests that, at least in certain populations where the MEFV mutations are frequent, these mutations may be acting as one of the susceptibility factors for PAN.[26,27] Additionally, there are reports of PAN occurring in siblings within families, which may add weight to the genetic hypothesis.[28] Notably, mutations in the gene encoding adenosine deaminase 2 (ADA2) result in a syndrome of intermittent fevers, early-onset lacunar strokes, and other neurovascular manifestations; livedoid rash, hepatosplenomegaly, and systemic PAN-like vasculopathy have been recently described by two independent groups.[29,30]

Clinical Features

Systemic PAN is characterized by constitutional symptoms such as malaise, fever (no specific pattern), weight loss, and a variety of different skin manifestations, diffuse myalgia, abdominal pain, arthralgia, and, on occasion, arthritis.[2,4,13] Other clinical features including ischemic heart and testicular pain, renal involvement (hematuria, proteinuria, and hypertension), and neurological features (focal defects, hemiplegia, visual loss, mononeuritis multiplex, and organic psychosis) may occur.[2,4,13]

Skin lesions are variable and may rarely resemble those of HSP but can also be necrotic and associated with peripheral gangrene (Figs. 34-1 and 34-2).[2,4,13] Livedo reticularis is also a characteristic feature, and occasionally fixed tender subcutaneous nodules overlying affected arteries are present in both upper and lower limbs.[2,4,13] Skin infarctions may also be seen in this systemic form of the disease and can affect any part of the body.[2,4,13] The clinical features at presentation for the largest

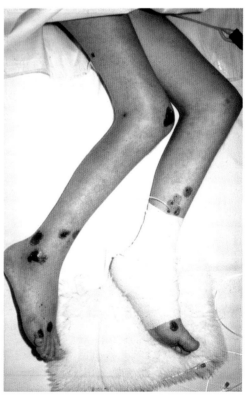

FIGURE 34-2 Necrotic lesions on the legs of a child with polyarteritis nodosa. Livedo reticularis is also present. (From L.H. Fraiser, S. Kanekal, J. Keher, Cyclophosphamide toxicity, Drugs 42 (1991) 781–795 by permission of Oxford University Press.)

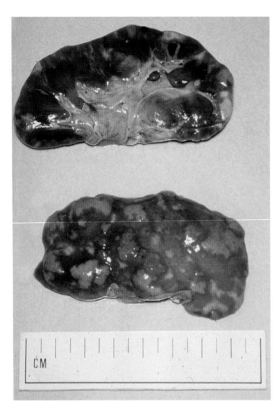

FIGURE 34-3 Postmortem appearances of the kidneys from a child with widespread aggressive polyarteritis nodosa, showing extensive areas of infarction secondary to the renal arterial necrotizing vasculitis.

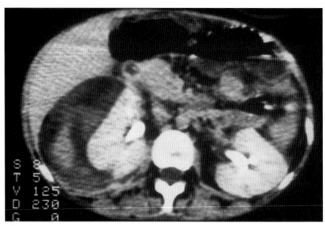

FIGURE 34-4 Abdominal computed tomography scan undertaken on a teenager with long-standing polyarteritis nodosa that was resistant to treatment, showing bilateral perirenal hematomata due to rupture of affected renal vessels.

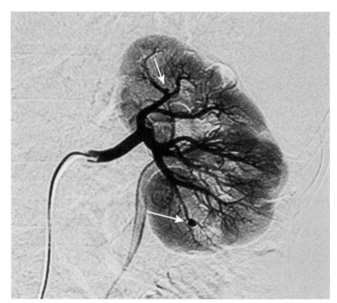

FIGURE 34-5 Aneurysms in branches of the renal artery in an angiogram from a child with polyarteritis nodosa. (Courtesy Dr. B. Peynircioglu.)

reported cohort of systemic PAN (69 children) were as follows: fever (87%), myalgia (83%), skin (88%), renal (19%), severe gastrointestinal (GI) (10%), and neurological involvement (10%).[13] Similar frequencies of clinical manifestations were recently reported in smaller studies from India and Croatia.[14,15] If the diagnosis and prompt treatment are delayed, widespread infarction can occur in affected viscera[2,4,13,31] (Fig. 34-3). In some patients, rupture of arterial aneurysms can cause peritoneal bleeding with perirenal hematomata being a recognized manifestation of this phenomenon, particularly in patients with both PAN and familial Mediterranean fever[2,4,13,31] (Fig. 34-4).

The differential diagnosis of PAN depends on the spectrum of organ involvement.[4] Other forms of vasculitis such as Kawasaki disease and secondary vasculitides need to be considered.[2] Infections such as bacterial endocarditis with microembolism also need to be excluded.[2] The autoinflammatory syndromes may also mimic certain features of PAN.[2,4] The diagnosis of PAN can only be secured by a combination of histopathological demonstration of necrotizing vasculitis and/or radiological demonstration of aneurysms and other angiographic typical findings.

Laboratory Investigations

Leukocytosis and thrombocytosis are frequent, along with elevated erythrocyte sedimentation rate (ESR) and C-reactive protein (CRP) levels.[2,4,13] Mild anemia may occur as well.[2,4,13] ANCA and antinuclear antibody (ANA) are typically negative in PAN.[2,4,13] Recently, there has also been some interest in measurement of circulating endothelial microparticles and circulating endothelial cells as markers of endothelial inflammatory damage in PAN and other vasculitides, and circulating endothelial progenitor cells that might point to evidence of endothelial repair.[32] Urinalysis findings may reflect renal arterial

involvement.[31] Proteinuria, hematuria, and even a decrease in renal function may occur.[13,31]

Radiological Investigations

Demonstration of aneurysms reflecting the necrotizing vasculitis of renal, celiac, mesenteric, or arteries in other parts of the body is a part of the diagnosis[9,33,34] (Fig. 34-5). Brogan et a. have shown that changes other than aneurysms may also suggest a diagnosis of PAN.[9] The most reliable nonaneurysmal signs were perfusion defects, the presence of collateral arteries, and delayed emptying of small renal arteries.[9] The authors indicated that the sensitivity of the diagnosis of PAN increased with the presence of these features.[9] If there is suspicion of cerebral vasculitis, cerebral arteriography may be required and can be done at the same examination. The dose of contrast agent administered requires careful consideration, particularly in small children.[2] Conventional angiography remains the overall gold standard, though future progress in imaging may improve the sensitivity of noninvasive imaging. Magnetic resonance angiography (MRA) and especially computerized tomography angiography (CTA) have emerged as alternative, noninvasive techniques to delineate vasculitic lesions in PAN.[35,36] However, MRA fails to detect small aneurysms or microaneurysms, although it can demonstrate large intrarenal and extrarenal aneurysms and stenosis or occlusions of the renal arteries or their branches, and areas of ischemia and infarction.[36,37] Of note, MRA may overestimate vascular stenotic lesions, particularly in small children.[36,37] CTA may also be able to reveal larger aneurysms and occlusive lesions and demonstrate areas of renal cortical ischemia and infarction, but concerns regarding the significant radiation exposure and its lack of sensitivity for the detection of vasculitic changes affecting smaller arteries in comparison to catheter arteriography limit its use.[2,35]

Indirect evidence of the presence of medium-sized vessel vasculitis affecting the renal arteries may be obtained by demonstrating patchy areas within the renal parenchyma of decreased isotope uptake on Tc-99m dimercaptosuccinic acid scanning of the kidneys.[2] These findings are not specific for vascular ischemia but in the context of a vasculitic illness, they are very suggestive, particularly if there is no history or evidence of another cause. They may be useful if diagnosis of PAN is still suspected but not confirmed on histology and/or angiography.[2]

The characteristic histopathological changes of PAN are fibrinoid necrosis of the walls of medium or small arteries with a marked inflammatory response within or surrounding the vessel wall.[2,13,38] The lesions tend to be focal and segmental.[2,13,38,39] There may be thrombosis and fibrinoid necrosis in association with necrotizing vasculitis; while sectoral involvement contributes to the blow-out type of aneurysms[2,13,38,39] (Fig. 34-6). Arteries in any organ system can be involved.[2,13,38,39] Biopsies of the muscle, sural nerve, kidney, liver, testis, or the GI tract may provide the diagnostic lesion.[2,13,23,38,39] Renal manifestations are usually secondary to medium-sized vessel involvement; true glomerulonephritis is uncommon and when present suggests polyangiitis overlap.[13] Immunofluorescence studies usually reveal no immune deposition.[2,13,23,38,39]

Management

The treatment of PAN requires the administration of high-dose corticosteroid with an additional cytotoxic agent such as cyclophosphamide

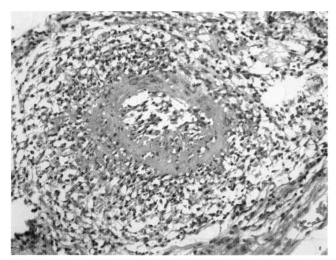

FIGURE 34-6 Biopsy of an intestinal wall artery in polyarteritis nodosa showing transmural fibrinoid necrosis and inflammatory infiltrate (hematoxylin-eosin stain,, original magnification ×200). (Courtesy Dr. D. Orhan.)

to induce remission, typically for the first 3 to 6 months.[2,4,13] There are no evidence-based data for the dose and administration of these therapeutic agents in children with PAN.[2,4,13] However, oral prednisone at a dose of 1 to 2 mg/kg is recommended with intravenous pulses in the case of more extensive disease.[2,4,13] Cyclophosphamide used to be given orally at a dose of 2 mg/kg/day; however, the authors recommend intravenous administration of 500 mg/m[2] possibly with a Euro-Lupus protocol.[2,4,13] Empirically, aspirin (2 to 5 mg/kg/day) has also been given as an antiplatelet agent by some clinicians.[2,4,13] When streptococcal infection is implicated, penicillin should be given in addition to the above induction of remission therapy regimen.[2,4,13,20] Disease activity and treatment response can be assessed using a modified Birmingham Vasculitis Activity Score—the Paediatric Vasculitis Activity Score (PVAS)—that has been recently validated.[40] PVAS also allows objective standardized definitions of clinical remission and relapse to be applied in a clinical trial setting and also in routine clinical practice, in line with the adult version of the tool.[40] Remission is defined as the absence of any clinical signs or symptoms of active vasculitis, as supported by laboratory evidence of normal CRP and ESR values and a PVAS of 0 of 63 (assigned retrospectively for every clinic visit), for two evaluations at least 1 month apart and with adherence to the prednisolone regimen.[13] Thus PVAS may now guide the management and treatment in PAN patients.

Once remission is achieved maintenance therapy with daily or alternate-day prednisone or prednisolone at doses of 0.2 to 0.4 mg/kg/day and oral azathioprine at a dose of 1 to 2 mg/kg/day is frequently utilized for an additional 12 to 18 months.[2,4,13] Adjunctive plasma exchange can be used during the induction phase of treatment in life- or organ-threatening situations.[41] Use of biological agents, including anti–tumor necrosis factor-α (anti–TNF-α) (intravenous infliximab 6 mg/kg every 6 to 8 weeks; subcutaneous adalimumab at 24 mg/m[2] for 2 weeks if body weight is less than 30 kg or 40 mg every 2 weeks if greater than 30 kg), and even rituximab (two doses at 750 mg/m[2] given 2 weeks apart) has also been described for children with systemic PAN, particularly those who do not respond to standard therapy (those who failed treatment with cyclophosphamide and steroids given for 6 months) or because of concern regarding cumulative toxicity.[42,43] PVAS as described above can be used to monitor efficacy and response to these biological therapies.

Notably, short-term complications, such as infections and corticosteroid-induced side effects, remain a concern for children with PAN receiving standard therapy.[2,4,13] Furthermore, late complications associated with cyclophosphamide therapy include malignancy and infertility at high doses.[44] Clinical trials in adults suggest that mycophenolate mofetil (MMF) could be a less toxic alternative to cyclophosphamide, with comparable efficacy, in the treatment of systemic lupus erythematosus and ANCA-associated vasculitis.[45,46] In that context, a multicenter, open-label, randomized controlled trial (RCT) of MMF versus cyclophosphamide for the induction of remission of childhood PAN (the MYPAN trial) is currently being developed as an RCT.

PAN associated with hepatitis B infection is now classified separately as a secondary vasculitis[7] and requires a different therapeutic approach because conventional treatment with glucocorticoids and cyclophosphamide allows the virus to replicate, facilitating evolution toward chronic hepatitis and liver cirrhosis.[2,47-49] The recommended approach is to combine plasma exchange and antiviral treatment with corticosteroids to control acute manifestations, then to stop the corticosteroids to enhance immunological clearance of hepatitis B virus–infected hepatocytes, and to favor seroconversion from positive hepatitis B e antigen to a positive anti–hepatitis B e antigen.[2,47-49]

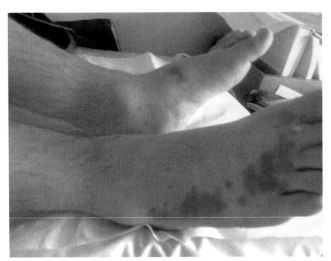

FIGURE 34-7 Cutaneous polyarteritis nodosa: painful purpuric and nodular lesions on the feet and a livedo pattern on the legs.

Outcome

Unlike some other vasculitides such as granulomatosis with polyangiitis, PAN appears to be a condition in which permanent remission can be achieved.[2,13] However, if treatment is delayed or inadequate, life-threatening complications can occur.[2,13] The relapse rate in a UK-based cohort of 69 children with PAN who were still receiving maintenance therapy was 35%.[13] Gastrointestinal involvement was associated with increased risk of relapse ($P = 0.03$), whereas a longer time to induce remission ($P = 0.022$) and increased cumulative cyclophosphamide dose, albeit with significant toxicity ($P = 0.005$), were associated with lower relapse risk.[13] In comparison with the almost 100% mortality seen in the presteroid era, in a recent case series by Eleftheriou et al.,[13] demonstrated reduced mortality rates to 4%.

CUTANEOUS POLYARTERITIS NODOSA

Cutaneous PAN is a form of vasculitis affecting small- and medium-sized vessels essentially limited to the skin.[50-53] It is characterized by the presence of fever and nodular, painful, nonpurpuric lesions with or without livedo reticularis (Fig. 34-7) occurring predominantly in the lower extremities, and with no systemic involvement except for myalgia, arthralgia, and nonerosive arthritis.[50-53] The skin features are similar to the systemic disease; however, infarcts are not present in cutaneous disease.[50-53] In a recent international survey of childhood vasculitis, approximately one third of children identified as having PAN were categorized as having cutaneous PAN.[4] The clinical course is characterized by periodic exacerbations and remissions that may persist for many years and occasionally throughout childhood.[50-53] The duration of the disease is quite variable and may last for years. Skin biopsy shows necrotizing nongranulomatous small- and medium-sized vessel vasculitis similar to that seen in systemic disease but confined to the skin; tests for ANCA are negative, and the condition is often associated with serological or microbiological evidence of streptococcal infection.[50-53] Nonrecurring cutaneous PAN has been observed in neonates born to mothers with chronic cutaneous PAN.[54] There has been much discussion as to whether the condition should be classed as a separate entity or as a part of the spectrum of PAN.[2,50] The condition remains essentially localized to the skin, although a proportion of cases appear to evolve into full-blown PAN in time, and clinicians need to be mindful of this possibility.[2,50] The distinction is difficult, and patients with greater systemic involvement or who show a lack of response to standard treatment may need to be further evaluated and possibly treated as if they had PAN.[2,50] A careful follow-up to establish any systemic involvement is warranted. Furthermore, if there is any complaint of ischemic pain in a child with elevated acute phase reactants, visceral angiography is indicated.

Treatment

Cutaneous PAN can respond to nonsteroidal antiinflammatory drugs, but it may require oral steroids in moderate doses to achieve remission.[50-53] Because the disease is not expected to have systemic involvement, some physicians are reluctant to give steroids; however, they are effective in suppressing the disease. When streptococcal infection is implicated, penicillin may need to be added to standard therapy.[50-53] Some clinicians recommend continuing prophylactic penicillin throughout childhood because relapses are common and occur in up to 25% of cases in association with further streptococcal infections.[20,50-53]

In circumstances where there has been lack of response to standard treatment or concerns about possible steroid toxicity,[51] some success has also been reported with the use of methotrexate, colchicine, intravenous immunoglobulin (IVIG), azathioprine and dapsone, cyclophosphamide, pentoxifylline, and chloroquine.[2,50,55-57]

SUMMARY

Systemic PAN and its localized form, cutaneous PAN, are well-recognized forms of vasculitis affecting children. Developments in investigative procedures and therapeutic approaches have resulted in improvements in diagnosis and treatment such that the current outlook for the majority of affected children is good.[4,13] However, those diagnosed late or with severe systemic disease still have a consequential morbidity and mortality. Hopefully, newer characterization of the etiopathogenetic mechanisms and genetic predispositions will lead to better and safer treatment. RCTs linked to prospective long-term follow-up studies are now urgently needed in order to provide evidence base for the management of children with PAN.

REFERENCES

Entire reference list is available online at www.expertconsult.com.

CHAPTER 35

Kawasaki Disease

Mary Beth Son, Robert P. Sundel

HISTORICAL BACKGROUND

Kawasaki disease (KD) is one of the most common vasculitides of childhood. It has the potential to cause severe complications, significant morbidity, and even mortality. Expeditious treatment can largely prevent these complications, underscoring the importance of early and accurate diagnosis. The diagnosis is based on clinical criteria (Box 35-1), and in the absence of a diagnostic test, correct identification of KD can be as exacting a challenge today as it has been for more than 40 years.

This vasculitis bears the name *Kawasaki disease* because of the highly detailed description of this illness in 50 children by Tomisaku Kawasaki in 1967.[1] Scattered case reports of young children who died of ruptured or thrombosed coronary artery aneurysms have appeared in the medical literature since 1871.[2,3] A clinical syndrome comprising most of the components of what is today recognized as KD was described by Munro-Faure in 1959[4] and by Itoga in 1960,[5] and an even earlier fatal inflammatory vasculopathy primarily affecting young boys, infantile polyarteritis nodosa (IPN), likely represents extreme cases of the same disorder.[6]

DEFINITION AND DIAGNOSTIC CRITERIA

KD is a self-limited vasculitis of unknown etiology characterized by fever, rash, conjunctivitis, oral mucositis, extremity changes, cervical lymphadenopathy, and, in a proportion of cases, dilation or aneurysms of the coronary and other arteries.

Criteria for the diagnosis of KD are shown in Box 35-1.[7] More recently proposed criteria include perineal rash in the criterion for changes in the extremities, and recognition that, in the presence of fever and coronary artery changes demonstrated by echocardiography, fewer than four criteria suffice to make the diagnosis of KD.[7,8] Muta and colleagues[9] showed that fewer cases of KD were missed when children were included whose fevers were abrogated with intravenous immunoglobulin (IVIG) within 5 days of the onset of fever.[10]

None of these guidelines has 100% sensitivity and specificity for the diagnosis of KD. If a child has the characteristic clinical features and develops coronary artery aneurysms, the diagnosis is certain. Children who do not meet the criteria may have an incomplete or atypical form of KD (discussed later). Alternatively, some patients who fulfill all criteria may have other conditions. In a study of patients referred because of possible KD, Burns and colleagues[11] found that the standard clinical diagnostic criteria for KD were fulfilled in 18 (46%) of 39 patients in whom other diagnoses were established. Furthermore, Benseler et al. found that in a consecutive series of children diagnosed with KD, up to one third had concurrent, identifiable infections,[12] including Group A streptococcal tonsillitis, viral illnesses, pneumonia, and gastroenteritis.

More concerning from the perspective of trying to prevent disease sequelae is that many children who develop coronary artery aneurysms never meet criteria for KD.[13] Witt et al. found in a single center study of 127 patients treated for KD that 36% did not meet the criteria for KD. Furthermore, the KD cases that did not meet the criteria for diagnosis had a significantly higher proportion of coronary artery abnormalities as compared to those cases that did meet criteria (20% vs. 7%, $P < 0.05$).[13] Sudo et al. utilized epidemiological data from the twentieth nationwide survey of KD in Japan and found that the prevalence of coronary artery lesions 1 month after disease onset tended to be higher in the cases with one or two principal criteria as compared with those cases that had five to six criteria (7.4% vs. 2.5% $P < 0.05$).[14] Consistent with this, a recent meta-analysis of over 20 studies of patients with KD found that incomplete KD is a risk factor for coronary artery abnormalities.[15]

The youngest patients are the least likely to meet the classic criteria, and unfortunately they also have the highest risk of developing coronary artery abnormalities.[16] Rosenfeld et al. found that up to 60% of children younger than 12 months old developed aneurysms in one series.[17] For this reason, the diagnosis of KD should be considered in any infant with prolonged, unexplained fever, and there should be a low threshold for performing echocardiography in this age group. Conversely, in older children, treating KD is seldom an emergency, especially when patients present symptoms after only 5 or 6 days of fever. Observation of children older than 6 months who do not fulfill criteria may be the best course of action. The mean duration of fever in children with untreated KD is 12 days,[18] much longer than typical viral illnesses, so the persistence of fever or development of additional signs of KD can be an indicator for treatment.

EPIDEMIOLOGY

Although worldwide in distribution, the incidence of KD is highest in Japan and is steadily increasing over time, although the reasons behind this increase are unclear. In 2010, the annual incidence rate recorded in Japan was 239.6 per 100,000 children aged up to 4 years, which is higher than during any of the three epidemics of KD in Japan in 1979, 1982, and 1986. Children of Japanese descent who reside outside Japan also face a higher risk of KD than do Caucasian children.[19] The incidence is increasing in South Korea as well, with the second highest worldwide incidence of 134.4/100,000 children younger than 5 years of age in 2011.[20] Rates in Taiwan[21] and China[22] are also high.

The epidemiology of KD in the United States differs from countries in Asia in that there are fewer cases (20.8/100,000 children <5 years in

Fever for more than 5 days (4 days if treatment with intravenous immuno-globulin eradicates fever) plus at least four of the following clinical signs not explained by another disease process:
- Bilateral conjunctival injection (80% to 90%)*
- Changes in the oropharyngeal mucous membranes, including one or more of injected and/or fissured lips, strawberry tongue, injected pharynx (80% to 90%)
- Changes in the peripheral extremities, including erythema and/or edema of the hands and feet (acute phase) or periungual desquamation (convalescent phase) (80%)
- Polymorphous rash, primarily truncal; nonvesicular (>90%)
- Cervical lymphadenopathy with at least one node >1.5 cm (50%)

*Numbers in parentheses indicate the approximate percentage of children with Kawasaki disease who demonstrate the criterion.

2006) and the incidence does not seem to be rising over time.[23] As assessed by hospital admissions in the U.S., children of Asian or Pacific Island ancestry have the highest incidence (30.3/100,000 <5 years). The incidence was intermediate for African Americans (17.5/100,00 <5 years) or children of Hispanic origin (15.7/100,000 <5 years), and lowest for whites (12/100,000 <5 years).[23] In one large area of Great Britain, the annual incidence rate was 5.5 cases per 100,000 for children younger than 5 years old; the incidence for children of Asian ancestry was more than double that for Caucasian and African or Afro-Caribbean children.[24]

KD is an illness of early childhood. Seventy-seven percent of affected patients are younger than 5 years old, with an average age of approximately 3 years,[23] although there are reports of KD occurring in older children[25] and adults.[26-28] KD is more common in boys than in girls (male-to-female ratio of 1.36:1 to 1.62:1).[29,30]

In Japan, the highest incidence occurs between 6 and 11 months old.[31] In North America, the peak age at onset of KD is between 2 and 3 years old. In a recent Australian study of the years 2000 through 2009, the mean age of diagnosis was 4.2 years.[32] The reasons for the geographic differences in age at onset are unclear.[33]

Several reports document a seasonal incidence of KD.[33-35] Burns et al. established a global seasonal pattern of KD with a peak in disease in January through March in the extratropical Northern Hemisphere.[35] In Japan, the disease occurs most frequently in winter and spring months, with a nadir in October.[31] In a study from Taiwan, the highest incidence was in the summer.[36] In North America, cases have tended to occur between November and May.[37] There were no seasonal variations in the incidence of KD in a study from western Australia.[32] Although epidemics of KD were documented in Japan up to 1987, none has occurred since then.[38]

In Japan, siblings of affected children have a risk of contracting KD that is approximately 10 times higher than the risk in the general population,[39] but cases among children sharing the same home in other countries are uncommon.[34] Dergun and colleagues[40] reported 18 families in the United States with 24 affected members, including 9 sibling pairs. Second and even third attacks have been reported in a range of 1.5% to 3% of cases.[31,36]

ETIOLOGY AND PATHOGENESIS

The cause of KD remains unknown. Many of its epidemiological and clinical manifestations suggest an infectious origin. If an infectious

agent does indeed cause KD, the putative organism would appear to be of very low communicability, or predominantly responsible for subclinical infections. Repeated attempts to identify a particular infectious trigger have been unsuccessful.[41]

A predominance of immunoglobulin A (IgA)-secreting plasma cells in the blood vessel walls of children with fatal KD has suggested to Rowley and colleagues that an organism that gained entry through mucosal surfaces underlies the disease.[42] No single pathogen is regularly demonstrable, although associations with Epstein–Barr virus (EBV),[43] rotavirus,[44] other viruses,[45,46] and with bacteria[47,48] have been reported. An association with a coronavirus[49] was not confirmed.[50] It is nonetheless a possibility that the vascular injury in KD may be the result of a direct cell-mediated attack on endothelial cells that are infected with an unidentified pathogen.[51]

Other investigators have proposed that the vasculitis in KD is caused by either conventional antigens or superantigens that trigger an immune response to endothelial cells, rather than by direct infection of the vessels.[52] Superantigens are produced by several bacteria, notably certain strains of Staphylococcus and Streptococcus, and are capable of stimulating large numbers of T cells in an antigen-nonspecific manner by interaction with the β chain of the T-cell receptor. Overrepresentation of T cells bearing Vβ2 among lymphocytes in coronary artery aneurysms, intestinal mucosa,[53,54] and peripheral blood[55] from patients with KD supports the hypothesized role of superantigens in the pathogenesis. A variety of additional circumstantial evidence[52,56-58] and a murine model of Lactobacillus casei–induced vasculitis lend credence to this theory.[59] Further, children with KD have unique reactions to mycobacterial antigens,[60-62] which may also function as superantigens, including recall reactions at the site of a previous bacillus Calmette–Guérin immunization.[61] Nonetheless, the only human illness definitively ascribed to superantigens is toxic shock syndrome, and different groups have published conflicting evidence regarding the isolation of superantigen-producing organisms, the detection of superantigen proteins, and the presence of an immunological signature of superantigen activity in patients with KD.[55,63,64]

Additional clues to the cause of KD may come from humoral factors, including antiendothelial cell antibodies, circulating immune complexes,[65] and antineutrophil cytoplasm antibodies (ANCAs) that are demonstrated by some researchers in a proportion of patients,[65,66] but not by others.[67,68] For example, findings from a murine model indicated that B cells may not be necessary for coronary arteritis.[69] However, genome-wide association studies have implicated single nucleotide polymorphisms (SNPs) in the B lymphoid tyrosine kinase and CD40 genes as evidence that B cells may play a pathogenic role in KD.[70,71]

Recent studies have demonstrated that regulation of T-cell activation may determine susceptibility to and severity of KD.[59] Onouchi et al. identified a functional SNP in the inositol 1,4,5-triphosphate 3-kinase C (IPTKC) gene on chromosome 19 through linkage disequilibrium mapping. ITPKC acts as a negative regulator for T-cell activation, and the SNP was associated with risk for developing KD and coronary artery lesions.[72] Supportive evidence for the role of T cells in KD has recently been provided via an animal model of KD, in which mice are injected intraperitoneally with Lactobacillus casei cell wall extract. T-cell costimulation was identified as a critical regulator of susceptibility to and severity of coronary arteritis in this model.[59]

In the absence of confirmed evidence of a single etiological agent, a reasonable working hypothesis is that KD represents a stereotyped, pathological immune response to one or a variety of environmental and/or infectious triggers. It may be a form of reactive vasculopathy, like polyarteritis nodosa or Henoch–Schönlein purpura, with an inflammatory response developing in sterile tissues as a result of immune activation.[73] Presumably, certain individuals are predisposed by virtue of their genetic constitution. The strong predilection for childhood onset may reflect the presence of developmental antigens that are targets for the inflammatory response only early in life, subtle maturational defects in immune responsiveness,[74] or the timing of exposure to environmental triggers.

GENETIC BACKGROUND

In Japan, approximately 1% of patients with KD have a history of an affected sibling,[75] and concordance for KD was 13.3% in dizygotic twins and 14.1% in monozygotic twins.[76] Similarly, in Japan there is a significantly increased frequency of a history of KD in the parents of children with the disease.[77] These observations indicate that there is a genetic predisposition to this disease, although the fact that affected twin pairs became ill within 2 weeks of each other also suggests an important role for an environmental agents.

The exact genetic factors that may underlie the disorder are unknown. Reported genetic associations have been reviewed by Hata and Onouchi.[78] Candidate genes include those at the histocompatibility locus and those for other proteins involved in immunoregulation. Human leukocyte antigen (HLA) genes for B5, B44, Bw51, DR3, and DRB3*0301 have been associated with KD in Caucasians; Bw54, Bw15, and Bw35 in the Japanese; and Bw51 in Israelis.[79] Onouchi and colleagues[80] concluded that HLA polymorphisms contributed little to the pathogenesis of KD. However, a recent study identified an SNP that achieved genome-wide significance in the HLA-DQB2-HLA-DOB locus.[81] There has been no reported association of any HLA antigen with the risk of coronary artery disease.[82]

Polymorphisms of the tumor necrosis factor (TNF)-α gene *(TNF),*[83] the *IL 18* gene,[84] the *HLA E* gene,[85] and the gene for angiotensin-converting enzyme[86,87] have also been associated with KD, but their pathogenic significance is disputed. A separate report implicated polymorphisms of the mannose-binding lectin (MBL) in the pathogenesis of KD.[88] MBL binds to n-acetyl glucosamine and mannose present on the surface of many microbes. This interaction results in activation of complement (C3) independent of antibody. Levels of MBL are determined by polymorphisms of the MBL 2 gene and its promoters. Higher expression of MBL is associated with lower incidence of coronary artery lesions in patients under 1 year old, but it has the opposite effect in older patients. This apparent paradox is congruent with the belief that MBL is important in protecting the very young child from infectious diseases.[88]

The gene controlling expression of inositol 1,4,5-triphosphate 3-kinase *(ITPKC)* has been identified as a susceptibility gene not only for KD, but also for coronary artery disease.[72] This enzyme is strongly expressed by peripheral blood mononuclear cells and has an important role in inflammation by decreasing interleukin (IL)-2 expression. The functional polymorphism ITPKC 3 is significantly increased in patients with KD and coronary artery disease in Japanese and American populations.[89] An SNP in the *caspase-3* gene on chromosome 4 has also been associated with risk for IVIG resistance and coronary artery abnormalities,[90] which may be due to its role in apoptosis. An SNP in the *FAM167A-BLK* gene is a recently identified locus that is significantly associated with a risk for KD.[70,81] It is of interest, as previous studies have reported an association between SNPs in this region and autoimmune diseases, including rheumatoid arthritis[91] and systemic lupus erythematosus.[92,93] There have also been reports of associations of functional SNPs in immunoglobulin receptor pathways[81,94] and in the gene for *CD40.*[71,81]

CLINICAL MANIFESTATIONS

Disease Course

The course of untreated KD may be divided into three phases (Fig. 35-1): An acute, febrile period lasting for 10 to 14 days is followed by a subacute phase of approximately 2 to 4 weeks. This ends with a return to normal of the platelet count and erythrocyte sedimentation rate (ESR). The subsequent convalescent or recovery period lasts months to years, during which time vessels undergo healing, remodeling, and scarring.

Acute Febrile Phase

The onset of fever in KD is characteristically abrupt, sometimes preceded by symptoms of an upper respiratory or gastrointestinal illness. Baker and colleagues[95] studied the symptoms in the 10 days prior to diagnosis of KD in 198 patients. They reported that irritability occurred in 50%, vomiting in 44%, decreased food intake in 37%, diarrhea in 26%, and abdominal pain in 18%. Cough was reported in 28%, and 19% had rhinorrhea. In addition, 19% reported weakness, and 15% reported arthralgia or arthritis. Perineal desquamation may be another early sign of KD.[96] Over the next 3 to 4 days, cervical adenitis, conjunctivitis, changes in the buccal and oral mucosa, a pleomorphic rash, and erythema and edema in the hands and feet develop. The manifestations occur in no particular order and can fluctuate in the first 7 to 10 days of illness. Accordingly, a thorough medical history is important for identifying subtle or transient manifestations of KD. Untreated, the clinical signs of KD subside after an average of 12 days. If myocarditis occurs, it often does so early and may be manifested by tachycardia, an S3 gallop, and perhaps signs of congestive heart failure.[97] Pericarditis, abdominal pain, ascites, and hydrops of the gallbladder also may occur at this time.

Subacute Phase

After the acute phase, the child may be entirely asymptomatic if given IVIG. During this period, desquamation of the skin and specifically, periungual desquamation of the digits,[98] may be the only clinically apparent residual feature. One in 13 children may develop arthritis of one or several joints during the late acute and subacute phases.[99] Coronary artery aneurysms most commonly first develop during the subacute phase or occasionally earlier, but rarely later in children treated with IVIG. The irritability that can be quite prominent in the acute phase diminishes and resolves completely during the subacute phase.

Convalescent Phase

Most children are asymptomatic during the convalescent phase. The acute phase response has usually returned to normal, unless there are complications. Horizontal ridging of the nails (Beau lines), characteristic of many acute inflammatory conditions, may appear during this period.

Clinical Characteristics of the Classification Criteria
Fever

Fever, often exceeding 40°C (104°F), is the hallmark of KD. The fever is typically persistent and minimally responsive to antipyretic agents, tending to remain above 38.5°C (101.3°F) during most of the acute phase of the illness. It reflects elevated levels of TNF-α and IL-1, which are thought to mediate the underlying vascular inflammation.[100] The diagnosis must be suspect in the absence of fever, though brief temperature spikes may be missed by fatigued or inexperienced parents.

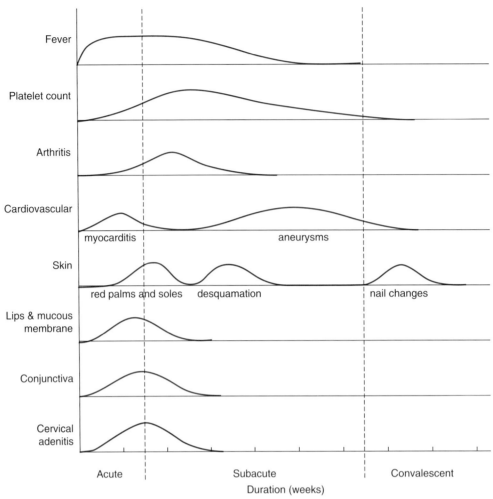

FIGURE 35-1 Kawasaki disease can be viewed as an illness with acute, subacute, and recovery phases. The temporal characteristics outlined here are typical of the course of the disease. (Adapted from Kawasaki T, Acute febrile mucocutaneous syndrome with lymphoid involvement with specific desquamation of the fingers and toes in children, *Arerugi* 16 (3) (1967) 178–222. [Article in Japanese].)

Conjunctivitis

Bilateral, nonexudative bulbar conjunctivitis occurs in more than 85% of patients with KD. Conjunctival injection typically spares the limbus, which is the zone immediately around the cornea. However, the characteristic of limbal sparing is not required for conjunctival erythema to qualify as a diagnostic criterion. Inflammation of the palpebral conjunctiva is not prominent. Purulent discharge is especially unusual[101] and suggests an alternative diagnosis.

Other ocular abnormalities also may occur, although they are not part of the diagnostic criteria. During the first week of illness, about three fourths of children are photophobic, a consequence of anterior uveitis,[102] which peaks between 5 and 8 days of illness and is more common in children over 2 years old. Ocular inflammation usually resolves without specific therapy or sequelae. In exceptional instances, there may be posterior synechiae, scleral[100] or conjunctival[103] scarring, changes in the retina and vitreous,[104] or even blindness.[105]

Changes in the Lips and Oral Mucosa

Swollen, vertically cracked red lips and a strawberry tongue are characteristic of KD; the latter is caused by sloughing of filiform papillae and prominence of the large hyperemic fungiform papillae (Fig. 35-2).

Diffuse erythema of the oropharynx is also seen. Vesicles, ulcers, or tonsillar exudate suggest a viral or bacterial infection rather than KD.

Exanthem

The cutaneous manifestations of KD are protean. Although the rash usually begins on the trunk, there is often a perineal confluence during the first days of the illness, followed by desquamation in the diaper area by day 6 in many cases.[96] Macular, morbilliform, or targetoid lesions of the trunk and extremities are most characteristic. The rash is seldom pruritic, and vesicular or bullous lesions are rare (Fig. 35-3). Psoriasis has been reported in several children with KD.[106]

Lymphadenopathy

Anterior cervical lymphadenopathy occurs during the acute phase of the disease, is usually unilateral, and may appear to involve only a single node. However, ultrasonography or computed tomographic imaging of the neck typically reveals grapelike clusters of enlarged nodes similar to those seen in EBV infections rather than the isolated adenopathy typical of bacterial adenitis.[107] Occasionally, a node enlarges rapidly and may be mistaken for infectious lymphadenitis. After 3 or 4 days, it usually shrinks with or without specific therapy.

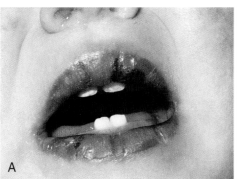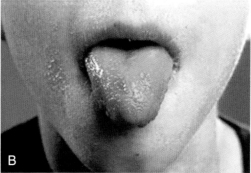

FIGURE 35-2 **A,** The intense reddening, swelling, and vertical cracking of the lips are characteristic of Kawasaki disease (KD). **B,** The strawberry tongue of acute KD with hypertrophied papillae on an erythematous base and the peeling of the facial skin.

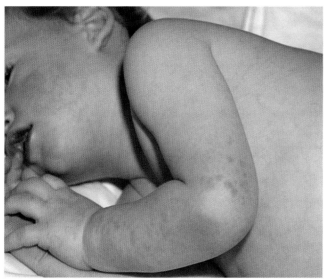

FIGURE 35-3 The nonspecific polymorphous rash is seen on the face arms and chest of this 2-year-old boy with acute Kawasaki disease.

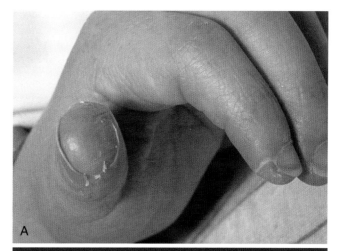

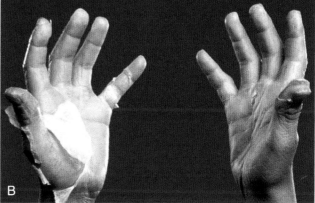

FIGURE 35-4 **A**, Desquamation of the skin of the tips of the thumb and finger seen during the subacute phase of Kawasaki disease. **B**, Desquamation of the skin of the hand occurs later in the subacute and early recovery phase of the disease. In many children, the degree of desquamation is much less than is depicted here.

Diffuse lymphadenopathy and splenomegaly are not typical of KD and should raise suspicions of a viral illness.

Extremity Changes

Indurated edema of the dorsum of the hands and feet and a diffuse red-purple erythema of the palms and soles occur early and last for 1 to 3 days. Sheetlike desquamation typically occurs 10 days or more after the start of the fever. It characteristically begins at the tips of the fingers followed by the toes, just below the distal edge of the nails (Fig. 35-4). Flaky desquamation may occur elsewhere, but acral skin peeling usually occurs late in the course of KD and may be absent or inapparent.[98] Consequently, it is more useful for retrospective confirmation of the diagnosis rather than for making therapeutic decisions.

Incomplete Kawasaki Disease

Signs and symptoms in children who do not meet criteria for KD tend to parallel those of children who fulfill the diagnostic criteria.[108] Incomplete KD is seen more frequently in young infants and older children, which is a critical observation as these groups of children are also at higher risk for coronary artery lesions.[25,31,109,110] A particularly high level of suspicion is needed in infants younger than 1 year old. In a retrospective review of 45 cases of KD, 5 (45%) of 11 infants had

incomplete disease, compared with 4 (12%) of 33 older children.[111] In this study, coronary artery complications occurred in three older children (9%) but in seven infants (64%), including all five with incomplete disease.[111] In view of these data, the American Heart Association (AHA) has suggested additional markers for identification of children who do not meet the classic criteria for KD but who might nonetheless be at increased risk for developing coronary artery aneurysms (Fig. 35-5).[7] Reports suggest that the algorithm recommended by the AHA committee performs well in reducing the number of children who are not treated for KD but who ultimately develop aneurysms.[112]

Other Clinical Manifestations of Kawasaki Disease

Table 35-1 shows other clinical manifestations of KD.

Cardiovascular Disease

At onset, there is nearly always tachycardia, typically commensurate with the degree of fever. Early myocarditis occurs in at least one third[113] to half[114] of patients, and pericarditis also may occur.[115] Myocardial involvement often leads to decreased contractility, commonly manifested by an S3 gallop that may become more prominent with hydration. Tachycardia out of proportion to the fever is also found in children with significant myocarditis. Such children may be misdiagnosed with viral myocarditis. In more severe cases, myocardial involvement may progress to dysrhythmias and signs of congestive heart failure.[116] Children with prominent KD-associated myocarditis tend to respond briskly to treatment with IVIG, and long-term

EVALUATION OF SUSPECTED INCOMPLETE KAWASAKI DISEASE (KD)[1]

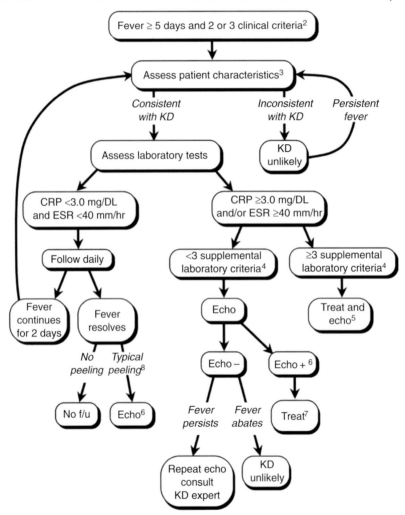

FIGURE 35-5 Evaluation of suspected incomplete Kawasaki disease. [1]In the absence of gold standard for diagnosis, this algorithm cannot be evidence based but rather represents the informed opinion of the expert committee. Consultation with an expert should be sought anytime assistance is needed. [2]Infants 6 months old on day 7 of fever without other explanation should undergo laboratory testing and, if evidence of systemic inflammation is found, an echocardiogram, even if the infants have no clinical criteria. [3]Characteristics suggesting disease other than Kawasaki disease include exudative conjunctivitis, exudative pharyngitis, discrete intraoral lesions, bullous or vesicular rash, or generalized adenopathy. Consider alternative diagnoses. [4]Supplemental laboratory criteria include albumin 3.0 g/dL, anemia for age, elevation of alanine aminotransferase, platelets after 7 d 450 000/mm³, white blood cell count 15 000/mm³, and urine 10 white blood cells/high-power field. [5]Can treat before performing echocardiogram. [6]Echocardiogram is considered positive for purposes of this algorithm if any of 3 conditions are met: z score of LAD or RCA 2.5, coronary arteries meet Japanese Ministry of Health criteria for aneurysms, or 3 other suggestive features exist, including perivascular brightness, lack of tapering, decreased LV function, mitral regurgitation, pericardial effusion, or z scores in LAD or RCA of 2–2.5. [7]If the echocardiogram is positive, treatment should be given to children within 10 d of fever onset and those beyond day 10 with clinical and laboratory signs (CRP, ESR) of ongoing inflammation. [8]Typical peeling begins under nail bed of fingers and then toes. (American Heart Association, Diagnosis, treatment, and long-term management of Kawasaki disease. Circulation 110 (2004) 2747–2771.)

TABLE 35-1 Manifestations of Kawasaki Disease

ORGAN SYSTEM	COMMON	UNCOMMON	FINDING SUGGESTS ALTERNATE DIAGNOSIS
Skin	Targetoid, urticarial, morbilliform rashes, livedo reticularis	Psoriasiform rash	Pustular, vesicular rashes
Lungs	Pleural effusion	Nodules, interstitial infiltrates	
Urinary tract	Urethritis, pyuria	Hematuria, proteinuria, orchitis	
Nervous system	Irritability, lethargy, anterior uveitis, sensorineural hearing loss	Seizure, stroke, cranial nerve palsy	
Gastrointestinal system	Diarrhea, vomiting, hydrops of gallbladder, hepatomegaly	Intestinal hemorrhage, ruptured viscus	
Hematological system	Anemia, thrombocytosis, leukocytosis	Thrombocytopenia, consumptive coagulopathy, hemophagocytic syndrome	Lymphocytosis*
Reticuloendothelial system	Anterior cervical lymphadenopathy	Posterior cervical, axillary lymphadenopathy	Diffuse lymphadenopathy, splenomegaly
Mucosa	Mucositis, glossitis, conjunctivitis		Discrete oral lesions, exudative conjunctivitis
Musculoskeletal system	Extremity edema, arthritis	Raynaud phenomenon	
Cardiac system	Tachycardia, gallop rhythm, myocarditis, pericarditis	Coronary artery aneurysm, aortic root dilation, valvulitis	

*Except during the convalescent phase.

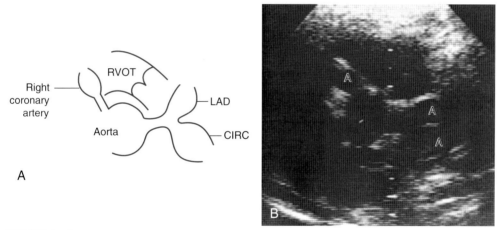

FIGURE 35-6 Echocardiographic demonstration of aneurysms of three coronary arteries in a child with Kawasaki disease. *A*, Aneurysms; *CIRC*, circumflex; *LAD*, left anterior descending coronary artery; *RVOT*, right ventricular outflow tract. (Courtesy Dr. Dennis Crowley.)

abnormalities of cardiac contractility are very uncommon in children treated appropriately during the acute phase of KD.[117] Tacke et al. performed cardiac magnetic resonance (MR) imaging in patients and controls at a median of 11.6 years following diagnosis of KD and found that only those with severe coronary artery pathology had evidence of cardiac dysfunction.[118]

Recently, there has been increasing awareness of a shocklike syndrome that can occur with KD (KD shock syndrome [KDSS]).[119] Kanegaye and colleagues identified 13 children with systolic hypotension, which is a 20% or greater decrease in baseline systolic blood pressure, or clinical signs of poor perfusion from a cohort of 187 consecutive patients with KD at a single center.[119] They found that a third of the children with KDSS had impaired left ventricular systolic function and nearly two thirds had coronary artery abnormalities. IVIG resistance was also seen more commonly in the patients with KDSS. A Taiwanese group performed a case control study of

9 patients with KDSS compared with 27 season-matched controls and also found that the cases had a higher risk for coronary artery dilation.[120]

The most significant and characteristic complication of KD, the development of coronary artery aneurysms in up to 25% of untreated patients, makes KD the leading cause of acquired heart disease among children in the developed world (Figs. 35-6 and 35-7). Frank aneurysms are unusual early in the course of disease, but the lack of tapering seen on echocardiograms is typical, and coronary artery dimensions may be increased in the first 5 weeks after the disease first manifests. Interestingly, Muniz et al. compared coronary artery dimensions of febrile patients with non-KD illnesses to KD patients, and found that the non-KD febrile controls exhibited enlarged coronary artery dimensions, although not to the same degree as the KD cases.[121] Similarly, Bratincsak found that no febrile controls had coronary artery diameters more than 2.5 standard deviations above the mean for age, size,

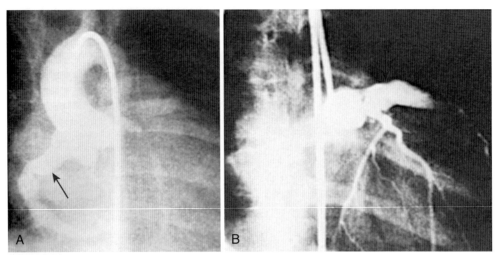

FIGURE 35-7 A, Angiography of the coronary vessels in a 7-month-old boy with Kawasaki disease shows a huge aneurysmal dilation of the right coronary artery (*arrow*). **B,** Aneurysm of the left coronary artery in a 3-year-old girl with Kawasaki disease (*arrow*). (Courtesy Dr. Zuidi Lababidi.)

and gender, a diameter typically reached by more than 10% of children with KD.[122]

The Japanese Ministry of Health (JPH) criteria[123,124] use angiography or echocardiography to define coronary arteries as abnormal if the internal lumen diameter is greater than 3 mm in children younger than 5 years old or greater than 4 mm in children at least 5 years old. In addition, vessels are considered aneurysmal if the internal diameter of a segment measures at least 1.5 times that of an adjacent segment or the coronary artery lumen is clearly irregular. Aneurysms can be defined as small (an internal diameter of <5 mm), medium (an internal diameter of 5 to 8 mm) or giant (an internal diameter >8 mm) per the JPH.

Although coronary artery dimensions in normal children have been shown to increase linearly with body surface area (BSA) or length,[125] the JPH criteria are not based on body size. Evaluation of coronary arteries in KD using age-, size-, and sex-adjusted indices (z scores) suggests that the incidence of abnormalities is higher than was generally recognized.[126] Among patients classified as having normal coronary arteries by the JPH criteria, 27% had at least one BSA-adjusted coronary artery dimension more than 2 standard deviations above the mean. Of note, z scores are available only for the left main coronary artery, the left anterior descending artery, and the right coronary artery. Other coronary vessels can be assessed using the JPH criteria. Even children whose vessel dimensions are within the "normal" range may demonstrate a decrease in coronary artery diameter as they convalesce from KD.[127] Some experts think that a z-score-based system of classifying aneurysms may be more discriminating, with a giant aneurysm defined as a z score of 10 or higher.

Coronary aneurysms may cause morbidity early in the course due to rupture or thrombosis, resulting in sudden death or myocardial infarction.[128] Development of *de novo* coronary artery abnormalities more than 2 weeks after the end of the acute illness is unusual.

Although involvement of the coronary arteries is the most characteristic manifestation of the vasculitis of KD, other medium-sized muscular arteries also may be involved. Aneurysms of brachial and femoral arteries may be palpable clinically or demonstrable angiographically (Fig. 35-8). In severe cases, peripheral arterial obstruction may lead to ischemia and gangrene. Visceral arteries are usually spared, although there are reports of gastrointestinal obstruction[129] and acute abdominal catastrophe[130] occurring because of vasculitis. Such complications generally arise in children with other signs of severe vasculitis, including aneurysms in coronary and peripheral arteries.

Central Nervous System Complications

One of the most consistent clinical observations of children with KD, particularly in infants and very young children, is their extreme irritability. This probably represents the effect of aseptic meningitis and associated headache.[131] Cerebrovascular accident[132,133] and facial nerve paralysis[134] have also been reported.

Musculoskeletal Disease

Arthritis was observed by Gong and colleagues[99] in 7.5% of 414 children with KD. Arthritis was oligoarticular in 55% and polyarticular in 45%. Joints most commonly affected were (in order of decreasing frequency) knee, ankle, wrist, elbow, and hip. Joint pain was often severe, but responded to IVIG and high-dose aspirin in most instances. It may occur at any time during the disease course but has been described most commonly during the recovery phase. Arthritis in KD ultimately resolves, leaving no residua.

Respiratory Tract Disease

Cough, coryza, hoarseness, and otitis media frequently occur early in the course of the disease, and suggest a viral upper respiratory tract infection. Approximately one third of children have some degree of sensorineural hearing loss when tested within 30 days of fever onset. Salicylate toxicity may be responsible for transient cases, but sensorineural hearing loss of unclear etiology rarely may persist after aspirin is discontinued.[135-137]

Gastrointestinal Tract Disease and Other Abnormalities

Abdominal pain is common, and approximately one fourth of children with KD have profuse, watery diarrhea during the acute febrile period. Abdominal distention may mimic mesenteric vasculitis or intussusception, and children with KD can present with an acute surgical abdomen, although this is rare.[130] Segmental bowel wall thickening has been described in children with KD and abdominal pain, presumably reflecting visceral arteritis.[138] The relatively common occurrence of hydrops of the gallbladder demonstrated by ultrasonography[139] may aid in the diagnosis of incomplete KD. Occasionally, the gallbladder becomes large enough to be seen as a bulge in the anterior abdominal

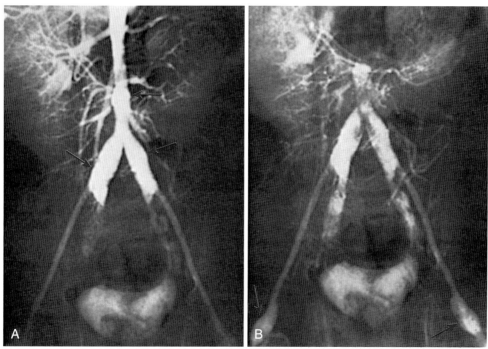

FIGURE 35-8 Angiographic study of a 2-year-old boy with severe Kawasaki disease resulting in multiple aneurysms of the coronary, axillary, iliac, and femoral arteries. The study revealed large aneurysms of the aorta and iliac arteries (**A**) and the femoral arteries (**B**; *arrows*). Aneurysms that were palpable in the axilla and groin in this patient later resolved. (Courtesy Dr. G. Culham.)

wall. The specificity of gallbladder distension is limited, however, and a dilated, engorged gallbladder may be seen in cases of streptococcal and staphylococcal infections, among other mimics of KD. Hepatosplenomegaly may occur in the absence of heart disease, or it may reflect cardiac failure.

Genitourinary Tract Involvement

Kidney and genitourinary tract involvement is uncommon but reported in KD.[140] A study of 50 children with KD from Taiwan[141] revealed hematuria (>5 red blood cells per high-power field [RBC/HPF]) in 6 patients, proteinuria (>100 mg/dL) in 5, and leukocyturia (>10 white blood cells per high-power field [WBC/HPF]) in 19. Renal ultrasonography was abnormal in five patients, and dimercaptosuccinic acid single photon emission computed tomography (DMSA SPECT) revealed inflammatory lesions in 26 children. Although renal function remained normal, scarring was demonstrated in 46% on repeated DMSA SPECT. Sterile pyuria is one of the supplemental laboratory criteria in the algorithm for suspected incomplete KD. Burns et al. compared pyuria in KD cases versus febrile controls without urinary tract infections. They found that pyuria was neither sensitive nor specific for KD, but that the magnitude of pyuria in KD was significantly higher than in febrile controls (42 WBC/μL vs. 12 WBC/μL).[142]

Scrotal pain and swelling due to testicular inflammation are characteristic of pediatric vasculitides, including Henoch–Schönlein purpura, polyarteritis nodosa, and KD.[143] Meatitis and dysuria also occur frequently during the acute phase of KD, and priapism has been described.[144] Hemolytic-uremic syndrome, immune complex–mediated glomerulonephritis, and acute interstitial nephritis have each been reported in a few cases.[145,146] Acute renal failure is a rare complication most commonly ascribed to complications of treatment with certain preparations of IVIG.[147]

BOX 35-2 Differential Diagnosis of Kawasaki Disease

Infectious Conditions
Adenovirus
Measles
Parvovirus
Human herpesviruses (HHV) (e.g., herpes simplex virus, cytomegalovirus, HHV-6, HHV-7)
Rocky Mountain spotted fever
Leptospirosis
Streptococci
Staphylococci

Immune System Reactions
Stevens–Johnson syndrome
Toxin-mediated diseases (toxic shock syndrome)
Serum sickness

Rheumatic Diseases
Systemic-onset juvenile idiopathic arthritis
Polyarteritis nodosa

DIFFERENTIAL DIAGNOSIS

The differential diagnosis of KD includes viral and bacterial infections, toxin-mediated diseases, systemic-onset juvenile idiopathic arthritis and Stevens–Johnson syndrome (Box 35-2). Viral illnesses such as measles (especially when atypical or occurring after vaccination), EBV, and adenovirus infections share many of the signs of mucocutaneous involvement, but they typically have less evidence of systemic inflammation and generally lack the extremity changes of KD. Toxin-mediated illnesses, especially scarlet fever, staphylococcal scalded skin syndrome, and toxic shock syndrome lack the ocular and articular involvement typical of KD. Drug reactions, such as those in Stevens–Johnson syndrome or serum sickness, may mimic KD but have subtle differences in the ocular and mucosal manifestations. In particularly severe or prolonged KD, the possibility of a chronic vasculitis such as polyarteritis nodosa[148] must be considered carefully. A lack of renal involvement and presence of mucocutaneous changes favor the diagnosis of KD over polyarteritis nodosa.

PATHOLOGY

The signs and symptoms of KD are due to a systemic necrotizing vasculitis with fibrinoid necrosis of the medium-sized muscular arteries; the coronary arteries are the predominant sites of involvement.[149] Disruption of the lamina elastica is characteristic of the aneurysms. Fujiwara documented early neutrophilic infiltrate in all layers of the heart, including the valves. Inflammation begins in the microvasculature (i.e., arterioles, capillaries, vasa vasorum, and venules) and subsequently spreads to larger vessels, especially the coronary arteries.[150] In these lesions, infiltrating cells are mostly macrophages and IgA-secreting plasma cells,[42] findings that may be unique to KD.[151] Endothelial cells express a variety of markers of activation, presumably as a result of the high levels of proinflammatory cytokines that characterize the acute phase of disease.[152] Some children have a lymphocytic myocarditis, with endomyocardial biopsy demonstrating cellular infiltrates or myofibrosis that may persist for years in untreated cases.[153]

Evolution of the cardiac lesions was detailed in the study by Fujiwara and Hamashima.[150] Pericarditis, myocarditis, and endocarditis were universal findings early in the disease, but diminished as fibrosis of the myocardium became the predominant lesion in children whose death occurred 40 days or more after onset. Coronary artery vasculitis predominated early in the disease but was absent in those who died after 28 days of illness. Aneurysms, thrombosis, and stenosis did not appear until 12 days of disease or later.

In a study of 262 children, Suzuki and colleagues[154] documented an equal frequency of aneurysms in the right and left coronary arteries, but a higher propensity for development of segmental stenosis and occlusions in the right coronary artery.

Using light and electron microscopy, Orenstein et al. reviewed autopsy and cardiac transplant tissues from KD patients, and described three phases to the arteriopathy of KD that differ in some ways from prior descriptions.[155] The first phase is characterized by a neutrophilic necrotizing arteritis that begins in the endothelium and can cause saccular aneurysms as the process moves through the walls of the arteries to the adventitia in the first 2 weeks of illness. This is followed by a subacute or chronic vasculitis driven by lymphocytes, plasma cells, and eosinophils that may last weeks to years and results in fusiform aneurysms. During the subacute or chronic vasculitis, smooth muscle cells may be converted to myofibroblasts that cause progressive stenosing lesions, leading to thrombosis.[155]

LABORATORY EXAMINATION

There are no specific diagnostic tests for KD, but at onset, evidence of inflammation is manifested by elevation of C-reactive protein (CRP) and ESR, leukocytosis, and a left shift in the white blood cell (WBC) differential count. Toxic granulation of neutrophils is more frequent in children with KD than in those with other febrile illnesses.[156] Occasionally, significant neutropenia occurs early[157]; this may be a marker for particularly severe disease. Thrombocytopenia and anemia may

herald the onset of macrophage activation syndrome (see Chapter 49).[158] Although platelet counts may be normal at the onset of disease, by the second week of illness they characteristically rise and may reach 1,000,000/mm^3 (reactive thrombocytosis) in the most severe cases. Children with KD often present with a normocytic, normochromic anemia; hemoglobin concentrations greater than 2 standard deviations below the mean for age are found in half of patients within the first 2 weeks of illness.[11]

Sterile pyuria is of urethral origin and therefore is missed on urinalyses obtained by bladder aspiration or catheterization. The WBCs are mononuclear and are not detected by dipstick tests for leukocyte esterase. Measurement of liver enzymes often reveals elevated transaminase levels or mild hyperbilirubinemia due to intrahepatic congestion. A few children develop obstructive jaundice from hydrops of the gallbladder or hepatic vasculitis.

Cerebrospinal fluid (CSF) analysis typically displays a mononuclear pleocytosis with normal glucose and protein. In a chart review of 46 children with KD, 39% were documented to have elevated CSF WBC counts.[131] The median count was 22.5 cells/mm^3 with 6% neutrophils and 91.5% mononuclear cells, although cell counts as high as 320/mm^3 with up to 79% neutrophils were reported. Arthrocentesis of involved joints typically demonstrates synovial fluid WBC counts of 50 to 300,000 WBC/mm^3 consisting primarily of neutrophils.

Children with KD develop significant perturbations in serum lipid profiles beginning during the subacute phase of illness. These abnormalities include elevated concentrations of triglycerides and low-density lipoproteins, and depressed levels of high-density lipoproteins.[159] They are most likely caused by widespread endothelial injury, and persistent abnormalities in lipid profiles are more likely in those children with coronary artery abnormalities. Ou et al. found that 1 year after the onset of KD, children with coronary artery aneurysms were more likely to have depressed high-density lipoprotein cholesterol levels and elevated high-sensitivity CRP levels than those KD patients who had normal coronary arteries.[160] As with other sequelae of KD, normalization may take years in untreated children but typically occurs within weeks or months after IVIG therapy.

ANCAs[161] and antibodies to endothelial cells[162] may be present late but not early in the disease.[67] Consequently, they have unclear pathological significance and are of little diagnostic value. Other autoantibodies are usually absent. Elevated levels of von Willebrand factor antigen indicate the presence of damaged endothelium.[163] Activation products of C3 and C4 have been demonstrated on erythrocytes (C3g) and in the plasma (C4d),[164] suggesting the participation of complement in at least some of the manifestations of the disease.

TREATMENT

General Approach

The child with suspected or definite KD should be admitted to the hospital for observation, monitoring of cardiac status, and management of systemic manifestations (Box 35-3). Initial evaluation of the heart should include an electrocardiogram to identify dysrhythmias, signs of ischemia, or myocarditis. A baseline echocardiogram should be performed to detect coronary artery vasculitis, ectasia, or aneurysms and to document biventricular function. If the diagnosis is relatively certain (even if diagnostic criteria are not met), and other diagnoses have been considered and excluded, treatment should be initiated with aspirin and IVIG without further delay.

Goals of Therapy

In addition to control of the acute inflammation and its symptoms, the goal of therapy is to prevent long-term sequelae and, most

BOX 35-3 Initial Evaluation and Management of Kawasaki Disease

Evaluation

- General physical exam
- Cardiac status (ECHO, ECG)
- CNS status
- Hematological and inflammatory parameters (CBC, differential, platelet count, ESR, CRP)
- Fluid and electrolyte status (AST, ALT, bilirubin, electrolytes, BUN, creatinine); urinalysis
- Ophthalmological status
- Monitor cardiac status
- Monitor CRP (ESR) and platelet count at 2-week intervals until stable, then 1-month intervals until normal
- Repeat echocardiogram at 6 to 8 weeks

Treatment

- Aspirin:
  - If patient is febrile: 80 to 100 mg/kg/day in four doses
  - If patient is afebrile: 3 to 5 mg/kg/day in one dose
- IVIG: 2 g/kg administered over 8 to 12 hours with premedications
- Keep in hospital until afebrile for 24 hours or if there are complications
- If fever persists, repeat IVIG once
- If inadequate clinical response, consider corticosteroids (2 mg/kg/day, or 30 mg/kg/dose, or infliximab 5 mg/kg [see discussion in this chapter])
- Maintain low-dose aspirin until ESR and platelet count are normal if there have been no coronary artery abnormalities; for 2 years if coronary abnormalities have resolved; "forever" if coronary artery disease persists

ALT, Alanine transaminase; *AST*, aspartate transaminase; *BUN*, blood urea nitrogen; *CNS*, central nervous system; *CRP*, C-reactive protein; *ECG*, electrocardiogram; *ECHO*, echocardiogram; *ESR*, erythrocyte sedimentation rate; *IVIG*, intravenous immunoglobulin.

importantly, coronary artery abnormalities. The consequences of failure to appropriately treat a child with KD are so important that, within reason and after very careful evaluation, error on the side of premature or unnecessary therapy is preferable to delayed or missed therapy for a child for whom the diagnosis is uncertain. The American Academy of Pediatrics and the AHA recommend that children with KD should be treated with aspirin and IVIG during the first 10 days of the illness.[7,165]

Treatment strategies also depend on the presence of coronary artery dilation, given the long-term morbidity associated with this complication. Approximately half of coronary artery aneurysms demonstrated by echocardiogram regress to normal lumen diameter via myointimal proliferation in 1 to 2 years after illness onset, usually in aneurysms smaller than 6 mm in diameter.[166] However, persistent vasodilatory abnormalities have been observed in arteries where aneurysms resolved.[167] Giant coronary artery aneurysms, with an internal diameter larger than 8 mm, are associated with the highest risk of morbidity and mortality. Up to one third of such aneurysms become obstructed, leading to myocardial infarction, dysrhythmias, or sudden death.[168] Treatment with IVIG decreases the incidence of giant aneurysms by more than 98% and the overall incidence of aneurysms by 85%.[18,169]

Acute phase reactants and platelet counts do not return to normal for up to 2 months after apparently successful treatment with IVIG, suggesting that vasculitis and endothelial inflammation may not fully resolve, even when fever is controlled. IVIG-resistant KD requires additional therapy, and questions remain whether initial treatment should

be more robust than IVIG alone, at least for some children at high risk of responding incompletely to IVIG, aiming for anatomically and functionally normal vessels in everyone.

Aspirin

Aspirin was the first medication to be used for treatment of KD because of its antiinflammatory and antithrombotic effects.[170] Antiinflammatory regimens using high-dose (>80 mg/kg/day)[7] or lower-dose (30 to 50 mg/kg/day)[170] aspirin have been recommended during the acute phase of the illness. After the fever resolves, the dose is usually reduced to an antiplatelet range of 3 to 5 mg/kg/day. These doses, well below the antiinflammatory level, have the effect of inhibiting platelet adhesion to endothelium by curtailing platelet release of thromboxane A_2 without suppressing prostacyclin production by endothelial cells.[171] This effect is thought to be beneficial in preventing thrombosis when platelet counts are elevated, although no studies have demonstrated such a benefit clinically. In the event of aspirin sensitivity, another antiplatelet agent, such as dipyridamole, should be considered in patients at particular risk of developing thromboses. Unless coronary artery abnormalities are detected by echocardiogram, aspirin is discontinued after results of laboratory studies return to normal, usually within 2 months of disease onset.

A meta-analysis found that high-dose and lower-dose aspirin regimens were associated with a similar incidence of coronary artery abnormalities at 30 and 60 days after disease onset.[172] Lee et al. enrolled 51 children with KD and treated them with standard doses of IVIG but without concomitant use of acetylsalicylic acid (ASA) in the acute phase, and compared them to a historical control group treated with IVIG plus high-dose ASA. The ASA-treated group had shorter duration of fever as compared to the no-ASA group, but there was no difference in IVIG resistance (17.1% vs. 15.7%, P = 1.000) or the development of coronary artery lesions (7.8% vs. 3.9%, P = 0.514).[173] A retrospective study by Hsieh et al. had similar findings, although the duration of fever was not different in the no-ASA group.[174] Although the necessity of using high-dose aspirin might be questioned because of the rapid response to IVIG, all of the trials showing the benefit of IVIG were conducted with children who also were receiving antiinflammatory doses of aspirin. There have been no published comparisons of aspirin with other antiinflammatory agents, and it is unclear whether salicylates are uniquely efficacious for this condition. For other complications, such as treatment of prolonged arthritis, alternative antiinflammatory agents may be used. The AHA warns against prescribing ibuprofen in children, as they require protection from thrombosis because ibuprofen antagonizes the antiplatelet effects of low-dose aspirin.[7,175]

The risks of aspirin appear to be similar to those reported in other settings: chemical hepatitis, transient hearing loss, and, rarely, Reye syndrome.[176] These risks may be increased in KD. Aspirin-binding studies have suggested that the hypoalbuminemia of children with KD predisposes them to toxic levels of free salicylate, despite measured (bound) values within the therapeutic range.[177]

Intravenous Immunoglobulin

Furusho and co-workers[178] first reported that high-dose IVIG appeared to decrease the incidence of coronary artery abnormalities. Newburger and colleagues[18] verified these findings in a 19-month, randomized, controlled clinical trial in 168 children with KD. Half of the children received IVIG (400 mg/kg/day on 4 consecutive days) plus high-dose aspirin (100 mg/kg/day), and half of the children received aspirin alone. IVIG reduced the incidence of coronary artery abnormalities by 78%, and no child suffered serious adverse effects from the therapy, thereby confirming the remarkable therapeutic potential of IVIG.

The initial IVIG treatment regimen was based on then-current protocols for treating immune thrombocytopenic purpura. The question of whether this protocol was optimal for KD was addressed in 1991.[179] Children were randomized to receive the traditional four-dose regimen or a single dose of 2 g/kg of IVIG infused over 8 to 12 hours. Children receiving the larger, single dose fared better. Meta-analyses have documented a dose-response benefit of IVIG therapy in the range of 200 mg/kg to 2 g/kg.[180]

IVIG is most effective in reducing the risk of coronary artery disease when administered within 10 days of the onset of fever. Unfortunately, the diagnosis may remain in doubt as this deadline approaches. In ambiguous cases, the physician may be guided by the epidemiology of the disease. More than 50% of infants with KD present atypically (i.e., do not fulfill diagnostic criteria), and they have a very high incidence of aneurysms. Thus, empiric treatment in very young children warrants serious consideration.[6]

The mechanism of action of IVIG is uncertain, with studies adding induction of neutrophil apoptosis[181] and reversal of inhibited lymphocyte apoptosis[182] to a long list of immunomodulatory effects of IVIG (Box 35-4). The response is generally prompt, and temperature returns to normal in many children even before the end of the IVIG infusion, with rapid clearing of the rash, mucositis, and conjunctivitis. Irritability and emotional lability, however, may persist for up to several weeks before resolving.

The greatest long-term concern about IVIG use is potential transmission of blood-borne pathogens. Technical deficiencies in production led to more than 100 cases of hepatitis C in recipients of a single brand of IVIG in 1994, although none was a child with KD.[183] No cases of IVIG-transmitted infections have been reported since the institution, in 1995, of current purification and processing practices, and no cases of IVIG-transmitted human immunodeficiency virus (HIV) have ever been reported. Overall, the cost-benefit analysis documents that IVIG treatment of KD is one of the most cost-effective medical therapies available, leading to impressive short- and long-term savings.[184]

Infusion reactions (fever, rash, nausea, and hypotension) occasionally accompany IVIG administration and are best managed by slowing the rate of infusion and administering diphenhydramine. With no viable alternative therapies, aggressive premedication with

corticosteroids, or even use of a different brand of IVIG, is preferable to foregoing immunoglobulin. Rarely, a child might develop congestive heart failure during or after infusion of the IVIG because of the high solute load and subsequent increase in intravascular volume. Slowing the infusion rate and administration of furosemide are usually the only treatments required. Treatment with IVIG leads to improvement in myocardial contractility and is almost invariably adequate therapy.[7] Hemolysis is uncommon, but occasionally it may be severe, requiring transfusion.[185] Headache up to 72 hours after the infusion is common, especially in older patients. Such children may require low-dose opiates for relief.[186]

Virtually all data concerning the role of IVIG are limited to treatment during the first 10 days of illness. This is not to say that treatment after 10 days of illness is ineffective or contraindicated; it is merely inadequately studied. In a report of 16 children with coronary artery aneurysms treated a mean of 17 days after the onset of fever, echocardiogram showed there was a trend toward resolution of abnormalities.[187] The American Academy of Pediatrics cautiously recommends IVIG for children beyond the tenth day of illness with "manifestations of continuing inflammation," and such an approach appears prudent.[165] Questions have arisen concerning very early treatment of KD.[188] Tse and colleagues,[189] on the other hand, reported that IVIG given on or before the fifth day of illness resulted in fewer coronary artery abnormalities at the 1-year follow-up assessment. Thus, decisions about the optimal date for treating with IVIG are best made based on a patient's clinical status and the certainty of the diagnosis of KD rather than anticipated advantages of administration on a particular day of disease.

Prediction of IVIG Resistance

The clinical importance of predicting which children will suffer from cardiac sequelae from KD has led to the creation of several risk scores for IVIG resistance. In a retrospective series from Japan, Fukunishi and colleagues[190] found higher serum levels of CRP, lactate dehydrogenase, and bilirubin to be predictive of failure to respond to IVIG. More recently, Kobayashi and colleagues reported on several factors that were associated with decreased responsiveness to IVIG, and therefore increased risk of coronary artery abnormalities: hyponatremia; elevated hepatic transaminase and CRP; a high percentage of bands on the WBC count differential; a platelet count of 300,000 or less; short duration between fever onset and diagnosis (4 days or less); and being younger than 12 months of age at onset.[191] Egami et al.[192] and Sano et al.[193] have also constructed risk scores for IVIG resistance utilizing similar parameters. Unfortunately, application of these risk scores did not accurately identify all children at risk for IVIG resistance and coronary artery abnormalities in a North American cohort.[194] In a Canadian study, Han and colleagues[188] could not identify any difference in laboratory parameters between responders and nonresponders. Confirming the importance of controlling inflammation in KD, Mori and co-workers[195] reported that a rise in the WBC count and CRP level after IVIG infusion are independent predictors of coronary artery abnormalities.

Glucocorticoids

Glucocorticoids, the preferred initial treatment for other forms of vasculitis, were considered unsafe in KD for many years following the early descriptions of the disease. This is based primarily on a study[196] that demonstrated an extraordinarily high incidence of coronary artery aneurysms (11 of 17 patients) in a group that received oral prednisolone at a dose of 2 to 3 mg/kg/day for at least 2 weeks, followed by 1.5 mg/kg/day for an additional 2 weeks. Interestingly, seven patients in the same study received prednisolone plus aspirin, and none developed aneurysms. In fact, no subsequent study has indicated that corticosteroids are harmful when used either with IVIG or as an alternative to IVIG therapy. Corticosteroids in KD have been studied both as primary therapy and "rescue" therapy, and doses have ranged from pulse doses of 30 mg/kg (maximum of 1 g) to conventional antiinflammatory doses (2 mg/kg/day).

Potential benefits of corticosteroids as rescue therapy in KD have been reported. Initially, two retrospective analyzes supported the use of corticosteroids in children who were unresponsive to two doses of IVIG or who relapsed after such therapy.[197,198] Hashino and colleagues[199] also found a beneficial effect of glucocorticoids in KD in a prospective trial. Children who had failed to respond to two doses of IVIG were randomized to receive a third dose of IVIG or pulse-dose methylprednisolone. Patients who received methylprednisolone had a significantly shorter duration of fever, and although transient coronary artery dilation was associated with glucocorticoid therapy, there was no overall difference in the incidence of coronary artery abnormalities between groups. Recently, Kobayashi et al.[200] retrospectively reviewed 359 consecutive KD patients over 12 years who failed to respond to first-line therapy of IVIG. They compared outcomes of children who received a second dose of IVIG versus a second dose of IVIG plus prednisolone versus prednisolone as monotherapy (maximum dose of 2 mg/kg/day for all children receiving steroids). They found that outcomes were better in the IVIG + prednisolone group with decreased need for subsequent treatments (aOR 0.16, 95% confidence interval [CI] 0.09-0.31), and fewer coronary artery abnormalities at 1 month (aOR 0.40, 95% CI 0.18-0.91) than the IVIG group. However, the treatment regimens were selected arbitrarily in this retrospective study. A prospective study is likely needed to assess the role of corticosteroids as rescue therapy.

Might steroids be more effective if administered earlier in the course of KD? Shinohara and colleagues[201] retrospectively reviewed the results in almost 300 patients with acute KD seen between 1982 and 1998 who were treated before the tenth day of illness. All patients received aspirin, dipyridamole, and propranolol. The addition of prednisolone therapy, either alone or with IVIG, was associated with a significantly shorter duration of fever and a lower prevalence of coronary artery aneurysms. No adverse reactions were recorded for any therapy. A prospective study suggested benefit as well: Inoue[202] reported that the frequency of coronary artery abnormalities in children treated with IVIG plus prednisolone at a dose of 2 mg/kg/d was lower than in those treated with IVIG alone. Three other studies[197,203,204] have shown that children treated with intravenous methylprednisolone (IVMP) (or dexamethasone) plus IVIG had a faster resolution of fever, more rapid improvement in the markers of inflammation, and a shorter length of hospitalization than those who received IVIG alone. Two of these studies had insufficient statistical power to detect a potential benefit of glucocorticoid therapy on coronary artery outcomes. The third trial, by Newburger and colleagues, found no significant difference in the frequency or severity of coronary artery lesions between treatment groups at the 1- or 5-week follow-up. Interestingly, however, post hoc analysis suggested that children who ultimately failed to respond to an initial dose of IVIG were less likely to develop coronary artery aneurysms if their initial therapy had included IVMP.

Following up on this finding, the Osaka Kawasaki Disease Study Group[205] conducted a comparative trial of IVIG versus IVIG + IVMP in children with KD who were regarded as being at high risk to be nonresponse to IVIG.[193] Patients were given heparin (10 U/kg/hour) for 48 hours beginning 2 hours before receiving IVMP (30 mg/kg), followed by IVIG (2 g/kg). Aspirin (30 mg/kg/d) was started at the end of the heparin infusion and reduced to 10 mg/kg/day after resolution of fever. Therapy was effective in 44% of those given IVIG alone

compared with 66% of those receiving both IVIG and IVMP. Coronary artery abnormalities, including aneurysms, were significantly less frequent in the IVIG + IVMP group (24%) compared with the IVIG-alone group (46%).

In a meta-analysis of eight studies, Wooditch and Aronson concluded that the incidence of coronary artery aneurysms was reduced by the addition of corticosteroids to therapeutic regimens that included aspirin.[198] However, a subsequent meta-analysis of four studies that evaluated primary treatment of KD with corticosteroids found that IVIG resistance was less common in those treated with steroids as primary therapy (OR 0.48, 95% CI 0.24-0.95), but coronary outcomes did not differ.[206]

The most definitive trial to date regarding corticosteroids in combined primary therapy with IVIG was the RAISE trial by Kobayashi et al. in 2012.[207] There were 248 patients were enrolled in this multicenter, prospective, randomized, open label, blinded end points trial. All patients enrolled had a Kobayashi score or 5 or greater,[191] and therefore were considered to be at high risk for IVIG resistance. Of note, patients on day 9 or later of illness were excluded, as were patients with coronary artery abnormalities on baseline echocardiogram. Patients were randomized to standard therapy with IVIG and ASA versus IVIG plus prednisolone at a dose of 2 mg/kg/day. The corticosteroid was initially given intravenously for 5 days, which was changed to oral dosing if the patient's fever abated, and then tapered following normalization of the CRP. The primary end point of the trial was defined as coronary artery abnormalities per JPH criteria seen on two-dimensional (2D) echocardiography in the steroid versus IVIG alone groups at weeks 1, 2, or 4. A significant difference in coronary artery abnormalities between the groups at the interim analysis, favoring administration of steroids with IVIG (3% [n = 4] vs. 23% [n = 28], $P < 0.0001$), led to early termination of the study. Secondary end points included incidence of coronary artery abnormalities at week 4, z scores of coronary arteries, incidence of need for rescue therapy, duration of fever after enrollment, and serum CRP concentrations at weeks 1 and 2. All secondary end points were also met, a remarkable achievement. Of note, although the overall incidence of coronary artery abnormalities in the IVIG group was high at 23% during the study period, as would be expected in this group of high-risk patients, the maximum z scores were relatively low, between 2.26 and 2.32.[207]

Challenges in determining the optimal use of corticosteroid treatment in KD remain. An accurate, easily applicable risk score has not been constructed to effectively stratify children with KD in North America and Europe who are at increased risk of developing coronary artery abnormalities. Furthermore, it remains unclear whether corticosteroids are best used as intensification of primary therapy for all KD patients at a time when the vascular walls of the arteries may be particularly vulnerable, or as rescue therapy for children who fail conventional therapy and are at higher risk for coronary artery abnormalities.

Anti-TNF Agents

Levels of TNF-α are markedly increased in children with KD, especially in those who develop coronary artery lesions.[208,209] As such, infliximab, a monoclonal antibody to TNF-α, has been the subject of trials in children with KD, both as rescue therapy as well as primary therapy.

A prospective randomized multicenter comparison of the effectiveness of IVIG (2 g/kg) and infliximab (5 mg/kg) in children who had not responded to an initial infusion of IVIG[210] showed that both agents were equally safe and well tolerated. Hirono and colleagues[211] also found that infliximab was effective in controlling fever but did not completely prevent coronary artery changes, although single case reports document resolution of aneurysms following infliximab therapy in some patients.[212,213] A retrospective two-center comparison of KD patients resistant to initial therapy with IVIG who were treated with either methylprednisolone (30 mg/kg) or infliximab (5 mg/kg) found that infliximab-treated patients had less fever and fewer days in the hospital, but there were no differences in coronary artery outcomes between the treatment groups.[214]

Recently, Tremoulet et al. explored the utility of administering infliximab (5 mg/kg) as primary therapy with IVIG.[215] There were 196 patients enrolled in a phase 3, randomized, double-blind, placebo-controlled trial at two centers. The primary end point of a difference in IVIG resistance between patients receiving combined therapy with IVIG and infliximab, and those receiving IVIG alone, was not met (11.2% vs. 11.3%, $P = 0.81$). Patients treated with infliximab had fewer days of fever and reduced inflammatory markers. The z score of the left anterior descending artery was significantly decreased in the infliximab group as compared with the placebo group at week 2 ($P = 0.45$). However, coronary outcomes at week 5 did not differ between treatment groups. There were no serious adverse events attributed to infliximab during the trial. At this time, the use of infliximab in the treatment of patients with KD remains essentially center-dependent, though convincing evidence of a beneficial effect on coronary artery outcomes is lacking.

Other Therapeutic Approaches

Therapies that are effective in other forms of vasculitis have been used in KD. Pentoxifylline was alleged to be effective in preventing coronary artery aneurysms,[216] but demonstration of flaws in the analysis of the data in this study[217] led to the conclusion that it is ineffective. Similarly, the human trypsin inhibitor, Ulinastatin, has been the subject of studies from Japan. Its efficacy in preventing coronary artery disease in KD is not convincing.[218]

The recent data regarding the potential role of T cells in KD[59,72] have led researchers to prescribe cyclosporine, a potent suppressor of T-cell activity through the nuclear factor of activated T-cells (NFAT) pathway. Suzuki et al.[219] studied 28 patients treated with cyclosporine A (CyA, 4 to 8 mg/kg/day) for refractory KD, defined as persistent fever after two doses of IVIG. The fevers of 18 of 28 patients subsided within 3 days of starting CyA. Four patients developed aneurysms, one of which was a giant aneurysm. Hyperkalemia occurred in nine patients, but no serious adverse events were reported. Tremoulet et al. also evaluated the use of calcineurin inhibitors in IVIG-resistant KD.[220] All 10 patients had already received rescue therapy in the form of an additional dose of IVIG (10 patients), pulsed methylprednisolone (3 patients), and infliximab (4 patients). Following treatment with a calcineurin inhibitor, all 10 patients reported the subsidence of fever. Seven of the patients experienced rapid resolution of the fever within 24 hours of starting treatment. Four of the patients had developed coronary artery aneurysms prior to therapy with a calcineurin inhibitor; all improved thereafter.

The use of statins has been explored in patients with significant cardiovascular sequelae from KD, given their potential beneficial effects on vascular reactivity and remodeling as well as their antiinflammatory effects.[221,222] A very small study of 11 KD patients with coronary artery aneurysms treated with simvastatin for 3 months reported a significant reduction in the high-sensitivity (hs)-CRP level and improvement in flow-mediated dilation.[223] Niedra et al. evaluated the safety of atorvastatin by following 20 patients with coronary artery aneurysms for a median of 2.5 years while treated with atorvastatin (5 to 10 mg daily).[224] Almost half of the patients had at least one episode of hypocholesterolemia, and two required a lowered dose. Mild transaminitis occurred in seven of the patients; only one patient had increased creatine phosphokinase level. They concluded that use of atorvastatin was safe with close monitoring.[224]

The potential role for cyclophosphamide[225] in KD is extremely limited, but it may be useful in cases with persistent active disease that is unresponsive to conventional therapy. In fact, children with prolonged inflammation ascribed to KD may be similar to children with polyarteritis nodosa, in which longer-term immunosuppression with cyclophosphamide is standard therapy.[226] A dramatic response to plasmapheresis in refractory cases of KD also has been reported,[227] but the technical limitations and potential hazards of this therapy are considerable. It should be reserved for children with active inflammation who have failed all available medical interventions, including multiple doses of IVIG, intravenous methylprednisolone, and TNF inhibition. There have been conflicting reports of the efficacy of abciximab, a monoclonal antibody that inhibits platelet glycoprotein IIb/IIIa receptor. In one study,[228] there was an increased resolution of aneurysms in patients with KD who received abciximab compared with those who received conventional treatment. However, a second study[229] could not duplicate these findings.

TREATMENT OF RELAPSES

Fever returns within 48 hours of treatment with IVIG in 10% to 20% of children, indicating failure to suppress the underlying inflammatory process. Because prolonged fever is an independent risk factor for the development of coronary artery aneurysms, current treatment protocols generally recommend retreatment with a second dose of IVIG (2 g/kg).[6] Those who fail to respond to a second dose—up to one third of patients in some studies[230]—are at extremely high risk of developing coronary artery aneurysms.[199] As noted above, use of corticosteroids appears to have the most convincing evidence of benefit in children resistant to IVIG, although definitive evidence for preference of one regimen over another is lacking. Therapeutic strategies include intravenous methylprednisolone (30 mg/kg/day for 1 to 3 days)[188] prednisolone at 2 mg/kg/day,[200] or infliximab (5 mg/kg).[231] Regardless of which approach is selected, treatment should continue until fever resolves and the CRP is normal. Frequent monitoring of the coronary arteries should be pursued until children have fully recovered.

PREVENTION AND MANAGEMENT OF THROMBOSES

The risk of thrombosis of coronary or other arteries depends on the degree of vascular damage. In all patients with KD, irrespective of the demonstration of coronary artery abnormalities, low-dose (3 to 5 mg/kg/day) aspirin should be continued until the ESR and platelet counts have normalized. Children with coronary artery abnormalities demonstrated by echocardiography are often treated with antithrombotic agents, such as low-dose aspirin, for as long as the abnormalities persist (Table 35-2). Children with large aneurysms are given warfarin or low-molecular-weight heparin to induce anticoagulation.

When injured coronary arteries become obstructed (risk level V), in addition to anticoagulation, various therapies have been attempted to restore circulation. Should the obstruction occur within 6 weeks of the onset of illness, control of vascular inflammation with IVIG and other agents is an essential prerequisite to arterial reperfusion. Thereafter, treatments may include thrombolytic therapy for arterial thrombosis or vasodilators if tissue viability is primarily threatened by vasospasm. Urokinase, streptokinase, and tissue-type plasminogen have all been used for the lysis of coronary artery thromboses. Similarly, peripheral arterial obstruction may be corrected by thrombolysis,

TABLE 35-2   Recommendations for Long-Term Follow-Up

RISK LEVEL	PHARMACOLOGICAL THERAPY	PHYSICAL ACTIVITY	FOLLOW-UP AND DIAGNOSTIC TESTING	INVASIVE TESTING
I (no coronary artery changes at any stage of illness)	None beyond first 6-8 weeks	No restrictions beyond first 6-8 weeks	Cardiovascular risk assessment counseling at 5-year intervals	None recommended
II (transient coronary artery ectasia disappears within first 6-8 weeks)	None beyond first 6-8 weeks	No restrictions beyond first 6-8 weeks	Cardiovascular risk assessment counseling at 3- to 5-year intervals	None recommended
III (1 small to medium coronary artery aneurysm/major coronary artery)	Low-dose aspirin (3-5 mg/kg aspirin/day), at least until aneurysm regression documented	For patients <11 years old, no restriction beyond first 6-8 weeks; patients 11-20 years old, physical activity guided by biennial stress test, evaluation of myocardial perfusion scan; contact or high-impact sports discouraged for patients taking antiplatelet agents	Annual cardiology follow-up with echocardiogram + electrocardiogram, combined with cardiovascular risk assessment, counseling; biennial stress test/ evaluation of myocardial perfusion scan	Angiography, if noninvasive test suggests ischemia
IV (≥1 large or giant coronary artery aneurysm, or multiple or complex aneurysms in same coronary artery, without obstruction)	Long-term antiplatelet therapy and warfarin (target international normalized ratio 2.0-2.5) or low-molecular-weight heparin (target: antifactor Xa level 0.5-1.0 U/mL) should be combined in giant aneurysms	Contact or high-impact sports should be avoided because of risk of bleeding; other physical activity recommendations guided by stress test/evaluation of myocardial perfusion scan outcome	Biannual follow-up with echocardiogram + electrocardiogram; annual stress test/evaluation of myocardial perfusion scan	First angiography at 6-12 months or sooner if clinically indicated; repeated angiography if noninvasive test, clinical, or laboratory findings suggest ischemia; elective repeat angiography under some circumstances
V (coronary artery obstruction)	Long-term low-dose aspirin; warfarin or low-molecular-weight heparin if giant aneurysm persists; consider use of β-blockers to reduce myocardial O$_2$ consumption	Contact or high-impact sports should be avoided because of risk of bleeding; other physical activity recommendations guided by stress test/myocardial perfusion scan outcome	Biannual follow-up with echocardiogram and electrocardiogram; annual stress test/evaluation of myocardial perfusion scan	Angiography recommended to address therapeutic options

From Newburger, Takahashi, Gerber, et al., Diagnosis, treatment and long-term management of Kawasaki disease: a statement for health professionals from the committee on rheumatic fever, endocarditis and Kawasaki disease. Council on Cardiovascular Disease in the Young: American Heart Association, Pediatrics 114 (2004) 1708–1733.

after which perfusion is maintained with heparin followed by a chronic oral anticoagulant regimen. If these treatments fail, a variety of invasive approaches have been suggested, including percutaneous transluminal coronary angioplasty[232] and coronary artery bypass grafting.[233] A small number of children with particularly severe coronary artery disease due to KD have required cardiac transplantation.[234]

MONITORING CARDIAC STATUS

There is no universal agreement about the timing and frequency of echocardiographic monitoring of patients with KD. Most protocols take into account the development of coronary artery aneurysms, which occur most frequently between the second and the eighth weeks after the onset of fever. It is recommended that the initial echocardiogram be obtained at the time a diagnosis of KD is suspected, and that each child with KD have a repeat echocardiography at 2 weeks and 6 weeks following illness.[235] Patients should also have repeated clinical examinations during the first 2 months to detect dysrhythmias, congestive heart failure, valvular insufficiency, or myocarditis.[236] Further

follow-up is individualized, with more frequent studies performed in children with demonstrated coronary artery abnormalities (see Table 35-2).

Children whose coronary arteries have always been normal (risk level I) or are normal by echocardiographic criteria 1 to 2 months after the acute illness (risk level II) are regarded as healthy, and no further intervention is recommended after the 8-week follow-up assessment. In view of possible chronic abnormalities in endothelial function, however, many physicians consider a history of KD to be a risk factor for the development of coronary artery disease later in life.[237] They counsel modification of other atherosclerotic risk factors and continue to monitor children once every 5 years.

Single small- to medium-sized aneurysms (risk level III) usually resolve as determined by echocardiographic criteria, although this is not always the case. Healing occurs by fibrointimal proliferation, often accompanied by calcification, and vascular reactivity does not return to normal despite a grossly normal appearance.[238] This point is highlighted by a report of the sudden death of a 3½-year-old child 3 months after the child's dilated coronary arteries had regained a normal echocardiographic appearance.[239] Autopsy revealed obliteration of the lumen of the left anterior descending coronary artery due to fibrosis, with evidence of ongoing active inflammation in the epicardial arteries. Such reports emphasize the need for confirmation of complete response to therapy in children who have had KD.

Giant aneurysms with an internal diameter of at least 8 mm represent a significant risk for morbidity and mortality, including a 35% chance of infarction (risk level IV).[168] These children are followed more closely and are treated with more aggressive antithrombotic and anticoagulation regimens.

DISEASE COURSE AND PROGNOSIS

Although standard therapy with IVIG and aspirin given within the first 10 days of illness greatly improves outcomes, approximately 5% of children still develop coronary artery aneurysms, and more children demonstrate coronary artery ectasia.[7]

The mortality rate has dropped steadily as the diagnosis and treatment have improved. Currently, the rate is about 0.1% in the United States and Japan.[239,240] Recurrent disease after full recovery from a first episode of KD is rare, but it does occur. In Japan, the recurrence rate is 3.6%,[31] with a higher incidence of cardiac complications during the second episode.[241] In the United States, the rate of recurrence is lower.

There have been two recent studies from Japan of long-term outcomes in KD cases complicated by giant coronary artery aneurysms. Suda et al. reviewed the case records of 76 patients with giant coronary artery aneurysms and found that the 30-year survival rate was 88%. However, there was a nearly 60% cumulative coronary intervention rate at 25 years from onset, indicating that these patients carry significant morbidity in terms of multiple procedures.[242] Tsuda reported similar survival rates in patients with giant coronary artery aneurysms followed for up to 3 decades, and noted that the long-term outcomes were worse for those patients with involvement of both the right coronary and the left coronary arteries.[243]

As mentioned previously, whether children with normal coronary artery dimensions throughout their illness are at higher risk for atherosclerotic disease later in life remains an area of ongoing research. Studies to date have been conflicting.[244-248] However, when standardized mortality ratios were calculated in 2009 for individuals in Japan who were diagnosed with KD during the years 1982–1992 and who had no cardiac sequelae, the mortality ratios of the KD patients showed no increases as compared to the general population.[249] Definitive data regarding long-term outcomes in KD patients who always have normal coronary arteries will likely be established as the KD cohorts in Japan reach middle age.

REFERENCES

1. T. Kawasaki, Acute febrile mucocutaneous syndrome with lymphoid involvement with specific desquamation of the fingers and toes in children, Arerugi 16 (1967) 178–222, [Article in Japanese].
7. J.W. Newburger, M. Takahashi, M.A. Gerber, et al., Diagnosis, treatment, and long-term management of Kawasaki disease: a statement for health professionals from the Committee on Rheumatic Fever, Endocarditis, and Kawasaki Disease, Council on Cardiovascular Disease in the Young, American Heart Association, Pediatrics 114 (2004) 1708–1733.
8. S. Ozen, N. Ruperto, M.J. Dillon, et al., EULAR/PReS endorsed consensus criteria for the classification of childhood vasculitides, Ann. Rheum. Dis. 65 (2006) 936–941.
11. J.C. Burns, W.H. Mason, M.P. Glode, et al., Clinical and epidemiologic characteristics of patients referred for evaluation of possible Kawasaki disease. United States Multicenter Kawasaki Disease Study Group, J. Pediatr. 118 (1991) 680–686.
12. S.M. Benseler, B.W. McCrindle, E.D. Silverman, et al., Infections and Kawasaki disease: implications for coronary artery outcome, Pediatrics 116 (2005) e760–e766.
17. E.A. Rosenfeld, K.E. Corydon, S.T. Shulman, Kawasaki disease in infants less than one year of age, J. Pediatr. 126 (1995) 524–529.
18. J.W. Newburger, M. Takahashi, J.C. Burns, et al., The treatment of Kawasaki syndrome with intravenous gamma globulin, N. Engl. J. Med. 315 (1986) 341–347.
23. R.C. Holman, E.D. Belay, K.Y. Christensen, et al., Hospitalizations for Kawasaki syndrome among children in the United States, 1997-2007, Pediatr. Infect. Dis. J. 29 (2010) 483–488.
42. A.H. Rowley, S.T. Shulman, B.T. Spike, et al., Oligoclonal IgA response in the vascular wall in acute Kawasaki disease, J Immunol. 166 (2001) 1334–1343.
55. P.A. Brogan, V. Shah, L.A. Clarke, et al., T cell activation profiles in Kawasaki syndrome, Clin. Exp. Immunol. 151 (2008) 267–274.
56. P.A. Brogan, V. Shah, N. Klein, M.J. Dillon, Vbeta-restricted T cell adherence to endothelial cells: a mechanism for superantigen-dependent vascular injury, Arthritis Rheum. 50 (2004) 589–597.
59. R.S. Yeung, Kawasaki disease: update on pathogenesis, Curr. Opin. Rheumatol. 22 (2010) 551–560.
69. D.J. Schulte, A. Yilmaz, K. Shimada, et al., Involvement of innate and adaptive immunity in a murine model of coronary arteritis mimicking Kawasaki disease, J Immunol. 183 (2009) 5311–5318.
71. Y.C. Lee, H.C. Kuo, J.S. Chang, et al., Two new susceptibility loci for Kawasaki disease identified through genome-wide association analysis, Nat. Genet. 44 (2012) 522–525.
72. Y. Onouchi, T. Gunji, J.C. Burns, et al., ITPKC functional polymorphism associated with Kawasaki disease susceptibility and formation of coronary artery aneurysms, Nat. Genet. 40 (2008) 35–42.
81. Y. Onouchi, K. Ozaki, J.C. Burns, et al., A genome-wide association study identifies three new risk loci for Kawasaki disease, Nat. Genet. 44 (2012) 517–521.
89. D. Burgner, S. Davila, W.B. Breunis, et al., A genome-wide association study identifies novel and functionally related susceptibility Loci for Kawasaki disease, PLoS Genet. 5 (2009) e1000319.
95. A.L. Baker, M. Lu, L.L. Minich, et al., Associated symptoms in the ten days before diagnosis of Kawasaki disease, J. Pediatr. 154 (2009) 592–595 e592.
108. C. Manlhiot, E. Christie, B.W. McCrindle, et al., Complete and incomplete Kawasaki disease: two sides of the same coin, Eur. J. Pediatr. 171 (2012) 657–662.
109. T. Sonobe, N. Kiyosawa, K. Tsuchiya, et al., Prevalence of coronary artery abnormality in incomplete Kawasaki disease, Pediatr Int. 49 (2007) 421–426.
112. E.S. Yellen, K. Gauvreau, M. Takahashi, et al., Performance of 2004 American Heart Association recommendations for treatment of Kawasaki disease, Pediatrics 125 (2010) e234–e241.
117. A.M. Moran, J.W. Newburger, S.P. Sanders, et al., Abnormal myocardial mechanics in Kawasaki disease: rapid response to gamma-globulin, Am. Heart J. 139 (2000) 217–223.
118. C.E. Tacke, S. Romeih, I.M. Kuipers, et al., Evaluation of cardiac function by magnetic resonance imaging during the follow-up of patients with Kawasaki disease, Circ Cardiovasc Imaging. 6 (2013) 67–73.
119. J.T. Kanegaye, M.S. Wilder, D. Molkara, et al., Recognition of a Kawasaki disease shock syndrome, Pediatrics 123 (2009) e783–e789.
121. J.C. Muniz, K. Dummer, K. Gauvreau, et al., Coronary artery dimensions in febrile children without Kawasaki disease, Circ Cardiovasc Imaging. 6 (2013) 239–244.
124. Report of the Subcommittee on Standardization of Diagnostic Criteria and Reporting of Coronary Artery Lesions in Kawasaki Disease. Tokyo, Japan: Research Committee on Kawasaki Disease, Ministry of Health and Welfare, 1984.
126. A. de Zorzi, S.D. Colan, K. Gauvreau, et al., Coronary artery dimensions may be misclassified as normal in Kawasaki disease, J. Pediatr. 133 (1998) 254–258.

128. H. Kato, E. Ichinose, T. Kawasaki, Myocardial infarction in Kawasaki disease: clinical analyzes in 195 cases, J. Pediatr. 108 (1986) 923–927.

142. H. Shike, J.T. Kanegaye, B.M. Best, et al., Pyuria associated with acute Kawasaki disease and fever from other causes, Pediatr. Infect. Dis. J. 28 (2009) 440–443.

155. J.M. Orenstein, S.T. Shulman, L.M. Fox, et al., Three linked vasculopathic processes characterize Kawasaki disease: a light and transmission electron microscopic study, PLoS ONE 7 (2012) e38998.

159. J.W. Newburger, J.C. Burns, A.S. Beiser, J. Loscalzo, Altered lipid profile after Kawasaki syndrome, Circulation 84 (1991) 625–631.

160. C.Y. Ou, Y.F. Tseng, C.L. Lee, et al., Significant relationship between serum high-sensitivity C-reactive protein, high-density lipoprotein cholesterol levels and children with Kawasaki disease and coronary artery lesions, J. Formos. Med. Assoc. 108 (2009) 719–724.

167. M. Iemura, M. Ishii, T. Sugimura, et al., Long term consequences of regressed coronary aneurysms after Kawasaki disease: vascular wall morphology and function, Heart 83 (2000) 307–311.

168. H. Kato, T. Sugimura, T. Akagi, et al., Long-term consequences of Kawasaki disease. A 10- to 21-year follow-up study of 594 patients, Circulation 94 (1996) 1379–1385.

173. G. Lee, S.E. Lee, Y.M. Hong, S. Sohn, Is high-dose aspirin necessary in the acute phase of kawasaki disease? Korean Circ J. 43 (2013) 182–186.

174. K.S. Hsieh, K.P. Weng, C.C. Lin, et al., Treatment of acute Kawasaki disease: aspirin's role in the febrile stage revisited, Pediatrics 114 (2004) e689–e693.

178. K. Furusho, T. Kamiya, H. Nakano, et al., High-dose intravenous gammaglobulin for Kawasaki disease, Lancet 2 (1984) 1055–1058.

179. J.W. Newburger, M. Takahashi, A.S. Beiser, et al., A single intravenous infusion of gamma globulin as compared with four infusions in the treatment of acute Kawasaki syndrome, N. Engl. J. Med. 324 (1991) 1633–1639.

185. R. Berard, B. Whittemore, R. Scuccimarri, Hemolytic anemia following intravenous immunoglobulin therapy in patients treated for Kawasaki disease: a report of 4 cases, Pediatr Rheumatol Online J. 10 (2012) 10.

189. S.M. Tse, E.D. Silverman, B.W. McCrindle, R.S. Yeung, Early treatment with intravenous immunoglobulin in patients with Kawasaki disease, J. Pediatr. 140 (2002) 450–455.

191. T. Kobayashi, Y. Inoue, K. Takeuchi, et al., Prediction of intravenous immunoglobulin unresponsiveness in patients with Kawasaki disease, Circulation 113 (2006) 2606–2612.

194. L.A. Sleeper, L.L. Minich, B.M. McCrindle, et al., Evaluation of Kawasaki disease risk-scoring systems for intravenous immunoglobulin resistance, J. Pediatr. 158 (2011) 831–835 e833.

195. M. Mori, T. Imagawa, K. Yasui, et al., Predictors of coronary artery lesions after intravenous gamma-globulin treatment in Kawasaki disease, J. Pediatr. 137 (2000) 177–180.

197. R.P. Sundel, A.L. Baker, D.R. Fulton, J.W. Newburger, Corticosteroids in the initial treatment of Kawasaki disease: report of a randomized trial, J. Pediatr. 142 (2003) 611–616.

198. A.C. Wooditch, S.C. Aronoff, Effect of initial corticosteroid therapy on coronary artery aneurysm formation in Kawasaki disease: a meta-analysis of 862 children, Pediatrics 116 (2005) 989–995.

200. T. Kobayashi, T. Kobayashi, A. Morikawa, et al., Efficacy of intravenous immunoglobulin combined with prednisolone following resistance to initial intravenous immunoglobulin treatment of acute Kawasaki disease, J. Pediatr. 163 (2013) 521–526.

202. Y. Inoue, Y. Okada, M. Shinohara, et al., A multicenter prospective randomized trial of corticosteroids in primary therapy for Kawasaki disease: clinical course and coronary artery outcome, J. Pediatr. 149 (2006) 336–341.

204. J.W. Newburger, L.A. Sleeper, B.W. McCrindle, et al., Randomized trial of pulsed corticosteroid therapy for primary treatment of Kawasaki disease, N. Engl. J. Med. 356 (2007) 663–675.

206. G. Athappan, S. Gale, T. Ponniah, Corticosteroid therapy for primary treatment of Kawasaki disease—weight of evidence: a meta-analysis and systematic review of the literature, Cardiovasc J Afr. 20 (2009) 233–236.

207. T. Kobayashi, T. Saji, T. Otani, et al., Efficacy of immunoglobulin plus prednisolone for prevention of coronary artery abnormalities in severe Kawasaki disease (RAISE study): a randomised, open-label, blinded-endpoints trial, Lancet 379 (2012) 1613–1620.

210. J.C. Burns, B.M. Best, A. Mejias, et al., Infliximab treatment of intravenous immunoglobulin-resistant Kawasaki disease, J. Pediatr. 153 (2008) 833–838.

212. R.J. Brogan, D. Eleftheriou, J. Gnanapragasam, et al., Infliximab for the treatment of intravenous immunoglobulin resistant Kawasaki disease complicated by coronary artery aneurysms: a case report, Pediatr Rheumatol Online J. 7 (2009) 3.

215. A.H. Tremoulet, S. Jain, P. Jaggi, et al., Infliximab for intensification of primary therapy for Kawasaki disease: a phase 3 randomised, double-blind, placebo-controlled trial, Lancet 383 (2014) 1731–1738.

217. M.C. Nash, A.M. Wade, No evidence for use of pentoxifylline in acute Kawasaki disease, Eur. J. Pediatr. 155 (1996) 258.

218. S. Iwashima, M. Seguchi, T. Matubayashi, T. Ohzeki, Ulinastatin therapy in Kawasaki disease, Clin. Drug Investig. 27 (2007) 691–696.

220. A.H. Tremoulet, P. Pancoast, A. Franco, et al., Calcineurin inhibitor treatment of intravenous immunoglobulin-resistant Kawasaki disease, J. Pediatr. 161 (2012) 506–512 e501.

223. S.M. Huang, K.P. Weng, J.S. Chang, et al., Effects of statin therapy in children complicated with coronary arterial abnormality late after Kawasaki disease: a pilot study, Circ. J. 72 (2008) 1583–1587.

225. C.A. Wallace, J.W. French, S.J. Kahn, D.D. Sherry, Initial intravenous gammaglobulin treatment failure in Kawasaki disease, Pediatrics 105 (2000) E78.

231. J.C. Burns, W.H. Mason, S.B. Hauger, et al., Infliximab treatment for refractory Kawasaki syndrome, J. Pediatr. 146 (2005) 662–667.

235. J.W. Newburger, M. Takahashi, M.A. Gerber, et al., Diagnosis, treatment, and long-term management of Kawasaki disease: a statement for health professionals from the Committee on Rheumatic Fever, Endocarditis and Kawasaki Disease, Council on Cardiovascular Disease in the Young, American Heart Association, Circulation 110 (2004) 2747–2771.

236. D.R. Fulton, J.W. Newburger, Long-term cardiac sequelae of Kawasaki disease, Curr. Rheumatol. Rep. 2 (2000) 324–329.

Entire reference list is available online at www.expertconsult.com.

Antineutrophil Cytoplasmic Antibody Associated Vasculitis

David A. Cabral, Kimberly Morishita

Antineutrophil cytoplasmic antibody (ANCA)-associated vasculitis (AAV) is a group of vasculitides characterized by small- to medium-sized blood vessel inflammation, clinically overlapping features, and the presence of ANCA. This group of vasculitides includes granulomatosis with polyangiitis (GPA), formerly Wegener's granulomatosis; eosinophilic granulomatosis with polyangiitis (EPGA), formerly Churg–Strauss syndrome; and microscopic polyangiitis (MPA). These conditions are rare in childhood and adolescence. Consequently, most knowledge about them comes from small case series or has been adapted from studies of adults. However, early diagnosis and treatment are critical to minimize morbidity and improve outcomes.

ANTINEUTROPHIL CYTOPLASMIC ANTIBODIES

The relatively recent identification of autoantibodies of clinical and pathogenic significance has led to subclassification of small-vessel vasculitis under the rubric of AAV.[1] ANCAs are a heterogeneous group of autoantibodies that bind to antigens in the primary granules of neutrophils and the lysosomes of monocytes. ANCAs are detected by immunofluorescence microscopy in predominantly cytoplasmic (cANCA), perinuclear (pANCA), or indeterminate or atypical patterns (Fig. 36-1).[2] The target antigen of cANCA is PR3, a serine protease that is physiologically inhibited by α1-antitrypsin. The predominant target antigen of pANCA is myeloperoxidase (MPO), which is naturally inhibited by ceruloplasmin, but other targets include elastase, cathepsin G, lactoferrin, lysozyme, and beta-glucuronidase.[3] Antibodies to targets PR3 and MPO, respectively called PR3-ANCA or MPO-ANCA, are found in AAV, so-called renal limited vasculitis, and in certain drug-induced vasculitis syndromes.[4-6] The presence of either has been used in classification algorithms to distinguish GPA and MPA from polyarteritis nodosa (PAN),[7] but the different specificities of ANCA do not clearly differentiate among AAV. PR3-ANCA (cANCA) is highly sensitive for GPA,[8] although it should be noted that nearly 50% of patients with localized disease are ANCA negative.[9] It is also found in up to 30% of patients with MPA and perhaps less than 5% of patients with EGPA. ANCA, almost invariably MPO-ANCA, is found in up to 70% of patients with MPA[10] but may also be found in about 10% of patients with GPA.[11,12] ANCA, predominantly MPO-ANCA, is found in up to 40% of patients with EGPA.[13-15]

Recent genome-wide studies suggest that GPA and MPA are genetically distinct subsets of AAV.[17] However, the associations with identified single nucleotide polymorphisms (SNPs) were stronger with "PR3-ANCA versus MPO-ANCA" rather than the traditional "GPA versus MPA" phenotype. Recent clinical studies have also supported this notion in that ANCA serotype,[18] or ANCA serotype linked with specific organ involvement,[19] has been shown to be more relevant prognostically than traditional GPA or MPA phenotypes. Even if these findings are confirmed, classifying patients according to ANCA serotype alone would leave many small-vessel vasculitis ANCA-negative patients unclassifiable. The role of ANCA in the pathogenesis of AAV needs to account for ANCA-negative patients and the conflicting results of studies that associate active or relapsing GPA with rising ANCA titers.[20-22]

ANCAs may be naturally occurring nonpathogenic autoantibodies[23,24] that may become pathogenic because of defects in regulatory T cells,[25] or their induction may relate to molecular mimicry[26] or epigenetic modifications of target antigens.[27] Mechanistically, *in vitro* experiments demonstrate that ANCA-activated neutrophils can in themselves cause endothelial damage[28,29] but also cause a cascade of other detrimental inflammatory processes.[30] The most compelling argument for a direct pathogenic role for ANCA is in MPA. Animal studies have shown that immunization with MPO, or the passive transfer of anti-MPO antibodies in both mouse[31] and rat[32] models, result in the development of necrotizing and crescentic glomerulonephritis, granulomatous inflammation, and systemic necrotizing vasculitis. There are two case reports of transplacental transfer of MPO-ANCA from mother to newborn causing neonatal MPA[33,34]; however, in another report, an infant born to an affected mother remained healthy despite persistence of transferred MPO-ANCA for several weeks.[35] The overlapping clinical features of MPA with GPA and EGPA likely reflect the small-vessel vasculitis component of the diseases, whereas the differences reflect the presence of an additional granulomatous inflammatory process in GPA and eosinophilia and granulomatous inflammation in EGPA.[1,36] Herein is part of the difficulty in attempts to successfully develop a robust PR3-ANCA vasculitis animal model similar to the MPO-ANCA animal models.[37,38]

GRANULOMATOSIS WITH POLYANGIITIS

Granulomatosis with polyangiitis (GPA) is a chronic vasculitis involving small- to medium-sized arteries. It is characterized by granulomatous inflammation of the upper and lower respiratory tracts; necrotizing, pauci-immune glomerulonephritis; and vasculitis that frequently involves other organs. McBride first described the condition in 1897 as a midfacial granuloma syndrome,[39] but the complete picture was not described until the 1930s.[40,41] We now know that the disease can involve multiple organs and is life-threatening. GPA, previously known as Wegener's granulomatosis, was renamed in April 2011 with a reported consensus recommendation of the American College of Rheumatology (ACR), American Society of Nephrology, and the

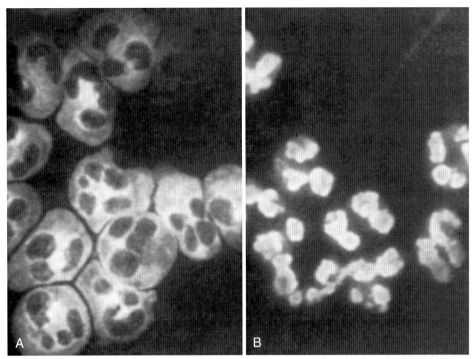

FIGURE 36-1 Indirect immunofluorescence microscopy staining patterns produced by antibodies directed at neutrophil cytoplasmic antigens (ANCAs) with a cytoplasmic staining pattern (cANCA) **(A)** and those with a perinuclear staining pattern (pANCA) **(B)** on alcohol-fixed neutrophils.[16]

European League against Rheumatism (EULAR).[42] Although GPA is most common in later life,[43-45] and rare in childhood, it may be one of the most common forms of vasculitis seen by pediatric rheumatologists.[46-48]

Classification

The ACR classification criteria for vasculitis[36] and GPA[49] and the subsequent Chapel Hill Consensus Conference (CHCC) disease definitions,[50] were derived primarily from adult data. Because of the poor performance of ACR criteria in classifying children with vasculitis, notably GPA,[51] a pediatric-specific adaptation of ACR criteria, the EULAR/PRINTO/PRES criteria, were developed using pediatric data (see Chapter 32). The EULAR/PRINTO/PRES criteria and the ACR criteria are compared in Table 36-1. The pediatric criteria for GPA had improved sensitivity compared to the adult-based ACR criteria (93% vs 83%),[52] but there are some limitations to their application. Neither pediatric nor adult systems have criteria for MPA, and in one report, pediatric patients classified as having GPA according to ACR criteria could be described as having MPA according to the CHCC definitions.[53] When both the ACR and pediatric-specific criteria were applied to a cohort of 155 pediatric patients with AAV and unclassified vasculitis, the sensitivities of the systems when applied to GPA patients were 62% and 77%, respectively.[54] These differences in sensitivities might be because this last study challenged the ability of the EULAR/PRINTO/PRES criteria to distinguish GPA from MPA, in comparison with the validation cohort where there were extremely few MPA patients among a much wider spectrum of vasculitides.

Epidemiology

Recent population studies suggest a stable incidence of 0.8 to 1.2 per 100,000 persons in some regions,[55-57] and a 23-year UK study demonstrates a cyclical pattern with peaks of incidence in 1996-1998 and 2005.[58] The rising incidence between the 1970s and 1990s, described

for some regions[45,59-61] in earlier studies, may only partly be explained by improved case recognition after the introduction of ANCA testing in the 1980s.[56,61] Regional differences of GPA have been described with higher incidences in both Norway and areas of the UK compared to Spain and Japan.[62,63] A study in New Zealand similarly describes a higher incidence in higher latitudes.[64]

Much less is known about the incidence of GPA in children and adolescents. American[43] and Norwegian[44] population studies from the 1980s and 1990s, respectively, estimated incidences of 0.6 and 0.8 per 100,000 persons per year. In these studies 3.3% and 7% of patients had disease onset before 20 years or 16 years of age, respectively, for calculated annual incidences of 0.02 and 0.06. A recent Canadian study demonstrated an increase in the incidence of childhood GPA from 0.28 to 0.64 per 100.000 per year in southern Alberta between 2003 and 2008.[65]

In the general population, the peak incidence of GPA is in the sixth decade,[44,45,66] and males outnumber females 1.6:1.[44] In the pediatric population, the disease occurs in the second decade of life, with a female preponderance.[51,53,67,68]

Pathogenesis

The cause of GPA is unknown, although it is likely a multifactorial disease.[30,69] As with many other polygenic systemic autoimmune diseases, GPA is probably the result of interactions between genetic factors predisposing to loss of self-tolerance and triggering environmental exposures.[70] Epidemiological studies describing Caucasian predisposition[53,71] suggest genetic factors play some role. However, the infrequent reported familial occurrences,[72-75] relatively late mean age at onset of GPA in the general population, and the variations in incidence related to season or latitude, for example, argue for the importance of environmental and nongenetic factors. The vast majority of genetic-association studies of AAV have been in relation to SNPs, and the variants most strongly and reproducibly associated with GPA have

TABLE 36-1   Comparison of the American College of Rheumatology and the Pediatric Specific European League Against Rheumatism/Pediatric Rheumatology International Trials Organisation/Pediatric Rheumatology European Society Criteria for Classification of Granulomatosis with Polyangiitis

ACR CRITERIA[51]		EULAR/PRINTO/PRES CRITERIA[52]	
A patient is said to have GPA when two of the following four criteria are present:		A patient is said to have GPA when three of the following six criteria are present:	
	Descriptors		*Descriptors*
1 **Nasal or oral inflammation**	*Painful or painless oral ulcers or purulent or bloody nasal discharge*	**Upper airway involvement**	*Chronic purulent or bloody nasal discharge, or recurrent epistaxis/crusts/granulomata*
			Nasal septal perforation or saddle-nose deformity
			Chronic or recurrent sinus inflammation
2 **Abnormal chest X-ray**	*Nodules, fixed infiltrates, or cavities*	**Pulmonary involvement**	*Chest X-ray or CT scan showing the presence of nodules, cavities, or fixed infiltrates*
3 **Abnormal urinalysis**	*Red blood cell casts or Microhematuria: >5 RBC/high-power field*	**Renal involvement**	*Proteinuria >0.3 g/24 hours or greater than 30 mmol/mg of urine albumin/creatinine ratio on a spot morning sample*
			Hematuria or red blood cell casts: >5 red blood cells per high-power field, or red blood cell casts in urinary sediment, or >2+ on dipstick
			Necrotizing pauci-immune glomerulonephritis
4 **Granulomatous inflammation**	*Granulomatous inflammation within wall of artery or in perivascular or extravascular area of artery or arteriole*	**Granulomatous inflammation**	*Granulomatous inflammation within wall of artery or in perivascular or extravascular area of artery or arteriole*
5		**Laryngo tracheo bronchial stenosis**	*Subglottic, tracheal, or bronchial stenosis*
6		**ANCA**	*ANCA positivity by immunofluorescence or by ELISA (MPO/p or PR3/c ANCA)*

ACR, American College of Rheumatology; *EULAR,* European League Against Rheumatism; *GPA,* Granulomatosis with polyangiitis; *PRINTO,* Pediatric Rheumatology International Trials Organisation; *PRES,* Pediatric Rheumatology European Society.

been found in human leukocyte antigen (HLA), protein tyrosine phosphatase nonreceptor type 22 (PTPN22), and cytotoxic T-lymphocyte antigen 4 (CTLA4) genes.[76-85]

Since GPA was first described[40,41] researchers have unsuccessfully looked for exogenous agents that might stimulate granuloma formation in the airway. An association between primary systemic vasculitis or GPA and crystalline silica exposure and farming has been shown by some[86-88] but not by others.[89] A role for an infectious trigger has been proposed by many and supported by a number of observations: increased rates of chronic nasal carriage of *Staphylococcus aureus* in patients with GPA compared with non-GPA patients[90]; reduced risk of relapse in GPA patients who are on antibacterial maintenance treatment against *S. aureus*[91]; high frequency of respiratory tract infections preceding or accompanying onset or flares of GPA[92,93]; and increased antibody levels against several other infectious agents in patients with GPA have been reported.[94] Several mechanisms linking infection to autoimmunity in AAV have been proposed.[69,95]

The presence of ANCAs implicates neutrophils as key effector cells in GPA. The predominant antigenic target of ANCA in GPA is PR3. Patients with GPA have an increased percentage of neutrophils expressing PR3 on their membranes as compared to healthy individuals,[96] and among patients with GPA increased membrane expression of

PR3 is associated with severity[97] and rate of relapse.[98] Success in studies of B-cell depletion therapy with rituximab argues for a pathogenic role of autoantibodies,[99-101] as well as the observation that activated B lymphocytes are increased in patients with GPA compared with healthy controls and are higher in patients with active disease than in those individuals in remission.[102] Although autoantibodies probably play some role in GPA pathogenesis, the characteristic presence of granulomas suggest a more complex process with a predominance of Th-1 cells in the cell-mediated hypersensitivity model of disease.[103,104] Arguably, inflammation of the upper airways by *S. aureus*, other pathogens, or environmental exposure induces cytokine production.[90,105,106] Elucidation of the intricate immune pathways and processes continues, and recently a role for Th-17 cells in the pathogenesis of GPA[107] and other autoimmune disease has also been proposed.[108,109]

Clinical Manifestations

The triad of upper and lower respiratory tract inflammation and renal disease is characteristic of childhood GPA as described in the five largest pediatric series.[51,53,67,68,110,111] The largest cohort describes 130 patients[111] collected within A Registry for Children with Vasculitis: e-entry (ARChiVe) and includes patients accumulated since the earlier report of 65 patients.[53] The median age at diagnosis was 14.9 years (range 4 to 19) and the median interval from symptom onset to diagnosis was 4.8 months (range 0 to 67). At disease onset, the most common features were constitutional symptoms including fatigue, weight loss, and fever, then followed by pulmonary (81%); renal (79%); and ear, nose, and throat (ENT) (75%) manifestations. Less frequently involved were the musculoskeletal system (64%), skin (55%), gastrointestinal tract (39%), nervous system (27%), and eyes (30%). The frequencies of other clinical features according to organ system as described in the two most recent large pediatric series are listed in Table 36-2. Features of MPA patients in the largest cohort are listed for comparison. In contrast to the adult experience[71,112] and two smaller pediatric series,[113,114] so-called limited or localized GPA defined by the absence of kidney disease occurred in a minority of children at the time of diagnosis[67,68,110,111] and was even less frequent in follow-up, as the frequency of renal disease may accumulate with time.[68] The spectrum of pulmonary manifestations in the ARChiVe cohort included chronic cough (61%), shortness of breath (49%), and hemoptysis or alveolar hemorrhage (42%). Pulmonary function tests were abnormal in 61% of the 67 patients tested. Upper respiratory tract signs and symptoms at presentation were as common as lower respiratory tract features and in follow-up were reported in 91% and 96% of patients, respectively.[67,68] One study reported that subglottic stenosis was five times as common in pediatric-onset GPA compared with adults, and this feature was subsequently included in the EULAR/PRES classification criteria.[68] In the ARChiVe cohort, subglottic stenosis was no more frequent than otitis/mastoiditis or hearing loss, and less frequent than nasal and sinus involvement. Its inclusion as a classification criterion reflected its specificity. In a cohort of 28 patients from the Cleveland Clinic, a quaternary referral center for vasculitis, airway stenosis with careful screening at diagnosis occurred in 36% of children, increasing to 50% at follow-up; among the 14 patients with airway stenosis, the tracheobronchial tree was involved in 5.[110] Damage to the nasal cartilage, characteristic of long-standing disease, may result in a saddle-nose deformity, similar to that seen in relapsing polychondritis (Fig. 36-2). Renal involvement as manifested by significantly elevated serum creatinine was found in 36% of the patients in the ARChiVe cohort and 28% of patients in the Toronto cohort[67,111]; renal dialysis was necessary in 13% of the ARChiVe cohort and 20% in the Toronto cohort.

Diagnosis

The diagnosis of GPA is based on a combination of clinical features (e.g., pulmonary-renal vasculitis syndrome), the presence of serological markers (specifically ANCA, and most commonly PR3-ANCA or cANCA), and characteristic histopathological findings (pauci-immune granulomatous inflammation of predominantly small to medium arteries, capillaries or small veins, or pauci-immune glomerulonephritis). If GPA is suspected, it is crucial to take a careful and specific history of upper respiratory tract involvement and consider formal otolaryngological assessment.[110] Because one third of adult patients initially have asymptomatic renal and pulmonary involvement, it is crucial to examine fresh-spun urinary sediment, and look for pulmonary changes both radiographically and with pulmonary function testing.[71] A decrease in the diffusion capacity of carbon monoxide (DL$_{CO}$) may be the earliest sign of pulmonary hemorrhage. If the disease is limited to a single organ system, tissue diagnosis is desirable to confirm the diagnosis and exclude other diseases. The differential diagnoses include infections (notably mycobacteria, fungi, or helminths, which may also be associated with granulomatous vasculitis),[115,116] neoplastic disease,[117] sarcoidosis[118] and in young children, chronic granulomatous disease. Pulmonary manifestations in

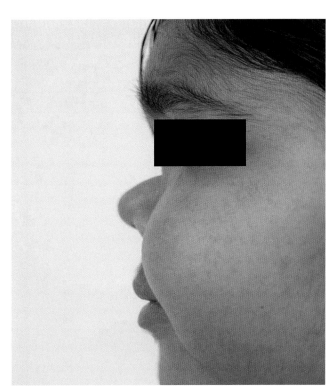

FIGURE 36-2 Saddle-nose deformity in a girl with erosive sinusitis and granulomatosis with polyangiitis.

ANCA-positive ulcerative colitis patients have also mimicked GPA.[119] Other forms of vasculitis that can manifest as pulmonary-renal syndromes, such as antiglomerular basement membrane (anti-GBM) disease, systemic lupus erythematosus, mixed connective tissue disease, or PAN, should also be considered. Guided kidney biopsy is now a relatively safe procedure with a high yield, and the finding of pauci-immune glomerulonephritis together with characteristic serology provides a relatively secure diagnosis. GPA can be more readily distinguished from MPA by the presence of upper airway disease including saddle-nose deformity, nasal septal perforation, subglottic stenosis, dacryocystitis, proptosis associated with periorbital tumor, characteristic lung nodules (distinguished from hemorrhage), or the presence of granuloma in biopsy specimens. Characteristic histological features may be patchy in the lungs, and the yield from biopsies may be low especially with fine needle aspirations, but are better with transbronchial or open lung procedures.[120,121] Frequent involvement of the upper respiratory tract in patients with GPA (e.g., trachea, ears, nose, sinuses, and eyes) may offer sites for relatively noninvasive biopsy procedures; however, the yield from such sites is disappointingly low.[122] When the disease is isolated to these sites, a definitive diagnosis may be difficult, and the diagnostician may need to rely on nonspecific or incomplete histopathological confirmation, serological findings, and the combined expertise of multiple disciplines including the otorhinolaryngologist, ophthalmologist, pathologist, radiologist, and rheumatologist. The need for tissue diagnosis in such cases may be influenced by disease severity, the need to embark upon toxic chemotherapy, and the need to exclude other diseases.

Laboratory Examination

White blood cell counts may be elevated particularly in generalized disease, and associated with normochromic normocytic anemia, thrombocytosis, and markedly elevated erythrocyte sedimentation

TABLE 36-2 Presenting Manifestations (Reported as Percentages) in Children with Granulomatosis with Polyangiitis and Microscopic Polyangiitis from the US/Canadian Multicenter ARChiVe Cohort (n = 152) and from the Toronto Hospital for Sick Children (n = 25) with 33 Months Median Follow-up Data for HSC Cohort

| | ARCHIVE[b] (N = 152)[111] | | HSC[a] (N = 25)[67] | |
| | ONSET | ONSET | ONSET | ANY TIME |
CLINICAL FEATURE	GPA (N = 130)	MPA (N = 22)	GPA	GPA
Constitutional/General	88	100	96	96
Malaise, fatigue	87	86	NR	NR
Fever	55	46	72	76
Weight loss	46	46	56	60
Pulmonary	81	41	80	84
Hemoptysis/alveolar hemorrhage	42	14	44	48
Nodules	54[d]	18[e]	44	52
Abnormal pulmonary function tests	61[f]	43[g]	NR	NR
Fixed pulmonary infiltrates	34[d]	0[e]	16	24
Oxygen dependency	20	9	NR	NR
Pleurisy	13	0	8	8
Requiring ventilation	11	5	16	20
Renal	79	82	88	88
Abnormal urinalysis	75	73	88	88
Biopsy proven glomerulonephritis	22	27	64	64
Elevated serum creatinine	36	89	28	44
Ear, Nose, Throat	75	18	84	96
Nasal involvement	52	0	40[h]	60
Sinusitis	48	0	44	56
Otitis/mastoiditis	17	0	24	24
Subglottic involvement	12	0	4	4
Hearing loss	12	0	16	16
Oral ulcers	13	0	28	32
Eyes	30	18	52	60
Nonspecific red eye	10	0	NR	NR
Conjunctivitis	12	9	44	56
Scleritis	8	0	12	12
Cutaneous	55	45	32	48
Palpable purpura/petechia	29	23	32	40
Gastrointestinal	39	68	12	16
Nonspecific abdominal pain	25	36	NR	NR
Chronic nausea	13	41	NR	NR
Musculoskeletal	64	62	NR	NR
Arthralgia/myalgia	52[i]	55	64	76
Arthritis	22[i]	9	32	44
Nervous system	27	27	8	12
Severe headache	15	18	NR	NR
Dizziness	6	5	NR	NR
Cardiovascular	5	7	12+	16
Venous thrombosis	2	0	12	16

[a]Hospital for Sick Children (HSC), Toronto ON, Canada.
[b]A Registry for Children with Vasculitis: e-entry (ARChiVe); patients met two or more of the American College of Rheumatology classification criteria for GPA.
[c]NR, frequency not reported.
[d]Of 125 patients who had imaging (chest radiograph and/or chest computed tomography).
[e]Of 17 patients who had imaging.
[f]Of 67 patients tested.
[g]Of 7 tested.
[h]Nasal involvement features were reported separately, with epistaxis occurring in 40% and nasal ulcers in 24% of children at disease onset.
[i]Arthralgias and arthritis at disease onset were not reported separately.

rates (ESRs) or C-reactive protein levels.[71,115] In early disease, or in disease limited to a single or few systems, these tests may be normal or only slightly abnormal. Proteinuria, microscopic hematuria, and red blood cell casts in a fresh urine sample indicate glomerular disease.[49,115] Gross hematuria is uncommon.[68] Elevation of blood urea nitrogen and serum creatinine levels indicates the presence of significant renal disease.

Antinuclear antibodies of unknown specificity are present in 20% to 36% of children tested.[53,67] Rheumatoid factors are present in approximately 50% of adult and pediatric patients.[67,92] Children with GPA may be at risk for thrombosis because of antiphospholipid antibodies and factor V Leiden mutations.[123] Antiphospholipid antibodies were evident at presentation in 6 (18%) of 34 children tested in one series but were not associated with venous thrombosis.[53] The antibodies were present in two of nine children in another series who had venous thrombosis.[67]

ANCAs of any kind (cANCA, pANCA, PR3-ANCA, or MPO-ANCA) were present in 98% of 124 children with GPA who were tested. Either cANCA or PR3-ANCA was present in 73%, and either pANCA or MPO-ANCA was present in 29%.[111] Similar frequencies of ANCA positivity were found in other pediatric series[67,110] and relatively recent adult series,[8,44] although rates of cANCA positivity were lower and pANCA positivity were higher in the ARChiVe cohort.[111] While cANCA and anti-PR3 are highly sensitive and specific for GPA, pANCA and anti-MPO antibodies may occur especially in so-called renal limited GPA[124] and in Chinese patients with multisystem GPA.[125]

von Willebrand factor antigen (vWFAg), a nonspecific marker of endothelial injury, has been shown to be elevated in other forms of vasculitis during active disease and may be elevated in AAV.[126-129] Other potential biomarkers of vascular inflammation and injury include matrix metalloproteinase-3 (MMP-3), tissue inhibitor of metalloproteinase-1, pentraxin3 (PTX3), and CXL13 (B-cell attracting chemokine 1).[130-132]

Pathology

The full histological spectrum of GPA includes necrotizing granulomas of the upper and/or lower respiratory tract, with necrotizing or granulomatous vasculitis involving predominantly small arteries and veins (commonly in the lungs but also in some other systemic organs), and focal segmental necrotizing glomerulonephritis.[133] Granulomata characterize the disease and show acute and chronic inflammation with central necrosis and histiocytes, lymphocytes, and giant cells; eosinophils may be present in small numbers that should not be confused with the large numbers found in specimens from EGPA patients[121] (Fig. 36-3). The granulomas may be discrete, confluent, or poorly formed with scattered giant cells; at times, lung specimens demonstrate nonspecific inflammation.[121] Renal glomeruli are infiltrated with lymphocytes and histiocytes (Fig. 36-4). The earliest renal change may be glomerular thrombosis[134] but the most commonly reported renal lesions are extracapillary proliferation (with or without fibrinoid necrosis) and crescent formation found in a focal and segmental pattern, followed by necrotizing glomerulonephritis.[135,136] Renal granulomata are rare.[137] Immunofluorescence microscopy is characteristic of a pauci-immune pattern with scanty deposition of immunoglobulins and complement.[135] Dense subendothelial deposits are visible on electron microscopy.[138]

Imaging

Approximately 78% of children with GPA have abnormalities on chest radiographs, with nodules being more common than fixed infiltrates[67,111] (Fig. 36-5). Cavitations, pleural effusions, and pneumothoraces may also occur. Although these gross abnormalities are readily

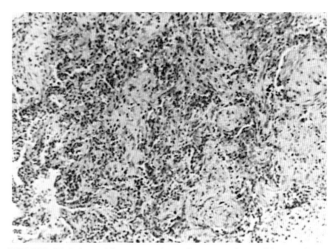

FIGURE 36-3 Lung biopsy specimen from a patient with granulomatosis with polyangiitis. Necrotizing granulomata and fibrous tissue have obliterated the normal alveolar architecture. Hematoxylin-eosin stain, magnification ×480.

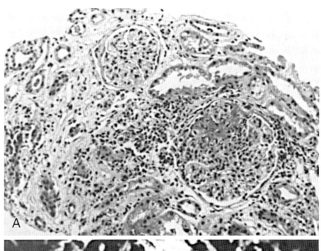

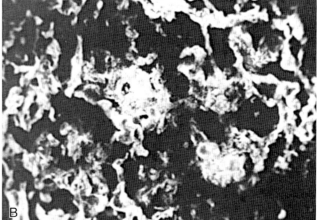

FIGURE 36-4 **A,** Renal biopsy specimen from a child with granulomatosis with polyangiitis. The glomerulus on the right shows areas of hypercellularity and fibrinoid necrosis with interstitial inflammation. Hematoxylin-eosin stain, magnification ×480. **B,** Positive immunofluorescent stain for fibrin in a renal biopsy specimen from a patient with granulomatosis with polyangiitis. Magnification ×480.

detectable on conventional radiography,[139,140] high-resolution computed tomography (CT) is more effective at detecting other characteristic changes such as small nodules; linear opacities; focal low attenuation infiltrates[139,141]; and fluffy centrilobular, perivascular densities[142] (Fig 36-6). The CT halo sign (a rim of ground-glass opacity surrounding the pulmonary lesion) is seen in up to 15% of adult cases and is usually the result of hemorrhage.[143] Sinus radiographs or CT may demonstrate thickening of the sinus lining, opacification of the frontal or maxillary sinuses, or bony thickening, cavitation, and destruction[144] (Fig 36-7). However, magnetic resonance imaging (MRI)

is superior in defining highly active mucosal disease. MRI is also helpful in visualizing soft tissue changes that involve the nose, orbits, mastoids and upper airways (i.e., subglottic stenosis), and the characteristic patterns that have been described.[145-147] Several case reports and a recent retrospective study also suggest a role for 18-F-fluorodeoxy-glucose positron emission tomography (PET)/CT scans as an imaging modality in GPA, especially for delineating disease distribution and guiding biopsies of active lesions.[148-151]

Treatment

Prior to the aggressive use of glucocorticoids and cyclophosphamide (CYC) for the treatment of GPA, the disease was fatal in the majority of pediatric[152] and adult patients.[153] Oral CYC originally prescribed together with glucocorticoids for more than 2 years, often regardless of disease severity, induced remission in more than 90% of adult[71,154] and pediatric patients.[68] Although this strategy was lifesaving,[71,115,154] disease relapses were frequent, and CYC-related toxicity and morbidity

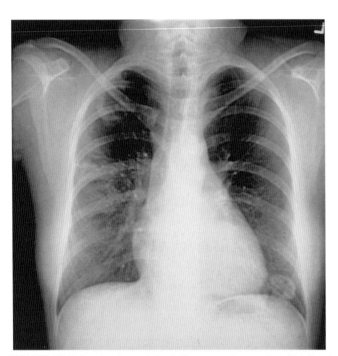

FIGURE 36-5 Patchy, lower lobe infiltrates and several well-defined granulomata (*left*, lower lobe; *right*, upper and middle lobes) are evident in the lung of an adolescent with granulomatosus with polyangiitis.

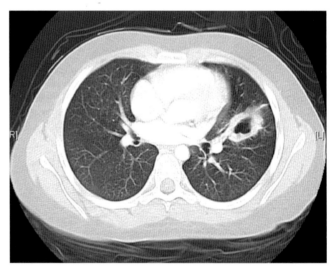

FIGURE 36-6 Cavitating lung disease and main bronchus stenosis in a child with granulomatosis with polyangiitis.

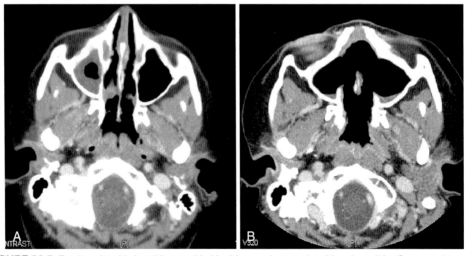

FIGURE 36-7 Erosive sinusitis in a 12-year-old girl with granulomatosis with polyangiitis. Computed tomography of the sinuses in (A) September 2008 and (B) October 2009 showing almost complete destruction of the medial walls of the maxillary sinuses bilaterally.

TABLE 36-3 Classification Schemes for Staging (Subclassifying) Granulomatosis with Polyangiitis

European Vasculitis Network (EUVAS) Scheme[162]

SUBGROUP	ORGAN INVOLVEMENT
Localized	Confined to upper and/or lower respiratory tract
Early systemic	Any organ system except renal, and no imminent vital organ failure
Generalized	Renal with serum creatinine level <500 µmol/L and/or other imminent vital organ failure
Severe renal	Renal with serum creatinine level >500 µmol/L
Refractory	Progressive disease despite standard therapy with glucocorticoids and cyclophosphamide

Vasculitis Clinical Research Consortium (VCRC) Scheme[163]

SUBGROUP	DEFINITION
Limited	No red blood cell casts in urine
	If hematuria is present, serum creatinine is ≤1.4 mg/dL, and creatinine rise is no greater than 25% above baseline
	If pulmonary involvement, PO$_2$ in room air >70 mm Hg and O$_2$ saturation >92%
	Pulmonary hemorrhage may be included provided there is no evidence of progression
	No other critical organ involvement requiring immediate institution of maximal therapy
Severe	Any patient whose disease is not classifiable as limited

(infections, bone marrow failure, infertility, hemorrhagic cystitis, and bladder cancer) was high.[9,71,154,155] The clinical challenge, and aim of ongoing clinical trials in adults described below, is to balance the risks associated with current or emerging therapies, against the damage associated with either *undertreating* aggressive disease[156] or *overtreating* less aggressive disease.[71,157-160] Thus in considering strategies to reduce CYC burden,[161] criteria have been developed for subclassifying or "staging" patients according to disease severity (Table 36-3).[162,163] It has been recommended that treatment be based on disease severity and be divided into two phases described as *remission induction* and *remission maintenance*.[163-165] The following sections and Tables 36-4 and 36-5 summarize the conclusions from several clinical trials in adults. It should be noted that the large majority of trials have evaluated cohorts under the rubric of AAV. These trials have included both GPA and MPA patients, but not patients with EGPA. There have been no trials in children.

Remission induction: Administering CYC for 3 to 6 months only, until remission is achieved and then switching to less aggressive therapy for remission maintenance, has been the predominant strategy used to reduce the CYC cumulative burden. The European Vasculitis Study Group (EUVAS) designed and tested a regimen to administer the CYC by intermittent intravenous pulses every 2 to 3 weeks (see Table 36-6) as an alternative to oral induction therapy that uses 50% less CYC.[178,179] In the CYCLOPS (Daily Oral Versus Pulsed Cyclophosphamide) trial, the intravenous EUVAS protocol was not inferior to daily oral therapy at inducing remission and was associated with lower rates of leukopenia and infection.[167] However, during a median of 4.3 years of follow-up, the rate of relapse was higher in the pulsed group compared to the oral daily group.[180] Of note, for patients who fail to achieve remission

on an intravenous CYC regimen, subsequently switching to oral CYC can be an effective rescue treatment (WEGENT trial).[181]

Glucocorticoids remain a cornerstone of therapy for remission induction and maintenance of remission, but they also carry a toxicity burden. There are no clinical trials examining their role, but their use is integral in all studies evaluating other immunosuppressive treatments for GPA. In critically ill patients, high-dose intravenous methylprednisolone can be used initially.[182] Otherwise, for remission induction prednisone should be started at a dose of 1 to 2 mg/kg/day to a maximum of 60 mg in two or three divided doses to be given for a minimum of 2 weeks (Table 36-6). Reduction in therapy to twice daily and/or to a single daily dose should take place over 4 to 6 weeks. Dose reductions of about 10% to 15% should be on a regular schedule every 2 to 4 weeks as long as the patient remains well with no evidence of worsening disease activity, ultimately aiming to establish the patient on a prolonged low "maintenance" dose, for at least 12 months.[183] In one study where glucocorticoids were withdrawn rapidly[177] and another study where maintenance therapy of any kind was discontinued at 12 months,[166] relapse rates were high.

Several other agents are being used or are being evaluated for use as an alternative to CYC for remission induction. For those patients with less severe GPA (non–life-threatening or non–organ-threatening), methotrexate effectively induces remission,[71,157,160,184] and in the randomized NORAM (Nonrenal Wegener's Granulomatosis Treated Alternatively with Methotrexate) trial, it was not inferior to CYC at inducing remission in patients without significant renal disease.[166] For both CYC and methotrexate, remission rates were 93.5% and 89.8%, respectively; comparable but high relapse rates of 46.5% and 69.5% suggest the need for more prolonged maintenance therapy.

Rituximab, a monoclonal antibody that binds to the CD20 antigen on the surface of activated B cells, is being increasingly used and evaluated for the treatment of AAV. In the RAVE (Rituximab in ANCA-Associated Vasculitis) trial, 197 patients with newly diagnosed or relapsing GPA or MPA were randomized to receive either rituximab or oral CYC for remission induction.[101] Rituximab was not inferior to CYC at inducing remission by 6 months (64% vs. 53%, respectively), and for the 100 patients with relapsing disease, rituximab was superior to CYC (67% vs. 42%).[101] In the RITUXVAS trial (Rituximab versus Cyclophosphamide in ANCA-Associated Renal Vasculitis), newly diagnosed patients with ANCA-associated renal vasculitis were assigned to receive rituximab plus one or two doses of intravenous CYC or intravenous CYC for 3 to 6 months followed by azathioprine.[168] By 12 months both groups had achieved high remission rates (the rituximab group, 76%; the CYC-only group, 82%), but rituximab was not found to be superior to intravenous CYC for remission induction in newly diagnosed ANCA-associated renal vasculitis. Adverse event rates in both groups were similar.[168] Longer-term studies evaluating the safety and efficacy of rituximab are still needed.

Preliminary results from a trial comparing mycophenolate mofetil with pulse CYC (MYCYC trial) for inducing remission by 6 months in AAV suggest that mycophenolate mofetil is not inferior to CYC; however, subsequent risk of relapse appears higher with mycophenolate mofetil.[172]

For patients with pulmonary hemorrhage, intensive care unit management with ventilatory support and even extracorporeal membrane oxygenation (ECMO) may be required for initial life support.[53] For such patients there may be a role for plasmapheresis in addition to other aggressive immunosuppressive therapy.[185] The routine role for plasma exchange in remission induction in GPA remains unclear.[186] When used in conjunction with standard CYC and glucocorticoid therapy, renal survival improved in a small randomized trial of 32 patients,[171] and when compared to methylprednisolone pulse therapy

TABLE 36-4   Summary of Randomized Controlled Trials for Remission-Induction in Adults with AAV

TRIAL	TYPE OF PATIENTS (STAGE)	TREATMENT	CONCLUSION
NORAM[166]	GPA or MPA (early systemic)	MTX versus oral daily CYC	MTX not inferior to CYC for remission induction
CYCLOPS[167]	GPA or MPA (generalized)	IV pulse CYC versus oral daily CYC	IV pulse CYC not inferior to oral CYC for remission induction, higher relapse rates with IV pulse CYC
RAVE[101]	GPA or MPA (generalized)	Rituximab versus oral daily CYC	Rituximab not inferior to CYC for remission induction; rituximab better than CYC for relapsing disease
RITUXVAS[168]	AAV with renal disease (generalized)	Rituximab versus IV pulse CYC	Rituximab not inferior to CYC for remission induction
MEPEX[169,170]	AAV with severe renal disease (severe)	Plasma exchange versus IV pulse methylprednisolone (3 doses); both groups received oral daily CYC	Early renal outcomes better in plasma exchange group but rates of ESRD, mortality, and relapse were similar at 4-year follow-up
Plasma exchange for remission induction in GPA[171]	GPA with moderate to severe renal disease (generalized and severe)	Plasma exchange plus standard immunosuppression versus standard immunosuppression	Improved renal survival in plasma exchange group, no difference in mortality rates
MYCYC[172]	GPA and MPA (generalized)	MMF versus IV CYC	Noninferiority of MMF was not demonstrated (preliminary results)
PEXIVAS (http://clinicaltrials.gov/ct2/show/ NCT00987389)	AAV (severe)	Plasma exchange versus no plasma exchange (both groups receive CYC or rituximab), two glucocorticoid regimens will also be trialed	Currently enrolling

CYC, Cyclophophamide; *CYCLOPS,* daily oral versus pulsed cyclophosphamide trial; *IV,* intravenous; *MEPEX,* methylprednisolone versus plasma exchange trial; *MMF,* mycophenolate mofetil; *MTX,* methotrexate; *MYCYC,* mycophenolate versus cyclophosphamide for remission induction trial; *NORAM,* nonrenal Wegener's granulomatosis treated alternatively with methotrexate trial; *PEXIVAS,* plasma exchange and glucocorticoid dosing in ANCA-Associated Vasculitis trial; *RAVE,* rituximab in AAV trial; *RITUXVAS,* rituximab versus cyclophosphamide in ANCA-associated renal vasculitis trial.
Adapted from Schonermarck et al. Ref. 172.

TABLE 36-5   Summary of Randomized Controlled Trials for Remission-Maintenance in Adults with AAV

TRIAL	TYPE OF PATIENTS	TREATMENT	CONCLUSION
CYCAZAREM[173]	GPA or MPA (generalized)	Azathioprine versus oral daily CYC	No difference in relapse rates
IMPROVE[174]	GPA or MPA (generalized)	MMF versus azathioprine	More relapses with MMF
WEGENT[175]	GPA or MPA (generalized)	MTX versus azathioprine	Similar adverse event rate and relapse rates
LEM[176]	GPA (generalized)	MTX versus leflunomide	Study terminated prematurely due to higher than expected relapse rates in MTX group; trend toward more adverse events in leflunomide group
WGET[177]	GPA (limited or severe)	Etanercept plus standard therapy versus placebo plus standard therapy (CYC or MTX)	Etanercept is not effective for remission maintenance (no difference in relapse rates between groups) and high rate of treatment-related complications including cancers in the etanercept group
REMAIN (http://www.vasculitis.nl/media/ documents/remain.pdf)	GPA or MPA (generalized)	Azathioprine for 18-24 months versus 4 years following remission induction	Currently enrolling
MAINRITSAN (http://clinicaltrials.gov/ct2/show/ NCT00748644)	GPA or MPA (generalized)	Rituximab versus azathioprine for remission maintenance	Study complete, results pending

CYC, Cyclophosphamide; *CYCAZAREM,* cyclophosphamide versus azathioprine during remission in AAV trial; *IMPROVE,* international mycophenolate mofetil protocol to reduce outbreaks of vasculitis trial; *LEM,* leflunomide versus methotrexate in the therapy of AAV trial; *MAINRITSAN,* maintenance of remission using rituximab in systemic AAV trial; *MMF,* mycophenolate mofetil; *MTX,* methotrexate; *REMAIN,* randomized trial of prolonged remission-maintenance therapy in systemic vasculitis trial; *WEGENT,* comparison of methotrexate or azathioprine as maintenance therapy for AAV trial; *WGET,* Wegener's granulomatosis etanercept trial.
Adapted from Schonermarck et al. Ref. 172.

TABLE 36-6 Recommended Therapy of Granulomatosis with Polyangiitis Adapted from EULAR Recommendations

PHASE	DRUG	REGIMEN
Induction (3-6 mo)	Prednisone PLUS	1-2 mg/kg/day PO in two or three divided doses (max, 60 mg); (exceptionally ill patients initially receive methylprednisolone, 30 mg/kg/day [max, 1 g] for 1-3 days IV)
	Cyclophosphamide PLUS	15 mg/kg IV every 2 weeks for three doses and then three weekly (alternatively, 0.5-1.0 g/m² monthly IV pulses have been traditionally used following NIH SLE protocol) or 2 mg/kg/day PO
	Plasma exchange	For selected patients with rapidly progressive severe renal disease, can be used as an adjunct to cyclophosphamide and prednisone
	OR Methotrexate	0.5-1 mg/kg SC once weekly (max, 25-30 mg) (for early systemic/localized disease without renal disease)
Maintenance (minimum 18-24 mo)	Prednisone PLUS	After 4 weeks, prednisone is consolidated and tapered as long as the patient remains well
	Methotrexate OR	0.5-1 mg/kg SC once weekly (max, 25-30 mg)
	Azathioprine OR	2 mg/kg/day PO
	Leflunomide	10-20 mg once daily (weight dependent)
Refractory	Rituximab	375 mg/m²/week for 4 weeks (alternatively 500 mg/m²/dose 2 weeks apart for two doses [max, 1 gram per dose] is also being used as a convenient schedule)
	Infliximab	5-10 mg/kg IV every 1-2 months
	Intravenous immunoglobulin	2 g/kg monthly
	Mycophenolate mofetil	300-600 mg/m²/dose twice daily (max, 3 g/day)

in the MEPEX (Methylprednisolone versus Plasma Exchange) trial, there was reduced dialysis dependency and end-stage renal disease (ESRD).[169] However, there did not seem to be improved overall survival in either study,[171] and in a median 4-year follow-up of patients from the latter study[170] there were no differences in ESRD. The PEXIVAS (Plasma Exchange and Glucocorticoid Dosing in the Treatment of ANCA-Associated Vasculitis) trial is an international randomized controlled trial that is currently enrolling patients and will further examine the role of plasma exchange in the treatment of GPA.[170]

Remission Maintenance

Relapse rates following remission induction are high, but in view of toxicity, long-term remission maintenance therapy with CYC is no longer an acceptable option. Azathioprine used for at least 18 months following remission induction was shown to be not inferior to CYC for remission maintenance in a large randomized trial[187] and has been adopted as a standard of care for adult patients with AAV. Several other drug regimens have been compared to azathioprine, but none have proved to be significantly better.[174,175,177] A summary of the major trials and their outcomes are shown in Table 36-4. Methotrexate may be considered as an alternative; however, it should be used with caution in patients with impaired renal function.[175] Leflunomide has also been shown to be effective in remission maintenance in GPA but may be associated with more adverse effects than methotrexate.[188] Mycophenolate mofetil appears to be less effective than azathioprine for remission maintenance.[174] Trials evaluating optimal duration of maintenance therapy as well as the use of rituximab for remission maintenance are currently underway (European Vasculitis Study Group. Clinical Trial Protocol: REMAIN, http://www.vasculitis.nl/media/documents/remain.pdf (2006); US National Library of Medicine. Clinicaltrials.gov, http://clinicaltrials.gov/ct2/show/NCT00748644 (2013); US National Library of Medicine. Clinicaltrials.gov, http://clinicaltrials.gov/ct2/show/NCT01697267).

Localized Disease

Trimethoprim sulfamethoxazole alone or in combination with glucocorticoids may be considered for remission induction for select cases of localized GPA, especially when limited to the upper respiratory tract[186,189-191]; however, rates of relapse may be high for patients who receive trimethoprim sulfamethoxazole alone.[9,192] Trimethoprim sulfamethoxazole may have a role as an adjunctive remission-maintenance treatment for patients in limiting the rate of relapse of disease of the ear, nose, and throat.[91,193] For patients with nasal disease and chronic nasal carriage of *Staphylococcus aureus*, treatment with topical antibiotics might help limit relapse at that site.[90] Certain disease manifestations such as tracheal and subglottic stenosis may develop or persist despite optimal systemic immunosuppression and may require other treatments such as intralesional glucocorticoid injections, tracheostomy, stent placement, endoscopic dilatation, and laser surgery followed by mitomycin-C application.[110,194-197]

Refractory Vasculitis

A small proportion of patients will have disease that persists or progresses despite standard therapy.[198] Several studies support the role of rituximab for refractory disease.[99,100,199-203] Other treatments that may be beneficial but which require further study include antithymocyte globulin; alemtuzumab (monoclonal antibody against CD52); stem-cell transplantation; 15-deoxyspergualin; and tumor necrosis factor antagonists.[204-210] Of note, the use of etanercept is contraindicated in the treatment of GPA following the results of the Wegener's Granulomatosis Etanercept Trial (WGET), where 6 out of 91 (7%) patients who received etanercept plus standard therapy developed solid tumors; those who received standard therapy alone developed no tumors.[177]

Current Recommendations

In 2008 EULAR provided recommendations for the management of primary small- and medium-vessel vasculitis in adults[164] based on the results of clinical trials at that time. Intravenous CYC (15 mg/kg [max 1.2 g] every 2 weeks for three pulses followed by three to six pulses every 3 weeks), combined with high-dose glucocorticoids, is recommended for remission induction in life-threatening or organ-threatening generalized primary small- and medium-vessel vasculitis. Plasma exchange is recommended for select patients with rapidly progressive severe renal disease. Methotrexate combined with glucocorticoids is recommended for remission induction in non–organ-threatening or non–life-threatening AAV. For remission maintenance therapy, a combination of low-dose glucocorticoids and either azathioprine, leflunomide, or methotrexate is recommended. Prophylactic treatment against *Pneumocystis jiroveci* with trimethoprim sulfamethoxazole on alternative days was recommended for patients being treated with CYC.[211,212]

The EULAR recommendations were intended for use in adults, and currently there are no pediatric-specific recommendations. In the absence of any pediatric clinical trials, current treatment in children is largely based on adult recommendations and summarized in Table 36-6. In ARChiVe, the majority of pediatric patients in the United States and Canada are given CYC and glucocorticoids for remission induction, but maintenance therapy is not reported. The most common treatment alternative to CYC in this series[53] and other single-center case series[67,213] was methotrexate. Plasma exchange and rituximab in refractory disease have also been reported in case reports or case series of children with GPA,[214,215] and rituximab for refractory disease.[216] The case series of Fowler et al. focuses on local and systemic treatment of airway disease.[110]

Disease Measurement Tools

Staging disease severity and measuring disease activity and damage are an important part of clinical practice and an essential part of conducting clinical trials. Various tools have been developed and used in adult patients with AAV, including the disease severity scales described above, the Birmingham Vasculitis Activity Score (BVAS) and the Vasculitis Damage Index (VDI).[217-220] Such tools have become widely established in adult AAV and are accepted by the Outcome Measures in Rheumatology Clinical Trials (OMERACT) initiative.[221] When the performance of BVAS was examined in pediatric AAV patients in ARChiVe, there was a weak correlation with disease activity by physician's global assessment (PGA), and only a moderate correlation with ESR and treatment decision.[222] In the same cohort of patients, the EUVAS and WGET adult severity subclassification systems were adapted to pediatrics and applied retrospectively. They were found to have a strong correlation with physician choice of treatment; however, they have not been prospectively used to guide therapy.[223] Recently, a pediatric tool based on modifications to the BVAS—the Pediatric Vasculitis Activity Score (PVAS)—was developed and preliminarily validated.[224] Further validation of this tool on an independent dataset and the development of a pediatric adapted tool for assessing damage are planned.

Clinical Course and Outcome/Prognosis

Prognosis arguably depends in part on the clinical state or stage of disease at diagnosis, which in turn may be influenced by the interval from symptom onset to diagnosis. The 1-year mortality of adult patients with untreated GPA was approximately 80%,[92,225] whereas more recent studies report 5-year mortality rates of treated patients on the order of 10% to 25%.[71,154,226] The cause of death of 28 adult patients with GPA in a long-term follow-up of subjects used in development of the ACR classification criteria were as follows: infection (29%), cardiac disease (18%), renal failure (18%), and malignancy (14%).[227] Twenty-two children younger than 15 years of age died of the disease

in the United States in a 10-year period ending in 1988.[43] In adults treated with prednisone and CYC over 90% of patients responded completely or partially; however, more than 50% relapsed within 5 years.[71,154] Similar rates of remission and relapse are reported in two pediatric series.[67,68] The pediatric series reported 23 and 25 patients who were followed for a mean of 8.7 years and a mean of 2.7 years, respectively. In the former series reported by Rottem and associates, one patient died of severe lung disease and cor pulmonale, and one died of sepsis.[68] No patients died in the series reported by Akikusa and associates.[67]

Reports of long-term morbidity from adult cohorts describe an increased risk of cardiac disease and cardiovascular related events (cardiovascular death, stroke, coronary artery disease, and myocardial infarction).[228,229] The identified increased risk of malignancy in patients with AAV[230] is lower in studies of more contemporary cohorts, and this might be attributable to the reduced cumulative exposure to CYC.[231] No patient developed malignancy in either pediatric series.[67,68] Other important morbidities in both adult and pediatric patients include osteoporosis, chronic kidney disease, ESRD, infertility, cystitis, diabetes, and avascular necrosis.[68,214,232]

For pediatric GPA there is an increasingly high rate of ENT involvement accumulating with time described in general follow up series.[67,68,233] In two of the series, approximately half of patients developed ENT manifestations including hearing impairment, nasal septal, or upper airway deformities over the course of their disease.[68,233] Two additional single-center case series from 2011[234] and 2013[110] each with 28 children having GPA, focused primarily on ENT disease and airway stenoses. In the 2011 study, during followup seven children (25%) developed airway stenosis, predominantly subglottic, but also tracheal, bronchial, with multilevel involvement in four children. In the 2013 study, 14 children (50%) reported the same conditions, with three children developing multilevel airway stenosis. Both studies recommended a multidisciplinary treatment approach involving ENT, pulmonology, and rheumatology, and described the need for several surgical interventions and biological therapy.

MICROSCOPIC POLYANGIITIS

Microscopic polyangiitis (MPA) was originally described as a subset of PAN, but with time MPA has become increasingly recognized as a distinct entity among the systemic vasculitides because of the presence of necrotizing glomerulonephritis,[235] the frequent involvement of predominantly small vessels in the lungs and kidneys,[236] and the high frequency of association with ANCA, specifically anti-MPO-ANCA.

Definition and Disease Classification

MPA is described as a small-vessel vasculitis in both adult[1,50] and pediatric[237] nomenclature. Within this small-vessel disease category the 2012 CHCC[1] groups MPA with AAV. It is defined as a necrotizing vasculitis, with few or no immune deposits, predominantly affecting small vessels (i.e., capillaries, venules, or arterioles), although arteritis of the small- and medium-sized arteries may be present.[50] Necrotizing glomerulonephritis and pulmonary capillaritis are common, and granulomatous inflammation is absent. The most recent classification initiatives for vasculitis in adults[36] and in children[52] did not include criteria for classifying MPA. As a result, it is inevitable that patients defined as having MPA might also be concurrently classified as having GPA[54] or PAN.[238] Watts et al.[7] criticized the poor performance of existing criteria[36,50,239] in classifying adult patients with PAN or any of the ANCA-associated vasculitides into mutually exclusive categories. To address this issue, they proposed a classification algorithm that has been adopted by the European Medicines Agency (EMA). The concept of the algorithm is to apply the different criteria in a stepwise approach, first defining EGPA patients in whom the criteria are most specific, and subsequently and sequentially applying elements of different criteria to the remaining patients to classify each into a single category for study purposes.

Epidemiology

Epidemiological data on MPA are limited because of its origins as a subset of PAN and because it is now frequently described collectively with the other AAVs. There are, however, genetically distinct differences between the AAV subsets that associate somewhat better with ANCA specificity (MPO versus PR3) than clinical phenotype (MPA versus GPA).[17] Following the CHCC description of MPA, Watts et al. estimated a regional UK incidence of 3.6 cases per million compared with the incidence of PAN of 2.4 cases per million.[238] Mohamed et al., using an algorithm to uniquely classify patients, described the following prevalence figures of primary systemic vasculitis in southern Sweden per million inhabitants: GPA, 160; MPA, 94; PAN, 31; and EGPA, 14.[240] By survey, pediatric rheumatologists in the United States and Canada recognize MPA among their patients as frequently as PAN and about half as frequently as GPA.[48] In ARChiVe, with over 250 patients, there were 22 patients with MPA and 130 patients with GPA.[111] The average age of onset in adults is around 50 years, and the male-to-female ratio ranges from 1.0 to 1.8:1.[236,240,241] In the limited pediatric case series, the mean age of onset in children ranges from 9 to 12 years.[111,242-245] Except for the Turkish study,[244] in which the sex ratio was equal, more than 68% of patients were female.

Pathogenesis

Seventy-five percent of patients have pANCA with specificity for MPO.[1,10,124] ANCA likely has a key role in the pathogenesis of MPA, as discussed above. Genetic associations include HLA-DRB1*0901 in a Japanese population[246] and HLA-DQ in a large European cohort.[17] Unlike GPA, MPA has no strong association with any infectious triggers, but it has been associated with certain drug exposures such as propylthiouracil[247] and hydralazine.[248,249] In northern Europe, GPA is much more common than MPA, whereas the opposite is true in southern Europe.[250] In addition, MPA is more common than GPA in Japan and China.[63,251] This further suggests a role for genetic and/or environmental factors.

Clinical Manifestations

Reports on clinical manifestations of MPA in both adults[10,236,241,252,253] and children[242-245] should be interpreted with the understanding that MPA is often described collectively with other types of vasculitis.[244] Additionally, MPA is not always defined by criteria that are mutually exclusive of diseases such as GPA, EGPA, or PAN.[7] Clinical manifestations of MPA in children are described in three retrospective case series of 21, 7, and 26 patients from Japan,[242] Serbia,[245] and Turkey, respectively,[244] and also in 22 patients in ARChiVe[111] classified according to the EMA algorithm and listed in Table 36-2. General features such as fever, weight loss, myalgias, and arthralgias were present in more than 86%.[111,242,245] Renal involvement, including hypertension, hematuria, proteinuria, and even renal failure (in 33% of patients at time of diagnosis),[242] occurred in 100% of patients[242,244,245] in series reported from departments of nephrology and in 82% of patients in ARChiVe.[111] Pulmonary involvement occurred in 17% to 62% of patients.[242,244,245] In the Japanese series one third of patients had hemoptysis as a presenting manifestation and about half had pulmonary hemorrhage at some time.[242] In the adult series, pulmonary involvement ranges from mildly bloody sputum or episodic cough, pleuritic chest pain, and

dyspnea to massive pulmonary hemorrhage occurring in 25% to 72% of patients.[10,236,241,252,253] Pulmonary manifestations most frequently occur as part of a pulmonary-renal syndrome, but lung disease may rarely be present without kidney involvement. Skin manifestations are predominantly purpura but also ulcers, and are present in 38% to 100% of pediatric patients; in adults the predominant skin manifestation is purpura (often palpable),[10,236,241,252,253] but other lesions such as petechiae, livedo reticularis, ulcers, urticaria, and erythema occur.[254-257] Other less frequent manifestations include central nervous system disease (convulsions, severe headaches), gastrointestinal symptoms (abdominal pain and gastrointestinal bleeding), and ocular symptoms (episcleritis and conjunctivitis).[242,244,245] Peripheral neuropathy was not described in adult and pediatric series where PAN was actively excluded.[111,242,245]

Pathology

Pauci-immune necrotizing vasculitis predominantly affecting small vessels and necrotizing glomerulonephritis define MPA (see above).[1,50] Patients with ANCA-associated glomerulonephritis without other organ manifestations may have renal histopathology that is indistinguishable from MPA. In the Japanese series, 10 of 21 children with MPA had necrotizing crescentic glomerulonephritis from a total of 31 kidney biopsies; in 22 of these biopsies crescents were found in more than 50% of the glomeruli. Extraglomerular vasculitis was present in four cases.[242]

Diagnosis and Differential Diagnosis

Patients presenting with renal disease and ANCA-associated glomerulonephritis should be clinically assessed for extrarenal manifestations of MPA. One third of patients with anti-GBM disease may have both anti-GBM antibodies and ANCA[258]; they are differentiated from MPA by immunofluorescence microscopy of a renal biopsy. GPA may be distinguished from MPA by the presence of granulomatous inflammation, upper respiratory tract involvement (specifically nasal septal perforation and/or saddle-nose deformity), chest imaging findings of nodules, nodular infiltrates, or cavitation representing granulomatous inflammation rather than capillaritis. GPA may more frequently have PR3-ANCA rather than MPO-ANCA.[242] PAN may be distinguished by the absence of MPO-ANCA, rapidly progressive glomerulonephritis and lung hemorrhage, and the presence of microaneurysms and other abnormal angiographic findings.[236,259,260] Other small-vessel vasculitides such as Henoch–Schönlein purpura and cryoglobulinemic vasculitis may present similarly but are distinguished by their clinical course and/or histopathology showing well-defined or prominent immune complex deposits, and immunoglobulin A (IgA) in the case of Henoch–Schönlein purpura.

Laboratory Examination

As with the other AAV, nonspecific measurements of inflammation (increased ESR and C-reactive protein, anemia, thrombocytosis, and hypoalbuminemia), and characterization of urinalysis and renal function are useful for following disease activity and course. The presence of pANCA in 75% of patients with MPA is useful diagnostically, depending on the prior clinical probability of systemic vasculitis and the MPO specificity.[50] In the most recent pediatric series, ANCA of any specificity was found in 95% of patients.[111] During the course of the disease, the relationship of ANCA titers with disease activity, relapse, or mortality risk is not consistent.[242,261,262]

Treatment

There are no clinical trials in pediatrics to guide therapy for MPA, but treatment principles and practices are used that are based on studies in adults in which MPA and GPA are collectively treated with common regimens (Table 36-5). In the pediatric MPA series, most patients initially received glucocorticoids and/or CYC, intravenously or orally, in various regimens. Plasmapheresis was used for some pediatric patients[111,242,244,245] and rituximab was included in initial treatment of 2 of 22 patients in ARChiVe. Patients receiving CYC seem to do better than patients receiving corticosteroids alone.[10,244] As described above for GPA immunosuppressive agents other than CYC are used when disease is staged as less severe according to classification schemes (Table 36-3),[162,163] or if there are no poor prognostic factors (i.e., significant renal disease, cardiomyopathy, central nervous system or gastrointestinal involvement) that have been established for adult patients with PAN, EGPA,[263] and MPA.[264] Massive pulmonary hemorrhage is also a bad prognostic sign.

Course of the Disease and Prognosis

Of the 30 patients in the Japanese[242] and Serbian[245] series, only one patient died 3 months after diagnosis, from cytomegalovirus infection. In the Turkish[244] series of 26 patients (including 2 patients with PAN), in which only 13 patients received CYC, there were nine deaths, four due to renal failure, two from central nervous system disease, two from massive gastrointestinal hemorrhage, and one from cardiac failure. Follow-up in these series ranged from less than 6 months to 10 years. Among the 64 patients (including 10 with ANCA-associated necrotizing crescentic glomerulonephritis), 25 developed ESRD. A shorter duration between disease onset and treatment is associated with a better outcome: patients treated early after disease onset had renal lesions showing focal segmental necrosis on kidney biopsies, whereas those with a later diagnosis and treatment had a predominance of circumferential fibrosis and/or crescents.[245] Among the 30 Japanese patients, the 10 diagnosed early through a school-based urine screening program for hematuria and proteinuria had a more favorable renal outcome than the other 20 patients.[242]

EOSINOPHILIC GRANULOMATOSIS WITH POLYANGIITIS

Eosinophilic granulomatosis with polyangiitis (EGPA), the new name for Churg–Strauss syndrome (CSS), was also known as allergic granulomatosis and angiitis.[1] This rare necrotizing vasculitis, originally described in 1951 by Churg and Strauss, was distinguished from PAN by its involvement of predominantly small rather than medium-sized vessels, and by the presence of extravascular granuloma and eosinophilic infiltration.[265] Clinically, EGPA is characterized by severe asthma or allergic rhinitis, skin disease, and vasculitis that commonly involves the cardiovascular system, kidneys, nervous system, and gastrointestinal tract. Because of the high frequency of associated ANCA, specifically anti-MPO-ANCA,[266] it is described as an ANCA-associated small-vessel vasculitis.

Definition and Disease Classification

A patient meets the 2012 CHCC definition of EGPA if he or she is found to have eosinophil-rich and necrotizing granulomatous inflammation, usually of the respiratory tract, and necrotizing vasculitis predominantly affecting small to medium vessels, associated with asthma and eosinophilia.[1] The ACR classification criteria for EGPA aim to distinguish this disease from the other vasculitides and are not diagnostic criteria (Table 36-7). There are no pediatric-specific classification criteria for EGPA. The criteria proposed by Lanham et al. require a patient to have asthma, peripheral blood eosinophilia, and systemic vasculitis in two or more extrapulmonary sites.[239]

TABLE 36-7   American College of Rheumatology Criteria for Classification of Eosinophilic Granulomatosis with Polyangiitis Syndrome

CRITERION*	DESCRIPTION
Asthma	History of wheezing or diffuse high-pitched rales on expiration
Eosinophilia	Eosinophils >10% of differential white blood cell count
History of allergy	History of seasonal allergy (e.g., allergic rhinitis) or documented allergies, including food, contactants, and others (except for drug allergies)
Mononeuropathy or polyneuropathy	Mononeuropathy, multiple mononeuropathies or polyneuropathy (i.e., glove/stocking distribution) attributable to a systemic vasculitis
Pulmonary infiltrates	Migratory or transitory pulmonary infiltrates on radiographs attributable to a systemic vasculitis
Paranasal sinus abnormality	History of acute or chronic paranasal sinus pain or tenderness, or radiographic opacification of the paranasal sinuses
Extravascular eosinophils	Biopsy including artery, arteriole, or venule, showing accumulation of eosinophils in extravascular areas

*For classification purposes, a patient is said to have EGPA if at least four of these criteria are present. The presence of any four or more criteria has a sensitivity of 85% and a specificity of 99.7%.

Epidemiology

EGPA is a rare disease with an estimated annual incidence of one to three cases per million, and similarly to GPA, there may be an increasing frequency in higher latitudes and rural areas, which suggests environmental influences.[62,250,267] The mean age of diagnosis is 50 years,[239,268] and it is rare in children. In a report of 117 children with AAV from 30 US and Canadian centers, 2 children had EGPA compared with 76 with GPA and 17 with MPA.[53] Gendelman et al.[269] reported nine children with EGPA, together with children from other recent case reports and the 33 collected cases reviewed and reported by Zwerina et al.[270] Among the identified 47 reported cases of childhood EGPA, the mean age was 12 years with a 3:1 female preponderance.[269] There is no clear male or female predominance in adult studies.[13-15,239,268] Various vaccinations, inhaled allergens, infectious agents, and drugs (e.g., omalizumab, macrolides, carbamazepine, and quinine) have been implicated as triggers.[271] Cysteinyl leukotriene receptor antagonists (montelukast) said to be pathogenic in precipitating EGPA when given to some asthma patients was likely to have unmasked an underlying EGPA or EGPA-like syndrome when it effectively reduced the patient's corticosteroid requirement.[272]

Pathogenesis

The etiology of EGPA remains poorly understood. There is likely a pathogenic role for eosinophils[273,274] with their procoagulant properties accounting for the propensity for cardiovascular complications.[275] Interleukin-5 (IL-5) identified on peripheral blood mononuclear cells from EGPA patients[276] is a key cytokine for the induction and promotion of hypereosinophilia. Th-2 responses predominate over Th-1 with upregulation of IL-4, IL-13, and IL-5, and they are of relevance for current or future targeted therapy. Also, low levels of T-regulatory (Treg) cells have been associated with relapses[277,278]; a favorable balance of Treg cells might be achieved by IL-2[279] or IL-5[280] therapy. In contrast, IL-5 blockade reduces hypereosinophilia.[281] ANCA likely has a pathogenic role[13] when present, but it is found in a minority of adult patients in some adult series (31% to 73%)[13,15,268,282] and pediatric patients (25%).[269] EGPA may include more than one disease entity,[283] with a recognized ANCA-positive phenotype in which patients may more frequently have glomerulonephritis; alveolar hemorrhage; ear, nose, throat, and peripheral nerve involvement; and biopsy-proven vasculitis.[13,268] By comparison, ANCA-negative patients more frequently have cardiac involvement.[13,14,268] Genetic factors may also play a role in the pathogenesis of EGPA. HLA-DRB4 and HLA-DRB1*07 have been found to be more prevalent in patients with EGPA as compared with healthy controls.[284,285] Polymorphisms in the IL-10 gene were associated with the ANCA-negative subset of EGPA.[286]

Clinical Manifestations

EGPA usually has a very prolonged prodromal course of many years, which consists of asthma and other allergic manifestations such as chronic allergic rhinitis and nasal polyposis.[239] This is followed by an eosinophilic phase with eosinophilia and pulmonary infiltrates, and then vasculitis.[239] These three phases do not always occur sequentially, and asthma may occasionally follow the onset of vasculitis.[282,287] Among the collected reports of 47 pediatric cases,[269,270] presenting features were asthma in 91% of individuals, pulmonary involvement with non-fixed infiltrates in 83%, sinusitis in 75%, skin involvement in 67%, cardiac disease in 45% (cardiomyopathy, 34%; pericarditis, 26%), gastrointestinal involvement in 47%, peripheral neuropathy (mononeuritis multiplex) in 40%, arthralgia in 27%, myalgia in 22%, and kidney disease in 13%. Other organs occasionally involved include lymph nodes, orbits, salivary glands, mammary glands, testicles, and the thymus. Compared with 383 adult patients described in the French vasculitis study group cohort,[268] the above frequencies for asthma and arthralgia were the same. Peripheral neuropathy (51%), renal disease (21%), and myalgia (39%) were more frequent in the adult cohort, but each of the other organ systems listed above was approximately twice as frequently involved in children. This pediatric series is a collection of case reports or small case series with potential selection bias for severe or interesting cases.

Asthma is the hallmark of the disease in both adults and children, and usually requires steroids for treatment. The severity and frequency of asthma attacks may increase during the prodromal phase prior to the onset of vasculitis, with the patient becoming dependent on steroids for its treatment.[15,288] The presence of skin manifestations in a majority of patients reflects the involvement of small vessels; the specific manifestations resemble those of the other small-vessel vasculitides and include petechiae or palpable purpura that may be necrotic, digital ischemia, cutaneous nodules, papules that may look urticarial, maculopapular rash, livedo reticularis, ulcers, and bullae.[289] Cardiac disease, predominantly because of cardiomyopathy, was an important cause of mortality in both the pediatric[269,270] and adult series.[15,268] Renal disease is generally mild and rarely progresses,[239,287] although it may occasionally.[290] Hypertension, ocular involvement, and pseudotumor cerebri occur in some patients.[291] Peripheral neuropathy, usually mononeuritis multiplex but also polyneuropathy, occurs more frequently in lower limbs, and is an important cause of morbidity.[292,293] The spectrum of gastrointestinal manifestations include abdominal pain, nausea, vomiting, diarrhea, acute abdominal bleeding or perforation—some of these features likely resulting from small-vessel vasculitis that involves the mesentery or small or large bowel.[15,294]

Pathology

The characteristic histopathological findings in specimens from any involved site are angiitis and extravascular necrotizing granulomas usually with eosinophilic infiltrates.[133] The angiitis may be granulomatous or nongranulomatous, and involve arteries and veins, as well as pulmonary and systemic blood vessels.[133] The so-called Churg–Strauss granuloma describes the skin nodules and papules over the extensor surfaces of joints. The histological pattern of palisading granulomas with central necrosis are not unique to EGPA but also occur in GPA, systemic lupus erythematosus, and other diseases.[295] Similarly, many of the skin manifestations and the associated histopathology of leukocytoclastic vasculitis with or without eosinophils are not unique to EGPA.[289]

Diagnosis and Differential Diagnosis

Ultimately the diagnosis of EGPA, like the other systemic vasculitides, is made on the basis of clinical and histopathological features. EGPA should be considered in patients with chronic asthma, fever, a deteriorating clinical course, and eosinophilia. There may also be features suggestive of vasculitis at other extrapulmonary sites[239] and also as described above (Table 36-7). Diagnosis should ideally be confirmed histopathologically with biopsy of renal, skin, or lung tissue, and show eosinophilic infiltration of granulomas and vasculitis. The main differential diagnoses are other hypereosinophilic syndromes[296] and other vasculitides. When extrapulmonary features are not prominent, conditions that need to be excluded are parasitic infections, drug reactions, acute and chronic eosinophilic pneumonia, allergic bronchopulmonary aspergillosis, and idiopathic hypereosinophilic syndrome. It has been proposed by the European Society EGPA Task Force that that this last disorder, when involving multiple organs with no evidence of vasculitis, be called *hypereosinophilic asthma with systemic manifestations* (HASM).[297] This task force has also proposed mutually exclusive diagnostic criteria for EGPA and HASM.[297] Among the chronic vasculitides, EGPA needs to be distinguished, particularly from GPA and MPA, in the presence of ANCA.

Laboratory Examination

Elevation of acute phase reactants accompanies active disease. Peripheral blood eosinophilia (with eosinophils accounting for 10% or more of leukocytes) and elevation of serum levels of IgE are typical. Serum IgG4 levels may correlate with disease activity.[298] Chest radiographs or CT of the chest may reveal diffuse pulmonary infiltrates (Fig. 36-8), and pulmonary function tests may demonstrate poor lung diffusing capacity and low PO_2. ANCAs, most commonly anti-MPO, are found in less than 50% of patients.[13,15,268,270,282] Examination of bronchopulmonary lavage fluid may be useful in confirming the presence of eosinophilic inflammation[299,300] and in excluding infectious and other pathologies. Transbronchial biopsy is less invasive than transthoracic biopsy for obtaining lung specimens.[301] Electrocardiogram and echocardiogram can be used to evaluate for cardiac disease, and the role of other diagnostic investigations such as cardiac MRI is being studied.[302-304]

Treatment

There are no clinical trials in adults or pediatrics to help guide therapy. The principles of treatment should be similar to those described for GPA. Systemic glucocorticoid therapy, initially at high doses, is the mainstay of treatment.[269,270] The need for, and choice of, an additional immunosuppressive agent should be determined by the severity of the disease. The disease might be considered severe if it is life- or organ-threatening, and in the presence of some defined prognostic risk factors (i.e., renal insufficiency, proteinuria greater than 1 g/day,

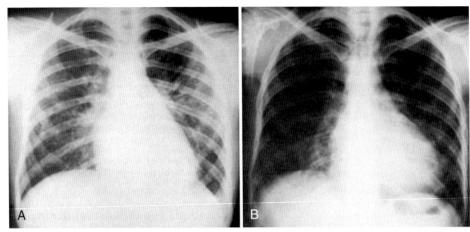

FIGURE 36-8 Chest radiographs of a young man with eosinophilic granulomatosis with polyangiitis. **A,** The initial film demonstrates an enlarged cardiac silhouette and relatively normal pulmonary fields. **B,** The film was taken during an acute episode of left- and right-sided heart failure. Notice the cardiac enlargement and disappearance of the normal pulmonary vascular markings, indicating acute pulmonary hypertension and cor pulmonale, which, in this case, is due to vasculitis.

cardiomyopathy, central nervous system or gastrointestinal involvement),[263] induction treatment with CYC may be warranted. These prognostic factors can be formally used to obtain a Five Factor Score (FFS), which is a prognostic scoring system used to define disease severity in EGPA and PAN.[263] An FFS of 0 is given when none of these factors is present. An FFS of 1 indicates that one factor is present, and was associated with a 25.9% 5-year mortality rate. An FFS of 2 or higher was associated with a 45.95% 5-year mortality rate in a cohort of 342 patients with EGPA and PAN.[263] Alternative immunosuppressants for less severe or steroid-dependent disease include methotrexate, azathioprine, mycophenolate mofetil,[305-307] interferon-α,[308] and intravenous gamma globulin.[309] EGPA has not been included in the clinical trials of rituximab. Successful use of rituximab has been described in several cases of EGPA with refractory disease,[200,310,311] but there is also a report of ineffectiveness.[312] Some pilot studies targeting IL-5 with mepolizumab have been promising.[313,314]

Course of the Disease and Prognosis

When first described, EGPA seemed to be universally fatal.[265] More recent mortality rates have ranged from being no higher than the general population[282] to 40%.[15,268,287,315] Increasing mortality was related to increasing age[315] and the presence of risk factors described above.[263] The most frequent cause of death in both adults and children is due to cardiac involvement,[239,268,270] but other causes include infections, cancers, and severe asthma or other terminal respiratory events.[268] In the literature review of 47 pediatric patients the mortality was 13%.[269] A majority of patients in long-term remission may require continuing treatment with corticosteroids (oral or inhaled) because of residual asthma.[15]

REFERENCES

1. J.C. Jennette, R.J. Falk, P.A. Bacon, et al., 2012 revised International Chapel Hill Consensus Conference nomenclature of vasculitides, Arthritis Rheum. 65 (2013) 1–11.
4. X. Bosch, A. Guilabert, J. Font, Antineutrophil cytoplasmic antibodies, Lancet 368 (2006) 404–418.
7. R. Watts, S. Lane, T. Hanslik, et al., Development and validation of a consensus methodology for the classification of the ANCA-associated vasculitides and polyarteritis nodosa for epidemiological studies, Ann. Rheum. Dis. 66 (2007) 222–227.
10. L. Guillevin, B. Durand-Gasselin, R. Cevallos, et al., Microscopic polyangiitis: clinical and laboratory findings in eighty-five patients, Arthritis Rheum. 42 (1999) 421–430.
15. L. Guillevin, P. Cohen, M. Gayraud, et al., Churg-Strauss syndrome. Clinical study and long-term follow-up of 96 patients, Medicine (Baltimore) 78 (1999) 26–37.
17. P.A. Lyons, T.F. Rayner, S. Trivedi, et al., Genetically distinct subsets within ANCA-associated vasculitis, NEJM 367 (2012) 214–223.
18. S. Lionaki, E.R. Blyth, S.L. Hogan, et al., Classification of antineutrophil cytoplasmic autoantibody vasculitides: the role of antineutrophil cytoplasmic autoantibody specificity for myeloperoxidase or proteinase 3 in disease recognition and prognosis, Arthritis Rheum. 64 (2012) 3452–3462.
20. M.M. Boomsma, C.A. Stegeman, M.J. van der Leij, et al., Prediction of relapses in Wegener's granulomatosis by measurement of antineutrophil cytoplasmic antibody levels: a prospective study, Arthritis Rheum. 43 (2000) 2025–2033.
30. J.C. Jennette, R.J. Falk, P. Hu, H. Xiao, Pathogenesis of antineutrophil cytoplasmic autoantibody-associated small-vessel vasculitis, Annu. Rev. Pathol. 8 (2013) 139–160.
36. J.F. Fries, G.G. Hunder, D.A. Bloch, et al., The American College of Rheumatology 1990 criteria for the classification of vasculitis. Summary, Arthritis Rheum. 33 (1990) 1135–1136.
42. R.J. Falk, W.L. Gross, L. Guillevin, et al., Granulomatosis with polyangiitis (Wegener's): an alternative name for Wegener's granulomatosis, Arthritis Rheum. 63 (2011) 863–864.
45. R.A. Watts, S.E. Lane, G. Bentham, D.G. Scott, Epidemiology of systemic vasculitis: a ten-year study in the United Kingdom, Arthritis Rheum. 43 (2000) 414–419.
48. N.M. Wilkinson, J. Page, A.G. Uribe, et al., Establishment of a pilot pediatric registry for chronic vasculitis is both essential and feasible: a Childhood Arthritis and Rheumatology Alliance (CARRA) survey, J. Rheumatol. 34 (2007) 224–226.
49. R.Y. Leavitt, A.S. Fauci, D.A. Bloch, et al., The American College of Rheumatology 1990 criteria for the classification of Wegener's granulomatosis, Arthritis Rheum. 33 (1990) 1101–1107.
50. J.C. Jennette, R.J. Falk, K. Andrassy, et al., Nomenclature of systemic vasculitides. Proposal of an international consensus conference, Arthritis Rheum. 37 (1994) 187–192.
51. V.M. Belostotsky, V. Shah, M.J. Dillon, Clinical features in 17 paediatric patients with Wegener granulomatosis, Pediatr. Nephrol. 17 (2002) 754–761.

52. N. Ruperto, S. Ozen, A. Pistorio, et al., EULAR/PRINTO/PRES criteria for Henoch-Schönlein purpura, childhood polyarteritis nodosa, childhood Wegener granulomatosis and childhood Takayasu arteritis: Ankara 2008. Part I: overall methodology and clinical characterisation, Ann. Rheum. Dis. 69 (2010) 790–797.

53. D.A. Cabral, A.G. Uribe, S.M. Benseler, et al., Classification, presentation and initial treatment of Wegener's granulomatosis in childhood, Arthritis Rheum. 60 (2009) 3413–3424.

54. A.G. Uribe, A.M. Huber, S. Kim, et al., Increased sensitivity of the European medicines agency algorithm for classification of childhood granulomatosis with polyangiitis, J. Rheumatol. 39 (2012) 1687–1697.

56. E. Ntatsaki, R.A. Watts, D.G. Scott, Epidemiology of ANCA-associated vasculitis, Rheum. Dis. Clin. North Am. 36 (2010) 447–461.

65. S. Grisaru, G.W. Yuen, P.M. Miettunen, L.A. Hamiwka, Incidence of Wegener's granulomatosis in children, J. Rheumatol. 37 (2010) 440–442.

67. J.D. Akikusa, R. Schneider, E.A. Harvey, et al., Clinical features and outcome of pediatric Wegener's granulomatosis, Arthritis Rheum. 57 (2007) 837–844.

68. M. Rottem, A.S. Fauci, C.W. Hallahan, et al., Wegener granulomatosis in children and adolescents: clinical presentation and outcome, J. Pediatr. 122 (1993) 26–31.

69. C.G. Kallenberg, Pathogenesis of PR3-ANCA associated vasculitis, J. Autoimmun. 30 (2008) 29–36.

71. G.S. Hoffman, G.S. Kerr, R.Y. Leavitt, et al., Wegener granulomatosis: an analysis of 158 patients [see comments], Ann. Intern. Med. 116 (1992) 488–498.

90. C.A. Stegeman, J.W. Tervaert, W.J. Sluiter, et al., Association of chronic nasal carriage of Staphylococcus aureus and higher relapse rates in Wegener granulomatosis, Ann. Intern. Med. 120 (1994) 12–17.

92. A.S. Fauci, B.F. Haynes, P. Katz, S.M. Wolff, Wegener's granulomatosis: prospective clinical and therapeutic experience with 85 patients for 21 years, Ann. Intern. Med. 98 (1983) 76–85.

101. J.H. Stone, P.A. Merkel, R. Spiera, et al., Rituximab versus cyclophosphamide for ANCA-associated vasculitis, NEJM 363 (2010) 221–232.

112. J.H. Stone, Limited versus severe Wegener's granulomatosis: baseline data on patients in the Wegener's granulomatosis etanercept trial, Arthritis Rheum. 48 (2003) 2299–2309.

115. A.S. Fauci, B.F. Haynes, P. Katz, S.M. Wolff, Wegener's granulomatosis: prospective clinical and therapeutic experience with 85 patients for 21 years, Ann. Intern. Med. 98 (1983) 76–85.

164. C. Mukhtyar, L. Guillevin, M.C. Cid, et al., EULAR recommendations for the management of primary small and medium vessel vasculitis, Ann. Rheum. Dis. 68 (2009) 310–317.

165. B. Hellmich, O. Flossmann, W.L. Gross, et al., EULAR recommendations for conducting clinical studies and/or clinical trials in systemic vasculitis: focus on anti-neutrophil cytoplasm antibody-associated vasculitis, Ann. Rheum. Dis. 66 (2007) 605–617.

166. K. de Groot, N. Rasmussen, P.A. Bacon, et al., Randomized trial of cyclophosphamide versus methotrexate for induction of remission in early systemic antineutrophil cytoplasmic antibody-associated vasculitis, Arthritis Rheum. 52 (2005) 2461–2469.

167. K. de Groot, L. Harper, D.R. Jayne, et al., Pulse versus daily oral cyclophosphamide for induction of remission in antineutrophil cytoplasmic antibody-associated vasculitis: a randomized trial, Ann. Intern. Med. 150 (2009) 670–680.

168. R.B. Jones, J.W. Tervaert, T. Hauser, et al., Rituximab versus cyclophosphamide in ANCA-associated renal vasculitis, NEJM 363 (2010) 211–220.

175. C. Pagnoux, A. Mahr, M.A. Hamidou, et al., Azathioprine or methotrexate maintenance for ANCA-associated vasculitis, NEJM 359 (2008) 2790–2803.

180. L. Harper, M.D. Morgan, M. Walsh, et al., Pulse versus daily oral cyclophosphamide for induction of remission in ANCA-associated vasculitis: long-term follow-up, Ann. Rheum. Dis. 71 (2012) 955–960.

184. C.A. Langford, C. Talar-Williams, M.C. Sneller, Use of methotrexate and glucocorticoids in the treatment of Wegener's granulomatosis. Long-term renal outcome in patients with glomerulonephritis, Arthritis Rheum. 43 (2000) 1836–1840.

186. U. Schonermarck, W.L. Gross, K. de Groot, Treatment of ANCA-associated vasculitis, Nat. Rev. Nephrol. 10 (2014) 25–36.

187. D. Jayne, N. Rasmussen, K. Andrassy, et al., A randomized trial of maintenance therapy for vasculitis associated with antineutrophil cytoplasmic autoantibodies, N. Engl. J. Med. 349 (2003) 36–44.

213. B.S. Gottlieb, L.C. Miller, N.T. Ilowite, Methotrexate treatment of Wegener granulomatosis in children, J. Pediatr. 129 (1996) 604–607.

217. A.R. Exley, P.A. Bacon, R.A. Luqmani, et al., Development and initial validation of the Vasculitis Damage Index for the standardized clinical assessment of damage in the systemic vasculitides, Arthritis Rheum. 40 (1997) 371–380.

218. R.A. Luqmani, P.A. Bacon, R.J. Moots, et al., Birmingham Vasculitis Activity Score (BVAS) in systemic necrotizing vasculitis, QJM 87 (1994) 671–678.

220. C. Mukhtyar, R. Lee, D. Brown, et al., Modification and validation of the Birmingham Vasculitis Activity Score (version 3), Ann. Rheum. Dis. 68 (2009) 1827–1832.

221. P.A. Merkel, S.Z. Aydin, M. Boers, et al., The OMERACT core set of outcome measures for use in clinical trials of ANCA-associated vasculitis, J. Rheumatol. 38 (2011) 1480–1486.

222. K. Morishita, S.C. Li, E. Muscal, et al., Assessing the performance of the Birmingham Vasculitis Activity Score at diagnosis for children with antineutrophil cytoplasmic antibody-associated vasculitis in A Registry for Childhood Vasculitis (ARChiVe), J. Rheumatol. 39 (2012) 1088–1094.

223. K. Morishita, J. Guzman, P. Chira, et al., Do adult disease severity subclassifications predict use of cyclophosphamide in children with ANCA-associated vasculitis? An analysis of ARChiVe study treatment decisions, J. Rheumatol. 39 (2012) 2012–2020.

224. P. Dolezalova, F.E. Price-Kuehne, S. Ozen, et al., Disease activity assessment in childhood vasculitis: development and preliminary validation of the Paediatric Vasculitis Activity Score (PVAS), Ann. Rheum. Dis. 72 (2013) 1628–1633.

232. J. Robson, H. Doll, R. Suppiah, et al., Damage in the anca-associated vasculitides: long-term data from the European Vasculitis Study group (EUVAS) therapeutic trials, Ann. Rheum. Dis. (2013).

233. N. Arulkumaran, S. Jawad, S.W. Smith, et al., Long-term outcome of paediatric patients with ANCA vasculitis, Pediatr. Rheumatol. Online J. 9 (2011) 12.

237. S. Ozen, N. Ruperto, M.J. Dillon, et al., EULAR/PReS endorsed consensus criteria for the classification of childhood vasculitides, Ann. Rheum. Dis. 65 (2006) 936–941.

263. L. Guillevin, F. Lhote, M. Gayraud, et al., Prognostic factors in polyarteritis nodosa and Churg-Strauss syndrome. A prospective study in 342 patients, Medicine (Baltimore) 75 (1996) 17–28.

264. M. Gayraud, L. Guillevin, P. le Toumelin, et al., Long-term followup of polyarteritis nodosa, microscopic polyangiitis, and Churg-Strauss syndrome: analysis of four prospective trials including 278 patients, Arthritis Rheum. 44 (2001) 666–675.

265. J. Churg, L. Strauss, Allergic granulomatosis, allergic angiitis, and periarteritis nodosa, Am. J. Pathol. 27 (1951) 277–301.

268. C. Comarmond, C. Pagnoux, M. Khellaf, et al., Eosinophilic granulomatosis with polyangiitis (Churg-Strauss): clinical characteristics and long-term followup of the 383 patients enrolled in the French Vasculitis Study Group cohort, Arthritis Rheum. 65 (2013) 270–281.

269. S. Gendelman, A. Zeft, S.J. Spalding, Childhood-onset eosinophilic granulomatosis with polyangiitis (formerly Churg-Strauss syndrome): a contemporary single-center cohort, J. Rheumatol. 40 (2013) 929–935.

270. J. Zwerina, G. Eger, M. Englbrecht, et al., Churg-Strauss syndrome in childhood: a systematic literature review and clinical comparison with adult patients, Semin. Arthritis Rheum. 39 (2009) 108–115.

271. C. Pagnoux, P. Guilpain, L. Guillevin, Churg-Strauss syndrome, Curr. Opin. Rheumatol. 19 (2007) 25–32.

Entire reference list is available online at www.expertconsult.com.

Central Nervous System Vasculitis

Adam Kirton, Susanne M. Benseler

INTRODUCTION

Vasculitis of the vessels of the central nervous system (CNS) may occur as part of a systemic vasculitis, result from infectious or neoplastic disease, metabolic diseases, medication, or radiation therapy,[1] or be restricted to the CNS, so-called primary CNS vasculitis. Calabrese and colleagues first systematically reviewed primary CNS vasculitis in adults, proposed diagnostic criteria, and suggested a clinical approach.[2] In 2001, Lanthier and colleagues described two children with CNS vasculitis and distinguished between small- and large-vessel vasculitis.[3] Gallagher and colleagues described angiographic findings in four children with primary CNS vasculitis.[4] In 2006, Benseler and colleagues described angiographic findings in 62 children with primary CNS vasculitis[5] and 4 children with normal angiographs but histological evidence of small-vessel vasculitis.[6]

This chapter is concerned with primary CNS vasculitis and some of the inflammatory brain diseases that may be important in differential diagnosis.

DEFINITION AND CLASSIFICATION

Primary CNS angiitis is, by definition, inflammation of vessels of the brain that is not associated with vasculitis of any other organ. The diagnosis of childhood-onset primary angiitis of the CNS (cPACNS) is commonly based on the Calabrese criteria proposed for adult PACNS[2] (Table 37-1), modified to include children with predominant psychiatric features or development-related phenotypes.

The classification of cPACNS depends on the size of involved vessels, which determines the presence or absence of angiographic changes (Table 37-2). Small-vessel vasculitis (SV-cPACNS) involves vessels throughout the brain and meninges that are not primary branches of the circle of Willis; large-vessel vasculitis primarily targets major arteries such as the anterior, middle and posterior cerebral arteries, and the vertebral and cerebellar arteries.

EPIDEMIOLOGY

No epidemiological data are available for SV-cPACNS or inflammatory brain diseases in general. An estimated 40% to 60% of arterial ischemic strokes (AIS) in children are thought to be related to CNS vasculitis.[7,8] The incidence of childhood AIS is estimated at 3.3 to 7.9 per 100,000 children per year[9-11] with a male predominance.[12] Boys are more commonly affected with large–medium vessel cPACNS consistent with the male predominance of childhood AIS in general.[5,12] In contrast, small-vessel vasculitis is more commonly seen in females.[6] In the cohort reported by Benseler et al.[5] the mean age at diagnosis was 7.2 years (range 0.7 to 17.6 years).

ETIOLOGY AND GENETIC FACTORS

The trigger for inflammation targeting the cerebral vessels remains unknown. Viral studies have been uniformly uninformative and the histopathology of the affected tissue is nonspecific. No specific genetic associations have been identified in cPACNS, but predisposing immune dysregulations such as complement deficiencies and T-cell killing defects (perforin deficiencies) are shown to be associated with inflammatory brain diseases.[13]

CLINICAL MANIFESTATIONS

Large-Vessel cPACNS

The Toronto series demonstrated that the anterior CNS is most commonly affected by large-vessel cPACNS. One third of children had inflammation of both anterior and posterior vessels. A small subgroup of children had inflammation affecting only the posterior basilar system, and they had progressive disease. Patients within this category appear to be different from those with the previously described nonprogressive posterior circulation vasculopathy that predominantly affected teenage boys.[5] A comparison of the clinical presentation of large- and small-vessel cPACNS is shown in Table 37-3. Children with large/medium vessel cPACNS usually present with focal deficits and headache. They may have fine motor deficit, cranial neuropathies, movement disorders, and other symptoms corresponding to the stenosis of specific cerebral vessels and their vascular distributions. A recent large study of AIS in children supported the belief that inflammatory vessel disease was a leading cause.[14] AIS can take many forms, some of which are described below.

The syndrome of unilateral, large–medium arteriopathy is the leading cause of childhood stroke. A representative example is shown in Fig. 37-1. Common features reported[15-18] include unilateral arteriopathy of the large vessels of the anterior circulation including the distal internal carotid artery and proximal segments of the middle and anterior cerebral arteries, and distinct angiographic appearance with focal, segmental stenosis often with alternating areas of narrowing and dilation with a "banding" or "striated" appearance. Features of other arteriopathies such as dissection or moyamoya are absent. Serial arterial imaging demonstrates fluctuations over days to weeks. This syndrome typically occurs in healthy, school-aged children, and has high recurrence rates and poor outcomes. Indirect evidence that this syndrome is caused by vasculitis includes a temporal association with nonspecific symptoms of infection, and imaging markers such as vessel-wall enhancement.[19] However, definitive evidence of an inflammatory pathophysiology cannot usually be obtained as the affected arteries are not amenable to biopsy and postmortem studies are lacking.

TABLE 37-1 Proposed Diagnostic Criteria for cPACNS

A newly acquired neurological and/or psychiatric deficit PLUS
Angiographic and/or histological evidence of CNS vasculitis in the absence of any systemic condition known to be associated with or mimic CNS vasculitis.

TABLE 37-2 Classification of Childhood Primary Angiitis of the CNS (cPACNS)

CATEGORY	ANGIOGRAPHIC CHARACTERISTICS
Small-vessel cPACNS	Normal
Large-vessel cPACNS	Arterial stenoses, dilations, occlusions
Progressive	New lesions seen 3 months or more after initial imaging
Nonprogressive	No new lesions 3 months or more after initial imaging

TABLE 37-3 Clinical Characteristics at Diagnosis of Large-Vessel and Small-Vessel cPACNS

	LARGE-VESSEL cPACNS ANGIOGRAPHY POSITIVE	SMALL-VESSEL cPACNS ANGIOGRAPHY NEGATIVE
	N = 144	N = 58
Reduced level of consciousness	5%	38%
Focal Deficit		
Hemiparesis	72%	14%
Focal gross motor deficit	88%	22%
Focal fine motor deficit	90%	54%
Gait abnormality	86%	62%
Hemisensory deficit	64%	18%
Language deficit	52%	78%
Cranial nerve deficit	64%	14%
Optic neuritis	0%	10%
Ataxia, chorea, dystonia	14%	17%
Diffuse Deficit		
Cognitive dysfunction	42%	69%
Memory deficit	32%	64%
Behavior abnormality	38%	66%
Concentration deficit	34%	64%
Seizures		
Focal	10%	69%
Generalized	4%	33%
Status epilepticus	0%	24%

Data from Ref. 5.

The syndrome described above closely resembles childhood stroke diagnoses such as transient cerebral arteriopathy (TCA) and focal cerebral arteriopathy (FCA). TCA diagnosis requires angiography (within 3 months) showing unilateral focal or segmental stenosis or occlusion of the distal internal carotid or proximal middle cerebral artery (MCA) and anterior cerebral artery (ACA), and lack of progression at 6 months.[18,20,21] FCA criteria share the same features as those of TCA,[15,16] but do not require determination of progression at 6 months, allowing more immediate diagnosis. Postvaricella angiopathy (PVA) shares many of these features and is discussed below. It is therefore possible that cPACNS, TCA, and FCA represent the same disease or closely related conditions within a spectrum.[5,6] Bilateral large-vessel arteriopathy without collaterals[16] accounts for only 20% of cases of cPACNS,[6,22,23] and may be part of the spectrum with unilateral disease, or may fall within a spectrum of other bilateral arteriopathies such as fibromuscular dysplasia or moyamoya disease,[21] or be difficult to determine.

Progressive large/medium vessel cPACNS is uncommon. Clinical presentation is less acute, typically with longer-standing, nonfocal, diffuse neurological symptoms such as neurocognitive decline, seizures, or headaches. Imaging often reveals multifocal, bilateral parenchymal lesions with multiple, bilateral stenoses of the large vessels on angiography.[5,24] Antemortem tissue diagnosis is not possible due to large intracranial artery involvement. Diagnosis relies on neuroimaging, specifically angiography, which cannot definitively implicate inflammatory pathophysiology or immediately differentiate a progressive from nonprogressive prognosis. Long-term surveillance and outcome studies are required to better understand the natural history and predictors of monophasic versus chronic or progressive forms of large/medium vessel cPACNS.

Small-Vessel cPACNS

Primary angiitis of the small cerebral blood vessels provides more direct pathological evidence of vascular inflammation. Unlike large-vessel disease, direct examination of affected vessels is often possible via brain biopsy; in fact, the diagnostic yield for a diagnostic brain biopsy was 69% in one single-center series.[1,25] Clinical presentations are distinct from typical stroke syndromes that feature acute onset of focal neurological deficits. Small-vessel cPACNS more often develops with more gradual, subacute onset of generalized signs and symptoms including headache, behavioral changes, school failure or cognitive decline, or seizures.[26,27] When stroke occurs, patterns are varied and do not conform to large-vessel territories. Lesions can mimic many other diseases and may include hemorrhage in a small percentage of cases.[28] As magnetic resonance angiography (MRA) or computed tomography angiography (CTA) cannot assess distal arterial branches, such noninvasive arterial imaging is typically normal. Conventional angiography can demonstrate abnormalities in small order arteries but is often normal. Accordingly, small-vessel cPACNS has also been referred to as angiography-negative CNS vasculitis.[24]

With such varied clinical presentations and limited diagnostic tools that are both nonspecific and insensitive, diagnosis of small-vessel cPACNS is often challenging. Original criteria for adult PACNS proposed by Calabrese[2] focused on a very similar small-vessel syndrome. These have therefore been reasonably extrapolated for use in children.[27] The modified pediatric criteria include the following: (1) unexplained acquired neurologic deficits that remain unexplained after thorough evaluation, (2) classic angiographic or histopathological features of CNS angiitis, and (3) absence of systemic vasculitis or other condition explaining or mimicking the angiographic or pathological features.

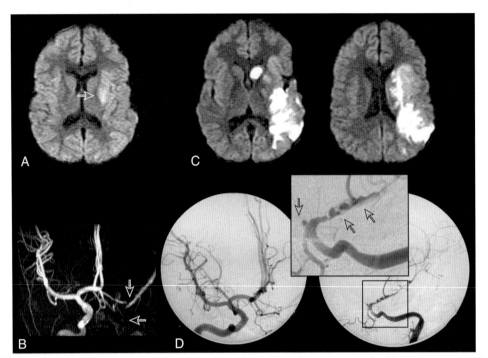

FIGURE 37-1 Large-vessel cPACNS. A healthy 5-year-old child presented with acute onset right hemiparesis. **A,** Diffusion MRI at 6 hours shows restricted diffusion limited to the left putamen. **B,** MRA shows loss of flow in the left ICA and proximal MCA. **C,** Following clinical deterioration with dysphasia and worsening weakness on day 2, repeat diffusion MRI shows new restricted diffusion throughout the MCA territory including the caudate nucleus and frontal, parietal, and temporal lobes. **D,** Conventional angiography (left ICA injection) demonstrates severe irregularity of the distal ICA and proximal MCA with alternating striae or "bands" of narrowing (the right ICA is normal). Years later, the child has moderate hemiparesis, language dysfunction, learning delays, and epilepsy.

DIFFERENTIAL DIAGNOSIS OF CNS VASCULITIS

Large-Vessel Vasculitis

An increasingly complex list of nonvasculitic and nonstroke conditions must be considered in the differential diagnosis of large-vessel CNS vasculitis. Arterial dissection is an important cause of childhood stroke that is often atraumatic and may extend intracranially with imaging features similar to large/medium vessel cPACNS, TCA, or FCA.[29] A recent description of four children with presumed FCA and suspected vasculitis found pathological and wall imaging evidence of intracranial dissection.[30] Additional noninflammatory childhood arteriopathies are increasingly well defined, including moyamoya disease or syndrome,[31] postradiation vasculopathy,[32] and an expanding list of congenital arteriopathies. Unique pediatric forms of fibromuscular dysplasia (FMD) associated with childhood stroke are described, often associated with systemic arteriopathy and renovascular hypertension.[33] Reversible cerebral vasoconstriction syndrome (RCVS; sometimes called Call–Fleming syndrome) has been described in children and may mimic vasculitis.[34]

Small-Vessel Vasculitis

Angiography-negative small-vessel vasculitis has a distinctly different differential diagnosis that has to be carefully, yet promptly, explored before considering invasive diagnostic strategies such as brain biopsy[35,36] (Table 37-4). Many conditions resemble the less specific clinical and imaging presentations of small-vessel cPACNS, including demyelinating diseases (such as acute disseminated encephalomyelitis and multiple sclerosis); other autoimmune disorders such as anti–N-methyl-D-aspartate (anti-NMDA) receptor encephalitis; toxin exposures; inborn errors of metabolism; hypertensive crisis (posterior reversible encephalopathy syndrome); neoplasia including CNS lymphoma; sarcoidosis; and others.[36] An increasing number of autoimmune encephalitides may have similar presentations, but distinguishing features include normal angiography and distinct serum and CNS antibodies and/or brain biopsy pathology.[37]

DIAGNOSTIC WORK UP

A framework for the diagnostic workup of childhood stroke and vasculitis is summarized in Table 37-5. Investigations should be selected from this exhaustive list on the basis of diagnostic probability based on clinical findings.

Clinical Evaluation

Children with cPACNS can show a broad spectrum of focal and diffuse deficits and psychiatric symptoms. A recent study identified clusters of characteristic clinical findings for large- and small-vessel cPACNS.[26] Overall, children with large-vessel cPACNS most commonly display stroke features; headaches are equally common.[5] Progressive disease is frequently associated with constitutional symptoms and diffuse deficits such as cognitive decline, and behavior or personality changes. The most common clinical phenotype of small-vessel disease is seizures or even status epilepticus. Presence of seizures at diagnosis was recently shown to be a risk factor associated with higher disease activity as measured by physician global assessment over time.[38]

TABLE 37-4 Differential Diagnosis of Small-Vessel Primary CNS Vasculitis in Children

CNS Vasculitis Complicating Other Diseases
Infections
- Bacterial *(Mycobacterium tuberculosis, Mycoplasma pneumoniae, Streptococcus pneumoniae)*
- Viral (Epstein–Barr virus, cytomegalovirus, enterovirus, varicella-zoster virus, hepatitis C virus, parvovirus B19, West Nile virus)
- Fungal *(Candida albicans, Actinomyces, Aspergillus)*
- Spirochete *(Borrelia burgdorferi, Treponema pallidum)*

Rheumatic and Inflammatory Diseases
- Systemic vasculitis such as granulomatosis with polyangiitis, microscopic polyangiitis, Henoch–Schönlein purpura, Kawasaki disease, polyarteritis nodosa, Behçet disease
- Systemic lupus erythematosus, juvenile dermatomyositis, morphea
- Inflammatory bowel disease
- Autoinflammatory syndromes
- Hemophagocytic lymphohistiocytosis
- Neurosarcoidosis

Other
- Drug-induced vasculitis
- Malignancy-associated vasculitis

Nonvasculitis Inflammatory Brain Diseases
Demyelinating Diseases
- Multiple sclerosis, acute demyelinating encephalomyelitis (ADEM), optic neuritis, and transverse myelitis

Antibody-Mediated Inflammatory Brain Disease
- Anti-NMDA-receptor encephalitis, neuromyelitis optica (NMO), antibody-associated limbic encephalitis (antibodies against LGI, AMP, AMP-binding protein), Hashimoto encephalopathy, celiac disease and pediatric autoimmune neuropsychiatric disorders associated with streptococcal infections (PANDAS)

T-Cell Associated Inflammatory Brain Disease
- Rasmussen's encephalitis

Other
- Febrile infection-related epilepsy syndrome (FIRES)

Noninflammatory Vasculopathies
- Hemoglobinopathies (sickle cell disease), thromboembolic disease
- Radiation vasculopathy, graft-versus-host disease
- Metabolic and genetic diseases such as cerebral autosomal dominant arteriopathy with subcortical infarcts and leukoencephalopathy (CADASIL), mitochondrial encephalopathy lactic acidosis and strokelike episodes (MELAS)
- Malignancy (lymphoma)

Modified from Ref. 36.

TABLE 37-5 Diagnostic Investigations in Childhood CNS vasculitis

History	Neurological review of systems (focal, headaches, seizures, other)
	Past medical history
	Family history
	Infectious exposures/risk factors for stroke
	History of skin, ophthalmologic, joint involvement, recurrent fevers
Physical examination	Vital signs, peripheral pulses
	General and neurological examinations
	Rheumatologic assessment
	Neuropsychological assessment
Laboratory investigation	*Markers of Inflammation:* CBC, CRP, ESR, IgG, C3, vWF
	Prothrombotic Markers: Protein S, C, antithrombin III, fibrinogen, plasminogen, homocysteine; factor V Leiden, prothrombin gene mutations, lupus anticoagulant
	Autoantibodies: ANA, ENA, dsDNA, ANCA, APL, ACL (depending on the differential diagnosis: NMDAR, VGKC, GAD, GABA)
	Infectious serology: B. burgdorferi, VDRL, HIV, VZV
Lumbar CSF analysis	Opening pressure, cell count, protein, glucose, IgG, oligoclonal bands
	Cryptococcal antigen, VDRL, appropriate viral serology
	Paired serum and CSF B. burgdorferi and VZV serology
	Bacterial, fungal, TB cultures
	Specific autoantibodies depending on the differential diagnosis
Neuroimaging	CT/CTA
	MRI/MRA with gadolinium and vessel wall imaging
	Cerebral angiography
	Brain SPECT
	PET/CT
	Doppler ultrasound
Tissue biopsies	Brain and overlying meninges
	Skin, nerve, muscle as indicated

ACL, Anticardiolipin antibodies; *ANA,* antinuclear antibodies; *ANCA,* antineutrophil cytoplasmic antibodies; *APL,* antiphospholipid antibodies; *C3,* complement component 3; *CBC,* complete blood count; *CRP,* C-reactive protein; *CSF,* cerebrospinal fluid; *CT,* computed tomography; *CTA,* computed tomography angiography; *dsDNA,* double-stranded DNA antibody; *ELISA,* enzyme-linked immunosorbent assay; *ENA,* extractable nuclear antibody; *ESR,* erythrocyte sedimentation rate; *GABA,* γ-aminobutyric acid; *GAD,* glutamate decarboxylase; *HIV,* human immunodeficiency virus; *IgG,* immunoglobulin G; *LAC,* lupus anticoagulant; *MRA,* magnetic resonance angiography; *MRI,* magnetic resonance imaging; *NMDAR,* N-methyl-D-aspartate receptor; *PET,* positron emission tomography; *SPECT,* single-photon emission computed tomography; *TB,* tuberculosis; *VDRL,* Venereal Disease Research Laboratory; *VGKC,* voltage-gated calcium channel; *vWF,* von Willebrand factor; *VZV,* varicella-zoster virus.

Laboratory Investigations

Elevation of inflammatory markers is more common in small-vessel cPACNS and virtually absent in large/medium vessel disease. A single-center, retrospective study of 62 children with cPACNS found elevated erythrocyte sedimentation rates (ESRs) in 51%, elevated C-reactive protein (CRP) levels in 74%, and elevated serum levels of immunoglobulin G (IgG) in 35%.[5] These biomarkers were not associated with outcome or progression. A single-center cohort of 39 patients with cPACNS[39] documented that two thirds of both angiography negative and angiography positive patients had elevated von Willebrand factor (vWF) levels closely correlating with disease activity. Abnormalities in levels of tumor necrosis factor (TNF)-α, interleukin (IL)-2, IL-6, and IL-8[40] may be useful in assessing activity of cPACNS. Antinuclear antibodies are usually absent but variably elevated in a minority of patients[3,4]; antineutrophil cytoplasmic antibodies are absent.

Cerebrospinal Fluid

Cerebrospinal fluid (CSF) analysis can be very informative in the diagnosis of small-vessel cPACNS and the exclusion of many mimics, most notably infection. CSF inflammatory markers such as cell count and protein are typically normal in large/medium cPACNS.[3,4] In contrast, a significant proportion of children with small-vessel disease have mild to moderately elevated cell counts with lymphocyte-predominant pleocytosis or raised protein levels in the CSF.[41] Cytospins may be important in suspected malignancies or CNS manifestations of hemophagocytosis syndromes.[42] Elevated opening pressures and raised CSF protein have been described in both forms of cPACNS.[43,41] The presence of oligoclonal bands supports the intrathecal synthesis of antibodies more suggestive of autoimmune disorders.

Neuroimaging

Modern neuroimaging has revolutionized the ability to diagnose cPACNS. The threshold for magnetic resonance imaging (MRI) imaging of children with possible cPACNS needs to be low. Angiography-negative cases may have distinct parenchymal MRI abnormalities,[5,22,23] including supratentorial, asymmetrical, anterior circulation lesions of the white matter or deep gray structures. The presence of multifocal, bilateral, and gray matter lesions, combined with multiple, bilateral, or distal vessel stenosis are predictors of progressive disease.

Advanced cerebral vascular imaging modalities have increased the sensitivity of detecting childhood arteriopathies. CTA and MRA can confirm and often characterize arteriopathy in most children with large-vessel disease, providing excellent images of first- and second-order cerebral arteries. Conventional angiography can add additional details while helping to exclude other causes such as dissection or moyamoya, and it is safe for children.[44] Vascular imaging features suggesting inflammation and large-vessel vasculitis include stenosis or occlusion without evidence of dissection or chronic arteriopathies. Vessel-wall enhancement on MR angiograms performed with gadolinium is also suggestive of vasculitis. Banding or striae may be unique features of large- or medium-vessel vasculitis (Fig. 37-1). Isolated, alternating areas of stenosis and dilation in very distal arterial beds may rarely be seen in small-vessel cPACNS.

Noninvasive vascular imaging is preferred for ongoing surveillance or syndromes with high recurrence risk. Comparisons of MRA to conventional angiography suggest sensitivity and specificity for known abnormalities were 70% and 98%, respectively.[23] Only 71% of children with abnormal conventional angiography had detectable MRA changes.[23] Conventional angiography is clearly more sensitive and specific than MRA. New vessel wall MRA techniques including high resolution anatomical and blood sensitive sequences may help demonstrate

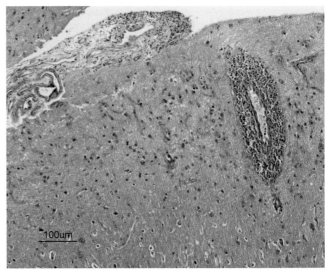

FIGURE 37-2 Elective nonlesional brain biopsy in a 5-year-old child with primary small vessel vasculitis. Masson stain demonstrates intramural and perivascular mononuclear infiltrates in small muscular arteries of the cortical gray matter and the leptomeninges (magnification ×400).

arterial pathology in adult vasculitis.[19,45-48] Such approaches are not yet well described in children. Case reports of FCA suggest possible reversible wall enhancement,[49] although some periarterial enhancement is detected in normal children.[50] It is important to note that without a gold standard diagnostic test for large-vessel vasculitis, there are no validated imaging markers of inflammation in childhood stroke.[51] MRI changes in children with postvaricella CNS vascular complications have been described.[52]

Tissue Pathology

Histological evidence of vascular inflammation is the diagnostic gold standard in small-vessel vasculitis[41] (Fig. 37-2). In this cPACNS subtype, vessel imaging, including conventional angiography, is by definition normal, although brain lesions are commonly identified by MRI. Targeting the biopsy site must balance the benefits of sampling MRI-proven lesions with the relative eloquence of the affected area. It is uncertain if nonlesional biopsies carry a lower diagnostic yield.[41] Biopsies are typically taken from noneloquent areas such as the anterior temporal lobe in the nondominant hemisphere. Leptomeningeal enhancement on MRI is also suggestive of disease and an appropriate site to biopsy. Used properly, brain biopsy has vastly advanced the recognition and understanding of small-vessel, angiography-negative cPACNS,[25] and helped to exclude other diagnoses.[53]

Brain biopsies should be an adequate size ($1 \times 1 \times 2$ cm³), include all layers (meninges, gray and white matter), and processing should include a snap-frozen section for electron microscopy. The biopsy should be obtained within 2 weeks of initiating treatment because long-term and high-dose immunosuppressive therapy confounds the vasculitis-specific histological findings and may impair wound healing after surgery.

Histopathological findings in childhood cPACNS are distinctly different from adult studies. By definition, vasculitis implies direct invasion of one or more layers of the vessel wall by inflammatory cells. In small-vessel cPACNS, a nongranulomatous, lymphocytic infiltration of small vessels is the most typical finding.[16,43] Additional cell populations have been described including macrophages, polymorphonuclear cells, and occasional eosinophils. Microglia activation, often termed *micro-*

glial nodules, is commonly seen in children with long-standing inflammatory disease.

TREATMENT

Hutchinson and colleagues[54] reported the results of a treatment protocol in 19 children with small-vessel cPACNS. Induction therapy over the first 6 months of treatment used a combination of prednisone (beginning at 2 mg/kg/day, maximum 60 mg/day), and intravenous cyclophosphamide (500 to 750 mg/m^2 every 4 weeks for a total of seven infusions, with cotrimoxazole prophylaxis. During the subsequent 18 months, maintenance therapy consisted of continuing tapering of the prednisone dose, mycophenolate mofetil (MMF) (800 to 1200 mg/m^2/day, maximum 2000 mg/day) or azathioprine (2 to 5 mg/kg/day, maximum 150 mg/day). Of the 19 children, 2 failed induction therapy, and 3 were continuing to receive induction therapy at the time of the study. Of the 14 children who completed the induction phase, 9 were maintained on azathioprine, and 5 received MMF. Seven of the children maintained on azathioprine were switched to MMF either because of disease flare (five children) or intolerance of azathioprine (two children). As a result, the authors recommend maintenance therapy with MMF rather than azathioprine. The primary outcome of this study was the pediatric stroke outcome measure (PSOM). At 24 months, PSOM scores in the normal or mild deficit range were observed in 9 of 13 children being evaluated, and moderate or severe deficits were present in 4 children. Sen et al.[55] studied three children with cPACNS whose disease had flared while on maintenance azathioprine or methotrexate and were subsequently treated with MMF with good effect. The use of biologics to treat cPACNS has not been reported, but Salvarani and colleagues reported the successful use of rituximab in an adult with PACNS.[56]

OTHER INFLAMMATORY BRAIN DISEASES

Several inflammatory brain diseases may mimic small-vessel cPACNS.[26]

Infections

Infections with influenza A, parainfluenza, enterovirus, Epstein–Barr virus, varicella zoster, cytomegalovirus, and herpes simplex virus are important viral causes of encephalitis, which may be characterized by altered mental status, seizures or focal neurological signs similar to those seen in small-vessel cPACNS.[57] Mycoplasma pneumoniae upper respiratory tract infection may be followed by rapidly progressive encephalitis characterized by decreased level of consciousness, psychiatric symptoms, and seizures[58]; the MRI typically shows bilateral posterior thalamic lesions.[58] Treatment includes antimicrobial therapy, intravenous immunoglobulin, and/or corticosteroids.[59]

Demyelinating Inflammatory Brain Diseases

The most common demyelinating brain disease in childhood are acute disseminated encephalomyelitis (ADEM), and multiple sclerosis.[26] ADEM is often preceded by a prodrome, and rapidly progresses over hours to weeks. The most common signs are ataxia, cranial nerve palsy hemiparesis, seizures, and impaired consciousness. The course of multiple sclerosis is relapsing and remitting and much more prolonged. It is characterized by long tract signs, optic neuritis, and brain stem dysfunction.

Immunologically Mediated Inflammatory Brain Diseases

Antibodies reacting with *N*-methyl-D-aspartate receptor (NMDAR) are associated with a very distinct disease course.[60-62] Children develop behavioral changes, memory loss, psychosis, orofacial dyskinesia, movement disorders, seizures, alteration of speech leading to mutism, and autonomic dysfunction and hypoventilation if not treated.

McKeon and colleagues reported a syndrome (neuromyelitis optica [NMO]) characterized clinically by optic neuritis (83%), transverse myelitis (78%) and/or episodic encephalopathic signs, ataxia, seizures, and vomiting (45%).[63] All had antibodies to water channel aquaporin 4 (anti-NMO antibodies). MRI studies showed widespread lesions. The presence of anti-NMO antibodies should lead to the consideration of Sjögren syndrome in the differential diagnosis.[64] Treatment with rituximab was reported to reduce the frequency of attacks and improve long-term outcome.[65]

Rasmussen's encephalitis is a T-cell–mediated[66] parenchymal inflammatory brain disease usually appearing in childhood as intractable focal seizures.[67,68] Typically, only one brain hemisphere is involved. The etiology of Rasmussen's encephalitis is unknown. Surgical resection of the affected tissue may be required to halt ongoing seizures.

REFERENCES

1. J. Elbers, S.M. Benseler, Central nervous system vasculitis in children, Curr. Opin. Rheumatol. 20 (2008) 47–54.
2. L.H. Calabrese, A.J. Furlan, L.A. Gragg, T.J. Ropos, Primary angiitis of the central nervous system: diagnostic criteria and clinical approach, Cleve. Clin. J. Med. 59 (1992) 293–306.
3. S. Lanthier, A. Lortie, J. Michaud, et al., Isolated angiitis of the CNS in children, Neurology 56 (2001) 837–842.
4. K.T. Gallagher, B. Shaham, A. Reiff, et al., Primary angiitis of the central nervous system in children: 5 cases, J. Rheumatol. 28 (2001) 616–623.
5. S.M. Benseler, E. Silverman, R.I. Aviv, et al., Primary central nervous system vasculitis in children, Arthritis Rheum. 54 (2006) 1291–1297.
6. S.M. Benseler, G. deVeber, C. Hawkins, et al., Angiography-negative primary central nervous system vasculitis in children: a newly recognized inflammatory central nervous system disease, Arthritis Rheum. 52 (2005) 2159–2167.
7. R. Askalan, S. Laughlin, S. Mayank, et al., Chickenpox and stroke in childhood: a study of frequency and causation, Stroke 32 (2001) 1257–1262.
8. H. Fullerton, J.K. Lynch, G. deVeber, The call for multicenter studies of pediatric stroke, Stroke 37 (2006) 330–331.
9. G. deVeber, E.S. Roach, A.R. Riela, et al., Stroke in children: recognition, treatment and future directions, Semin. Pediatr. Neurol. 7 (2000) 309–317.
10. M. Giroud, M. Lemesle, J.B. Gouyon, et al., Cerebrovascular disease in children under 16 years of age in the city of Dijon France: a study of incidence and clinical features from 1985-1993, J. Clin. Epidemiol. 48 (1995) 1343–1348.
11. J.K. Lynch, D.G. Hirtz, G. deVeber, et al., Report of the National Institute of Neurological Disorders and Stroke workshop on perinatal and childhood stroke, Pediatrics 109 (2002) 116–123.
13. D. Moshous, O. Feyen, P. Lankisch, et al., Primary necrotizing lymphocytic central nervous system vasculitis due to perforin deficiency in a four-year-old girl, Arthritis Rheum. 56 (2007) 995–999.
14. M.T. Mackay, M. Wiznitzer, S.L. Benedict, et al., Arterial ischemic stroke risk factors: the international pediatric stroke study, Ann. Neurol. 69 (2011) 130–140.
15. C. Amlie-Lefond, T.J. Bernard, G. Sébire, et al., Predictors of cerebral arteriopathy in children with arterial ischemic stroke: results of the International Pediatric Stroke Study, Circulation 119 (2009) 1417–1423.
16. T.J. Bernard, M.J. Manco-Johnson, W. Lo, et al., Towards a consensus-based classification of childhood arterial ischemic stroke, Stroke 43 (2012) 371–377.
17. A. Mineyko, A. Kirton, Mechanisms of pediatric cerebral arteriopathy: an inflammatory debate, Pediatr. Neurol. 48 (2013) 14–23.
18. G. Sébire, H. Fullerton, E. Riou, G. deVeber, Toward the definition of cerebral arteriopathies of childhood, Curr. Opin. Pediatr. 16 (2004) 617–622.

19. W. Küker, S. Gaertner, T. Nagele, et al., Vessel wall contrast enhancement: a diagnostic sign of cerebral vasculitis, Cerebrovasc. Dis. 26 (2008) 23–29.

20. S. Chabrier, G. Rodesch, P. Lasjaunias, et al., Transient cerebral arteriopathy: a disorder recognized by serial angiograms in children with stroke, J. Child Neurol. 13 (1998) 27–32.

21. K.P. Braun, M.M. Bulder, S. Chabrier, et al., The course and outcome of unilateral intracranial arteriopathy in 79 children with ischaemic stroke, Brain 132 (Pt 2) (2009) 544–557.

22. D. Eleftheriou, T. Cox, D. Saunders, et al., Investigation of childhood central nervous system vasculitis: magnetic resonance angiography versus catheter cerebral angiography, Dev. Med. Child Neurol. 52 (2010) 863–867.

23. R.I. Aviv, S.M. Benseler, G. DeVeber, et al., Angiography of primary central nervous system angiitis of childhood: conventional angiography versus magnetic resonance angiography at presentation, AJNR Am. J. Neuroradiol. 28 (2007) 9–15.

24. T. Cellucci, S.M. Benseler, Central nervous system vasculitis in children, Curr. Opin. Rheumatol. 22 (2010) 590–597.

25. S. Venkateswaran, C. Hawkins, E. Wassmer, Diagnostic yield of brain biopsies in children presenting to neurology, J. Child Neurol. 23 (2008) 253–258.

26. T. Cellucci, P.N. Tyrrell, M. Twilt, et al., Distinct phenotypic clusters in childhood inflammatory brain diseases: implications for diagnostic evaluation, Arthritis Rheum. 66 (2014) 750–756.

27. M. Twilt, S.M. Benseler, The spectrum of CNS vasculitis in children and adults, Nat. Rev. Rheumatol. 8 (2011) 97–107.

28. K. Pistracher, V. Gellner, S. Riegler, et al., Cerebral haemorrhage in the presence of primary childhood central nervous system vasculitis—a review, Childs Nerv. Syst. 28 (2012) 1141–1148.

31. R.M. Scott, E.R. Smith, Moyamoya disease and moyamoya syndrome, N. Engl. J. Med. 360 (2009) 1226–1237.

32. M. Omura, N. Aida, K. Sekido, et al., Large intracranial vessel occlusive vasculopathy after radiation therapy in children: clinical features and usefulness of magnetic resonance imaging, Int. J. Radiat. Oncol. Biol. Phys. 38 (1997) 241–249.

33. A. Kirton, M. Crone, S. Benseler, et al., Fibromuscular dysplasia and childhood stroke, Brain 136 (2013) 1846–1856.

35. M. Twilt, S.M. Benseler, Childhood inflammatory brain diseases: pathogenesis, diagnosis and therapy, Rheumatology 53 (2014) 1359–1368.

36. P. Gowdie, M. Twilt, S.M. Benseler, Primary and secondary central nervous system vasculitis, J. Child Neurol. 27 (2012) 1448–1459.

38. T. Cellucci, P.N. Tyrrell, S. Sheikh, S.M. Benseler, Childhood primary angiitis of the central nervous system: identifying disease trajectories and early risk factors for persistently higher disease activity, Arthritis Rheum. 64 (2012) 1665–1672.

39. T. Cellucci, P.N. Tyrrell, E. Pullenayegum, S.M. Benseler, von Willebrand factor antigen–a possible biomarker of disease activity in childhood central nervous system vasculitis?, Rheumatology (Oxford) 51 (2012) 1838–1845.

40. D. Yürürer, S. Teber, G. Deda, et al., The relation between cytokines, soluble endothelial protein C receptor, and factor VIII levels in Turkish pediatric stroke patients, Clin. Appl. Thromb. Hemost 15 (2009) 545–551.

41. J. Elbers, W. Halliday, C. Hawkins, et al., Brain biopsy in children with primary small-vessel central nervous system vasculitis, Ann. Neurol. 68 (2010) 602–610.

42. K. Deiva, N. Mahlaoui, F. Beaudonnet, et al., CNS involvement at the onset of primary hemophagocytic lymphohistiocytosis, Neurology 78 (2012) 1150–1156.

43. R. Yaari, I.A. Anselm, I.S. Szer, et al., Childhood primary angiitis of the central nervous system: two biopsy-proven cases, J. Pediatr. 145 (2004) 693–697.

44. I.M. Burger, K.J. Murphy, L.C. Jordan, et al., Safety of cerebral digital subtraction angiography in children: complication rate analysis in 241 consecutive diagnostic angiograms, Stroke 37 (2006) 2535–2539.

45. W. Küker, Cerebral vasculitis: imaging signs revisited, Neuroradiology 49 (2007) 471–479.

46. W. Küker, Imaging of cerebral vasculitis, Int. J. Stroke 2 (2007) 184–190.

47. S. Aoki, N. Hayashi, O. Abe, et al., Radiation-induced arteritis: thickened wall with prominent enhancement on cranial MR images report of five cases and comparison with 18 cases of Moyamoya disease, Radiology 223 (2002) 683–688.

48. R.H. Swartz, S.S. Bhuta, R.I. Farb, et al., Intracranial arterial wall imaging using high-resolution 3-tesla contrast-enhanced MRI, Neurology 72 (2009) 627–634.

49. E.T. Payne, X.C. Wei, A. Kirton, Reversible wall enhancement in pediatric cerebral arteriopathy, Can. J. Neurol. Sci. 38 (2011) 139–140.

50. A. Mineyko, A. Kirton, D. Ng, X.C. Wei, Normal intracranial periarterial enhancement on pediatric brain MR imaging, Neuroradiology 55 (2013) 1161–1169.

51. A. Mineyko, A. Narendran, M.L. Fritzler, et al., Inflammatory biomarkers of pediatric focal cerebral arteriopathy, Neurology 79 (2012) 1406–1408.

52. G. Chiang, T. Panyaping, G. Tedesqui, et al., Varicella zoster CNS complications. A report of four cases and review of the literature, Neuroradiol. J. 27 (2014) 327–333.

53. J.T. Lie, Malignant angioendotheliomatosis (intravascular lymphomatosis) clinically simulating primary angiitis of the central nervous system, Arthritis Rheum. 35 (1992) 831–834.

54. C. Hutchinson, J. Elbers, W. Halliday, et al., Treatment of small vessel primary CNS vasculitis in children: an open label cohort study, Lancet Neurol. 9 (2010) 1078–1084.

55. E.S. Sen, V. Leone, N. Abinun, et al., Treatment of primary angiitis of the central nervous system in childhood with mycophenolate mofetil, Rheumatology 49 (2010) 806–811.

56. C. Salvarani, R.D. Brown Jr., J. Huston 3rd, et al., Treatment of primary CNS vasculitis with ritiximab: case report, Neurology 82 (2014) 1287–1288.

58. L.J. Christie, S. Honarmand, D.F. Talkington, et al., Pediatric encephalitis: what is the role of Mycoplasma pneumoniae?, Pediatrics 120 (2007) 305–313.

59. F. Daxboeck, A. Blacky, R. Seidl, et al., Diagnosis, treatment, and prognosis of Mycoplasma pneumoniae childhood encephalitis: systematic review of 58 cases, J. Child Neurol. 19 (2004) 865–871.

60. J. Dalmau, A.J. Gleichman, E.G. Hughes, et al., Anti-NMDA-receptor encephalitis: case series and analysis of the effects of antibodies, Lancet Neurol. 7 (2008) 1091–1098.

61. N. Luca, T. Daengsuwan, J. Dalmau, et al., Anti-N-methyl-D-aspartate receptor encephalitis: a newly recognized inflammatory brain disease in children, Arthritis Rheum. 63 (2011) 2516–2522.

62. M.J. Titulaer, L. McCracken, I. Gabilondo, et al., Treatment and prognostic factors for long-term outcome in patients with anti-NMDA receptor encephalitis: an observational cohort study, Lancet Neurol. 12 (2013) 157–165.

63. A. McKeon, V.A. Lennon, T. Lotze, et al., CNS aquaporin-4 autoimmunity in children, Neurology 71 (2008) 93–100.

64. M. Morreale, P. Marchione, P. Giacomini, et al., Neurological involvement in primary Sjögren syndrome. A focus on central nervous system, PLoS ONE 9 (2014) e84605.

65. A. Jacob, B.G. Weinshenker, I. Violich, et al., Treatment of neuromyelitis optica with rituximab: retrospective analysis of 25 patients, Arch. Neuro. 65 (2008) 1443–1448.

67. T. Rasmussen, J. Olszewski, D. Lloydsmith, Focal seizures due to chronic localized encephalitis, Neurology 8 (1958) 435–445.

68. C.G. Bien, H. Widman, H. Urbach, et al., The natural history of Rasmussen's encephalitis, Brain 125 (2002) 1751–1759.

Entire reference list is available online at www.expertconsult.com.

CHAPTER 38

Other Vasculitis

Philip J. Hashkes

COGAN SYNDROME

Cogan syndrome was first described in 1945 by Dr. David Cogan, an ophthalmologist, who described four patients who developed near simultaneously interstitial keratitis and vestibular-auditory symptoms, which led to deafness in three women.[1] Later reports, in particular a series of 60 patients seen at the Mayo Clinic,[2] widened the scope of this syndrome to include features of systemic and large-vessel vasculitis with classic and atypical presentations. There are reports on about 30 pediatric cases with a maximum of 3 from individual centers,[3-24] of which 23 were summarized in 2012.[3]

There is no formal definition or classification of this syndrome. Historically, classic cases were defined as patients with interstitial keratitis who developed both ocular and vestibular-auditory symptoms within 2 years. Patients with ophthalmological manifestations other than interstitial keratitis or with more than 2 years between the development of ocular and vestibular-auditory symptoms were considered to have "atypical" syndrome. Signs of large-vessel vasculitis, particularly of the proximal aorta and aortic valve insufficiency, were also considered "atypical."

Most cases occur in young adulthood with rare cases in childhood. The median onset in childhood is approximately 11 years of age, with the youngest reported case at 6 months of age.[3,15] Nearly two thirds of childhood cases are in males, whereas in adults there is no gender predilection. In adults there is no ethnic predilection. Familial cases are rare. Adult series reported human leukocyte antigen (HLA) associations with A9, Bx17, Bw35, and Cw4.[25]

The etiology is unknown. However, similarities to syphilitic keratitis have led to searches for infectious etiologies. Studies from the National Institutes of Health (NIH) found serologic evidence for infection by *Chlamydia trachomatis* in many patients, but this has not been replicated by other investigators. Other investigated organisms included other species of *Chlamydia* and *Borrelia burgdoferi*. The Mayo Clinic series found that smoking rates among patients were twice that of the general population.[2]

The pathogenesis is considered to be autoimmune. Usually relatively protected from the immune system, the eye and inner ear may develop an immune response to various undetermined insults resulting in T- and B-lymphocyte activation and the formation of autoantibodies. However, most adult studies did not find evidence of autoantibody formation to antigens of the inner ear, including to 68 kDa, frequently found in idiopathic progressive bilateral sensorineural hearing loss.[26,27] Other adult studies found in some patients with Cogan syndrome antibodies to the density-enhanced protein tyrosine phosphatase 1 (DEP-1) expressed on endothelial cells, which has a peptide with partial homology to the SS-A antigen.[26]

No specific pathology has been found in eye and inner ear structures. Large-vessel vasculitis resembles that of Takayasu's arteritis and polyarteritis nodosa.

Clinical Manifestations

Often the disease onset is preceded by an infection, most commonly an upper respiratory infection. There does not appear to be significant differences between adult and childhood disease. The median time from onset to diagnosis is about 8 months. Table 38-1 details the proportion of children with ocular, vestibular-auditory, musculoskeletal, and systemic symptoms at onset and at follow-up.[3-24] Signs of large-vessel vasculitis, particularly proximal aortitis and aortic valve insufficiency, are present in 10% to 15% of children.

More than 50% of the children have multisystem disease with approximately 25% of cases involving two systems; in approximately 20% of the cases, only one system is involved. The interval between development of ocular and vestibular-auditory symptoms is generally less than 2 years. However, several children were already deaf by the time ocular symptoms started.

Investigations

Acute phase reactants are usually elevated but can be normal in patients with isolated ocular and vestibular-auditory disease. Autoantibodies are usually negative, but in a few patients antiphospholipid antibodies and antineutrophil cytoplasmic antibodies may be found, the latter in a perinuclear pattern. Repeated audiometry testing is crucial, with hearing loss noted initially in the high and low frequencies, similar to Ménière's syndrome. Brain stem auditory evoked potentials are abnormal in advanced disease.

Echocardiography may demonstrate aortic valve insufficiency with thickening and proximal aortitis. Inner ear magnetic resonance imaging (MRI) with gadolinium may show cochlear enhancement. Proximal aorta MRI is useful to search for evidence of aortitis. Calcific obliteration of cochlear and vestibular structures can be found in computed tomography.

Differential Diagnosis

The association of interstitial keratitis with vestibular-auditory inflammatory disease can be seen in many other conditions. Infections include *Chlamydia*, Lyme disease,[10] and congenital syphilis. Inflammatory diseases include sarcoidosis, polyangiitis with granulomatosis, relapsing polychondritis, Behçet disease, Sjögren syndrome, Susac syndrome, and antiphospholipid antibody syndrome. Other conditions include lymphoma, Vogt–Kouangi–Harada syndrome, mitochondrial cytopathies, and Whipple disease.

TABLE 38-1 Features of Pediatric Cogan Syndrome (N = 30 cases)

	ONSET	LAST FOLLOW-UP
Median age (years)	10.5 (range 0.5-18)	12.5 (range 1-16)
Systemic features	12 (40%)	0
Musculoskeletal symptoms	13 (43.3%)	0
Ocular	28 (93.3%)	3 (10%)
Interstitial keratitis	17 (56.7%)	1 (3.3%)
Uveitis	7 (23.3%)	1 (3.3%)
Conjunctivitis/episcleritis	6 (20%)	1 (3.3%)
Vestibular/auditory	21 (70%)	14 (46.7%)
Vertigo/nausea/dizziness	10 (33.3%)	1 (3.3%)
Sensorineural hearing loss	14 (46.7%)	4 (13.3%)
Deafness	2 (6.7%)	7 (23.3%)
Tinnitus/hyperacusia	8 (26.7%)	2 (6.7%)
Cardiovascular	4 (13.3%)	4 (13.3%)

Other manifestations: rash, 3 (10%); abdominal/chest pain, 3 (10%); splenomegaly, 2 (6.7%); liver dysfunction, 2 (6.7%).

Treatment and Outcome

There are no controlled therapeutic trials. However, early diagnosis and institution of high-dose corticosteroids (between 1 and 2 mg/kg/day) is crucial to save hearing or prevent further loss of hearing.[2,15] It is often hard to wean corticosteroids, and steroid-sparing medications are often necessary, methotrexate being the most commonly used in children.[3,17] Other options used in children include mycophenolate mofetil, leflunomide, azathioprine, cyclosporine A, and cyclophosphamide (the latter mainly in cases of large-vessel vasculitis).[9,19,20] In adults anti-tumor necrosis factor (TNF) agents have been used with some success.[28] Ocular corticosteroid drops are commonly used. Cochlear implants are beneficial in patients with established deafness.[3,21]

Only about 30% patients achieve complete, damage-free remission. Ocular outcomes are usually excellent with rare permanent damage. However, permanent partial hearing loss or deafness residua occur in nearly 50% of childhood cases. Delayed diagnosis of more than 2 months was the most important factor related to a poor outcome in pediatric cases.[3] Aortic valve damage is usually not reversible, although it rarely leads to the need for surgical replacement. Only one case of death, from subarachnoid hemorrhage, was seen in childhood cases.[3]

IMMUNE COMPLEX SMALL-VESSEL VASCULITIS

Antiglomerular Basement Membrane Disease

Antiglomerular basement membrane (GBM) disease, formerly called Goodpasture syndrome, is one of the pulmonary-renal syndromes[29] resulting from antibodies to the non-collagenous-1 (NC1) domain alpha 3 chain of type IV collagen in alveolar and glomerular basement membranes.[30]

Clinically and histologically the disease is similar to microscopic polyangiitis (see Chapter 36).[29] Overlap cases with both anti-GBM and perinuclear antineutrophil cytoplasmic antibodies (pANCAs) with specificity for myeloperoxidase have been reported in children, with a worse prognosis than isolated anti-GBM disease.[31] Immunofluorescence demonstrating a linear deposition of IgG along the capillary basement membrane can differentiate between the two conditions.

This disease predominantly affects young men and has been reported in approximately 25 children and adolescents.[29,32-40] Anti-GBM disease has occurred after therapy with D-penicillamine, in cases of heavy metal and hydrocarbon exposure, and in patients with a variety of rheumatic diseases.[39]

Treatment includes corticosteroids, plasmapheresis, and immunosuppressive agents.[32,34,41-43] Recently, rituximab has shown promise.[44] The survival rate is about 90%, but many children progress to end-stage renal disease. In children, the disease is almost always monophasic.[32,34,40]

CRYOGLOBULINEMIC VASCULITIS

This disease is defined by the Chapel Hill Consensus Conference as vasculitis with immune deposits in capillaries, venules, or arterioles of the skin and kidney associated with cryoglobulins in the serum.[45] The two types of cryoglobulins seen in children are type II (monoclonal immunoglobulin M [IgM] rheumatoid factor [RF]) and type III (polyclonal IgM RF). Clinically, both resemble other forms of leukocytoclastic vasculitis.[45,46] The most common and earliest manifestation is distal extremity purpura (>75%), often precipitated by exposure to cold, which can lead to ulceration. Other manifestations include musculoskeletal disease, more arthralgia (~67%) than frank arthritis (~10%),[47] polyneuropathy, Raynaud phenomenon, and liver enzyme abnormalities. Renal involvement with hypertension occurs later in the disease course (~50%), mainly in the form of membranoproliferative glomerulonephritis.[48,49]

Laboratory findings include low C4 levels and positive RF (both >65%), hematuria, proteinuria, and mixed type II or III cryoglobulins in the serum. Pathology shows leukocytoclastic vasculitis with deposits of IgM, IgG, and complement seen by immunofluorescence.[50]

Cryoglobulinemic vasculitis is rare in children.[49,51-55] In one series (n = 18), children had a significantly higher prevalence of prolonged fever, arthralgia, arthritis, and cutaneous involvement compared with adults.[51] The etiology is primarily secondary to hepatitis C infection (see below).[50,56] Hepatitis B, chronic salmonella infections, and other conditions such as DiGeorge syndrome, sickle-cell anemia, thalassemia, and even Henoch–Schönlein purpura (HSP) have been associated with childhood cryoglobulinemia.[48,57-60] One case of symptomatic cryoglobulinemia in an infant was related to transplacental transmission.[61] Traditional treatment includes combinations of corticosteroids, cyclophosphamide, plasmapheresis, and intravenous immunoglobulin (IVIG).[62,63] Recently, the efficacy of rituximab has been demonstrated.[64,65] Progressive renal disease is the principal cause of long-term morbidity.[45]

Cryofibrinogenemia, secondary to infection or in one instance occurring in three family members, can cause similar clinical and pathological phenomena to cryoglobulinemia.[66-68]

URTICARIAL VASCULITIS

Urticarial vasculitis (UV) should be suspected in children with individual lesions lasting in one location for 24 hours or longer, with associated purpura, fever, arthralgia/arthritis, and glomerulonephitis.[69-72] UV is a very rare cause of chronic urticaria in children (<1%).[73] It can present with normal[72,74] or decreased complement levels (hypocomplementemic).

Hypocomplementemic UV (HUV), first described in the 1970s,[69] tends to be more severe than normocomplementemic UV.[72,75] Diagnostic criteria include recurrent urticaria and low complement levels as major criteria and at least two minor criteria, including demonstration of venulitis on skin biopsy, arthritis, ocular inflammation, abdominal

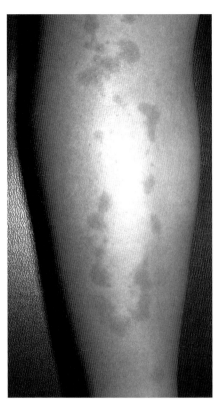

FIGURE 38-1 Linear bands of urticarial lesions in a 6-year-old girl with hypocomplementemic urticarial vasculitis. These lesions were transient and recurrent.

pain, positive C1q antibodies, and glomerulonephritis.[72] Positive antinuclear antibody (ANA) and double-stranded DNA antibodies are exclusion criteria.

UV occurs mostly in girls at all ages and can even occur in infants.[75-87] Children have recurrent episodes of urticaria associated more with a burning sensation than pruritus. The urticaria resolves over 2 to 4 days, leaving residual pigmentation (Fig. 38-1).[71,72] Other skin lesions include purpura, papules, and vesicles. Fever, nausea, vomiting, and abdominal pain may accompany cutaneous exacerbations (~25%). Arthralgias occur in approximately 60% of patients, and arthritis, usually of small joints, in approximately 30%. Arthritis episodes are short with no long-term residua. Pulmonary disease (e.g., cough, dyspnea, hemoptysis) occurs in approximately 30% of patients and clinical glomerulonephritis in approximately 15%. Less commonly, uveitis and episcleritis, fever, angioedema, Raynaud phenomenon, pseudotumor cerebri, and seizures are seen. In children, rapidly progressive glomerulonephritis and pulmonary hemorrhage have been described.[75,77,78,83,84]

HUV has been associated with systemic lupus erythematosus (SLE),[74,81,88,89] Sjögren syndrome, hepatitis B and C antigenemia (cryoglobulinemia), drug reactions, and excessive exposure to sun.[90] In fact, many patients subsequently develop full-blown SLE.

The pathogenesis of this condition is thought to result from the binding of IgG C1q antibodies to immune complexes with activation of the classic complement pathway.[88] Levels of C3, C4, and C1q are reduced in 18% to 50% of patients; the complement level often parallels the severity of the disease.[88] In two Turkish families with an autosomal recessive inheritance pattern, loss of function mutations in *DNASE1L3* (deoxyribonuclease 1-like 3), a protein coding gene, were the cause of HUV.[91] Skin biopsy documents a leukocytoclastic vasculitis, predominantly venulitis, with the deposition of IgM and C3 in

affected vessels.[71,74,90] Various types of renal lesions including mesangial, focal, membranoproliferative, and membranous glomerulonephritis are seen in approximately 50% of children.

Management consists of supportive measures and treatment of any associated disorders. Antihistamines, dapsone, hydroxychloroquine, colchicine, and indomethacin have been used with variable success.[71,92] Corticosteroids, IVIG, or other immunosuppressive drugs may be required in children with severe disease, especially those with crescentic glomerulonephritis.[93] The course of the disease depends on the associated disorders and extent of systemic involvement.

Normocomplementemic UV can also accompany other forms of vasculitis (for example, early HSP) and can be seen as part of neutrophilic urticaria such as the cryopyrin-associated periodic syndromes and Schnitzler syndrome.

VASCULITIS ASSOCIATED WITH SYSTEMIC DISEASE

Vasculitis may occur as part of systemic inflammatory diseases, mainly due to immune complex deposition, but also in part a result of accelerated atherosclerosis related to vascular inflammation.

Vasculitis in Juvenile Idiopathic Arthritis

Small- and medium-sized vessel vasculitis, first described in children and adolescents by Ansell in 1978,[94] is a rare phenomenon in patients with RF-positive polyarthritis juvenile idiopathic arthritis (JIA) and is associated with a poor prognosis. The most common findings are nailfold and digital cutaneous vasculitis, representing microinfarctions.[94,95] Digital and leg ulcers, scleritis, keratitis, mononeuritis multiplex, and aortic valve insufficiency are among other features.[95] The prevalence of this complication appears to have decreased dramatically, perhaps due to earlier aggressive therapy. Long-standing ankylosing spondylitis (almost always in adulthood) is associated with proximal aortitis with valve insufficiency.

Vasculitis Related to Systemic Lupus Erythematosus and Other Systemic Autoimmune Diseases

Leukocytoclastic vasculitis may occur in SLE, and present as palpable purpura, nodules, punctuate erythema, urticaria, livedo reticularis, panniculitis, and chilblains/pernio (see below).[96-99] Ulcerative skin lesions tend to be painful and are most frequently found on fingers or toes. Resistant ulcers have been associated with complement deficiencies.[81,100] Vasculitis can be the cause of several of the severe and life-threatening features related to SLE, especially central nervous system involvement (see Chapter 23). In dermatomyositis and scleroderma, fibroproliferative and thrombotic vasculopathy, rather than vasculitis, are the hallmarks of vascular involvement and the base for Raynaud phenomenon. Skin ulcers and gastrointestinal involvement in dermatomyositis and renal/pulmonary artery involvement in scleroderma indicate a poor prognosis (see Chapters 26 and 27).[101] Sarcoidosis is also associated with vasculitis (all vessel sizes), particularly in patients with central nervous system, aorta, and renal vessel involvement.[102] A variety of skin lesions are seen in sarcoidosis, including leukocytoclastic vasculitis (see Chapter 39).[102]

Familial Mediterranean Fever and Vasculitis

Approximately 5% to 7% of patients with familial Mediterranean fever (FMF) develop HSP, often prior to the development of classic FMF attacks (see Chapter 47). Ten percent of HSP patients in ethnic groups with high prevalence of FMF were found to have asymptomatic

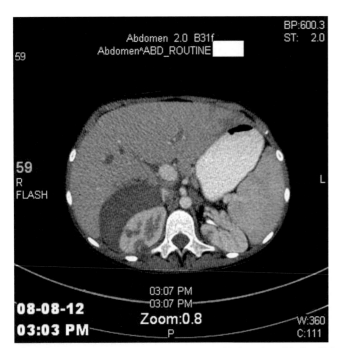

FIGURE 38-2 Abdominal CT of a 12-year-old female with familial Mediterranean fever (FMF) showing bilateral renal infarcts and right perinephric hematoma, characteristic of FMF-related polyarteritis nodosa.

homozygous mutations in the *MEFV* gene and 17% to 34% had heterozygote mutations.[103,104] The course of HSP in FMF patients is more "inflammatory," with higher fever and inflammatory markers, than idiopathic HSP.

Polyarteritis nodosa (PAN) is also more common among patients with FMF, especially in children.[103,105-108] Perinephric hematoma is a characteristic finding (Fig. 38-2). The course of PAN is usually milder than in idiopathic disease.[106]

Paraneoplastic Vasculitis

Lymphoproliferative disease is rarely (1% to 3%) accompanied by a paraneoplastic vasculitis, within 12 months of onset.[109] The most common type (45% to 60%) is leukocytoclastic vasculitis of the skin with arthralgia/arthritis. There are rare cases of PAN, granulomatosis with polyarteritis, Sjögren syndrome, and HSP. Occasionally, vasculitis precedes the diagnosis or can be the first sign of a relapse. Treatment is aimed primarily at the malignancy with careful use of corticosteroids. Lymphocytic lymphoma and Waldenström macroglobulinemia, both rare in children, can result in a cryoglobulinemic vasculitis (the latter type I).[109] Atrial myxoma can mimic vasculitis, through systemic symptoms and emboli dissemination.[110-112] Leukemia vasculitis is a result of direct invasion of dermal blood vessels.

VASCULITIS ASSOCIATED WITH PROBABLE ETIOLOGY

Viral-Induced Vasculitis

The various types of viral-induced vasculitis are summarized in Ref. 113.

Hepatitis B Virus

Shortly before the icteric phase of hepatitis B, 5% to 15% of patients develop an immune complex small-vessel vasculitis. Features include fever, a polymorphic rash (purpura, urticaria, maculopapular rash),

symmetric and predominantly small-joint arthritis, myalgia, and nephritis.[114-117] Low levels of C3, C4 (~40%), and RF (~25%) can be found. The presence of liver enzyme abnormalities, hepatitis B surface antigen (HBsAg) and IgM anti-hepatitis B core (HBc) antibodies is diagnostic. These features self-remit without specific treatment within 2 to 3 weeks, with the appearance of jaundice.

Hepatitis B–related PAN is extremely rare in childhood.[117] PAN usually occurs during the first year after infection and has a similar presentation to idiopathic disease but perhaps a more severe course.[116,118] Treatment consists of combined antiviral and immunosuppressive medications.[116-118] The disease is usually monophasic for those that attain remission.[118]

Hepatitis C Virus Cryoglobulinemic Vasculitis

Cryoglobulins are found in 40% to 50% of patients with hepatitis C, although cryoglobulinemic vasculitis, is seen in less than 5% of patients. However, hepatitis C infection is responsible for 80% to 90% of cases of cryoglobulinemic vasculitis. Clinical and laboratory manifestations are similar to other causes of cryoglobulinemic vasculitis (see above).[45,56,119-123]

Treatment of mild disease includes combination of antiviral therapy with low-dose corticosteroids.[124] In severe disease plasmapheresis, cyclophosphamide and rituximab are added to corticosteroids.[124] Recent data suggest that rituximab as monotherapy or in combination with antiviral therapy may lead to complete remission in more than 60% of cases.[125] Interferon-α use should be delayed in severe disease as it may initially worsen vasculitis.[124]

Other Viruses

Parvovirus B19 is associated with a small-vessel vasculitis that occurs during the second phase of an acute infection.[126-129] Clinical features include fever, purpuric rash and polyarthritis. Resolution of symptoms usually occurs within days to few weeks. IVIG has been beneficial in persistent cases.

Vasculitis has been reported in 1% to 2% of infections with human immunodeficiency virus (HIV) type 1.[130] The most common presentation is a PAN-like disease. Rarely HIV-related vasculitis presents as leukocytoclastic, large vessel, central nervous system (CNS), or Kawasaki disease.[130-132] In one series, 33% of cases of adult Kawasaki disease were associated with HIV.[131] Immunosuppressive treatment should be as "light" and short as possible and needs to be coordinated with HIV specialists.

Varicella-zoster (VZ) infection of the face and neck has been associated with medium to large-vessel CNS vasculitis 4 to 6 weeks following infection.[133-135] The estimated prevalence in children is 1 in 6500. Ipsilateral involvement of the carotid, anterior, and middle cerebral arteries is most common. The disease is usually monophasic but recurrent or progressive cases have been described. VZ is one of the most common causes of acute retinal vasculitis.[136] Purpura fulminans is a form of vasculitis associated with severe varicella infection.[137-139] Rare cases of vasculitis related to hepatitis A, influenza A, cytomegalovirus, Epstein-Barr virus and herpes simplex virus have been reported, some in immunocompromised patients.[113,140-144]

OTHER INFECTIONS

Bacterial infections can cause vasculitis either as part of the infection, secondary to sepsis or as a postinfectious immune complex process.[145-148]

The most common is related to *Neisseria* infections. Isolated infected vesicular and purpura lesions, occasionally leading to bullae and ulceration are seen in the early phase of gonococcal infections.

These usually occur on the volar aspect of the wrists but can occur elsewhere. Widespread purpura is seen both in acute and chronic (the latter most commonly seen in Australia) meningococcal infections.[149,150] An immune complex vasculitis including purpura, arthritis, and peripheral neuropathy can occur 5 to 9 days from the start of a meningococcal infection, following initial improvement after start of antibiotic treatment.[151,152] Rickettsial disease, particularly Rocky Mountain spotted fever, is associated with distal small-vessel vasculitis. Case reports or series of vasculitis related to a variety of other bacterial infections have been reported.[153-161] Most are associated with small-vessel vasculitis, but other size vessel involvement may occur in rare instances, including aortitis and coronary arteritis.[162-164] Aortitis is a major feature of tertiary syphilis. Cat scratch disease (*Bartonella henselae*) is associated with leukocytoclastic vasculitis and can resemble HSP.[165,166] Infectious endocarditis can result in immune complex small-vessel vasculitis in the skin (Osler and Janeway nodes), retina, kidney, and spleen. Neonatal necrotizing enterocolitis can also cause an immune complex vasculitis.[167] Leukocytoclastic vasculitis can be a feature of mycobacterium and salmonella infections related to IL-12 receptor deficiency.[168,169]

DRUG-ASSOCIATED VASCULITIS/ HYPERSENSITIVITY VASCULITIS

The terminology used to describe leukocytoclastic vasculitis resulting from a drug reaction remains confusing. The American College of Rheumatology (ACR) criteria define hypersensitivity vasculitis (Table 38-2)[170] as palpable purpura, with or without a maculopapular rash, precipitated by a medication or other agent, and a biopsied lesion characterized by a neutrophilic perivascular or extravascular infiltration in small vessels (such as those affected in HSP).[171,172] The pediatric vasculitis classification suggested by Ozen and colleagues refers to hypersensitivity vasculitis under the subheading "other vasculitis."[173] Historically, it was termed *serum sickness* because this immune complex–mediated vasculitis was encountered after the administration of heterologous antiserum to treat or prevent specific infections such as diphtheria and tetanus.[174] It has since been superseded in frequency by many other drugs, notably cefaclor, penicillin, quinolones, allopurinol, thiazide diuretics, nonsteroidal antiinflammatory drugs (NSAIDs), phenytoins, antithyroid drugs, and, rarely, vaccines, streptokinase, hematopoietic growth factors, recombinant human growth hormone, cytokines, and monoclonal antibodies.

A report of serum sickness–like arthritis in Finland estimated its frequency at 4.7 cases per 100,000 children younger than 16 years of age, establishing it as one of the most common causes of acute arthritis in childhood.[175] In that study, the arthritis was transient, usually lasting only a few weeks, and most commonly affected the ankles, metacarpophalangeal joints, wrists, and knees (Fig. 38-3). In another study, hypersensitivity vasculitis comprised 11% of cases of childhood cutaneous vasculitis versus 40% in adults.[176]

The clinical syndrome typically begins 7 to 14 days after primary exposure to the antigen and is characterized by fever, polyarthralgia, occasional frank arthritis with a patchy discoloration over affected joints, myalgia, lymphadenopathy, and a rash. The rash may be purpuric, linear, urticarial, bullae, livedo, or ecchymotic, and is distributed symmetrically, predominantly over the lower legs, although the trunk and arms may be involved. Lesions can progress to ulcers and tend to be at the same stage of development. Other system involvement is frequent, most commonly renal, but occasionally also the pulmonary, liver, gastrointestinal, and nervous system vasculature (Fig. 38-4). A study that compared the clinical features of HSP and hypersensitivity vasculitis found that transient arthralgias and oligoarthritis, myalgias, cutaneous nodules, ulcerations, livedo, gangrene, and eosinophilia were more common in patients with hypersensitivity vasculitis. Gastrointestinal bleeding, hematuria, and palpable purpura were frequent in those individuals with HSP.[171]

TABLE 38-2 Criteria for the Diagnosis of Hypersensitivity Vasculitis

CRITERION	DEFINITION
Age at onset >16 years	Development of symptoms after 16 years of age
Medication at disease onset	Medication that may have been a precipitating factor was taken at the onset of symptoms
Palpable purpura	Slightly elevated purpuric rash over one or more areas; does not blanch with pressure and not related to thrombocytopenia
Maculopapular rash	Flat and raised lesions of various sizes over one or more areas of the skin
Biopsy, including arteriole and venule	Histological changes showing granulocytes in a perivascular or extravascular location

For purposes of classification, a patient is said to have hypersensitivity vasculitis if at least three of these criteria are present. The presence of any three or more criteria has a diagnostic sensitivity of 71.0% and specificity of 83.9%. The age criterion is not applicable for children.
From L.H. Calabrese, B.A. Michel, D.A. Bloch, et al. (1990) The American College of Rheumatology 1990 criteria for the classification of hypersensitivity vasculitis, Arthritis Rheum. 33: 1108–1113.

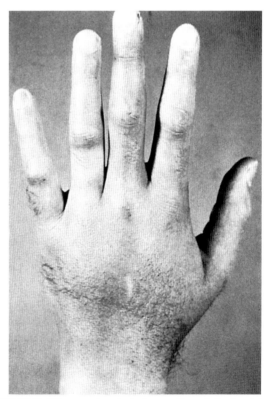

FIGURE 38-3 Diffuse and periarticular swelling of the hand in a boy with acute serum sickness.

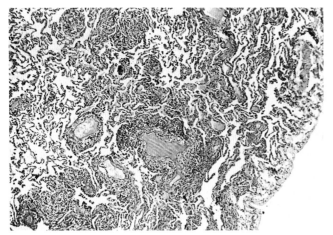

FIGURE 38-4 Hypersensitivity vasculitis is demonstrated in a lung biopsy specimen from a young drug addict with a short history of increasing dyspnea on exertion, and purpura. This section shows prominent infiltration by inflammatory cells and eosinophils of the alveolar walls and around the blood vessels. Hematoxylin-eosin stain.

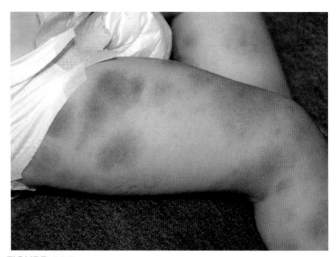

FIGURE 38-5 Acute hemorrhagic edema of infancy with purpura, ecchymosis, and edema of thigh.

Leukocytosis is frequent and is sometimes accompanied by eosinophilia and circulating immune complexes.[175] Elevated acute phase reactants are not a necessary feature. IgG antibodies to the putative antigen may be demonstrable. Hematuria may be found. Antineutrophil cytoplasmic antibodies are occasionally found, especially in cases related to propylthiouracil and hydralazine use. Biopsy of a cutaneous lesion confirms that small venules and capillaries are the predominantly involved vessels. Histopathology findings consist of large numbers of polymorphonuclear cells and eosinophils as well as monocytes with various immunofluorescence patterns.

Removal of the precipitating agent, if identified, is the first step of therapy. In the absence of systemic features, management is usually symptomatic, because the course, although often acute, is self-limited. The duration in patients with isolated skin disease is generally less than 1 month, but it can be longer in those with systemic involvement. Antihistamines and NSAIDs can alleviate cutaneous symptoms and arthralgias. Corticosteroid and other immunosuppressive therapy may be indicated in children with severe cutaneous symptoms or systemic vasculitis. Drug rechallenge is not recommended following recovery.

CYSTIC FIBROSIS

Cystic fibrosis patients can develop a transient recurrent pruritic and painful nodular and purpuric rash, mainly over the ankles and lower legs.[177-181] Histologically, panniculitis and small-vessel vasculitis are usually found, mainly venulitis.[177] The pathogenesis is considered to be immune complex deposition often related to exacerbations of chronic pulmonary infections. Antineutrophil cytoplasmic antibodies with specificity mainly for bactericidal or permeability-increasing protein, but also proteinase 3, are found in more than 50% of these patients.[182-184] The clinical significance and association with vasculitis is unclear. Other autoantibody tests are negative. NSAIDs, chloroquine, and occasionally low-dose corticosteroids are usually beneficial.[185] Colchicine has been used successfully (personal communication).

OTHER VASCULITIDES AND VASCULOPATHIES

Acute Hemorrhagic Edema of Infancy

Acute hemorrhagic edema of infancy (AHEI) is a leukocytoclastic vasculitis in infants and toddlers, usually younger than 2 years of age,[140,142,186-199] and represents 2.5% to 7% of HSP cases.[195,196] It is characterized by a purpuric/ecchymotic rash with pronounced edema, predominantly over the face, ears, and limbs (Fig. 38-5). There is debate about whether this entity represents a mild form of HSP or is a separate entity, as IgA deposits are seen only in 10% to 35% of biopsy specimens.[195,197] Most cases are triggered by an upper respiratory infection,[195,196] but other viral or vaccine triggers have been implicated.[140,142,199] Patients rarely have joint (~3%), gastrointestinal (~3%) or renal (~2.5%) involvement, although in one series, 33% of patients had systemic involvement.[189] Systemic involvement is more common in older infants.[197] Rare cases of severe involvement have been reported.[198] Corticosteroids were used in approximately 4% of patients.[197] AHEI has an excellent prognosis, with resolution without treatment usually within 10 to 21 days,[190,195,197] although in one series the median resolution was as long as 10 months.

Erythema Elevatum Diutinum

Erythema elevatum diutinum (EED) is a low-grade form of leukocytoclastic vasculitis localized in the dermal papillae and subepidermal spaces.[200-208] EED occurs most frequently in adults, although rare pediatric cases have been reported (first by Bury in 1889) in children as young as 3 years of age.[201,206] The clinical presentation is highly characteristic with persistent, symmetrical, yellow, red, or brown papules, nodules, and plaques affecting mainly the extensor surfaces of the extremities, the ears, trunk, and buttocks. Atypical presentations with vesiculobullous, hemorrhagic, and ulcerative lesions have occasionally been reported.[208] Arthralgia is sometimes present. The course is chronic with a slow-healing, fibrotic phase. Histopathologically, the presence of collections of neutrophils in association with nuclear dust is typical.[204] The cause is unknown, whereas the pathogenesis is considered to be the consequence of an immune complex reaction triggered by bacterial and viral agents and drugs.[203,207] In some pediatric cases an association with systemic diseases has been reported,[205,206] and in several others, streptococcal infection has been implicated as the trigger.[204,208] Dapsone may be beneficial.[203,204]

Soter Syndrome (Cutaneous Necrotizing Venulitis)

This rare syndrome includes dermal nodules, urticaria, palpable purpura, arthralgia, flexion contractures of the fingers and toes, abdominal pain, and, rarely, glomerulonephritis.[209-213] Skin lesions can be induced by physical stimuli of cold or trauma. Elevated acute phase reactants are characteristic. Some patients have hypocomplementemia (mainly C1q, C4).[210] Massive degranulation of the mast cells, followed by the infiltration of neutrophils and eosinophils, results in the development of venular endothelial cell necrosis, immune complex and fibrin deposits, and venulitis.[214] HLA associations with A11 and BW35 were found in more than 25% of patients.[215]

Livedoid Vasculopathy

Livedoid vasculopathy (or *livedoid vasculitis* as it is sometimes mistakenly called) is characterized by ulceration of the lower extremities.[216] In its late stages, it can progress to the cutaneous features described as *atrophie blanche*. The condition can mimic leukocytoclastic vasculitis clinically, but histologically an occlusive vasculopathy is observed with thrombosis within dermal blood vessels and endothelial proliferation. The disease is more common in middle-aged females but is also described in children. Sometimes a defined prothrombotic state is identified, such as factor V Leiden mutation, decreased protein C or S, and antiphospholipid antibodies, although this is by no means a universal feature of the condition.[217,218] Livedo may be a presenting symptom of the newly described vasculopathy related to deficiency of adenosine deaminase 2 associated with early-onset stroke with fever and PAN phenotypes.[219,220] Other conditions associated with livedo in children include trisomy 21 and drug reactions.[221-223] Corticosteroids are usually ineffective and may even worsen the condition. Treatment is aimed at prevention of thrombosis with low molecular weight heparin, warfarin, or antiplatelet agents, such as dipyridamole or low-dose aspirin. Vasodilators, such as calcium channel blockers, may be useful to maintain perfusion in the superficial skin vessels.

Susac Syndrome (Retinocochleocerebral Vasculopathy)

Susac syndrome, first described in 1979,[224] is a vasculopathy of unknown cause, characterized by the clinical triad of encephalopathy, branch retinal artery occlusions, and sensorineural hearing loss.[224-231] There is pathological similarity to dermatomyositis, with findings of a microangiopathy affecting the precapillary arterioles of the brain, retina, and inner ear. Antibodies against the endothelium, found in some patients, support the hypothesis of an autoimmune endotheliopathy.[232]

Young females are predominantly affected (20-40 years old), but cases in children as young as 7 years of age have been reported.[228] Clinically, patients' symptoms may include headache, visual disturbances, hearing loss, and multifocal neurological manifestations—particularly long-tract signs, psychiatric features, confusion, memory loss, and other cognitive changes. Dementia may ensue.

Acute phase reactants are usually normal. Elevated levels of factor VIII and von Willebrand factor antigen reflect endothelial activation. Coagulation tests are normal. Cerebral fluid analysis often shows mild pleocytosis and elevated protein levels.[229] Multifocal supratentorial white matter involvement is commonly seen on MRI, with almost pathognomonic involvement of the corpus callosum.[233] Central callosal holes develop as active lesions resolve. Deep gray (~70%) and leptomeningeal involvement (~33%) are common. The "string of pearls" studding of the internal capsules is characteristic. Retinal arteries are best evaluated with fluorescein angiography, which shows the pathognomonic multifocal fluorescence retinal artery branch occlusions.[233]

In order to prevent irreversible damage early diagnosis and combination aggressive therapy is recommended with corticosteroids and immunosuppressive medications (azathioprine, mycophenolate mofetil, cyclophosphamide).[234-236] IVIG appears to be especially effective. The beneficial use of infliximab and rituximab has been reported.[236] Plasma exchange may be useful in severe cases; antiplatelet agents are usually added.

Long-term outcome usually shows stabilization with therapy. Existing hearing loss does not improve with treatment.[237] However, vision outcome is usually good despite continued retinal changes on fluorescein angiography. MRI lesions diminish over time but do not fully normalize; there is poor correlation between MRI and clinical outcomes.[237]

Köhlmeier–Degos Syndrome (Malignant Atrophic Papulosis)

Köhlmeier–Degos syndrome is a rare, often fatal (~50% mortality within 2-3 years) progressive occlusive vasculopathy of unknown cause affecting primarily the cutaneous, gastrointestinal, renal, and CNS small- and medium-sized arteries, which results in progressive occlusion by fibrosis, leading to infarction.[238-246] Papular skin lesions (2-15 mm) are characteristic with central porcelain white atrophy surrounded by telangiectasia. Rarely, episodic fever and organomegaly have been reported.[240] It occurs primarily in young to middle-aged men but has been reported in children, adolescents, and even in toddlers as young as 17 months of age.[239-245] In rare instances, an association with SLE was reported.[247] In general, no effective treatment exists for the systemic manifestations, although IVIG was effective in one case.[248] Vasodilators may improve skin lesions. Treprostinil and eculizumab have been tried with variable effectiveness.[249,250]

Mucha–Habermann Disease

Mucha–Habermann disease, also known as pityriasis lichenoides et varioliformis acuta (PLEVA), is a rare, idiopathic dermatosis characterized by erythematous and scaly papules. At presentation, the dermatitis has the appearance of chronic or recurrent papular and chickenpox-like lesions that become atrophic and scarred. In severe cases the rash is accompanied by fever, joint pain, and swelling. Lesions become hemorrhagic, necrotic, and ulcerate (Fig. 38-6). Mucosal surfaces may be involved. About 50% of the 60 described cases are in children.[251-254] Histologically, lesions are characterized by hyperkeratosis, acanthosis, and degeneration of the basal layer. Mononuclear infiltration obscures the dermoepidermal interface with a perivascular lymphocytic inflammation of capillaries and venules of the upper dermis (more than frank vasculitis). The prognosis in children is generally good with no fatalities reported (there is a 15% mortality in adults). Some children develop chronic arthritis, and one child later developed severe acrosclerosis and scleroderma.[251] Corticosteroids are the primary treatment with methotrexate showing promise in children as a steroid-sparing medication.[252,253] Other treatments include erythromycin, ultraviolet irradiation, infliximab, cyclosporine, dapsone, acyclovir, and IVIG.[252]

Sweet's Syndrome (Acute Febrile Neutrophilic Dermatosis)

Sweet's syndrome consists of an inflammatory perivasculitis (with a dermal and perivascular infiltrate of mature neutrophils) characterized clinically by spiking fever and crops of tender, raised, pseudovesicular, erythematous plaques or nodules on the face and extremities, and sometimes on the trunk.[255-266] About 15% of cases occur in childhood, and Sweet's syndrome has been described in at least 20 infants younger than 6 months old.[264] Arthritis occurs in approximately 33% of patients.[256,259] Multifocal osteomyelitis has also been reported in children.[258-260] Sweet's syndrome may occur secondary to infections, drugs, premalignancy/malignancy (especially hematological) and its treatment, SLE, Behçet syndrome, immunodeficiency, or miscellaneous disorders.[264] Similar skin pathology can be seen in

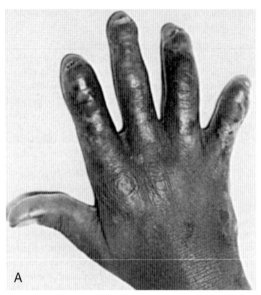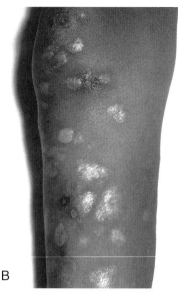

A   B

FIGURE 38-6 An 11-year-old black girl with destructive acrosclerosis and Mucha–Habermann disease. **A**, Hand. **B**, Forearm. The characteristic cutaneous lesions of Mucha–Habermann disease are visible, along with advanced ischemic digital changes.

neutrophilic autoinflammatory disorders, among them the chronic atypical neutrophilic dermatosis with lipodystrophy and elevated temperature (CANDLE) syndrome, Majeed syndrome, and deficiency of IL-1 receptor antagonist (DIRA).[264,267-269] Although absence of leukocytoclastic vasculitis is considered a diagnostic criterion, in one series some degree of vasculitis was found in as many as 74% of cases.[261] Untreated courses of idiopathic disease usually last up to 2 months and may respond to a brief course of corticosteroids.[263]

Stevens–Johnson Syndrome

Stevens–Johnson syndrome is a severe, systemic, widespread form of mucocutaneous erythema multiforme and merges into toxic epidermal necrolysis (depending on the surface area involved).[270-272] Numerous erosive, vesiculobullous, hemorrhagic, and papular lesions develop acutely on the mucosa and skin of the face, hands, trunk, and feet. Anal, genital, and ocular orifices are often affected, and scarring may result.[273] Onset is usually abrupt and is associated with fever, profound constitutional symptoms, and the appearance of periarticular swelling and pain or frank arthritis. The respiratory and gastrointestinal tracts can be involved in severe disease. The etiology is usually infectious (often mycoplasma, herpes simplex)[274] or related to drug exposure,[275] especially anticonvulsive medications,[276] sulfa and penicillin antibiotics, NSAIDs, and even acetaminophen and corticosteroids, but not vaccines.[277] Treatment is mainly supportive, preferably in a burn unit when severe.[271,277-279] The use of corticosteroids, IVIG, plasma exchange, and other medications is still controversial,[280-283] although it appears that in children, unlike adults, mortality may be decreased with the use of IVIG.[283] Mortality in children is rare, but nearly 20% of affected individuals may develop recurrent episodes.[284,285]

Mimics of Vasculitis

Because the diagnosis of vasculitis is often based on imaging alone, it is important to recognize the mimics of vasculitis. Optimal therapy is dependent on the correct diagnosis in order to minimize exposure to unnecessary immunosuppression. Hypercoagulable states such as antiphospholipid antibody syndrome, thrombotic thrombocytopenia purpura, and hemolytic uremic syndrome can cause widespread clots in any blood vessel, and thus mimic systemic vasculitis. Table 38-3 outlines some of the genetic and developmental mimics.[286-298]

Other conditions include thromboangiitis obliterans (Buerger disease), Schamberg's purpura, and chilblains/pernio.

Buerger disease is a chronic, inflammatory thrombotic, segmental obliterative vasculopathy, mainly involving the infrapopliteal and infrabrachial medium- and small-sized arteries, and is strongly associated with tobacco exposure (smoking and oral); therefore it is more common in males. It is extremely rare in childhood. Treatment consists of smoking cessation, pain relief, platelet inhibitors, vasodilators, pneumatic compression, and perhaps spinal cord stimulation and sympathectomy.[299]

Schamberg's disease, a subtype of pigmented purpuric dermatosis, is characterized by the extravasation of erythrocytes and marked hemosiderin deposits in the dermis. Clinically, patients present with nonpalpable, nonpainful purpura mainly over the lower extremities.[300-304] In some cases the etiology is allergic contact dermatitis.[300]

Chilblains/pernio is associated with SLE,[97-99] but more often represents a cold injury.[305-307] Patients show painful and pruritic purpuric papules, nodules, and occasionally ulcers. The toes and fingers are cyanotic, cold, and swollen, with prolonged capillary refill time, although nailfold capillary microscopy is normal.[305-312] The avoidance of cold, and drying and warming the extremities with use of vasodilators (topical and systemic) are beneficial.[312,313] A genetic form of chilblains/pernio, Aicardi–Goutières syndrome, is an autosomal recessive autoimmune disease with early onset progressive encephalopathy related to mutations in the *TREX1* and the AGS5 gene *SAMHD1*.[314-317]

Various medications and recreational drugs can mimic vasculitis; some of these mimics are related to vasospasm and others are a result of drug-induced blood vessel damage resulting in inflammation. The classic example is cocaine inhalation, which can result in nasal features that mimic granulomatosis with polyangiitis. Other medications or drugs include ergotamines, amphetamines, vinyl chloride, various chemotherapy agents (bleomycin, vincristine, carboplatin), and even methylphenidate and dextroamphetamine.[318]

TABLE 38-3 Selected Genetic and Developmental Noninflammatory Mimics of Vasculitis

CONDITION	CAUSE	VASCULAR MANIFESTATIONS	CLINICAL AND OTHER MAJOR MANIFESTATIONS	TREATMENT	COMMENT
*Middle aortic syndrome[286-291]	Unknown, developmental disorder	Stenosis of abdominal aorta, renal and visceral arteries	Hypertension, abdominal angina	Hypertensive medications, surgery[†]	Possibly burned out Takayasu's arteritis?
Fibromuscular dysplasia	Unknown	Stenosis/string of beads, mainly renal artery	Hypertension	Hypertensive medications, surgery[†]	
Marfan's syndrome[292,293]	Autosomal dominant mutations in fibrillin 1 gene	Ascending and thoracic aortic aneurysms and dissection	Mitral valve prolapse, hypermobility, scoliosis, arachnodactyly, high-arched palate, ectopic lentis, dural ectasia	β blockers, surgery[†]	
Ehlers–Danlos type IV[294]	Autosomal dominant mutations in type III procollagen gene	Aneurysms of aorta, other large- (carotid) and medium-sized arteries	Velvety skin, dolls face, mild hypermobility, aorta dissection, visceral rupture	β blockers, surgery[†]	
Loey–Dietz syndrome[295,296]	Autosomal dominant mutations in transforming growth factor β receptor gene (1 or 2)	Aorta and other large and medial artery aneurysms, and tortuosity	Cleft palate, craniosynostosis, congenital heart defects, bifid uvula, learning disability	Surgery[†]	
Grange syndrome[297]	Familial, gene not found, transmission unclear	Multiple artery stenosis and aneurysms ("beading")	Hypertension, brachysyndactyly, bone fragility, congenital heart defects, learning disability	Surgery[†]	
Segmental arterial[298] mediolysis	Unknown	Gastrointestinal and central nervous system medium-sized artery ectasia and aneurysm	Hemorrhage	Surgery[†]	

*Differential diagnosis includes neurofibromatosis. Williams syndrome, mucopolysaccharidoses.
[†]Surgery includes angioplasty with balloon or stents, bypass grafts, anastomoses, endarterectomies, aneurysm repair, embolization, and other vascular manipulations.

TAKAYASU ARTERITIS

Takayasu arteritis (TA) is a rare, chronic, granulomatous vasculitis affecting the aorta and its main branches. In addition to angiographic abnormalities, the patient should have at least one of five additional criteria: (1) decreased peripheral artery pulse(s) and/or claudication of extremities; (2) blood pressure difference between limbs of >10 mm Hg; (3) bruits over aorta and/or its major branches; (4) systolic/diastolic hypertension (greater than 95th percentile for height); and (5) ESR >20 or CRP above upper normal limit. Autoantibodies are generally not present. Although corticosteroids are the mainstay of therapy, many patients require additional immunosuppression. A full discussion of TA is available online at www.expertconsult.com.

REFERENCES

3. I. Pagnini, M.E. Zannin, F. Vittadello, et al., Clinical features and outcome of Cogan syndrome, J. Pediatr. 160 (2012) 303–307.
26. C. Lunardi, C. Bason, M. Leandri, et al., Autoantibodies to inner ear and endothelial antigens in Cogan's syndrome, Lancet 360 (2002) 915–921.
39. S.R. Williamson, C.L. Phillips, S.P. Andreoli, et al., A 25-year experience with pediatric anti-glomerular basement membrane disease, Pediatr. Nephrol. 26 (2011) 85–91.
40. A. Bayat, K. Kamperis, T. Herlin, Characteristics and outcome of Goodpasture's disease in children, Clin. Rheumatol. 31 (2012) 1745–1751.
44. U.A. Syeda, N.G. Singer, M. Magrey, Anti-glomerular basement membrane antibody disease treated with rituximab: A case-based review, Semin. Arthritis Rheum. 42 (2013) 567–572.

51. Y.T. Liou, J.L. Huang, L.S. Ou, et al., Comparison of cryoglobulinemia in children and adults, J. Microbiol. Immunol. Infect. 46 (2013) 59–64.
61. V. Laugel, J. Goetz, S. Wolff, et al., Neonatal management of symptomatic transplacental cryoglobulinaemia, Acta Paediatr. 93 (2004) 556–558.
91. Z.B. Ozçakar, J. Foster 2nd, O. Diaz-Horta, et al., DNASE1L3 mutations in hypocomplementemic urticarial vasculitis syndrome, Arthritis Rheum. 65 (2013) 2183–2189.
95. A. Sayah, J.C. English 3rd, Rheumatoid arthritis: a review of the cutaneous manifestations, J. Am. Acad. Dermatol. 53 (2005) 191–209.
102. S.R. Fernandes, B.H. Singsen, G.S. Hoffman, Sarcoidosis and systemic vasculitis, Semin. Arthritis Rheum. 30 (2000) 33–46.
103. H. Ozdogan, N. Arisoy, O. Kasapcapur, et al., Vasculitis in familial Mediterranean fever, J. Rheumatol. 24 (1997) 323–327.
106. S. Ozen, E. Ben-Chetrit, A. Bakkaloglu, et al., Polyarteritis nodosa in patients with Familial Mediterranean Fever (FMF): a concomitant disease or a feature of FMF?, Semin. Arthritis Rheum. 30 (2001) 281–287.
109. M.D. Wooten, H.E. Jasin, Vasculitis and lymphoproliferative diseases, Semin. Arthritis Rheum. 26 (1996) 564–574.
113. D. Vassilopoulos, L.H. Calabrese, Virally associated arthritis 2008: clinical, epidemiologic, and pathophysiologic considerations, Arthritis Res. Ther. 10 (2008) 215.
125. D. Saadoun, M. Resche-Rigon, D. Sene, et al., Rituximab combined with Peg-interferon-ribavirin in refractory HCV-associated cryoglobulinemia vasculitis, Ann. Rheum. Dis. 67 (2008) 1431–1436.
126. C.M. Magro, M.R. Dawood, A.N. Crowson, The cutaneous manifestations of human parvovirus B19 infection, Hum. Pathol. 31 (2000) 488–497.
127. H.W. Lehmann, P. von Landenberg, S. Modrow, Parvovirus B19 infection and autoimmune disease, Autoimmun. Rev. 2 (2003) 218–223.

135. H.J. Fullerton, M.S. Elkind, A.J. Barkovich, et al., The vascular effects of infection in pediatric stroke (VIPS) study, J. Child Neurol. 26 (2011) 1101–1110.

152. C.A. Goedvolk, I.A. von Rosenstiel, A.P. Bos, Immune complex associated complications in the subacute phase of meningococcal disease: incidence and literature review, Arch. Dis. Child. 88 (2003) 927–930.

168. N. Kutukculer, F. Genel, G. Aksu, et al., Cutaneous leukocytoclastic vasculitis in a child with interleukin-12 receptor beta-1 deficiency, J. Pediatr. 148 (2006) 407–409.

175. I. Kunnamo, P. Kallio, P. Pelkonen, et al., Serum-sickness-like disease is a common cause of acute arthritis in children, Acta Paediat. Scand. 75 (1986) 964–969.

176. R. Blanco, V.M. Martínez-Taboada, V. Rodríguez-Valverde, et al., Cutaneous vasculitis in children and adults. Associated diseases and etiologic factors in 303 patients, Medicine (Baltimore) 77 (1998) 403–418.

180. M.L. Bernstein, M.M. McCusker, J.M. Grant-Kels, Cutaneous manifestations of cystic fibrosis, Pediatr. Dermatol. 25 (2008) 150–157.

183. A. Sedivá, J. Bartůnková, I. Kolárová, et al., Antineutrophil cytoplasmic autoantibodies (ANCA) in children with cystic fibrosis, J. Autoimmun. 11 (1998) 185–190.

190. I. Krause, A. Lazarov, A. Rachmel, et al., Acute haemorrhagic oedema of infancy, a benign variant of leucocytoclastic vasculitis, Acta Paediatr. 85 (1996) 114–117.

197. E. Fiore, M. Rizzi, M. Ragazzi, et al., Acute hemorrhagic edema of young children (cockade purpura and edema): a case series and systematic review, J. Am. Acad. Dermatol. 59 (2008) 684–695.

203. S.I. Katz, J.I. Gallin, K.C. Hertz, et al., Erythema elevatum diutinum: skin and systemic manifestations, immunologic studies, and successful treatment with dapsone, Medicine (Baltimore) 56 (1977) 443–455.

204. S.M. Wilkinson, J.S. English, N.P. Smith, et al., Erythema elevatum diutinum: a clinicopathological study, Clin. Exp. Dermatol. 17 (1992) 87–93.

212. N.A. Soter, Chronic urticaria as a manifestation of necrotizing venulitis, N. Engl. J. Med. 296 (1977) 1440–1442.

217. B.R. Hairston, M.D. Davis, M.R. Pittelkow, et al., Livedoid vasculopathy: further evidence for procoagulant pathogenesis, Arch. Dermatol. 142 (2006) 1413–1418.

225. J.O. Susac, Susac's syndrome: the triad of microangiopathy of the brain and retina with hearing loss in young women, Neurology 44 (1994) 591–593.

230. J. Dörr, S. Krautwald, B. Wildemann, et al., Characteristics of Susac syndrome: a review of all reported cases, Nat Rev Neurol. 9 (2013) 307–316.

231. M. García-Carrasco, C. Mendoza-Pinto, R. Cervera, Diagnosis and classification of Susac syndrome, Autoimmun. Rev. 13 (2014) 347–350.

245. A. Kelly, P. Riley, N. Sebire, et al., Degos disease: a rare occlusive vasculopathy mimicking polyarteritis nodosa, Arch. Dis. Child. 94 (2009) A80–A81.

246. A. Theodoridis, E. Makrantonaki, C.C. Zouboulis, Malignant atrophic papulosis (Köhlmeier-Degos disease)—a review, Orphanet J. Rare Dis. 8 (2013) 10.

253. B.S. Perrin, A.C. Yan, J.R. Treat, Febrile ulceronecrotic Mucha-Habermann disease in a 34-month-old boy: a case report and review of the literature, Pediatr. Dermatol. 29 (2012) 53–58.

261. G. Ratzinger, W. Burgdorf, B.G. Zelger, et al., Acute febrile neutrophilic dermatosis: a histopathologic study of 31 cases with review of literature, Am. J. Dermatopathol. 29 (2007) 125–133.

262. T. Hospach, P. von den Driesch, G.E. Dannecker, Acute febrile neutrophilic dermatosis (Sweet's syndrome) in childhood and adolescence: two new patients and review of the literature on associated diseases, Eur. J. Pediatr. 168 (2009) 1–9.

272. M. Atanasković-Marković, B. Medjo, M. Gavrović-Jankulović, et al., Stevens-Johnson syndrome and toxic epidermal necrolysis in children, Pediatr. Allergy Immunol. 24 (2013) 645–649.

277. U. Raucci, R. Rossi, R. Da Cas, et al., Stevens-Johnson syndrome associated with drugs and vaccines in children: a case-control study, PLoS ONE 8 (2013) e68231.

283. Y.C. Huang, Y.C. Li, T.J. Chen, The efficacy of intravenous immunoglobulin for the treatment of toxic epidermal necrolysis: a systematic review and meta-analysis, Br. J. Dermatol. 167 (2012) 424–432.

285. Y. Finkelstein, G.S. Soon, P. Acuna, et al., Recurrence and outcomes of Stevens-Johnson syndrome and toxic epidermal necrolysis in children, Pediatrics 128 (2011) 723–728.

294. M. Pepin, U. Schwarze, A. Superti-Furga, et al., Clinical and genetic features of Ehlers-Danlos syndrome type IV, the vascular type, N. Engl. J. Med. 342 (2000) 673–680.

296. B.L. Loeys, U. Schwarze, T. Holm, et al., Aneurysm syndromes caused by mutations in the TGF-beta receptor, N. Engl. J. Med. 355 (2006) 788–798.

303. A. Torrelo, C. Requena, I.G. Mediero, et al., Schamberg's purpura in children: a review of 13 cases, J. Am. Acad. Dermatol. 48 (2003) 31–33.

307. S. Padeh, M. Gerstein, S. Greenberger, et al., Chronic chilblains: the clinical presentation and disease course in a large paediatric series, Clin. Exp. Rheumatol. 31 (2013) 463–468.

309. T.D. Simon, J.B. Soep, J.R. Hollister, Pernio in pediatrics, Pediatrics 116 (2005) e472–e475.

314. G. Rice, T. Patrick, R. Parmar, et al., Clinical and molecular phenotype of Aicardi-Goutieres syndrome, Am. J. Hum. Genet. 81 (2007) 713–725.

Entire reference list is available online at www.expertconsult.com.

CHAPTER 39

Pediatric Sarcoidosis

Carlos Daniel Rosé, Carine Wouters

Pediatric sarcoidosis comprises a spectrum of childhood granulomatous inflammatory conditions with the hallmark being the presence of noncaseating epithelioid giant cell granulomas in a variety of tissues and organ systems. The finding in 2001 of a mutation in the nucleotide-binding oligomerization domain 2/caspase activation recruitment domain 15 *(NOD2/CARD15)* gene among patients with a history of familial granulomatous arthritis constituted a major advance and revealed the complexity and heterogeneity of the spectrum of pediatric sarcoidosis.[1]

Blau syndrome and early-onset sarcoidosis constitute the familial and sporadic forms of a pediatric disease characterized by a triad of polyarthritis, uveitis, and rash; and a unique association with mutations in or near the central NOD/NACHT domain of the *NOD2* gene.[1-5] The term *pediatric granulomatous arthritis* (PGA) proposed for both conditions[6,7] falls short in describing the systemic and visceral manifestations that have been documented in a number of patients with PGA.

Many children with sarcoidosis are *NOD2* mutation negative and tend to exhibit systemic and visceral manifestations at presentation. Within this group, the authors identified a distinct entity, infantile-onset panniculitis, with uveitis and systemic granulomatosis.[8]

The form of sarcoidosis observed in adults, characterized mainly by interstitial pulmonary involvement and hilar adenopathy, can also be seen in the pediatric age group but is limited to older children. Certain clinical symptom complexes of granulomatous inflammation, including Löfgren and Mikulicz syndromes, can occur in children. Granulomatous inflammation can be seen secondary to immunodeficiencies, in the context of malignancies and some systemic vasculitides or with certain drug therapies.

EPIDEMIOLOGY

Scarce data exist on the epidemiology of pediatric sarcoidosis. A Danish National Registry study included 48 children within a cohort of 5536 patients with sarcoidosis, resulting in a calculated overall incidence for childhood sarcoidosis of 0.29 per 100,000 per year. The incidence ranged from 0.06 per 100,000 per year for children younger than 5 years old to 1.02 per 100,000 per year for children 14 to 15 years old.[9,10]

An earlier international registry reported on 53 pediatric patients, of whom 14 had a family history, which yielded a ratio of 1 : 5 for familial to sporadic forms.[11] The International Registry of Pediatric Sarcoidosis, established in 2005, shows no gender difference or geographic predominance; the majority of patients exhibiting the classic triad of arthritis, uveitis, and rash have disease onset before reaching 5 years old.[5]

ETIOPATHOGENESIS

The familial cases manifesting the classic clinical triad and an autosomal dominant transmission pattern have been termed *Blau syndrome* (BS).[12] Using linkage analysis of the original pedigree, the susceptibility locus for BS was mapped to a region of chromosome 16, which was found to contain a gene associated with Crohn's disease (CD) called *IBD1*.[13,14] The *IBD1* gene was later found to be *NOD2*.[15] In 2001, Miceli and colleagues identified mutations within the NOD/NACHT domain of the *NOD2* gene in four French families with the Blau phenotype.[1] This seminal work revealed that NOD2 substitutions associated with BS were located in a different domain of the protein than those associated with CD. Wang and colleagues reported *NOD2* mutations in 50% of 10 pedigrees with the BS phenotype.[16] Later, identical mutations were reported among patients with early-onset sarcoidosis (EOS), a sporadic disease with the same phenotype of granulomatous arthritis, uveitis, and rash. Currently, BS and EOS are considered to be the same disease.[4,5] Conversely, mutations in *NOD2* are not found in variant forms of pediatric sarcoidosis that display a more heterogeneous phenotype, nor are they found in adult sarcoidosis, yet certain NOD2 polymorphisms are reportedly associated with severe pulmonary sarcoidosis.[7,17,18,19]

The *NOD2* gene encodes a 1,040 amino-acid protein composed of three main functional domains: two amino-terminal caspase recruitment domains (CARDs), a central nucleotide binding oligomerization domain (NOD/NACHT), and carboxyterminal leucine-rich repeats (LRRs). An expanding number of mutations causing amino-acid substitutions in and near the NOD domain have been documented.[20,21] Substitutions R334W (arginine to glutamine in position 334) and R334Q (arginine to tryptophan) are by far the most common. Yet mutations in position 802 (LRR region) were seen at least in one patient with BS. Variants associated with CD are concentrated in the carboxyterminal LRR region; although CD and BS/EOS have very different phenotypes, they are both characterized by the presence of giant cell granulomas.

The NOD2 protein is a member of a growing family of NOD-like receptor cytosolic proteins comprising different functional domains and implicated in pathways of inflammation and apoptosis. The two amino-terminal CARD domains of NOD2 have an important role in the mediation of nuclear factor (NF)-κB activation and secretion of proinflammatory cytokines, resulting from CARD–CARD interactions between NOD2 and a pivotal downstream kinase protein receptor-interacting serine/threonine kinase (RICK) also known as RIP2 or CARDIAK. The centrally located NOD domain mediates self-oligomerization of NOD2 proteins and activation of downstream effector molecules. The LRR region is structurally related to the LRR

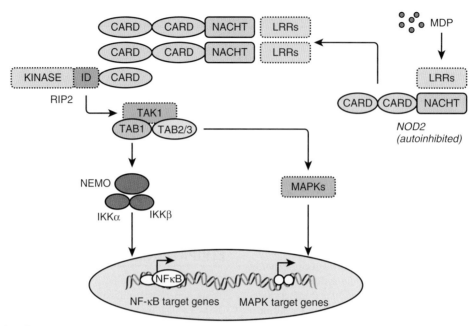

FIGURE 39-1 NOD2 is expressed inside epithelial cells, granulocytes, monocytes, macrophages and dendritic cells in a monomeric and autoinhibited state. Upon recognition of muramyldipeptide (MDP), NOD2 unfolds, oligomerizes through its NOD domain, and recruits RIP2 kinase through CARD–CARD interaction, causing its autophosphorylation. Activated RIP2 recruits TAK1 complex, allowing NF-κB and MAP kinase activation and production of proinflammatory cytokines.

regions of the Toll-like receptors, which are molecules of the innate immune system indispensable for the "sensing" of molecular motifs specific to pathogens, such as lipopolysaccharide. Studies have shown that the moiety recognized by NOD2 is actually muramyldipeptide, a building block of peptidoglycan found in both Gram-positive and Gram-negative bacterial cell walls. NOD2 is expressed constitutively in monocytes, granulocytes, dendritic cells, and in Paneth cells in the villous crypts of the small intestine.[22,23]

The downstream effects of *NOD2* mutations and their relationship with the clinical phenotype are largely unknown. The *NOD2* mutations associated with BS involve residues located in the NOD domain and reportedly act as constitutively active *NOD2* mutants, which are gain-of-function variants consistent with the autosomal-dominant nature of the disease (Fig. 39-1). Using transfection systems, a constitutive NF-κB activation through an abnormal stabilization of the active conformation in the mutated NOD2 protein has been suggested, although these findings have not been replicated to date.[24,25] Conversely, experiments using patients' circulating mononuclear cells could not confirm the expected upregulation and release of interleukin (IL)-1 and other proinflammatory cytokines, an *in vitro* phenomenon poorly understood that somewhat contradicts the notion of a gain-of-function effect on the mutations and activation of NF-κB.[26]

The pathological hallmark of sarcoidosis is the presence of noncaseating epithelioid granulomas thought to result from an exaggerated immune-inflammatory response to a persistent unidentified antigen. The granulomas consist of a central cluster of monocytes/macrophages in various stages of activation, epithelioid cells aligned in a way reminiscent of epithelial cells, and multinucleated giant cells (Fig. 39-2). A corona of mostly CD4+ T lymphocytes, scattered CD8+ T lymphocytes, and plasma cells surrounds the central region. Immunohistochemistry studies in adult sarcoidosis have demonstrated the presence of T-helper (Th)-1 type lymphokines (IL-2, interferon [IFN]-γ) and proinflammatory cytokines (IL-1, tumor necrosis factor [TNF]-α, IL-6) *in situ*.[27]

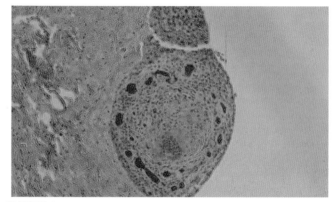

FIGURE 39-2 Synovial biopsy showing a typical noncaseating epithelioid cell granuloma with multinucleated giant cells.

Blau granulomas display a distinct morphology characterized by large polycyclic granulomas with dense lymphocytic coronas. They reflect an exuberant inflammatory response that is in line with a gain-of-function mutation in *NOD2*. Using immunohistochemistry, a predominance of CD68+ macrophages and CD4+ T lymphocytes, an abundant inflammatory cytokine expression *in situ* is typically observed. A prominent expression of IFN-γ is in accordance with an important role for Th1 lymphocytes in granulomatous inflammation. This is seen in association with a very high expression of IL-6, TGF-β, and IL-17, as well as an increased expression of IL-23 receptor on granuloma cells. These findings are suggestive of activation of the Th17 lymphocyte axis in Blau granulomas.[28] Of interest, a role for both Th1 and Th17 cells in adult sarcoidosis has recently been reported as well.[29]

In Blau granulomas, widespread extensive emperipolesis (cell-in-cell phenomenon) of lymphocytes within multinucleated giant cells,

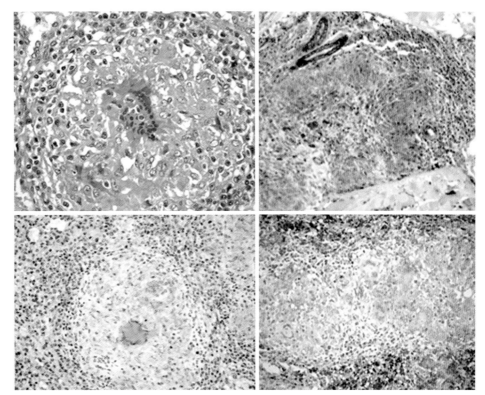

FIGURE 39-3 Morphological and immunohistochemical characteristics of Blau granulomas. Clockwise from *top left*: Hematoxylin-eosin staining showing prominent lymphocyte corona, emperipoletic lymphocytes, and multinucleated giant cells death with fragmented cytoplasm and pyknotic nuclei. Using immunohistochemistry dense staining was observed for IFN-γ (*top right*), IL-6 (*bottom left*), and IL-17 (*bottom right*).

associated with multinucleated giant cell death, was seen as well, a finding of interest in view of the recently reported role of NOD2 in autophagy (Fig. 39-3).[28]

The relationship between the formation and persistence of inflammatory granulomas and the effect of *NOD2* mutations on inflammatory and apoptosis pathways remains to be elucidated.

CLINICAL FEATURES

Sarcoidosis Associated With *NOD2* Mutation

NOD2 mutation–associated sarcoidosis comprises patients with either BS or EOS manifesting a consistent clinical phenotype with polyarthritis, dermatitis, and uveitis (Fig. 39-4). In recent years, because of the availability of genetic testing, a more protean clinical picture than initially conceived has been observed. That this form of sarcoidosis is different from the better-known adult form should not be forgotten.

The initial manifestations include the typical exanthema followed within months by a symmetrical polyarthritis. Ocular involvement tends to occur toward the second year. The median age at onset in the International Blau Registry was 26 months, with two unusual cases showing an age at onset of 2 months and 14 years old.[7]

Cutaneous Involvement

The rash varies in color from pale pink with varied degrees of tan to intense erythema. The lesions appear on the trunk, mainly dorsally, and extend to the face and limbs with accentuation of the tan color on extensor surfaces, where it may become scaly brownish over time (see Fig. 39-4A). The lesions are tiny (5 to 7 mm), round, and barely palpable. At onset, the rash often shows a very fine desquamation, which

may lead to confusion with atopic dermatitis. Over the course of years the rash waxes and wanes. With time, the desquamation predominates, and, in adolescence, it may mimic ichthyosis vulgaris.

Subcutaneous nodules, often located in the lower limbs, are the second most common dermatological manifestation and may be clinically indistinguishable from erythema nodosum.[7] The nodules are mildly tender and resolve without atrophy or pigmentation, even in patients with recurrent episodes. Erysipelas-like lesions have been observed as well, and in one case an urticarial rash showed typical histological features of leukocytoclastic vasculitis.[30]

Articular Disease

The majority of patients will report a polyarticular symmetrical, generalized, or additive arthritis, affecting large and small peripheral joints and tendon sheaths. The joints most frequently involved comprise wrists, knees, ankles, and proximal interphalangeal (PIP) joints. A characteristic feature of both synovitis and tenosynovitis is the exuberance of the swelling. The distal flexor tendons of the digits, the extensor and peroneal compartments, and the flexor groups of the carpus can reach significant size. The anserine tendon sheath diameter can reach 1 cm in some cases. The synovial outpouching can acquire a cystic appearance in the dorsum of the carpus and tarsus. Despite the prominent "boggy" synovitis, pain and morning stiffness appear to be moderate and are overall well tolerated. Except for the PIP joints, where a characteristic flexion contracture described as "camptodactyly" can be seen, the range of motion is relatively well preserved, at least in childhood (see Fig. 39-4, *B*). The course of the arthritis is variable, and erosive changes are mostly modest. However, limited joint mobility and joint contractures may develop with time; ulnar deviations, wrist subluxations, and joint space narrowing have been described.[12,31] It

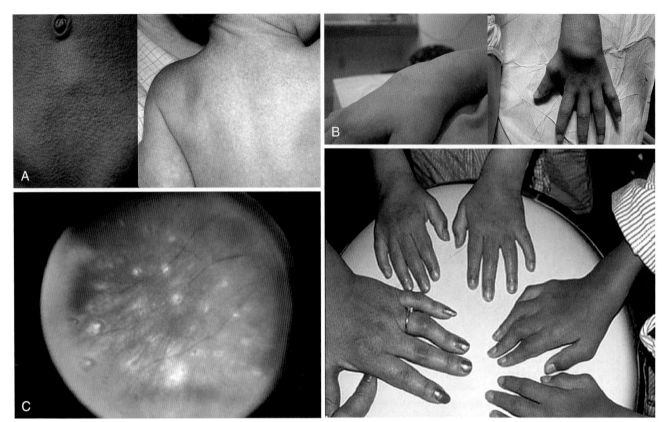

FIGURE 39-4 Clinical triad typical of *NOD2*-associated pediatric sarcoidosis. **A,** Cutaneous features with fine maculopapular erythematous/tan eruption with ichthyosiform appearance (*right*). **B,** Typical "boggy" synovitis with preserved range of motion and cystlike synovial swelling. In the image directly below, a family with *NOD2*-associated polyarthritis and PIP contractures causing camptodactyly. **C,** Multifocal choroiditis characteristic of granulomatous panuveitis.

appears that in addition to the postinflammatory sequelae on radiograph there are a number of other abnormalities suggestive of dysplastic changes. There are limited data on the functional effects of BS arthritis over time. In a recent study it was noted that between one quarter and one third of patients show moderate or severe pain, and moderate to severe functional impairment after a mean follow-up of 16 years.[32]

Ocular Disease

An insidious granulomatous iridocyclitis and posterior uveitis can evolve into a severe destructive panuveitis. Of the clinical triad elements, the ocular disease exhibits the most somber functional prognosis. It tends to start within the first 2 years of disease, and initially there is little to no redness or photophobia. Over time, characteristic iris nodules, focal synechiae, cataract, increased intraocular pressure, and clumpy keratic precipitates at the limbus ensue. Nodules may also occur in the conjunctivae and, in this location, offer an early diagnostic clue and biopsy site. A description of the slit-lamp appearance of sarcoid uveitis compared with juvenile idiopathic arthritis (JIA)-associated uveitis was published by Lindsley and Godfrey.[33] Posterior involvement includes vitritis, multifocal choroiditis, retinal vasculopathy, and optic nerve edema (see Fig. 39-4, *C*). Significant visual loss is observed in 20% to 30% of the affected individuals.[7,11,12,31] Ocular disease can be difficult to control. A prospective study on the natural course of the disease showed persistent vitreous inflammation in 60% of patients and anterior segment activity in 30% despite aggressive therapy during the years of disease course.[32]

Visceral Involvement

As our understanding of the disease spectrum evolves, it has become apparent that the clinical phenotype is not restricted to the classic triad. Among patients with sarcoidosis and associated *NOD2* mutations, a myriad of clinical manifestations including granulomatous and interstitial nephritis, chronic renal insufficiency, small-vessel vasculitis, interstitial pneumonitis, peripheral and mediastinal (excluding hilar) lymphadenitis, pericarditis, cranial neuropathy (VII cranial nerve), and parotitis have been documented.[6,30,33a] Visceral manifestations have been described in patients with BS before the *NOD2* mutation was known.[34-37] Systemic manifestations including prolonged fever have been reported at the onset and may recur during first few years of the disease.[6,38] Large-vessel vasculopathy has been reported in past studies,[39-41] and in one *NOD2* mutated family studied by Wang,[16] but it was not confirmed in more recent series.[6,7,38] Severe arterial hypertension without demonstrable vascular involvement by digital imaging has been observed in 25% of patients who had extra-triad manifestations. The mechanism is unknown, but renal vasculopathy was suggested.[38]

Until recently, no cases of asymptomatic mutation carrying have been observed; however, one family with a mutation E383K in four asymptomatic members has been reported.[38,42]

Sarcoidosis Without *NOD2* Mutation

Sarcoidosis with wild-type *NOD2* constitutes a heterogeneous group of granulomatous inflammatory disorders with protean manifestations. Within this group, two distinct subsets have been identified,

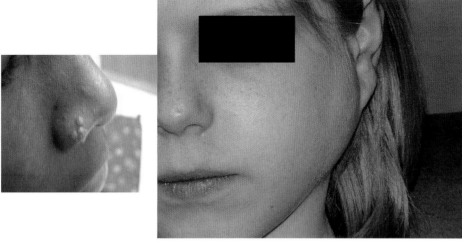

FIGURE 39-5 Clinical signs in sarcoidosis with wild-type *NOD2*. **Left,** Typical maculopapular lesion consisting of multiple noncaseating granulomas on nose. **Right,** Mikulicz syndrome with parotid and lacrimal gland involvement in a girl presenting with sicca symptoms.

including infantile-onset panniculitis with systemic granulomatosis and pediatric-onset adult sarcoidosis.

Infantile-Onset Panniculitis With Uveitis and Systemic Granulomatosis

Four infants with a unique phenotype, including recurrent lobular nonlipophagic panniculitis, severe systemic involvement with persistent fever, hepatosplenomegaly, and granulomatous inflammation affecting joints, eyes, internal organs, and the CNS, have been described. The disease course is progressive, although a partial response to anti-TNF agents can be seen. This condition has been considered a new clinical and pathological entity.[8]

Pediatric-Onset "Adult-Type" Sarcoidosis

Overall, this form of sarcoidosis is characterized primarily by systemic features: pulmonary and lymph node involvement, rather than articular disease. The incidence increases with age and tends to cluster in early adolescence. A review of published pediatric sarcoidosis cohorts reveals the presence of systemic features (malaise, fever, weight loss) at presentation in 60% to 98% of patients; lung involvement in 90% to 100%; hilar adenopathy in 40% to 67% and peripheral adenopathy in 71% to 76%, and 71% to 76% of patients, respectively. Hepatomegaly and splenomegaly were seen in up to 43% of patients; mild elevation of liver enzymes is common, but severe sarcoid hepatitis rarely occurs. A liver biopsy may show granulomas but also cholestatic, necroinflammatory, and vascular changes. Cutaneous manifestations including erythema nodosum, erythematous macules, papules, and plaques were observed in 25% to 42% of patients (Fig. 39-5); eye involvement was seen in 23% to 51%; and uveitis, the most common ocular manifestation, was observed in 25%. Neurological manifestations, mainly CNS involvement, was seen in 23% of patients.[10,43,44]

Some particular presentations of adult sarcoidosis can rarely be observed in older children as well. Löfgren syndrome is characterized by an acute onset of arthritis (mainly of the ankles), erythema nodosum, and hilar adenopathy, and occurs in 9% to 34% of adult sarcoidosis patients.[44,45] The authors have observed one case of Mikulicz syndrome (parotid and lacrimal gland enlargement) with granulomatous inflammation on a lacrimal gland biopsy in a child who later developed interstitial pneumonitis (Fig. 39-5).

Particular Features of Organ Involvement in Pediatric-Onset Adult Sarcoidosis

Neurosarcoidosis in children develops differently from the way it develops in adults. Seizures as the manifestation of sarcoid encephalopathy are common in prepubertal children, whereas cranial nerve palsy, the most common neurological complication among adults, is less frequent and only seen at an older age. A review of 29 pediatric cases of neurosarcoidosis by Baumann and colleagues showed that masslike lesions on imaging are more common than previously recognized; additional features were leptomeningeal enhancement and multifocal T2 hyperintense magnetic resonance imaging (MRI) lesions within cortical gray and subcortical white matter. Cerebrospinal fluid analysis characteristically reveals a mild lymphocytosis, mildly elevated protein, and increased immunoglobulins with oligoclonal banding. Evidence of hypothalamic dysfunction is also common with patients showing growth failure, diabetes insipidus, and failure of sexual maturation.[46]

Renal sarcoidosis deserves attention because of the risk of renal dysfunction and coexistent calcium metabolism abnormalities. In a review of 15 pediatric case series, the frequency of a decreased creatinine clearance was 26% to 45%. Mild to moderate proteinuria and sediment changes (especially leukocyturia) were noted in 31% of patients. Hypercalciuria was found in 47% and hypercalcemia in 21% of patients. Pathology most often showed interstitial and granulomatous nephritis; tubulopathy, glomerular, and vascular changes were rarely seen.[47] In fact, the same pattern of interstitial nephritis with renal failure was documented by Meiorin and colleagues in a child with proven *NOD2* mutation, suggesting that similar renal manifestations are seen in both *NOD2* mutation related and unrelated forms.[30]

Symptomatic sarcoid myositis is rare in children and adults, although asymptomatic granulomatous involvement has been detected in up to 80% of muscle biopsy specimens.[48] Three distinct clinical patterns reported in children comprise an acute inflammatory myositis with myalgia and increased muscle enzymes,[49] a long-lasting myopathy with progressive muscle weakness,[50] and a nodular myopathy with palpable muscle nodules.[51]

Similarly, although clinically recognized cardiac involvement is uncommon, autopsy studies demonstrate granulomatous infiltration of the myocardium in as many as 27% of adults. The most common clinical manifestations in adults include conduction and rhythm disturbances. Heart failure and sudden death are rare but have been described as well.[52] Death from multiorgan failure and chronic congestive heart failure 10 years after disease onset has been reported in a child; autopsy revealed sarcoid granulomas throughout the myocardium.[34]

The cumulative clinical manifestations in a cohort of 75 patients with sarcoidosis in the International PGA Registry are presented in Fig. 39-6. In *NOD2*-associated sarcoidosis, the majority of patients display a typical clinical triad of skin, joint, and eye involvement, but incomplete forms and extended manifestations are observed (see Fig. 39-6, *A*). Conversely, a tremendous heterogeneity in clinical manifestations is seen in sarcoidosis with wild-type *NOD2,* although specific subgroups may be identified (see Fig. 39-6, *B*).

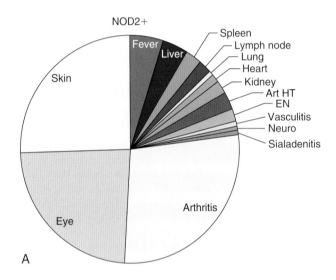

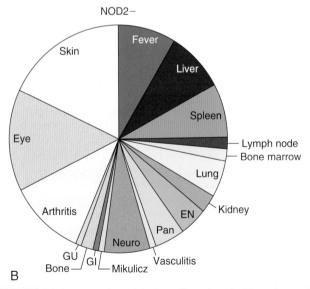

FIGURE 39-6 Cumulative clinical manifestations in 75 patients with pediatric sarcoidosis recruited through the International PGA Registry. **A,** The large majority of patients with *NOD2*-associated sarcoidosis display a clinical triad with skin, joint, and eye involvement, although incomplete forms and extended manifestations exist. **B,** A large heterogeneity of clinical manifestations is typical of sarcoidosis with wild-type *NOD2*.

Secondary Granulomatous Inflammatory Diseases

Children with primary immunodeficiency disorders can develop granulomatous inflammation without an identifiable infectious cause. These granulomas have been described in association with ataxia telangiectasia, common variable immunodeficiency, Wiscott–Aldrich syndrome, chronic granulomatous disease, immunoglobulin (Ig)-A deficiency, X-linked hypogammaglobulinemia, and severe combined immunodeficiency, hypomorphic RAG mutation, Rothmund–Thomson syndrome, cartilage hair hypoplasia.[53] The mechanism is unknown, and the extent of organ involvement varies, although lymphatic nodes, skin, lung, liver, and spleen are reportedly the main sites involved.[54,55] The etiology of granulomas in children with primary immunodeficiencies remains to be elucidated.

Histopathological features of granulomatous lesions are heterogeneous, and these can include the following: (1) sarcoidosis-like granulomas, mainly composed of epithelioid cells associated with few lymphocytes and giant cells arranged in well-circumscribed nodules; (2) poorly defined tuberculoid granulomas with numerous giant multinucleated cells associated with some lymphocytes and few epithelioid cells; and (3) histiocytic palisading granulomas with a central necrobiotic area.[56]

Immunohistochemical studies have documented a predominance of CD8[+] T cells and a lower CD4[+]/CD8[+] ratio in these granulomas as compared with the findings in sarcoidosis.[56,57]

A rare form of chronic granulomatous cheilitis (Miescher syndrome) in children with noncaseating giant cell granulomas in the inflammatory infiltrate is considered a monosymptomatic variant of the Melkersson–Rosenthal syndrome, a nongranulomatous disorder of unknown etiology comprising a triad of recurrent orofacial swelling, relapsing facial paralysis, and a fissured tongue.[58]

Malignant and histiocytic disorders that are related can show a granulomatous infiltrate and hence be confused with primary sarcoidosis. This has been observed in patients with Hodgkin disease and non-Hodgkin T-cell lymphomas, seminoma of the testis, and ovarian dysgerminoma.[59,60] In Hodgkin disease, granulomas may be seen in the liver and spleen, tissues that otherwise exhibit no evidence of Hodgkin disease. Lymphomas can be seen in patients with a previous diagnosis of sarcoidosis—the so-called sarcoidosis lymphoma syndrome.[61]

Langerhans cell histiocytosis (LCH) is a heterogeneous disease, characterized by accumulation of dendritic cells with features similar to epidermal Langerhans cells in various organs. The LCH cell, the hallmark of the lesion, is characterized by the expression of CD1a and CD207. The diagnostic Langerhans cell can be masked by an admixture of eosinophils, T cells, macrophages, and osteoclast-like multinucleate giant cells.[62,63] By virtue of this complex cellular composition, bone lesions in particular have been called granulomatous, although usually a classic, walled-off granuloma structure is lacking.[64]

Granulomatous inflammation of the lungs, and less frequently lymph nodes, skin, and bone marrow, has been observed in patients receiving anti-TNF therapy for nongranulomatous inflammatory diseases. This is an emerging entity probably related to the anti-TNF agent, but it is still poorly understood.[65,66]

DIAGNOSIS

Laboratory Parameters

There is no laboratory test that indicates a diagnosis of sarcoidosis. The sedimentation rate and acute phase reactants reflect clinical disease activity. Peripheral blood cell counts are usually within normal limits, although mild anemia, leucopenia, or lymphopenia can be seen. Hypergammaglobulinemia is often present, but autoantibodies are absent. Elevation of angiotensin converting enzyme (ACE) is not consistent, and the value of serum ACE levels in diagnosing and managing sarcoidosis remains unclear. ACE levels are influenced by ACE gene polymorphisms, and physiological values vary according to age, with a higher normal range of serum values seen in children.[12] Hypercalciuria and hypercalcemia result from overproduction of 25-hydroxy vitamin D-1 α-hydroxylase, which converts 25-hydroxy vitamin D to 1,25-dihydroxy vitamin D, by sarcoid macrophages. Hypercalciuria can lead to nephrocalcinosis and nephrolithiasis.

Pathology

The diagnosis of sarcoidosis is confirmed by the finding of characteristic noncaseating epithelioid and giant cell granulomas, which can be documented in biopsies of skin, synovium, conjunctiva, lymph nodes, or any involved tissue. It has to be noted that asymptomatic granulomatous inflammation has been observed in various organs including liver, skeletal muscle, and myocardium.[35,48,52]

Genetic Testing

In early publications the frequencies of *NOD2* mutation among patients who exhibited the clinical triad of dermatitis, arthritis, and uveitis varied between 50% in familial forms[16] and 90% in sporadic forms.[25] The authors of the present chapter found *NOD2* mutations in 98% of the patients of the International PGA Registry who exhibited the classic triad phenotype with either a sporadic or a familial form. The recent discovery of *NOD2* mutations in a few asymptomatic individuals of a large family and the finding of extended clinical manifestations suggest the interference of supplementary modulating genes in the clinical phenotype. *NOD2* genetic analysis is becoming standard in the diagnostic workup in patients with suspected BS.

DIFFERENTIAL DIAGNOSIS

The diagnosis of sarcoidosis in a child with granulomatous inflammation requires a concerted effort to exclude chronic infections, notably mycobacteria and fungi, by appropriate staining and cultures. Various primary immunodeficiency disorders can present with granulomatous inflammation without an identifiable infectious cause, and should be excluded by evaluation of neutrophil function and analysis of circulating lymphocyte subsets and serum levels of immunoglobulins.

Pediatric sarcoidosis needs to be differentiated from other systemic inflammatory disorders in children, such as CD, and necrotizing granulomatous vasculitides, notably Wegener granulomatosis, Churg–Strauss syndrome, and lymphomatoid granulomatosis. Wegener granulomatosis often is associated with granulomatous inflammation of the upper respiratory tract; careful examination of tissue will reveal signs of small-vessel vasculitis. CD can display a wide array of extraintestinal manifestations seen in sarcoidosis, including erythema nodosum, uveitis, arthritis, and vasculitis.[67]

NOD2 mutation–associated sarcoidosis bears a resemblance to other causes of polyarthritis with uveitis in children, especially JIA and Behçet syndrome. The cutaneous rash in patients with the classical phenotype is commonly confused with atopic dermatitis or with ichthyosis vulgaris. The presence of fever and visceral involvement in *NOD2*-associated sarcoidosis can evoke systemic-onset JIA as well.[6]

PROGNOSIS

Until recently there were limited data on the outcome of *NOD2* mutation–associated sarcoidosis in children. EOS is reportedly not always a benign disease with possible dissemination and vital organ involvement occurring at a later stage.[34] Articular and ocular disease remain active after years in a number of patients, and functional impairment both ocular and articular is seen in one third to two thirds of patients.[32] Severe hypertension and visceral involvement, including glomerulonephritis with renal failure and interstitial pneumonitis, have been observed in patients from the International PGA Registry, indicating the necessity of careful surveillance throughout the course of disease.[38] Ocular disease can be relentless and causes visual loss in more than one third of patients. Uveitis severity is variable even among patients with the same *NOD2* substitution, suggesting the influence of additional genetic factors. Arthritis seems to be nondestructive, especially during the first years, but as the disease progresses, flexion deformities, camptodactyly, and erosions can be observed. The outcome of pediatric sarcoidosis with wild-type *NOD2* is very variable. The large majority of patients with adult-type sarcoidosis enter into remission within 2.2 (0.5 to 5.9) years after disease onset. By contrast, chronic active inflammation and organ damage involving lung, eye, CNS, and/or kidney have been noted in up to one fifth of patients. The outcome is worse in patients with severe lung or organ involvement at presentation, CNS or multiorgan involvement, or eye disease.[44]

Infantile-onset panniculitis with systemic granulomatosis is a separate entity with a potentially fatal course; two out of six affected children died before age 15 because of widespread visceral organ inflammation.[8]

TREATMENT

Evidence-based data on the optimal treatment of pediatric sarcoidosis are scarce. Moderate- to low-dose daily corticosteroid therapy is effective in controlling uveitis and joint disease, but the side effects of prolonged use may become unacceptable. Methotrexate at a dosage of 10 to 15 mg/m² once weekly is effective in suppressing disease activity and allowing corticosteroid tapering.[68,69] The introduction of anti-TNF monoclonal antibody agents may constitute a major therapeutic advance in the treatment of pediatric sarcoidosis.[70,71] Infliximab (5 to 10 mg/kg every 4 to 8 weeks) was found to effectively control chronic arthritis and visceral manifestations; however, the effect on uveitis activity may be less convincing.[7] The experience with IL-1 antagonists (e.g., anakinra) is minimal and associated with variable results.[6,26] A case of a 4 year old with intractable uveitis who responded to Canakinumab was recently reported.[72]

At present there is no evidence for an effective treatment for all patients with Blau syndrome. In a currently ongoing prospective Blau cohort study,[32] more than two thirds of Blau patients received medical therapy for several years, often combining systemic steroids, and immunosuppressive and/or biological drugs to control both uveitis and arthritis. TNF antagonists were the most commonly used biological therapy and seemingly useful in achieving partial control of articular disease. The observation of persistently active disease in a majority of Blau patients in this study underlines the need for development of effective targeted therapies.

REFERENCES

1. C. Miceli-Richard, S. Lesage, M. Rybojad, et al., CARD15 mutations in Blau syndrome, Nat. Genet. 29 (2001) 19–20.
2. E.B. Blau, Familial granulomatous arthritis, iritis, and rash, J. Pediatr. 107 (1985) 689–693.
3. A.F. North Jr., C.W. Fink, W.M. Gibson, et al., Sarcoid arthritis in children, Am. J. Med. 48 (1970) 449–455.

4. N. Kanazawa, S. Matsushima, N. Kambe, et al., Presence of a sporadic case of systemic granulomatosis syndrome with a CARD15 mutation, J. Invest. Dermatol. 122 (2004) 851–852.

5. C.D. Rosé, T.M. Doyle, G. McIlvain-Simpson, et al., Blau syndrome mutation of CARD15/NOD2 in sporadic early onset granulomatous arthritis, J. Rheumatol. 32 (2005) 373–375.

6. J.I. Arostegui, C. Arnal, R. Merino, et al., NOD2 gene-associated pediatric granulomatous arthritis: clinical diversity, novel and recurrent mutations, and evidence of clinical improvement with interleukin-1 blockade in a Spanish cohort, Arthritis Rheum. 56 (2007) 3805–3813.

7. C.D. Rose, C.H. Wouters, S. Meiorin, et al., Pediatric granulomatous arthritis: an international registry, Arthritis Rheum. 54 (2006) 3337–3344.

8. C.H. Wouters, T.M. Martin, D. Stichweh, et al., Infantile onset panniculitis with uveitis and systemic granulomatosis: a new clinicopathologic entity, J. Pediatr. 151 (2007) 707–709.

9. K.E. Byg, N. Milman, S. Hansen, Sarcoidosis in Denmark 1980–1994. A registry-based incidence study comprising 5536 patients, Sarcoidosis Vasc. Diffuse Lung Dis. 20 (2003) 46–52.

10. A.L. Hoffmann, N. Milman, K.E. Byg, Childhood sarcoidosis in Denmark 1979–1994: incidence, clinical features and laboratory results at presentation in 48 children, Acta Paediatr. 93 (2004) 30–36.

11. C.B. Lindsley, R.E. Petty, Overview and report on international registry of sarcoid arthritis in childhood, Curr. Rheumatol. Rep. 2 (2000) 343–348.

12. C. Wouters, C.D. Rosé, A.M. Prieur, Rhumatologie Pédiatrique, Flammarion Médecine-Sciences, Paris, 2009.

13. G. Tromp, H. Kuivaniemi, S. Raphael, et al., Genetic linkage of familial granulomatous inflammatory arthritis, skin rash, and uveitis to chromosome 16, Am. J. Hum. Genet. 59 (1996) 1097–1107.

15. J.P. Hugot, M. Chamaillard, H. Zouali, et al., Association of NOD2 leucine-rich repeat variants with susceptibility to Crohn's disease, Nature 411 (2001) 599–603.

16. X. Wang, H. Kuivaniemi, G. Bonavita, et al., CARD15 mutations in familial granulomatosis syndromes: a study of the original Blau syndrome kindred and other families with large-vessel arteritis and cranial neuropathy, Arthritis Rheum. 46 (2002) 3041–3045.

20. Infevers: The Registry of Hereditary Auto-inflammatory Disorders Mutations, fmf.igh.cnrs.fr/infevers, 2014.

21. C.D. Rose, T.M. Martin, C.H. Wouters, Blau syndrome revisited, Curr. Opin. Rheumatol. 23 (2011) 411–418.

22. N. Inohara, G. Nunez, NODs: intracellular proteins involved in inflammation and apoptosis, Nat. Rev. Immunol. 3 (2003) 371–382.

23. N. Inohara, M. Chamaillard, C. McDonald, G. Nuñez, NOD-LRR proteins: role in host-microbial interactions and inflammatory disease, Annu. Rev. Biochem. 74 (2005) 355–383.

24. M. Chamaillard, D. Philpott, S.E. Girardin, et al., Gene-environment interaction modulated by allelic heterogeneity in inflammatory diseases, Proc. Natl. Acad. Sci. U.S.A. 100 (2003) 3455–3460.

25. N. Kanazawa, I. Okafuji, N. Kambe, et al., Early-onset sarcoidosis and CARD15 mutations with constitutive nuclear factor-kappaB activation: common genetic etiology with Blau syndrome, Blood 105 (2005) 1195–1197.

26. T.M. Martin, Z. Zhang, P. Kurz, et al., The NOD2 defect in Blau syndrome does not result in excess interleukin-1 activity, Arthritis Rheum. 60 (2009) 611–618.

28. C.E. Janssen, C.D. Rose, G. De Hertogh, et al., Morphologic and immunohistochemical characterization of granulomas in the nucleotide oligomerization domain 2-related disorders Blau syndrome and Crohn disease, J. Allergy Clin. Immunol. 129 (2012) 1076–1084.

29. M. Facco, A. Cabrelle, A. Teramo, et al., Sarcoidosis is a Th1/Th17 multisystem disorder, Thorax 66 (2011) 144–150.

30. S.M. Meiorin, G. Espada, C.E. Costa, et al., Granulomatous nephritis associated with R334Q mutation in NOD2, J. Rheumatol. 34 (2007) 1945–1947.

31. C. Wouters, C.D. Rose, Childhood sarcoidosis, in: R. Cimaz, T. Lehman (Eds.), Pediatrics in Systemic Autoimmune Diseases. vol. 6 ed, Elsevier, Amsterdam, 2008.

32. C.D. Rosé, S. Pans, I. Castels, et al., Blau syndrome: cross-sectional data from a multicentre study of clinical, radiological and functional outcomes, Rheumatology (2014) doi:10.1093/rheumatology/kew437; First published on line November 20, 2014.

33. M.L. Becker, T.M. Martin, T.M. Doyle, C.D. Rosé, Interstitial pneumonitis in Blau syndrome with documented mutation in CARD15, Arthritis Rheum. 56 (2007) 1292–1294.

37. D.A. Jabs, J.L. Houk, W.B. Bias, F.C. Arnett, Familial granulomatous synovitis, uveitis, and cranial neuropathies, Am. J. Med. 78 (1985) 801–804.

38. C.D. Rosé, J.I. Arostegui, T.M. Martin, et al., NOD2-associated pediatric granulomatous arthritis, an expanding phenotype: study of an international registry and a national cohort in Spain, Arthritis Rheum. 60 (2009) 1797–1803.

42. F.T. Saulsbury, C.H. Wouters, T.M. Martin, et al., Incomplete penetrance of the NOD2 E383K substitution among members of a pediatric granulomatous arthritis pedigree, Arthritis Rheum. 60 (2009) 1804–1806.

43. E.N. Pattishall, E.L. Kendig Jr., Sarcoidosis in children, Pediatr. Pulmonol. 22 (1996) 195–203.

44. N. Milman, A.L. Hoffmann, Childhood sarcoidosis: long-term follow-up, Eur. Respir. J. 31 (2008) 592–598.

46. R.J. Baumann, W.C. Robertson Jr., Neurosarcoid presents differently in children than in adults, Pediatrics 112 (2003) e480–e486.

47. R. Coutant, B. Leroy, P. Niaudet, et al., Renal granulomatous sarcoidosis in childhood: a report of 11 cases and a review of the literature, Eur. J. Pediatr. 158 (1999) 154–159.

48. F. Fayad, F. Liote, F. Berenbaum, et al., Muscle involvement in sarcoidosis: a retrospective and followup studies, J. Rheumatol. 33 (2006) 98–103.

49. M.M. Jamal, A.M. Cilursu, E.L. Hoffman, Sarcoidosis presenting as acute myositis. Report and review of the literature, J. Rheumatol. 15 (1988) 1868–1871.

50. G.A. Rossi, E. Battistini, M.E. Celle, et al., Long-lasting myopathy as a major clinical feature of sarcoidosis in a child: case report with a 7-year follow-up, Sarcoidosis Vasc. Diffuse Lung Dis. 18 (2001) 196–200.

51. E.N. Pattishall, G.L. Strope, S.M. Spinola, F.W. Denny, Childhood sarcoidosis, J. Pediatr. 108 (1986) 169–177.

52. K.J. Silverman, G.M. Hutchins, B.H. Bulkley, Cardiac sarcoid: a clinico-pathologic study of 84 unselected patients with systemic sarcoidosis, Circulation 58 (1978) 1204–1211.

53. C.D. Rose, B. Neven, C. Wouters, Granulomatous inflammation: the overlap of immune deficiency and inflammation, Best Pract. Res. Clin. Rheumatol. 28 (2014) 191–212.

54. L.J. Mechanic, S. Dikman, C. Cunningham-Rundles, Granulomatous disease in common variable immunodeficiency, Ann. Intern. Med. 127 (1997) 613–617.

55. D.F. Arnold, J. Wiggins, C. Cunningham-Rundles, et al., Granulomatous disease: distinguishing primary antibody disease from sarcoidosis, Clin. Immunol. 128 (2008) 18–22.

56. D. Moshous, I. Meyts, S. Fraitag, et al., Granulomatous inflammation in cartilage-hair hypoplasia: risks and benefits of anti-TNF-α mAbs, J. Allergy Clin. Immunol. 128 (2011) 847–853.

57. M. de Jager, W. Blokx, A. Warris, et al., Immunohistochemical features of cutaneous granulomas in primary immunodeficiency disorders: a comparison with cutaneous sarcoidosis, J. Cutan. Pathol. 35 (2008) 467–472.

58. R.M. Greene, R.S. Rogers 3rd, Melkersson-Rosenthal syndrome: a review of 36 patients, J. Am. Acad. Dermatol. 21 (1989) 1263–1270.

59. H. Brincker, Coexistence of sarcoidosis and malignant disease: causality or coincidence?, Sarcoidosis 6 (1989) 31–43.

60. E.W. Leatham, R. Eeles, M. Sheppard, et al., The association of germ cell tumours of the testis with sarcoid-like processes, Clin. Oncol. (R. Coll. Radiol.) 4 (1992) 89–95.

61. P.R. Cohen, R. Kurzrock, Sarcoidosis and malignancy, Clin. Dermatol. 25 (2007) 326–333.

62. L. Schmitz, B.E. Favara, Nosology and pathology of Langerhans cell histiocytosis, Hematol. Oncol. Clin. North Am. 12 (1998) 221–246.

63. R. Haupt, M. Minkov, I. Astigarraga, et al., Langerhans cell histiocytosis (LCH): guidelines for diagnosis, clinical work-up, and treatment for

patients till the age of 18 years, Pediatr. Blood Cancer 60 (2013) 175–184.

64. R.M. Egeler, A.G. van Halteren, P.C. Hogendoorn, et al., Langerhans cell histiocytosis: fascinating dynamics of the dendritic cell-macrophage lineage, Immunol. Rev. 234 (2010) 213–232.

65. E. Toussirot, E. Pertuiset, B. Kantelip, D. Wendling, Sarcoidosis occuring during anti-TNF-alpha treatment for inflammatory rheumatic diseases: report of two cases, Clin. Exp. Rheumatol. 26 (2008) 471–475.

66. M. Ramos-Casals, P. Brito-Zeron, M.J. Soto, et al., Autoimmune diseases induced by TNF-targeted therapies, Best Pract. Res. Clin. Rheumatol. 22 (2008) 847–861.

67. C.D. Rose, T.M. Martin, Caspase recruitment domain 15 mutations and rheumatic diseases, Curr. Opin. Rheumatol. 17 (2005) 579–585.

68. M.C. Iannuzzi, B.A. Rybicki, A.S. Teirstein, Sarcoidosis, N. Engl. J. Med. 357 (2007) 2153–2165.

69. R.P. Baughman, D.B. Winget, E.E. Lower, Methotrexate is steroid sparing in acute sarcoidosis: results of a double blind, randomized trial, Sarcoidosis Vasc. Diffuse Lung Dis. 17 (2000) 60–66.

70. A. Brescia, G. Mcllvain-Simpson, C. duPont, Infliximab therapy for steroid-dependent early onset sarcoid arthritis and Blau syndrome, Arthritis Rheum. 46 (2014) S313.

71. N. Milman, C.B. Andersen, A. Hansen, et al., Favourable effect of TNF-alpha inhibitor (infliximab) on Blau syndrome in monozygotic twins with a de novo CARD15 mutation, APMIS 114 (2006) 912–919.

72. G. Simonini, Z. Xu, R. Caputo, et al., Clinical and transcriptional response to the long-acting interleukin-1 blocker canakinumab in Blau syndrome-related uveitis, Arthritis Rheum. 65 (2013) 513–518.

Entire reference list is available online at www.expertconsult.com.

40 CHAPTER

Behçet Disease

Seza Ozen

INTRODUCTION AND HISTORICAL REVIEW

In 1937, the Turkish dermatologist Hulusi Behçet[1] described the syndrome that bears his name, which manifests with the clinical triad of aphthous stomatitis, genital ulceration, and uveitis. Superficial thrombophlebitis was identified as the fourth criterion in 1946.[2] Matteson[3] identified even earlier reports of this condition, including those from Japan. The history of Behçet disease (BD) has been reviewed by Kaklamani and colleagues.[4]

DEFINITIONS AND CLASSIFICATIONS

In the nomenclature of the revised Chapel Hill Consensus Conference (CHCC 2012), BD is described as a vasculitis that can affect arteries or veins of any size, and is characterized by recurrent oral and/or genital aphthous ulcers accompanied by cutaneous, ocular, articular, gastrointestinal, and/or central nervous system inflammatory lesions.[5]

Several sets of diagnostic criteria have been proposed. Those of the International Study Group (ISG)[6] are most widely used and are listed in Table 40-1. If only one of the criteria is present along with recurrent oral ulcerations, the term *incomplete Behçet disease* is applied. Criteria proposed by Mason and Barnes[7] (Table 40-2) and O'Duffy and Goldstein[8] emphasize the broader spectrum of disease. The ISG criteria have a specificity of 96% and sensitivity of 91%; the Mason and Barnes criteria have a specificity of 84% and sensitivity of 86%.[9] All criteria have been applied to the diagnosis of BD in children, although none have been validated in this age group.

EPIDEMIOLOGY

Incidence and Prevalence

The occurrence of BD varies markedly throughout the world. The highest prevalence occurs along the historical route of the Silk Route from Japan to the eastern edge of the Mediterranean Sea and through areas of the former Ottoman Empire.[10] However, BD is by no means confined to these areas. It is rarely reported in children from India,[11] and more commonly identified in children from Europe[12] and North America, reflecting emigration patterns in the 20th century. A recent report from France showed that among adult vasculitides, BD was much more common than expected, with higher frequencies than those for other rare vasculitides.[13] BD is undoubtedly more common in Turkey and other parts of the Middle East, where an overall prevalence of 1 in 250 persons has been reported,[14] compared with a prevalence of fewer than 1 in 100,000 persons in the UK.[15] Ozen and co-workers[16] have proposed that the prevalence in children is not more than 10 cases per 100,000 in Turkey. The frequency of BD in French

children younger than 15 years of age is approximately 1 case in 600,000. One third were of North African origin.[17]

Several reviews document BD in childhood and adolescence.[12,18-25] An international study of the clinical features of BD in 86 children from France, Turkey, Iran, and Saudi Arabia used the ISG criteria.[12] Eighteen Greek children who met the ISG criteria for BD were described by Vaiopoulos and colleagues in 1999.[19] There have also been series reported from Greece,[19] Saudi Arabia,[20] Turkey,[21] Korea,[22] Japan,[23] and Israel.[24] Recently a large international registry has been established to assess the pediatric features and develop new criteria for children.[25]

Sex Ratio and Age at Onset

In most series, boys and girls are affected with equal frequency, in contrast to BD in adults, in which men are affected almost twice as frequently as women. The age at onset of disease ranges widely. Overall, 5.4% to 7.6% of all patients experience onset of BD in childhood.[26] BD has been reported in neonates born to mothers with BD[27,28] and in one newborn with no maternal history of the disease.[29]

GENETIC BACKGROUND

There is substantial evidence supporting the genetic basis for BD. The increased sibling and twin recurrence rate, familial cases, the high frequency of the disease among people along the historic Silk Road, and evidence for genetic anticipation all support genetic contribution in the pathogenesis.[30-32] In an international study of BD in European children,[25] 12.3% had a family member with the disease, suggesting a genetic burden in early-onset BD. The frequency of BD among North African immigrants to France was comparable with rates reported from North Africa and Asia, and was not related to age at immigration.[13]

The human leukocyte antigen (HLA) molecule B*5101 is the strongest genetic association with BD. It is likely that B51 confers significant risk (odds ratio [OR] 3.49-5.78), particularly in patients with a family history of the disease.[33,34] Large genome-wide association studies (GWAS) have further shown an association with interleukin (IL)-10 and *IL23R/IL12RB2* genes.[35,36] IL-10 is an antiinflammatory cytokine, whereas IL-23 is crucial for the inflammatory Th17 pathway. In order to identify further susceptibility loci in BD, a cohort of 1209 Turkish patients was reevaluated with a GWAS of 779,465 single nucleotide polymorphisms (SNPs).[37] This analysis identified new associations, such as STAT4 (a transcription factor in a signaling pathway related to cytokines such as IL-12, type I interferons [IFNs] and IL-23) and two SNPs in endoplasmic reticulum aminopeptidase (ERAP1)1 that were confirmed in different ethnic groups.[37] Furthermore, an epistatic interaction with ERAP1 and major histocompatibility

TABLE 40-1 Criteria of the International Study Group for the Diagnosis of Behçet Disease

CRITERION	DESCRIPTION
Recurrent oral ulceration	Minor aphthous, major aphthous, or herpetiform ulceration recurring at least three times in one 12-month period, observed by physician or patient
Plus two of the following:	
Recurrent genital ulcers	Aphthous ulceration or scarring observed by physician or patient
Eye lesions	Anterior uveitis, posterior uveitis, or cells in vitreous on slit-lamp examination, or retinal vasculitis observed by an ophthalmologist
Skin lesions	Erythema nodosum observed by physician or patient; pseudofolliculitis or papulopustular lesions; acneiform nodules observed by physician in postadolescent patient not on corticosteroid treatment
Pathergy	Skin reaction to a needle prick observed by physician 24-48 hours afterward

From Ref. 6.

TABLE 40-2 Mason and Barnes Criteria for a Diagnosis of Behçet Disease

MAJOR CRITERIA*	MINOR CRITERIA
Buccal ulceration	Gastrointestinal lesions
Genital ulceration	Thrombophlebitis
Eye lesions	Cardiovascular lesions
Skin lesions	Arthritis
	Central nervous system lesions
	Family history of Behçet disease

*Diagnosis requires the presence of at least three major criteria or two major plus two minor criteria.
From R.M. Mason, C.G. Barnes, Behçet's syndrome with arthritis, Ann. Rheum. Dis. 28 (1969) 95–103.[7]

complex (MHC) class I region was identified: homozygosity for the putative ERAP1 conferred a threefold risk in HLA-B51 positive patients, whereas the risk was 1.48 for those who were HLA-B51 negative.[37] It is interesting that persons of Japanese origin living in the United States, or those of Turkish origin living in Germany, have been reported to have a lower incidence of BD than persons living in Japan or Turkey. This suggests an environmental impact on the genetic predisposition.[38,39]

ETIOLOGY AND PATHOGENESIS

The cause of BD is not known. Microbial agents have been suggested that trigger the disease through inducing an aberrant immune response in a genetically predisposed individual. Evidence for a microbial cause of BD is reviewed by Verity and colleagues.[40] Lehner[41] has suggested that immunity to microbial heat-shock proteins that share homology with human 65 kD mitochondrial heat-shock protein may be important in pathogenesis. There are several studies suggesting a role for herpes simplex virus type 1, parvovirus B19, and streptococci; however, no microbial cause has been established.

In addition to the evidence for involvement of the adaptive immune system, neutrophils and the inflammation mediated by the innate immune also play a major role in BD. The involvement of the innate immune system, the absence of autoimmune features, and the episodic nature of the disease course has led to the suggestion that BD as an autoinflammatory disease of multifactorial origin.[42]

The genetic findings provide new insight in the pathogenesis of the disease. HLA-B51 is known to have a low affinity for peptides and may therefore have a larger peptide repertoire.[33] In fact the long-standing suggestions of the role of triggering infections may be linked to the behavior of HLA-B51 (see below).[31] Recent data summarized by Gül and Ohno[33] suggest that the slow folding of HLA-B51 loaded with a peptide may play a critical role just as suggested for HLA-B27 in ankylosing spondylitis (AS). ERAP1, an endoplasmic reticulum–expressed aminopeptidase, functions in processing and loading of peptides onto MHC class I molecules. When HLA class I molecules bind the peptide

of the microbe, they need to fold. Unfolded protein response (UPR) leads to endoplasmic stress and the triggering of inflammation through the IL-23/IL-17 pathway in BD.[43] ERAP is also associated with the pathogenesis of AS, and misfolding of HLA-B27 has been shown to activate the IL-23/IL-17 axis.[43] Furthermore, a number of studies in sera and cell culture of BD patients have clearly shown that IL-17 is important in the inflammation of BD.[44,45] Thus the presence of the critical SNPs in ERAP1 may lead to an unfolded protein response of HLA-B51, with the trigger of a variety of infectious agents leading to an inflammation led by Th17 cells.

CLINICAL MANIFESTATIONS

One of the most characteristic features of the disease is the heterogeneity of the clinical presentation. The clinical presentations differ among geographies: gastrointestinal disease is increased in patients from Asia, and vascular disease is more common among those from the Middle East and the eastern Mediterranean.[46] Symptoms tend to occur in clusters, such as, for example, the acne/arthritis/enthesitis cluster or the vasculitis cluster (venous thrombi and pulmonary arterial disease), suggesting that more than one pathological pathway is involved.[46] The heterogeneity of BD poses problems not only in classification of the disease, but in genetic and treatment studies as well.

The clinical manifestations of BD often emerge over a period of several years. In a study of 40 Korean children, the mean interval between the first and the second major manifestations was 7 years.[22] The usual course of BD in any organ system is that of exacerbations and remissions, with the overall activity generally declining with time. The frequencies of the major and minor manifestations are given in Table 40-3.

Mucocutaneous Disease

Most BD patients have oral ulceration; it usually occurs at disease onset and may persist for much of the course of the disease.[12,23,25] Crops of extremely painful ulcers appear on the lips, tongue, palate, and elsewhere in the gastrointestinal tract (Fig. 40-1). They last for 3 to 10 days (sometimes longer), recur at various intervals, and heal without scarring. The exception to this is neonatal disease, in which extensive scarring may result.[28] Recurrent, painful ulcerations of the glans penis, prepuce, scrotum, and perianal area in the male, and of the vulva and vagina in the female are characteristic. These ulcers usually occur after oral ulcers and may heal with scarring, unlike oral ulcers.

Other skin lesions occur in more than 90% of children with BD.[12,22] These include erythema nodosum, purpura (which may be palpable), papulopustular (acneiform) lesions, ulcers, or folliculitis.[24,25] Pathergy,

TABLE 40-3	Behçet Disease in Childhood							
CRITERIA (%)								
STUDY	N	M:F	ONSET (AGE)	OU	GU	SKIN	UVEITIS	PATHERGY
Lang et al.[18]	37	19:18	8.7	100	75	84*	30	?
Bahabri et al.[20]	12	7:5	11.5	100	65	83*	92	57
Koné-Paut et al.[12]	65	33:32	8.4	100	96	92*	45	80
Eldem et al.[21]	20	15:5	15.1	100	65	35*	80	?
Kim et al.[22]	40	16:24	10.6	100	82	72*	27	?
Fujikawa and Suemitsu[23]	31	14:17						
Uziel et al.[24]	15	7:8	6.6*	100	33	100*	53	40
Total	220	111:109						

*Includes pathergy.
GU, Genital ulceration; *M:F*, sex ratio; *OU*, oral ulceration.

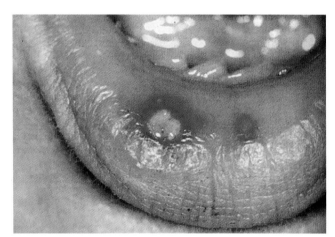

FIGURE 40-1 Oral aphthous lesion in a girl with Behçet disease.

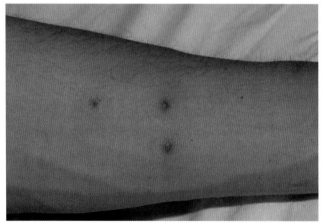

FIGURE 40-2 Pathergy photo and legend.

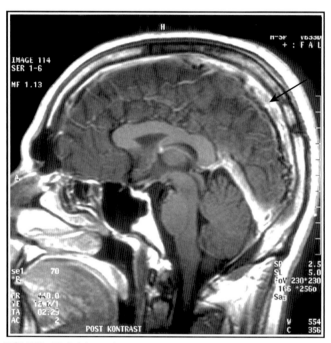

FIGURE 40-3 Magnetic resonance imaging demonstrates sagittal sinus thrombosis in a patient with Behçet disease. (Courtesy of Dr. A. Dinc.)

an unusual cutaneous pustular reaction occurring 24 to 48 hours after a needle puncture of the dermis, is highly characteristic but not pathognomonic of the syndrome[47] (Fig. 40-2). Pathergy test positivity varies considerably from one series to another and occurs most commonly (50% to 70%) in patients from the Middle East.[4]

Ocular Disease

Eye lesions occur in 30% to 61% of children with BD.[12,20-25] The typical eye involvement is in the form of a chronic relapsing bilateral posterior and anterior uveitis.[48] The basic retinal lesion is a vasculitis. In a series of 20 children, posterior uveitis was the most common ocular manifestation, occurring in 11 patients, although anterior uveitis occurred in 3 patients, and 2 had papilledema.[21] BD should be considered in the differential diagnosis of a child presenting with isolated anterior uveitis. The eye may be painful and red. Hypopyon may occur, and severe uveitis may lead to blindness. In older studies, it was reported that blindness was common in untreated patients. Complications may include glaucoma and cataracts. Corneal ulceration, cystoid macular edema, retinal vasculitis, retinal detachment, and retrobulbar neuritis are rare events. Ocular disease is much more common in boys than girls.[12,21]

Central Nervous System Disease

The reported frequency of central nervous system (CNS) disease in children varies from 5% to 15% (Fig. 40-3).[12,23,25] It may be parenchymal or nonparenchymal (vascular).[49] Neurologic involvement may present as an encephalomyelitis (e.g., pyramidal, extrapyramidal, cerebellar, spinal cord abnormalities, seizures) or aseptic meningitis. The nonparenchymal involvement is usually a benign intracranial hypertension with papilledema and is often due to dural sinus thrombosis.[25,49-51] Several of the neurologic manifestations may occur simultaneously. The most common CNS disorder in adults is meningoencephalitis with headache and pleocytosis of the cerebrospinal fluid.[50] In children, however, cerebral venous sinus thrombosis is most common.

Neuro-BD develops in 5% to 15% of affected children.[12] In a recent report of 26 children with neuro-BD, 11 presented with neurological abnormalities although not all fulfilled the criteria of BD at onset.[49] The leading feature was cerebral venous sinus thrombosis. In these children, abnormalities of the coagulation pathway should also be considered. Parenchymal involvement was rare; only two patients had brainstem lesions, whereas one had spinal cord involvement.[49] The outcome was much better than in adults; only two had sequelae (one with bilateral optic atrophy). Mora et al.[51] reviewed pediatric neuro-BD: 13 of the 53 children neuro-BD was diagnosed at presentation, and cerebral venous sinus thrombosis was again common. Seventy-five percent had headaches, whereas patients with parenchymal involvement showed encephalomyelitis, seizures, cranial nerve palsy, hemiparesis, mental changes, and meningitis.[51]

Musculoskeletal Disease

Polyarthritis or oligoarthritis occurs in 50% to 75% of children with BD.[12,24] It most commonly affects the knees, ankles, wrists, and elbows but may occur in other joints as well.[12,24] The disease is usually oligoarticular, but polyarthritis may be observed.[12] The disease does not usually result in erosions or joint destruction. Although an association with sacroiliac arthritis has been reported in adults, this has not been observed in childhood.[12,46,52]

Acute, localized myositis is uncommon; it is rarely multifocal[53] and has been reported in only a few children.[18,53] Generalized myositis may also occur.[53] It may be confused with vasculitis or venous thrombosis.[18]

Vascular Disease

The vasculitis of BD is unique in that it is the only vasculitis that involves both the arterial and venous systems and can affect a vessel of any size. Hence it is described as "variable vessel vasculitis" in the CHCC 2012 classification.[5] It is characteristically associated with arterial or venous thromboses and aneurysms or occlusions in arteries of any size.[5] Superficial or deep venous thromboses are common in adults but occur only in 5% to 15% of children.[12] Most thromboses develop in veins, especially those of the lower extremities. Arteritis and arterial aneurysms may occur,[54-56] and involvement of the pulmonary artery and central retinal artery has been reported.[55-57] Pulmonary artery thrombosis is rare, but it is one of the most severe features of the disease and is associated with high morbidity and mortality.[57] A recent series of 47 patients with pulmonary artery aneurysms or thrombosis showed that peripheral venous thrombosis was present in 36 of 47 (77%) patients, and intracardiac thrombi in 12 of the 36 (33%) patients.[57] Patients who develop superficial thrombophlebitis were more likely to develop major venous occlusions. A recent study has assessed the features of 21 children and adolescents with vascular involvement in BD: 4 had anticardiolipin antibodies and 2 had protein C deficiency.[55] Cerebral sinuses were a common site of thrombosis.[54,55]

Gastrointestinal Disease

Gastrointestinal manifestations are characterized by exacerbations and remissions. Diarrhea, abdominal pain, and ulceration of the ileum, cecum, and colon[12,23,24] appear to be more common in Japanese patients.[46,58] Gastrointestinal tract lesions histologically indistinguishable from those of Crohn's disease or ulcerative colitis may develop in patients with BD.[59] Hepatic vein occlusion may result in Budd–Chiari syndrome.[59]

Renal Disease

Renal involvement is rare but probably more common than was initially recognized. The most common manifestations are amyloidosis and a wide spectrum of glomerulonephritides, but renal artery disease, renal vein thrombosis, and interstitial nephritis are also documented.[60] Renal involvement may occur in the form of vascular disease, including renal artery aneurysms or renal vein thrombosis.[60]

Other Uncommon Manifestations

A number of cardiac complications (e.g., endocarditis, myocarditis, pericarditis, arrhythmias) have been reported in adults but are rare in children. Dilatation of the proximal aorta, atrial septal aneurysm, mitral valve prolapse, and mitral valve regurgitation were the most common vascular abnormalities reported in one survey.[61] Pulmonary abnormalities in BD have been reviewed by Erkan and colleagues.[62] Recurrent dyspnea, cough, chest pain, and hemoptysis suggest pulmonary hemorrhage.

PATHOLOGY

The underlying pathological lesion is an occlusive vasculitis in arterioles and veins. In the skin, the lesions may be necrotizing but do not exhibit fibrinoid degeneration.[6] Inflammation in the synovium is nonspecific, with a predominantly neutrophil infiltration. Muscle biopsies have demonstrated a wide range of abnormalities, from perivascular infiltrates and fibrosis to muscle necrosis.[18]

There is some controversy regarding the histopathology of the pathergy reaction. A serial study of the lesion revealed a superficial and deep perivascular mixed inflammatory cell infiltrate, with neutrophils peaking at 24 hours.[63] True vasculitis was not reported to be present in this study. However, leukocytoclastic vasculitis and a neutrophilic vascular reaction with endothelial swelling have also been reported.[64] The differences in the reported series may be explained by the variability of the immune response or by ethnic factors or timing.

LABORATORY INVESTIGATIONS

There is no laboratory test that indicates a diagnosis of BD. There is a generalized increase in acute phase reactants with active disease. Autoantibodies are not expected to be present in BD; however, there has been one report of antibodies to ocular and oral mucosal antigens.[65]

Anticardiolipin antibodies are uncommon,[55] and one study[66] suggests there is no primary pathogenic role of these antibodies in BD. Elevated levels of von Willebrand factor antigen and decreased thrombomodulin levels were associated with vasculitis and active disease. Concentrations of protein C and protein S were normal.[67] The pathogenic significance of elevated serum levels of cytokines, including tumor necrosis factor (TNF) receptor in serum, awaits further evaluation.[68] However, recent studies suggest a clear role of IL-17 in the pathogenesis of BD,[45,46] supported by the GWAS highlighting the importance of the IL-23/IL-17 pathway.

Neutrophils are prominent infiltrating cells in the skin and eye lesions of BD, and inconsistent abnormalities of their function have been reported. Carletto and colleagues[69] studied neutrophil function in 15 adults and found that although superoxide production and adhesion were normal, migration was significantly increased in patients with active disease compared with those with inactive disease or with the control subjects. Enhanced migration into inflammatory sites facilitates their participation in the leukocytoclastic vasculitis or neutrophilic vasculitis that may occur in BD and may be at least partly responsible for pathergy. In other studies,[70] levels of reactive oxygen species were increased. The role of neutrophil abnormalities in the pathogenesis of BD requires further study. Synovial fluid analysis is also characterized by a predominance of neutrophils (15,000/ml; 1.5×10^8) and low glucose levels.[71] The frequency of HLA-B51 varies from population to population and is not one of the diagnostic criteria.

RADIOLOGICAL EXAMINATIONS

The most important imaging studies are angiography to delineate the extent and character of the vascular lesions and magnetic resonance imaging (MRI) to evaluate the effects of disease on the CNS. Magnetic resonance angiography is an alternative to direct angiography, although it is less accurate for imaging smaller arteries.[72] In a study of 98 adult patients,[73] brain stem or basal ganglia lesions were demonstrated by MRI, especially during an attack. Similar findings were evident by single photon emission computed tomography.[74]

DIFFERENTIAL DIAGNOSIS

The differential diagnosis depends on the leading clinical features. Other causes of uveitis need to be considered for eye involvement; the presence of retinal vasculitis and accompanying features will help in the differentiation. It may be challenging to differentiate the gastrointestinal involvement from that of inflammatory bowel disease. The lesions in BD are most frequently in the ileum (rarely in the rectum) and appear as typical ulcers. The CNS disease may need to be differentiated from thrombotic lesions in a patient with genetic predispositions. Vasculitis may mimic other vasculitides because it can involve any size artery. Involvement of veins sets BD apart from other vasculitides, however.[75] Autoinflammatory disorders such as periodic fever, aphthous stomatitis, pharyngitis, adenitis syndrome (PFAPA) may be a consideration in the early or incomplete presentation of BD (see Chapter 47). The typical features of BD—family history, ethnicity, and the presence of HLA-B51—may help guide the physician.

TREATMENT

BD is difficult to treat, and therapy depends largely on the site and severity of involvement. There are no controlled studies evaluating treatment of BD in children, and physicians must therefore depend on the experience gained in treating adults.[76] European League Against Rheumatism (EULAR) recommendations for the management of adult BD have recently been published and will be discussed in the following sections. Whether they are entirely appropriate for pediatric patients is not certain.

Oral and Genital Ulcers

Topical treatment with sucralfate suspension or topical corticosteroids should be the first line of treatment for ulcers.[76] During the acute stage of ulceration, a short course of oral prednisone helps provide fast relief. For severe ulceration, thalidomide is very useful, but the high risk of peripheral neuropathy and its contraindication during pregnancy limits its usefulness.[77] A number of regimens have been used. An initial dose of thalidomide of 50 mg/day for adolescents is reduced to 50 mg twice per week if the patient responds. Alternatively, the drug may be started in a dose up to 1 mg/kg/day and tapered to 1 mg/kg taken 2 days each week or every other day.

There is little evidence regarding the efficacy of the thalidomide analog lenalidomide. Dapsone (100 mg/day) has been reported to have a beneficial effect on mucocutaneous lesions.[78]

Long-term colchicine administration was effective in controlling the frequency and severity of oral and genital ulceration in one study.[79] A double-blind study with adults with BD showed that colchicine significantly reduced the frequency of genital ulcers, erythema nodosum, and arthritis among women, and arthritis among men.[79] There are no controlled trials of the use of penicillin or other antibiotics to treat oral ulcers in children with BD.

In published reports summarized by Arida et al.,[80] anti-TNF agents (especially infliximab) have been shown to be very effective in approximately 90% of adults with resistant oral and genital ulcerations and skin lesions. The response was prompt and complete in 20%, partial in 70%, and with monthly infusions (in the case of infliximab), sustained for a median follow-up of 16 months.

Ocular Inflammation

Eye disease should be managed in conjunction with an experienced ophthalmologist. Azathioprine (2 mg/kg/day) has been beneficial in trials surveyed in the Cochrane Controlled Trials Register,[81] and it is one of the first choices of treatment for the severe uveitis of BD.[82] The addition of cyclosporine to glucocorticoids has been recommended for the treatment of sight-threatening uveitis in adults.[83] The EULAR recommendations state that the patient with inflammatory eye disease that affects the posterior segment should receive azathioprine and systemic corticosteroids. If the disease is resistant, cyclosporine or infliximab should be added.[76] Combination therapies with azathioprine and interferon or methotrexate have been successful for severe uveitis.[84] Short-term chlorambucil therapy may be useful in treatment of intractable ocular disease,[85] but its potential toxicity has relegated it to a questionable role in the management of ocular BD.

Biologics have assumed an important place in the management of resistant ocular inflammation.[86] In prospective studies of adults with ocular BD that was refractory to topical corticosteroids and systemic methotrexate, cyclosporine, or azathioprine, infliximab resulted in a complete resolution of ocular involvement in 65% of patients and a partial response in 24%. The addition of methotrexate, cyclosporine, or azathioprine to infliximab yielded an even better response. Adalimumab treatment resulted in remission in all of the patients in whom it was given; etanercept was effective in 60%.[80] It is also effective for severe panuveitis.[84,87] In a case series of 19 patients with BD, prompt sustained remission of uveitis was achieved by treatment with adalimumab.[88] An open label pilot study with an IL-1–regulating antibody, XOMA 052 (gevokizumab) reported that complete resolution of intraocular inflammation that had been resistant to azathioprine and/or cyclosporine was achieved in 4 to 21 days (median 14 days), with a long duration of response.[89]

Treatment of Other Manifestations

Prednisone is usually chosen as the initial therapy for other manifestations of BD. Methylprednisolone may be given intravenously initially at 10 to 20 mg/kg per dose, depending on the severity of the disease, or prednisone may be given orally in a dose of 1 to 2 mg/kg/day, followed by reducing the dose by 0.2 mg/kg each day or every other day. Steroid-sparing or alternative immunosuppressive treatment options include sulfasalazine, which has been reported to benefit the associated gastrointestinal disease.[84] Treatment with low-dose methotrexate,[90] azathioprine, anti-TNF agents, or cyclophosphamide may be tried for CNS disease.[76]

There are no controlled data to guide the management of vasculitis in BD. The venous thrombosis reflects vascular inflammation, and the author treats patients with immunosuppressives, although there is no firm evidence to support their use. Immunosuppressives such as cyclophosphamide, interferon, methotrexate, azathioprine, and TNF antagonists have been recommended. Similarly, there are no controlled data on the use of anticoagulants.[76] Desbois et al.[91] retrospectively analyzed the effect of immunosuppression in 296 BD patients with venous thrombosis. In multivariate analysis, the use of immunosuppressive agents was found to prevent relapse of venous thrombosis ($P = 0.00021$), and there was a trend toward prevention of relapse with the use of glucocorticoids.[91] Although a retrospective study, these data confirm the need for steroids and immunosuppressives for these patients. There is no consensus on the use of anticoagulation for the thrombosis of BD. An international survey showed that rheumatologists in the United States and Israel were more likely to use anticoagulants than those from Turkey.[92] Among 21 pediatric patients, 5 were treated with anticoagulants and 3 with antiplatelet therapies.

A systematic review has analyzed 113 papers reporting a total of 390 BD patients treated with anti-TNF drugs.[80] This review showed high response rates in patients with resistant mucocutaneous, ocular, gastrointestinal, and CNS involvement; however, information from randomized placebo-controlled studies was limited. There has been an increase in the number of case reports of the use of other biologics such as anti-IL-6 and anti-IL-1 agents in adult BD.[93,94]

COURSE OF DISEASE AND PROGNOSIS

BD tends to run a very long, relapsing course. A young age at onset and male sex are both indicators of a prolonged disease course. The ocular and CNS manifestations in particular can be extremely incapacitating.[24] Potentially fatal lesions include occlusion or aneurysms of arteries supplying the CNS or heart; pulmonary hemorrhage; and bowel perforation.[58,94] In a recent series of BD patients with pulmonary artery aneurysms, 26% of the patients were dead at 7 years after onset in spite of treatment with corticosteroids and cyclophosphamide or azathioprine.[95] Embolization of large pulmonary aneurysms has met with limited success.[96] Improved endovascular techniques will surely decrease this high mortality. In a series of 65 patients with BD, the overall mortality rate was 3%.[12] The frequency of postoperative complications such as poor wound healing may be increased in BD patients because of an exaggerated inflammatory response to simple penetrating trauma. However, this is not a contraindication to surgery.

REFERENCES

5. J.C. Jennette, R.J. Falk, P.A. Bacon, et al., 2012 revised International Chapel Hill Consensus Conference Nomenclature of Vasculitides, Arthritis Rheum. 65 (2013) 1–11.
6. International Study Group for Behçet's Disease, Criteria for diagnosis of Behçet's disease, Lancet (1990) 1070–1080.
12. I. Koné-Paut, S. Yurdakul, S.A. Bahabri, et al., Epidemiological features of Behçet's syndrome in children: an international collaborative survey of 86 cases, J. Pediatr. 132 (1998) 721–725.
13. A. Mahr, L. Belarbi, B. Wechsler, et al., Population-based prevalence study of Behçet's disease: differences by ethnic origin and low variation by age at immigration, Arthritis Rheum. 58 (2008) 3951–3959.
14. G. Hatemi, Y. Yazici, H. Yazici, Behcet's syndrome, Rheum. Dis. Clin. North Am. 89 (2013) 245–261.
25. I. Koné-Paut, M. Darce-Bello, F. Shahram, et al., Registries in rheumatological and musculoskeletal conditions. Paediatric Behçet's disease: an international cohort study of 110 patients. One-year follow-up data, Rheumatology 50 (2010) 184–188.
29. Y.S. Chang, Y.H. Yang, B.L. Chiang, Neonatal Behçet's disease without maternal history, Clin. Rheumatol. 30 (2011) 1641–1645.
30. S. Ozen, F.K. Eroglu, Pediatric-onset Behçet disease, Curr. Opin. Rheumatol. 25 (2013) 636–642.
34. G. Hatemi, E. Seyahi, I. Fresko, V. Hamuryudan, Behçet's syndrome: a critical digest of the recent literature, Clin. Exp. Rheumatol. 30 (3 Suppl. 72) (2012) S80–S89.
35. N. Mizuki, A. Meguro, M. Ota, et al., Genome-wide association studies identify IL23R-IL12RB2 and IL10 as Behçet's disease susceptibility loci, Nat. Genet. 42 (2010) 703–706.
36. E.F. Remmers, F. Cosan, Y. Kirino, et al., Genome-wide association study identifies variants in the MHC class I, IL10, and IL23R-IL12RB2 regions associated with Behçet's disease, Nat. Genet. 42 (2010) 698–702.
37. Y. Kirino, G. Bertsias, Y. Ishigatsubo, et al., Genome-wide association analysis identifies new susceptibility loci for Behçet's disease and epistasis between HLA-B*51 and ERAP1, Nat. Genet. 45 (2013) 202–207.
40. D.H. Verity, G.R. Wallace, R.W. Vaughan, M.R. Stanford, Behçet's disease: from Hippocrates to the third millennium, Br. J. Ophthalmol. 87 (2003) 1175–1183.
42. S. Ozen, J. Frenkerl, N. Ruperto, M. Gattorno, Eurofever progress towards better care for autoinflammatory diseases, Eur. J. Pediatr. 170 (2011) 449–452.
43. M.L. DeLay, M.J. Turner, E.I. Klenk, et al., HLA-B27 misfolding and the unfolded protein response augment interleukin-23 production and are associated with Th17 activation in transgenic rats, Arthritis Rheum. 60 (2009) 2633–2643.
44. K. Hamzaoui, Th17 cells in Behçet's disease: a new immunoregulatory axis, Clin. Exp. Rheumatol. 29 (2011) S71–S76.
45. X. Liu, P. Yang, C. Wang, et al., IFN-alpha blocks IL-17 production by peripheral blood mononuclear cells in Behçet's disease, Rheumatology (Oxford) 50 (2010) 293–298.
46. H. Yazici, S. Ugurlu, E. Seyahi, Behçet Syndrome: is it one condition? Clin. Rev. Allergy Immunol. 43 (2012) 275–280.
48. A. Reiff, S. Kadayıfcılar, S. Ozen, Inflammatory eye diseases in childhood, Rheum. Dis. Clin. North Am. 39 (2013) 801–832.
49. D. Uluduz, M. Kurtuncu, Z. Yapici, et al., Clinical characteristics of pediatric-onset neuro-Behçet disease, Neurology 77 (2011) 1900–1905.
51. P. Mora, C. Menozzi, J.G. Orsoni, et al., Neuro-Behçet's disease in childhood: a focus on the neuro-ophthalmological features, Orphanet J. Rare Dis. 8 (2013) 18.
53. H. Sarui, T. Maruyama, I. Ito, et al., Necrotising myositis in Behçet's disease: characteristic features on magnetic resonance imaging and a review of the literature, Ann. Rheum. Dis. 61 (2002) 751–752.
54. B. Krupa, R. Cimaz, S. Ozen, et al., Pediatric Behcet's disease and thromboses, J. Rheumatol. 38 (2011) 387–390.
55. S. Ozen, Y. Bilginer, N. Besbas, et al., Behçet disease: treatment of vascular involvement in children, Eur. J. Pediatr. 169 (2010) 427–430.
56. D. Saadoun, B. Asli, B. Wechsler, et al., Long-term outcome of arterial lesions in Behçet disease: a series of 101 patients, Medicine (Baltimore) 91 (2012) 18–24.
57. E. Seyahi, M. Melikoglu, C. Akman, et al., Pulmonary artery involvement and associated lung disease in Behçet disease: a series of 47 patients, Medicine (Baltimore) 91 (2012) 35–48.
59. Y. Bayraktar, E. Ozaslan, D.H. van Thiel, Gastrointestinal manifestation of Behçet's disease, J. Clin. Gastroenterol. 30 (2000) 144–154.
60. T. Akpolat, M. Akkoyunlu, I. Akpolat, et al., Renal Behçet's disease: a cumulative analysis, Semin. Arthritis Rheum. 31 (2002) 317–337.
61. C. Gürgün, E. Ercan, C. Ceyhun, et al., Cardiovascular involvement in Behçet's disease, Jpn. Heart J. 43 (2002) 389–399.
62. F. Erkan, A. Gül, E. Tasali, Pulmonary manifestations of Behçet disease, Thorax 56 (2001) 572–578.
66. S. Tokay, H. Direskeneli, S. Yurdakul, T. Akoglu, Anticardiolipin antibodies in Behçet's disease: a reassessment, Rheumatology (Oxford) 40 (2001) 192–195.
67. S. Demirer, N. Sengül, M.A. Yerdel, et al., Haemostasis in patients with Behçet's disease, Eur. J. Vasc. Endovasc. Surg. 19 (2000) 570–574.
72. T. Akpolat, M. Danaci, U. Belet, et al., MR imaging and MR angiography in vascular Behçet's disease, Magn. Reson. Imaging 18 (2000) 1089–1096.

73. G. Akman-Demir, S. Bahar, O. Coban, et al., Cranial MRI in Behçet's disease: 134 examinations of 98 patients, Neuroradiology 45 (2003) 851–859.

74. F. Nobili, M. Cutolo, A. Sulli, et al., Brain functional involvement by perfusion SPECT in systemic sclerosis and Behçet's disease, Ann. N. Y. Acad. Sci. 966 (2002) 409–414.

75. S. Ozen, The spectrum of vasculitis in children, Best Pract. Res. Clin. Rheumatol. 16 (2002) 411–425.

76. G. Hatemi, A. Silman, D. Bang, et al., EULAR recommendations for the management of Behçet disease, Ann. Rheum. Dis. 67 (2008) 1656–1662.

77. J.A. Kari, V. Shah, M.J. Dillon, Behçet's disease in UK children: clinical features and treatment including thalidomide, Rheumatology (Oxford) 40 (2001) 933–938.

78. K.E. Sharquie, R.A. Najim, A.R. Abu-Raghif, Dapsone in Behçet's disease: a double blind placebo controlled cross over study, J. Dermatol. 29 (2002) 267–279.

79. S. Yurdakul, C. Mat, Y. Tüzün, et al., A double-blind trial of colchicine in Behçet's syndrome, Arthritis Rheum. 44 (2001) 2686–2692.

80. A. Arida, K. Fragiadaki, E. Giavri, P.P. Sfikakis, Anti-TNF Agents for Behçet's disease: analysis of published data on 369 patients, Semin. Arthritis Rheum. 41 (2011) 61–70.

81. A. Saenz, M. Ausejo, B. Shea, et al., Pharmacotherapy for Behçet's syndrome, Cochrane Database Syst. Rev. 2 (2004) CD001084.

82. H. Yazici, H. Pazarli, G.G. Barnes, et al., A controlled trial of azathioprine in Behçet's syndrome, N. Engl. J. Med. 322 (1990) 281–285.

86. N.R. Benitah, L. Sobrin, G.N. Papaliodis, The use of biologic agents in the treatment of ocular manifestations of Behcet's disease, Semin. Ophthalmol. 26 (2011) 295–303.

87. P.P. Sfikakis, Behçet's disease: a new target for anti-tumour necrosis factor treatment, Ann. Rheum. Dis. 61 (Suppl. 2) (2002) ii51–ii53.

88. D. Perra, M.A. Alba, J.L. Callejas, et al., Adalimumab for the treatment of Behçet's disease. Experience in 19 patients, Rheumatology (Oxford) 51 (2012) 1825–1831.

89. A. Gül, I. Tugal-Tutkun, C.A. Dinarello, et al., Interleukin-1β-regulating antibody XOMA 052 (gevokizumab) in the treatment of acute exacerbations of resistant uveitis of Behçet's disease: an open-label pilot study, Ann. Rheum. Dis. 71 (2011) 563–536.

91. A.C. Desbois, B. Wechsler, M. Resche-Rigon, et al., Immunosuppressants reduce venous thrombosis relapse in Behçet's disease, Arthritis Rheum. 64 (2012) 2753–2760.

92. O.E. Tayer-Shifman, E. Seyahi, J. Nowatzklym, F. Ben-Chitrit, Major vessel thrombosis in Behçet's disease. The dilemma of anticoagulant therapy— the approach of rheumatologists from different countries, Clin. Exp. Rheumatol. 30 (2012) 735–740.

95. H. Yazici, F. Esen, Mortality in Behçet's syndrome, Clin. Exp. Rheumatol. 26 (2008) S138–S140.

96. E. Seyahi, M. Melikoglu, K. Akman, et al., Pulmonary artery involvement and associated lung disease in Behçet syndrome. A series of 47 patients, Medicine (Baltimore) 91 (2012) 35–48.

Entire reference list is available online at www.expertconsult.com.

CHAPTER | 41

Infectious Arthritis and Osteomyelitis

Ronald M. Laxer, James Wright, Carol B. Lindsley

Musculoskeletal infection can be considered a medical emergency, and as such it is critically important for rheumatologists to make a diagnosis quickly. Accurate diagnosis is essential to successful treatment, which is often shared among multiple specialists. New and emerging pathogens have changed the nature of musculoskeletal infections as well as some of the management strategies.

SEPTIC ARTHRITIS

Definition and Classification

Arthritis related to infection can be regarded as septic, reactive, or postinfectious.[1] *Septic arthritis* occurs when a viable infectious agent is present or has been present in the synovial space. Although direct bacterial infection of the joint constitutes the most widely recognized form of septic arthritis, direct infection with viruses, spirochetes, or fungi also occurs. *Reactive arthritis* is a response to an infectious agent that is or has been present in some other part of the body, usually the upper airway, gastrointestinal tract, or genitourinary tract. By definition, viable infectious agents are not recoverable from the synovial space in patients with reactive arthritis, which may be regarded as an immune-related disorder resulting from immunological cross-reactivity between articular structures and infectious antigens. The reactive arthritis group merges pathogenically with diseases such as the spondyloarthritides. *Postinfectious arthritis* may be considered a special type of reactive arthritis in which immune complexes containing nonviable components of an initiating infectious agent may be present in the inflamed joint. Lyme disease is discussed in Chapter 42, the reactive arthritides in Chapter 43, and rheumatic fever and poststreptococcal arthritis in Chapter 44. In chronic arthritides, which are currently considered aseptic, concerted investigations for infectious agents that use the most powerful techniques of molecular biology may yet demonstrate the causative agent in the joint space. Such techniques have isolated viral antigen or living virus from synovial fluid lymphocytes or membrane and have also demonstrated *Borrelia* organisms in patients with Lyme disease. Although the study of infectious agents, such as viruses, as possible initiators of some forms of arthritis in children has attracted much attention, it is important to remember that intraarticular and systemic bacterial infections remain the most important curable causes of arthritis in childhood.

EPIDEMIOLOGY

Sex Ratio and Age at Onset

Septic arthritis is slightly less common in girls than in boys, who account for 55% to 62% of patients in reported series.[2-4] Septic arthritis is found most often in the very young[5] and the very old; it may occur in the neonate and is most common in children younger than 2 years old. It diminishes in frequency throughout childhood.[6,7]

Familial and Geographical Clustering

There does not appear to be a genetic predisposition to septic arthritis. Typical cases of presumed septic arthritis in which no pathogen is identified tend to occur in the summer and fall,[8] but geographical clustering has not been reported. In spirochetal arthritis, such as Lyme disease, there are marked geographic and seasonal outbreaks.

Etiology and Pathogenesis

A wide range of microorganisms can cause septic arthritis in children; *Staphylococcus aureus* and non-group A and B streptococci are most common overall.[7,9-11] However, different organisms are more common at some ages and in certain circumstances (Table 41-1). *Haemophilus influenzae* type B had been the most common infection identified in children younger than 2 years old, but vaccination of infants for *H. influenza* has almost eliminated infection with this organism in those areas that routinely and effectively immunize.[10,12-15] *Streptococcus pneumoniae* is a frequent cause of infection in children younger than 2 years old and is common in the older child.[16,17] After a child reaches 2 years old, *S. aureus* is the most frequently occurring organism.[10] Group A streptococci and enterococci account for a small proportion of all cases of septic arthritis in childhood and are most prevalent in the age group of 6 to 10 year olds. *Salmonella* arthritis constitutes approximately 1% of all cases of septic arthritis, and it is commonly associated with sickle cell disease.[18] Infection with *Mycobacterium tuberculosis* is an unusual cause of septic monoarthritis in childhood. Other rare causes of infectious arthritis in children include *Streptobacillus moniliformis* (rat-bite fever), *Pseudomonas aeruginosa*, *Bacteroides* species, *Campylobacter fetus*, *Serratia* species, *Corynebacterium pyogenes*, *Neisseria meningitis*, *Pasteurella multocida*, and *Propionibacterium acnes*. *Kingella kingae* is emerging as an important pathogen in children with septic arthritis[19-22] and may account for a significant portion of culture-negative cases.[23] Most infections with this organism

TABLE 41-1   Common Microorganisms Involved in Septic Arthritis and Osteomyelitis

AGE	ORGANISMS
Neonate	Group B *Streptococcus*
	Staphylococcus aureus
	Gram-negative bacilli
Infant	*Staphylococcus aureus*
	Streptococcus species
	Haemophilus influenzae
Child	*Staphylococcus aureus*
	Streptococcus pneumoniae
	Group A *Streptococcus*
	Kingella kingae (some areas)
Adolescent	*Staphylococcus aureus*
	Streptococcus pneumoniae
	Group A *Streptococcus*
	Neisseria gonorrhoeae

TABLE 41-2   Extraarticular Sites of Infection in Children With Septic Arthritis

SITES OF INFECTION	NELSON AND KOONTZ[2] N = 117 (%)	WELKON ET AL.[8] N = 95 (%)	SPEISER ET AL.[3] N = 86 (%)
Osteomyelitis	12	12	26
Meningitis	4	4	11
Cellulitis, abscess	—	—	9
Respiratory tract	19	—	9
Middle ear	—	20	3
Urine	—	—	1
Genital tract	4	—	1
Pericardium	—	—	1
Pleura	—	—	1

occur in children younger than 5 years old, and 60% occur in children younger than 2.[24] In infants less than 60 days old, the most common causative organisms are *S. aureus* (40% to 50%) or group B *Streptococcus* (20% to 25%).[3,6,25] Enterobacteriaceae, gonococcus, and *Candida* species are also rarely pathogens in the neonate. Finally, methicillin-resistant *Staphylococcus aureus* (MRSA), a particularly virulent organism, although prevalent in southern United States, is increasing worldwide.[26]

Septic arthritis usually results from hematogenous spread from a focus of infection elsewhere in the body.[27] Direct extension of an infection from overlying soft tissues (e.g., cellulitis, abscess), bone (e.g., osteomyelitis),[28] or traumatic invasion of the joint accounts for only 15% to 20% of cases. In the hips, shoulders, ankles, and elbows, the joint capsule overlies a portion of the metaphysis, the usual site for osteomyelitis. As a result, if a focus of underlying osteomyelitis breaks through the metaphysis, it can enter the joint and result in septic arthritis.

Joint damage, one of the dreaded sequelae of infection, can result from several mechanisms. Proliferation of bacteria in the synovial membrane results in accumulation of polymorphonuclear (PMN) leukocytes and the inflammatory effects outlined in Chapters 3 and 4. In septic arthritis, synovial fluid contains high levels of proinflammatory cytokines (tumor necrosis factor [TNF]-α, interleukin [IL]-1β)[29] that mediate cartilage damage by metalloproteinases.[30] The ensuing damage to cartilaginous surfaces of the bone and the supporting structures of the joint may be severe and permanent if treatment is not urgently initiated.

Although trauma or extraarticular infection preceding onset of septic arthritis is common in case histories, knowledge of the etiological significance of these factors is incomplete.[31] In one series, upper respiratory tract infections preceded septic arthritis in approximately 50% of patients, and approximately one third of the patients had received antibiotics within 1 week of onset.[8] A history of a mild, nonpenetrating injury to the affected extremity was elicited in approximately one third of patients. However, all of these studies reflect frequent events in a child's life, and after onset of serious disease, they are especially prone to recall bias. Intravenous (IV) drug users are at particular risk for septic arthritis of the sacroiliac and sternoclavicular joints, usually caused by Gram-negative organisms.[32] Other recognized risk factors include prosthetic joints, diabetes, alcoholism, recent intraarticular steroids in patients who have a systemic infection, and

cutaneous ulcers.[33] Chronic inflammatory arthritis, including juvenile idiopathic arthritis (JIA), may predispose to joint infection.[34]

Clinical Manifestations

Septic arthritis is usually accompanied by systemic signs of illness (e.g., fever, vomiting, headache)[35] and may be a component of a more generalized infection that might include meningitis, cellulitis, osteomyelitis, or pharyngitis.[36] Joint pain is usually severe, and the infected joint and periarticular tissues are swollen, hot, and sometimes erythematous, unless muted by partial antibiotic treatment. Passive and active motion of the joint is severely, often completely, restricted (e.g., in the young child this may present as pseudoparalysis). Osteomyelitis frequently accompanies bacterial arthritis, and the presence of bone pain and point tenderness (as opposed to joint pain) should alert the examiner to this possibility. Other sites of hematogenous spread, although less common, are nonetheless important (Table 41-2).[2,3,8]

Affected Joints

The joints of the lower extremities are the most common sites of infection, and knees, hips, ankles, and elbows account for 90% of infected joints in children. Septic arthritis affecting the small joints of the hands or feet is rare (Table 41-3).[3,4,6] Pyogenic sacroiliac joint disease can occur.[37]

Multiple Infected Joints

Although septic arthritis is most often a monoarthritis, two or more joints are infected simultaneously or during the course of the same illness in a few children. In the large clinical experience reported by Fink and Nelson,[6] septic arthritis was monoarticular in 93.4% of patients but affected two joints in 4.4%, three in 1.7%, and four in 0.5%. Multijoint septic arthritis is usually part of generalized septicemia such as with staphylococcus aureus.

Geographical variation exists with up to 24% multisite involvement reported in some studies.[38] Certain immune deficiencies, such as chronic granulomatous disease or acquired immunodeficiency syndrome (AIDS), may predispose to septic arthritis in multiple joints.

Diagnosis

A systematic review concluded that in the absence of positive cultures in either the synovial fluid or the blood, the overall clinical judgment of an experienced clinician is superior to laboratory or radiological investigations for the diagnosis of septic arthritis.[39] Recently, a European group used the Delphi technique to achieve consensus on criteria for the definitive diagnosis of septic arthritis.[40] However, the group was

TABLE 41-3 Frequency of Infected Joints in Septic Arthritis

INFECTED JOINT	FINK AND NELSON[6] N = 591 (%)	WELKON ET AL.[8] N = 95 (%)	SPEISER ET AL.[3] N = 86 (%)	WILSON AND DI PAOLA[4] N = 61 (%)	OVERALL N = 833 (%)
Knee	40	46	30	29	39
Hip	23	25	29	40	25
Ankle	13	15	17	21	14
Elbow	14	5	11	3	12
Shoulder	4	4	2	3	4
Wrist	4	—	1	1	3
PIP, MCP, MTP	1	—	10	—	2
Other	1	5	—	1	1

MCP, Metacarpophalangeal; *MTP,* metatarsophalangeal; *PIP,* proximal interphalangeal.

unable to reach consensus on criteria for "probable diagnosis" (eTable 41-4). Guidelines for the management of suspected septic arthritis have been published for adults and may be applicable to the older child as well.[41] It is essential that every child with acute unexplained monoarthritis undergo aspiration of the affected joint immediately, because septic arthritis continues to be associated with considerable morbidity and mortality.[15,42,43]

If an anaerobic organism or mycobacterium is suspected, enriched culture medium and special anaerobic culture conditions are necessary. Children in whom septic arthritis is considered should also have cultures of blood and of any potential source of infection (e.g., cellulitis, abscess, and cerebrospinal fluid) performed. Rapid antigen latex agglutination tests for *H. influenzae,* group B and C streptococci, *Neisseria meningitidis,* and *S. pneumoniae* are available in most clinics. The polymerase chain reaction (PCR) has proved useful in detecting evidence of infectious agents in synovial fluid,[44-47] and real-time PCR may be even more beneficial in the investigation of culture-negative septic arthritis,[20,48] especially *Kingella.*[22]

In a group of children with septic arthritis in whom the bacterial agent was identified,[6] Fink and Nelson reported that synovial fluid was culture positive in 307 (79%) of 389 patients.[3,4,8] The remaining 21% had positive cultures from sites other than the joint: blood (10%), cerebrospinal fluid (3.8%), blood and cerebrospinal fluid (2.3%), and the vagina (1.3%). Initial inoculation of synovial fluid into blood culture bottles may increase the yield of some organisms, especially *Kingella kingae.*[21] Although an organism can be identified in one third to two thirds or more of patients by the culturing of all appropriate sites, no causative organisms are ever identified in a significant number of children with pyogenic arthritis.[49] In these patients, the diagnosis of septic arthritis is based on a typical history and the demonstration of frank pus by arthrocentesis. The gross appearance is used to judge the presence (or absence) of pus. As indicated in the next section, although synovial fluid analysis may help, cloudy fluid that precludes reading typed words through a test tube and clinical findings suggest septic arthritis, which may help direct therapy.

Synovial Fluid Analysis

The characteristics of the synovial fluid depend somewhat on the duration and severity of the disease and previous administration of antibiotics. Synovial fluid may appear normal, turbid, or grayish green with bloody streaks. The synovial fluid white blood cell (WBC) count is often markedly elevated, with 90% polymorphonuclear leukocytes (PMN) leukocytes. Speiser and colleagues[3] reported that synovial WBC counts in septic arthritis were less than 50,000/mm[3] (50×10^9/L) in 15% of children; 50,000 to 100,000/mm[3] (50×10^9

to 100×10^9/L) in 34%, and more than 100,000/mm[3] (100×10^9/L) in 51%. Fink and Nelson[6] found a relatively low WBC count (less than 25,000/mm[3] or 25×10^9) in one third of their patients.

The protein content is high (more than 2.5 g/dL) in septic arthritis and the glucose concentration, compared with plasma glucose, is usually low, although it may be normal. A Gram stain identifies the organism in half of untreated patients but in only one fifth of those who have received antibiotics. A Gram stain provides rapid confirmation of bacterial infection and tentative identification of the organism (if the findings are positive), permitting rational antibiotic therapy. Special procedures such as counterimmunoelectrophoresis, latex agglutination, or evaluation by PCR may sometimes identify bacterial antigens in a culture-negative fluid (i.e., blood, urine, or cerebrospinal fluid). These techniques have the advantage of providing antigenic identification much more rapidly than cultures, but they do not provide antibiotic sensitivities. Use of real-time PCR to identify *Kingella kingae* toxin substantially increases the detection of this organism not identified in routine culture.[50]

Blood Studies

At least two blood cultures should always be performed for a child suspected of having septic arthritis. An elevated WBC count with a predominance of PMNs and bands and a markedly elevated erythrocyte sedimentation rate (ESR) or C-reactive protein (CRP) level, although of limited help in specific diagnosis, provide a baseline whereby the efficacy of subsequent treatment can be judged. CRP is a better predictor of septic arthritis than the ESR. If the CRP value is less than 1 mg/dL, the likelihood that the patient does not have septic arthritis was 87% in one study.[51] Concentrations of other acute phase reactants are usually increased, but provide no additional useful information.

Radiological Examination

A number of imaging techniques may be helpful in evaluating a child with septic arthritis[52-56] Plain radiographs are not diagnostic but might be helpful in excluding other disorders. They may show an underlying osteomyelitis as the etiology of the septic arthritis and may demonstrate only increased soft tissue and capsular swelling. Juxtaarticular osteoporosis reflects inflammatory hyperemia and is evident within several days after onset of infection. Cartilage loss and narrowing of the joint space and subluxation are late findings that develop as the disease progresses. These changes are followed by marginal erosions and eventually by ankylosis (Fig. 41-1, *A, E*).[55] Computed tomography (CT) and especially magnetic resonance imaging (MRI) are additional confirmatory techniques.

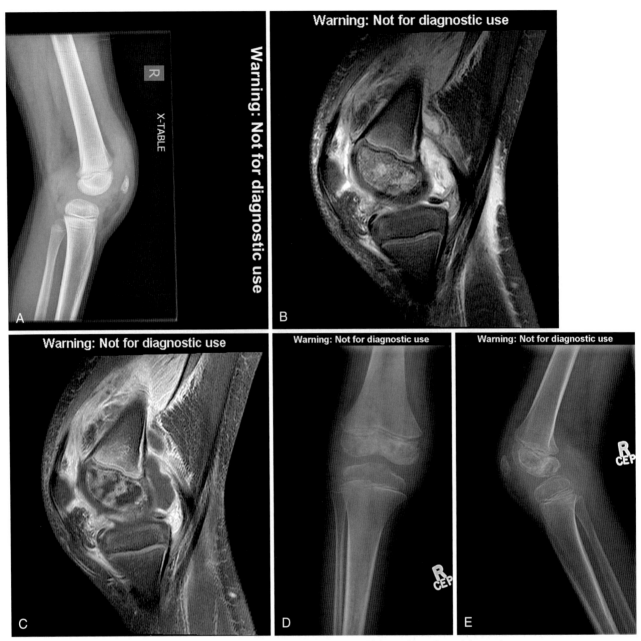

FIGURE 41-1 A, Lateral view of the right knee in a 6-year-old boy with pain and fever demonstrates a large joint effusion. MRI obtained a few days later confirms a large joint effusion with diffuse synovial thickening on the sagittal STIR image **(B)**. The sagittal T1 fat-saturated image post-gadolinium **(C)** shows avid enhancement of the thickened synovium with nonenhancing pockets of fluid. There is also abnormal enhancement of the distal femoral epiphysis in keeping with osteomyelitis with bone abscess (*arrow*). AP **(D)** and lateral **(E)** radiographs of the right knee following treatment shows resolution of the joint effusion with patchy sclerosis in the distal femoral epiphysis indicating ongoing healing from osteomyelitis. (Courtesy Dr. Jennifer Stimec.)

Computed Tomography

The role of CT is generally limited, as other imaging techniques are usually sufficient in children. It may be especially helpful for the evaluation of sacroiliac and sternoclavicular joints. It is also helpful, in combination with ultrasound, to guide aspirations and biopsies.

Ultrasonography

Detection of joint fluid by ultrasound can help guide fluid aspiration. The sonographic detection of an effusion in the hip of a child treated

for osteomyelitis of the femur often indicates the presence of septic arthritis of the joint.[55] Color Doppler may show increased capsular vascularity. In children, ultrasound is the imaging modality of choice for guidance during aspiration or biopsy whenever possible. It may be used in isolation or combination with other imaging modalities.

Radionuclide Scans

During the first few days of disease, when plain radiographs show only soft tissue changes, 99mTc-MDP scans reflect hyperemia of the infected area on blood flow studies and increased uptake of the isotope on both sides of the joint.[56] Occasionally, decreased uptake may occur if significant accumulation of intraarticular fluid impedes local blood flow. This technique is useful in the early detection of joint or bone inflammation or infection, but it does not differentiate the two with certainty and cannot differentiate septic arthritis from synovitis from other causes (e.g., JIA). It is helpful in differentiating septic arthritis from osteomyelitis and soft tissue infection, and in the detection of multifocal joint infections.[57] Radionuclide scans with gallium-67 or the patient's indium-111-labeled granulocytes or monoclonal antibodies may be helpful but are not routinely needed. It is possible that 2-deoxy-2-[^{18}F] fluoro-D-glucose positron emission tomography (FDG-PET)/CT may have an important role in the diagnosis of difficult cases because PET is a relatively fast, whole-body imaging modality and can be used to find infectious foci outside of the bone or joint.[57] It may be particularly helpful for infections of the vertebrae. In general, however, this modality has been replaced by MRI, which provides more detailed information without radiation exposure. PET positivity may help indicate which focus to approach for potential biopsy or aspiration.

Magnetic Resonance Imaging

Delineation of soft tissue structures by MRI is superior to that provided by CT.[54,55] Changes may be seen as soon as 24 hours following infection. Synovial enhancement is detected in virtually all patients. Signal-intensity alterations in the bone marrow are characteristic, but not diagnostic of, septic arthritis (i.e., low intensity on fat-suppressed, gadolinium-enhanced, T1-weighted, spin-echo images, and high signal intensity on fat-suppressed, T2-weighted, fast spin-echo images)[58] (Fig. 41-1, B, C). Articular cartilage and growth cartilage are depicted along with other fibrous structures, muscle, blood vessels, and synovial fluid. An abnormal collection of fluid or debris, often displacing the joint capsule, eroding into other tissues, or, in children, even leading to subluxation, supports the possibility of septic arthritis. Fat-suppressed, gadolinium-enhanced MRI is 100% sensitive and 79% specific for the diagnosis of septic arthritis in adults.[59] MRI may be most helpful in children who do not respond to therapy in the predicted fashion to look for unresolved or other sites of infection in adjacent sites. As technology improves, MRI-guided biopsies or aspirations or other image fusion techniques are becoming useful diagnostic methods when the abnormality is only visible on MRI.

Treatment

The child with septic arthritis requires hospitalization and consultation with an orthopedic surgeon and usually a specialist in infectious diseases. Nonsteroidal antiinflammatory drugs (NSAIDs) may be used to help minimize the effects of inflammation, to control fever, and to contribute to pain relief. IV dexamethasone has been shown to reduce the duration of symptoms and minimize joint damage in a randomized, double-blind study, but it is rarely, if ever, used.[60,61] A clinical practice guideline for the management of septic arthritis in children has been proposed.[62] It was demonstrated that this approach was effective in minimizing the use of bone scans, in minimizing the rate of joint drainage, in accelerating the change to oral antibiotic administration, and in shortening the duration of hospital stay. There were no differences in outcomes such as readmission to the hospital, recurrence of infection, or the development of residual joint damage.

Antibiotics

In a child with septic arthritis, health care professionals should obtain cultures of blood, joint fluid and any other potential site of infection. IV antibiotics should then be administered as promptly as possible.

TABLE 41-5 **Recommended Empiric Antibiotic Therapy by Age***	
<3 months	Cefotaxime + nafcillin/oxacillin (if >1 week in NICU, consider using vancomycin)
>3 months	If CA-MRSA <10%: nafcillin/oxacillin or cefazolin
	If CA-MRSA >10%: clindamycin (check for resistance) or vancomycin

*Every effort should be made to secure cultures and adjust therapy accordingly. Linezolid is an alternative to vancomycin or clindamycin if MRSA is a concern. If *Kingella kingae* is suspected, use cefazolin.

The main issue that may influence the first dose is the timing of joint aspiration. In general, aspiration is preferred to identify organisms, but if any delay is anticipated, antibiotic treatment should be started as soon as blood cultures are obtained. The choice of antibiotic depends on the presence of predisposing factors; the age of the child; and the organisms suspected because of the Gram stain or rapid antigen detection tests (although it is hazardous to narrow initial treatment based solely on these results because either can be wrong). If the Gram stain and results of rapid antigen detection are negative or not available, an approach based on age (as outlined in Table 41-5) is suggested.[37] For uncomplicated osteoarticular infection in infants and children, clindamycin was as effective as cephalosporin.[63] The demonstration of an organism or antigen may support or contradict the generalizations outlined in this table and should influence the physician in selection of the initial antibiotic treatment.[42,64]

Although monitoring intravenous antibiotic efficacy with serum bactericidal titer can be performed, it is seldom used unless response to therapy has been unsatisfactory. After satisfactory control—based on a combination of clinical signs such as absence of fever and improved movement of the affected joint plus laboratory parameters such as reduction of the WBC, ESR, and CRP—of the infectious process with IV antibiotic administration is achieved, treatment by the oral route in the hospital or on an outpatient basis may be appropriate.[65-67] Trials have suggested that the duration of treatment can be shortened to 10 days in total.[63,68] Home IV antibiotic programs may also be effective in reducing the hospital stay, but they may be associated with complications in up to 30% of children.[69] Such programs should be undertaken only after careful consideration and consultation with an expert in pediatric infectious disease. The criteria for conversion from IV to oral therapy are uncertain. Although many criteria have been suggested, such as resolution of fever, significant decrease in pain, improvement in range of motion, and falling laboratory measures of inflammation, the most useful assessment is when the child starts to move the limb voluntarily with a reducing or absent fever.

If the cultures are negative, IV antibiotics should be continued for a minimum of 21 days.[1] If the child's clinical state is improving (i.e., temperature returning to normal, pain diminishing, range of motion improving) and the WBC count and ESR/CRP are falling, the initial antibiotics chosen should be maintained. If the patient does not appear to be responding, clinicians need to consider that the drug, dose, route, and compliance are appropriate, and the possibility of the reaccumulation of joint fluid or another site of infection. Because of various patterns of antibiotic susceptibility and resistance, guidelines regarding antibiotic choice and duration of treatment are constantly changing, and the physician is urged to review the most current recommendations. This is especially important with the rise in the incidence of community-acquired Methicillin-resistant *Staphylococcus aureus* (CA-MRSA), which requires specific antibiotic management. As noted previously, the total duration of therapy is controversial but in uncomplicated septic arthritis in a child who responds rapidly, 10 days is probably sufficient.[63]

Aspiration and Drainage

The usefulness of repeated aspiration and drainage of an infected joint has been hotly debated. There is no dispute that an initial diagnostic arthrocentesis must be performed. Any joint that appears to be under pressure from an effusion can probably benefit from aspiration, if only for pain relief. Studies of the importance of repeated aspirations under other circumstances, however, have failed to show a consistent benefit. Open drainage is no better than closed needle aspiration (except for specific joints such as the hip and shoulder) and is attended by significantly increased morbidity. It is not known whether irrigation of the joint at the time of aspiration provides additional benefit with improved outcome. Occasionally, arthroscopic examination is indicated. Intraarticular administration of antibiotic is unnecessary because therapeutic synovial fluid antibiotic levels are readily achieved,[70] and it may induce chemical synovitis in the infected joint.

Special Cases
Neonatal Septic Arthritis

In addition to *S. aureus,* group B *Streptococcus* and Gram-negative bacteria can be the offending organisms in the neonate.[71] Infections with these organisms are rare but potentially extremely serious in this age group. They may have a subtle presentation and can occasionally be bilateral, and they are much more likely to occur in association with osteomyelitis than in older children. Most affected newborns show no fever, toxemia, or leukocytosis.[72,73] Any infant who has swelling in the region of the thigh or holds the leg flexed, abducted, or externally rotated, or refuses to use the upper limb must be investigated promptly. Problems in early recognition of disease undoubtedly contribute to the often disastrous outcome of this involvement.[74]

Septic Hip Joint

Septic arthritis of the hip is such an important problem that it merits special attention.[75,76] Because the risks of missing this diagnosis are so high, there must a very low threshold for hip aspiration to establish the diagnosis.[62] The femoral head is intracapsular, and the arterial supply passes through the ligamentum teres into the intracapsular space. Increased intracapsular pressure can therefore interrupt the blood supply to the femoral head, with disastrous consequences to its viability, leading to the subsequent development of avascular necrosis.[77] Metaphyseal osteomyelitis readily leads to septic arthritis of the hip joint in the infant because nutrient blood vessels pass from the metaphysis through the epiphyseal growth plate and terminate in the distal ossification center.

Septic arthritis of the hip joint is most common in infants and very young children; 70% of patients are 4 years old or younger.[78] The typical clinical picture is that of an infant or young child who may have an unexplained fever, is irritable, and refuses to move a leg, bear weight, or walk. Any movement of the hip is extremely painful, and the affected leg is held in a position of partial flexion, abduction, and external rotation at the hip. Occasionally, the child has lower abdominal pain or tenderness, sometimes with paralytic ileus.

The most common differential diagnosis for septic arthritis of the hip in the younger child is transient synovitis or irritable hip syndrome. Transient or toxic synovitis of the hip is an idiopathic disorder often preceded by a nonspecific upper respiratory tract infection. It occurs most commonly in boys (70%) between 3 and 10 years old.[79] Pain in the hip, thigh, or knee may be of sudden or gradual onset

and lasts for an average of 6 days. Bilateral involvement occurs in approximately 4% of cases. There is loss of internal rotation of the hip, and the hip may be held in the flexed, abducted position. The ESR and WBC count are usually normal.[79,80] Radiographs often appear normal or may document widening of the joint space with lateral displacement of the femoral head because of effusion. These findings can be confirmed by CT or ultrasound studies.[79] Radionuclide scanning may demonstrate a transient decrease in uptake of technetium 99m phosphate. Signal intensity is normal with MRI and differentiates toxic synovitis of the hip from a septic process,[58] which is usually the principal differential diagnosis.[81] After a diagnostic ultrasound scan to confirm the presence of fluid, the hip joint should be aspirated to exclude bacterial sepsis if the diagnosis is uncertain.[82] The ability to weight bear and move the hip voluntarily, and the absence of elevated inflammatory markers, all suggest transient synovitis of the hip. The synovial fluid has a normal or minimally increased cell count but may be under high pressure. After aspiration, the pain and range of motion are dramatically improved, at least temporarily. Treatment includes the use of analgesics or NSAIDs, bed rest, and skin traction with the hip in 45° flexion to minimize intracapsular pressure.[79] Long-term sequelae include Legg–Calvé–Perthes disease, which appears in about 1.5% of cases at some point in the future.[83,84] The only other long-term sequela is the development of coxa magna, which fortunately is of no clinical significance. Recurrences are often accompanied by low-grade fever. Although prediction rules tend not to function well in the general population,[85] possible criteria used to differentiate septic arthritis from irritable hip syndrome include refusal to bear weight; a fever of 38.5°C; ESR greater than 40 mm/hour; and WBC greater than 12×10^9/L.[86] Another study suggested refusal to bear weight and CRP greater than 20 mg/L were highly predictive of septic arthritis.[87]

In very young or premature infants, a number of risk factors predispose to septic arthritis of the hip.[88] In a study of septic arthritis of the hip of 16 infants younger than 4 weeks old, 11 were premature, 7 had an umbilical catheter, and 12 had septicemia. In contrast, of 13 children between the ages of 1 month and 3 years with septic arthritis, none was premature or had an umbilical catheter, and only 5 were septicemic. A high frequency of preceding or accompanying osteomyelitis of the femur or pelvis has been observed. The association of septic arthritis of the hip and femoral venipuncture has been recorded[89] and may account in part for the high frequency of arthritis of this site in the premature neonate.

Management of septic arthritis of the hip requires open drainage to minimize intraarticular pressure.[90,91] Children are seldom immobilized, instead allowing early passive and active physiotherapy to prevent loss of range of motion. In the unusual circumstance of septic arthritis with subluxation or dislocation, older children require immobilization and neonates require a Pavlik harness for the hip. Prognosis is guarded even with the best treatment, especially in the neonate. The anatomy of the shoulder joint is not unlike that of the hip with respect to vascular supply. Septic arthritis of this joint, although rare, should be treated similarly.[92]

Gonococcal Arthritis

In reported series of septic arthritis in children and adolescents, disease caused by *N. gonorrhoeae* appears to be uncommon. When it occurs, it is most common in the adolescent, although it occasionally occurs in the neonate in association with disseminated infection.[93] It is more common in girls than in boys and is particularly likely just after menstruation or with pregnancy.[94] Gonococcal arthritis usually develops in patients with primary asymptomatic genitourinary gonorrhea or with a gonococcal infection of the throat or rectum. The patient presents with a systemic illness characterized by fever and chills.[95] A vesiculopustular rash, sparsely distributed on the extremities, commonly yields organisms on culture or Gram stain of the smear. Gonococcal arthritis may have an initial migratory phase and may be accompanied by tenosynovitis. In contrast to most patients with septic arthritis, those with gonococcal arthritis may present with a purulent arthritis of several joints. For a patient with suspected gonococcal arthritis, it is important to culture samples from the genital tract, throat, rectum, and any vesicles in addition to the affected joint. Special culture media with Thayer-Martin agar will help in isolating the organism. The possibility of sexual abuse should be considered and appropriately investigated.

Mycobacterial Arthritis

Tuberculous arthritis is seldom encountered in North America or Europe, although its frequency may be increasing because of immunosuppressive therapy, drug-resistant strains of tuberculosis, the human immunodeficiency virus (HIV) epidemic, and international travel.[96-98] Tuberculous arthritis is by no means rare in other parts of the world. Typically, arthritis arises on a background of pulmonary tuberculosis as indolent, chronic monoarthritis, often of the knee or wrist, which eventually results in extreme destruction of the joint and surrounding bones. It manifests as acute arthritis in rare instances.[99] Occasionally it may present as otherwise typical oligoarticular JIA in the absence of pulmonary disease.[100,101] If a patient suspected of having oligoarticular JIA fails to respond to intraarticular corticosteroid treatment, the suspicion of tuberculous monoarthritis should be raised, especially if there may be a relevant travel history or contact with people from endemic areas.

Joint infection occurs by hematogenous dissemination of the organism or from adjoining osteomyelitis. For example, hip arthritis can result from spinal infection where organisms track down to the iliopsoas muscle that communicates with the joint. Chronic draining fistulae may develop. Pott disease is a consequence of vertebral osteomyelitis (Fig. 41-2). Tuberculous dactylitis may occur with cystic expansion and destruction of bone (i.e., spina ventosa) (Fig. 41-3).[102] A family or environmental history of pulmonary tuberculosis and a positive purified protein derivative (Mantoux) skin test result suggest

the possibility of tuberculous arthritis. Although synovial fluid cultures are positive in approximately 75% of patients, synovial membrane biopsy and culture are preferred and confirm the diagnosis in almost all patients (Fig. 41-4). The synovial WBC count is classically less than 50,000/mm^3 (50×10^9/L), with a high proportion of mononuclear cells. Genus-specific PCR is invaluable in the diagnosis.[46] Rarely, a polyarthritis accompanies tuberculosis (i.e., Poncet's disease); it probably represents a reactive arthritis because culture of the inflamed joints fails to demonstrate tubercle bacilli.[103,104]

Another mycobacterial disease that can result in arthritis is leprosy, caused by *Mycobacterium leprae*. Although the most common clinical manifestations are rash and peripheral neuropathy, arthritis occurs in approximately 75% of cases.[105,106] Different types of arthritis in leprosy include Charcot joints, septic arthritis, acute polyarthritis, chronic arthritis, and tenosynovitis. Clinical differentiation from JIA may be

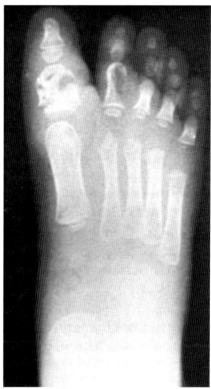

FIGURE 41-3 Advanced osseous destruction occurred in the foot of a child with tuberculous dactylitis (i.e., spinal ventosa).

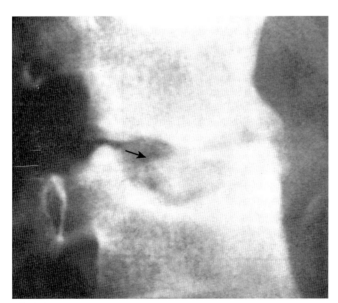

FIGURE 41-2 Pott disease of the vertebral column in an adolescent boy with pulmonary tuberculosis produced destruction of the disk space and vertebral end-plate erosion (*arrow*).

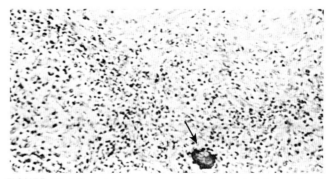

FIGURE 41-4 Synovial biopsy specimen of chronic inflammation in tuberculous joint disease in which a giant cell (*arrow*) is indicated.

difficult, especially if the possibility of leprosy is not considered in a nonendemic area; a high degree of clinical suspicion is required to make this diagnosis.[107] *Mycobacterium leprae* is not always easily identified in synovial biopsies.[108,109] Serologic testing may be helpful in confirming the diagnosis.[105] Additional cases of leprosy have been reported following the institution of anti-TNF therapy in patients with rheumatoid arthritis.[110]

Arthritis Associated With Brucellosis

Human *Brucella* infections are reported primarily from Europe,[111,112] Israel,[113] and South America,[114,115] with a substantial number of patients having arthritis. Cases that develop in North America are more likely to have been acquired elsewhere.[116] The species most frequently implicated are *Brucella melitensis*[112,114,115] and, less commonly, *Brucella canis*.[117] Unpasteurized milk is a source of infection.

The systemic illness is often mild in children but is usually characterized by undulant fever, gastrointestinal complaints, lymphadenopathy, and sometimes dermatitis. In 88 children from Israel,[113] the classic triad of fever (91%), arthralgia or arthritis (83%), and hepatosplenomegaly (63%) was characteristic of most patients. In a large series of cases from Peru,[114] almost one third were children, and one third had arthritis. In the neonate to 15-years-old age group, peripheral arthritis of a hip or knee was most common. In patients whose onset was after 15 years of age, sacroiliitis was the most common articular syndrome. Spondylitis and sacroiliac arthritis became predominant after children reached 15 years of age. Gomez-Reino and colleagues[112] found that periarthritis without effusion was most common and that small joints and the spine were not affected. Whether this reflects differences in the infecting organism or in ascertainment is not known. No association with human leukocyte antigen (HLA)-B27 has been demonstrated.[111] Synovial fluid WBC counts are only modestly elevated, with a slight predominance of mononuclear cells.[114,118] Joint fluid culture is positive for the organism in some patients. Tetracyclines, aminoglycosides, rifampin, and trimethoprim-sulfamethoxazole, often in combination, provide effective treatment of the acute infection, although permanent sequelae may result.[112,115]

Mycoplasma and Arthritis

Myalgia and arthralgia are common during pulmonary infection with *Mycoplasma pneumoniae*. Objective oligoarticular, polyarticular, or migratory arthritis has also been described.[119] Sensitive screening tests may uncover *Mycoplasma* as a cause of arthritis even in the absence of pneumonia.[120,121]

Bartonella Infection and Arthritis

There have been rare reports of *Bartonella henselae* infection causing arthritis in children (e.g., cat scratch disease).[122-124] In two children, the disease mimicked systemic JIA[123,124]; a third child had polyarthritis and subcutaneous nodules.[122] Arthropathy occurred in 3% of patients in an Israeli registry. It was characterized by large- and medium-sized monoarthritis, oligoarthritis, or polyarthritis (most commonly symmetric oligoarthritis), which was debilitating. Despite cat scratch disease being a disease of children and adolescents, in this series no patient under 20 years old had joint involvement. The arthropathy usually occurred concurrent with the lymphadenopathy. Erythema nodosum was more common in those with than without arthropathy.[125,126]

Arthritis in Immunocompromised Patients

Chronic inflammatory arthritis in patients with a primary immunodeficiency is discussed in Chapter 46. Typical septic arthritis has been reported infrequently in immunodeficient children.[127] *Mycoplasma*

is the most common cause of severe chronic erosive arthritis in patients with congenital immunodeficiency syndromes[128] and has been recovered from joints of patients with AIDS.[129] *Ureaplasma urealyticum* has been identified in patients with agammaglobulinemia.[130] *Candida albicans* is occasionally responsible for arthritis in immunosuppressed patients.[130,131] Patients with HIV have increased incidence of *Streptococcus pneumoniae* infection that requires broad-spectrum antibiotics.[132]

Course of the Disease and Prognosis

The outcome in septic arthritis is somewhat guarded because permanent damage may occur even with early and appropriate antibiotic treatment. The child usually recovers from the acute illness, but with the passage of time, reduction in range of motion, pain, and eventually degeneration of the surfaces of the affected joint may require surgical intervention. It is estimated that residual dysfunction occurs in 10% to 25% of children, although the changes (e.g., limited joint mobility, joint instability or chronic subluxation) may not be apparent until years later.[8] Recently, a simplified radiographic classification system has been developed to determine prognosis and to guide surgical management of the sequelae of septic arthritis of the hip.[133]

Related Disorders
Arthritis Associated With Acne

The association between arthritis and acne has been noted for decades. Most patients are male and have onset of musculoskeletal complications during adolescence. The syndrome includes severe truncal acne followed in several months by fever and arthralgia or arthritis, most often involving hips, knees, and shoulders. Myopathy may also accompany the disorder.[134] It is possible that this syndrome is another example of reactive arthritis. Although arthritis lasts for only a few months in some patients, recurrences over many years have been documented.[135,136] Treatment with NSAIDs and with antibiotics for control of the acne is indicated. Treatments for acne may also be associated with arthritis, such as minocycline-induced autoimmune phenomena[137] and isotretinoin causing an acute arthritis.[138-141] Infliximab for the treatment of arthritis has been reported to cause acne.[142] Some cases fall under the category of the pyogenic arthritis pyoderma gangrenosum acne (PAPA) syndrome, reviewed in Chapter 47. Recurrent attacks of acute episodes of monoarthritis and fever, resembling septic arthritis, may also be seen in patients with familial Mediterranean fever, also reviewed in Chapter 47.

Whipple Disease

Whipple disease, first described in 1907,[143] is rare in childhood, although primary infection with the causative organism may cause diarrhea and transitory fever in young children.[144] The disease[145] is caused by the bacterium *Tropheryma whipplei*, a ubiquitous organism present in the environment, and is characterized by abdominal pain, weight loss, diarrhea, and, in 65% to 90% of patients, arthralgias or arthritis that in most cases precedes other clinical signs by several years.[145-148] Whipple disease occurs 10 times more frequently in males than in females and is most common in middle age, although it has been identified in young children.[144,149,150] Migratory, peripheral joint pain and inflammation lasting hours to months occur over a period of many years, often in association with fatigue, weight loss, and anemia. Joint swelling with increased synovial fluid and restriction of range of motion may occur,[151] although residual deformity does not.[152] The joints most frequently affected are the ankles, knees, elbows, and wrists,[151,153] and spondylitis has been reported in 20% of cases.[152] Occasionally, arthritis or spondylodiscitis may be present in the absence of gastrointestinal symptoms, and Whipple disease should be considered in patients who are resistant to antirheumatic treatment.[154] A significant percentage of the population, especially those who work with soil or in sewage plants, may be asymptomatic carriers. Periodic acid–Schiff–positive material and bacteria are detectable in macrophages infiltrating the upper small intestine and lymph nodes. Other diagnostic tools include PCR, immunohistochemistry, and electron microscopy. These tests may also be diagnostic on synovial tissue.[153] Because it takes several months to culture the organism, cultures are not recommended as a diagnostic tool. Furthermore, patients with arthritis may not have gastrointestinal (GI) symptoms, and duodeno-jejunal biopsies will be negative. In such cases PCR is especially important. A genetic predisposition has been suggested based on the ubiquitous nature of the organism, but causative genes have not been identified. Antimicrobial therapy has greatly improved the outcome in this disease. In the absence of neurological involvement, the combination of doxycycline and hydroxychloroquine is the recommended first-line treatment. If there is neurological involvement, sulfadiazine should be added to this regimen.[145] The immune reconstitution syndrome has been reported in several patients following successful treatment.[155]

OSTEOMYELITIS

Although osteomyelitis, like septic arthritis, is most often encountered and treated by specialists in orthopedics and infectious diseases, its frequent association with septic arthritis and the diagnostic problems that it presents require that it be included in this discussion.[156,66,157-163]

Definition and Classification

Bacteria or, rarely, fungi may lead to an intraosseous infection. Historically, osteomyelitis has been classified as acute, subacute, or chronic, based on the duration of symptoms. This classification, based on duration of symptoms, is no longer useful in guiding treatment due to the emergence of MRSA. Classically, *acute osteomyelitis* is of recent onset and short duration (less than 2 weeks). It is most often hematogenous in origin but may result from trauma such as a compound fracture or puncture wound. It can be metaphyseal, epiphyseal, or diaphyseal in location. *Subacute osteomyelitis* is of longer duration and is usually caused by less virulent organisms. *Chronic osteomyelitis* results from ineffective treatment of acute osteomyelitis, or delay in treatment, and is characterized by necrosis and sequestration of bone.

Epidemiology

Acute osteomyelitis is somewhat less common than acute septic arthritis. An incidence of 16.7 cases of acute osteomyelitis per year was reported from an institution at which acute septic arthritis occurred at a rate of 28.4 cases per year.[6] However, osteomyelitis may be more common than septic arthritis in developing countries of the world.[164] An incidence rate of 8 per 100,000 children per year has been reported in high-income countries.[165] Although its incidence may be declining in many parts of the world, that is not necessarily the case everywhere.[166] Acute osteomyelitis occurs twice as often in boys as in girls[6,164,167] and is more common in younger children. It can occur in the neonate.[71]

Etiology and Pathogenesis

S. aureus (50% to 80%) and the group A streptococci (5% to 10%) are the predominant organisms at all ages.[6,168] CA-MRSA has emerged as an important pathogen.[169,170,171] Up to 15% of children with CA-MRSA who carry the genes encoding Panton–Valentine leukocidin *(pvl)* have multiple sites of infection.[172] These organisms are also associated with chronic osteomyelitis. *Kingella kingae* is also an important cause of osteomyelitis, especially in younger children, and specific

microbiological techniques may be needed to detect it.[22] Even before specific immunization, *H. influenzae* seldom caused osteomyelitis (2% to 10%) and should now be even less common.[13,173] In certain circumstances, specific or unusual organisms (15%) are found. For example, infection of the calcaneus or other bone in the foot associated with a puncture wound through athletic footwear is likely caused by *P. aeruginosa*.[27,31,174,175] Osteomyelitis caused by *S. pneumonia*[16,176] usually occurs in children with associated diseases such as sickle cell anemia,[177-179] asplenia,[159,180] or hypogammaglobulinemia,[160,181] although it has been observed in young infants without underlying disease.[182] *Salmonella* osteomyelitis is a complication of sickle cell anemia but also occurs in children without sickle cell anemia.[183] In the neonate, group B streptococci,[184,185] Gram-negative organisms,[186-188] and *Candida* in addition to *S. aureus* are all potential causes of osteomyelitis. *B. melitensis* uncommonly results in osteomyelitis, but when it does, it has a predilection for the vertebral bodies.[117] Tuberculous osteomyelitis may take various forms and may mimic chronic pyogenic disease, Brodie abscess, tumor, or other types of granuloma.[189-191] *B. henselae* (the organism of cat scratch disease) has been identified as the causative agent in a few patients with osteomyelitis.[192-194]

Clinical Manifestations

Fever, bone pain, and tenderness with or without local swelling should suggest the possibility of osteomyelitis. Although a history of prior trauma is elicited in approximately one third of young patients, its significance is uncertain. In the infant, fever may be minimal, and localization of the pain may make it difficult to detect on physical examination.[195] Pseudoparalysis of a limb is often evident. The examiner may find clinical evidence of a preceding systemic infection. The site of the bone infection is usually metaphyseal, and bony tenderness is elicited by pressure near or over the infected area. The presence of a joint effusion adjacent to the site of bone infection may reflect septic arthritis or a sterile noninflammatory "sympathetic" effusion.[196] With delay in treatment or the presence of virulent organisms such as MRSA, the local signs, usually due to abscess formation, resemble cellulitis.

Osteomyelitis in children has a predilection for the metaphysis of rapidly growing bone. Many explanations have been suggested for this tendency. The anatomical differences in vasculature in this area in children and its easily compromised blood supply may in part explain the clinical observation (see Chapter 2). In one anatomical model, bacteremia and, in some cases, preceding microtrauma were sufficient to initiate disease.[197] The bones of the lower extremity are affected in 66% of patients; those of the upper extremity account for approximately 25%, but those of the skull, face, spine, and pelvis are the sites of infection in fewer than 10% (Table 41-6).[6,164,198-200] Fewer than 10% of children have two or more simultaneously infected bones; in some cases, five or more bones are involved as part of a severe septicemic illness, usually caused by staphylococci. This type of involvement must be distinguished from chronic recurrent multifocal osteomyelitis (see Chapter 48).

Acute osteomyelitis can be associated with the development of deep-vein thromboses (DVT).[201] In a series of 35 patients from Dallas who had osteomyelitis involving the proximal humerus, femur, proximal tibia or fibula, pelvis, or vertebrae, 10 had evidence of DVT based on imaging studies, although it was only symptomatic in one patient. In two patients, the DVT was related to a central catheter placed for long-term antibiotic therapy, whereas in the remaining eight, the DVT occurred in veins adjacent to the site of infection. The authors attributed the DVTs to the inflammatory response leading to localized endothelial damage and activation of the coagulation cascade. Compounding factors include the local edema, venous compression and immobility in patients with lower extremity involvement. Organisms with the *pvl* gene were more likely to be associated with DVTs.[202] Features that suggest methicillin-resistant versus methicillin-sensitive *Staphylococcus aureus* osteomyelitis include a temperature of higher than 38°C; hematrocrit at less than 34%; WBC greater than 12,000; and CRP greater than 13mg/L.[203]

Subacute Osteomyelitis

Compared with acute osteomyelitis, patients with subacute osteomyelitis, defined as disease duration between 2 weeks to 3 months,

TABLE 41-6 Affected Sites in Septic Osteomyelitis

BONE	OSTEOMYELITIS* (%)
Tibia	25
Clavicle	<1
Fibula	6
Spine	1
Femur	27
Metatarsus, metacarpus, phalanx	4
Radius	4
Pelvis	6
Humerus	11
Ulna	2
Sternum	<1
Mandible	<1
Scapula	<1
Rib	<1
Talus	1
Calcaneus	6

*Data from C.W. Fink, J.D. Nelson, Septic arthritis and osteomyelitis in children, Clin. Rheum. Dis. 12 (1986) 423, and from W.G. Cole, R.E. Dalziel, S. Leitl, Treatment of acute osteomyelitis in childhood, J. Bone Joint Surg. Br. 64 (1982) 218.

experience less pain, often have no fever, and have frequently received a course of antibiotics. Laboratory changes are less common, but radiographs are usually abnormal and may be confused with Ewing sarcoma or osteoid osteoma.[166] Brodie abscess, a unique form of subacute osteomyelitis, is usually of staphylococcal origin and may develop after a penetrating injury or more likely by hematogenous spread of an infection to the metaphysis. It is characterized clinically by tenderness with pain that may awaken the child at night. Radiographs demonstrate only soft tissue swelling early, but eventually metaphyseal osteolytic lesions are evident. They are most common in the proximal or distal ends of the tibia (Fig. 41-5).[204,205] Culture of the abscess may be negative. Treatment includes IV antibiotics, an NSAID, and immobilization.

Chronic Osteomyelitis

Chronic osteomyelitis develops when acute osteomyelitis has been inadequately treated, or it develops in states of impaired host or antibiotic resistance. Reduced blood flow leads to the formation of a sequestrum, which may be surrounded by a sleeve of periosteal new bone (involucrum). Complications of chronic osteomyelitis include growth plate arrest or stimulation, avascular necrosis, pathological fracture, septicemia, and if it becomes chronic, amyloidosis.[166]

Neonatal Osteomyelitis

Neonatal osteomyelitis merits special consideration.[72] Until a child reaches the age of approximately 18 months, metaphyseal blood vessels can cross over the open physis into the epiphysis, permitting infection to move across the growth plate. The thin cortical bone of newborns allows infection to spread rapidly into the subperiosteal region, and the relative immune deficient state of the newborn allows for rapid spread. The lack of a systemic inflammatory response often leads to a delay in diagnosis, and involvement of more than one site is common. Although *S. aureus* remains the most common organism responsible for neonatal osteomyelitis, especially in newborns with central lines, group B streptococci, Gram-negative bacteria, and *Candida albicans* may also be responsible.

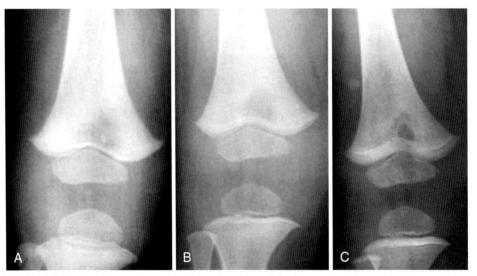

FIGURE 41-5 Brodie abscess is revealed in radiographs of the knee of a 16-month-old boy with acute hematogenous osteomyelitis inadequately treated 1 month earlier. **A,** Central sequestration with a surrounding, ill-defined lytic margin. The patient was appropriately treated with antibiotics at this stage. **B,** One month later, the sequestrum has been removed by osteoclasts. **C,** One month later, the radiograph shows a well-defined lesion with sclerotic borders. (Courtesy Dr. B. Wood.)

Diagnosis

As in septic arthritis, it is essential that every reasonable attempt be made to identify the organism and determine its antibiotic susceptibility.[159] Recently, a European group of experts arrived at a consensus definition of osteomyelitis.[40] A high index of suspicion for this diagnosis must be maintained in any child with unexplained pain, fever, limp, or lack of use of an extremity. Aspiration of subperiosteal pus, if present, can be used for diagnosis and, together with cultures of the blood, synovial fluid, or an infected wound, should yield an organism in approximately 70% to 80% of cases. Blood cultures alone are positive in 30% to 50% of infants and children with osteomyelitis.[206] A bone biopsy may be desirable or necessary if other sites of culture prove negative. The elevated WBC count, CRP, and ESR are nonspecific and provide little help with diagnosis; they are useful in assessing effectiveness of therapy.

Radiographic evaluation may delineate soft tissue swelling early, but osteopenia is not evident until days 10 to 14, and diagnostic findings may not be clear until days 10 to 21 (Fig. 41-6).[53] Radionuclide scanning (i.e., technetium 99m polyphosphonate or diphosphonate) provides a sensitive if nonspecific method for the early detection of increased blood flow and uptake in the infected bone (see Fig. 41-6C).[27,56,207] While a bone scan may be helpful in localizing osteomyelitis in the neonate or infection of the axial skeleton and in searching for subclinical areas of infection in multifocal osteomyelitis, it is seldom used. A positive result is not necessarily diagnostic of osteomyelitis, but a negative scan is unlikely for a child with bacterial osteomyelitis, except in the very early stages of the illness.

MRI is superior to other modalities in identifying changes in the marrow (see Fig. 41-6, D).[37,208-210] T1- or T2-weighted MR images and fat-suppression enhancement can confirm a focal area of increased inflammatory exudate (i.e., protons or water). A major advantage of MRI in early disease over plain radiographs, ultrasonography,[211-213] or CT is the delineation of soft tissue or subperiosteal pus.[214] Gadolinium does not add to diagnostic accuracy[215] except in the young child in whom it may detect involvement of nonossified growth cartilage.[203]

Treatment

As noted above, historically, acute osteomyelitis would respond to antibiotic therapy. However, with the emergence of MRSA the duration of symptoms may not be an accurate guide to disease severity. A more useful designation may be to consider osteomyelitis as *complicated* or *uncomplicated*. Complicated osteomyelitis presents with local findings of cellulitis, radiographic findings, or systemic toxicity with high fever, high WBC, and elevated ESR/CRP. While antibiotic care is needed in

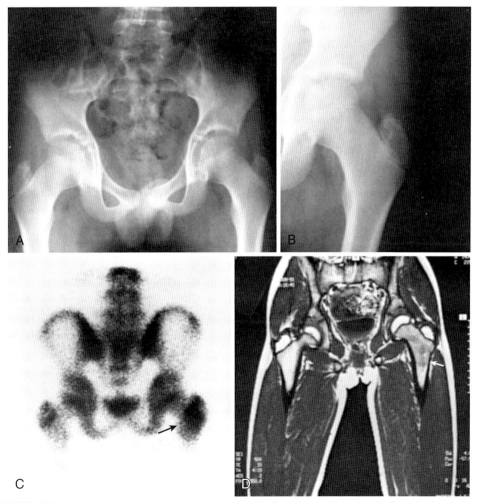

FIGURE 41-6 A, Anteroposterior radiograph of the pelvis of a 14-year-old body with fever and an irritable left hip. This X-ray film **(A)** and close-up film of the left hip **(B)** are normal. **C,** A bone scan documents increased uptake of technetium-99m in the area of the left proximal femur (*arrow*). **D,** MRI demonstrates an increased marrow signal in the same area of the left hip (*arrow*), which indicates acute osteomyelitis.

all cases, complicated osteomyelitis requires MR imaging and may need surgical therapy.[216,217]

Following a practice guideline in a nonrandomized retrospective study reduced the length of hospital stays and readmission rates.[218] While somewhat dependent on local prevalence, in the absence of specific indications to the contrary,[67] the initial antibiotic choices in many areas for the treatment of acute osteomyelitis should be effective against MRSA (see Table 41-5[219]). Screening of *S. aureus* for inducible clindamycin resistance with the D-test helps determine whether the patient should be treated with clindamycin or vancomycin.[220] Linezolid may become an important oral agent in the initial treatment and in the treatment of clindamycin-resistant MRSA, although studies to date are limited.[221] IV antibiotics for 4 to 6 weeks have been traditionally recommended with subsequent oral coverage if appropriate. Because of the complications that may occur from central venous catheters required to maintain IV access[222] for uncomplicated osteomyelitis, recent recommendations have included a shortened total course of 3 weeks of antibiotic treatment.[214,223-225] The decision to transition from IV to oral antibiotic is guided by the clinical response (e.g., the use of the limb and decreasing fever).[226]

Surgical treatment, which may be needed in complicated osteomyelitis,[227] includes drainage of subperiosteal and soft tissue abscesses and debridement of associated lesions. Surgery is also often needed for subacute and chronic osteomyelitis. Although early weight bearing is permitted with uncomplicated osteomyelitis, it must be avoided in complicated osteomyelitis to prevent risk of fracture.

Course of the Disease and Prognosis

The most dreaded complications of acute osteomyelitis are chronic osteomyelitis and impaired bone growth.[227] Chronic osteomyelitis or alternative sites of infection should be suspected in a child whose systemic symptoms have responded slowly or incompletely to antibiotics or in whom there is a late recurrence of pain at the affected site.

Differential Diagnosis and Related Disorders

Chronic recurrent multifocal osteomyelitis and synovitis, acne, pustulosis, hyperostosis, and osteomyelitis syndrome are discussed extensively in Chapter 48.

Diskitis

There is considerable dispute about whether diskitis is an infectious process. Infection of an intervertebral disk space from osteomyelitis of an adjoining vertebral body is rare.[228] However, acute diskitis unassociated with vertebral osteomyelitis is a self-limited inflammation of an intervertebral disk that may be caused by pathogens of low virulence, although bacteria or viruses are seldom recovered by aspiration. *S. aureus* and Enterobacteriaceae or *Kingella* organisms are responsible in some patients. Diskitis occurs throughout childhood, but one half of the cases manifest before the patient reaches 4 years of age (peak age, 1 to 3 years old).[229,230] The sex ratio is approximately equal, although one review observed that diskitis occurred more frequently in girls.[231]

Clinical signs may be subtle. Diskitis is characterized by vague back pain and stiffness, often resulting in a characteristic tripod position during sitting or other unusual posturing.[232] The child, who usually has a low-grade fever, often refuses to walk, stand, or bend over, and may complain of abdominal pain. Palpation of the spine may produce localized tenderness, usually in the lower lumbar region. The ESR is usually moderately elevated.

Plain radiographs of the affected area often appear normal until late in the disease (Fig. 41-7). A technetium 99m bone scan or MRI is valuable diagnostically. The L4-L5 interspace is most often affected (44%), followed by L3-L4 (37%), L2-L3 (7%), and L5-S1 (6%).[229-234] The cervical spine may also be involved. In one study, disk space narrowing occurred in 82% of children, and a bone scan was positive in 72%.[235] MRI may be valuable in differentiating infection from other conditions, including idiopathic disk calcification (Fig. 41-8).[236-238] Aspiration of the disk space or disk biopsy should not be routinely necessary. Immobilization provides symptomatic relief. With signs of systemic infection, IV antibiotics should be instituted until results of blood cultures are available.

ARTHRITIS CAUSED BY VIRUSES

With changing demographics and advances in clinical and laboratory virology, emerging viral infections are playing an increasingly important role in rheumatology worldwide.[239] Many of the reasons for this are listed in Box 41-1. A classification of viruses known to be associated with arthritis in humans is shown in Table 41-7.[240] The togaviruses account for most of the viral arthritides. In general, viral arthritides occur much more often in adults than in children.[241] Arthralgia is more common than objective arthritis, and both are usually migratory and of short duration (1 to 2 weeks), disappearing without residual joint disease. There are a number of potential mechanisms by which viruses may lead to arthritis, including targeting the cells of innate immunity and adaptive immunity, inducing the

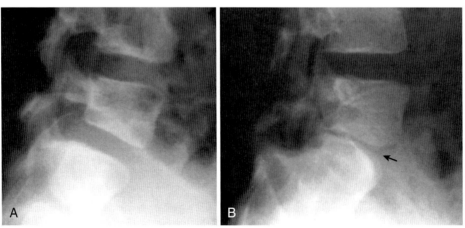

FIGURE 41-7 A, Normal disk space is demonstrated on a lateral view of the lumbar spine. **B,** Diskitis has caused collapse of the disk space (*arrow*).

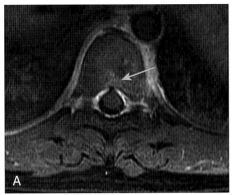
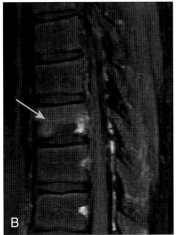
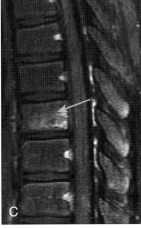

FIGURE 41-8 A 10-year-old male with back pain and diskitis. **A,** Axial T1-weighted fat-suppressed MR image postcontrast showing bone enhancement. **B,** Sagittal T1-weighted fat-suppressed MR image following contrast administration with increased signal on the inferior aspect of the vertebral body surrounding an area of decreased enhancement. **C,** Sagittal T2-weighted MR image showing increased signal intensity within the T7 vertebral body and narrowing of the adjacent inferior disk. (Courtesy Dr. P. Babyn.)

TABLE 41-7   Viruses That Cause Arthritis in Humans

VIRUS	COMMENT
Togaviruses	
Rubivirus	
Rubella	Global; most reports from North America and Europe
Alphaviruses	
Ross River	Australasia
Chikungunya	Africa, Asia
O'nyong-nyong	Africa
Mayaro	South America
Sindbis	Africa, Asia, Australia
Ockelbo	Sweden
Pogosta	Finland
Parvoviruses	B19 associated with fifth disease, aplastic crises
Hepadnaviruses	
Hepatitis B	Global
Hepatitis C	Global
Adenoviruses	
Adenovirus 7	Rare
Herpesviruses	
Epstein–Barr	Rare; suggested role in rheumatoid arthritis
Cytomegalovirus	Rare
Varicella-zoster	Rare
Herpes simplex	Rare
Paramyxoviruses	
Mumps	Rare
Enteroviruses	
Echovirus	Rare
Coxsackievirus B	Rare
Orthopoxvirus	
Variola virus (smallpox)	Nonexistent today
Vaccinia virus	Rare

Adapted from R.E. Petty, A.J. Tingle, Arthritis and viral infection, J. Pediatr. 113 (1998) 948.

BOX 41-1   Determinants of Emerging Viral Infections and Their Spread

- Viral Factors
  - Mutability
  - Mutational robustness
  - Transmissibility
  - Genetic composition (DNA/RNA)
  - Ability to infect multiple species
  - Short-lived versus persistent infection
  - Ability to elicit immune response in host
- Vector factors
  - Increased breeding
  - Migration
  - Increased extrinsic incubation rate
  - Decreased extrinsic incubation period
  - Altered biting behavior
  - Ability to harbor new pathogens
  - Environmental adaptability
- Human and ecological factors
  - Increased population density
  - Limited cultivable land
  - Decreased crop returns
  - Natural disasters
  - Strained health resources
  - Limited financial resources
  - Working conditions
  - Immune status and response

From Khasnis, Schoen, Calabrese (Ref. 239).

production of autoantibodies and T cell–mediated autoimmunity, or directly infecting synovial cells.[242] As arthritis is seldom the main symptom of viral disease, clues as to the etiology should be sought in the history, including travel to areas where alphaviruses and human T-cell leukemia virus type 1 (HTLV-1) may be common, a history of blood transfusions, IV drug abuse, recent vaccinations, or ongoing epidemics or exposures.

Small joints are most often affected by rubella, hepatitis B, and members of the alphavirus group (e.g., Ross River, chikungunya), whereas one or two large joints (usually the knees) are most often affected by mumps, varicella, and other viruses. In some viral arthritides, virus (e.g., rubella, varicella, herpes simplex, cytomegalovirus) can be isolated from the joint space; in others, only virus-containing immune complexes (e.g., hepatitis B, adenovirus 7) are found; and in still others, neither virus nor viral antigen can be recovered from the joint.[243] Whether this represents limitations of recovery and culture techniques or the fact that culture-negative viral arthritis is "reactive" rather than "septic" is unknown.

Rubella Virus

Rubella-associated arthropathy was recognized by Osler[244] and was one of the most commonly identified virus-associated arthritides in North America. Musculoskeletal symptoms after natural rubella infection are relatively common in young women. These symptoms are unusual in preadolescent children and in males, however, and are much less frequent after rubella immunization than after natural infection. Arthritis is more common after natural infection, and it is more severe and lasts longer.[245]

Arthralgia usually begins within 7 days of the appearance of the rash or 10 to 28 days after immunization. The joints of the fingers and, later, the knees are most frequently affected. Joint pain may be accompanied by warmth, erythema, and effusion, and tenosynovitis is common. Carpal tunnel syndrome has also been reported. These findings usually disappear within 3 to 4 weeks but occasionally persist for months or even years.

In a study of natural rubella infection in 37 teenage students, 52% of girls and 8% of boys developed objective arthritis,[245] and an additional 13% and 48%, respectively, experienced arthralgia. In a group of young women who received RA 27/3 rubella vaccine, 14% developed an acute polyarthritis. Arthralgia and arthritis are most common in adults, although approximately 25% of prepubertal females develop arthralgia, and 10% develop arthritis.[246,247] Chronic arthritis in 5% to 11% of adult women has been reported after vaccination.[248,249] It has been suggested that reinfection contributes to arthritis in susceptible hosts.[250,251] Rubella virus has been recovered from the synovial fluid of patients with rubella arthritis in many,[252,253] but not all, instances.[241,254] The virus was isolated from synovial or peripheral blood mononuclear cells in 7 of 19 children with juvenile rheumatoid arthritis but from no control subjects.[252] Other investigations have shown no association.[255]

Parvovirus

An arthropathy associated with parvovirus B19 was first reported in 1985. This agent, responsible for erythema infectiosum (i.e., fifth disease or slapped cheek syndrome), is sometimes accompanied by an arthritis not unlike that of rubella infection.[256-261]

Arthralgia, symmetrical joint swelling, and morning stiffness have been described in adults, especially women, after parvovirus B19 infection.[259] Carpal tunnel syndrome, hepatitis, and angioedema have been described. This syndrome may be more widespread than previously thought and may be considerably underdiagnosed. In some patients, symptoms have persisted for years. An early study of erythema infectiosum in 364 patients indicated that joint pain, most often affecting knees and wrists, was present during the first week in 77% of adults and 8% of patients younger than 20 years old.[262] Subsequently, it was determined that arthritis was most common in patients who were HLA-DR4 positive.[263] Whether or not a chronic arthritis results from parvovirus B19 infection is still controversial.[243,264]

Parvovirus infection is common and widespread. The parvovirus B19 genome consists of linear, 5.6-kD, single-stranded deoxyribonucleic acid (DNA). There is only one serotype of parvovirus B19. Human parvovirus B19 has been implicated as the causative agent in erythema infectiosum, aplastic crises, some cases of hemophagocytic syndrome, and hydrops fetalis.[265] Erythema infectiosum is a common exanthem of older children that lasts for a few days to a week and presents with a low-grade fever, an erythematous facial rash ("slapped cheeks"), and a lacy, reticular rash on the extremities. These manifestations often recur with malaise, irritability, and arthralgia.

The association of documented parvovirus B19 infection and arthritis is uncommon.[257,266-268] Joint symptoms tend to be mild and transient and generally appear in association with the exanthem. Nocton and associates[266] described acute arthritis in 20 children with parvovirus B19 infections. The arthritis was associated with constitutional symptoms in one half of the children and was of brief duration (less than 4 months) in 14. Six children had persistent arthritis lasting up to 13 months; criteria for a diagnosis of JIA would have been met in this group. Laboratory results were generally normal, except for serological evidence of the B19 infection. Usually, NSAID treatment will suffice, but for patients with persistent symptoms, intravenous immunoglobulin (IVIG) may be a treatment option.[269] Persistent parvovirus-associated arthritis has been reported as a presenting manifestation of common variable immune deficiency.[270] The seroprevalence of parvovirus B19 did not show an increase in patients with JIA compared with diseased or healthy controls in one large study.[271]

The precise relation of the viral infection to arthritis has not been clarified. The virus has not been grown from synovial fluid or blood from patients with joint symptoms, although B19-specific DNA has been identified by hybridization in the synovial fluid of adults[272] and by PCR amplification in synovial tissue.[273] However, Soderlund and colleagues[274] demonstrated genomic B19 DNA in the synovium of joints that had suffered trauma even more frequently than in the joints of those children with chronic arthritis. Inflammatory synovitis may not be identifiable by arthroscopy. Although infection gives rise first to immunoglobulin (Ig)-M antibodies[275] and then to IgG antibodies, there is no evidence that the arthropathy represents an immune complex disease. Demonstration of IgM antibodies, however, is essential to diagnosis. They are present 10 to 12 days after infection and usually disappear within 3 to 4 months. The prevalence of IgG antibodies in the general population is too high to be diagnostically helpful, unless a fourfold increase concurrent with the clinical symptoms is demonstrated.[276-278] Similarly, false-positive PCR results may occur because of persistence of B19 DNA.

Hepatitis B Arthritis–Dermatitis Syndrome

In adults, up to 20% of infections with hepatitis B virus are characterized by a period of rash and arthritis that resembles serum sickness.[279] The arthritis is often explosive in onset and often occurs in the preicteric phase of hepatitis B infections. In a review of reported cases of arthritis associated with hepatitis B infection,[280] the age of the patients ranged from 14 to 56 years, and the male-to-female ratio was 1.5:1. The dermatitis is characterized by a maculopapular rash, sometimes with petechiae or urticaria, and is most prominent on the lower extremities. The arthritis usually begins abruptly and symmetrically and affects the interphalangeal joints in 82% of patients, knees in 30%, and ankles in 24%. Although erythema and warmth are present, synovial effusions are uncommon. Joint symptoms last for 4 weeks on average, respond well to NSAIDs, and disappear without sequelae. The ESR is usually normal, although serum and synovial fluid complement levels are low in the early stages of the illness.[281] Synovial fluid has been reported to show a mononuclear cell predominance.[282] Electron microscopic evidence of hepatitis antigen in the synovial membrane has been reported.[283]

Hepatitis C

Hepatitis C virus is lymphotrophic and is associated two different types of arthritis. The first is a rheumatoid arthritis-like picture, although milder and rarely associated with erosions, and the second is an intermittent monoarticular or oligoarticular nondestructive arthritis affecting large- and medium-sized joints, often with mixed cryoglobulinemia.[241,284,285] Hepatitis C virus may coexist with JIA; although there is no evidence from pediatric studies, the use of anti–TNF-α agents appears to have an acceptable safety profile in adults with rheumatoid arthritis (RA).[286] As many of these patients may be rheumatoid factor positive, the presence of anti-CCP has been proposed as a useful tool in diagnosing true RA in the hepatitis C–infected individual.[287,288]

Alphaviruses

Epidemic polyarthritis caused by infection with one of the alphaviruses is the most common virus-associated arthritis in Australia, the islands of the South Pacific, Africa, and Asia.[289] These viruses are transmitted by arthropods, usually the mosquito, and incite an illness characterized by arthritis and a rash that may be macular, papular, vesicular, or purpuric. Although there are some virus-specific differences in these illnesses, they usually are mild in children and occur with equal frequency in males and females.

In Ross River virus disease, the wrist is most commonly affected and is often accompanied by tenosynovitis and enthesitis at the insertion of the plantar fascia into the calcaneus.[289,290] The synovial fluid is said to be highly characteristic, with a predominance of vacuolated macrophages and very few PMNs. In chikungunya, the knee is the most commonly involved joint, and back pain and myalgia are prominent. The arthritis lasts 1 to 2 weeks and is followed by complete recovery. However, recent outbreaks have resulted in a more chronic course, sometimes with an RA-like picture.[291] In an animal model of chikungunya arthritis, expressed genes were very similar to those expressed in RA, suggesting that these two disorders may share inflammatory processes that may inform therapy.[292] Diagnosis rests on the clinical presentation and an elevated level of antibodies to the specific virus. Viral antigen has not been recovered from synovial fluid.

Herpes Viruses

Four of the herpes viruses have been associated with arthritis. Herpes simplex virus type 1 has been isolated from the synovial fluid of one patient with arthritis and disseminated herpes simplex infection.[293] Epstein–Barr virus has long been thought by some investigators to have a primary role in the cause or pathogenesis of rheumatoid arthritis, although direct evidence is lacking.[294-296] Arthritis is a rare complication of infectious mononucleosis.[297-299] Cytomegalovirus is occasionally associated with arthritis and has been isolated from synovial fluid in one instance.[293]

Varicella-zoster infection is uncommonly complicated by arthritis.[300-307] However, there have been instances of bacterial septic arthritis complicating chickenpox.[305,308,309] Primary varicella arthritis is usually monoarticular with a lymphocyte predominance in the synovial fluid. It usually resolves within 1 week although occasionally a more chronic

but nonerosive arthritis may ensue.[310] Occasionally, chickenpox is associated with the emergence of psoriatic arthritis.[311] Acute monoarthritis has been reported in association with herpes zoster in two adults.[312,313]

Mumps Virus

The paramyxovirus (mumps) rarely causes arthritis. In a 1984 review[314] only 32 cases were well documented. Since then, two additional patients have been reported.[315,316] The male-to-female ratio is 3.6 : 1, and the peak age of occurrence is 21 to 30 years of age. Four patients younger than 11 years old and seven between the ages of 11 and 20 years have been described. Arthritis occasionally preceded parotitis, but usually followed by 1 to 3 weeks. In children, the arthritis was mild, affected few joints, and lasted 1 to 2 weeks. In postadolescent males, arthritis was often accompanied by orchitis and pancreatitis.[314] It is reported that the arthritis responds to ibuprofen or prednisone but not to aspirin.[314] The pathogenesis is unknown, and no attempts at recovery of mumps virus from synovium or synovial fluid have been reported. Arthritis has not occurred after mumps immunization.

Human Immunodeficiency Virus

The spectrum of rheumatic diseases that can accompany HIV infection has changed with the introduction of highly active antiretroviral (HAART) treatment. AIDS resulting from HIV infection may be complicated by septic arthritis, although this is now considered rare.[317] Virtually any organism can be responsible; *Streptococcus pneumonia* was identified more commonly in HIV-infected than noninfected pediatric patients with septic arthritis in South Africa, suggesting that treatment for this organism should be part of initial management in HIV-infected children. A number of stereotypical presentations of arthritis associated with HIV have been documented in adults.[318] These include reactive arthritis, psoriasiform arthritis, and an undifferentiated spondyloarthropathy,[319-323] often more severe than in patients without HIV infection. A similar picture has been observed in children infected with HIV. Of interest, reactive arthritis may relate to the mode of acquisition of HIV rather than the HIV itself. Studies in AIDS acquired via IV drug abuse show a much lower prevalence of reactive arthritis that in patients who acquired AIDS through sexual transmission, suggesting that the reactive arthritis might be due to sexually transmitted infections.[324] Arthralgias occur initially with viremia; lower extremity oligoarthritis or persistent polyarthritis can supervene later. A study of 270 patients concluded that the most frequent pattern of joint involvement was one of an acute onset, short duration, few if any recurrences, and no erosive sequelae.[325] The authors have observed chronic oligoarthritis in two young children with HIV infection (one transplacental and one related to blood products). Osteomyelitis may also occur; tuberculosis infection is a relatively common cause.[326] In addition to musculoskeletal infections, HIV infection can be associated with the diffuse infiltrative lymphocytosis syndrome and cutaneous and systemic vasculitis, including Kawasaki disease.[327] In the post-HAART era, there has been a decline in reactive, psoriatic, and infectious causes of musculoskeletal syndromes, but disorders such as osteoporosis, osteomalacia, and osteonecrosis have become more prevalent.[317] The immune reconstitution inflammatory syndrome (IRIS) may develop after institution of HAART.[328]

Other Viruses

There are reports of arthritis associated with adenovirus type 7 infections, although the virus was not isolated from the synovial fluid, and diagnosis was confirmed only on clinical and serological grounds.[325,329,330] Echoviruses[331-333] and coxsackieviruses type B[330,334] have been rarely implicated as the cause of arthritis. Smallpox (variola virus infection), now eradicated from the world, was often accompanied by arthritis, especially in children younger than 10 years old. Arthritis also followed cowpox vaccination.[335] HTLV-1 has been associated with a number of rheumatic disorders in adults, including arthritis and Sjögren's syndrome.[336] A 1998 report[337] outlined an outbreak of Sindbis virus–induced Pogosta disease (e.g., fever, rash, joint symptoms) in Finland.

ARTHRITIS ASSOCIATED WITH OTHER INFECTIONS

Fungal Arthritis

Arthritis caused by fungal infection is rare[338] and is almost unknown in children beyond the neonatal period. Fungi that have been reported as causing arthritis or osteomyelitis are *C. albicans*,[339] *Sporothrix schencii*,[340,341] *Actinomyces israelii*,[342] *Aspergillus fumigatus*,[343] *Histoplasma capsulatum*,[344] *Cryptococcus neoformans*,[344] *Blastomyces dermatitidis*,[345] *Coccidioides immitis*,[346] *Paracoccidioides brasiliensis*,[347] *Nocardia asteroides*,[348] and *Pseudallescheria boydii*.[349] Candidal arthritis,[339] usually associated with accompanying osteomyelitis, is most common in the newborn and infant in the pediatric population,[350,351] and occurs occasionally in immunocompromised patients[352,353] and in patients with prosthetic joints.[354] Newborns and infants with risk factors for candidemia who develop nonspecific localizing signs and symptoms must be evaluated for osteoarticular infection with *Candida*. Furthermore, laboratory signs of inflammation are not typically as high as in other forms of musculoskeletal infection, and therefore a high index of suspicion must be kept in mind for at-risk populations.

Sporotrichosis and Plant Thorn Synovitis

Infection with *Sporothrix schenckii* is a rare but significant occupational hazard of gardeners, night-crawler farmers, and field workers.[340,341] Monoarthritis or, less commonly, polyarthritis resembling RA, has been reported (Fig. 41-9). Synovial biopsy is often necessary to make the diagnosis (Fig. 41-10).

Synovitis caused by the penetration of a plant thorn into the joint space or surrounding structures is probably a reaction to the foreign material rather than an outright infection, although the circumstances of the injury may suggest the latter. The synovial effusion is inflammatory, and culture occasionally yields a relatively nonvirulent organism.

In the case of rose thorn penetration, *S. schenckii* is the probable cause. More commonly, the thorn of the palm tree or blackthorn is implicated. There are signs of local inflammation, and radiographs demonstrate periosteal new bone formation, a radiolucent defect in bone, or the presence of radiopaque foreign material. Ultrasound and MRI have replaced CT as the imaging modalities of choice.[355,356] Because this disorder may develop months after the initial injury, foreign-body synovitis may be ignored as a diagnostic possibility. Treatment should be directed at appropriate surgical exploration and removal of the foreign material.[357]

Arthritis Caused by Spirochetes
Lyme Disease

The geographical and temporal clustering of cases of what was thought to be juvenile RA in Old Lyme, Connecticut, led to the discovery and description of the cause, pathogenesis, and cure of Lyme disease. This epidemiological work is one of the most important developments of the past 3 decades in rheumatology and provides a model for approaching the question of the infectious cause of other chronic arthritides of childhood. Unfortunately, work on the development of a safe and effective vaccine has stalled.[358] Chapter 42 provides a complete discussion of classic Lyme disease.

Other Spirochetes and Arthritis

Arthritis rarely complicates leptospirosis (*Leptospira icterohemorrhagica*)[359] and syphilis (*Treponema pallidum*).[360,361] Congenital syphilis causes juxtaepiphyseal osteochondritis and periarthritis in infancy and syphilitic dactylitis in early childhood (Fig. 41-11). Clutton joints—relatively painless, recurrent, nonprogressive, symmetrical synovitis of the knees—develop later.[362]

Parasites and Arthritis

There have been case reports of arthritis accompanying a wide range of parasitic infestations,[363] including *Giardia intestinalis (lamblia)*,[364] *Endolimax nana*,[365] *Toxocara canis*,[366] schistosomiasis,[367] and others.[368] In general, the joint disease is presumably reactive or postinfectious rather than septic and pursues a benign course with a good prognosis. A case of leishmaniasis complicated anti–IL-1 treatment in a patient with systemic JIA.[369]

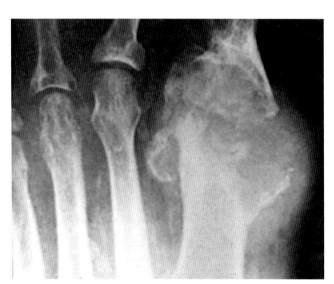

FIGURE 41-9 Destruction of the first metatarsophalangeal joint was caused by sporotrichosis.

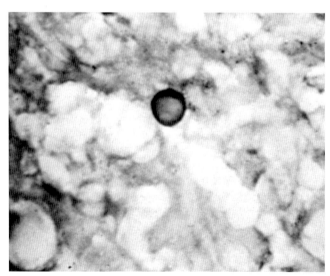

FIGURE 41-10 *Sporothrix schenckii* is identified in a Gram-stained preparation of the synovial fluid aspirate.

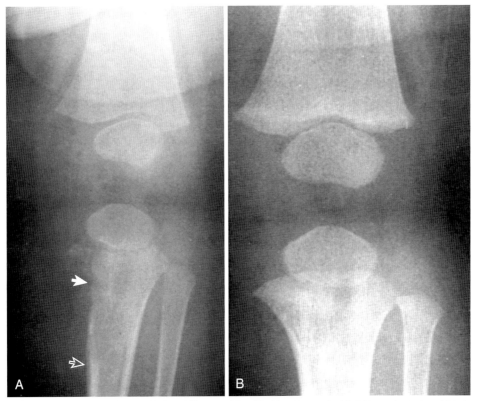

FIGURE 41-11 Lesions of congenital syphilis were identified in a 6-month-old girl brought to the child abuse clinic because of multiple fractures that occurred during the previous 10 days. Her rapid plasma reagin test result was 1:256. **A,** Bilateral, symmetrical, destructive metaphysitis lesions of the proximal ends of the tibiae (Wimberger sign) (*solid arrow*) and periosteal new bone apposition (*open arrow*) can be seen. **B,** With penicillin therapy, the lesions have almost healed 2 months later.

Musculoskeletal Manifestations of Systemic Bacterial Infections

Bacterial infection of ventricular shunts for the management of hydrocephalus may result in arthritis and nephritis.[370] Rheumatoid factors may be demonstrable in the sera of these patients. Meningococcemia is complicated by arthritis in up to 10% of cases.[371] It is usually oligoarticular and occurs most often during the recovery phase, when immune complexes can be demonstrated in the synovium.[372] It can also be complicated by acute septic arthritis in the early stage of the disease. *H. influenzae* type B meningitis may lead to a sterile arthritis.[373]

Infective endocarditis frequently causes arthralgia or arthritis[374,375] and signs suggesting vasculitis (e.g., Osler nodes, Janeway lesions, Roth spots). The musculoskeletal signs and symptoms (e.g., arthralgia, arthritis, myalgia, low back pain) may precede other manifestations of infective endocarditis by weeks.[375] The arthritis is characteristically polyarticular and symmetrical, affecting both large and small joints. An immune complex–mediated pathogenesis is thought to be responsible, and the presence of hypocomplementemia,[376] circulating immune complexes,[346] and sometimes rheumatoid factors[376] support this theory. Specificity of the rheumatoid factors is directed to the patient's IgG in combination with the infecting organism.

REFERENCES

6. C.W. Fink, J.D. Nelson, Septic arthritis and osteomyelitis in children, Clin. Rheum. Dis. 12 (2) (1986) 423–435.

13. A.W. Howard, D. Viskontas, C. Sabbagh, Reduction in osteomyelitis and septic arthritis related to Haemophilus influenzae type B vaccination, J. Pediatr. Orthop. 19 (6) (1999) 705–709.

20. S. Chometon, Y. Benito, M. Chaker, et al., Specific real-time polymerase chain reaction places Kingella kingae as the most common cause of osteoarticular infections in young children, Pediatr. Infect. Dis. J. 26 (5) (2007) 377–381.

22. P. Yagupsky, E. Porsch, J.W. St Geme 3rd., Kingella kingae: an emerging pathogen in young children, Pediatrics 127 (3) (2011) 557–565.

23. K.M. Kiang, F. Ogunmodede, B.A. Juni, et al., Outbreak of osteomyelitis/septic arthritis caused by Kingella kingae among child care center attendees, Pediatrics 116 (2) (2005) e206–e213.

26. K.Z. Vardakas, I. Kontopidis, I.D. Gkegkes, et al., Incidence, characteristics, and outcomes of patients with bone and joint infections due to community-associated methicillin-resistant Staphylococcus aureus: a systematic review, Eur. J. Clin. Microbiol. Infect. Dis. 32 (6) (2013) 711–721.

33. C.J. Mathews, G. Coakley, Septic arthritis: current diagnostic and therapeutic algorithm, Curr. Opin. Rheumatol. 20 (4) (2008) 457–462.

38. T.R. Nunn, W.Y. Cheung, P.D. Rollinson, A prospective study of pyogenic sepsis of the hip in childhood, J. Bone Joint Surg. 89 (1) (2007) 100–106.

39. C.J. Mathews, G. Kingsley, M. Field, et al., Management of septic arthritis: a systematic review, Ann. Rheum. Dis. 66 (4) (2007) 440–445.

40. A. Mitha, M. Boulyana, V. Hue, et al., Consensus in diagnostic definitions for bone or joint infections in children by a Delphi method with European French-speaking experts, Acta Paediatr. 101 (8) (2012) e350–e356.

46. I.M. van der Heijden, B. Wilbrink, L.M. Schouls, et al., Detection of mycobacteria in joint samples from patients with arthritis using a genus-specific polymerase chain reaction and sequence analysis, Rheumatology (Oxford) 38 (6) (1999) 547–553.

49. R.M. Lyon, J.D. Evanich, Culture-negative septic arthritis in children, J. Pediatr. Orthop. 19 (5) (1999) 655–659.

52. R.F. Buchmann, D. Jaramillo, Imaging of articular disorders in children, Radiol. Clin. North Am. 42 (1) (2004) 151–168, vii.

53. D. Jaramillo, S.T. Treves, J.R. Kasser, et al., Osteomyelitis and septic arthritis in children: appropriate use of imaging to guide treatment, AJR Am. J. Roentgenol. 165 (2) (1995) 399–403.

57. K.D. Stumpe, K. Strobel, Osteomyelitis and arthritis, Semin. Nucl. Med. 39 (1) (2009) 27–35.

59. M. Karchevsky, M.E. Schweitzer, W.B. Morrison, J.A. Parellada, MRI findings of septic arthritis and associated osteomyelitis in adults, AJR Am. J. Roentgenol. 182 (1) (2004) 119–122.

62. M.S. Kocher, How do you best diagnose septic arthritis of the hip? in: J.G. Wright (Ed.), Evidence-Based Orthopedics, Elsevier Saunders, Philadelphia, 2009, pp. 206–215.

73. A.C. Offiah, Acute osteomyelitis, septic arthritis and discitis: differences between neonates and older children, Eur. J. Radiol. 60 (2) (2006) 221–232.

74. R.R. Betz, D.R. Cooperman, J.M. Wopperer, et al., Late sequelae of septic arthritis of the hip in infancy and childhood, J. Pediatr. Orthop. 10 (3) (1990) 365–372.

79. H. Wingstrand, Transient synovitis of the hip in the child, Acta Orthop. Scand. Suppl. 219 (1986) 1–61.

81. M.S. Kocher, D. Zurakowski, J.R. Kasser, Differentiating between septic arthritis and transient synovitis of the hip in children: an evidence-based clinical prediction algorithm, J. Bone Joint Surg. Am. 81 (12) (1999) 1662–1670.

94. S.P. Brogadir, B.M. Schimmer, A.R. Myers, Spectrum of the gonococcal arthritis-dermatitis syndrome, Semin. Arthritis Rheum. 8 (3) (1979) 177–183.

116. M.W. Shen, Diagnostic and therapeutic challenges of childhood brucellosis in a nonendemic country, Pediatrics 121 (5) (2008) e1178–e1183.

126. E. Maman, J. Bickels, M. Ephros, et al., Musculoskeletal manifestations of cat scratch disease, Clin. Infect. Dis. 45 (12) (2007) 1535–1540.

129. M.S. Gilbert, L.M. Aledort, S. Seremetis, et al., Long term evaluation of septic arthritis in hemophilic patients, Clin. Orthop. Relat. Res. 328 (1996) 54–59.

130. B.I. Asmar, J. Andresen, W.J. Brown, Ureaplasma urealyticum arthritis and bacteremia in agammaglobulinemia, Pediatr. Infect. Dis. J. 17 (1) (1998) 73–76.

133. E. Forlin, C. Milani, Sequelae of septic arthritis of the hip in children: a new classification and a review of 41 hips, J. Pediatr. Orthop. 28 (5) (2008) 524–528.

145. X. Puéchal, Whipple's disease, Ann. Rheum. Dis. 72 (6) (2013) 797–803.

154. T. Schneider, V. Moos, C. Loddenkemper, et al., Whipple's disease: new aspects of pathogenesis and treatment, Lancet Infect. Dis. 8 (3) (2008) 179–190.

156. P. Christiansen, B. Frederiksen, J. Glazowski, et al., Epidemiologic, bacteriologic, and long-term follow-up data of children with acute hematogenous osteomyelitis and septic arthritis: a ten-year review, J. Pediatr. Orthop. B 8 (4) (1999) 302–305.

161. R.J. Scott, M.R. Christofersen, W.W. Robertson Jr., et al., Acute osteomyelitis in children: a review of 116 cases, J. Pediatr. Orthop. 10 (5) (1990) 649–652.

163. H. Peltola, M. Paakkonen, Acute osteomyelitis in children, N. Engl. J. Med. 370 (4) (2014) 352–360.

170. R.J. Gorwitz, A review of community-associated methicillin-resistant Staphylococcus aureus skin and soft tissue infections, Pediatr. Infect. Dis. J. 27 (1) (2008) 1–7.

171. J. Saavedra-Lozano, A. Mejías, N. Ahmad, et al., Changing trends in acute osteomyelitis in children: impact of methicillin-resistant Staphylococcus aureus infections, J. Pediatr. Orthop. 28 (5) (2008) 569–575.

187. L.T. Gutman, Acute, subacute, and chronic osteomyelitis and pyogenic arthritis in children, Curr. Probl. Pediatr. 15 (12) (1985) 1–72.

191. M.N. Wang, W.M. Chen, K.S. Lee, et al., Tuberculous osteomyelitis in young children, J. Pediatr. Orthop. 19 (2) (1999) 151–155.

196. M.H. Perlman, M.J. Patzakis, P.J. Kumar, P. Holtom, The incidence of joint involvement with adjacent osteomyelitis in pediatric patients, J. Pediatr. Orthop. 20 (1) (2000) 40–43.

200. P.N. Tyrrell, V.N. Cassar-Pullicino, S.M. Eisenstein, et al., Back pain in childhood, Ann. Rheum. Dis. 55 (11) (1996) 789–793.

203. L.P. Browne, R.P. Guillerman, R.C. Orth, et al., Community-acquired staphylococcal musculoskeletal infection in infants and young children: necessity of contrast-enhanced MRI for the diagnosis of growth cartilage involvement, AJR Am. J. Roentgenol. 198 (1) (2012) 194–199.

205. N.E. Green, R.D. Beauchamp, P.P. Griffin, Primary subacute epiphyseal osteomyelitis, J. Bone Joint Surg. Am. 63 (1) (1981) 107–114.

206. J.J. McCarthy, J.P. Dormans, S.H. Kozin, P.D. Pizzutillo, Musculoskeletal infections in children. Basic treatment principles and recent advancements, J. Bone Joint Surg. Am. 86-A (4) (2004) 850–863.

209. G.A. Mandell, Imaging in the diagnosis of musculoskeletal infections in children, Curr. Probl. Pediatr. 26 (7) (1996) 218–237.

216. J. Dartnell, M. Ramachandran, M. Katchburian, Haematogenous acute and subacute paediatric osteomyelitis: a systematic review of the literature, J. Bone Joint Surg. Br. 94 (5) (2012) 584–595.

217. S.N. Faust, J. Clark, A. Pallett, N.M. Clarke, Managing bone and joint infection in children, Arch. Dis. Child. 97 (6) (2012) 545–553.

218. L.A. Copley, M.A. Kinsler, T. Gheen, et al., The impact of evidence-based clinical practice guidelines applied by a multidisciplinary team for the care of children with osteomyelitis, J. Bone Joint Surg. Am. 95 (8) (2013) 686–693.

222. R. Ruebner, R. Keren, S. Coffin, et al., Complications of central venous catheters used for the treatment of acute hematogenous osteomyelitis, Pediatrics 117 (4) (2006) 1210–1215.

223. A. Karwowska, H.D. Davies, T. Jadavji, Epidemiology and outcome of osteomyelitis in the era of sequential intravenous-oral therapy, Pediatr. Infect. Dis. J. 17 (11) (1998) 1021–1026.

226. A.R. Howard-Jones, D. Isaacs, Systematic review of duration and choice of systemic antibiotic therapy for acute haematogenous bacterial osteomyelitis in children, J. Paediatr. Child Health 49 (9) (2013) 760–768.

228. F.L. Sapico, J.Z. Montgomerie, Pyogenic vertebral osteomyelitis: report of nine cases and review of the literature, Rev. Infect. Dis. 1 (5) (1979) 754–776.

236. M. Fernandez, C.L. Carrol, C.J. Baker, Discitis and vertebral osteomyelitis in children: an 18-year review, Pediatrics 105 (6) (2000) 1299–1304.

239. A.A. Khasnis, R.T. Schoen, L.H. Calabrese, Emerging viral infections in rheumatic diseases, Semin. Arthritis Rheum. 41 (2) (2011) 236–246.

240. R.E. Petty, A.J. Tingle, Arthritis and viral infection, J. Pediatr. 113 (5) (1988) 948–949.

242. R. Franssila, K. Hedman, Infection and musculoskeletal conditions: Viral causes of arthritis, Best Pract. Res. Clin. Rheumatol. 20 (6) (2006) 1139–1157.

266. J.J. Nocton, L.C. Miller, L.B. Tucker, J.G. Schaller, Human parvovirus B19-associated arthritis in children, J. Pediatr. 122 (2) (1993) 186–190.

280. R.D. Inman, Rheumatic manifestations of hepatitis B virus infection, Semin. Arthritis Rheum. 11 (4) (1982) 406–420.

285. I. Rosner, M. Rozenbaum, E. Toubi, et al., The case for hepatitis C arthritis, Semin. Arthritis Rheum. 33 (6) (2004) 375–387.

305. P. Schreck, P. Schreck, J. Bradley, H. Chambers, Musculoskeletal complications of varicella, J. Bone Joint Surg. Am. 78 (11) (1996) 1713–1719.

317. N. Patel, N. Patel, L.R. Espinoza, HIV infection and rheumatic diseases: the changing spectrum of clinical enigma, Rheum. Dis. Clin. North Am. 35 (1) (2009) 139–161.

324. E. Lawson, K. Walker-Bone, The changing spectrum of rheumatic disease in HIV infection, Br. Med. Bull. 103 (1) (2012) 203–221.

351. M.N. Gamaletsou, D.P. Kontoyiannis, N.V. Sipsas, et al., Candida osteomyelitis: analysis of 207 pediatric and adult cases (1970–2011), Clin. Infect. Dis. 55 (10) (2012) 1338–1351.

Entire reference list is available online at www.expertconsult.com.

CHAPTER 42

Lyme Disease

Hans-Iko Huppertz, Lawrence Zemel, Frank Dressler

Lyme arthritis was first described in 1977 by Steere and colleagues[1] in a cluster of children thought to have juvenile rheumatoid arthritis. They lived in and around Old Lyme, Connecticut. Subsequent studies documented that the disease was caused by the spirochete *Borrelia burgdorferi*[2,3] and that arthritis was only one of many possible manifestations of this infection, now known as *Lyme borreliosis* or *Lyme disease*.[4-6]

Clinical case descriptions of various manifestations of this disease date back more than a century. Acrodermatitis chronica atrophicans was described in Germany in 1883.[7] Erythema migrans, the early skin manifestation of Lyme borreliosis, was reported in Sweden in 1909.[8] The first case of neuroborreliosis and its association with a tick bite was observed in France in 1922.[9] Among the cases of lymphocytic meningitis and inflammatory polyneuritis studied by Bannwarth[10] in Germany in 1941, several patients described had "rheumatism," probably the first report of what is now called *Lyme arthritis*. Successful treatment with penicillin was described in 1946.[11] Erythema migrans was transferred by skin biopsy to healthy human volunteers in 1955.[12] These observations suggested an infectious cause.

DEFINITION AND CLASSIFICATION

Lyme disease is a complex disease with cutaneous, articular, neurological, and other manifestations that result from infection with the spirochete *B. burgdorferi* transmitted by the bite of a tick of the genus *Ixodes*. Various components of the disease (e.g., erythema migrans, arthritis, neuroborreliosis) may occur in isolation. The term *Lyme borreliosis* is often used in Europe; *Lyme disease* is the most frequent term used in North America. Lyme arthritis is usually responsive to antibiotics. The term *antibiotic-refractory Lyme arthritis* is used for patients who do not show clearance of Lyme arthritis following two courses of appropriate antibiotics.

EPIDEMIOLOGY

Geographical Distribution

Lyme disease has been documented only in the temperate zones of the northern hemisphere.[4,13] In North America, the disease is recognized most commonly in the northeastern, mid-Atlantic and north-central United States; it occurs less frequently on the West Coast and in southern Canada.[14] Lyme borreliosis is rare or absent in the other parts of the United States and Canada. In Europe, the disease is most common in central Europe but occurs endemically from southern Sweden to the northern Mediterranean and from Portugal to Russia. Although sporadic cases of Lyme disease have been reported in eastern Russia, China, Korea, and Japan, it appears to be much less common in Asia than in the endemic areas of North America or Europe. A recent review explores the drivers and mechanisms for changing geographic ranges of ticks and tick-borne pathogens.[15]

Incidence and Prevalence

The Centers for Disease Control and Prevention (CDC) have reported a rapid increase in the frequency of Lyme disease in the United States since 1982. Between 1992 and 2009, the incidence tripled, and a maximum of 29,959 confirmed cases were reported in 2009.[14] Case numbers were slightly smaller for the years 2010 to 2012, the last year for which a detailed analysis has been published. Recently, the CDC estimated that due to underreporting, the true U.S. incidence might be as high as 300,000 cases annually.[16] However, this figure may be inflated because it was based, in part, on patient self-reporting of a Lyme diagnosis and on laboratory diagnosis, so false-positive results may be included. The highest statewide incidence of reported confirmed cases was 111.2 cases per 100,000 persons of the general population in Delaware in 2009.[14] Throughout this period, the highest local incidence shifted from the island of Nantucket, Massachusetts, to Columbia County, New York, with a peak incidence of 962 per 100,000 during the years 2002 to 2006.[14] There has also been a geographical spread of cases both along the Northeastern seaboard as well as in the Midwestern states.[14]

Data from the Slovenian National Registry document a maximum annual incidence of Lyme disease of 309 cases per 100,000 persons in 2009 and subsequent declines to 244 and 274 for 2010 and 2011, respectively (F. Strle, personal communication, 2013). A study in southern Sweden reported an incidence of 69 cases per 100,000; Lyme arthritis was present in 7% of all cases.[17] In a population-based study in Würzburg, Germany, the incidence was 111 per 100,000, with higher rates among children younger than 16 years old.[18]

In a community-based Connecticut cohort study of 201 consecutive cases in children in whom Lyme disease had been newly diagnosed, 13 (6%) had arthritis, and 5% had facial palsy.[19] In Europe, Lyme arthritis and neuroborreliosis have been reported in similar frequencies, and in the Würzburg study, arthritis was more common.[18] Compared with adults, children more frequently had manifestations other than isolated erythema migrans.[18] Early onset of cutaneous disease and neural involvement are closely related to tick activity in the spring to autumn; there is no seasonal pattern for late manifestations, such as Lyme arthritis, because arthritis may occur a year or longer after tick exposure.[4,5,18,20]

Sex Ratio and Age at Onset

Both sexes are affected equally. Cases have been reported among all age groups, with peaks occurring in school-age children and people between 40 and 74 years old.[17,18]

GENETIC BACKGROUND

Although Lyme disease may affect several members of the same family, genetic factors appear to have a limited influence on its occurrence. Nonetheless, host factors influence the course of the disease. In American patients, the development of chronic Lyme arthritis and an antibiotic-refractory course have been associated with the presence of human leukocyte antigen (HLA)-DR4. HLA-DR2 is an additional risk factor, especially in patients who are HLA-DR4 negative.[21] These results have not been confirmed in European patients. A DR4-positive mouse model has been established.[22]

ETIOLOGY AND PATHOGENESIS

Etiology

Lyme disease is the most common vector-borne infection in North America and Europe and is transmitted by hard-bodied ticks of the genus *Ixodes*[4,23] (Fig. 42-1). Transmission by other ticks or flying hematophagous insects has been suggested but has not been proven. Ticks of the genus *Ixodes* include *Ixodes ricinus* in central Europe, *Ixodes persulcatus* in Eastern Europe and Asia, *Ixodes scapularis* in the northeastern and north-central United States and Ontario, Canada, and *Ixodes pacificus* in the western United States.[4]

To become active, ticks require a warm and humid environment and are affected by climatic variability.[24] Infection is acquired in tick habitats, including forests, shaded valleys, gardens, lawns, and inner-city parks. After gaining access to unprotected skin, ticks crawl to the preferred feeding locations in the popliteal region, thighs, groins, breasts, axillae, neck, or head. *Ixodes* ticks feed only once during each of the three stages of their life cycle. Most human infections occur after the painless bite of nymphs (Fig. 42-2). *Ixodes* ticks also transmit tick-borne encephalitis virus, *Ehrlichia*, *Anaplasma phagocytophila*, and

Babesia organisms. Coinfection of these organisms with *B. burgdorferi* has been reported in rare cases.[25-27] Infection with *Anaplasma* results in higher fever and more severe illness than in patients with early Lyme disease.[28] Recently, it was shown in Russia and in the United States that *Ixodes* ticks also transmit some relapsing fever *Borreliae* such as

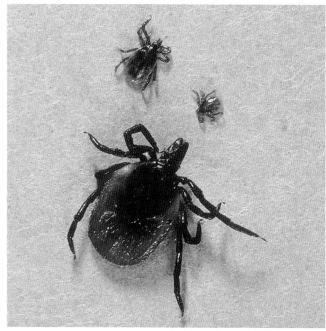

FIGURE 42-1 *Ixodes scapularis*, a member of the *Ixodes ricinus* complex. Clockwise, beginning at top: nymph, larva, and adult female.

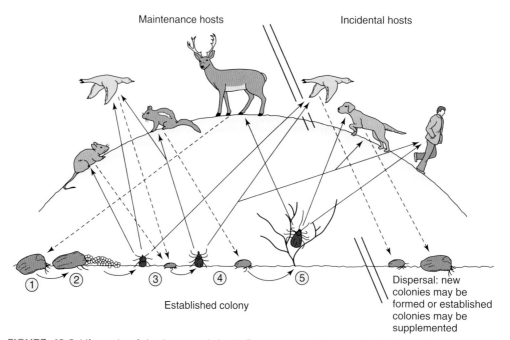

FIGURE 42-2 Life cycle of *Ixodes scapularis*: **1,** Engorged adult female. **2,** Adult female laying eggs. **3,** Questing and engorged larva. **4,** Questing and engorged nymph. **5,** Questing adult. A questing tick successfully finds a host (*solid arrows*). The tick engorges and drops from the host (*dashed arrows*). The tick develops to the next stage (*curved arrows*). (Redrawn from J.F. Anderson, L.A. Magnarelli, Avian and mammalian hosts for spirochete-infected ticks and insects in a Lyme disease focus in Connecticut, in: A.C. Steere, A.C. Malawista, J.E. Craft et al. (Eds.), First International Symposium on Lyme Disease, New Haven, CT. Yale J. Biol. Med. 57 (1984) 638.)

B. miyamotoi; clinical cases have been described in Russia, the United States, and Central Europe.[29-31]

Microbiology

Lyme disease is caused by infection with one of several species of *B. burgdorferi* sensu lato. These spirochetes have a protoplasmic cylinder surrounded by a cell membrane, a periplasmic flagellum, and an outer membrane.[32] They are microaerophilic and grow best at 33°C in a special liquid medium. They grow slowly, with doubling times between 12 and 24 hours. *B. burgdorferi* sensu lato has been subdivided into several species, of which only *B. burgdorferi* sensu stricto has been found to cause human disease in North America; *Borrelia garinii* and *Borrelia afzelii* also have been identified regularly in patients in Europe.[4,5] Two newer species, *Borrelia spielmanii* and *B. bavariensis,* have been isolated in Europe and associated with cases of erythema migrans.[33-35] In rare instances, these species may also cause Lyme arthritis. *Borrelia lusitaniae* was isolated from a 13-year-old girl with a vasculitis-like syndrome in Portugal.[36] The pathological potential of this species remains to be defined. In general, diversity in *B. burgdorferi* organisms has been greater in Europe and Asia than in North America. Concurrent infection with more than one species of *B. burgdorferi* was described in a patient with acrodermatitis and erythema migrans,[37] as was culture-confirmed reinfection in patients with several episodes of erythema migrans.[38] In all patients who had another erythema migrans following antibiotic treatment for the first episode, reinfection with a genetically different *B. burgdorferi* strain, and not relapse of disease by the strain causing the first episode, could be demonstrated.[39] These results demonstrate no evidence for persistent infection as a cause of human Lyme borreliosis after appropriate antibiotic treatment.

B. burgdorferi species differ genomically. Even within a species, different strains express proteins of different molecular weights as identified on gel electrophoresis. The major proteins identified in sonicates of *B. burgdorferi* are the 41-kD flagellar antigen; the 60-kD GroEL heat-shock protein; the three major outer surface proteins (Osp) OspA (30 to 32 kD), OspB (34 to 36 kD), and OspC (21 to 25 kD); the vlsE lipoprotein, the 39-kD BmpA protein; and the 83- to 100-kD antigen. Two membrane glycolipids of *B. burgdorferi* have recently been shown to lead to strong IgG responses in patients with Lyme arthritis.[40] The linear chromosome and plasmids of *B. burgdorferi* sensu stricto strain B31 as well as of 2 *B. afzelii* and 2 *B. garinii* strains and one strain each of *B. spielmanii, B. valaisiana,* and *B. bissettii* have been sequenced.[41-43]

The natural reservoirs of *B. burgdorferi* are mice and voles, although hedgehogs and birds may also serve this function. The life cycle of *Ixodes* ticks lasts 2 years (see Fig. 42-2).[44] The eggs hatch and larvae develop in the spring of the first year. The larvae feed once that summer on their preferred host (i.e., mice and voles) and so become infected with *B. burgdorferi.* The next spring, the larvae molt into nymphs, which feed on the preferred host before becoming mature ticks, at which time larger animals (e.g., deer) act as hosts. Humans are accidental hosts. Mating occurs while the female tick feeds. The female then detaches and lays her eggs on the ground.

Pathogenesis

Lyme arthritis provides a fascinating model for other arthritides because the causative organism and the clinical picture are well known. However, knowledge of the pathogenesis of this disease remains fragmented. *B. burgdorferi* excreted through tick salivary glands spread locally in the skin and can frequently be found at the advancing edge of erythema migrans. They attach to human cells by binding to various integrins, such as the fibronectin and vitronectin receptors.[45] Binding of the organism to platelets may play a role in its hematogenous spread.[46] Some of the molecular mechanisms involved in vascular interactions of *B. burgdorferi* have been described in a living mouse model.[47] *B. burgdorferi* organisms are presumed to reach the synovium through the bloodstream. It is probable that their presence in synovium is required at the onset of arthritis.

Survival of *B. burgdorferi* for decades in the lesions of acrodermatitis chronica atrophicans indicates that the spirochetes are able to evade the host immune response. There is also evidence that *B. burgdorferi* may survive intracellularly in endothelial cells, fibroblasts, and synovial cells.[48-50] *B. burgdorferi* use the mechanism of sequential variation of their outer surface proteins to attempt to evade the host immune response. This contributes to the survival of the organisms in spite of a strong antibody response. Arthritis appears to be largely due to the host inflammatory response.[51] Neutrophil-activating protein A is elevated in synovial fluid from patients with Lyme arthritis recruiting inflammatory cells into the joint cavity.[52] *B. burgdorferi* have stimulatory effects on B cells,[53] and a dominant T-helper cell 1 (Th1) response has been found in synovial fluid of patients with Lyme arthritis.[54,55] A Toll-like receptor 1 polymorphism has been associated with heightened Th1 inflammatory responses and antibiotic-refractory Lyme arthritis.[56] Higher numbers of regulatory T cells were implicated in contributing to antibiotic-responsive Lyme arthritis.[57] Recent work from the same group found higher expression of activation coreceptors and less effective inhibition of proinflammatory cytokines as well as more activated natural killer cells in patients with antibiotic-refractory Lyme arthritis.[58,59] A *B. burgdorferi*–specific CD8+ cytotoxic T-cell response has also been reported in patients with Lyme arthritis.[60] These cells were found only after the disappearance of arthritis.[60] *B. burgdorferi* also stimulate synovial γ/δ T cells from patients with Lyme arthritis, leading to high and prolonged expression of Fas ligand associated with cytolytic activity.[61,62] A number of cytokines are induced, including interleukin (IL)-1 and IL-6,[63,64] tumor necrosis factor,[65] CXCR3, CCR5, CXCL9,[66] and interferon (IFN)-γ, and IL-10.[67] The chemokine CXCL13 appears to be a key regulator of B cell recruitment in acute neuroborreliosis.[68]

Molecular mimicry may also play a role in the pathogenesis of some of the manifestations of Lyme disease. Sequence homologies have been identified between *B. burgdorferi* flagellin and human myelin basic protein, as well as cross-reactivity between flagellin and a human axonal protein.[69,70] Antibody reactivity to OspA and OspB occurred late in the course of infection in American patients with chronic Lyme arthritis.[71] Tick-specific borrelial antigens such as OspA and OspD were upregulated in American but not European patients with Lyme arthritis.[72] Th cells from patients with antibiotic-refractory Lyme arthritis demonstrated dominant recognition of an OspA peptide of *B. burgdorferi,*[73] and high levels of CXCL9 and IFN-γ were found in synovial fluid and tissue.[66] Human homologues of the borrelial T-cell epitope were found, but reactivity with the self-peptides was lower, implying that molecular mimicry is unlikely to be the critical mechanism.[74] The human leukocyte function-associated antigen-1 (LFA-1) was implicated as a candidate autoantigen in treatment-resistant Lyme arthritis.[75] However, later work cast doubt that LFA-1 was a relevant autoantigen.[76] Recently, endothelial cell growth factor, a novel human autoantigen, was implicated in the pathogenesis of antibiotic-refractory Lyme arthritis.[77] IL-17 and Th17 lymphocytes have an additional role in Lyme arthritis.[78,79]

CLINICAL MANIFESTATIONS

Many persons infected with *B. burgdorferi* are asymptomatic, and the risk of developing Lyme disease following a tick bite is low, even if the

TABLE 42-1 Major Clinical Manifestations of Lyme Disease in Children and Adolescents

ORGAN SYSTEM	EARLY LYME DISEASE	LATE LYME DISEASE
Skin	Erythema migrans Borrelial lymphocytoma*	Acrodermatitis chronica atrophicans*
Nervous system	Cranial nerve palsy Lymphocytic meningitis	Chronic encephalomyelitis*
Musculoskeletal system	Arthralgia	Arthritis
Other	Carditis*	

*Rare in childhood.

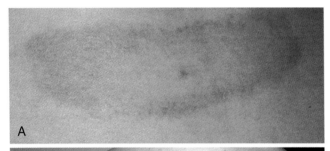

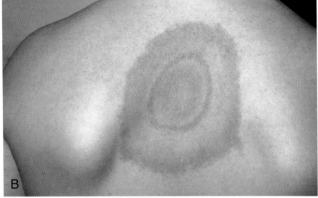

FIGURE 42-3 Erythema migrans. **A,** The site of the tick bite is visible near the center of the lesion. **B,** Typical "bull's-eye" lesion.

tick was infected by *B. burgdorferi*.[80] Very often, a tick bite is not recalled. In symptomatic patients, the cutaneous, nervous, and musculoskeletal systems are most frequently involved.[4,5] Symptoms of Lyme disease can be divided into early and late manifestations (Table 42-1). Early signs of infection become evident within days to weeks of the tick bite, whereas late organ involvement begins several months or even years later. Early symptoms are usually self-limiting, whereas late manifestations may become chronic and rarely lead to irreversible damage of involved organs. In most patients with the disease, only one organ system is affected.

Cutaneous Disease

The earliest and most common skin manifestation, *erythema migrans,* typically occurs days to several weeks after infection as an enlarging, warm, but usually painless, erythematous rash at the site of the bite, and it lasts for days or weeks (Fig. 42-3).[4,5,81] In its classic form, this lesion begins as a red macule or papule and expands peripherally with partial central clearing occurring later. Sometimes, the rash does not

clear; in other cases, the clearing is so complete that erythema migrans becomes a mere curved red streak. In children, the neck and head are the most frequently affected sites, and the erythema may look more cellulitic. It is also common in the groin, axilla, or thigh and may expand up to 30 cm. Secondary lesions can occur at sites distant from the tick bite. Erythema migrans may be accompanied by flulike symptoms of fever, chills, arthralgia, musculoskeletal pain, headaches, malaise, and fatigue. Lyme disease may also begin as a flulike illness in the absence of erythema migrans.[82]

Weeks to months after infection, *borrelial lymphocytoma,* also known as *lymphadenosis cutis benigna* (e.g., a purple swelling most commonly at an earlobe, the scrotum, or a nipple), is occasionally reported in European patients.[83] Recently, Lyme chondritis presenting as ear erythema has been distinguished from borrelial lymphocytoma.[84] *Acrodermatitis chronica atrophicans,* a late skin manifestation, rarely affects European children and then only years after infection.[81,85] In the early phase of acrodermatitis, the affected limb develops inflammatory changes with a red or bluish discoloration. Later, cutaneous atrophy becomes apparent. A peripheral neuropathy can accompany the skin lesion. Lymphocytoma and acrodermatitis are extremely uncommon in North America.

Nervous System Disease: Neuroborreliosis

Early neuroborreliosis most frequently presents as lymphocytic meningitis or a cranial nerve palsy weeks to months after infection.[86,87] It may be accompanied by fever, headache, nausea, vomiting, radicular paresthesias, or pain. In endemic areas Lyme meningitis may be the most common form of meningitis in childhood.[86,88] Unilateral or bilateral facial nerve palsy is the most common focal neurological manifestation, but cranial nerves III, IV, VI, and VIII may also be affected. Also, the optic nerves may be involved, but mostly secondary to increased intracranial pressure.[89] Signs of meningitis may be mild or absent in spite of increased protein and lymphocytes in the cerebrospinal fluid. A painful meningoradiculoneuritis is the most common neurological manifestation in European adults but is relatively uncommon in children. Months to years after infection, a small number of patients develop late neuroborreliosis, progressive encephalomyelitis, or an encephalopathy.[87,90] Other rare neurological manifestations include Guillain–Barré syndrome,[91,92] pseudotumor cerebri,[93,94] cerebral vasculitis,[95,96] and neurogenic bladder.[97]

Musculoskeletal Disease

After erythema migrans, arthritis is the most common manifestation of Lyme borreliosis in many series of pediatric patients and is more common in North America than in Europe.[4,5,22,98-100] There is little evidence that the musculoskeletal symptoms of Lyme borreliosis otherwise differ between Europe and North America. Myalgia, myositis, and enthesitis are uncommon, although *B. burgdorferi* have been identified in a few patients with enthesitis or nodular fasciitis.[101-103] Arthralgia and myalgia develop as early as days to weeks after infection, sometimes concurrent with erythema migrans or flulike symptoms. However, arthritis appears typically months to years after infection.[104]

The two largest series of pediatric patients with Lyme arthritis include 90 children from Connecticut[100] and 109 from Germany,[104] 62 of whom have been described in detail.[19] Monoarthritis of a knee occurred in approximately two thirds of all children.[19,100] Both knees or other large joints may also be affected.[19,100,104] Polyarticular involvement of small joints was rare. At onset, the arthritis was usually episodic, with relatively painless swelling lasting only a few days and disappearing without the need for therapy. Recurrent episodes of arthritis may become prolonged, and chronic arthritis (duration of more than 3 months) has been reported in up to 18% of patients.[19] Among 109 German children with Lyme arthritis, 70 had monoarthritis, 32 oligoarthritis, and 7 polyarthritis.[104] The pattern of oligoarticular involvement differed from that found in patients with early-onset oligoarticular juvenile idiopathic arthritis or juvenile spondyloarthritis.[104] However, ocular involvement with keratitis and anterior and intermediate uveitis may occur in children with Lyme arthritis.[105] Lyme arthritis may occasionally be confused with septic arthritis, especially when there is isolated hip involvement. In several studies, fever and complete refusal to bear weight on the affected joint were negative predictors for Lyme arthritis versus septic arthritis, whereas knee involvement, sedimentation rate less than 40, and absolute blood neutrophil count less than 10,000 were positive predictors.[106-109] Children are more likely than adults to show acute disease.[110]

Lyme arthritis was reported in a woman after autologous chondrocyte transplantation.[111] The investigators hypothesize that *B. burgdorferi* was asymptomatically present in the patient's joint before the chondrocyte transplant procedure. Myositis has only rarely been described in adult patients,[101] and only myalgia has been reported in children.[112] A dermatomyositis-like picture has also been described in a single adult patient.[113]

Other Manifestations

Involvement of other organ systems is much more uncommon. Carditis is rare in children and most commonly manifests as a reversible atrioventricular block.[114] A recent report documented three adult deaths from undetected lymphoplasmacytic pancarditis (Fig. 42-4).[115] Ocular involvement, including conjunctivitis, keratitis, iridocyclitis, intermediate uveitis, choroiditis, or optic neuritis, has been described in children with Lyme disease.[105,116,117] Even more uncommonly, patients may develop hepatitis.[118] There have been anecdotal reports of transplacental transmission of *B. burgdorferi*,[119] but this has not been confirmed in controlled studies.[120] The offspring of 5 of 19 pregnant women who had Lyme disease during pregnancy had one or more of the following abnormal outcomes: prematurity, syndactyly, rash, cortical blindness, developmental delay, or intrauterine fetal death.[121,122] Whether any of these complications is attributable to infection with

B. burgdorferi or with other spirochetes is not certain. There is no evidence that maternal infection presents a significant risk to the fetus.

PATHOLOGY

The synovitis of Lyme arthritis resembles that of juvenile idiopathic arthritis or juvenile rheumatoid arthritis, with villous hypertrophy, synovial cell hyperplasia, and infiltration of lymphocytes and plasma cells.[123] Lymphoid follicles may also be present. Endarteritis is a characteristic finding in patients with Lyme synovitis. In one study, spirochetes were detected in 2 of 17 synovia, mainly in a perivascular distribution.[123] Other studies using special silver stains have also identified *B. burgdorferi* in synovium or synovial fluid.[124,125] The organism has been recovered from the margins of erythema migrans lesions and cardiac tissue.[126-128] Although cardiomyopathy may result from the initial myocarditis, valvular endocarditis does not develop. Myositis may in part account for the myalgia and fatigue that occur in this disease, and DNA from *B. burgdorferi* has been identified in the muscle of such patients.[129]

LABORATORY EXAMINATION

Nonspecific Abnormalities

The erythrocyte sedimentation rate is elevated in half of the patients, especially during the early phase of Lyme arthritis. Meningoencephalitis causes mild cerebrospinal fluid lymphocytic pleocytosis, with a median cerebrospinal fluid (CSF) cell count of 160 cells/mm³, mostly lymphocytes.[130] The mean synovial fluid white blood cell count ranges from less than 5000/mm³ to greater than 100,000/mm³, with a predominance of neutrophils in samples with high cell counts.[19,109] Children have higher synovial cell counts than adults.[110]

Confirmation of Infection With *Borrelia burgdorferi*

Laboratory methods to document infection with *B. burgdorferi* include direct tests, such as culture or the polymerase chain reaction (PCR) to detect borrelial sequences, and indirect tests, such as serology (Table 42-2).[131] The latter tests are most frequently used and universally

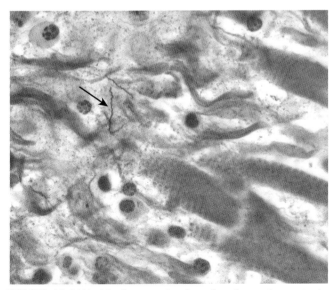

FIGURE 42-4 Warthin–Starry stain of cardiac tissue demonstrating *Borrelia burgdorferi* spirochetes *(arrow)* in one of three patients whose death was associated with Lyme carditis during November 12 to July 2013. (Ref. 115.)

TABLE 42-2 Laboratory Diagnosis of Lyme Arthritis

METHOD	ASSESSMENT
Culture of *Borrelia burgdorferi*	Requires weeks; rarely successful
Histochemistry using silver stain or monoclonal antibodies	Rarely successful in synovial tissue
Polymerase chain reaction for borrelial DNA	Efficiency varies widely: Urine, 5% to 30%; synovium, 6% to 90% (higher in membrane than in fluid)
Enzyme immunoassay or immunofluorescence assay using serum	High sensitivity, low specificity, rarely false negative, >10% false positive
Immunoblot using serum	Confirmatory test with high specificity; healthy blood donors <3% positive
Lymphocyte-proliferation assay with borrelial antigens	Sensitivity and specificity <80% Limited availability

All diagnostic tests bear the risk of false-negative or false-positive results. No test is of value in a patient with low pretest probability of having Lyme arthritis.

Adapted from H.I. Huppertz, Lyme arthritis, in: U. Wahn, R. Seger, V. Wahn, et al. (Eds.), Paediatrische Allergologie und Immunologie, fourth ed., Elsevier, Munich, 2005.

available. In spite of the standardization of the laboratory evaluation in North America, the approach suggested by the American College of Physicians[132,133] has not been widely adopted for European patients. Common problems with standardization of test procedures for the diagnosis of Lyme disease have been reviewed.[134]

Direct Methods to Detect Infection

Culture of *B. burgdorferi* usually takes 2 weeks to a few months, requires immediate suspension of the test material in special medium, and has high rates of recovery only from skin biopsies of patients with dermatological manifestations of the disease.[126] Culture of the organism from blood and especially from synovial fluid has been relatively unsuccessful. The possibility of obtaining positive cultures is better from the CSF of patients with early neuroborreliosis.[135] Methods such as silver staining of spirochetes in tissue specimens or staining with monoclonal antibodies are not routinely performed and are prone to artifacts.

The PCR can demonstrate DNA of *B. burgdorferi* in tissues or bodily fluids, including synovial fluid.[136-142] In a large North American study of synovial fluid from patients with Lyme arthritis,[136] PCR results were positive for 96% of patients not previously treated with antibiotics and 37% of those who had been treated. In a later study from the same group, borrelial sequences were undetectable in synovial specimens from patients with chronic Lyme arthritis after appropriate antibiotic therapy.[137]

Other groups have found a smaller percentage of positive PCR results in synovial fluid of patients with Lyme arthritis. The precise role of PCR in routine diagnosis remains unclear. False-positive or false-negative results may occur. Optimization of PCR includes using more than one primer pair, targeting genes situated on the bacterial chromosome and the plasmids, performing nested PCR, and analyzing synovial fluid and urine.[138] There is evidence that PCR of synovial tissue may have a higher positivity rate than in synovial fluid[141] and may remain positive in patients with ongoing arthritis whose synovial fluid is negative by PCR after antibiotic treatment.[142] *B. burgdorferi* in the skin lesions of patients with erythema migrans were active and viable, whereas the spirochetes in synovial fluid or tissue from Lyme arthritis patients were moribund or dead.[143] PCR results for urine may be positive in healthy humans whose sera contain *B. burgdorferi*–specific antibodies; urine testing for Lyme antigens is not an approved assay.[144]

Indirect Methods to Detect Infection

Specific antibodies can be demonstrated after *B. burgdorferi* infection by a variety of tests including enzyme immunoassay (EIA), immunofluorescence, hemagglutination, and Western blotting[145] (Fig. 42-5). It is recommended that a sensitive EIA be used as a screening test and that all results in the indeterminate or positive ranges be confirmed by Western blotting; this has been called *two-tier testing*.[146]

Typical IgM and IgG responses of patients with Lyme arthritis and the North American criteria for a positive IgG blot are shown in Fig. 42-5.[146,147] In early Lyme borreliosis, IgM blots are considered positive if at least two of the following three bands are present: 21-kD OspC, 39-kD BmpA, and 41-kD flagellin.[146,148] Antigens from different strains of *B. burgdorferi* have different molecular weights, and, for this reason, North American criteria cannot easily be applied in Europe or Asia, where there is greater strain diversity. Even so, a two-test approach is the best available method for diagnosis of Lyme disease in European children.[19] In a German pediatric Lyme arthritis study,[19] at least six specific bands were required for a positive IgG Western blot, similar to the American criteria. Commonly, patients with Lyme arthritis have 10 or more IgG bands (see Fig. 42-5), including the ones mentioned earlier. Specific blot-positivity criteria have been established for each

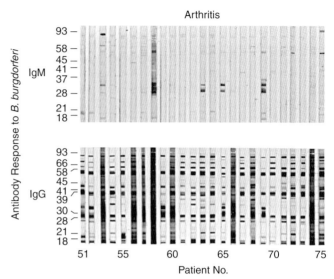

FIGURE 42-5 Western blots of immunoglobulin M (IgM) and IgG antibody responses of 25 patients with Lyme arthritis to a sonicated whole-cell lysate of *Borrelia burgdorferi* sensu stricto strain G39/40. Molecular masses (in kilodaltons) are indicated on the left side. Characteristic of Lyme arthritis, strong IgG responses against many antigens are demonstrated. In North America, the criteria for a positive IgG blot are the detection of at least 5 of the following 10 bands: 18 kD, 21-kD Osp C, 28 kD, 30 kD, 39-kD BmpA, 41-kD flagellin, 45 kD, 58 kD, 66 kD, and 93 kD. All patients met these criteria. A minority of patients also have IgM responses to a smaller number of antigens. Molecular masses depend on the strain used for testing. (Adapted from F. Dressler, J.A. Whalen, B.N. Reinhardt, et al., Western blotting in the serodiagnosis of Lyme disease, J. Infect. Dis. 167 (1993) 392.)

of the three pathogenic species in Europe, with different positivity criteria for each strain.[149,150] North American studies found that kinetic EIAs detecting IgG responses to recombinant *B. burgdorferi* antigen vlsE1 or to a conserved internal sequence of vlsE1 were equally sensitive and specific in assessing patients with Lyme arthritis and more sensitive in assessing patients with early skin or neurological manifestations of Lyme borreliosis.[151,152] There was also a cost-reduction with that strategy.[153] European studies have also shown the usefulness of EIAs or Western blots using recombinant vlsE1 peptide antigen in children with Lyme arthritis[154] or adults with neuroborreliosis.[155] In North American studies comparing two-tier testing with enzyme-linked immunosorbent assay (ELISA) and Western blot with a vlsE C6 peptide ELISA, both methods had similar sensitivity, but two-tier testing had slightly better specificity.[152,156] Using an IgG Western blot with a vlsE IgG band as the second-tier test improved sensitivity while maintaining the specificity of standard IgM and IgG two-tier testing.[157] Two recent studies have examined the use of American serologic assays for Lyme borreliosis acquired in Europe and found significantly less sensitivity.[158,159] European serologic tests performed well for Lyme disease acquired in the United States.[159]

Within the first weeks after infection, all serological results may be negative because specific IgM antibodies usually do not appear until 3 to 4 weeks after infection, and IgG antibodies cannot be detected until 4 to 8 weeks after infection. Frequently, an EIA may give false-positive results related to cross-reactive antibodies such as rheumatoid factors or after infection with Epstein–Barr virus[160] or other spirochetes, including *Treponema pallidum, Treponema denticola, Borrelia hermsii,* and leptospira.[161] Antibodies to *B. burgdorferi* occasionally are found in children with juvenile rheumatoid arthritis,[162,163]

BOX 42-1 Assessment of Patients with Suspected Lyme Arthritis

Patient living in or having visited an endemic area
Presence of arthritis documented
No other obvious cause of arthritis
Serology positive (enzyme immunoassay [EIA] and Western blot for IgG antibodies to *B. burgdorferi*):
  No further laboratory test needed
  Start therapy
Serology negative (EIA and Western blot):
  Rule out other diagnosis
  Refer for specialized evaluation

TABLE 42-3 Diagnosis of Lyme Arthritis Using a Clinical Score

CRITERION	SCORE*
Episodic arthritis	+4
Arthralgia before onset of arthritis	−3
Age at onset of arthritis	+0.3 × age (in years)
Initial arthritis in knee joint	+2
History of tick bite	+2
Number of joints involved	−0.4 × number of large joints affected

Scoring example: A 10-year-old boy without prior arthralgia or history of a tick bite developed arthritis in a knee. The arthritis resolved after 10 days but recurred after a 3-month interval.[†]

Episodic arthritis present	+4
No initial arthralgias	+0
Age at onset × 0.3	+3
Initial arthritis in knee	+2
No history of tick bite	+0
1 large joint affected	−0.4
Total score	+8.6

*If a criterion is recognized, its indicated value is added to or subtracted from the total score for the patient. If it is not identified, the item is scored as 0. Values of 6 or greater indicate the presence of Lyme arthritis, and values of 2.5 or less exclude the diagnosis.
†The patient's serum was later shown to contain IgG antibodies to *Borrelia burgdorferi* by enzyme immunoassay and immunoblot. He was treated with ceftriaxone for 2 weeks. Arthritis disappeared during therapy and did not recur in the subsequent 2 years of follow-up.
Adapted from H.I. Huppertz, W. Bentas, I. Haubitz, et al., Diagnosis of pediatric Lyme arthritis using a clinical score, Eur. J. Pediatr. 157 (1998) 304.

systemic lupus erythematosus,[164] and other illnesses (e.g., bacterial endocarditis, mumps, Rocky Mountain spotted fever, and other rickettsial diseases).

Serological tests cannot distinguish patients with active infection from those with a previous infection who have responded to therapy. In particular, about 10% of patients with late manifestations of Lyme disease continue to demonstrate an IgM response in addition to the IgG response. Because IgG titers tend to remain elevated for years,[165] serology cannot be used to monitor treatment success or failure. Contrary to claims that the rate of decline of antibodies to the conserved internal sequence of vlsE1 could be useful to monitor treatment efficacy, this was not true in German children with Lyme arthritis.[154] In an endemic area, serological tests should be performed only in patients with clinical signs suggestive of the disease; a positive result in a patient with a low pretest probability of Lyme disease is much more likely to represent a false-positive rather than a true-positive result.[134,166] Because of the rampant overtesting for Lyme disease, the American College of Rheumatology has recommended not testing for Lyme disease as a cause of musculoskeletal symptoms without an exposure history and appropriate examination findings.[167] Given these restrictions, serology is useful diagnostically in patients with suspected Lyme arthritis because virtually all patients are clearly IgG seropositive.[19,100] The diagnosis of Lyme arthritis must not be based on inappropriate Western blot testing of synovial fluid alone.[168] Box 42-1 provides a simplified overview of the laboratory evaluation.

DIAGNOSIS

Clinical characteristics of patients with arthritis that suggest a diagnosis of Lyme arthritis include residence in or travel to an endemic area, a previous tick bite, episodic oligoarthritis involving the knee joint, the absence of arthralgias preceding the onset of arthritis, and being of adolescent age at onset. Specific criteria have been combined to form a clinical diagnostic score that would confirm or exclude Lyme arthritis in two thirds of children with arthritis[169] (Table 42-3). For a diagnosis of Lyme arthritis, arthritis (i.e., swelling and effusion or painful limitation of motion in the absence of trauma) must be observed by a physician. Arthralgias alone or reports by the patient or the parents that the joint was swollen are not objective signs of arthritis in this context.

Frequently, however, the clinical presentation of Lyme arthritis may be indistinguishable from that of other rheumatic diseases of childhood with arthritis as a principal manifestation, making laboratory tests mandatory in all patients with arthritis living in or having traveled to an endemic area.[134] A recent review addressed a number of common misconceptions about the diagnosis and treatment of Lyme disease.[170]

The CDC established the following criteria for the diagnosis of Lyme disease[171]: the presence of erythema migrans larger than 5 cm in diameter, or at least one clinical sign (i.e., arthritis, meningitis, radiculoneuritis, mononeuritis, or carditis) and the presence of specific antibodies to *B. burgdorferi*.

These criteria were developed for epidemiological research and may not always be applicable in the clinical setting. For example, borrelial lymphocytoma may initially occur in the absence of specific antibodies. Moreover, the mere combination of an objective sign with specific antibodies may include chance associations between two frequent events: arthritis of some kind may affect 1 in 1000 children, and in endemic areas, the prevalence of antibodies to *B. burgdorferi* is high; 3% or more of healthy blood donors may be positive for specific antibodies to *B. burgdorferi*.[172] In a population-based survey among 5-year-old children in Sweden the seroprevalence of *Borrelia* IgG antibodies was 3.2%,[173] and in a nationwide German study among 1- to 17-year-old children and adolescents it was 4.8%.[174] Some high-risk populations, such as forestry workers, have a much higher incidence of seropositivity—up to 45%—without clinical evidence of Lyme disease.[175] Serology can provide evidence of current or prior infection but cannot absolutely confirm a pathogenic link between the infection and the clinical manifestation. The child may have been infected with *B. burgdorferi* as documented by serology; however, arthritis may result from other known or unknown causes. Overdiagnosis of Lyme disease in children has also been reported.[176]

Synovial fluid analysis is of little help in establishing a diagnosis of Lyme arthritis because the white blood cell count and type of cells vary greatly.[140,177] However, synovial fluid analysis can exclude septic arthritis and other infection-associated arthritides, yields material for testing by PCR, and confirms the presence of inflammation. Although a positive PCR result from an experienced laboratory may indicate a persistent infection, a negative result does not exclude the diagnosis. Synovial tissue may be more suitable than synovial fluid for PCR testing, especially after antibiotic treatment has failed to produce a remission of symptoms.[141,142]

A lumbar puncture should be performed in patients with suspected neuroborreliosis. Lymphocytic pleocytosis and elevated CSF protein levels are characteristic.[86,87] In the presence of neurological symptoms and CSF lymphocytic pleocytosis the serological standard in diagnosing neuroborreliosis in European adult patients remains the detection of intrathecal antibody production.[86,87,178] However, especially in children, specific antibody production frequently occurs only after several weeks to months of infection and has been less commonly demonstrable in American patients. Therefore intrathecal antibody production is not required for diagnosing early neuroborreliosis in children. Recent studies showed that the detection of the chemokine CXCL13 improves the diagnostic performance in children with early neuroborreliosis.[178-180] A clinical prediction rule of fewer than 7 days of headaches, fewer than 70% CSF mononuclear cells, and the absence of cranial nerve palsy has been used in American children to distinguish aseptic meningitis due to other causes from Lyme meningitis.[181]

TREATMENT

Antibiotic Regimens

Recommendations by the Infectious Diseases Society of America (IDSA) for the treatment of Lyme disease (Table 42-4) have been published and vary according to disease manifestations.[182] In the treatment of patients with erythema migrans or neuroborreliosis, amoxicillin is as effective as doxycycline.[183] Cephalosporins were only marginally better than penicillin G.[183-188] Cefuroxime axetil was equally efficacious as doxycycline in adults or as amoxicillin in children with erythema migrans.[189,190] Although doxycycline and ceftriaxone have been equally effective,[190] most macrolide antibiotics are inferior to these antibiotics.[191-194] However, clarithromycin was as effective as amoxicillin in children with erythema migrans.[195] It is not known whether these results are applicable to patients with Lyme arthritis, for whom a variety of antibiotics have been recommended, including parenteral penicillin G, oral penicillins, amoxicillin with or without probenecid, ceftriaxone, cefotaxime, cefuroxime, erythromycin, roxithromycin (plus cotrimoxazole), azithromycin, tetracycline, doxycycline, and others.[20,196] For Lyme arthritis, oral antibiotic therapy for 4 weeks with amoxicillin in young children or with doxycycline in adolescents has been recommended by the IDSA; however, controlled trials of oral versus intravenous antibiotics have not been performed. Oral treatment may be more convenient for the patient and more cost-effective but involves administration of up to 84 doses of amoxicillin. Intravenous treatment with ceftriaxone once daily for 14 days can be given as an outpatient and may be more convenient for some patients. Before the physician can conclude that antibiotic therapy has failed, at least two courses of sufficient duration and well-documented compliance are required. When confronted with failure of a treatment program with appropriate antibiotics, the correctness of a diagnosis of Lyme arthritis should be questioned and reconfirmed.

Among 51 German patients followed for at least 12 months after initiation of antibiotic treatment, 8 patients still had arthritis, and 4 had arthralgias.[197] Risk factors for a prolonged course of disease were female gender, age over 10 years, and intraarticular steroids given before antibiotic treatment.

Duration of therapy is a matter of debate. Because *B. burgdorferi* are slow-growing organisms, treatment should be continued for at least 10 days in early Lyme disease. In adults with erythema migrans, extension of treatment with doxycycline from 10 days to 20 days provided no additional benefit.[198] In a retrospective study of Swedish children with early neuroborreliosis, antibiotic treatment for 10 days was considered sufficient.[199] Even doxycycline courses of less than 10 days were effective in patients with early Lyme disease, including their long-term prognosis.[200] There is also no proof that treatment extending beyond 1 month is of any additional benefit. The success of antibiotic treatment must be determined clinically, because serological results remain positive for a long time after resolution of all manifestations.[165,201]

An approach to treatment is shown in Table 42-4. In young children, erythema migrans is treated with amoxicillin (50 mg/kg/day) in three divided doses for 10 days to 3 weeks. In children 9 years of age or older, doxycycline is given for 10 days to 3 weeks. Most doxycycline studies in Lyme disease have used 100 mg twice a day; however, it is likely that 200 mg once a day is equally effective. If erythema migrans resolves within a week, 10 days of treatment may be long enough; otherwise, a longer duration up to 3 weeks is recommended. In neuroborreliosis or Lyme carditis, ceftriaxone (50 mg/kg/day) is

TABLE 42-4	**Treatment Recommendations for Lyme Disease in Children and Adolescents**			
MANIFESTATION	**DRUGS***	**DOSAGE***		**DURATION**
Erythema migrans	Amoxicillin	50 mg/kg/day in 3 doses		10-21 days‡
	Doxycycline†	200 mg/day in 1 to 2 doses		10-21 days‡
	Clarithromycin	15 mg/kg/day in 2 doses		10-21 days‡
Neuroborreliosis and Lyme carditis	Ceftriaxone	50 to 100 mg/kg/day in 1 dose		2-4 weeks
	Cefotaxime	150 mg/kg/day in 3 doses		2-4 weeks
Lyme arthritis	Ceftriaxone	50 mg/kg/day in 1 dose		2-4 weeks
	Amoxicillin	50 mg/kg/day in 3 doses		4 weeks
	Doxycycline†	200 mg/day in 1 to 2 doses		4 weeks
	Cefuroxime	30 mg/kg/day in 2 doses		4 weeks
	Roxithromycin	5 mg/kg/day plus cotrimoxazole, 6 mg/kg/day in 2 doses each		4 weeks

Maximum daily dose of amoxicillin = 2 g; doxycycline = 200 mg; ceftriaxone = 2 g; cefotaxime = 6 g.
*Ceftriaxone and cefotaxime are administered intravenously; amoxicillin and doxycycline are taken orally.
†Doxycycline should not be administered to patients younger than 10 years old.
‡Continue treatment for another 10 days if erythema migrans is still present at the end of 10 days.

administered intravenously for 14 days. Because only one 20-minute infusion is required per day, treatment can be provided in an outpatient setting. Oral doxycycline is as effective as intravenous ceftriaxone for the treatment of European patients with neuroborreliosis.[202] Therefore the treatment recommendation by the European Federation of Neurological Societies includes, as an alternative, a 14-day oral course with doxycycline for children and adults with neuroborreliosis that is confined to the meninges, cranial nerves, nerve roots, or peripheral nerves.[178] Patients with Lyme arthritis also benefit from intravenous therapy, but they have been treated successfully with oral antibiotics, including amoxicillin or doxycycline, for 4 weeks. The latter approach to treatment is more convenient for most patients and more cost-effective than intravenous regimens, but it should not be used in patients with central nervous system neuroborreliosis, or carditis.[203] In case of allergy to penicillin or amoxicillin, cephalosporins are an option but may cross-react with penicillin allergy in rare instances. Macrolide antibiotics are recommended in children younger than 9 years, although many of these drugs are less effective than the β-lactam antibiotics.[191,204] Clarithromycin can be used in erythema migrans[195] or alternatively a combination of roxithromycin and cotrimoxazole.[205] Infection during pregnancy should be treated with antibiotics that do not pose a risk to the fetus (e.g., amoxicillin, intravenous penicillin G, or cephalosporins).

During antibiotic treatment, up to 10% of patients with arthritis develop a Jarisch–Herxheimer reaction, with fever; a nonpruritic, nonpalpable rash; and severe pain. This complication usually develops after the first few doses of antibiotics but may occur up to 10 days after beginning treatment. It must be distinguished from allergic reactions to the administered drug.[20] In the authors' experience, many reactions thought to be allergic are Jarisch–Herxheimer reactions. Whereas an allergic response to the antibiotic requires immediate interruption of administration of the drug, a Jarisch–Herxheimer reaction is a favorable, self-limited sign, and treatment can be continued.

Although nonsteroidal antiinflammatory agents are frequently given to patients with Lyme arthritis, often before the correct diagnosis is made, their efficacy has not been established; however, nonsteroidal antiinflammatory agents can be used as analgesics or after antibiotics have failed. Treatment failures in patients with Lyme arthritis or late neuroborreliosis are often associated with prior administration of glucocorticoids.[184] In such instances, repetition of antibiotic treatment with the same or another antibiotic is recommended. Intraarticular steroids, sulfasalazine, methotrexate, or arthroscopic synovectomy[204] with a further course of antibiotics (in that order) are treatment options. In addition, Steere has given hydroxychloroquine or infliximab in adult patients.[206] The total duration of arthritis was shortened in those patients with ongoing arthritis after antibiotic therapy in comparison to patients that were not treated with antibiotics.[206]

Chronic Lyme Disease

The term *chronic Lyme disease* has been used in a variety of individuals who can be divided into four groups.[207] Persons in the first group have medically unexplained symptoms without laboratory evidence of Lyme disease and become convinced that they have Lyme disease. Persons in the second group have an illness other than Lyme disease but prefer to believe that their illness is Lyme disease. Individuals in the third group are seropositive for previous *Borrelia burgdorferi* infection but never satisfied criteria for Lyme disease, and individuals in the last group are those patients who had Lyme disease, were treated, but continue to have symptoms.[207-209] Adding to the confusion regarding "chronic Lyme disease," the majority of advocacy Internet sites that purportedly contain Lyme education material were grossly inaccurate.[210]

Patients with "chronic Lyme disease" are frequently treated by so-called Lyme-literate doctors who employ alternative diagnostic strategies such as lymphocyte transformation assay, concentration of CD57-NK (natural killer) cells, or visual contrast sensitivity assay. These tests are based on alternative theories of pathogenesis of Lyme disease with a borrelial neurotoxin remaining in enterohepatic circulation and with a frequent persistent infection with *B. burgdorferi*. There is no evidence supporting these assumptions, and these diagnostic tests have been shown to be inferior to serology or show a complete lack of evidence and/or biological plausibility. Therefore these hypotheses have been labeled *antiscience*.[211] Unfortunately, the erroneous belief that a child has "chronic Lyme disease" may lead to Munchausen syndrome by proxy.[212]

"Lyme-literate" doctors believe that the infection is still present after standard courses of antibiotics, and requires unproven—and potentially dangerous—prolonged courses of antibiotics. In double-blind trials, prolonged courses of antibiotics showed no clinically meaningful improvement of the manifestations in "chronic Lyme disease" patients compared to placebo.[213] Prolonged antibiotics may produce untoward side effects, including death, alteration of the microbiome, and distraction of the patient from the real illness at hand, be it inflammatory or somatoform.

Prevention

Recommendations for the prevention of Lyme disease have been published by the American Academy of Pediatrics,[214] and the subject has been reviewed in detail.[215]

Avoidance of Tick Bites

Avoiding tick bites in endemic areas is difficult. Reduction of tick numbers on residential properties and gardens can be achieved through landscaping measures that create a drying barrier between forest and lawn, the use of acaricides, and the removal of deer from specified areas.[215] Appropriate clothing with light-colored long trousers tucked into socks makes it more difficult for ticks to attach to a human host. Tick repellents containing *N,N*-diethyl-*meta*-toluamide (DEET), or permethrin applied to clothing, especially the shoes and socks of a person who is walking, can reduce tick attachment for several hours.[23,216] DEET may also be applied directly to skin, but the use of repellents on skin should be limited because toxic side effects can occur. Other repellents have been used, including icaridin, IR3535, and citriodora, but results are controversial and depend on vector species, infection of the vector, additional components and concentration of the repellent, and possibly other, yet unknown conditions.[217] Many plant-based repellents provide only short duration protection.[217] Ticks should be removed promptly because *B. burgdorferi* organisms reside in the tick's midgut, and proliferation starts only after the host's blood has entered the tick's gut. Thereafter, *B. burgdorferi* spread by the acarial hemolymph to the tick's salivary glands. Because this takes 24 to 36 hours, a daily search for and removal of ticks is helpful in endemic areas.[23] There is evidence that *B. afzelii* may be transmitted more quickly than *B. burgdorferi* sensu stricto,[218] and there are reports of more rapid transmission in a few cases.[219] Ticks should be grasped with tweezers or fingernails as close to their point of attachment as possible and pulled steadily away from the skin to allow the tick to detach its mouth parts.[23] Mouth parts that remain in the skin do not pose a risk for further transmission of *B. burgdorferi* but may lead to a superficial bacterial infection. The site of the tick bite should be disinfected after the tick is removed. The removed tick should not be assessed for the presence of *B. burgdorferi* because the results of this test are of no therapeutic importance.[207] The use of prophylactic antibiotics after a tick bite is controversial. A single dose of 200 mg of doxycycline after *I. scapularis* bites was found to reduce the occurrence of erythema migrans.[220] Pooled data from four placebo-controlled trials suggest that in endemic areas of North America, one case of Lyme disease may be prevented for every 50 patients treated with antibiotics.[221] However, most tick bites remain unnoticed, and in most geographical areas, the frequency of antibiotic side effects exceeds the estimate of preventable disease manifestations. Failures of prophylactic treatment also have been described.[222,223] In the future the use of azithromycin cream might become available for prophylaxis at the site of a tick bite. This has been successful in mice[224]; human data are pending. Prompt antibiotic treatment of the early manifestations of Lyme disease usually prevents late manifestations such as arthritis.

Immunization

Two human vaccines have been developed with a recombinant fragment of OspA of *B. burgdorferi* sensu stricto. These vaccines were first evaluated in North American adults and were found to be safe. After three injections, vaccine efficacy in adults was 76% to 92%.[223,225] One of these vaccines was safe and efficacious in North American children,[226] and recommendations for the use of the vaccine were published.[227] However, these vaccines were never intended for use in Europe or Asia because of the greater strain variation on these continents. The only licensed vaccine was withdrawn from the American market due to economic reasons in 2002. A study of patients with a new onset of arthritis following Lyme disease vaccination found no evidence for an unusual OspA response or a more common occurrence of HLA alleles associated with treatment-resistant Lyme arthritis as compared with vaccinated and healthy controls.[228] A novel multivalent OspA vaccine potentially protecting against different *B. burgdorferi* species has been developed and successfully gone through phase I and II studies.[229]

COURSE OF THE DISEASE AND PROGNOSIS

The prognosis for children with erythema migrans or early neuroborreliosis is excellent when the disease has been promptly treated with appropriate antibiotics.[199,230-233] Even in children with Lyme arthritis who have not been treated, manifestations usually diminish and eventually disappear over time.[117] Among 90 children with Lyme arthritis treated with appropriate antibiotics, four had ongoing musculoskeletal complaints 7 years later.[100] Of 51 German children with Lyme arthritis examined 1 year after initiation of antibiotic treatment, 8 patients had chronic arthritis, and 4 had persistent arthralgias in joints previously affected by arthritis.[197] Of 99 children with Lyme arthritis, 76 responded fully to antibiotics.[233] Among the 23 who initially did not, spontaneous improvement occurred in 3, and successful treatment was possible with nonsteroidal antiinflammatory drugs in 6, intraarticular steroids in 4 or disease-modifying antirheumatic drugs in 5 patients. Another 5 patients were lost to follow-up, but none of the 94 patients with available follow-up data developed long-term arthritis.[234] Similarly, of 31 children with Lyme arthritis, 23 (74%) showed complete resolution of arthritis after one or two courses of antibiotics.[235] In rare cases, flares of arthritis in a previously affected joint have been observed several years after antibiotic treatment and the initial disappearance of arthritis. Among 94 children with Lyme arthritis, 39% had resolution of arthritis longer than 6 months after beginning antibiotic therapy, and 13% had resolution after more than 12 months.[236] In these studies, no clinical or laboratory feature could be identified to distinguish antibiotic-responsive patients from those with longer disease duration.

Erosion of cartilage is rare in children. Arthralgia in joints previously affected by arthritis may persist for several months, but children generally do not fulfill diagnostic criteria for fibromyalgia, and arthralgias usually do not restrict the physical or educational performance of adolescents. Late neurological complications have been described in untreated children with Lyme arthritis[117] but have not been observed after appropriate treatment.[237] However, transient neurocognitive abnormalities may occur.[90] Late development of keratitis has occurred in treated and in untreated children.[117] Lyme disease is not fatal in children, and in adults, reported deaths have been extremely rare.[238] Lyme disease rarely results in significant persistent organ damage, but coinfection with tick-borne encephalitis virus or with *Ehrlichia* or *Babesia* organisms may lead to a more severe disease course.[25,26,27]

A follow-up study of American adult patients found more musculoskeletal disease and verbal memory impairment in patients than in control groups.[239] An antibiotic-refractory course of Lyme arthritis in American adults has been associated with the DRB1*0401 and DRB1*0101 alleles[75,76] and the presence of antibodies to OspA. The risk of treatment failure seems to increase with increasing age and when intraarticular steroids were given before antibiotics.[184,197]

Up to 15% of patients with documented Lyme disease may continue to experience ongoing complaints after appropriate antibiotic therapy. This has been referred to as *post-Lyme syndrome* or later as one group of patients with "chronic Lyme disease."[182] Symptoms are similar to fibromyalgia, with fatigue, musculoskeletal pain, headache, and cognitive decline prominent. These complaints are usually self-limited, and respond to symptomatic therapies. For this group of patients, several well-conducted trials have shown that prolonged antibiotics are no more effective than placebo.[213]

Szer and colleagues[117] studied 46 American children (25 boys) with chronic Lyme arthritis with onset of disease between 1976 and 1979. None had been treated with antibiotics for the first 4 years of the disease. Almost all (98%) had arthralgias during the early phase, with a median time from disease onset to development of arthritis of 3 months (range, 2 to 24 months). The number of children with recurrent episodes declined each year. Older children tended to have arthritis of longer duration. At the end of the study, 12 children (31%) still had occasional brief episodes of joint pain. One child had marked fatigue, and two developed keratitis. All 46 children had persistently positive IgG antibody responses. IgM responses were more frequent, and IgG titers were higher in children with recurrent symptoms than in those who became asymptomatic.

REFERENCES

1. A.C. Steere, S.E. Malawista, D.R. Snydman, et al., Lyme arthritis. An epidemic of oligoarticular arthritis in children and adults in three Connecticut communities, Arthritis Rheum. 20 (1977) 7–17.
2. W. Burgdorfer, A.G. Barbour, S.F. Hayes, et al., Lyme disease—a tick-borne spirochetosis? Science 216 (1982) 1317–1319.
3. A.C. Steere, R.L. Grodzicki, A.N. Kornblatt, et al., The spirochetal etiology of Lyme disease, N. Engl. J. Med. 308 (1983) 733–740.
4. G. Stanek, G.P. Wormser, J. Gray, F. Strle, Lyme borreliosis, Lancet 379 (2011) 461–473.
5. A.C. Steere, Lyme disease, N. Engl. J. Med. 345 (2001) 115–125.
6. F. Dressler, P. Irigoyen, N. Ilowite, H.I. Huppertz, Lyme arthritis, in: S.K. Sood (Ed.), Lyme Borreliosis in Europe and North America: Epidemiology and Clinical Practice, John Wiley & Sons, Hoboken, NJ, 2011.
14. Centers for Disease Control and Prevention, Lyme Disease Data. <www.cdc.gov/lyme/stats> (accessed October 15, 2013).
18. H.I. Huppertz, M. Böhme, S.M. Standaert, et al., Incidence of Lyme borreliosis in the Würzburg region of Germany, Eur. J. Clin. Microbiol. Infect. Dis. 18 (1999) 697–703.

20. H.I. Huppertz, H. Karch, H.J. Suschke, et al., Lyme arthritis in European children and adolescents, Arthritis Rheum. 38 (1995) 361–368.
28. G.P. Wormser, M.E. Aguero-Rosenfeld, M.E. Cox, et al., Differences and similarities between culture-confirmed human granulocytic anaplasmosis and early Lyme disease, J. Clin. Microbiol. 51 (2013) 954–958.
32. A.G. Barbour, S.F. Hayes, Biology of Borrelia species, Microbiol. Rev. 50 (1986) 381–400.
47. M.U. Norman, T.J. Moriarty, A.R. Dresser, et al., Molecular mechanisms involved in vascular interactions of the Lyme disease pathogen in a living host, PLoS Pathog. 4 (10) (2008) e1000169.
50. H.J. Girschick, H.I. Huppertz, H. Rüssmann, et al., Intracellular persistence of Borrelia burgdorferi in human synovial cells, Rheumatol. Int. 16 (1996) 125–132.
51. A.C. Steere, L. Glickstein, Elucidation of Lyme arthritis, Nat. Rev. Immunol. 4 (2004) 143.
58. N.K. Vudattu, K. Strle, A.C. Steere, E.E. Drouin, Dysregulation of CD4+ CD25high T cells in the synovial fluid of patients with antibiotic-refractory Lyme arthritis, Arthritis Rheum. 65 (2013) 1643–1653.
79. D.T. Nardelli, S.M. Callister, R.F. Schell, Lyme arthritis: current concepts and a change in paradigm, Clin. Vaccine Immunol. 15 (2008) 21–34.
86. H.J. Christen, F. Hanefeld, H. Eiffert, et al., Epidemiology and clinical manifestations of Lyme borreliosis in childhood. A prospective multicentre study with special regard to neuroborreliosis, Acta Paediatr. Suppl. 386 (1993) 1–75.
100. M.A. Gerber, L.S. Zemel, E.D. Shapiro, Lyme arthritis in children: clinical epidemiology and long-term outcomes, Pediatrics 102 (1998) 905–908.
104. H.I. Huppertz, H. Michels, Pattern of joint involvement in children with Lyme arthritis, Br. J. Rheumatol. 35 (1996) 1016–1018.
105. H.I. Huppertz, D. Münchmeier, W. Lieb, Ocular manifestations in children and adolescents with Lyme arthritis, Br. J. Ophthalmol. 83 (1999) 1149–1152.
106. A. Thompson, R. Mannix, R. Bachur, Acute pediatric monoarticular arthritis: distinguishing lyme arthritis from other etiologies, Pediatrics 123 (2009) 959.
115. Centers for Disease Control and Prevention (CDC), Three sudden cardiac deaths associated with Lyme carditis—United States, November 2012-July 2013, MMWR Morb. Mortal. Wkly Rep. 62 (2013) 993–996.
116. T.M. Aaberg, The expanding ophthalmologic spectrum of Lyme disease, Am. J. Ophthalmol. 107 (1989) 77–80.
119. K. Weber, H.J. Bratzke, U. Neubert, et al., Borrelia burgdorferi in a newborn despite oral penicillin for Lyme borreliosis during pregnancy, Pediatr. Infect. Dis. J. 7 (1988) 286–289.
134. L.H. Sigal, Pitfalls in the diagnosis and management of Lyme disease, Arthritis Rheum. 41 (1998) 195–204.
135. M. Karlsson, K. Hovind-Hougen, B. Svenungsson, et al., Cultivation and characterization of spirochetes from cerebrospinal fluid of patients with Lyme borreliosis, J. Clin. Microbiol. 28 (1990) 473–479.
136. J.J. Nocton, F. Dressler, B.J. Rutledge, et al., Detection of Borrelia burgdorferi DNA by polymerase chain reaction in synovial fluid from patients with Lyme arthritis, N. Engl. J. Med. 330 (1994) 229–234.
138. S. Priem, M.G. Rittig, T. Kamradt, et al., An optimized PCR leads to rapid and highly sensitive detection of Borrelia burgdorferi in patients with Lyme borreliosis, J. Clin. Microbiol. 35 (1997) 685–690.
143. X. Li, G.A. McHugh, N. Damle, et al., Burden and viability of Borrelia burgdorferi in skin and joints of patients with erythema migrans or Lyme arthritis, Arthritis Rheum. 63 (2011) 2238–2247.
148. S.M. Engstrom, E. Shoop, R.C. Johnson, Immunoblot interpretation criteria for serodiagnosis of early Lyme disease, J. Clin. Microbiol. 33 (1995) 419–427.
149. U. Hauser, G. Lehnert, R. Lobentanzer, et al., Interpretation criteria for standardized Western blots for three European species of Borrelia burgdorferi sensu lato, J. Clin. Microbiol. 35 (1997) 1433–1444.
150. U. Hauser, G. Lehnert, B. Wilkske, Validity of interpretation criteria for standardized Western blots (immunoblots) for serodiagnosis of Lyme borreliosis based on sera collected throughout Europe, J. Clin. Microbiol. 37 (1999) 2241–2247.
151. R.M. Bacon, B.J. Biggerstaff, M.E. Schriefer, et al., Serodiagnosis of Lyme disease by kinetic enzyme-linked immunosorbent assay using recombinant vlsE1 or peptide antigens of Borrelia burgdorferi compared with 2-tiered testing using whole cell lysates, J. Infect. Dis. 187 (2003) 1187–1199.
152. G.P. Wormser, M. Schriefer, M.E. Aguero-Rosenfeld, et al., Single-tier testing with the C6 peptide ELISA kit compared with two-tier testing for Lyme disease, Diagn. Microbiol. Infect. Dis. 75 (2013) 9–15.
153. G.P. Wormser, A. Levin, S. Soman, et al., Comparative cost-effectiveness of two-tiered testing strategies for serodiagnosis of Lyme disease with noncutaneous manifestations, J. Clin. Microbiol. 51 (2013) 4045–4049.
156. A.C. Steere, G. McHugh, N. Damle, V.K. Sikand, Prospective study of serologic tests for Lyme disease, Clin. Infect. Dis. 47 (2008) 188–195.
157. J.A. Branda, M.E. Aguero-Rosenfeld, M.J. Ferraro, et al., 2-tiered antibody testing for early and late Lyme disease using only an immunoglobulin G blot with the addition of a VlsE band as the second-tier test, Clin. Infect. Dis. 50 (2010) 20–26.
158. J.A. Branda, F. Strle, K. Strle, et al., Performance of United States serologic assays in the diagnosis of Lyme borreliosis acquired in Europe, Clin. Infect. Dis. 57 (2013) 333–340.
159. G.P. Wormser, A.T. Tang, N.R. Schimmoeller, et al., Utility of serodiagnostics designed for use in the United States for detection of Lyme borreliosis acquired in Europe and vice versa, Med. Microbiol. Immunol. 203 (2014) 65–71.
161. V.P. Berardi, K.E. Weeks, A.C. Steere, Serodiagnosis of early Lyme disease: analysis of IgM and IgG antibody responses by using an antibody-capture enzyme immunoassay, J. Infect. Dis. 158 (1988) 754–760.
167. J. Yazdany, G. Schmajuk, M. Robbins, et al., Choosing wisely: the American College of Rheumatology's Top 5 list of things physicians and patients should question, Arthritis Care Res. (Hoboken) 65 (2013) 329–339.
168. S.S. Barclay, M.T. Melia, P.G. Auwaerter, Misdiagnosis of late-onset Lyme arthritis by inappropriate use of Borrelia burgdorferi immunoblot testing with synovial fluid, Clin. Vaccine Immunol. 10 (2012) 1806–1809.
170. J.J. Halperin, P. Baker, G.P. Wormser, Common misconceptions about Lyme disease, Am. J. Med. 126 (2013) 264.e1–264.e7.
171. M. Wharton, T.L. Chorba, R.L. Vogt, et al., Case definitions for public health surveillance, MMWR Recomm. Rep. 39 (RR–13) (1990) 1–43.
172. M. Böhme, S. Schweneke, E. Fuchs, et al., Screening of blood donors and recipients for Borrelia burgdorferi antibodies: no evidence of B. burgdorferi infection transmitted by transfusion, Infusionsther. Transfusionsmed. 19 (1992) 204–207.
173. B.H. Skogman, C. Ekerfelt, J. Ludvigsson, P. Forsberg, Seroprevalemce of Borrelia IgG antibodies among young Swedish children in relation to reported tick bites, symptoms and previous treatment for Lyme borreliosis: a population-based survey, Arch. Dis. Child. 95 (2010) 1013–1016.
174. M. Dehnert, V. Fingerle, C. Klier, et al., Seropositivity of Lyme borreliosis and associated risk factors: a population-based study in children and adolescents in Germany (KiGGS), PLoS ONE 7 (2012) e41321.
175. A. Lakos, Z. Igari, N. Solymosi, Recent lesson from a clinical and seroepidemiological survey: low positive predictive value of Borrelia burgdorferi antibody testing in a high risk population, Adv. Med. Sci. 57 (2012) 356–363.
177. H.I. Huppertz, H. Karch, J. Heesemann, Diagnostic value of synovial fluid analysis in children with reactive arthritis, Rheumatol. Int. 15 (1995) 167–170.
179. I. Tjernberg, A.J. Henningsson, I. Eliasson, et al., Diagnostic performance of cerebrospinal fluid chemokine CXCL13 and antibodies to the C6-peptide in Lyme neuroborreliosis, J. Infect. 62 (2011) 149–158.
180. H. Sillanpää, B.H. Skogman, H. Sarvas, et al., Cerebrospinal fluid chemokine CXCL13 in the diagnosis of neuroborreliosis in children, Scand. J. Infect. Dis. 45 (2013) 526–530.
181. K.A. Cohn, A.D. Thompson, S.S. Shah, et al., Validation of a clinical prediction rule to distinguish Lyme meningitis from aseptic meningitis, Pediatrics 129 (2012) e46–e53.
183. R.J. Dattwyler, D.J. Volkman, S.M. Conaty, et al., Amoxicillin plus probenecid versus doxycycline for treatment of erythema migrans borreliosis, Lancet 336 (1990) 1404–1406.
186. H.W. Pfister, V. Preac-Mursic, B. Wilske, et al., Cefotaxime versus penicillin G for acute neurologic manifestations in Lyme borreliosis. A prospective randomized study, Arch. Neurol. 46 (1989) 1190–1194.

188. E.M. Massarotti, S.W. Luger, D.W. Rahn, et al., Treatment of early Lyme disease, Am. J. Med. 92 (1992) 396–403.

189. R.B. Nadelman, S.W. Luger, E. Frank, et al., Comparison of cefuroxime and doxycycline in the treatment of early Lyme disease, Ann. Intern. Med. 117 (1992) 273–280.

190. S.C. Eppes, J.A. Childs, Comparative study of cefuroxime axetil versus amoxicillin in children with early Lyme disease, Pediatrics 109 (2002) 1173–1177.

195. T. Nizič, E. Velikanje, E. Ružić-Sabljić, M. Arnež, Solitary erythema migrans in children: comparison of treatment with clarithromycin and amoxicillin, Wien. Klin. Wochenschr. 124 (2012) 427–433.

200. T.J. Kowalski, S. Tata, W. Berth, et al., Antibiotic treatment duration and long-term outcomes of patients with early Lyme disease from a Lyme disease-hyperendemic area, Clin. Infect. Dis. 50 (2010) 512–520.

204. R.T. Schoen, J.M. Aversa, D.W. Rahn, et al., Treatment of refractory chronic Lyme arthritis with arthroscopic synovectomy, Arthritis Rheum. 34 (1991) 1056–1060.

205. R. Gasser, I. Wendelin, E. Reisinger, et al., Roxithromycin in the treatment of Lyme disease-update and perspectives, Infection 23 (Suppl. 1) (1995) S39–S43.

206. A.C. Steere, S.M. Angelis, Therapy for Lyme arthritis—strategies for the treatment of antibiotic-refractory arthritis, Arthritis Rheum. 54 (2006) 3079–3086.

207. H.M. Feder Jr., B.J. Johnson, S. O'Connell, et al., A critical appraisal of "chronic Lyme disease", N. Engl. J. Med. 357 (2007) 1422–1430.

208. H.I. Huppertz, P. Bartmann, U. Heininger, et al., Rational diagnostic strategies for Lyme borreliosis in children and adolescents: recommendations by the Committee for Infectious Diseases and Vaccinations of the German Academy for Pediatrics and Adolescent Health, Eur. J. Pediatr. 171 (2012) 1619–1624.

209. M. Johnson, H.M. Feder Jr., Chronic Lyme disease: a survey of Connecticut primary care physicians, J. Pediatr. 157 (2010) 1025–1029.

210. J.D. Cooper, H.M. Feder Jr., Inaccurate information about Lyme disease on the internet, Pediatr. Infect. Dis. 23 (2004) 1105–1108.

211. P.G. Auwaerter, J.S. Bakken, R.J. Dattwyler, et al., Antiscience and ethical concerns associated with advocacy of Lyme disease, Lancet Infect. Dis. 11 (2011) 713–719.

212. A.L. Hassett, D.C. Radvanski, S. Buyske, et al., Role of psychiatric comorbidity in chronic Lyme disease, Arthritis Care Res. 59 (2008) 1742–1749.

213. M.S. Klempner, P.J. Baker, E.D. Shapiro, et al., Treatment trials for post-Lyme disease symptoms revisited, Am. J. Med. 126 (2013) 665–669.

215. E.B. Hayes, J. Piesman, How can we prevent Lyme disease? N. Engl. J. Med. 348 (2003) 2424–2430.

216. N.J. Miller, E.E. Rainone, M.C. Dyer, et al., Tick bite protection in permethrin-treated summer clothing, J. Med. Entomol. 48 (2011) 327–333.

217. E. Lupi, C. Hatz, P. Schlagenhaut, The efficacy of repellents against *Aedes, Anopheles, Culex* and *Ixodes* spp.—a literature review, Travel Med. Infect. Dis. 11 (2013) 374–411.

219. E.D. Hynote, P.C. Mervine, R.B. Stricker, Clinical evidence for rapid transmission of Lyme disease following a tickbite, Diagnostic Microbiol. Infect. Dis. 72 (2012) 188–192.

220. R.B. Nadelman, J. Nowakowski, D. Fish, et al., Prophylaxis with single-dose doxycycline for the prevention of Lyme disease after an *Ixodes scapularis* tick bite, N. Engl. J. Med. 345 (2001) 79–84.

221. S. Warshafsky, D.H. Lee, L.K. Francois, et al., Efficacy of antibiotic prophylaxis for the prevention of Lyme disease: an updated systematic review and meta-analysis, J. Antimicrob. Chemother. 65 (2010) 1137–1144.

224. J. Piesman, A. Hojgaard, A.J. Ullmann, M.C. Dolan, Efficacy of an experimental azithromycin cream for prophylaxis of tick-transmitted Lyme disease spirochete infection in a murine model, Antimicrob. Agents Chemother. 58 (2014) 348–351.

225. L.H. Sigal, J.M. Zahradnik, P. Lavin, et al., A vaccine consisting of recombinant Borrelia burgdorferi outer-surface protein A to prevent Lyme disease, N. Engl. J. Med. 339 (1998) 216–222.

226. H.M. Feder Jr., J. Beran, C. van Hoecke, et al., Immunogenicity of a recombinant Borrelia burgdorferi outer surface protein A vaccine against Lyme disease in children, J. Pediatr. 135 (1999) 575–579.

227. Advisory Committee on Immunization Practices (ACIP), Recommendations for the use of Lyme disease vaccine. MMWR Recomm. Rep. 48 (RR–7) (1999) 1–17, 21–25.

231. J.C. Salazar, M.A. Gerber, C.W. Goff, Long-term outcome of Lyme disease in children given early treatment, J. Pediatr. 122 (1993) 591–593.

234. H.O. Tory, D. Zurakowski, R.P. Sundel, Outcomes of children treated for Lyme arthritis: results of a large pediatric cohort, J. Rheumatol. 37 (2010) 1049–1055.

235. S. Nimmrich, I. Becker, G. Horneff, Intraarticular corticosteroids in refractory childhood Lyme arthritis, Rheumatol. Int. 34 (2014) 987–994.

238. K.J. Kugeler, K.S. Griffith, L.H. Gould, et al., A review of death certificates listing Lyme disease as a cause of death in the United States, Clin. Infect. Dis. 52 (2011) 364–367.

The entire reference list is available online at www.expertconsult.com.

CHAPTER 43

Reactive Arthritis

Rubén Burgos-Vargas, Janitzia Vázquez-Mellado

The reactive arthritides constitute a group of diverse inflammatory arthropathies in which the joint and extraarticular manifestations are caused by a preceding extraarticular infection with specific bacteria. This chapter reviews arthritis related to enteric or genitourinary bacterial infections. Rheumatic fever, caused by a pharyngeal infection with *Streptococcus*, is discussed in Chapter 44.

DEFINITION AND EVOLVING CONCEPT

In this chapter, use of the term *reactive arthritis* (ReA) is restricted to the arthritides triggered by enteric infections, with one of the so-called arthritogenic bacteria (*Yersinia, Salmonella, Shigella,* or *Campylobacter*) and genitourinary infections with *Chlamydia trachomatis*.[1-3] Although ReA has predominantly occurred in individuals who are human leukocyte antigen (HLA)-B27 positive, a significant proportion of patients are HLA-B27 negative.

The finding of viable *Chlamydia* within the joints of patients with ReA challenges the idea that ReA is a nonseptic arthritis and raises the possibility that it can be considered to be an infectious arthritis[4] or an infectious nonsuppurative arthritis. The current hypothetical relation between ReA, spondyloarthritis (SpA), and septic arthritis as result of *Chlamydia* arthritis according to Gracey and Inman[5] is shown in Fig. 43-1. The triad of arthritis, conjunctivitis, and urethritis (or cervicitis) was called *Reiter's syndrome* in the past; currently the triad is still being recognized, but the eponym has been deleted from contemporary literature.

CLASSIFICATION AND DIAGNOSTIC CRITERIA

The diagnosis of ReA is a clinical challenge because it requires the demonstration of an infection preceding the appearance of arthritis. Diagnosis is currently based on the presence of lower limb, asymmetrical oligoarthritis, and clinical or laboratory evidence of a preceding infection. In 1995, a proposal for diagnostic criteria was developed in an expert's meeting in Berlin[6] (Boxes 43-1 and 43-2). Based on existing definitions and diagnostic criteria, Pacheco-Tena and colleagues[7] proposed alternative classification criteria. A preceding bacterial infection is most frequently documented serologically, but its actual value is still controversial.[8] In general, the value of diagnostic tests depends on the pretest probability of the diagnosis.[9]

EPIDEMIOLOGY

There appears to be a progressive decline in the number of publications dealing with ReA, perhaps reflecting a decreasing frequency of the disease. The prevalence of ReA appears related to that of HLA-B27 and probably to the rate of infections by arthritogenic bacteria in the general population.[10] However, ReA may occur in HLA-B27–negative patients, including the majority of those reported in series of arthritis triggered by *Salmonella* and *Yersinia*.

The frequency of arthritis following infection with arthritogenic organisms varies widely. In adults, rates of ReA following *Salmonella* infection ranged from 3.2%[3] and 4.4%[11] to 43%.[12] In a *Salmonella* outbreak in Germany,[13] no cases of ReA occurred among 286 infected children, although 6 children had brief arthralgia. In contrast, 20% of 207 children reported joint, eye, or mucocutaneous symptoms after an outbreak of *Salmonella typhimurium* phage type 135a in Australia.[12] ReA develops in 5% to 10% of children with *Yersinia*.[14,15] ReA occurred in 43% of adults infected; the role of HLA-B27 was considered to be of minor relevance. A foodborne outbreak of *Yersinia Pseudotuberculosis* O:1 led to ReA in 22% of infected adults; 67% of those adults who were tissue typed had HLA-B27, but none of 12 infected children did.[16] However, 42% of the children had erythema nodosum. In studies summarized by Keat,[3] ReA was estimated to occur in 1% of patients with sexually acquired infections. Recent studies suggest that the prevalence of *Chlamydia*-related ReA is underestimated and that it is the most common of the arthritogenic bacteria-related arthritides.[17] Keat reported that 2.4% of those with either *Shigella* or *Campylobacter* infections developed ReA. ReA has been also linked to *Mycoplasma*[18] and *Chlamydia pneumoniae*, which was responsible for approximately 10% of cases of ReA in a Finnish study.[19] HLA-B27 ReA has also been associated with *Clostridium difficile*.[20,21]

The relative frequency of ReA among patients in pediatric rheumatology clinics in the United States,[22,23] United Kingdom,[24] and Canada[25] ranged between 4.1% and 8.6%. This wide variation is consistent with differences in the stringency of diagnostic and classification criteria used in each study. Despite reports from other sources suggesting an increase in the recognition of ReA,[26-32] that does not seem to be the case today. Most cases of ReA occur in boys between the ages of 8 and 12 years, but sex and age distribution vary according to the causative organism. In an Italian study of children with *Yersinia*-triggered ReA, most cases occurred between the ages of 3 and 7 years, and there was a slight predominance of females.[31] Enteric infections are responsible for ReA at all ages, but ReA following genital infections with *Chlamydia* occurs more frequently during adolescence and in adults.

GENETIC BACKGROUND

Although the susceptibility to the primary infection is not related to any known genetic marker, it is considered that ReA occurs most frequently in individuals with HLA-B27. Moreover, the severity of joint pain after intestinal infections by *Salmonella, Shigella,* and *Yersinia* may

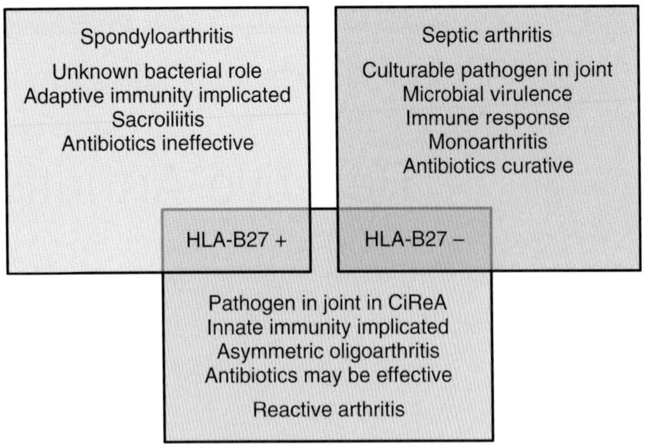

FIGURE 43-1 The relationship between spondyloarthritis, reactive arthritis, and septic arthritis. Reactive arthritis shares clinical and immunopathogenic features with both spondyloarthritis, of which it is considered a subset, and septic arthritis. Enteric-pathogen-associated reactive arthritis better represents spondyloarthritis, whereas Chlamydia-associated reactive arthritis represents a noncanonical septic arthritis. *CiRea, Chlamydia*-induced reactive arthritis. (Modified from Ref. 5, with permission from Nature Publishing Group.)

BOX 43-1 The Berlin Diagnostic Criteria for Reactive Arthritis

Typical Peripheral Arthritis
Predominantly lower limb, asymmetric oligoarthritis
Plus
Evidence of Preceding Infection
If there is a clear history of diarrhea or urethritis within the preceding 4 weeks, laboratory confirmation is desirable but not essential.
Where no clear clinical infection is identified, laboratory confirmation of infection is essential.
Exclusion Criteria
Patients with other known causes of monoarthritis or oligoarthritis (such as other defined spondyloarthropathies, septic arthritis, crystal arthritis, Lyme disease, and streptococcal reactive arthritis) should be excluded.

Modified from Ref. 6, with permission from the BMJ Publishing Group.

BOX 43-2 Laboratory Tests for Documenting Preceding Infection in Reactive Arthritis

Routine
Culture of stool and urethra
Serology: antibodies against specific arthritogenic bacteria
Research Studies
Urethral swab for detection of chlamydial DNA by polymerase chain reaction (PCR)*
Synovial fluid or synovial membrane biopsy for detection of bacterial DNA by PCR*
Immunofluorescence microscopy for detection of bacteria in synovial biopsy specimen†
Stimulation of synovial fluid lymphocytes with antigens from arthritogenic bacteria†

*A potential diagnostic test.
†Research tools, not suitable for routine diagnostic use.
Modified from Ref. 6, with permission from the BMJ Publishing Group.

ETIOLOGY AND PATHOGENESIS

Arthritogenic Bacteria

Several bacteria are involved in the etiology of ReA. In preadolescent patients, *Salmonella, Shigella, Yersinia,* or *Campylobacter* enteric infections precede the onset of arthritis in 80% of instances. *Shigella flexneri,*[41-45] *Yersinia enterocolitica,*[45] and *Salmonella enteritidis*[46] have all been isolated from children with the postdysenteric ReA conjunctivitis and urethritis triad. In at least two youths and three children, *Chlamydia trachomatis*[47] was identified in synovial fluid. Respiratory tract infection with *Mycoplasma pneumoniae*[18,48] has been associated with ReA in a few children.

Role of HLA-B27

The role of HLA-B27 in the pathogenesis of ReA is still unknown.[49] The arthritogenic peptide hypothesis[49-52] postulates that the HLA-B27 molecule is able to bind a unique bacterial or self-antigenic peptide (not yet identified, but supposedly present in the joints), which is then presented to an HLA-B27–restricted cytotoxic (CD8[+]) T cell.[53,54] CD8[+] T cells' cross-reaction with bacterial epitopes may then lead to inflammation and tissue damage. Several bacterial amino acid sequences homologous to HLA-B27 amino acid sequences have been described.[55-61] Most recently, analysis of the HLA-B*2705 peptidome identified a number of peptides derived from various sources, mainly cartilage or bone-related proteins such as osteoprotegerin, annexin 2, chondrocyte-derived metalloproteinase, and proteoglycans, which share certain homologies with human HLA-B27.

Three of the peptides related to cartilage or bone shared 6-8 amino acids with amino acid sequences from arthritogenic bacteria.[62]

Equally relevant is the B27 misfolding hypothesis, which refers to the accumulation of misfolded heavy chains of HLA-B27 in the endoplasmic reticulum mediated by the E3 ubiquitin ligase HRD1 (SYVN1) and the ubiquitin conjugating enzyme UBE2JL.[63,64] Endoplasmic reticulum (ER) stress signaling pathways may be activated by HLA-B27 upregulation and misfolded heavy chains.[63,64] Misfolding leads then to the activation of nuclear factor-κB and proinflammatory cytokines.[65] The HLA-B27–free heavy chain and homodimer hypothesis refers to abnormal B27 molecule folding and the formation of HLA-B27 homodimers.[66] Such homodimers may turn into receptors for humoral

---

be associated with the presence of HLA-B27.[33] Nonetheless, the frequency of HLA-B27 in children with ReA varies widely; in children with mild forms of *Yersinia-, Campylobacter-, Chlamydia-,* and *Mycoplasma pneumoniae*–related ReA, the frequency of HLA-B27 is similar to that of the population.[9,18,34]

Other associations have been reported in specific populations. An association with the tumor necrosis factor (TNF) c1 allele independent of B27 was reported in a predominantly adult Finnish population with ReA.[35] In a similar population, TAP2J, a polymorphism of transporters associated with antigen processing (TAP2), was more frequent in B27-positive patients with ReA.[36] An association between the Toll-like receptor 2 and ReA has been described after an outbreak of *S. enteritidis* in Canada.[37] Single nucleotide polymorphisms in the interferon (IFN)-γ gene (rs2430561 and rs1861493) appear to predispose the Dutch to ReA,[38] and solute carrier family 11 member A1 gene polymorphisms are increased in the Chinese.[39] In contrast, the chemokine receptor-5 (CCR5)-delta 32 mutation does not play a role in the susceptibility to ReA in patients with *Chlamydia trachomatis* infection.[40]

or cell-mediated responses mediated by class I HLA molecules or as proinflammatory targets, which lead to excessive cytokine production.[67-69] The deposition of β2 microglobulin in the synovium, and perhaps other tissues, induces inflammation.[70]

HLA-B27 modulates the production of cytokines and influences both bacterial invasion of cells and killing of bacteria.[71-80] As a result, intracellular survival of arthritogenic bacteria is prolonged. Arthritogenic bacteria invade the gut mucosa and replicate within polymorphonuclear cells and macrophages. Studies in murine fibroblasts transfected with B27, not replicated in human cells, indicated that the expression of this antigen inhibited cell invasion by arthritogenic bacteria.[71-80] Persistence of the organism within B27 cells was prolonged.[80,81] Various bacterial components (including lipopolysaccharide, DNA, and RNA) have been identified in both synovial fluid cells and synovial membranes of patients with ReA.[82-91] Regarding *Chlamydia*, a microorganism with both intracellular and extracellular life cycles, there is now clear evidence it may turn into a nonreplicative, nonculturable, but viable state within the cell.[4,5,92] In this sense, it is now possible to consider that *Chlamydia* ReA may actually be a form of septic arthritis.[4,5]

The antibody response against arthritogenic bacteria in ReA lasts longer than in infected patients who do not develop arthritis. Nevertheless, the role of antibodies in the pathogenesis of ReA is probably minimal. Additional findings suggest a role for heat-shock proteins[93,94] and bacterial peptidoglycan in the pathogenesis of ReA.[95]

CLINICAL MANIFESTATIONS

The course and severity of ReA vary considerably. Symptoms of infection usually precede the onset of arthritis, enthesitis, or extraarticular disease by 1 to 4 weeks. After an active period of weeks to months, the arthritis subsides and the patient then enters a sustained remission or a phase of recurrent disease activity, which may evolve into enthesitis-related arthritis or SpA, including ankylosing spondylitis.

Characteristics of the Primary Infection

An appreciation of the characteristics of the enteric or genitourinary infections, which trigger ReA, could possibly aid in the identification of the bacteria involved in the pathogenesis of the disease.

Shigella Enteritis

A period of high fever, with or without watery diarrhea, and cramping abdominal pain lasting 48 to 72 hours, may be followed in 7 to 21 days by the sudden onset of nonmigratory oligoarthritis (knees and ankles) lasting from several weeks to 3 or 4 months. Diagnosis requires a history, the presence of agglutinins to *Shigella flexneri* serotype 2 or 2a, and an attempt to isolate the organism from the stool. Because of the long interval between the diarrhea and the joint complaints, blood cultures are positive in less than 4% of patients.

Salmonella Infection

The acute onset of oligoarthritis, mostly in the knees and ankles, may follow an enteric infection with *Salmonella typhimurium* or *Salmonella enteritidis* by 1 to 3 weeks.[96,97] The enteric infection may be mild, but the onset of arthritis is usually accompanied by low-grade fever. Because *Salmonella* infection can also result in osteomyelitis and septic arthritis, it is important to make certain that the synovial fluid is sterile. The erythrocyte sedimentation rate (ESR) is usually elevated, and the leukopenia that may accompany the acute infection is generally followed by leukocytosis. Stool cultures are usually positive, even late in the disease course, but seroconversion to *Salmonella* H and O antigens occurs in only 50% of patients.

Yersinia Infection

ReA triggered by *Yersinia* may affect some children.[31,45,98] The interval between infection and onset of arthritis in 18 children with *Yersinia*-triggered ReA[31] was 7 to 30 days. The diarrhea preceding ReA was notably very mild, much more so than in the usual *Yersinia* enterocolitis. Contact with the organism is through infected drinking water or milk. *Yersinia enterocolitica* causes gastroenteritis in young children and a syndrome of abdominal pain similar to that of appendicitis in older children. In a study of children hospitalized because of *Yersinia* infection, 35% had arthritis lasting 3 to 22 months (average, 6.5 months).[15] Of those with arthritis, 85% had HLA-B27. *Yersinia* can occasionally cause septic arthritis.

Campylobacter Infection

In an epidemic outbreak of *Campylobacter jejuni* enteritis in Finland, 2.6% of patients—all adults—developed oligoarthritis or polyarthritis 4 days to 4 weeks after infection. Synovial fluid cultures were negative, and 33% of the patients with arthritis were positive for HLA-B27.[99]

Chlamydia Infection

Genitourinary tract infection with *Chlamydia trachomatis* is often asymptomatic but may cause dysuria, frequency, and a urethral or vaginal discharge. ReA may also be related to upper respiratory tract infections with *Chlamydia pneumoniae*.[19] Artamonov and colleagues[100] found evidence of nasopharyngeal infection in 45 of 52 children with ReA. Although the prevalence of HLA-B27 was higher than that in the control population (relative risk, 2.5), it was much lower than that in those who developed ReA after intestinal infection. *Chlamydia* infection is increasingly recognized in teenagers, and particularly in young adults.

Musculoskeletal Disease

Acute arthritis with marked pain and sometimes erythema over the affected joints is characteristic of ReA, but some children show only slight to moderate joint pain and swelling over several weeks.[15,31,45,47,97-106] Enthesitis may occur alone or with arthritis, tenosynovitis, or bursitis (Figs. 43-2 and 43-3). In other children, arthralgias appear before the onset of arthritis for a variable amount of time. The initial episode of arthritis usually affects the knees or ankles. The pattern of arthritis in the metatarsophalangeal (MTP) joints and the proximal and distal interphalangeal (IP) joints of the feet may be that of a dactylitis and may involve two or three joints in one or more digits in combination with tenosynovitis and bursitis. Arthritis of the small joints of the hands caused by *Yersinia* and *Salmonella* has also been described in ReA.[15,31,45,47,96-100]

The synovial fluid effusion is usually marked, but proliferative synovitis is uncommon. In addition to involvement of peripheral joints and entheses, there may be inflammation of joints of the axial skeleton resulting in spinal and sacroiliac pain, stiffness, and reduced mobility of the lumbar and cervical spine.

In a study of 11 children with ReA followed for 0.9 to 6.7 years, Hussein[101] observed recurrent episodes of arthritis in most patients: 4 children had severe arthritis, 5 had sacroiliitis, but none had significant disability. Cuttica and colleagues[102] found that, at a mean follow-up of 28.6 months, 18 of 26 children with the triad of arthritis, conjunctivitis, and urethritis developed oligoarthritis, 7 developed polyarthritis, and 1 developed monoarthritis, with axial symptoms in 6. Five patients followed for around 7 years developed radiographic sacroiliitis. Symptoms remitted in most patients, but some had either a sustained or a fluctuating course. In a group of nine Greek children with *Salmonella*-triggered ReA, disease was active at 4 to 13 months, and there were one

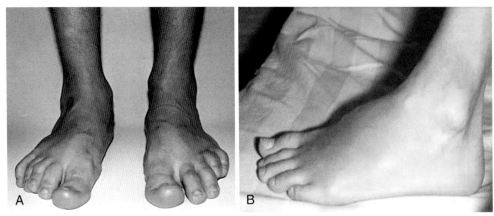

FIGURE 43-2 A, There is slight swelling of the midfoot and dactylitis involving the second right toe and the fourth and fifth left toes in an adolescent with *Salmonella*-triggered reactive arthritis of 6 months' duration. **B,** The foot of a teenage girl with post-*Yersinia* reactive arthritis showing swelling and erythema of the dorsum of the foot.

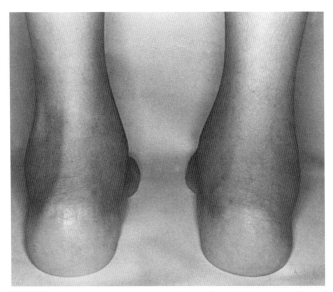

FIGURE 43-3 Achilles tendinitis and swelling of the retrocalcaneal bursa of the right foot of a patient with ReA.

to four recurrences in four patients during a period of 48 to 78 months, but there were no axial symptoms.[97]

Constitutional Signs and Symptoms

Apart from the infection itself, children with ReA may continue to have fever, weight loss, fatigue, and muscle weakness during active periods of disease.[103,104] Polyarthralgia, muscle pain, and joint stiffness affecting peripheral joints and the axial skeleton sometimes accompany these symptoms. Myocarditis and pericarditis have been described during the active phase of the disease in children with *Salmonella enteritidis*-triggered ReA.[105]

Mucocutaneous and Ocular Disease

Painless, shallow ulcers of the oral mucosa and palate are common and often asymptomatic. Aphthous stomatitis occurs in some patients. Urethritis and cervicitis are rare manifestations, occurring more frequently in adolescents with sexually acquired ReA caused by *Chlamydia*. These conditions are often mild, and girls tend to have no

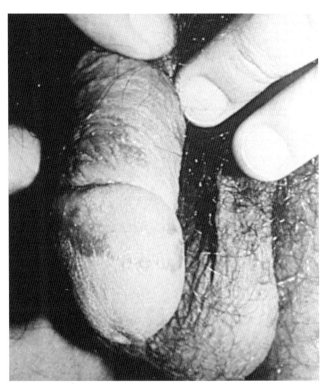

FIGURE 43-4 Circinate balanitis in an adolescent with *Chlamydia*-triggered reactive arthritis. The shallow ulcers on the glans penis are usually painless.

symptoms; they are detected only because of the presence of sterile pyuria. Diarrhea occurs in association with bacterial infection but may also be part of a generalized episode of mucositis.

Skin lesions in ReA include erythema nodosum in some children with *Yersinia*-triggered ReA, circinate balanitis (Fig. 43-4), and keratoderma blennorrhagicum (Fig. 43-5), with or without conjunctivitis or urethritis.[9,47,99,106] Keratoderma may be clinically and histologically indistinguishable from psoriasis. Mucocutaneous involvement in ReA tends to parallel disease activity in the peripheral joints.

Conjunctivitis occurs in about two thirds of children at onset. In *Yersinia*-triggered ReA, conjunctivitis may be purulent and severe.[100,107]

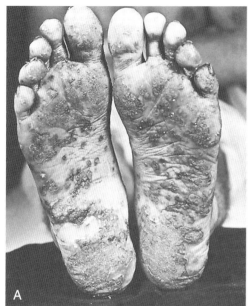
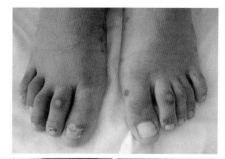
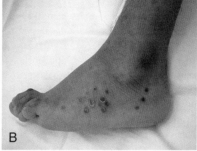
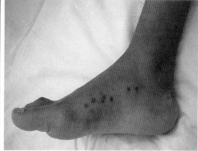

FIGURE 43-5 Keratoderma blennorrhagicum. **A,** This scaly eruption on the soles of the feet of an 18-year-old youth with reactive arthritis is difficult to distinguish from psoriasis. **B,** Dorsal, lateral, and medial aspects of the feet of a 16-year-old patient with chronic reactive arthritis. *Dorsal view:* While the third digit on the right foot shows some diffuse swelling and hyperpigmentation, the first toe looks more atrophic than its counterpart on the left foot. *Lateral view:* Midfoot and ankle swelling. *All views:* There is nail dystrophy of the first three digits in the right foot (clearly seen on the first toe) and multiple keratoderma blennorrhagic lesions. This patient had recurrent episodes of severe arthritis and enthesitis involving both feet but only recently skin lesions.

Acute iridocyclitis in these cases is characterized by flare and cells in the anterior chamber, small keratic precipitates, cells in the vitreous, and occasionally fibrinous exudates, posterior synechiae, and macular edema in a unilateral or bilateral pattern. Acute anterior uveitis has also been described in ReA triggered by *Salmonella typhimurium.*[101,108] Although there are few studies of the visual prognosis in children with ReA, the frequency of patients with permanent ocular sequelae appears to be low.

LABORATORY EXAMINATION

In the early inflammatory phase, there may be a slight decrease of hemoglobin and hematocrit, mild leukocytosis, and neutrophilia. The platelet count and serum levels of immunoglobulin M (IgM), IgG, and occasionally IgA may be elevated. The ESR and C-reactive protein (CRP) correlate with disease activity. In patients with severe disease—particularly in those with polyarthritis and polyenthesitis, fever, weight loss, fatigue, mucositis, or dermatitis—these laboratory abnormalities may be extreme. In particular, the hemoglobin concentration may fall to 8 to 10 g/dL, and the platelet count rise well above 400,000/mm³. The ESR and CRP values may remain elevated for a protracted period. Autoantibodies (e.g., rheumatoid factor, antinuclear antibodies) are usually absent. Synovial fluid analysis and culture helps to distinguish between ReA and septic arthritis.[109]

With the exception of epidemics and some isolated reports, the clinical and laboratory confirmations of infection as a trigger in children with ReA are seldom made. When available, cultures obtained at the time of the infection may be helpful. *Salmonella, Yersinia, Shigella,* and *Campylobacter* may be isolated from the gut during an episode of diarrhea, or *Chlamydia* may be cultured from the urethra, but negative results do not exclude the diagnosis of infection-related arthritis.

Because *Salmonella* and *Chlamydia* may also be present in asymptomatic carriers, these organisms can occasionally be cultured from patients who have arthritis not directly related to these organisms. Nonetheless, it is important to bear in mind that viable but nonculturable *Chlamydia* might be found in the joints of patients with arthritis. Electron microscopy, immunochemistry, and DNA studies might help in identifying extracellular elemental and intracellular replicative bodies and other constituents of *Chlamydia.*[82,86]

More frequently, ReA is diagnosed in the appropriate clinical setting because of the presence of high titers of serum antibodies against arthritogenic bacterial antigens.[4,5] Hemagglutination tests are useful in documenting recent infections with *Salmonella* or *Yersinia.*[15,31,45,47,97-100] Both the sensitivity and the specificity of circulating IgA and IgM antibodies to *Salmonella, Yersinia,* and *Campylobacter* detected by enzyme-linked immunoassay are acceptable, but results must be compared with those in the control population. IgG antibodies are useful if levels change significantly; a rising titer of IgA antibodies may be noted. Overall, the use of these types of tests and their interpretation are still somewhat controversial.[8]

Lymphoproliferation assays performed on cells from peripheral blood or synovial fluids also have some use as diagnostic tools.[6,8,9] Unfortunately, these tests are not easy to perform and often demonstrate nonspecific responses to several antigens.

Yersinia or *Chlamydia* antigens may be detected in intestinal or genital smears or biopsies. By using electron and immunofluorescence microscopy and immunohistochemistry, it has been possible to identify intraarticular chlamydial extracellular elemental bodies and intracellular replicative bodies,[81,84,85] *Yersinia* 60-kD heat-shock proteins and the urease β subunit,[85,86] and *Salmonella* lipopolysaccharide.[87] Likewise, bacterial DNA or RNA from several bacterial species, including *Chlamydia* sp., *Salmonella* sp., *Shigella* sp., and *Campylobacter* sp. has been identified in synovial fluid cells or the synovial membrane by PCR.[79-84] The role of these tests as diagnostic tools is restricted at present.

IMAGING STUDIES

Radiographic abnormalities early in the disease consist only of non-specific soft tissue swelling, juxtaarticular osteopenia, and (less frequently) slight periosteal irregularities at tendon attachments.[110] The occurrence of subchondral cysts; erosions; and sometimes extensive destruction of joints, such as the hips, proximal and distal IPs of the hands and feet, and less commonly, joints of the wrist indicate the severity of the synovitis that can occur in ReA. Ultrasonographic studies may delineate synovial sheath and tendon thickening and the accumulation of synovial fluid within the tendon sheath and bursae. Short tau inversion recovery (STIR) and T1 (with or with gadolinium or T2 fat-suppressed magnetic resonance imaging [MRI]) sequences may show bone edema, which is interpreted as inflammation, as well as synovitis, tenosynovitis, and bursitis. Various entheses, especially those at the attachment of the plantar fascia to the calcaneus, show erosions and marked bony proliferation and spur formation. These abnormalities may also be apparent in the navicular bone, greater trochanter, and ischium. Unilateral or bilateral subchondral cysts and bony erosions of the hip, metacarpophalangeal, MTP, and proximal IP joints of the hands and feet characterize more extensive and unremitting disease. An association between joint erosions and occult inflammation of the gut has been described in patients with ReA.[111] Symptomatic and radiographic involvement of the sacroiliac joint and spine are rare in children with ReA, but MRI of the sacroiliac joints may reveal acute and chronic changes.[112]

DIFFERENTIAL DIAGNOSIS

Differentiation of ReA from other types of arthritis is often difficult (Box 43-3). Reactive and infectious arthritides not associated with HLA-B27 have similar symptoms, although the primary site of infection is usually the upper airway. ReA is usually more painful and is associated with erythema of the overlying skin, a feature rarely seen in juvenile idiopathic arthritis (JIA). Specific clinical features, such as

---

BOX 43-3 Differential Diagnosis of Reactive Arthritis

Arthritis Related to Infection
Presumed viral arthritis (including transient synovitis of the hip)
Poststreptococcal arthritis (including rheumatic fever)
Lyme disease
Septic arthritis, tuberculosis, gonococcal arthropathy

Idiopathic Inflammatory Diseases
Juvenile idiopathic arthritis
Arthritis associated with Crohn's disease and ulcerative colitis
Synovitis, acne, pustulosis, hyperostosis, and osteomyelitis (SAPHO) syndrome
Behçet disease
Kawasaki disease

Orthopedic and Amplification Pain Syndromes
Legg–Calvé–Perthes disease, Osgood–Schlatter disease
"Growing pains"
Idiopathic pain syndromes (fibromyalgia, reflex sympathetic dystrophy)

---

rash, subcutaneous nodule, and lymphadenopathy, help differentiate diseases such as Kawasaki disease[113] and Lyme disease[114] from ReA. Early JIA and the arthritis of inflammatory bowel disease must also be considered. Laboratory test abnormalities, such as a positive synovial fluid culture or elevated antistreptolysin O titers suggest septic arthritis or rheumatic fever. The presence of elevated inflammatory indexes helps exclude orthopedic conditions.

TREATMENT

Disease activity, functional status, and quality of life should be evaluated in children with ReA. Although no specific instruments have been developed for this disease, the use of validated measures of health status designed for other chronic arthritides of childhood may be appropriate (Chapter 7).

There are no special nutritional recommendations for children with ReA. Any measure taken to avoid bacterial contamination of food, from slaughtering of the animals to refrigeration, cooking, and serving, is essential to avoid enteric infections. ReA is not only an epidemic disease but also endemic in some areas of the world. Programs that improve the sanitary conditions of the community to prevent the spread of infectious diseases are required. Counseling of the family about the risk of recurrences in case of enteric infections is advisable. This applies to adolescents with regard to the risk of sexually transmitted diseases.

Pharmacologic Therapy

The inflammatory manifestations of ReA require the administration of nonsteroidal antiinflammatory drugs (NSAIDs) in nearly all patients and glucocorticoids in some. The requirement for NSAIDs tends to be intermittent rather than constant. However, in patients in whom ReA becomes chronic, medications may include sulfasalazine. Except for the use of antibiotics in selected cases, there is no clear evidence that any drug alters the course of the disease.

Recommended doses and therapeutic regimens of NSAIDs in children with ReA are similar to those used in other forms of childhood arthritis. Because episodes of ReA tend to be self-limiting, lasting from 3 to 6 months, NSAIDs may be discontinued in many children with onset of a remission. Glucocorticoids may be required for children with severe and disabling polyarthritis and polyenthesitis. Enthesitis responds poorly and may require higher doses and longer courses of drug therapy than usual. Fever, fatigue, and anemia tend to disappear, and CRP and ESR levels tend to fall after several weeks of treatment. Glucocorticoid dose reduction and withdrawal in children with ReA are usually easily achieved.

The required doses of prednisone or prednisolone vary between 5 and 10 mg/day; doses of deflazacort vary between 6 and 24 mg/day. In certain patients, the intraarticular administration of triamcinolone hexacetonide or methylprednisolone and hydrocortisone produces rapid and sustained relief. There is no reported experience regarding the injection of synovial sheaths, bursae, or entheses in children with ReA. Injection of entheses may result in postinjection pain and local soft tissue calcification or atrophy.

Because of the possible occult nonspecific inflammation of the gut in patients with HLA-B27–associated arthritis, including ReA,[115,116] and their responsiveness to sulfasalazine,[117,118] this drug is often recommended in dosages ranging from 30 to 50 mg/kg/day (maximum 1.5 to 2.0 g/day in adolescents). The response to sulfasalazine in adults with ReA is as variable as it is when treating children. Some patients enter remission after 3 to 6 months of therapy, but this also may occur spontaneously. The frequency of adverse events ranges from 10% to 20% (see Chapter 12). Some beneficial effects of the drug have also been observed in patients with uveitis and skin manifestations, such as keratoderma blennorrhagicum. Because of limited response of SpA to methotrexate, this drug is not recommended for ReA. In contrast, its effects on iritis and keratoderma blennorrhagicum in children may be satisfactory. Uveitis usually responds to topical or systemic glucocorticoids, but severe, resistant ocular inflammation occasionally requires other immunosuppressive drugs (see Chapter 22).

No antibiotic regimen has been clearly efficacious in ReA.[119] Double-blind and open trials of various tetracycline derivatives (except for one using lymecycline) or ciprofloxacin have noted no significant differences when compared with placebo in the short and long term.[120,121] Compared with placebo, lymecycline[120] reduced the time to recover from arthritis in patients with *Chlamydia* but not in those with enteritis-related ReA. A recent study, focusing on *Chlamydia*-associated ReA showed that various combinations of doxycycline, rifampin, and azithromycin were more efficacious than placebo in a 6-month trial.[121] Antibiotic treatment, however, does not change the natural history of ReA.[122] In children, it has been suggested that amoxicillin alone or in combination with clavulanic acid may be useful.[123]

The use of TNF-α blockers, specifically infliximab, has been reported to be of benefit in adults with ReA,[124-126] although no data are yet available in children.

Physical Therapy and Rehabilitation

In the acute inflammatory phase, treatment of ReA is similar to that for other forms of chronic arthritis (Chapter 14). Rest, ice, hot packs, and ambulation aids may be useful. Custom-made insoles relieve pain caused by enthesitis at the heel and metatarsal heads and help preserve the longitudinal arch of the foot. The use of night resting splints helps avoid joint contractures associated with tendonitis or tenosynovitis. Both active and passive stretching of joints and muscle strengthening should be prescribed when inflammation is being controlled and pain permits. Children with chronic and recurrent ReA tend to develop fibrous ankylosis first, followed by bone ankylosis of the midtarsal joints and subluxation of the MTP joints, and therefore require special attention to insoles and shoes. Knee, hip, and axial disease benefits from activities such as biking and swimming.

Orthopedic Surgery

Arthroscopic synovectomy is potentially beneficial for children with recurrent synovitis of the knee or small joints of the hands and feet, although is seldom necessary. Early soft tissue release of contractures at the hip, knee, MTP, and IP joints increases functional capacity and may reduce the risk of severe impairment thereafter. Adolescents with severe hip or knee disease may require joint replacements in the long term.

COURSE OF THE DISEASE AND PROGNOSIS

The course of arthritis in children with ReA varies. Most children have only a single episode of monoarthritis or oligoarthritis. This is typical of ReA triggered by *Yersinia*[15,41,98] or *Campylobacter*.[99] Others have recurrent episodes of oligoarthritis or an extended form of disease affecting multiple joints and entheses. Although remission may still occur in these patients, many others evolve into enthesitis-related arthritis, SpA, or ankylosing spondylitis with sacroiliitis.

Children with ReA who have HLA-B27 have more severe involvement.[33,34] Extraarticular disease, including iridocyclitis and the triad of arthritis, conjunctivitis, and urethritis, also occurs more frequently among children with ReA who are HLA-B27 positive. In one report, three of five HLA-B27–positive children with *Salmonella*-triggered ReA developed psoriasis.[97] The number of joints involved at onset, the

presence of fever or anemia, and the number and duration of episodes of disease activity influence the outcome.

The prognosis of *Chlamydia*- or *Yersinia*-triggered ReA is less severe than that described after *Shigella* or *Salmonella* infection. Whether this is a direct influence of the infectious agent or represents different frequencies of association with HLA-B27 is uncertain.

REFERENCES

4. T. Hannu, R. Inman, K. Granfors, M. Leirisalo-Repo, Reactive arthritis or post-infectious arthritis? Best Pract. Res. Clin. Rheumatol. 20 (2006) 419–433.

5. E. Gracey, R.D. Inman, Chlamydia-induced ReA: immune imbalances and persistent pathogens, Nat Rev Rheumatol 8 (2011) 55–59.

6. G. Kingsley, J. Sieper, Third international workshop on reactive arthritis. An overview, Ann. Rheum. Dis. 55 (1996) 564–584.

7. C. Pacheco-Tena, R. Burgos-Vargas, J. Vázquez-Mellado, et al., A proposal for the classification of patients for clinical and experimental studies on reactive arthritis, J. Rheumatol. 26 (1999) 1338–1346.

8. T. Tuuminen, K. Lounamo, M. Leirisalo-Repo, A review of serological tests to assist diagnosis of reactive arthritis: critical appraisal on methodologies, Front Immunol 4 (2013) 418.

10. N. Hajjaj-Hassouni, R. Burgos-Vargas, Ankylosing spondylitis and reactive arthritis in the developing world, Best Pract. Res. Clin. Rheumatol. 22 (2008) 709–723.

11. R. Tuompo, T. Hannu, L. Mattila, et al., Reactive arthritis following Salmonella infection: a population-based study, Scand. J. Rheumatol. 42 (2013) 196–202.

12. A.T. Lee, R.G. Hall, K.D. Pile, Reactive joint symptoms following an outbreak of Salmonella typhimurium phage type 135a, J. Rheumatol. 32 (2005) 524–527.

13. M. Rudwaleit, S. Richter, J. Braun, et al., Low incidence of reactive arthritis in children following a salmonella outbreak, Ann. Rheum. Dis. 60 (2001) 1055–1057.

14. J.A. Hoogkamp-Korstanje, V.M. Stolk-Engelaar, Yersinia enterocolitica infection in children, Pediatr. Infect. Dis. J. 14 (1995) 771–775.

16. M. Vasala, S. Hallanvuo, P. Ruuska, et al., High frequency of reactive arthritis in adults after Yersinia pseudotuberculosis O:1 outbreak caused by contaminated grated carrots, Ann. Rheum. Dis. 73 (2014) 1793–1796.

17. J.D. Carter, R.D. Inman, Chlamydia-induced reactive arthritis: hidden in plain sight? Best Pract. Res. Clin. Rheumatol. 25 (2011) 359–374.

18. M. Harjacek, J. Ostojic, O. Djakovic Rode, Juvenile spondyloarthropathies associated with Mycoplasma pneumoniae infection, Clin. Rheumatol. 25 (2006) 470–475.

31. G. Taccetti, S. Trapani, M. Ermini, F. Falcini, Reactive arthritis triggered by Yersinia enterocolitica: a review of 18 pediatric cases, Clin. Exp. Rheumatol. 12 (1994) 681–684.

33. P. Schiellerup, K.A. Krogfelt, H. Locht, A comparison of self-reported joint symptoms following infection with different enteric pathogens: effect of HLA-B27, J. Rheumatol. 35 (2008) 480–487.

37. F.W. Tsui, N. Xi, S. Rohekar, et al., Toll-like receptor 2 variants are associated with acute reactive arthritis, Arthritis Rheum. 58 (2008) 3436–3438.

38. Y. Doorduyn, W. Van Pelt, C.L. Siezen, et al., Novel insight in the association between salmonellosis or campylobacteriosis and chronic illness, and the role of host genetics in susceptibility to these diseases, Epidemiol. Infect. 136 (2008) 1225–1234.

39. Y.J. Chen, C.H. Lin, T.T. Ou, et al., Solute carrier family 11 member A1 gene polymorphisms in reactive arthritis, J. Clin. Immunol. 27 (2007) 46–52.

40. J.D. Carter, A. Rehman, J.P. Guthrie, et al., Attack rate of Chlamydia-induced reactive arthritis and effect of the CCR5-Delta-32 mutation: a prospective analysis, J. Rheumatol. 40 (2013) 1578–1582.

49. R. Sorrentino, R.A. Böckmann, M.T. Fiorillo, HLA-B27 and antigen presentation: at the crossroads between immune defense and autoimmunity, Mol. Immunol. 57 (2014) 22–27.

50. R. Benjamin, P. Parham, Guilt by association: HLA-B27 and ankylosing spondylitis, Immunol. Today 11 (1990) 137–142.

51. M. Ramos, J.A. López de Castro, HLA-B27 and the pathogenesis of spondyloarthritis, Tissue Antigens 60 (2002) 191–205.

52. R.H. Scofield, W.L. Warren, G. Koelsch, et al., A hypothesis for the HLA-B27 immune dysregulation in spondyloarthropathy: contributions from enteric organism, B27 structure peptides bound by B27, and convergent evolution, Proc Natl Acad Sci USA 90 (1993) 9330–9334.

58. E. Frauendorf, H. von Goessel, E. May, et al., HLA-B27-restricted T cells from patients with ankylosing spondylitis recognize peptides from B*2705 that are similar to bacteria-derived peptides, Clin. Exp. Immunol. 134 (2003) 351–359.

59. J.J. Cragnolini, J.A. de Castro, Identification of endogenously presented peptides from Chlamydia trachomatis with high homology to human proteins and to a natural self-ligand of HLA-B27, Mol. Cell. Proteomics 7 (2008) 170–180.

60. K.P. Karunakaran, J. Rey-Ladino, N. Stoynov, et al., Immunoproteomic discovery of novel T cell antigens from the obligate intracellular pathogen Chlamydia, J. Immunol. 180 (2008) 2459–2465.

61. C. Alvarez-Navarro, J.J. Cragnolini, H.G. Dos Santos, et al., Novel HLA-B27-restricted epitopes from Chlamydia trachomatis generated upon endogenous processing of bacterial proteins suggest a role of molecular mimicry in reactive arthritis, J. Biol. Chem. 288 (2013) 25810–25825.

62. L. Ben Dror, E. Barnea, I. Beer, et al., The HLA-B*2705 peptidome, Arthritis Rheum. 62 (2010) 420–429.

63. R.A. Colbert, HLA-B27 misfolding: a solution to the spondyloarthropathy conundrum? Mol. Med. Today 6 (2000) 224–230.

64. R.A. Colbert, T.M. Tran, G. Layh-Schmitt, HLA-B27 misfolding and ankylosing spondylitis, Mol. Immunol. 57 (2014) 44–51.

66. N.S. Dangoria, M.L. DeLay, D.J. Kingsbury, et al., HLA-B27 misfolding is associated with aberrant intermolecular disulfide bond formation (dimerization) in the endoplasmic reticulum, J. Biol. Chem. 28 (2002) 23459–23468.

68. S. Kollnberger, L. Bird, M.Y. Sun, et al., Cell-surface expression and immune receptor recognition of HLA-B27 homodimers, Arthritis Rheum. 46 (2002) 2972–2982.

69. K. McHugh, P. Bowness, The link between HLA-B27 and SpA-new ideas on an old problem, Rheumatology (Oxford) 51 (2012) 1529–1539.

70. B. Uchanska-Ziegler, A. Ziegler, Ankylosing spondylitis: a beta2m-deposition disease? Trends Immunol. 24 (2003) 73–76.

71. M. Saarinen, P. Ekman, M. Ikeda, et al., Invasion of Salmonella into human intestinal epithelial cells is modulated by HLA-B27, Rheumatology (Oxford) 41 (2002) 651–657.

73. J.J. Cragnolini, N. García-Medel, J.A. de Castro, Endogenous processing and presentation of T-cell epitopes from Chlamydia trachomatis with relevance in HLA-B27-associated reactive arthritis, Mol. Cell. Proteomics 8 (2009) 1850–1859.

75. S. Vähämiko, M.A. Penttinen, K. Granfors, Aetiology and pathogenesis of reactive arthritis: role of non-antigen-presenting effects of HLA-B27, Arthritis Res. Ther. 7 (2005) 136–141.

77. K. Kapasi, R.D. Inman, ME1 epitope of HLA B27 confers class I–mediated modulation of gram-negative bacterial invasion, J. Immunol. 153 (1994) 833–840.

78. O. Ortiz-Alvarez, D.T. Yu, R.E. Petty, B.B. Finlay, HLA-B27 does not affect invasion of arthritogenic bacteria into human cells, J. Rheumatol. 25 (1998) 1765–1771.

79. H.-I. Huppertz, J. Heesemann, The influence of HLA B27 and interferon-gamma on the invasion and persistence of Yersinia in primary human fibroblasts, Med Microbiol Immunol 185 (1996) 163–170.

89. C. Pacheco-Tena, C. Alvarado De La Barrera, Y. López-Vidal, et al., Bacterial DNA in synovial fluid cells of patients with juvenile onset spondyloarthropathies, Rheumatology 40 (2001) 920–927.

94. M. Singh, N.K. Ganguli, H. Singh, et al., Role of 30 kDa antigen of enteric bacterial pathogens as a possible arthritogenic factor in post-dysenteric reactive arthritis, Indian J. Pathol. Microbiol. 56 (2013) 231–237.

95. R. Burgos-Vargas, A. Howard, B.M. Ansell, Antibodies to peptidoglycan in juvenile onset ankylosing spondylitis and pauciarticular onset juvenile arthritis associated with chronic iridocyclitis, J. Rheumatol. 13 (1986) 760–762.

99. T. Hannu, M. Kauppi, M. Tuomala, et al., Reactive arthritis following and outbreak of Campylobacter jejuni infection, J. Rheumatol. 31 (2004) 528–530.

102. R.J. Cuttica, E.J. Scheines, S.M. Garay, et al., Juvenile onset Reiter's syndrome. A retrospective study of 26 patients, Clin. Exp. Rheumatol. 10 (1992) 285–288.

106. D. Zivony, J. Nocton, D. Wortmann, N. Esterly, Juvenile Reiter's syndrome: a report of four cases, J. Am. Acad. Dermatol. 38 (1998) 32–37.

109. H.I. Huppertz, H. Karch, J. Heesemann, Diagnostic value of synovial fluid analysis in children with reactive arthritis, Rheumatol. Int. 15 (1995) 167–170.

110. E.M. Azouz, C.M. Duffy, Juvenile spondyloarthropathies: clinical manifestations and medical imaging, Skeletal Radiol. 24 (1995) 399–408.

114. S. Esposito, S. Bosis, C. Sabatini, et al., Borrelia burgdorferi infection and Lyme disease in children, Int. J. Infect. Dis. 17 (2013) e153–e158.

119. C.E. Barber, J. Kim, R.D. Inman, et al., Antibiotics for treatment of reactive arthritis: a systematic review and metaanalysis, J. Rheumatol. 40 (2013) 916–928.

121. J.D. Carter, L.R. Espinoza, R.D. Inman, et al., Combination antibiotics as a treatment for chronic Chlamydia-induced reactive arthritis: a double-blind, placebo-controlled, prospective trial, Arthritis Rheum. 62 (2010) 1298–1307.

122. K. Laasila, L. Laasonen, M. Leirisalo-Repo, Antibiotic treatment and long-term prognosis of reactive arthritis, Ann. Rheum. Dis. 62 (2003) 655–658.

124. K.S. Oili, H. Niinisalo, T. Korpilähde, J. Virolainen, Treatment of reactive arthritis with infliximab, Scand. J. Rheumatol. 32 (2003) 122–124.

125. H. Gill, V. Majithia, Successful use of infliximab in the treatment of Reiter's syndrome: a case report and discussion, Clin. Rheumatol. 27 (2008) 121–123.

126. M.D. Schafranski, Infliximab for reactive arthritis secondary to Chlamydia trachomatis infection, Rheumatol. Int. 30 (2010) 679–680.

Entire reference list is available online at www.expertconsult.com.

CHAPTER 44

Acute Rheumatic Fever and Poststreptococcal Reactive Arthritis

Khaled Alsaeid, Yosef Uziel

ACUTE RHEUMATIC FEVER

Introduction

Group A β-hemolytic streptococcus (GAS) is notorious for causing a myriad of human diseases associated with significant morbidity and mortality. GAS is the etiological agent for bacterial pharyngitis, impetigo, and the more invasive toxic shock syndrome and necrotizing fasciitis. Noninvasive complications of GAS are as important and range from diseases with a clear definition and causation, such as acute rheumatic fever (ARF), poststreptococcal glomerulonephritis, and poststreptococcal reactive arthritis (PSRA) to less defined ones as in Pediatric Autoimmune Neuropsychiatric Disorders Associated with Streptococcal Infections (PANDAS). The global burden of disease caused by GAS is large. Recent population-based data estimate that there are at least 517,000 deaths each year due to severe GAS diseases (examples include ARF, rheumatic heart disease (RHD), poststreptococcal glomerulonephritis, and invasive infections). It is estimated that worldwide there are at least 15.6 million people with rheumatic heart disease, with 282,000 new cases and 233,000 deaths attributed to this disease each year.[1]

Definition and Classification

ARF is a disease characterized by an inflammatory process that affects several organs. It is one of the few rheumatic diseases for which the cause has been identified—tonsillopharyngitis caused by group A β-hemolytic streptococcus (GAS). The streptococcal infection and the onset of the clinical manifestations of ARF are separated by a period of latency of 2 to 3 weeks. During this time, the patient is asymptomatic. The clinical presentations include arthritis, carditis, chorea, a characteristic rash, and subcutaneous nodules. Arthritis is the most common, but least specific, of these manifestations, whereas carditis is the most specific and serious. The pathological process underlying the inflammatory reaction in the various organs is a vasculitis mediated by an immune reaction to the streptococcal antigen. This nonpurulent complication of group A streptococcal disease can be prevented by appropriate treatment of the streptococcal pharyngitis.

Epidemiology

Incidence and Prevalence

ARF was prevalent worldwide until the middle part of the twentieth century. The advent of industrialization and improved public hygiene in Western Europe and North America was associated with a sharp decline in the incidence of this disease. During the early part of the twentieth century, incidence rates of 100 to 200 cases per 100,000 members of the general population were documented in the United States.[2] Although this rate still prevails in developing countries,[3] current estimates of the incidence of ARF in children in the United States document a markedly lower incidence rate of 0.5 to 3 cases per 100,000 children.[4] Between 1985 and 1990, a marked resurgence of the disease occurred in several areas of the United States.[5-14] This dramatic reappearance of what had been an increasingly rare disease was followed by a persistently higher rate in the incidence of ARF in these geographical areas.[15-17] However, the focal nature of these episodes has not significantly affected the overall prevalence of the disease in the United States. ARF cases are still reported from pockets in the developed countries especially in immigrant communities. Pastore reported an increase in the incidence of ARF in Trieste, Italy suggesting that ARF still occurs in industrialized counties.[18]

Age at Onset and Sex Ratio

The age-related incidence of ARF, like that of GAS pharyngitis, peaks between the ages of 6 and 15 years. Approximately 5% of all cases of ARF occur in children younger than 5 years of age.[19-21] Among adults at high risk for streptococcal pharyngitis, such as military recruits and persons working in crowded settings, the incidence of the disease is higher. There is no difference in the incidence of ARF between males and females.

Geographical and Racial Distribution

Once considered to be a disease of temperate climate, ARF is now more common in countries with tropical climates, particularly in developing countries. In the United States, the highest seasonal incidence is in the spring, following the peak season of streptococcal pharyngitis in the winter. In other countries, a season of peak frequency is less well defined.

Despite the decline of ARF in industrialized countries, its prevalence in developing areas of the world remains very high. Incidence rates per 100,000 population range from 23 in Kuwait, 35 in Iran, to 51 in India. It has been estimated that 95% of the nearly 20 million cases of rheumatic heart disease (RHD) in the world each year occur in developing countries.[22,23] Factors invoked in explaining the decreased incidence of the disease in the United States include less crowding in homes and schools and the increased availability of health care to children.[23,24] However, other factors may also be important because, in the United States, this disease has recently been occurring primarily in children from middle- to high-income families with ready access to medical care.[5]

Differences in the incidence of ARF among racial and ethnic groups have been described. In New Zealand, the disease is more common among the Maori population compared with local non-Maoris of

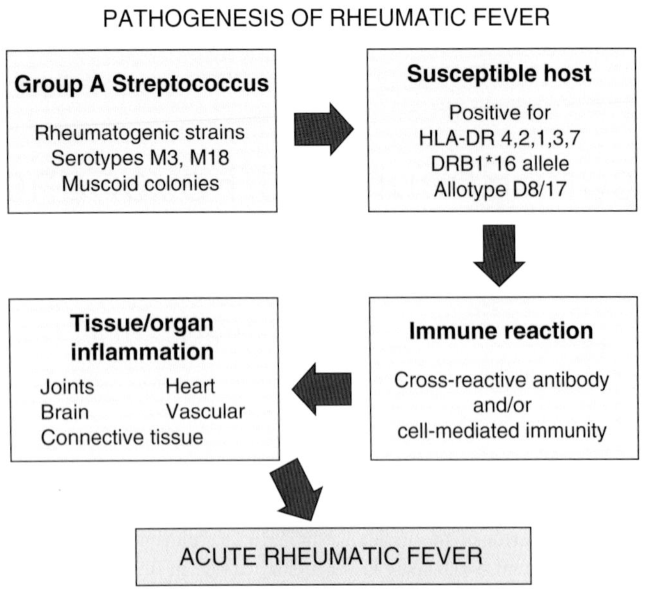

PATHOGENESIS OF RHEUMATIC FEVER

FIGURE 44-1 Interactions between the group A *Streptococcus* and the human host that lead to acute rheumatic fever. *HLA*, Human leukocyte antigen. (Adapted from E.M. Ayoub, Acute rheumatic fever, in: G.C. Emmanouilides, T.A. Riemenschneider, H.D., Allen, et al (Eds.), Moss and Adams' heart disease in infants, children, and adolescents, including the fetus and young adult, vol II, fifth ed., Williams & Wilkins, Baltimore, 1995.)

similar socioeconomic status.[25] ARF in the United States is more prevalent among African Americans and Hispanics than among whites.[4] Although genetic factors can account for these racial and ethnic differences, environmental factors may also be instrumental in explaining these observations.[3]

Etiology and Pathogenesis

ARF is a complication of a GAS tonsillopharyngitis in a predisposed human host; streptococcal pyoderma does not lead to this complication.[26] There is no experimental model for this disease. Specific factors that influence its evolution include the characteristics of the etiological organism, the site of the streptococcal infection, and a genetic predisposition of the host (Fig. 44-1). Less than 2% to 3% of previously healthy persons who acquire streptococcal pharyngitis develop ARF. This complication can be prevented by prompt identification and treatment of the streptococcal infection.

Etiological Agent

β-Hemolytic streptococci have been divided into 20 serogroups (A to H and K to V) by Lancefield[27] based on immunochemical differences in their cell-wall polysaccharide. The group A β-hemolytic *Streptococcus* is the most common bacterial pathogen associated with tonsillopharyngitis and is the only member of the group that can initiate ARF. Several cellular components and extracellular products produced by this streptococcus *in vivo* and *in vitro* have been identified.

The streptococcal bacterium consists of a cytoplasm enclosed in a membrane composed predominantly of lipoproteins. This structure is surrounded by a cell wall made up of three components. The primary component is a peptidoglycan that imparts rigidity to the cell wall. A complex of this component and the cell-wall polysaccharide elicits arthritis and a recurrent nodular reaction when injected into the skin of experimental animals.[28-30] Integrated into the peptidoglycan is the cell-wall polysaccharide or group-specific carbohydrate whose

immunochemical structure determines the serogroup specificity. This polysaccharide has been reported to share antigenic determinants with a glycopeptide present in mitral valve tissue.[31] Traversing through and extending outside the cell wall as hair-like fimbriae is the M protein, part of a mosaic that also includes the R and T proteins. The M protein is a coiled protein with an α-helical structure consisting of a free, distal, hypervariable amino terminus and a proximal carboxyl terminus anchored to the cell wall.[32] This protein is the type-specific antigen of the GAS.

More than 200 M proteins have been identified by differences in immunochemical composition of the variable amino terminus. A major biological property of the M protein is its capacity to inhibit phagocytosis of the streptococcus; this effect is neutralized by antibody to its amino terminal region. Immunity to GAS infections is therefore type specific, predicated on formation of antibodies to specific M proteins. Certain serotypes are associated with potential pathogenicity and virulence. Data procured during a resurgence of ARF confirmed that serotypes 3 and 18, particularly strains that produced mucoid colonies when cultured on blood agar, were primarily associated with the disease.[33,34] These two serotypes and the M1 serotype were also associated with severe, invasive group A streptococcal disease, including the streptococcal toxic shock syndrome.[35] Studies have indicated that bacterial strains that have conserved parts of the carboxyl terminal portion of the M-protein molecule exposed on their cell surface (class I strains) were associated with ARF, whereas strains that did not have this characteristic (class II) were not.[36] It was reported that phages and phage-like elements were the sources for variation in the genome of an M18 isolate, recovered from a patient with ARF, and an M1 strain.[37]

The pathogenetic importance of the M proteins is supported by data indicating that several epitopes of the M-protein molecule cross-react antigenically with human myocardium, myosin, and brain tissue, ostensibly leading to tissue inflammation.[38,39] M protein also functions as a "superantigen."[40] These findings indicate that this streptococcal molecule can induce an inflammatory response in certain tissues by eliciting "autoimmune" antibodies and tissue inflammation by nonspecific stimulation of cell-mediated immunity as a superantigen.

The cellular component of the GAS that has been implicated in the pathogenesis of arthritis is the hyaluronate capsule. Like the M protein, this moiety appears to carry epitopes that elicit antibodies that cross-react with human cartilage and synovial hyaluronate.[41] Some studies have documented that components of the M3 and M18 epitopes aggregate type IV collagen, a component of the human basement membrane. This reaction is effected in M3 strains by the production of a collagen-binding factor. M18 strains bind collagen through the hyaluronic acid capsule. Patients with ARF have higher levels of anti-collagen (IV) antibodies than controls;[42] mice immunized with recombinant M3 protein produce anti-collagen antibodies. In addition to the cellular components, extracellular products of the GAS have important biological activities and are of practical value in the diagnosis of GAS infections and their nonpurulent complications. Most of these products are proteins with enzymatic properties, and they possess specific biological and antigenic activity. The streptococcal pyrogenic exotoxins (SPEs) A, B, C, and F (i.e., the mitogenic factor) and streptococcal superantigen (SSA) are of particular interest because they act as superantigens that induce proliferation of T lymphocytes *in vitro* and the synthesis and release of several lymphokines *in vivo*.[38-44] This biological activity reflects the ability of SPEs to bind simultaneously to class II major human leukocyte antigens (HLA) of antigen-presenting cells and to the Vβ region of the T cell receptor. Production of these exotoxins is associated *in vivo* with a febrile response, alteration of membrane permeability, and enhancement of susceptibility to endotoxin-induced lethal shock.[45] Selective activation of lymphocytes has been ascribed to different SPEs. SPE A activates T cells bearing T cell receptor β-chain segments Vβ8, Vβ12, and Vβ14, whereas SPE B activates T cells bearing segments Vβ2 and Vβ8.[46] SPE B has been identified as a cysteine protease that inhibits phagocytosis and enhances dissemination of the organism *in vivo*. It also induces apoptosis of phagocytic cells.[47]

The frequencies of the SPE genes and their expression vary among group A streptococci; SPE A is found in 45% of strains, SPE B in almost all strains, and SPE C in 30% of strains. SPE A is expressed by 43% and SPE B by 76% of strains.[35,48,49] The frequencies of the SPE A genes and their products are similar among M1 and M3 serotypes.[48] The association of certain serotypes with various clinical manifestations of streptococcal infections, such as toxic shock syndrome, has been ascribed to the capacity of the infecting strain to produce one of the SPEs.[35,46,48] However, the ubiquity of the production of these toxins makes confirmation of the specificity of these associations questionable.[49]

Streptococcal Antibody Tests

The specific antigenicity of most of the streptococcal extracellular products led to the establishment of antibody tests for these products. These tests are used to confirm evidence of a GAS infection, primarily in patients with ARF and glomerulonephritis. The first and still most universally used is the antistreptolysin O (ASO) test, which was designed by Todd[50] to measure neutralizing antibodies to purified streptolysin O in patients with scarlet fever and ARF. This test proved helpful in providing evidence for antecedent group A streptococcal infection, particularly when throat cultures were negative. Subsequently, tests were developed to assay for antibodies to other streptococcal antigens (Table 44-1). The anti-DNase B test, which assays for antibodies to the most ubiquitous of four deoxyribonuclease isozymes produced by the group A streptococcus (A, B, C, and D), proved to be as reliable and reproducible as the ASO test. The other tests, which are no longer readily available, and the streptozyme test, which was widely used at one time, lacked standardization and reproducibility and should not be relied on for evidence of antecedent group A streptococcal infection.[51]

The pattern of the antibody response to the streptococcal antigens is illustrated in Figure 44-2. Antibodies peak approximately 2 to 3 weeks after the acute infection. Because of the period of latency

between the infection and the onset of the clinical manifestations of ARF, serum obtained at the time of clinical presentation should document the necessary evidence for antecedent group A streptococcal infection. However, as outlined in Table 44-2, only about 83% of patients with ARF mount an ASO response. Another streptococcal antibody test, such as anti-DNase B, can provide evidence for an antecedent streptococcal infection in patients in whom an ASO response has not been diagnostic.

Tests for antibodies to the cell-wall components of group A streptococci are available but not widely used. Determination of type-specific antibody to the different M proteins is employed in epidemiological studies to determine previous exposure or immunity to specific M serotypes. Testing for antibody to the group-specific carbohydrate is available in some laboratories. Because this antibody tends to persist for prolonged periods in patients with rheumatic valvular disease, it may help to confirm the rheumatic cause of mitral valve disease in a patient without a history of ARF.[52-55]

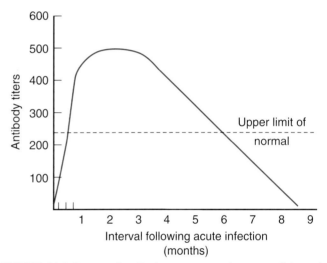

FIGURE 44-2 Pattern of antibody response to the extracellular antigens of the group A *Streptococcus* after tonsillopharyngeal infection in humans. (From E.M. Ayoub, Streptococcal antibody tests in rheumatic fever, Clin Immunol Newsletter 3 (1982) 107–111.)

TABLE 44-1 Group A Streptococcal Antigens and Corresponding Antibody Tests

STREPTOCOCCAL ANTIGEN	ANTIBODY TEST
Extracellular Product	
Streptolysin O	ASO
Streptokinase	Antistreptokinase
Hyaluronidase	Antihyaluronidase
DNase B	Anti-DNase B
NADase	Anti-NADase
Multiple antigens	Streptozyme
Cellular Component	
M protein	Type-specific antibody
Group-specific polysaccharide	Anti-A-carbohydrate

ASO, Antistreptolysin O; DNase B, deoxyribonuclease B; NADase, nicotinamide adenine dinucleotidase.
Adapted from E.M. Ayoub, Streptococcal antibody tests in rheumatic fever, Clin Immunol Newsletter 3 (1982) 107–111.

TABLE 44-2 Frequency of Patients with Acute Rheumatic Fever with Elevated Titers of Antistreptolysin O or Antideoxyribonuclease B

GROUP	ASO	ANTI-DNASE B	ASO AND ANTI-DNASE B
Normal controls	19%	19%	30%
Acute rheumatic fever	83%	82%	92%
Sydenham chorea (isolated)	67%	40%	80%

ASO, Antistreptolysin O; DNase B, deoxyribonuclease B.
Adapted from E.M. Ayoub, L.W. Wannamaker, Evaluation of the streptococcal deoxyribonuclease B and diphosphopyridine nucleotidase antibody tests in acute rheumatic fever and acute glomerulonephritis, Pediatrics 29 (1962) 527–538 and from E.M. Ayoub, L.W. Wannamaker, Streptococcal antibody titers in Sydenham's chorea, Pediatrics 38 (1966) 946–956.

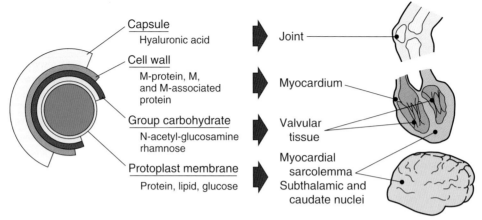

FIGURE 44-3 Group A streptococcal components and corresponding human tissues reported to exhibit immunological cross-reactivity. (From E.M. Ayoub, G.L. Schiebler, Acute rheumatic fever, in: V.C. Kelley (Ed.), Practice of pediatrics, vol. 8, Harper & Row, New York, 1985.)

Mechanism of Tissue Injury

Initial suggestions that tissue injury in ARF was caused by direct invasion by the streptococcus or the effect of its extracellular toxins were subsequently replaced by the theory that an immune mechanism was responsible for the inflammatory response in the affected organs. The potential role of an immunological process as the cause of tissue injury was predicated on the observation that the clinical manifestations of ARF occurred after a period of latency of about 3 weeks from the inciting GAS infection. Evidence for involvement of an immune mechanism in pathogenesis was first advanced by Kaplan and colleagues.[56,57] These investigators and others described the presence of common antigenic determinants among the cellular components of the group A streptococci and myocardial tissues. Structures that share cross-reactive antigenic determinants included components of the M protein and myocardial sarcolemma,[56-61] cell-wall carbohydrate and valvular glycoprotein,[31] streptococcal protoplast membrane and neuronal tissue of the subthalamic and caudate nuclei,[62,63] and the hyaluronate capsule and articular cartilage.[41] Based on these studies, it was concluded that antibodies, which formed against the streptococcal antigens, cross-reacted with the corresponding tissues and led to inflammation in the heart, joints, and brain (Fig. 44-3).[38,39]

As attractive as the process of "antigenic mimicry" is in explaining the inflammatory reaction in ARF, there are several flaws in this hypothesis. The most compelling of these arguments is the presence of high levels of cross-reactive antibodies in the sera of patients who do not have any manifestations of acute carditis or arthritis. An alternative explanation was provided by subsequent studies that documented a potential role for cell-mediated immunity in inducing tissue damage. These studies confirmed that peripheral blood lymphocytes from patients with acute rheumatic carditis were cytotoxic to human myocardial cells in tissue culture.[64] Addition of plasma from the same patients abrogated this cytotoxic effect. The latter observation suggested that the cross-reactive antibodies elicited by group A streptococci had a protective rather than a detrimental effect on the host. Based on these arguments, the prevalent hypothesis for explaining tissue injury in ARF is that an immunological mechanism involving the humoral or the cellular immune system may be responsible. An alternative hypothesis, albeit less established, is based on the observation that streptococcal M protein N-terminus domain binds to the CB3 region in collagen type IV. This binding seems to initiate an antibody response to the collagen and result in ground substance inflammation. These antibodies do not cross-react with M proteins, suggesting that

no molecular mimicry occurs in rheumatic fever. This alternative hypothesis shares similarity with collagen involvement in both Goodpasture syndrome and Alport syndrome.[65]

Genetic Background

Early postulates regarding the epidemiology of rheumatic fever suggested that persons who acquired this disease had a peculiar susceptibility to it. This postulate was based on the observation that 30% to 80% of patients who had had ARF developed a recurrence of the disease after subsequent group A streptococcal pharyngitis, whereas only about 2% of normal persons would develop ARF after such an infection.[66] Several studies documented the familial occurrence of the disease. Further evidence on the heritability of ARF is derived from twin studies. A recent systemic review by Engel of six twin studies on ARF included 465 pairs of twins. The pooled probandwise concordance risk for acute rheumatic fever was 44% in monozygotic twins and 12% in dizygotic twins, and the association between zygosity and concordance was strong (OR 6.39). The estimated heritability across all the studies was 60%.[67-68]

More substantial evidence for a genetic association was provided by Khanna and associates,[69] who reported that a B cell alloantigen, designated D8/17, was present in 99% of patients with ARF but in only 14% of normal controls; data that have been confirmed in subsequent studies.[70] A number of investigations have demonstrated associations of ARF with several class II human leukocyte antigens (HLA) such as DRB1*16 and DRB1*07,[71-82] (Table 44-3). These associations with rheumatic heart disease are more evident and consistent among clinically homogeneous patients.[80]

Initial reports of hyperresponsiveness to a number of streptococcal and nonstreptococcal antigens in ARF was not confirmed in subsequent studies.[83,84] An increased immune response to the group A streptococcal group-specific carbohydrate was demonstrated in patients with rheumatic valvular disease.[52-55,85] This response was associated with inheritance of HLA-DR2 and HLA-DR4 antigens.[71] This finding is relevant in view of data that indicate that the immune response to streptococcal cell-wall antigen is under genetic control in experimental animals and humans.[86-88]

Clinical Manifestations

Arthritis, carditis, Sydenham chorea (SC), erythema marginatum, and subcutaneous nodules constitute the major clinical manifestations of ARF (Fig. 44-4). A patient may present with only one, two, or more of

TABLE 44-3   Reported Associations of Histocompatibility Antigens-DR Antigens and Alleles with Rheumatic Fever

STUDY	LOCATION	NO. OF PATIENTS	ETHNICITY	HLA-DR ANTIGEN/ALLELE	PERCENT POSITIVE CONTROLS	PATIENTS
Ayoub et al.[71]	Florida, USA	24	White	DRB1*16	32	63
		48	African American	DR2	23	54
Anastasiou-Nana et al.[72]	Utah, USA	33	White	DR4	32	52
Jhinghan et al.[73]	New Delhi, India	134	Indian	DR3	26	50
Rajapakse et al.[74]	Riyadh, Saudi Arabia	40	Arab	DR4	12	65
Maharaj et al.[75]	Durban, South Africa	120	African American	DR1	3	13
Taneja et al.[76]	New Delhi, India	54	Indian	DQw2	32	63
Guilherme et al.[77]	San Paulo, Brazil	40	Brazilian (mulatto)	DR7	26	58
Ozkan et al.[78]	Istanbul, Turkey	107	Turkish	DR3	23	49
				DR7	33	57
Weidebach et al.[79]	Sao Paulo, Brazil	24	Brazilian (mulatto)	DR16	34	83
				DRw53		
Ahmed et al.[81]	Florida, USA	18	White	DRB1*16	4	15

HLA-DR, Human leukocyte antigens DR.
Adapted from E.M. Ayoub, Rheumatic fever, in: R.R. Rich (ed), Clinical immunology principles & practice, vol. 2, 2nd edn, Mosby, St Louis, 2001, pp. 1–7.

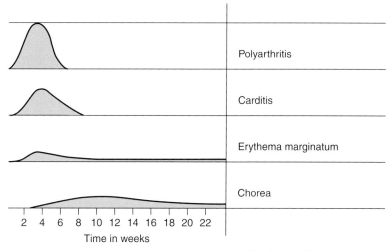

FIGURE 44-4 Major manifestations of acute rheumatic fever. This diagram illustrates the expected occurrence of each manifestation. The relative duration in weeks is indicated on the abscissa. The maximum clinical activity of each finding is represented by the peak of the shaded area. The expected frequency of each clinical manifestation is represented by the relative height of each shaded area. Polyarthritis and carditis usually are manifestations of acute disease. Chorea, although it may be an early manifestation, usually occurs about 3 months after the inciting episode of pharyngitis. It may be unaccompanied by other manifestations of the disease. Erythema marginatum is present for a longer period during and after the initial acute attack. This manifestation, although it is often associated with severe disease, is relatively uncommon in children.

these manifestations and with varying degrees of severity of each. Although the severity and frequency of these manifestations vary considerably from patient to patient, their overall frequencies in various populations are similar (Table 44-4). Minor manifestations of ARF include fever, arthralgia, abnormal acute phase reactants, and a prolonged PR interval.

Arthritis

Arthritis occurs in about 70% of patients. Although it is the most common of the major manifestations, it is relatively less specific than the other major criteria are because it is encountered in such a large number of other rheumatic diseases. As such, it is the most common cause of a misdiagnosis of ARF. Despite its lower specificity, the arthritis of ARF has characteristics that can help in its differentiation from that due to other causes. The arthritis primarily affects large joints, particularly the knees, ankles, wrists, and elbows. Small peripheral joints are only occasionally involved, and axial disease occurs rarely, if ever. The arthritis of ARF is characteristically migratory and additive; it is usually initially a monoarthritis but can be polyarticular.[89] Symptoms in an affected joint may resolve spontaneously within hours of onset, only to reappear in a different joint. The affected joint manifests the cardinal signs of inflammation with swelling, erythema, warmth, and pain. The latter symptom is the most prominent. It occurs at rest and is accentuated by passive or active movement of the joints. The

TABLE 44-4   Frequency of Major Manifestations of Acute Rheumatic Fever in U.S. and Non-U.S. Patients

MANIFESTATION	U.S. PATIENTS 1958-1962	1962-1980	1985-1989	NON-U.S. PATIENTS 1960-1980
Arthritis	75%	53%	65%	30-79%
Carditis	48%	78%	59%	41-93%
Sydenham chorea	16%	5%	20%	1-12%
Erythema marginatum	6%	2%	6%	0-16%
Subcutaneous nodules	7%	5%	5%	1-9%

Adapted from E.M. Ayoub, Resurgence of rheumatic fever in the United States: the changing pictures of a preventable disease, Postgrad. Med. 92 (1992) 133–142.

severity of pain induces guarding of the joints, which may lead to pseudoparalysis.

Carditis

Cardiac inflammation develops in more than 50% of the patients. The high frequency of this manifestation reported from developing countries probably reflects a bias toward hospitalization of patients with severe heart disease. Young children are more likely to develop moderate and severe carditis than older patients.[18] Carditis is the most common cause of morbidity and mortality. As with other manifestations, the severity of the carditis is highly variable.[90] In some patients, such as those with Sydenham chorea (SC), signs of carditis may be subtle, and cardiac involvement may be missed unless its diagnosis is pursued vigorously with echocardiographic examination.[91] Other patients may present with acute carditis and severe, life-threatening congestive heart failure. Carditis usually occurs in tandem with other major manifestations, such as arthritis. If it is not present initially, carditis may follow arthritis within 1 week; the onset of carditis beyond this interval is rare.

Pancarditis, inflammation involving the three layers of the heart, (endocardium, myocardium, and pericardium) was considered to be the hallmark of rheumatic heart disease (RHD). Recent research, however, indicates that the myocardium is not the primary target of inflammation in acute rheumatic fever as evidenced by the absence of an increase in markers of myocardial damage in patients with RHD. Additionally, myocardial biopsies fail to show evidence of myocarditis in such patients. Indeed, the main target and the site responsible for the pathological and clinical manifestations of RHD is predominantly the endocardium. Changes within the myocardium are mainly interstitial with little, if any, actual muscle tissue inflammation.[92]

Endocarditis, the major cause of morbidity and mortality in rheumatic carditis, affects principally valvular tissue and leads to the hallmark lesion of rheumatic carditis and valvular insufficiency. The valves most affected by rheumatic fever, in order, are the mitral and aortic valves. The tricuspid and pulmonary valves are rarely affected. In most cases, the mitral valve is involved with one or more of the other cardiac valves.

Mitral insufficiency or regurgitation is identified clinically by the presence on auscultation of a high-frequency, smooth, holosystolic, apical murmur. This murmur radiates to the left axilla and is best heard with the patient in a left lateral decubitus position. A mid- to late-diastolic flow murmur of relative mitral stenosis (i.e., Carey Coombs murmur) may be heard in patients with severe mitral insufficiency.

The murmur of aortic insufficiency is a high-frequency, diastolic murmur that starts with the aortic component of the second heart sound. It is best heard with the diaphragm of the stethoscope over the third left intercostal space with the patient in the upright position and leaning forward. The murmur of mild aortic insufficiency is faint and often difficult to hear. Murmurs of severe insufficiency are loud and accompanied by a diastolic thrill. In these patients, an increased pulse pressure due to aortic runoff is associated with bounding peripheral pulses (i.e., Corrigan pulse). Mitral and aortic valve stenoses result from valvular scarring and develop during the chronic stages of the disease.

Acute heart failure due to severe valvular insufficiency occurs in about 5% of children with ARF. The clinical manifestations vary greatly and include cough, chest pain, dyspnea, orthopnea, and anorexia. Tachycardia, cardiomegaly, and hepatomegaly with tenderness of the liver are present on physical examination.

Sydenham Chorea

Sydenham chorea (SC), also known as St. Vitus' dance, is a manifestation of inflammatory involvement of the basal ganglia and caudate nucleus of the central nervous system, which occurs in about 15% of patients. A higher frequency of SC was documented by several centers during the recent resurgence of ARF in the United States.[61] The latency period between the inciting streptococcal pharyngitis and the onset of clinical signs of chorea is longer than that of the other major manifestations of the disease, averaging 2 to 4 months, and sometimes extending to as long as 12 months.

A patient with SC presents with persistent involuntary and purposeless movements of the extremities, usually symmetric and with muscular incoordination. These movements are jerky and most prominent in the face, trunk, and distal extremities. These symptoms disappear during sleep. On examination, the patient grimaces and fidgets constantly. The protruded tongue darts in and out and resembles a bag of worms (i.e., wormian tongue). Speech is halting and explosive, and a steady tone cannot be maintained for even a short time. Extension of the arms above the head leads to pronation of the hands (i.e., pronator sign); extension of the arms anteriorly results in hyperextension of the fingers (i.e., spoon or dishing sign). When the patient is asked to squeeze the examiner's fingers, the examiner feels irregular contractions of the hand muscles (i.e., milkmaid's grip or milking sign). Handwriting, particularly drawing vertical straight lines, is clumsy and irregular because of the loss of fine muscle coordination. The patient has difficulty putting on clothes or buttoning a shirt. Such attempts lead to easy frustration and emotional upsets. Parents and teachers often complain about the child's clumsiness, inability to concentrate on tasks, or emotional lability. These symptoms usually resolve spontaneously in 2 to 3 weeks, but in severe cases they may persist for several months and sometimes for years.

A condition akin to SC, at least in pathophysiology, is pediatric autoimmune neuropsychiatric disorders associated with streptococcal infections (PANDAS). Though still an evolving concept in the mind of most pediatricians, this condition represents a subset of childhood obsessive-compulsive disorders (OCD) and tic disorders (TD) triggered by group A β-hemolytic streptococcus infections.[93] Physicians have long noted that up to 70% of these patients present with symptoms indistinguishable from classic OCD. In 1998, the National Institute of Mental Health characterized a group of children with a subset of OCD and TD and termed it PANDAS.[94] The clinical characteristics that define the PANDAS group are the presence of an OCD or a TD, prepubertal age at onset, abrupt onset, relapsing-remitting course, association with neurological abnormalities during exacerbations (e.g., adventitious movements or motor hyperactivity), and temporal association between symptoms exacerbation and GAS infection. In a systematic clinical evaluation of 50 children who met the diagnostic criteria for PANDAS, Swedo found that patients with PANDAS typically had a young age at illness onset and an abrupt onset of neuropsychiatric symptoms. GAS infection preceded 45 (31%) of 114 exacerbations of TD or OCD.[94] Antibrain and antibasal ganglia antibodies have been documented in children with PANDAS, further supporting this hypothesis.[95] It is not yet clear if prophylaxis with oral penicillin or azithromycin reduce streptococcal infections and neuropsychiatric exacerbations among children with PANDAS. In contrast to SC where carditis is highly prevalent (70% in some studies), carditis is not associated with PANDAS.[96] In fact, the discovery of carditis in a child with suspected PANDAS indicates Sydenham chorea of ARF, rather than PANDAS, as a diagnosis.

Erythema Marginatum

Erythema marginatum is characteristic of rheumatic fever and occurs in less than 5% of patients. This rash is nonpruritic and macular with a serpiginous erythematous border (Fig. 44-5). The individual lesions are about 0.4 cm in diameter and are usually located on the trunk and proximal inner aspects of the limbs, particularly where they join the trunk. The rash is rare on the face or other exposed areas. It is accentuated by warmth, such as the application of warm towels or a bath. Erythema marginatum is difficult to detect in patients with dark skin.

Subcutaneous Nodules

The subcutaneous nodules of ARF, which were most common in patients who developed chronic rheumatic heart disease and were a sign of severe involvement, now occur rarely. They are usually located on the extensor surfaces of the joints, particularly the elbows, knees, ankles, and knuckles, and occasionally on the occiput and spine. The overlying skin is not discolored. Their size varies from 0.5 to 2 cm, and they are firm, freely movable, painless and nontender. In many respects, they clinically and histologically resemble benign rheumatoid nodules.

Minor Manifestations of the Disease

The minor manifestations of fever, arthralgia, and elevated acute phase reactants are nonspecific and encountered in a number of other rheumatic diseases. The severity and duration of fever vary; the patient may have a temperature of 38.5°C (101°F) to 40°C (104°F) during the acute phase of the disease. Arthralgia (i.e., pain without objective changes in the joint) should be differentiated from arthritis. Elevated acute phase reactants are present during the acute stage of the disease. A prolonged PR interval on the electrocardiogram is another nonspecific finding. It occurs frequently in ARF but does not itself constitute a criterion for carditis; PR prolongation also does not correlate with the ultimate development of chronic rheumatic heart disease.

Pathology

The underlying pathology in ARF involves inflammation of the perivascular tissues in the joints, heart, brain, and skin, and is characterized by vasculitis that affects the smaller vessels and by proliferation of endothelial cells. This vasculitic process is reflected in the rash of ARF; inflammation of collagen occurs primarily in arthritis, valvulitis, and pericarditis. The synovitis of ARF is typified by a mononuclear cell infiltrate with fibrinoid degeneration. Joint cartilage is usually not involved.[97,98]

Inflammation of the heart, the most serious complication of the disease, characteristically and predominantly involves the endocardium and, to a lesser extent, the pericardium. Unlike other rheumatic diseases, such as systemic lupus erythematosus (SLE) or juvenile idiopathic arthritis (JIA), sole involvement of the pericardium is distinctly uncommon in ARF. The belief that pancarditis is characteristic of RHD is losing ground because laboratory and tissue evidence for actual myocardial inflammation is absent in most patients with RHD. Valvular endocarditis is the more common and characteristic inflammatory process and is the principal cause of chronic cardiac disease. Acute inflammation leads to valvular insufficiency and persistence of the inflammation results in scarring and stenosis (Fig. 44-6). The mitral valve is the most commonly involved, and mitral insufficiency is the

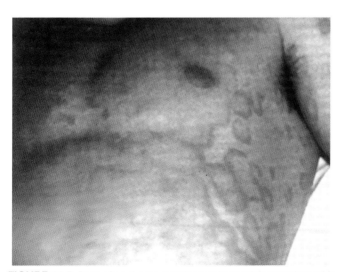

FIGURE 44-5 Rash of erythema marginatum in an adolescent boy with acute rheumatic fever occurred with its characteristic serpiginous and erythematous margins.

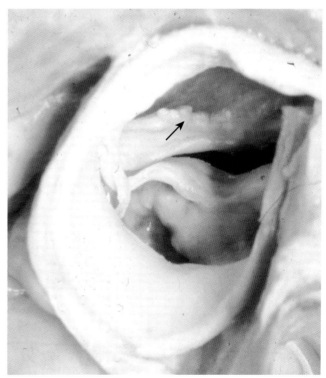

FIGURE 44-6 Chronic rheumatic valvular heart disease. Verrucal endocardial thickening was present along the line of closure of the valve leaflets *(arrow)*.

hallmark of rheumatic carditis. A review of the cardiac pathology by Roberts[98] indicated that isolated mitral valve disease was of rheumatic origin in 76% of cases, whereas aortic valve disease was ascribable to ARF in only 13% of cases. Serum cardiac troponin I, a sensitive and specific marker of myocardial injury, is not elevated in cases of ARF with cardiac involvement, indicating that congestive heart failure in ARF is related to valvular insufficiency rather than specific myocardial inflammation.[99]

The histological changes in acute rheumatic carditis are not specific, and the degree of abnormality does not necessarily correlate with the severity of carditis.[96,97] In the early stage, when dilatation of the myocardium is present, histological changes can be minimal. Despite this, cardiac function may be severely impaired and associated with a high rate of mortality. Progression of inflammation leads to an exudative and proliferative reaction in the myocardium, characterized by edematous changes followed by a cellular infiltrate of lymphocytes and plasma cells with few granulocytes. CD4 cells predominate in the lymphocytic infiltrate.[100] Degenerating collagen fibers are visible throughout the tissue as eosinophilic, granular deposits consisting of a mixture of fibrin, globulin, and other substances. This stage is followed by the formation of the Aschoff body.[101,102] This lesion consists of a perivascular infiltrate of large cells with polymorphous nuclei and basophilic cytoplasm arranged in a rosette around an avascular center of fibrinoid. The Aschoff body is pathognomonic of rheumatic carditis and occurs most commonly in patients with subacute or chronic carditis. It may develop in any area of the myocardium but is not present in other tissues.

Tissue edema and cellular infiltrates characterize the inflammation of valvular tissue. This inflammatory process also involves the chordae tendineae. Verrucae may form at the edge of the leaflets, preventing the valves from closing completely. Inflammation persisting for several years results in fibrosis and calcification of the valve that lead to stenosis.

The pathophysiology of SC is centered in the basal ganglia.[103] Magnetic resonance imaging volumetric studies have indicated focal striatal enlargement and response of the chorea to dopamine antagonists supporting this fact. Histological studies have documented cellular infiltration and neuronal loss in the basal ganglia as well as perivascular infiltration with lymphocytes.[104,105] Recent studies have shown IgG binding to neurons using immunohistochemistry, and have defined lysoganglioside as an important and potentially pathogenic antigen, further supporting a molecular mimicry hypothesis to SC.[106]

Subcutaneous nodules are characterized by a central area of fibrinoid necrosis surrounded by loosely demarcated zones of scattered mononuclear cells. Edema and vascular islands are present, but palisading of epithelioid cells is not well developed. Interstitial collagen fibers and scar formation occupy the outermost layers without formation of a capsule. The histology is not pathognomonic but resembles that of the Aschoff body. Descriptions of the pathological features of erythema marginatum are scant.

Diagnosis
Classification Criteria

There is no test for the definitive diagnosis of ARF. The diagnosis continues to be based on guidelines of clinical and laboratory criteria initially promulgated by T. Duckett Jones and subsequently revised by several committees of the American Heart Association (AHA). The latest modification of the Jones Criteria is outlined in Table 44-5.[107] These criteria were reaffirmed in 2002 by the American Heart Association Jones criteria workshop.[108] The purpose of these guidelines is to assist in the diagnosis of an initial attack of rheumatic fever and to minimize over-diagnosis. As stated under these guidelines, the

TABLE 44-5 Guidelines for the Diagnosis of an Initial Attack of Rheumatic Fever (Modified Jones Criteria, 1992)

MAJOR MANIFESTATIONS*	MINOR MANIFESTATIONS*
Carditis	Clinical
Polyarthritis	Fever
Sydenham chorea	Arthralgia
Erythema marginatum	Laboratory
Subcutaneous nodules	Elevated acute phase reactants:
	Erythrocyte sedimentation rate
	C-reactive protein level
	Prolonged PR interval

SUPPORTING EVIDENCE OF ANTECEDENT GROUP A STREPTOCOCCAL INFECTION*

Elevated or rising streptococcal antibody titers
Positive throat culture or rapid streptococcal antigen tests

*The presence of two major manifestations or of one major and two minor manifestations indicates a high probability of acute rheumatic fever, if supported by evidence of preceding group A streptococcal infection.
Adapted from A.S. Dajani, E.M. Ayoub, F.Z. Bierman, et al., Guidelines for the diagnosis of rheumatic fever: Jones Criteria, updated 1992, JAMA 87 (1992) 302–307.

presence of two major manifestations or one major plus two minor manifestations provides the basis for diagnosis of ARF, if supported by evidence of an antecedent GAS infection.

A positive throat culture or rapid antigen test can confirm an antecedent GAS pharyngitis. However, the period of latency between the inciting pharyngitis and the onset of ARF reduces the frequency of positive cultures to less than one third of patients.[109]

More reliable evidence can be obtained by the use of the streptococcal antibody tests listed in Table 44-1. Because of the latency period, serum obtained at the time of the initial evaluation of the patient coincides with the peak of the antibody response (see Fig. 44-2). An elevated ASO or anti-DNase B level is expected in about 85% of patients (see Table 44-2). When both tests are performed (considered by many to be a reasonable and conservative approach to diagnostic specificity), more than 90% of patients have an elevated titer for one of these tests. If the result of the ASO test is negative, a DNase B titer should be obtained. A four-fold (two tube) increase or decrease in titers should be demonstrated over time because normal children in many geographical areas may have elevated titers,[110] and it is useful to know the ASO titers in the normal population in the area in which the patient resides. Results of these antibody tests may be normal for most patients with chronic rheumatic heart disease, and a high proportion of patients with SC may have normal ASO or anti-DNase B titers (see Table 44-2). Neither the ASO nor the other streptococcal antibody tests are diagnostic of ARF; they provide supportive evidence for antecedent streptococcal infection.

The three acute phase reactants most commonly used in diagnosis are the peripheral blood leukocyte count, the erythrocyte sedimentation rate (ESR), and the C-reactive protein (CRP) level. The leukocyte count is the most variable and least dependable. It is normal in about one half of the patients with ARF. The ESR is markedly elevated in patients with acute disease but may be normal with severe congestive failure.[111] The CRP level is also elevated in patients with acute disease,[112] and unlike the ESR, its concentration is not affected by congestive heart failure. These tests are most useful in following the course of the disease and its response to treatment. Serum cardiac troponin 1 levels, known to be associated with myocardial injury, are not elevated in active rheumatic carditis.[99,113]

The role of Doppler echocardiography in making the diagnosis of ARF in the acute stage is controversial. According to the modified Jones criteria and the latest American Heart Association workshop on Jones criteria, Doppler echocardiographic abnormalities without concomitant clinical findings, namely subclinical carditis, are not considered in the diagnosis of rheumatic fever due to the lack of reference standards to differentiate between physiological regurgitation and minimal regurgitation resulting from subclinical valvulitis. In certain regions of the world where populations are at increased risk of rheumatic fever, such as the Maori and Pacific people in New Zealand and the aboriginal Australians, echocardiography has a central role in the diagnosis of rheumatic carditis. Australian criteria and the New Zealand guidelines for rheumatic fever diagnosis suggest that subclinical carditis, namely echocardiographic valvulitis without clinical findings, should be accepted as carditis for the diagnosis of rheumatic fever.[114] The World Heart Foundation (WHF) has published its guidelines concerning Doppler echocardiography in the diagnosis of rheumatic carditis. Its guidelines are based on both valve morphology as well as Doppler estimation of magnitude of valvular regurgitation. The following three categories are defined on the basis of assessment by 2D, continuous wave, and color Doppler echocardiography: definite RHD, borderline RHD, and normal. Four subcategories of definite RHD and three subcategories of borderline RHD exist, which reflect the various disease patterns. Although these guidelines may aid in the diagnosis and assessment of severity of rheumatic carditis, the question of subclinical carditis remains debatable.[115] In a recent review, 16.8% of 1700 patients with rheumatic fever had subclinical carditis. About half of patients with subclinical carditis improved while the remainder either remained unchanged or worsened over time.[116] Other studies useful in diagnosis include chest radiography and electrocardiography. A chest radiograph can detect cardiac enlargement or pericardial fluid. These findings are best confirmed by echocardiographic studies, which can also define the presence of myocarditis by assessing myocardial contractility and the nature and extent of valvular lesions. Electrocardiography is most useful in confirming abnormalities in conduction and rhythm during acute rheumatic carditis.

Differential Diagnosis

Other rheumatic diseases account for most of the disorders misdiagnosed as ARF. ARF can be confused with systemic JIA without carditis (see Chapter 16). Characteristics indicating a diagnosis of JIA rather than ARF include an onset of oligoarticular arthritis in a child before the age of 5 years old; absence of erythema of the joint; a protracted, recurrent course with an incomplete response to nonsteroidal antiinflammatory drug (NSAID) therapy; and in particular, the absence of evidence for antecedent group A streptococcal infection.

Poststreptococcal reactive arthritis (PSRA) poses some difficulty in differentiation from ARF. Clinical findings that should assist in the diagnosis of this disorder are discussed later in this chapter. Other conditions in which joint involvement is common include SLE, Kawasaki disease, mixed connective tissue disease, other reactive arthritides, and serum sickness.[117] Infectious arthritis, particularly gonococcal arthritis, and brucellosis in endemic areas, may present a problem in differential diagnosis. Leukemia and sickle cell disease with bone crises can rarely be mistaken for ARF.

Patients with carditis and pericarditis may develop secondary infections with a variety of bacterial, viral, rickettsial, or mycoplasmal agents. Endocardial involvement occurs in patients with bacterial endocarditis and in patients with SLE and Libman-Sacks endocarditis. A murmur and systolic clicks are present in patients with mitral valve prolapse. Some children with Kawasaki disease develop clinically obvious myocarditis and valvular disease during the early stages of illness. In these patients, the lack of evidence for antecedent group A streptococcal infection allows an initial differentiation from ARF.

Differentiation of Sydenham chorea (SC) from other neurological disorders requires careful evaluation.[118] Imaging studies of the central nervous system are not consistent and may be normal for patients with SC. Increased signal intensity on T-2 weighted images involving the basal ganglia may be seen. Other neurological conditions that may be confused with SC include congenital or acquired "habitual" tick disorders, PANDAS, and other obsessive-compulsive behaviors.[119] ASO and anti-DNase B tests should provide evidence for antecedent streptococcal infection in more than 80% of children with SC. Chorea is also a characteristic symptom in children with the antiphospholipid antibody syndrome (see Chapter 24).

TREATMENT

The initial treatment of ARF should address the eradication of streptococci (Table 44-6). Patients with ARF should be promptly evaluated for cardiac involvement. Subsequent management includes prophylaxis to prevent recurrence of streptococcal infections and treatment of residual cardiac disease.[120]

Eradication of Streptococci

Patients should receive a streptococcal eradicating regimen of antimicrobials even if their throat culture or rapid antigen test is negative.[121] Penicillin is the primary agent of choice administered intramuscularly as a single dose or orally for 10 days. The intramuscular route is preferable in children with cardiac involvement because of its greater dependability and efficacy. Patients allergic to penicillin should receive one of the following: a narrow spectrum cephalosporin, clindamycin, azithromycin, or clarithromycin. Tetracyclines or sulfonamides should not be used to treat group A streptococcal pharyngitis.

Treatment of Clinical Manifestations

Carditis. Acute carditis requires immediate attention.[122] For mild to moderate carditis, aspirin is administered in a dose of 80 to 100 mg/kg/day in four divided doses. This schedule is maintained for 4 to 8 weeks, depending on clinical response, and then is reduced gradually and discontinued during the next 4 weeks. Other NSAIDs have not yet been recommended by the expert committee of the American Heart Association.

Glucocorticoid therapy is reserved for patients with severe carditis and congestive heart failure, particularly those with pancarditis, in whom it may be lifesaving. The use of glucocorticoids, rather than aspirin in patients with heart failure, is also justified to avoid solute overload from aspirin. It should be emphasized that neither form of therapy has been demonstrated to influence the subsequent evolution of valvular disease.[123-125] Unlike most rheumatic diseases, the use of intravenous methylprednisone as a single antiinflammatory agent is inferior to conventional treatment with oral prednisone in the control of severe rheumatic carditis.[126] Prednisone is given orally in a dose of 2 mg/kg once daily. The duration of daily steroid therapy should rarely exceed 2 weeks, and the drug should be tapered and withdrawn during the next 2 to 3 weeks. One week before termination of therapy, aspirin should be instituted (following the regimen described earlier) to avoid the rebound of symptoms and acute phase reactants that occurs when steroid therapy is abruptly terminated.

TABLE 44-6 Antibiotic Regimens for Primary Prevention (Streptococcal Eradication) and Secondary Prevention of Rheumatic Fever

ANTIBIOTIC	DOSE	ROUTE	DURATION
Primary Prevention			
Benzathine penicillin G	600,000 U for patients <27 kg 1,200,000 U for patients >27 kg	Intramuscular	Single dose
Penicillin V	<27 kg 250 mg 2 to 3 times daily >27 kg 500 mg 2 to 3 times daily	Oral	10 days
For individuals allergic to penicillin			
Narrow-spectrum cephalosporins	Variable	Oral Or	10 days
Clindamycin	20 mg/kg/day 3 times daily	Oral Or	10 days
Azithromycin	12 mg/kg once daily	Oral Or	5 days
Clarithromycin	15 mg/kg/day twice daily	Oral	10 days
Secondary Prevention			
Benzathine penicillin G	600,000 U for patients <27 kg 1,200,000 U for patients >27 kg	Intramuscular	Every 4 weeks*
Penicillin V	250 mg twice daily	Oral	
Sulfadiazine	0.5 g once daily <27 kg 1.0 gm daily >27 kg	Oral	
For individuals allergic to penicillin and sulfadiazine			
Macrolide or azalide	Variable	Oral	

*May be given every 3 weeks in high-risk situation.
Adapted from M.A. Gerber, R.S. Baltimore, C.B. Eaton, et al., Prevention of rheumatic fever and diagnosis and treatment of acute streptococcal pharyngitis: a scientific statement from the American Heart Association Rheumatic Fever, Endocarditis, and Kawasaki Disease Committee of the Council on Cardiovascular Disease in the Young, the Interdisciplinary Council on Functional Genomics and Transitional Biology, and the Interdisciplinary Council on Quality of Care and Outcomes Research, Circulation 119 (2009) 1541–1551.

The ESR and CRP levels are essential in monitoring the response to antiinflammatory therapy. In patients with heart failure and a falsely low ESR, a rise in this test result may occur with recovery; the CRP level is more reliable in monitoring the response in these patients. Ancillary therapy for cardiac failure includes the judicious use of drugs to treat congestive heart failure.

The recommendation for complete bed rest for patients with acute carditis, overly emphasized in the past, led to prolonged confinement in bed and cardiac neurosis, and should be discouraged. Gradual resumption of normal activity should be allowed after the acute carditis subsides. Echocardiographic follow-up is predicated on the type and severity of the initial carditis and its response to therapy.[127]

Arthritis. The arthritis characteristically pursues a self-limited course, rarely lasting more than 1 week in any one joint. A hallmark of the arthritis in this disease is its exquisite sensitivity to salicylates. A dose of aspirin of 50 to 75 mg/kg/day given in three to four divided doses is usually effective. This therapy continues for no more than 2 weeks and is thereafter gradually withdrawn. A rapid resolution of the fever and a decline in the ESR usually parallel resolution of the arthritis. A lack of improvement of the arthritis within about 5 days of salicylate therapy should prompt a reconsideration of the correctness of the diagnosis. Other NSAIDs were found to be as effective as aspirin with less side effects.[128] Steroids should not be used in patients with isolated arthritis.

Chorea. Mild manifestations of SC require only bed rest and avoidance of physical and emotional stress. Although anticonvulsant drugs may help control severe symptoms, the response to these agents is unpredictable. Phenobarbital, haloperidol, carbamazepine, and valproate have been used with varying success. Antiinflammatory agents are not needed for the treatment of chorea.

Prophylaxis of Rheumatic Heart Disease

Medical management after the acute stage of the disease centers on prevention of recurrences of rheumatic fever and continued treatment of residual heart disease, including prevention of bacterial endocarditis. Antimicrobial prophylaxis against streptococcal pharyngitis has proved highly effective in reducing recurrences of rheumatic fever and in preventing cumulative heart damage.

Regimens for streptococcal prophylaxis recommended by the American Heart Association are outlined in Table 44-6. Because recurrences of rheumatic fever are most common during the 5 years after the initial attack, intramuscular benzathine penicillin prophylaxis is preferable and should be given once monthly in areas of low incidence of rheumatic fever and every 3 weeks in areas in which this disease is endemic. Oral prophylaxis, when good compliance is confirmed, is acceptable for patients without cardiac involvement. Although sulfonamides are ineffective in eradicating streptococcal infections, these agents are frequently used clinically and appear to be as effective, if not more effective, than oral penicillin for prophylaxis against recurrent streptococcal infections.

Current recommendations protocols of the American Heart Association on rheumatic fever prophylaxis are based on the risk of reinfection and the development of streptococcal pharyngitis.[129] This risk is highest in school-aged children, in persons working in crowded conditions, military recruits, and those in close contact with children, such as parents, teachers, and health care providers. Therefore, patients with carditis should receive prophylaxis well into adulthood, preferably for life, whereas it may be discontinued at the age of 21 years in those with no cardiac involvement (although all such patients should receive prophylaxis for a minimum of 5 years regardless of age).[130] Prophylaxis should be continued after surgical valve repair.

Endocarditis Prophylaxis

Current recommendations for bacterial endocarditis prophylaxis are limited to RHD patients with prosthetic valve replacement, those with a history of endocarditis or those who had a heart transplant. There is no evidence to indicate the routine administration of supplemental doses of antibiotics routinely to all children with RHD prior to surgical or dental procedure. If endocarditis prophylaxis is indicated, then non-penicillin antibiotics are preferred because patients with RHD are already on penicillin prophylaxis, and α-hemolytic streptococci are likely to have developed resistance to penicillin.[121]

Course of the Disease and Prognosis

Major morbidity in rheumatic fever is associated exclusively with the degree of cardiac damage. Severe carditis, which leads to chronic residual valvular disease (see Fig. 44-6), primarily occurs in children in developing countries. The availability of cardiac surgery has alleviated, to a considerable extent, the crippling effect of this complication. Mortality is rare and occurs predominantly in patients with pancarditis. A better understanding of the relationship of streptococcal infection to the occurrence of initial attacks and recurrences of rheumatic fever has led to the institution of prophylactic regimens that have prevented subsequent attacks of the disease and reduced the cumulative heart damage produced by these exacerbations. The study by Tompkins and colleagues[131] emphasizes the singular value of prophylaxis by confirming that signs of rheumatic valvular disease resolve in about 80% of patients who receive continuous, long-term prophylaxis. This information is of particular importance in encouraging patients with rheumatic heart disease to adhere to the prescribed regimen of prophylaxis.

Rheumatic arthritis is self-limited. A rare form of nonerosive but deforming arthropathy ascribed to rheumatic fever (i.e., Jaccoud arthritis) has been reported in adults but has not been reported in children.[132] It is more commonly associated with SLE. SC and erythema marginatum are also self-limited with no permanent residua. Patients who escape severe heart disease and are adherent with prophylaxis can be assured of a benign course and a good prognosis.

Group A Streptococcal Vaccines

The huge burden of illnesses caused by the various types of group A streptococcal (GAS) organisms on health and economies of developed and underdeveloped communities alike has created great interest in the development of an effective means of preventing group A streptococcal diseases. Mass vaccination, theoretically, may be the most effective means of prevention. Several vaccines against GAS have been developed. M protein, the known virulence factor for GAS and the determinant of serotype, has been the target of such vaccines. Because the M protein is encoded for by the *emm* gene, the various GAS M-serotypes correspond to different emm types. Figure 44-7 shows the structure of the M protein with its A, B, C, and D repeat regions. The A repeat region varies between serotypes and contains the highly variable serotype-specific amino acid sequence of M protein at the N terminus. The B repeat region varies from serotype to serotype, whereas the C repeat region contains a conserved sequence shared among all of the serotypes. Two main vaccines have been investigated; the N-terminal M protein based multivalent vaccine (26-valent extended to a 30-valent vaccines) and conserved M protein vaccine.

The multivalent vaccine consists of fused recombinant peptides from the N-terminal region of M proteins from multiple different emm types of GAS.[133] The first effective vaccine is a 26-valent vaccine,[133-135] which has been shown to be safe and immunogenic in humans.[133] Functional opsonic antibodies were induced against all emm types of GAS in the vaccine. The 26-valent vaccine was reformulated into a 30-valent vaccine to increase "coverage" of circulating emm types in the United States, Canada, and Europe as well as developing countries.[135] In preclinical studies, the 30-valent vaccine has also been shown to induce functional opsonic antibodies against all emm types of GAS represented in the vaccine. Although antibodies produced by the vaccine were shown to cross-opsonize a proportion of nonvaccine emm types of GAS it is important to note that vaccines may not be suitable for regions where strains other than the 30 included in the vaccine are circulating.

Conserved M protein vaccines contain antigens from the conserved C repeat portion of the M protein such as the chimeric peptide J8.[136] Laboratory studies have shown that such vaccines produce protective antibodies.[137] These vaccines have the clear advantage of being composed of single antigens. Limited data available for the J8 peptide indicate that its structure is highly conserved among multiple emm types of GAS and across regions.

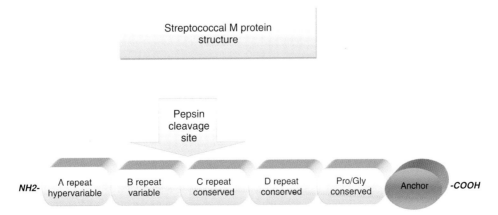

FIGURE 44-7 Proposed model of the M protein. The NH2 terminal of the M protein exhibits hypervariability and confers type specific immunity against the specific M serotype. Vaccines made against epitopes in this end are type specific. The COOH terminal is well conserved between the different M-proteins. A vaccine prepared against epitopes in this conserved region offers broad coverage against GAS.

An important limitation to GAS vaccines is related to its efficacy in preventing some of the serious complications of GAS, such as toxic shock syndrome where strains causing this disease where found not to express the M-protein. Another limitation, although still theoretical, is the possibility that the vaccine itself my trigger an autoimmune process, thus causing arthritis or carditis due to molecular mimicry.

POSTSTREPTOCOCCAL REACTIVE ARTHRITIS

Definition and Classification

The occurrence of arthritis after GAS infection in children who did not fulfill criteria for the diagnosis of ARF was described first by Crea and Mortimer in 1959.[138] Subsequently, many other studies reported on this entity, which was designated poststreptococcal reactive arthritis (PSRA).[81,139-150]

PSRA is distinct from ARF. In PSRA, arthritis appears relatively shortly after the infection. The arthritis is additive and persistent, and can also involve small joints, or the axial skeleton. Furthermore, although the arthritis of ARF responds dramatically to acetylsalicylic acid or NSAIDs, the response to this therapy in PSRA is much more modest.[148]

Epidemiology

Although it is difficult to assess accurately, the incidence of this disease in North-Central Florida was estimated to be one to two cases per 100,000 children at risk per year; 17 of 455 patients with rheumatic diseases encountered over a period of 2 years had PSRA.[81,151] This incidence was twice that for ARF during the same period.[148] The age distribution of PSRA appears to be bimodal; with a peak at ages 8 to 14 years, and another at age 21 to 37 years. In contrast, ARF has a single peak incidence in childhood around 12 years.[149] Both genders are equally affected.

Etiology and Pathogenesis

Evidence for GAS infection should be documented in all patients. In contrast to ARF, in which throat cultures or rapid antigen tests are positive in only one third of patients, results are positive in about 75% of patients with PSRA. This difference can be ascribed to the shorter latency (less than 10 days) for this disease.[142-143,146] Streptococcal pharyngitis is associated with an ASO and an anti-DNase B response in most patients.[81]

Genetic Background

There are conflicting results addressing the association of PSRA with HLA class II alleles. Ahmed et al. found an increased frequency of HLA DRB1*01 in patients with PSRA compared with healthy controls and patients with ARF.[81] In contrast, Simonini et al. did not find significant differences in frequency of various HLA DRB1 alleles (including DRB1*01 and 16) between 25 patients with ARF, 34 with PSRA and healthy controls.[152]

Studies of the relationship of PSRA with HLA-B27 failed to document a significant association[81] only three of 18 (16.7%) white American patients were positive. This frequency contrasts with reactive arthritis in which about 50% of patients are HLA-B27 positive.[153]

Clinical Manifestations

In addition to pharyngitis present in 66% of patients,[80,151] approximately 30% report the occurrence of low-grade fever, and a few describe a nonscarlatinal rash that precedes onset of the arthritis. About one half of the children complain of morning stiffness of varying duration.

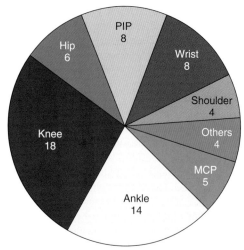

FIGURE 44-8 Frequency of joint involvement in patients with post-streptococcal reactive arthritis. Values represent the number of patients with involvement of that joint. *MCP*, Metacarpopharyngeal; *PIP*, proximal interphalangeal. (From S. Ahmed, E.M. Ayoub, J.C. Scornik, et al., Poststreptococcal reactive arthritis: clinical characteristics and association with HLA-DR alleles, Arthritis Rheum 41 (1998) 1096–1102.)

Arthritis

PSRA arthritis is additive and persistent, and can involve large joints, small joints, axial skeleton, and entheses.[148,154] Most patients present with arthritis involving one or more joints. About 10% complain only of arthralgia. The arthritis is nonmigratory in 70% to 80% and involves joints of the lower extremities in almost all patients. One-half of the patients also have arthritis involving the upper extremities.[81] The frequency of joint involvement is illustrated in Figure 44-8. Barash et al. described migratory arthritis in 79% of 159 pediatric ARF patients compared with 33% of 68 PRSA patients;[148] the arthritis was symmetrical in 40% of those with ARF, and 22% of those with PRSA. van Bemmel et al. described 60 adult patients with PSRA.[155] Small joints were involved in 23% of the patients; large joints were involved in 58%; both large and small joints were affected in 18%. Symmetric distribution was found in 60%. Involvement of upper limb joints was found in 18%, lower limb in 50%, and both in 32%.

Mackie et al.[149] conducted a systematic search on Medline using strict inclusion criteria. They identified 188 adult and pediatric cases of PSRA published in the literature between 1982 and 2002. Eighty-two percent had non-migratory arthritis, 23% monoarthritis, 37% oligo-arthritis, and 37% polyarthritis. Forty-one percent had symmetrical arthritis. The most frequently involved joints were knee, ankle, wrist, and hip. Nine patients had tenosynovitis.

Carditis

There are conflicting reports regarding heart involvement in PSRA.[81,141,143,149-150,155-157] One of 12 pediatric patients with PSRA developed ARF with valvulitis 18 months after the initial episode.[141] Ahmed et al. described carditis in 1 of 25 pediatric PSRA patients 9 month from the onset of arthritis.[81] Two of 40 pediatric patients with PSRA[150] who had normal baseline echocardiograms may have developed cardiac disease at 12 months of follow-up (left ventricular systolic dysfunction, mitral, tricuspid and pulmonary insufficiency). With the exception of the reports cited above, in contrast, in a more recent studies the incidence of late cardiac disease in PSRA patients appears to be negligible or not at all. Van Bemmel et al. described 60 adult PSRA patients who were not treated with antibiotic prophylaxis.

After a median follow-up of 8.9 years, there was no increased risk of valvular heart disease compared with the matched control group of 120 patients who were referred for atypical chest pain, palpitations, or syncope without murmur and had echocardiography.[155] Simonini described 52 children with PSRA, none of whom developed any clinical or echocardiographic evidence of cardiac involvement after a median follow-up of 8 years.[156] Barash et al. described 152 pediatric patients with PSRA, none of whom had late cardiac involvement.[148] In a late outcome follow-up study, no cardiac involvement was found in a large cohort a children.[157]

The 2009 American Heart Association (AHA) scientific statement recommends that patients with PSRA should be observed carefully for several months, for clinical evidence of carditis[121] and be treated with prophylactic penicillin during this time.

Diagnosis and Differential Diagnosis

Proposed criteria for the diagnosis of PSRA are in listed in Box 44-1.[151] The differential diagnosis includes most of the same arthritides outlined for ARF. The similarity in cause, and in some of the clinical manifestations of both diseases, poses unresolved difficulty in differentiating these two entities. However, as outlined in Table 44-7, clinical and laboratory differences should permit the separation of this entity from ARF and other reactive arthritides in most children. Recently, Barash et al. suggested a regression mathematical formula based on four diagnostic discriminators; ESR, CRP, days until resolution of arthritis, and recurrence of arthritis. This model can help to differentiate ARF from PSRA[148]

Laboratory Examination

The ESR and CRP are elevated in 75% of cases, but to a lesser degree than in ARF. The leukocyte count is normal in most patients. The ASO level is elevated in 88% and the anti-DNase B in 80% of patients. At least one of these antibodies is elevated in almost all patients at the time of presentation or shortly thereafter.[81,139] Because of the shorter period of latency between the streptococcal infection and the onset of arthritis, these patients have a higher frequency of positive throat cultures or rapid antigen tests for GAS than patients with ARF.

Treatment

NSAIDs (e.g., naproxen, ibuprofen, and tolmetin) are the principal drugs used in treatment. Aspirin probably offers no particular advantage. The value of disease-modifying drugs, such as methotrexate, has not been assessed. Physical therapy should be instituted for relief of joint pain and stiffness. In some patients the arthritis is poorly responsive to NSAIDS. In this case, a short course of low dose corticosteroids is very effective.

As recommended for patients with GAS pharyngitis and its complications, antimicrobial therapy should be prescribed at the time of initial diagnosis to eradicate streptococci from the tonsillopharyngeal tissue (see Table 44-6).

Antimicrobial prophylaxis to prevent recurrences, and possibly subsequent cardiac disease, has been recommended by some investigators, but this issue is controversial.[158]

The American Heart Association suggests secondary prophylaxis be given for up to 1 year after the onset of symptoms and, if there is no evidence of carditis thereafter, the prophylaxis is discontinued. If valvular disease is detected, the patient should be classified as having had ARF and should continue to receive secondary prophylaxis. However, the effectiveness of this strategy is not well established. The level of evidence for this recommendation is C ("only consensus opinion of experts, case studies, or standard of care") and IIb ("usefulness/efficacy- less well established by evidence/opinion").[121]

Course of the Disease and Prognosis

PSRA is an acute, self-limited disease. Unlike the arthritis of ARF, the course of the arthritis in PSRA might be protracted, lasting days to months, with a mean duration of 2 months from onset to resolution.[81]

BOX 44-1   Proposed Criteria for the Diagnosis of Poststreptococcal Reactive Arthritis

A. Characteristics of the arthritis
  1. Acute-onset arthritis; symmetrical or asymmetrical; usually nonmigratory; can affect any joint
  2. Persistent or recurrent
  3. Poorly responsive to aspirin or nonsteroidal antiinflammatory drugs
B. Evidence of antecedent group A streptococcal infection
C. Does not fulfill the modified Jones Criteria for the diagnosis of acute rheumatic fever

Adapted from E.M. Ayoub, S. Ahmed, Update on complications of Group A streptococcal infections, Curr Probl Pediatr 27 (1997) 90–101.

TABLE 44-7   Clinical and Laboratory Differences Between Poststreptococcal Reactive Arthritis and Acute Rheumatic Fever

	PSRA	ARF
Age	Bimodal: 8-14 years and 21-37 years	5-15 years with peak incidence around 12 years
Disease Onset Poststreptococcal Infection	7-10 days	10-28 days
Joint Involvement	Additive and persistent; large, small and axial joints	Migratory, transient; mainly large joints
Acute Phase Reactants	Moderately elevated	Markedly elevated
Response of Arthritis to Acetylsalicylic Acid or NSAID Treatment	Poor to moderate	Dramatic
Genetic Markers	Increased frequency of HLA DRB1*01	Increased frequency of the HLA DRB1*16 allele
Carditis	Conflicting reports, but uncommon	Major diagnostic criteria, between 60-70%
Antibiotic Prophylaxis	Antibiotic prophylaxis for one year if echocardiogram is normal	Long-term secondary antibiotic prophylaxis

ARF, Acute rheumatic fever; HLA, human leukocyte antigen; NSAID, nonsteroidal antiinflammatory drugs; PSRA, poststreptococcal reactive arthritis.
(Adapted from Y. Uziel, L. Perl, J. Barash, P.J. Hashkes, Post-streptococcal reactive arthritis in children: a distinct entity from acute rheumatic fever, Pediatr Rheumatol Online J 9 (2011) 32.)

Some patients continue to have arthralgia for several months after remission of the arthritis. This prolonged course is not altered significantly by the administration of NSAIDs or antimicrobials, but responds to corticosteroids.

Acknowledgment

This chapter is dedicated to the memory of Elia Ayoub, MD.

REFERENCES

2. G.H. Stollerman, Rheumatogenic group A streptococci and the return of rheumatic fever, Adv. Intern. Med. 35 (1990) 1–25.

3. A.C. Steer, J.R. Carapetis, T.M. Nolan, et al., Systematic review of rheumatic heart disease prevalence in children in developing countries: the role of environmental factors, J. Paediatr. Child Health 38 (2002) 229–234.

4. M. Markowitz, The decline of rheumatic fever: role of medical intervention. Lewis W. Wannamaker Memorial Lecture, J. Pediatr. 106 (1985) 545–550.

5. L.G. Veasy, S.E. Wiedmeier, G.S. Orsmond, et al., Resurgence of acute rheumatic fever in the intermountain area of the United States, N. Engl. J. Med. 316 (1987) 421–427.

9. S.P. Griffiths, W.M. Gersony, Acute rheumatic fever in New York City (1969 to 1988): a comparative study of two decades, J. Pediatr. 116 (1990) 882–887.

17. L.G. Veasy, L.Y. Tani, H.R. Hill, Persistence of acute rheumatic fever in the intermountain area of the United States, J. Pediatr. 124 (1994) 9–16.

22. K.B. Tibazarwa, J.A. Volmink, B.M. Mayosi, Incidence of acute rheumatic fever in the world: a systematic review of population-based studies, Heart 84 (2008) 1534–1540.

24. L. Gordis, The virtual disappearance of rheumatic fever in the United States: lessons in the rise and fall of disease. T. Duckett Jones memorial lecture, Circulation 72 (1985) 1155–1162.

26. L.W. Wannamaker, Differences between streptococcal infections of the throat and of the skin (second of two parts), N. Engl. J. Med. 282 (1970) 78–85.

31. I. Goldstein, B. Halpern, L. Robert, Immunologic relation between streptococcus A polysaccharide and the structural glycoproteins of heart valve, Nature 213 (1967) 44–47.

34. J.C. Smoot, E.K. Korgenski, J.A. Daly, et al., Molecular analysis of group A streptococcus type emm18 isolates temporally associated with acute rheumatic fever outbreaks in Salt Lake City, Utah, J. Clin. Microbiol. 40 (2002) 1805–1810.

36. D. Bessen, K.F. Jones, V.A. Fischetti, Evidence for two distinct classes of streptococcal M protein and their relationship to rheumatic fever, J. Exp. Med. 169 (1989) 269–283.

37. J.C. Smoot, K.D. Barbian, J.J. Van Gompel, et al., Genome sequence and comparative microarray analysis of serotype M18 group A Streptococcus strains associated with acute rheumatic fever outbreaks, Proc. Natl. Acad. Sci. U.S.A. 99 (2002) 4668–4673.

39. E.M. Ayoub, E. Kaplan, Host-parasite interaction in the pathogenesis of rheumatic fever, J. Rheumatol. Suppl. 30 (1991) 6–13.

41. J. Sandson, D. Hamerman, R. Janis, et al., Immunologic and chemical similarities between the streptococcus and human connective tissue, Trans. Assoc. Am. Physicians 81 (1968) 249–257.

45. D.L. Stevens, Streptococcal toxic-shock syndrome: spectrum of disease, pathogenesis, and new concepts in treatment, Emerg. Infect. Dis. 1 (1995) 69–78.

52. B.A. Dudding, E.M. Ayoub, Persistence of streptococcal group A antibody in patients with rheumatic valvular disease, J. Exp. Med. 128 (1968) 1081–1098.

53. E.M. Ayoub, S.T. Shulman, Pattern of antibody response to the streptococcal group A carbohydrate in rheumatic patients with or without carditis, in: S.E. Read, J.B. Zabriskie (Eds.), Streptococcal disease and the immune response, Academic Press, New York, 1980.

55. E.M. Ayoub, Immune response to group A streptococcal infections, Pediatr. Infect. Dis. J. 10 (1991) S15–S19.

56. M.H. Kaplan, M. Meyeserian, An immunological cross-reaction between group-A streptococcal cells and human heart tissue, Lancet 1 (1962) 706–710.

62. G. Husby, I. van de Rign, J.B. Zabriskie, et al., Antibodies reacting with cytoplasm of subthalamic and caudate nuclei neurons in chorea and acute rheumatic fever, J. Exp. Med. 144 (1976) 1094–1110.

70. L. Harel, A. Zeharia, Y. Kodman, et al., Presence of the d8/17 B-cell marker in children with rheumatic fever in Israel, Clin. Genet. 61 (2002) 293–298.

79. W. Weidebach, A.C. Goldberg, J.M. Chiarella, et al., HLA class II antigens in rheumatic fever: analysis of the DR locus by restriction fragment-length polymorphism and oligotyping, Hum. Immunol. 40 (1994) 253–258.

80. Y. Guedez, A. Kotby, M. El Demellawy, et al., HLA class II associations with rheumatic heart disease are more evident and consistent among clinically homogeneous patients, Circulation 99 (1999) 2784–2790.

81. S. Ahmed, E.M. Ayoub, J.C. Scornik, et al., Poststreptococcal reactive arthritis: clinical characteristics and association with HLA-DR alleles, Arthritis Rheum. 41 (1998) 1096–1102.

82. V. Stanevicha, J. Eglite, A. Sochnevs, et al., HLA class II associations with rheumatic heart disease among clinically homogeneous patients in children in Latvia, Arthritis Res. Ther. 5 (2003) R340–R346.

89. J.R. Carapetis, B.J. Currie, Rheumatic fever in a high incidence population: the importance of monoarthritis and low grade fever, Arch. Dis. Child. 85 (2001) 223–227.

90. R.V. Williams, L.L. Minich, R.E. Shaddy, et al., Evidence for lack of myocardial injury in children with acute rheumatic carditis, Cardiol. Young 12 (2002) 519–523.

94. S.E. Swedo, H.L. Leonard, M. Garvey, et al., Pediatric autoimmune Neuropsychiatric disorders associated with streptococcal infections: clinical description of the first 50 cases, Am. J. Psychiatry 155 (1998) 264–271.

95. P. Pavone, R. Bianchini, E. Parano, et al., Anti-brain antibodies in Pandas versus uncomplicated streptococcal infection, Pediatr. Neurol. 30 (2004) 107–110.

96. L.A. Snider, V. Sachdev, J.E. MaCkaronis, et al., Echocardiographic findings in the PANDAS subgroup, Pediatrics 114 (2004) e748–e751.

99. M. Gupta, R.W. Lent, E.L. Kaplan, et al., Serum cardiac troponin I in acute rheumatic fever, Am. J. Cardiol. 89 (2002) 779–782.

103. P.C. Faustino, M.T. Terreri, A.J. da Rocha, et al., Clinical, laboratory, psychiatric and magnetic resonance findings in patients with Sydenham chorea, Neuroradiology 45 (2003) 456–462.

110. S. Sethi, K. Kaushik, K. Mohandas, et al., Anti-streptolysin O titers in normal healthy children of 5-15 years, Indian Pediatr. 40 (2003) 1068–1071.

112. Z. Golbasi, O. Ucar, T. Keles, et al., Increased levels of high sensitive C-reactive protein in patients with chronic rheumatic valve disease: evidence of ongoing inflammation, Eur. J. Heart Fail. 4 (2002) 593–595.

113. B. Oran, H. Coban, S. Karaaslan, et al., Serum cardiac troponin-I in active rheumatic carditis, Indian J. Pediatr. 68 (2001) 943–944.

114. J.R. Carapetis, A. Brown, N.J. Wilson, K.N. Edwards, On behalf of the Rheumatic Fever Guidelines Writing Group: An Australian guideline for rheumatic fever and rheumatic heart disease: an abridged outline, MJA 186 (2007) 581–586.

117. H.M. Sondheimer, A. Lorts, Cardiac involvement in inflammatory disease: systemic lupus erythematosus, rheumatic fever, and Kawasaki disease, Adolesc. Med. 12 (2001) 69–78.

120. S.T. Shulman, Acute streptococcal pharyngitis in pediatric medicine: current issues in diagnosis and management, Paediatr. Drugs 5 (2003) 13–23.

121. M.A. Gerber, R.S. Baltimore, C.B. Eaton, et al., Prevention of rheumatic fever and diagnosis and treatment of acute streptococcal pharyngitis: a scientific statement from the American Heart Association Rheumatic Fever, Endocarditis, and Kawasaki Disease Committee of the Council on Cardiovascular Disease in the Young, the Interdisciplinary Council on Functional Genomics and Transitional Biology, and the Interdisciplinary Council on Quality of Care and Outcomes Research, Circulation 119 (2009) 1541–1551.

123. United Kingdom and United States Joint Report, The treatment of acute rheumatic fever in children: a cooperative clinical trial of ACTH, cortisone and aspirin, Circulation 11 (1955) 343–371.

124. United Kingdom and United States Joint Report, The evolution of rheumatic heart disease in children: five year report of a cooperative clinical trial of ACTH, cortisone and aspirin, Circulation 22 (1960) 503–515.

125. United Kingdom and United States Joint Report, The natural history of rheumatic fever and rheumatic heart disease: ten-year report of a cooperative clinical trial of ACTH, cortisone, and aspirin, Circulation 32 (1965) 457–476.

127. F.E. Figueroa, M.S. Fernandez, P. Valdes, et al., Prospective comparison of clinical and echocardiographic diagnosis of rheumatic carditis: long term follow up of patients with subclinical disease, Heart 85 (2001) 407–410.

130. Committee on Infectious Diseases American Academy of Pediatrics, Red Book 2012 Report of the Committee on Infectious Diseases, Twenty-ninth ed., AAP, Elk Grove Village, IL, 2012.

131. D.G. Tompkins, B. Boxerbaum, J. Liebman, Long-term prognosis of rheumatic fever patients receiving regular intramuscular benzathine penicillin, Circulation 45 (1972) 543–551.

139. Y. Uziel, L. Perl, J. Barash, et al., Post-streptococcal reactive arthritis in children: a distinct entity from acute rheumatic fever, Pediatr Rheumatol Online J 9 (2011) 32.

147. E.M. Ayoub, H.A. Majeed, Poststreptococcal reactive arthritis, Curr. Opin. Rheumatol. 12 (2000) 306–310.

148. J. Barash, E. Mashiach, P. Navon-Elkan, et al., Differentiation of post-streptococcal reactive arthritis from acute rheumatic fever, J. Pediatr. 153 (2008) 696–699.

149. S.L. Mackie, A. Keat, Poststreptococcal reactive arthritis: what is it and how do we know?, Rheumatology (Oxford) 43 (2004) 949–954.

151. E.M. Ayoub, S. Ahmed, Update on complications of group A streptococcal infections, Curr. Probl. Pediatr. 27 (1997) 90–101.

155. J.M. van Bemmel, V. Delgado, E.R. Holman, et al., No increased risk of valvular heart disease in adult poststreptococcal reactive arthritis, Arthritis Rheum. 60 (2009) 987–993.

156. G. Simonini, A. Taddio, R. Cimaz, et al., No evidence yet to change American Heart Association recommendations for poststreptococcal reactive arthritis: comment on the article by van Bemmel, Arthritis Rheum. 60 (2009) 3516–3518.

157. Y. Uziel, Y. Kwint, A. Matitiahu, et al., Late cardiac assessment in children who were diagnosed with post streptococcal reactive arthritis – a long term study, Pediatric Rheumatology 11 (Suppl. 2) (2013) O27. 5 December 2013.

Entire reference list is available online at www.expertconsult.com.

Musculoskeletal Manifestations of Systemic Disease

Ross E. Petty, Carol B. Lindsley

Many nonrheumatic systemic disorders cause musculoskeletal signs or symptoms, most commonly arthralgia, arthritis, myalgia, or bone pain. Sometimes these are trivial; however, occasionally they are the presentations of the underlying disease. This chapter outlines some systemic disorders that may present in the guise of a rheumatic disease. Rheumatic manifestations of malignancies are discussed in Chapter 50. It is not our intent to describe comprehensively the clinical and laboratory manifestations or management of such disorders, which can be found in standard textbooks dealing with the specific diseases.

DISORDERS RELATED TO VITAMIN DEFICIENCY OR EXCESS

A number of disorders in which there is a deficiency or excess of certain vitamins result in signs or symptoms that suggest a rheumatic disease.

Rickets and Osteomalacia

Rickets and osteomalacia are diseases associated with defective ossification of bone matrix. Rickets is a disease of the physis, and occurs only in children. Osteomalacia is a disease affecting the other sites of bone formation and occurs in both children and adults.[1,2] Rickets has many causes, which can be identified as being either calcipenic (mostly related to deficiency of the active form of vitamin D [1,25-dihydroxyvitamin D_3] or calcium deficiency), or phosphopenic (mostly resulting from renal wasting of phosphate) (Table 45-1).

Most cases of rickets worldwide result from exclusion from the sun for social or cultural reasons, or from insufficient dietary intake of vitamin D.[3,4] Vitamin D–deficiency rickets is seldom encountered in developed countries, but may occur in infantile and adolescent forms in the rest of the world.[1,5] It may also develop in the presence of sufficient dietary vitamin D, when there is impaired absorption because of celiac disease, inflammatory bowel disease, scleroderma, or liver disease. Maternal vitamin D insufficiency can influence fetal bone development as early as 19 weeks' gestation.[6] Some types (i.e., hypophosphatemic rickets and rickets associated with hypophosphatasia) are associated with defective mineralization and are classified as osteochondrodysplasias, as discussed in Chapter 53. Disorders such as cystinosis that result in renal tubular acidosis, may present as rickets with pain in the joints and metaphyseal enlargement (Fig. 45-1). Administration of some anticonvulsant medications interferes with vitamin D metabolism and, in children deprived of sunlight, may also be a cause.

The normal source of vitamin D_3 in humans is the skin in which ultraviolet rays of sunlight convert 7-dehydrocholesterol into the vitamin prohormone.[7] This compound is subsequently transformed to the 25-hydroxy form in the liver and then to active 1,25-dihydroxyvitamin in the kidney (Fig. 45-2). A deficiency of 1,25-dihydroxyvitamin D_3 may result from a nutritional deficiency, from hepatic failure to convert vitamin D to 25-hydroxyvitamin D, or from failure of the kidney to convert 25-hydroxyvitamin D to 1,25-dihydroxyvitamin D_3.

Hypophosphatemic vitamin D–resistant rickets, when expressed in infancy, leads to short stature, bowing of the legs, and ectopic calcification.[2,8] This disorder is inherited as an X-linked recessive or autosomal dominant trait, although sporadic cases occur. The basic defect is impaired parathormone-dependent proximal renal tubular reabsorption of phosphate. A low serum phosphate concentration with a normal calcium level is characteristic.

Type I vitamin D–dependent rickets is an autosomal recessive defect in renal 1-α–hydroxylase that results in failure of hydroxylation of 25-hydroxyvitamin D to 1,25-dihydroxyvitamin D_3. The onset of typical features of rickets occurs before the age of 2 years. Type II vitamin D–dependent rickets is rare and characterized by defective intracellular interaction between 1,25-dihydroxyvitamin D_3 and its receptor. Symptoms of rickets begin in early infancy. Alopecia and absence of eyelashes occur frequently in this disorder.[9]

Hypophosphatasia, a rare autosomal recessive disorder caused by a mutation in the gene for tissue-nonspecific alkaline phosphatase (TNSALP), presents in infancy as severe rickets and fractures.[2,10] Band keratopathy, proptosis, and papilledema develop. There may be early loss of teeth. Chondrocalcinosis and pseudogout may be associated features. There is a marked depression in the concentration of serum alkaline phosphatase. Treatment with nonsteroidal antiinflammatory drugs may lead to symptomatic improvement.[11] Recent reports have noted an association between hypophosphatasia and chronic recurrent multifocal osteomyelitis (chronic nonbacterial osteomyelitis) in at least four children.[12,13]

The child with rickets presents with joint pain and tenderness over the bones. Rickets can occasionally mimic inflammatory arthritis.[14] Bowing of the long bones and splaying of the rib cage are characteristic features. Proximal muscle weakness, particularly of the lower extremities, is occasionally prominent. Defective bone growth results from suppression of calcification and maturation of epiphyseal cartilage. The result is a wide, frayed, irregular zone of uncalcified osteoid at the epiphyseal line—the rachitic metaphysis (Fig. 45-3).

Scurvy

Ascorbic acid (vitamin C) is required for the formation of normal collagen and chondroitin sulfate.[15] Vitamin C is neither synthesized nor stored in the body, and in the malnourished child a deficiency of

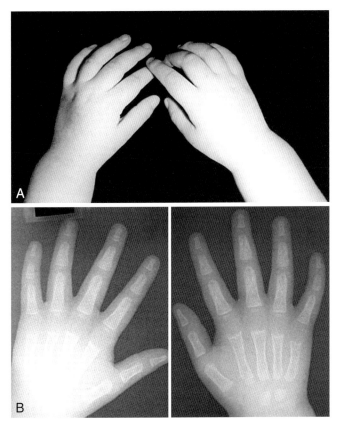

FIGURE 45-1 Cystinosis. An 18-month-old girl presented with joint pain primarily involving the large joints and profound muscle weakness due to cystinosis. **A,** Hands demonstrate swelling predominantly in the metaphyseal area of the radius and ulna, but not in the wrist joint proper. **B,** Radiographs document metaphyseal resorption that is typical of rickets.

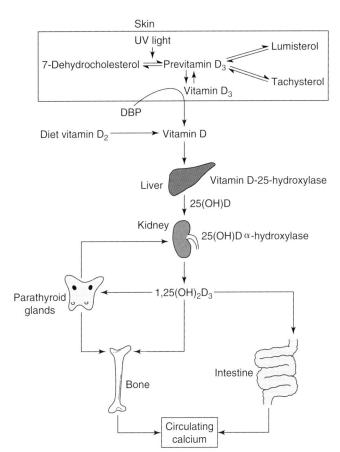

FIGURE 45-2 Metabolism of vitamin D. Previtamin D_3 is formed in the skin and isomerizes to vitamin D_3 or other biologically inert isomers. Vitamin D binding protein (DBP) has an affinity only for vitamin D_3, which is translocated to the circulation. Vitamin D is then hydroxylated in the liver and kidney to the active metabolite, $1,25(OH)_2D_3$. (From A.K. Bhalla, Osteoporosis and osteomalacia, in: P.J. Maddison, D.A. Isenberg, P. Woo, D.N. Glass (Eds.), Oxford Textbook of Rheumatology, Oxford University Press, Oxford, England, 1993, p. 1005.)

TABLE 45-1	**Causes of Rickets**
TYPE	**CAUSE OR BIOCHEMICAL ABNORMALITY**
Vitamin D deficiency	Exclusion from light or insufficient dietary vitamin D
Calcium deficiency	Impaired calcium absorption in celiac disease, inflammatory bowel disease, scleroderma, or liver disease
Vitamin D resistance	Impaired parathormone-dependent proximal renal tubular reabsorption of phosphate
Vitamin D dependence	
Type 1	Defect in renal 1-α-hydroxylase
Type 2	End-organ unresponsiveness to 1, 25-dihydroxyvitamin D_3
Hypophosphatasia	Decreased serum alkaline phosphatase

dietary vitamin C may lead to scurvy with poor collagen synthesis and intradermal, gingival, and subperiosteal hemorrhage.[16] Subperiosteal hemorrhage results in severe bone pain in the arms and legs; the child, usually an infant, assumes the flexed posture of pseudoparalysis and is irritable when picked up. Synovitis is rare, but hemarthroses may occur. In severe cases "scorbutic beads," resulting from subluxation of the sternum at the costochondral junctions, may be visible on physical examination. Radiographs demonstrate subperiosteal new bone apposition. Treatment with oral or parenteral vitamin C results in definite improvement within 2 weeks.[15-17]

Hypervitaminosis A

A large number of physiological functions, organogenesis, and embryogenesis are affected by vitamin A and the derivative retinoids.[18] Excess intake of vitamin A or retinoids causes pain in the extremities, irritability, apathy, alopecia, and delayed growth.[19] Cortical hyperostosis (e.g., metatarsal bones, ulnas, spine) is a typical radiographic finding. Abnormal epiphyseal growth and periosteal new bone apposition occur occasionally.

DISORDERS RELATED TO ENVIRONMENTAL FACTORS

Kashin-Beck Disease

An endemic progressive osteoarthropathy primarily affecting children between the ages of 5 and 15 years, has a prevalence of 1% to 2% in affected areas of Tibet, northwestern China, northeastern Russia, and North Korea.[20] It is unassociated with systemic or visceral manifestations. The etiology is uncertain, but it may result from *Fusarium* mycotoxins in fungus-infected grain or from selenium or iodine deficiency.[21-24] Experimental animals fed grain infected with *Fusarium* species develop a similar form of epiphyseal dysplasia.[21] There is depletion of aggregating proteoglycan (aggrecan),[25] which results in an epiphyseal dysplasia from a zonal necrosis of chondrocytes of the epiphyses and metaphyses.[26] These abnormalities increase in severity as long as the child lives in the endemic area and eats foods made with

the contaminated grain. Excessive amounts of iron in the water and diet may contribute further to the polyarthritis. A genetic influence has been proposed in humans[27] and in a murine model.[28] Differences in gene expression by osteoarthritis cartilage and cartilage from adults with Kashin–Beck disease imply different pathogenic mechanisms.[29]

Kashin–Beck disease causes symmetric polyarthritis and progressive enlargement and limitation of motion involving multiple joints (i.e., elbows, interphalangeal joints, wrists, knees, and ankles).[30,31] In the school-age child, morning stiffness, aching, and muscle weakness are the initial symptoms. Joint effusions and laboratory indices of inflammation are absent early in the disease. The eventual dwarfing, epiphyseal deformity, and short digits resemble those encountered in the lysosomal storage diseases. Radiographic findings include irregular erosions of the small bones of the hands and feet. Treatment with selenium may be beneficial.[32] Although iodine supplementation may be important,[33] iodine deficiency is not thought to be a causative factor.

Mseleni Joint Disease

Mseleni joint disease is a chronic polyarthritis that affects a large proportion of the Tsonga population of the Mseleni area of northern Zululand on the eastern seaboard of South Africa.[34-36] Onset of joint pain in childhood or adolescence is the first symptom of the disease. Restriction of movement and limitation of mobility develop at a variable rate. Mild stunting of growth is common, and a few patients develop severe dwarfing (Table 45-2). The life span is not shortened. Characteristic radiographic abnormalities include irregularity of the surface, density, and shape of the epiphyses that progresses to a secondary osteoarthritis; in the hips, which bear the brunt of the disease, protrusio acetabuli occurs in females (Fig. 45-4). Short metacarpals, ulna, and radius, and a deformity of the distal end of the ulna are also present. The diagnosis is usually obvious in the geographic and racial context, but the clinical presentation may suggest cretinism, brucellosis, hemochromatosis, alkaptonuria, and Legg–Calvé–Perthes disease at different stages of its development. Hips, knees, and ankles are the predominant sites of involvement in 66% of women, 25% of men, 7% of girls, and 4% of boys. Hands, wrists, shoulders, and elbows are less commonly affected. Neither a genetic nor an environmental cause has been identified. Handigodu, an idiopathic familial arthropathy found in a small area of southern India, closely resembles Mseleni joint disease, both clinically and radiographically.[37]

Fluorosis

Fluorosis is endemic in certain areas of the world, particularly Asia and Africa, and results in chronic rheumatic symptoms in children.[38] High levels of fluoride may occur naturally in the water supply or may result from pollution. Radiologically identified skeletal fluorosis was reported in 8% of children living in households with indoor coal-burning stoves

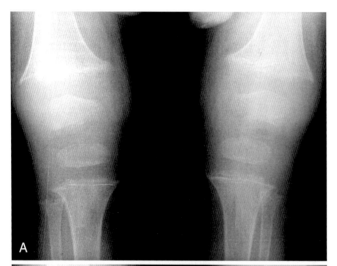
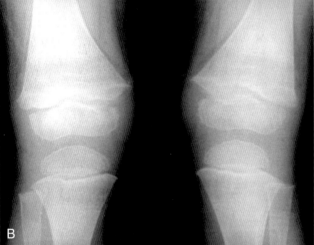

FIGURE 45-3 Vitamin D–deficient rickets in a toddler. **A,** Radiographs of knees demonstrate rachitic metaphyseal changes, indistinct cortices, and poorly defined trabeculation. The zone of provisional calcification is almost absent, the axial height of the epiphyseal plate is markedly increased, and cupping is evident. **B,** X-ray films taken 6 months later demonstrate progressive healing with replacement of vitamin D.

TABLE 45-2	Mseleni Joint Disease and Kashin–Beck Disease	
CHARACTERISTIC	**MSELENI JOINT DISEASE**	**KASHIN–BECK DISEASE**
First noted	6 yr to adult	6-10 yr
Inherited	Probably not	Probably not
Sex ratio	More females	More males
Stunting of growth	Slight to severe	Moderate
Posture	Lumbar lordosis, genu valgum	Lumbar lordosis, neck extended, knees flexed
Precocious osteoarthritis	Yes	Yes
Radiology	Fragmented epiphyses, flared metaphyses, brachymetacarpia, protrusio acetabuli, platyspondyly	Dysplastic interphalangeal, wrist, knee, ankle joints intraarticular loose bodies

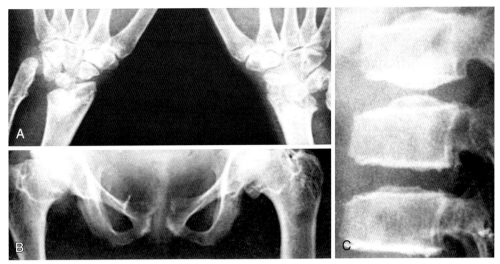

FIGURE 45-4 Mseleni joint disease. **A,** Irregularity and deformity of the distal ends of the ulna and radius with distraction of the radius from the ulna. **B,** Marked deformation of the femoral heads. **C,** Platyspondyly. (Courtesy Dr. G. Lockitch.)

in southern China,[39] and in 4.4% of children in an area of Tanzania with high water fluoride content.[40] Dental fluorosis is an early sign of toxicity. Knee pain is often an early symptom, followed by limb, hand, or characteristic spinal abnormalities that suggest a chronic inflammatory arthropathy. Radiographs demonstrate increased bone density and later show calcification of the spinal ligaments, intervertebral disks, and entheses.[41] Cord compression can result from narrowing of the spinal canal. There is a marked periosteal reaction in the long bones.

METABOLIC DISEASES

Abnormalities of Uric Acid Metabolism

Gout

The term gout refers to a group of disorders characterized by hyperuricemia and deposition of monosodium urate monohydrate crystals in tissues. Its major clinical manifestations include an acute monoarthritis, most commonly in the first metatarsophalangeal joint; chronic erosive arthritis associated with subcutaneous periarticular deposits of urate (tophi); and nephrolithiasis, often leading to chronic renal failure.

Serum urate levels increase normally at puberty, particularly in males, from approximately 3.5 mg/dL (0.21 mmol/L) in childhood to an upper limit of 7 mg/dL (0.42 mmol/L) in adult males, and 6 mg/dL (0.36 mmol/L) in adult females. Above these concentrations, the serum becomes saturated with urate.

Gout may result from increased production or decreased excretion of uric acid (Box 45-1). Diagnosis is confirmed by demonstration with compensated polarized light microscopy of negatively birefringent, needle-shaped monosodium urate crystals in synovial fluid (Fig. 45-5). Ultrasound, magnetic resonance imaging, and dual-energy CT have also been used to demonstrate urate in tophi.[42] Treatment of the acute attack with nonsteroidal antiinflammatory drugs (NSAIDs) such as indomethacin, or with colchicine, is usually effective. Short-term corticosteroids may be needed. After the acute episode has subsided, allopurinol is the drug of choice for prevention of recurrences.[43]

Gouty arthropathy is rare in children. Treadwell identified 66 patients younger than 20 years who were reported between 1769 and

---

BOX 45-1   Causes of Hyperuricemia and Gout

Increased Uric Acid Production
Primary
Lesch–Nyhan syndrome
Becker syndrome (phosphoribosyl pyrophosphate synthetase superactivity)

Secondary
Glycogenosis type I (glucose-6-phosphate dehydrogenase deficiency)
Myeloproliferative disorders
Lymphoproliferative disorders
Severe psoriasis
Gaucher disease
Cytotoxic drugs
Hypoxia
Chronic hemolysis
Secondary polycythemia

Decreased Uric Acid Excretion
Reduced glomerular filtration rate
Reduced fractional urate excretion
Down syndrome
Lead nephropathy
Analgesic nephropathy
Amyloidosis
Sickle cell anemia
Sarcoidosis
Hypothyroidism
Hyperparathyroidism
Increased levels of organic acids
Type I glycogen storage disease
Maple syrup urine disease
Drugs
Diuretics
Salicylates (low dose)
Levodopa

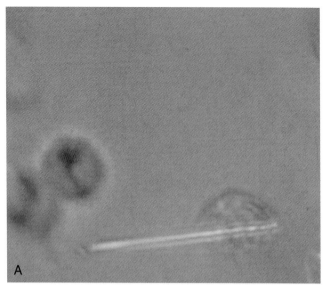

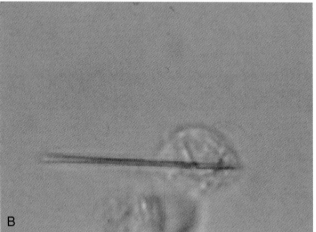

FIGURE 45-5 Urate crystals visualized with a polarizing microscope. A bright needle-shaped crystal of sodium urate monohydrate **(A)** shows negative birefringence **(B)** when viewed with a compensated polarized light microscope.

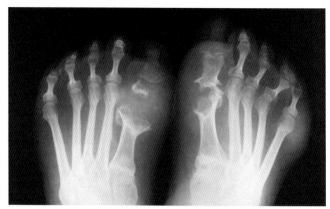

FIGURE 45-6 Radiograph of the forefeet of an adolescent boy with gout. Note destructive changes in the first metatarsophalangeal joints. Soft tissue swellings adjacent to these joints and the right fifth metatarsophalangeal joint are sites of tophi. (Photograph courtesy Dr. Jorge Jaimes).

TABLE 45-3	Lesch–Nyhan Syndrome
Clinical characteristics	Progressive development of choreoathetosis, spasticity, and mental retardation with self-mutilation
Genetics	X-linked recessive
Biochemical defect	Deficiency of hypoxanthine-guanine phosphoribosyltransferase
Laboratory findings	Hyperuricemia and uric acid crystalluria

1960 and added two additional cases.[44] In many early publications, the exact diagnosis is in doubt. The onset of gouty arthritis in a 14-year-old boy as a result of chronic compensated hemolysis of unknown cause has been described.[45] Yarom and colleagues[46] reported two children with marked hyperuricemia, mild renal failure, and acute, episodic, painful swelling of one joint, often the first metatarsophalangeal joint, knee, ankle, elbow, or a proximal interphalangeal joint of the hand. The authors have seen two unrelated boys with gout presenting as polyarthritis. Gout has also been reported in children with glycogen storage disease,[47] malignancy,[48] renal failure,[49,50] and in an adolescent with juvenile idiopathic arthritis (JIA).[51] Typical radiographic changes in a teenage boy are shown in Fig 45-6.

An exceptionally large group of children and youth with juvenile gout has been reported in Taiwan.[52] Juvenile gout accounted for 543 patients, 1.9% of all patients with the disease, and occurred in children as young as 8 years of age; 97% were male. Although greater than one half of the patients had a paternal history of gout, there is as yet no genetic explanation for this disease or for the uniquely high prevalence of gout in this age group in Taiwan.

Lesch–Nyhan Syndrome

The Lesch–Nyhan syndrome, first described in 1967 as an X-linked recessive disorder of uric acid metabolism and central nervous system dysfunction, results from a deficiency of the enzyme hypoxanthine-guanine phosphoribosyltransferase (HPRT) resulting in an overproduction of uric acid and uric aciduria. (Table 45-3).[53-56] There is a range of clinical phenotypes,[57] the most severe of which is characterized by developmental delay, choreoathetosis, and spasticity beginning in the first year of life. These abnormalities progress, and by 2 to 4 years of age, the child develops self-mutilation (lips, fingers). With rare exceptions,[58,59] affected boys do not develop acute gouty arthritis, at least not until the adolescent or adult years. Severity of the disorder is determined by the degree of HPRT deficiency resulting from unique mutations in each family.[56] Variants of Lesch–Nyhan syndrome have much less neurologic disease, but more frequent gout and nephrolithiasis and its complications. Lesch–Nyhan variants have been called the Kelley–Seegmiller syndrome, although Torres et al[57] present arguments against the appropriateness of this eponym.

Treatment with allopurinol, which blocks the conversion of xanthine and hypoxanthine to uric acid, effectively prevents the rheumatic complaints but does not alter the central nervous system disease, for which there is no effective therapy.

Phosphoribosyl Pyrophosphate Synthetase Superactivity

An X-linked mutation resulting in excessive activity of phosphoribosyl pyrophosphate synthetase (PPRPS), the enzyme that converts ribose-5-phosphate to PP-ribose-phosphate, results in increased purine production and is a rare cause of gout in children and young adults, sometimes with neurologic deficits and sensorineural deafness.[60,61] Allopurinol effectively controls this disorder.

Glucose-6-Phosphatase Deficiency

Glycogen storage disease type I (von Gierke disease) may be associated with the onset of gouty arthritis[62,63] or tendinitis[47] in childhood. Children with this disorder are stunted and have marked hepatomegaly, progressive mental retardation, abnormalities of platelet function, and hypoglycemia. Hyperuricemia results from increased catabolism of adenosine triphosphate and decreased urate excretion. Other types of glycogen storage disease and other metabolic disorders may have musculoskeletal manifestations, especially myopathy.[64-66]

Calcium Pyrophosphate Deposition Disease

Crystals of calcium pyrophosphate dihydrate (CPPD) in synovial fluid and joint structures are associated with a chronic inflammatory and degenerative joint disease (pseudogout).[67] The wrists, knees, shoulders, and ankles are most commonly affected. Synovial fluid CPPD crystals are positively birefringent when viewed through a compensated polarized light microscope and are shorter than urate crystals. The disease occurs almost exclusively in older adults. It has rarely been noted in adolescence.[68] Chondrocalcinosis, is a term that refers to the radiologic appearance of CPPD crystals in hyaline cartilage and fibrocartilage. Radiographs demonstrate linear calcifications in the menisci of the knee and in other cartilaginous structures, such as the triangular cartilage of the wrist.[69] In descriptions of familial chondrocalcinosis, however, there have been rare reports of adolescents in whom the disorder presented as an acute, self-limited polyarthritis, often precipitated by exercise or trauma.[70] The characteristics of the clinical disease have varied, however, depending on the kindred, age at onset, severity, and the presence of an associated osteoarthritis or chondrodysplasia.

Ochronosis

Ochronosis (alkaptonuria) is an autosomal recessive defect in homogentisic acid oxidase resulting in the accumulation of homogentisic acid in tissues, pigmentation of cartilage (e.g., ears, sclerae, heart valves), calcification and ossification of the intervertebral disks, accelerated osteoporosis and osteoarthritis, and vascular disease.[71] Black urine or staining of the diapers is often the sign that prompts referral of the child with this metabolic defect. Arthritis related to ochronosis has not been reported in children.

Hyperlipoproteinemia

Defects in lipoprotein metabolism are associated with a high risk of premature atherosclerosis, coronary artery disease, and musculoskeletal abnormalities. Articular and tendinous swelling accompany essential familial hypercholesterolemia and hypertriglyceridemia; both of these conditions are autosomal dominant traits.[72-74] In type II hyperlipoproteinemia (familial hypercholesterolemia), the Achilles, patellar, and extensor tendons of the hands are the principal locations of xanthomata.[75,76] These lesions are associated with recurrent episodes of an acute migratory polyarthritis. In type IV hyperlipoproteinemia (hypertriglyceridemia), the hands, knees, and ankles are primarily affected by mild chronic or migratory oligoarthritis.[77] The onset is often acute, and fever and an elevated white blood cell count may occur. The arthritis is self-limited but may be misdiagnosed as acute rheumatic fever, especially if the tendon xanthomata are mistaken for nodules.

Xanthomata of the tendons also occur in sitosterolemia, a syndrome resulting from accumulation of sterols derived from vegetable sources. The xanthomata initially appear in childhood and usually involve the extensor tendons of the hands and, later, the patellar, Achilles, and plantar tendons. Plasma sterol levels are elevated, and cholesterol levels may be increased.[78,79]

TABLE 45-4	Sphingolipidoses	
DISORDER	**GENETICS**	**MUSCULOSKELETAL ABNORMALITIES**
Farber disease	AR	Painful red masses along tendons at wrists, elbows, knees, and ankles
Gaucher disease	AR	Osteoporosis with pathological fractures of femur and vertebrae
Fabry disease	XR	Recurrent fever and severe distal arthritis with burning pain; rash

AR, Autosomal recessive; *XR*, x-linked recessive.

Sphingolipidoses

In the sphingolipidoses, lipid accumulates in cells as a result of specific enzyme deficiencies.[80] Of the many different sphingolipidoses, three have prominent musculoskeletal signs and symptoms (Table 45-4). Farber lipogranulomatosis is an autosomal recessive disorder marked in the neonatal period by a hoarse cry and irritability.[81,82] Painful red masses develop along tendon sheaths and over pressure points, as well as around the joints, especially the wrists, small joints of the hands and feet, elbows, knees, and ankles.[83] Nodules have also been described in conjunctivae, ears, and nares. Epiglottal and laryngeal swelling results in repeated pulmonary infections, leading to death by about 2 years of age. Delayed motor development and mental retardation are prominent. The basic process underlying this disease is the cytoplasmic accumulation of a glycolipid ceramide in fibroblasts, histiocytes, macrophages, and neurons, attributable to a deficiency of lysosomal acid ceramidase. The central nervous system, retina, respiratory tract, heart, liver, spleen, lymph nodes, synovium, and bone are all affected to various degrees. Radiographic changes in the skeleton consist of osteoporosis, juxtaarticular erosions, and disruption of the normal trabecular pattern.

In Gaucher disease, an autosomal recessive disorder, glucocerebroside accumulates in the reticuloendothelial cells of the bone marrow, spleen, liver, lymph nodes, and viscera as a result of deficiency of glucocerebrosidase. Hepatosplenomegaly and pathological fractures of the femur or vertebrae suggest the diagnosis. Premature osteoarthritis of weight-bearing joints is an important feature of the juvenile form of this disease.[84] One of the diagnostic hallmarks of Gaucher disease is widening of the distal femur. Characteristic areas of rarefaction and osteoporosis are visible in the peripheral and axial skeleton, including the skull.

Fabry disease is characterized by the progressive accumulation of birefringent deposits of triglycosylceramide in the endothelial, perithelial, and smooth muscle cells of blood vessels, and in ganglion and perineural cells of the autonomic nervous system. The disease results from an X-linked recessive deficiency of α-galactosidase A, resulting in the intralysosomal accumulation of glycosphingolipids.[85] The disease most often becomes evident in boys around 6 years of age and in girls one or two years later.[86] Children often present with chronic pain and recurrent episodes of fever and severe burning pain in the extremities, particularly the hands and feet, diarrhea or abdominal pain, hypohidrosis, and heat and cold intolerance. Osteoporosis and osteonecrosis may occur especially in weight-bearing joints such as the hips. A typical rash consisting of purple papules, *angiokeratoma corporis diffusum universale*, accompanies the other features of Fabry disease. Enzyme activity may be assayed in skin fibroblasts and leukocytes. Female heterozygotes may develop milder forms of this disorder. Renal, cardiac, or cerebral disease leads to death in the mid-adult years in

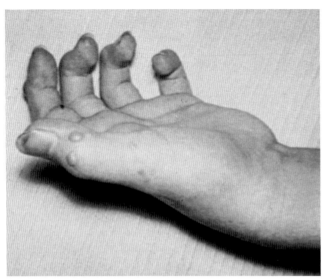

FIGURE 45-7 Multicentric reticulohistiocytosis in a 14-year-old boy. There is marked swelling and subluxation of the wrist and swelling of the distal interphalangeal joints of the fingers and the interphalangeal joint of the thumb. Cutaneous nodules are visible over the thumb.

untreated patients. Recombinant α-galactosidase enzyme replacement therapy and renal allograft transplantation, if renal failure has developed, correct the metabolic defect.[87] A diagnostic algorithm has been suggested.[88] A number of other rare disorders present in a manner similar to that of the diseases discussed earlier, but they have not been clearly identified as involving a lysosomal degradative enzyme. One such entity, multicentric reticulohistiocytosis, or lipoid dermatoarthritis, is a rare, mutilating, symmetric polyarthritis.[89,90] An important diagnostic clue is the presence of clear histiocytic cutaneous nodules (Fig. 45-7). Stiffness and contractures appear early, and the joints (with a predilection for the interphalangeal and metacarpophalangeal joints) are swollen and tender. Biopsy of the lesions of the skin, mucous membranes, or synovium demonstrates lipid-laden histiocytes and foamy multinucleated giant cells. Most described cases have been in adults and are not familial. The disease has been associated with a number of autoimmune disorders and malignancies.[89]

HEMATOLOGIC DISORDERS

Hemoglobinopathies

Homozygous sickle cell disease[91,92] and β-thalassemia[93-95] cause severe musculoskeletal manifestations as a result of skeletal changes that accompany hematopoietic expansion of the bone marrow and repeated episodes of avascular necrosis. Sickle cell anemia is an autosomal dominant trait and occurs almost exclusively in black children. Acute arthritis and long bone pain may be severe and incapacitating during sickle cell crises. In the infant, dactylitis and periostitis of the small bones of the hands may cause painful swollen extremities and the hand-foot syndrome.[96] Each acute episode lasts 1 to 3 weeks and is characterized by diffuse, symmetric, painful swelling of the hands or feet. Osteonecrosis may occur in any bone and leads to marked abnormalities of growth and deformity. The hip is particularly vulnerable and is the usual site of the septic arthritis caused by *Salmonella* or other species to which these children are unduly susceptible. Differentiation of sickle cell bone infarction from osteomyelitis is sometimes difficult and is aided by scintigraphy, ultrasonography, and magnetic resonance imaging.[97]

The thalassemias are a group of heterogeneous syndromes of inherited hypochromic anemias of differing severity. Thalassemia minor is characterized by anemia, hepatosplenomegaly, and recurrent brief episodes of joint pain, swelling, and effusion, especially in the ankles.[98] Bone pain was frequently reported in patients with β-thalassemia.[99] Deferiprone, an iron chelating agent used to treat patients with thalassemia has been associated with arthritis.[100] Musculoskeletal manifestations of the chronic anemias have been recently reviewed.[101]

Hemophilia

Recurrent intraarticular hemorrhage is a hallmark of classic hemophilia A (i.e., factor VIII deficiency) and is one of the most important causes of morbidity in this X-linked recessive coagulopathy.[102] The frequency of episodes of hemarthrosis is related to the plasma concentration of factor VIII; hemarthroses almost invariably occur in children with levels below 5% of normal.[103] A similar association is found in von Willebrand disease.[104] The presence of inhibitors is associated with greater risk for hemarthroses.[105] Iron deposition within the synovium is central to the pathogenesis of the proliferative synovitis that characterizes hemophilic arthropathy.[106]

Hemarthrosis can occur even before the child starts walking, and the frequency of episodes increases during the early childhood years. The knees, elbows, and ankles are most commonly affected, and bleeding into the small joints of the hands, feet, or spine is unusual.[107] Hemorrhage into soft tissues, especially muscle, may mimic hemarthrosis.[108,109] Acute hemarthrosis is signaled by onset over a few minutes to an hour of increasing pain, a feeling of fullness in the joints, and loss of range of motion. The joint is warm and distended. Resorption of the hemarthrosis takes place over several days with effective factor VIII replacement. Intraarticular bleeds, however, tend to be recurrent, and lead to secondary proliferation of synovium with hemosiderosis that produces a diffuse increase in the density of the soft tissues on radiographs and characteristic MRI findings that are highly suggestive of the diagnosis. These debilitating changes may develop in as little as 1 to 2 years. Radiographic abnormalities range from changes in the density of soft tissues to epiphyseal overgrowth, widening of the femoral intercondylar notch, osteoporosis, subchondral cyst formation and bony sclerosis, squaring of the patella, narrowing of the joint space, and eventually, osteoarthritis (Fig. 45-8).[110,111] Intensive physical therapy with strengthening of the muscles around affected joints helps to prevent hemarthroses.[112] Management of the acute bleed consists of factor VIII replacement,[106,113] application of ice to the affected joint, splinting, and rest. Agents that affect coagulation (e.g., NSAIDs) should be avoided. Joint aspiration has only a limited therapeutic role and must be preceded by factor VIII administration.[110] Arthrocentesis accompanied by intraarticular glucocorticoid is sometimes dramatically effective in reducing the severity and frequency of hemarthroses,[114] as is prophylactic administration of factor VIII. The current practice of prophylactic factor VIII replacement has dramatically reduced the incidence and severity of hemarthroses.[115,116] Surgical or radiosynovectomy has a place in treating the older child with early destructive changes.[117]

A recent study from two hemophilia centers demonstrated marked reduction (70% and 83%) bleeding frequency following radiosynovectomy.[118]

DISORDERS OF ENDOCRINE AND EXOCRINE GLANDS

Diabetes Mellitus

With the exception of diabetes mellitus, musculoskeletal disease is rarely associated with endocrinopathies in childhood. Grgic and

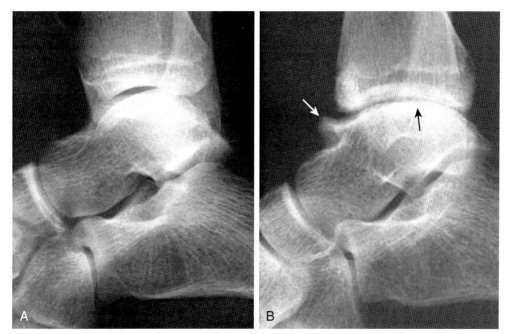

FIGURE 45-8 Hemophilic arthropathy. **A,** Normal ankle. **B,** Recurrent hemarthroses resulted in arthritis characterized by a loss of joint space and development of a talar osteophyte. (Courtesy Dr. R. Cairns.)

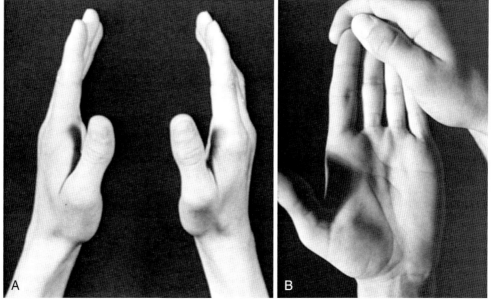

FIGURE 45-9 Diabetic cheiroarthropathy with soft tissue contractures that limit extension of the metacarpophalangeal and interphalangeal joints of the hands **(A)** and flexor tendon contractures in the palm **(B)**. In this 16-year-old boy, multiple flexion contractures without evidence of intraarticular or muscle inflammation had failed to respond to physical therapy over a 2-year period. A diagnosis of insulin-dependent diabetes mellitus was made, and 2 months after institution of insulin therapy, flexion contractures were considerably improved.

others[119] described a syndrome of juvenile-onset insulin-dependent diabetes mellitus, short stature, and contractures of the finger joints: diabetic cheiroarthropathy or stiff-hand syndrome (Fig. 45-9). In this survey of 229 diabetics aged 7 to 18 years, 29% had flexion contractures of one or more joints of the fingers, most often the proximal interphalangeal joints of the fifth or fourth fingers. In a few children, flexion contractures occurred in other joints (e.g., wrists, elbows, ankles, toes, knees), and spinal motion was decreased. In most instances, the child was unaware of any joint limitations and had no pain. Functional disability was uncommon. The prevalence of joint contractures increased from less than 10% in those with diabetes for less than 1 year to close to 50% in children with disease for longer than 9 years. However, there did not appear to be a correlation with the severity of the diabetes or adequacy of its control. Tightening of the skin over the distal phalanges mimicked the acrosclerosis of scleroderma.[120] The precise relation of diabetes mellitus to contractures is unknown. Studies have demonstrated increased glycosylation of collagen in this syndrome.[120] Perhaps increased cross-linking of collagen leads to the contractures. Magnetic resonance imaging demonstrates thickening of the tendon sheaths.[121] NSAIDs have no beneficial effect on this disorder. The frequency of inflammatory arthritis may be increased in children with diabetes mellitus. A case report describes a girl with JIA, type 1 diabetes, and Hashimoto thyroiditis.[122] Other musculoskeletal complications of diabetes mellitus (adhesive capsulitis, Dupuytren contracture, trigger finger, carpal tunnel syndrome, neuropathic (Charcot) joint, muscle infarction) have not been reported in children.[123] Occasionally, hemochromatosis occurs with diabetes mellitus and leads to an arthropathy that results in a characteristic bony enlargement of the second and third metacarpophalangeal joints; other joints are affected less commonly.[124] This disorder has not been documented in childhood. Juvenile hemochromatosis, unrelated to diabetes, is a rare autosomal recessive disorder (1q21) that results in iron overload lending to hypogonadism and cardiomyopathy.[125,126] Diabetic osteopathy is characterized by pain and osteoporosis of the distal metatarsal heads that may progress to erosion or even complete resorption of the ends of the bones. The cause of this phenomenon is unknown, and the disorder has not been recorded in childhood. These and other musculoskeletal complications of diabetes mellitus have been recently reviewed.[127]

Pancreatitis with Arthritis

Acute or chronic pancreatitis or pseudocyst formation from trauma to the pancreas may be accompanied by disseminated fat necrosis, leading to the development of subcutaneous nodules and osteolytic lesions resembling multicentric osteomyelitis or arthritis.[128] The nodules are tender, erythematous, widely disseminated, and similar to those of erythema nodosum. They are often accompanied by systemic illness and fever. Joint pains and effusions may develop 2 to 3 weeks later. The arthropathy is usually self-limited and remits spontaneously. Soft tissue swelling is evident on radiographs, which show multiple sites of periosteal new bone apposition and diaphyseal lytic lesions. Because the bony lesions are delayed in appearance by a few months, the initiating abdominal trauma may have been forgotten. Diagnosis is confirmed during the acute illness by elevation of the serum lipase and amylase concentrations. A bone scan may demonstrate increased uptake of isotope in the metaphyses or diaphyses because of the infarctions that have resulted from the disseminated intravascular fat.

Disorders of Other Endocrine Glands

Hyperparathyroidism is rare in children; in adults, it may be characterized by fever, abdominal pain, musculoskeletal pain, osteoporosis,[129] mental disturbances, and headaches. Elevation of serum parathormone levels confirms the diagnosis. Pseudohypoparathyroidism and pseudopseudohypoparathyroidism are classified as forms of acromelic dysplasia.

Hyperthyroidism and hypothyroidism can be associated with diffuse musculoskeletal pain and muscle weakness, although these disorders and their complications appear to be rare in childhood. Robazzi reported 40% of JIA patients had either subclinical hypothyroidism or positive tests for antithyroid antibodies.[130] Hashimoto thyroiditis can complicate systemic lupus erythematosus,[131] and autoimmune hyperthyroidism (i.e., Graves disease) is occasionally associated with JIA. Thyroid acropachy is a rare form of hyperostosis of the phalanges, metacarpals, and metatarsals that is associated with hyperthyroidism, pretibial myxedema, exophthalmos, and clubbing.[132]

CYSTIC FIBROSIS

Musculoskeletal complaints occur frequently in children and adults with cystic fibrosis,[133] possibly related to reduced range of motion,[134]

and objective inflammatory joint disease occurs in a small proportion of children.[135] Cystic fibrosis–associated arthropathy is estimated to occur in from 2 to 8.5% of patients with cystic fibrosis.[135,136] The cystic fibrosis–associated arthropathy described by Newman and Ansell[137] was an episodic arthritis lasting 1 to 10 days and recurring at intervals of weeks to months in three boys and two girls, aged 2 to 20 years. One or more joints were affected during each episode. A pruritic nodular rash occurred in all five children. Results of serologic studies for rheumatoid factors and antinuclear antibodies were negative, and radiographs demonstrated no abnormalities. The cause and pathogenesis of this self-limited arthropathy are unknown, but it may be a reaction to chronic bacterial infection in the lung. Management usually requires nonsteroidal antiinflammatory drugs, but for patients in whom the arthritis becomes chronic, disease modifying agents may be indicated.[138] Currently, there are no randomized controlled trials of nonsteroidal antiinflammatory drugs or disease modifying agents in cystic fibrosis.

Secondary hypertrophic osteoarthropathy occurs in approximately 5% of children with cystic fibrosis.[139] Patients infected with *Pseudomonas aeruginosa* may be more vulnerable to hypertrophic osteoarthropathy.[138] The probably coincidental occurrence of rheumatoid factor–positive JIA[140] and sarcoidosis[141] has been reported in patients with cystic fibrosis.

CELIAC DISEASE

Musculoskeletal complications of celiac disease are quite common in adults. Lubrano et al[142] described arthritis in 26% of patients compared to 7.5% of controls, and noted that this complication was more common in patients on a regular diet, than in those on a gluten-free diet. Arthritis occurred in peripheral joints in 19 patients, in joints of the axial skeleton in 15, and in both in 18 patients. It is usually nonerosive and nondeforming. Stagi and colleagues[143] reported the incidence of IgA antitissue transglutaminase antibodies in 10 of 151 children with JIA (6.6%). Seven children had oligoarticular JIA; three had polyarticular JIA. The diagnosis of celiac disease was confirmed by intestinal biopsy. In a study of 74 children with celiac disease, synovitis (most commonly joint effusion) was detected by ultrasound in 11% of children on a gluten-free diet, and 50% of those on a gluten-containing diet; the manifestations were improved by a gluten-free diet.[144] Alpigiani et al[142] also noted an increased prevalence of celiac disease in 108 children with JIA studied over a 13-year period. Improvement in joint disease following institution of a gluten-free diet in at some patients.[145] Iqbal studied 356 adult patients with celiac disease and found no increase in the rate of spondyloarthritis, but did find increased occurrence of thyroiditis, SLE, IDDM, and psoriasis.[146]

HYPEROSTOSIS

Hyperostosis, the abnormal subperiosteal or endochondral deposition of bone, may be primary or secondary.

Primary Hyperostosis
Pachydermoperiostosis

Pachydermoperiostosis is a rare autosomal dominant disorder characterized by onset (usually in adolescent boys) of spade-like enlargement of the hands and feet, sometimes accompanied by pain along the distal long bones.[147-149] In addition to the cylindrical enlargement of the digits, forearms, and lower legs, there may be minimal joint effusions, coarsening of the facial features, excessive oiliness of the skin, and occasionally gynecomastia, female hair distribution, striae, and acne.

It is caused by a mutation in the gene encoding the major enzyme for the degradation of prostaglandins.[150]

Familial infantile cortical hyperostosis (Caffey disease)

This rare disorder presents before 4 months of age with fever; irritability; abnormal acute phase indices; and swelling, tenderness, erythema, or altered contour of the mandible, shoulder girdles, and long bones.[151]A more severe, sometimes lethal form of the disease with prenatal onset has been reported.[152] Bone involvement tends to be asymmetric. The ribs and clavicles are often involved by marked cortical thickening with altered bone shape. The cause is unknown, although the condition appears to be inflammatory and may be triggered by an infection. It usually has a self-limited course of weeks to months, after which it subsides without sequelae. Short-term treatment with glucocorticoids may be considered for the infant with severe disease and marked systemic symptoms. There appears to be a familial but nongenetic basis.

The Goldbloom syndrome is a form of idiopathic, periosteal new bone formation associated with fever, constitutional symptoms, severe pain in the extremities, elevated serum immunoglobulin levels, and an increased erythrocyte sedimentation rate.[153,154] Radiographs demonstrate typical periosteal new bone apposition along the long bones. The child may develop limited motion in contiguous joints and refuse to walk if the lower extremities are involved. The disorder runs a chronic course over several months; a spontaneous recovery is expected. NSAIDs are sometimes useful for symptomatic control. There is no known cause, but the disorder may follow an infectious disease or viral syndrome.

Secondary Hyperostosis

Hypertrophic osteoarthropathy (secondary hyperostosis) is characterized by clubbing of the fingers and toes, painful subperiosteal apposition of new bone along the shafts of the long bones, and occasionally, arthritis. In children, it most commonly complicates suppurative lung disease, primary or secondary tumors of the lung, pleura, or mediastinum, and may occur in inflammatory bowel disease, or thyroid disease. Radiographs are characterized by a distinctive apposition of periosteal new bone along the shafts of long bones, soft tissue swelling, and joint effusions. Bone scintigraphy demonstrates increased isotope uptake in the areas of new bone formation. Asymptomatic, isolated clubbing can occur in children with cyanotic congenital heart disease. Familial clubbing can develop without associated systemic disease and is usually asymptomatic. Secondary hyperostosis is seen in several unrelated disorders[155] (Box 45-2).

BOX 45-2   Causes of Secondary Hypertrophic Osteoarthropathy

Malignant metastases to chest (lungs, pleura, mediastinum)
Osteosarcoma
Neuroblastoma
Lymphoma
Chronic suppurative pulmonary disease
Cystic fibrosis
Cyanotic congenital heart disease
Gastrointestinal disease
Inflammatory bowel disease
Biliary cirrhosis or ductal atresia
Thyroid acropachy

REFERENCES

1. R.M. Shore, R.W. Chesney, Rickets part 1, Pediatr. Radiol. 43 (2013) 140–151.
2. R.M. Shore, R.W. Chesney, Rickets part 2, Pediatr. Radiol. 43 (2013) 152–172.
3. S.A. Abrams, Nutritional rickets: an old disease returns, Nutr. Rev. 60 (2002) 111–115.
6. P. Mahon, N. Harvey, S. Crozier, et al., Low maternal vitamin D status and fetal bone development, J. Bone Miner. Res. 25 (2010) 14–19.
7. M.F. Holick, Vitamin D: a millennium perspective, J. Cell. Biochem. 88 (2003) 296–307.
11. H.J. Girschick, P. Schneider, I. Haubitz, et al., Effective NSAID treatment indicates that hyperprostaglandanism is affecting the clinical severity of childhood hypophosphatasia, Orphanet J. Rare Dis. 1 (2006) 24.
13. M.P. Whyte, D. Wenkert, W.H. McAlister, et al., Chronic recurrent multifocal osteomyelitis mimicked in childhood hypophosphatasia, J. Bone Miner. Res. 24 (2009) 1493–1505.
14. H. Demirbilek, D. Aydogdu, A. Ozön, Vitamin-D-deficient rickets mimicking ankylosing spondylitis in an adolescent girl, Turk. J. Pediatr. 54 (2012) 177–179.
15. O. Fain, Musculoskeletal manifestations of scurvy, Joint Bone Spine 72 (2005) 124–128.
17. P. Rosati, F. Nibbi, S. Mancini, et al., A child with painful legs, Lancet 365 (2005) 1438.
18. S. Perrotta, B. Nobili, F. Rossi, et al., Vitamin A and infancy. Biochemical, functional, and clinical aspects, Vitam. Horm. 66 (2003) 457–591.
20. L.-Y. Sun, L.-J. Yuan, Y. Fu, et al., Prevalence of Kashin-Beck disease among Tibetan children in Aba Tibetan and Qiang Autonomous Prefecture: a three year epidemiological survey, World J. Pediatr. 8 (2012) 140–144.
24. R. Moreno-Reyes, F. Mathieu, M. Boelaert, et al., Selenium and iodine supplementation of rural Tibetan children affected by Kashin-Beck osteoarthropathy, Am. J. Clin. Nutr. 78 (2003) 137–144.
25. J. Cao, S. Li, Z. Shi, et al., Articular cartilage metabolism in patients with Kashin-Beck disease. An endemic osteoarthropathy in China, Osteoarthritis Cartilage 16 (2008) 680–688.
29. C. Duan, X. Guo, X.-D. Zhang, et al., Comparative analysis of gene expression profiles between primary knee osteoarthritis and an osteoarthritis endemic to northwestern China, Kashin-Beck disease, Arthritis Rheum. 62 (2010) 771–780.
32. K. Zou, G. Liu, T. Wu, L. Du, Selenium for preventing Kashin-Beck osteoarthopathy in children—a meta-analysis, Osteoarthritis Cartilage 17 (2009) 144–1512.
36. V.E. Gibbon, J.S. Harington, C.B. Penny, V. Fredlund, Mseleni joint disease: a potential model of epigenetic chondrodysplasia, Joint Bone Spine 77 (2010) 399–404.
39. X. Qin, S. Wang, M. Yu, et al., Child skeletal fluorosis from indoor burning of coal in southwestern China, J. Environ. Pub. Health 2009 (2009) 969764.
40. H.G. Jarvis, P. Heslop, J. Kisima, et al., Prevalence and aetiology of juvenile skeletal fluorosis in the south-west of the Hai district in Tanzania: a community-based prevalence and case-control study, Trop. Med. Int. Health 18 (2013) 222–229.
47. C. Carves, A. Duquenoy, F. Toutain, et al., Gouty tendinitis revealing glycogen storage disease type Ia in two adolescents, Joint Bone Spine 70 (2003) 149–153.
52. S.Y. Chen, M.L. Shen, Juvenile gout in Taiwan associated with family history and overweight, J. Rheumatol. 34 (2007) 308–2311.
57. R.J. Torres, J.G. Puig, H.A. Jinnah, Update on the phenotypic spectrum of Lesch-Nyhan disease and its attenuated variants, Curr. Rheumatol. Rep. 14 (2012) 189–194.
59. H.K. Ea, T. Bardin, H.A. Jinnah, et al., Severe gouty arthritis and mild neurologic symptoms due to F199C, a newly identified variant of the hypoxanthine guanine phosphoribosyltransferase, Arthritis Rheum. 60 (2009) 2201–2204.
61. A.P.M. De Brouwer, J.A. Duley, J. Christodoulou, Phosphoribosylpyrophosphatase synthetase superactivity. Gene Reviews (internet), 2013.

63. J.Y. Chou, D. Matern, B.C. Mansfield, et al., Type I glycogen storage diseases: disorders of the glucose-6-phosphatase complex, Curr. Mol. Med. 2 (2002) 121–143.
64. W. Zhang, C. Bao, Y. Gu, S. Ye, Glycogen storage disease manifested as gout and myopathy: three case reports and review of the literature, Clin. Rheumatol. 27 (2008) 671–674.
65. M.L. Burr, J.C. Roos, A.J.K. Östör, Metabolic myopathies: a guide and update for clinicians, Curr. Opin. Rheumatol. 20 (2008) 639–647.
68. T. Fuchsberger, T. Pillukat, J. Van Schoonhoven, K.J. Promersberger, Acute and chronic calcium pyrophosphate dihydrate deposition disease in young patients, Handchir. Mikrochir Plast. Chir. 44 (2013) 181–183.
71. E. Cetinus, I. Cever, C. Kural, et al., Ochronotic arthritis: case reports and review of the literature, Rheumatol. Int. 25 (2005) 465–468.
79. D.-M. Niu, K.-W. Chong, J.H. Hsu, et al., Clinical observations, molecular genetic analysis, and treatment of sitosterolemia—in infants and children, J. Inherit. Metab. Dis. 33 (2010) 437–444.
84. G.M. Pastores, Musculoskeletal complications encountered in the lysosomal storage disorders, Best Pract. Res. Clin. Rheumatol. 22 (2008) 937–947.
86. R.J. Hopkin, T. Bissler, M. Banikazemi, et al., Characterization of Fabry disease in 352 pediatric patients in the Fabry registry, Pediatr. Res. 64 (2008) 550–555.
89. A.D. Islam, S.M. Nagawe, G.S. Cheema, et al., Multicentric reticulohistiocytosis. A rare yet challenging disease, Clin. Rev. Allergy Immunol. 45 (2013) 281–289.
91. J. Fixler, L. Styles, Sickle cell disease, Pediatr. Clin. North Am. 49 (2002) 1193–1210.
92. V.C. Ejindu, A.L. Hine, M. Mashayekhi, et al., Musculoskeletal manifestations of sickle cell disease, Radiographics 27 (2007) 1005–1021.
94. M.G. Vogiatzi, E.A. Macklin, E.B. Fung, et al., Bone disease in thalassemia: a frequent and still unresolved problem, J. Bone Min. Res. 24 (2009) 543–557.
99. M.G. Vogiatzi, E.A. Macklin, E.B. Fung, et al., Bone disease in thalassemia: a frequent and still unresolved problem, J. Bone Min. Res. 24 (2009) 543–557.
101. C. Martinoli, L. Bacigalupo, G.L. Forni, et al., Musculoskeletal manifestations of chronic anemias, Semin. Musculoskelet. Radiol. 15 (2011) 269–280.
102. M.N.D. De Minno, P. Ambrosino, M. Franchini, et al., Arthropathy in patients with moderate hemophilia A. A systematic review of the literature, Semin. Thromb. Hemost. 39 (2013) 723–731.
106. W.K. Hoots, Pathogenesis of hemophilic arthropathy, Semin. Hematol. 43 (2006) S18–S22.
111. A. Jelbert, S. Vaidya, N. Fotiadis, Imaging and staging of hemophilic arthropathy, Clin. Radiol. 64 (2009) 1119–1128.
117. K.L. Vanderhave, M.S. Caird, M. Hake, et al., Musculoskeletal care of the hemophilia patient, J. Am. Acad. Orthop. Surg. 20 (2012) 553–563.

118. A.G. Rampersad, A.D. Shapiro, E.C. Rodrigues-Merchan, et al., Radio-synovectomy: review of the literature and report from two hemophilia treatment centers, Blood Coagul. Fibrinolysis 24 (2013) 465–470.
121. G. Khanna, P. Ferguson, MRI of diabetic cheiroarthropathy, A. J. R. 188 (2007) 494–495.
123. I.A. Al-Hamood, Rheumatic conditions in patients with diabetes mellitus, Clin. Rheumatol. 32 (2013) 527–533.
126. C. Camaschella, A. Roetto, M. De Gobbi, Juvenile hemochromatosis, Semin. Hematol. 39 (2002) 242–248.
127. A. Del Rosso, M. Cerenic, F. De Giorgio, et al., Rheumatological manifestations in diabetes mellitus, Curr. Diabet. Rev. 2 (2006) 455–466.
132. V. Fatourechi, Thyroid dermopathy and acropachy, Best Prac Res. Clin Endo Metab 26 (2012) 553–565.
133. A.-K. Koch, S. Brömme, B. Wallschläger, et al., Musculoskeletal manifestations and rheumatic symptoms in patients with cystic fibrosis (CF)—No observations of CD-specific arthropathy, J. Rheumatol. 35 (2008) 1882–1891.
134. A. Mandrusiak, D. Giraud, J. MacDonald, et al., Muscles length and joint range of motion in children with cystic fibrosis compared to children developing typically, Physiother. Can. 62 (2010) 141–146.
136. E. Botton, A. Saraux, H. Laselve, et al., Musculoskeletal manifestations in cystic fibrosis, Joint Bone Spine 70 (2003) 327–335.
137. A.J. Newman, B.M. Ansell, Episodic arthritis in children with cystic fibrosis, J. Pediatr. 94 (1979) 594–596.
144. A. Iagnocco, F. Ceccarelli, M. Mennini, et al., Subclinical synovitis detected by ultrasound in children affected by coeliac disease: a frequent manifestation improved by a gluten-free diet, Clin. Exp. Rheumatol. 32 (1) (2014) 137–142.
145. M.G. Alpigiani, R. Haupt, S. Parodi, et al., Coeliac disease in 108 patients with juvenile idiopathic arthritis: a thirteen-year follow-up study, Clin. Exp. Rheumatol. 26 (2008) 162.
146. T. Iqbal, M.A. Zaidi, G.A. Wells, J. Karsh, Celiac disease arthropathy and autoimmunity study, J. Gastroenterol. Hepatol. 28 (2013) 99–105.
147. M. Castori, L. Sinibaldi, R. Mingarelli, et al., Pachydermoperiostosis: an update, Clin. Genet. 68 (2005) 477–486.
150. S. Uppal, C.P. Diggle, I.M. Carr, et al., Mutations in 15 hydroxy prostaglandin dehydrogenase cause primary hypertrophic osteoarthropathy, Nature Genet. 40 (2008) 789–793.
151. H. Nistala, O. Mäkitie, H. Jüppner, Caffey disease: new perspectives on old questions, Bone 60 (2014) 246–251.
155. C. Pineda, M. Martinez-Lavin, Hypertrophic osteoarthropathy. What a rheumatologist should know about this uncommon condition, Rheum. Dis. Clin. North Am. 39 (2013) 383–400.

Entire reference list is available online at www.experconsult.com.

CHAPTER 46

Immunodeficiencies and the Rheumatic Diseases

G. Elizabeth Legger, Nico M. Wulffraat, Joris M. van Montfrans

Although infections are the most common, and usually the earliest, clinical manifestations of primary immunodeficiencies, autoimmune diseases (as well as malignancies) often occur in immunodeficient patients. Knowledge of the genetic basis of immunodeficiencies has greatly increased recently, and the molecular defects underlying these diseases are now becoming more clear. Monogenic primary immunodeficiencies in particular provide information on genes and mechanisms involved in immune tolerance. This chapter focuses on genetically determined primary immunodeficiencies in which autoimmune disorders may occur. The compartments of the immune system will be considered in turn: the innate immune system (mainly complement system and phagocytes) and the adaptive system (B and T cells).

DISORDERS OF INNATE IMMUNITY ASSOCIATED WITH RHEUMATIC DISEASES

There is an increasing awareness of the association of rheumatic diseases with abnormalities of phagocytic cell function or complement, and other disorders of innate immunity. (Table 46-1). The function and interactions of key cells and molecules of the innate immune system are covered in detail in Chapter 3.

RHEUMATIC DISEASES ASSOCIATED WITH DISORDERS OF PHAGOCYTES

Chronic Granulomatous Disease

Chronic granulomatous disease (CGD) is a rare inherited primary immunodeficiency of phagocytic leukocytes characterized by recurrent life-threatening bacterial, fungal, and yeast infections especially of airways, lymph nodes, subcutaneous tissues, liver, and bones. It has an annual incidence of 1 in 250,000.[1] The disorder results from absence or malfunction of the reduced form of the nicotinamide adenine dinucleotide phosphate (NADPH) oxidase enzyme system that produces superoxide in the phagolysosome of phagocytic cells (neutrophils, monocytes, macrophages, and eosinophils). This oxidase enzyme system is required for the production of microbicidal oxygen metabolites: deficiency renders the phagocytes unable to kill ingested microorganisms. NADPH oxidase consists of several subunits, each encoded by a separate gene, and mutations in all these genes have been described in CGD.[1] Evaluation of superoxide production in phagocytic cells is the cornerstone of diagnosis. Subsequent genetic analysis is made, guided by mode of inheritance and NADPH-related protein expression or by gene panel analyses. The majority of patients (70%) suffer from

the X-linked form of the disease caused by mutations in *CYBB*, the gene that encodes the β-subunit of cytochrome b558, also called gp91phox. Mutations in three other subunits of cytochrome b558 cause autosomal recessive forms of CGD. These include α-subunit of cytochrome b558 (p22phox), which is needed for stabilization of the cytochrome in the plasma membrane of phagocytes, and the cytoplasmic proteins p47phox and p67phox that translocate to the cytochrome during cell activation, a process needed for induction of the bactericidal enzymatic activity after phagocytosis of microorganisms.[2] The molecular basis of CGD has been extensively reviewed.[2,3] Clinical variability in CGD is considerable: the degree of residual respiratory burst activity correlates relatively well with the genetic cause of CGD.[4] The course and outcome of the disease depends on time of diagnosis and is worse in children diagnosed with X-linked form of disease.[5] A European study reported an overall survival of approximately 62% at 30 years in X-linked CGD patients, versus an overall survival of approximately 81% in autosomal recessive (AR)-CGD patients. Treatment of CGD consists of antimicrobial prophylaxis and recombinant human IFN-γ.[1,6,7] In the more severe cases, stem cell transplantation or gene therapy can be performed.[7,8] Siblings of affected patients should be screened because timely diagnosis enables adequate prophylactic antimicrobial regimes (mainly antibacterial [e.g., co-trimoxazole] and antifungal [e.g., itraconazole]). These or comparable prophylactic measures reduce the morbidity and mortality of patients with CGD.[9]

Suppurative and granulomatous infections in CGD patients are established soon after birth, initially at body surfaces in contact with bacteria and fungi (e.g., skin, airways, and gut).[1] Thus, the major clinical manifestations of CGD are pyoderma, pneumonia, gastrointestinal involvement, lymphadenitis, liver abscesses, and osteomyelitis.[1,10,11] In contrast to healthy children, in whom osteomyelitis usually involves the metaphyseal areas of long bones, patients with CGD more often develop infections of the small bones of the hands and feet, and multiple sites are often involved.[1,11] Aspiration of pus is mandatory for identification of the pathogenic microorganism. A variety of bacterial pathogens have been isolated from the lesions of CGD.[1] *Staphylococcus aureus*, *Staphylococcus epidermidis*, and enterobacteria predominate. Common Gram-negative organisms include *E. coli*, *Salmonella*, *Pseudomonas*, *Klebsiella*, *Proteus*, *Serratia marcescens*, *Arizona*, and *Legionella*. Infections with *Nocardia* and *Mycobacteria* are of particular importance. Fungal pathogens isolated most commonly in CGD are *Aspergillus* species and, to a lesser extent, *Candida albicans*. The response to viral pathogens is normal, and parasitic infections, except for *Pneumocystis carinii*, are rare.

Patients with CGD may be considerably shorter than expected based on parental height.[12] This phenomenon is not fully explained.

TABLE 46-1   Disorders of Innate Immunity Associated With Rheumatic Disease

DISORDERS OF INNATE IMMUNITY	RHEUMATIC DISEASE ASSOCIATION
Phagocytic Defects	
Chronic granulomatous disease	DLE, SLE, polyarthritis
Chédiak–Higashi disease	HLH
Complement Disorders	
Deficiency of C1q	SLE-like, GTN
Deficiency of C1r	SLE, DLE, GTN
Deficiency of C1s	SLE, DLE
Deficiency of C1 INH	HANE, SLE, DLE
Deficiency of C4	SLE, Sjögren syndrome, JIA
Deficiency of C2	SLE, DLE, PM, HSP, vasculitis, GTN, Hodgkin disease, JIA, RA
Deficiency of C3	SLE, vasculitis, GTN, arthralgias, SLE
Deficiency of C5	SLE
Deficiency of C6	SLE, DLE
Deficiency of C7	SLE, sclerodactyly, RA, vasculitis
Deficiency of C8	SLE, JIA
Mutations of MBL gene	Kawasaki, SLE, Sjögren syndrome
Uncontrolled complement activation	Atypical hemolytic uremic syndrome

DLE, Discoid lupus erythematosus; *GTN,* glomerulotubulonephritis; *HANE,* hereditary angioneurotic edema; *HSP,* Henoch-Schönlein purpura; *JIA,* juvenile idiopathic arthritis; *PM,* polymyositis; *RA,* rheumatoid arthritis; *SLE,* systemic lupus erythematosus. (Adapted in part from S. Ruddy, Complement deficiencies and rheumatic diseases, in: W.N. Kelley, E.D. Harris Jr, S. Ruddy, C.B. Sledge, (Eds.), Textbook of Rheumatology, fourth ed., WB Saunders, Philadelphia, 1993, p. 1283.)

Infections often suppress growth temporarily, but catch-up growth is normal. Protein-calorie malnutrition due to CGD-related inflammatory bowel disease may explain the shorter stature in a number of patients. Patients typically have a normal pubertal growth spurt. The skin and oral mucosa were studied in an unselected series of nine carriers of X-linked CGD. The carrier state was established by functional tests on peripheral blood polymorphonuclear (PMN) leukocytes *in vitro.* Three carriers had discoid lupus erythematosus (DLE)-like skin lesions, which were histopathologically consistent with DLE. Four patients had experienced photosensitivity in childhood. Seven patients had recurrent aphthous-like stomatitis, which should be distinguished from the recurrent aphthous stomatitis seen in otherwise healthy individuals.[13-15] Occasionally, other rheumatic complaints are noted, and some mothers of patients with CGD have autoantibodies to nuclear antigens. A few cases of children with CGD who developed convincing clinical, serologic, and pathological evidence of SLE have been described.[15-18] However, the frequency of defects in neutrophil function among patients with DLE who lack a family history of CGD appears to be very low.[17] The pathogenesis of the cutaneous lesions of lupus in patients with CGD or carriers of mutations in CGD-related genes is unknown. It has been proposed that a partial defect in bactericidal ability leads to chronic antigen persistence and immune activation, possibly provoking autoantibody formation. Ultraviolet irradiation seems to be an environmental trigger.

Chédiak–Higashi Syndrome

The rare Chédiak–Higashi syndrome (less than 500 cases reported worldwide) is an autosomal recessive disorder caused by mutations in

the *CHS1* gene, which expresses the lysosomal trafficking regulator protein (LYST) on chromosome 1q42. The LYST protein plays a crucial role in intracellular trafficking of lysosomes involved in breakdown of phagocytosed bacteria. The disease is characterized by susceptibility to bacterial infection beginning in early childhood, partial oculocutaneous albinism, progressive neurological deterioration, and is associated with the presence of large cytoplasmic granules in neutrophils. The hemophagocytic lymphohistiocytosis syndrome (HLH), resulting from a defective immune response caused by the defects affecting intracellular trafficking,[19,20] is observed in the so-called accelerated phase of Chédiak–Higashi syndrome. This phase occurs in over 80% of patient with the disease.[21] Apart from HLH, other immune dysregulation disorders are rare. A genotype-phenotype relation in Chédiak–Higashi syndrome has been described: null mutations lead to a more severe, early-onset phenotype, whereas patients with missense mutations (associated with partial conservation of the LYST protein) present more frequently in adolescence or adulthood.[22]

RHEUMATIC DISEASES ASSOCIATED WITH COMPLEMENT DEFICIENCIES

Primary genetic deficiencies of complement are inherited as autosomal recessive traits, with the exception of C1 esterase inhibitor deficiency (causing hereditary angioneurotic edema (HANE), an autosomal dominant disease) and properdin deficiency, an X-linked disorder. The heterozygous state of deficiencies of complement can usually be detected by measuring the specific complement protein in serum. The clinical manifestations of complement deficiencies vary and partly relate to the specific component of the complement cascade that is deficient.[23-29] Some patients are asymptomatic, but most suffer from rheumatic diseases, particularly syndromes resembling SLE, a predisposition to vasculitis and to a Henoch–Schönlein-like disease.[30,31] The clinical findings include early onset of skin lesions resembling discoid lupus, alopecia, photosensitivity, and mild renal and pleuropericardial involvement. The two other main clinical presentations are increased susceptibility to infection (repeated bacterial infections with pathogens such as *Streptococcus pneumoniae* and *Neisseria meningitidis* and viral infections) and angioedema (in the case of HANE).[32,33] Frequent infections are the predominant manifestation of deficiencies of C3 and factors I and H, the absence of which leads to consumption of C3. C3 deficiency leads to infections with encapsulated bacteria such as *S. pneumoniae,* underlining the importance of C3 as a mediator of opsonization. Deficiencies of components of the membrane attack complex C5-C8 particularly predispose to recurrent infections with *Neisseria* species.[29,34,35] Systemic lupus erythematosus-like rheumatic disorders are the major clinical manifestations of classical pathway complement deficiencies.[26,29,30,36] The frequency and severity of disease vary with each deficiency. Systemic lupus erythematosus (SLE) was observed in 28 of 30 C1q-deficient individuals, 12 of 16 with C4 deficiency, approximately 40% with C2 deficiency, but in only 4 of 24 patients with C3 deficiency.[31] These observations imply a physiological protective activity of the early activation of the classical complement pathway against the development of the immune complex–mediated syndrome SLE. The mechanism by which complement deficiencies lead to SLE-like disorders might be the same as that proposed in SLE, through failure of effectively removing immune complexes from the circulation. Binding of C1 to immune complexes activates the classical complement pathway, resulting in the cleavage of C4 and C3 to C4b and C3b, leading to two important effects.[29,36] First, binding of C3b (and, to a lesser extent, C4b) promotes the solubility of immune complexes. Second, immune complexes are bound via C3b and C4b to CR1 receptors on peripheral blood cells (mainly erythrocytes) and transported to the liver and spleen, where immune complexes are transferred to macrophages.[37,38] The fact that erythrocytes transport immune complexes in SLE is demonstrated by the depression of CR1 numbers in active disease. This defect is also found in other diseases that are accompanied by complement fixation on red blood cells, whether by immune complexes or by red blood cell antibodies.[37,38] It has been proposed that failure of the mononuclear phagocytic system to remove immune complexes effectively allows immune complexes to deposit in tissue, causing inflammation and release of autoantigens, which in turn stimulate the production of autoantibodies and the production of more immune complexes. Specific autoantibodies are formed against defined antigens such as DNA, histones, and nonhistone proteins in the DNA nucleoprotein particle.[26,29] There is a less frequent disease association with C2 deficiency than with deficiencies of C1 and C4; in C2-deficient subjects, complement fixation proceeds as far as C4, which, to some degree, subserves functions otherwise carried out by fixed C3. Lesser degrees of defective complement function, either genetic or acquired, may also predispose to SLE.[39,40] In the case of the relatively common heterozygous C4 deficiency, the SLE-like phenotype is associated with deficiency of C4A (C4AQ0 allele) (relative risk, 2-5) but not the C4B allele.[37] The hypothesis that complement component deficiency itself is not responsible for the increased incidence of SLE, but that it is merely a marker for a true susceptibility gene, seems unlikely because C1q (encoded on chromosome 1), C1r and C1s (on chromosome 12), and C4 and C2 (in the major histocompatibility complex [MHC] on chromosome 6) are all associated with the same disease. Even for the MHC-linked complement loci, the concept that complement is simply a marker for another disease locus within the MHC seems to be excluded because C2 deficiency in whites is nearly always found as part of one particular haplotype (A10, B18, C4A2B4, DR2), whereas the complete C4 deficiency haplotypes are variable and quite different. Finally, C1 inhibitor deficiency, which results in a secondary subtotal deficiency of C2 and C4, is also associated with an increased incidence of autoimmune immune complex disease.[27,29,37,41] The frequency of complement deficiencies in the general population is low. C2 deficiency is the most frequently recognized component deficiency.[30,31] Heterozygous deficiency for C2 is estimated to be 1% of the population and the prevalence of homozygous C2-deficient individuals is of the order of 1/20,000 in Western Europe.[30] Nevertheless, particularly in children with early-onset SLE-like disease and in instances of familial SLE, hereditary primary deficiencies of complement should be considered.

C1 Deficiency

The absence of C1q is the most common abnormality of the first component of complement[38] and the strongest genetic risk factor for SLE. About 30 patients with homozygous C1q deficiency have been reported, of whom 28 suffered from SLE, one had discoid lupus alone, and a 38-year-old male was healthy.[42] A number of characteristic clinical features of SLE are associated with C1q deficiency.[42] Disease onset tends to be early, (median age at onset, 7 years; range, 6 months to 42 years). Skin rash was present in 25 cases. The SLE may be severe; six patients had central nervous system disease (five of six with grand mal seizures) and 11 had glomerulonephritis. Seventeen of 23 patients had antinuclear antigen (ANA), and autoantibodies to extractable nuclear antigens were reported in 10 patients (anti-ribonucleoprotein (RNP) in 6; anti-Sm in 6; anti-Ro in 4). Anti-dsDNA antibodies are unusual in the context of C1q deficiency. Therapy with hydroxychloroquine, disease-modifying antirheumatic drugs (DMARDS) and/or oral steroids may relieve some symptoms.[43] Thalidomide may benefit the skin lesions.[44] Inherited deficiency of C1r, often with a concomitant deficiency of C1s, has been reported in eight children, five of whom had

SLE and many of whom also had multiple episodes of upper respiratory tract infections, skin infections, meningitis, unexplained fevers, and glomerulonephritis[38,45] HANE, caused by a deficiency in C1q esterase inhibitor (gene locus *SERPING1*, coded for on chromosome 11), is associated with a Sjögren-like or lupus-like disease in some families.[23,45,46] HANE presents with episodic attacks of swelling that may affect the face, extremities, genitals, gastrointestinal tract, and upper airways. Swelling of the intestinal mucosa may lead to vomiting and painful, colic-like intestinal spasms that may mimic intestinal obstruction. Airway edema may be life threatening. The authors have observed a girl with familial C1q esterase deficiency, who developed classical discoid lupus erythematosus (DLE) with anti-Ro and anti-La antibodies in the absence of ANA antibodies or dsDNA antibodies.

C2 Deficiency

C2 deficiency is the most common genetic deficiency of complement.[47-49] Heterozygous C2 deficiency occurs in approximately 1% of the normal population; 1.4% of adults with rheumatoid arthritis, 3.7% of children with juvenile idiopathic arthritis (JIA) and 6% of patients with SLE.[48] About 60% of homozygous and 13% of heterozygous C2-deficient individuals have been found to have associated autoimmune disease, most commonly SLE. These patients usually exhibit a restricted set of clinical manifestations, including sun-sensitive skin lesions, alopecia, febrile episodes, arthritis, and renal disease. The SLE-like disease, particularly in association with heterozygous C2 deficiency, tends to be mild, with less clinically significant nephritis but more florid cutaneous lesions.[33,45] Steinsson and colleagues successfully treated a 43-year-old woman with homozygous C2 deficiency and SLE with infusions of fresh-frozen plasma and were able to discontinue previously required medications (prednisone and azathioprine).[50]

C3 Deficiency

Almost all reported patients with homozygous C3 deficiency have been infants or young children with severe bacterial infections (meningitis, pneumonitis, peritonitis, and osteomyelitis).[45,51,52] Other associations described in children have included SLE, vasculitis, arthralgia, and glomerulonephritis. Successful renal transplantation in a C3-deficient patient with glomerulonephritis has been reported.

C4 Deficiency

Deficiencies in C4A have been associated with autoimmune disease and C4B with an increased susceptibility to infections.[39,36] At least seven homozygous C4-deficient children have been recorded.[29,40,45,53] Five had SLE, one had glomerulonephritis, and three had serious infections. SLE is associated with an extended human leukocyte antigen (HLA) haplotype that includes the C4A null allele.[40,53] Gilliam et al. demonstrated partial C4 deficiencies in five JIA patients.[54]

Atypical Hemolytic Uremic Syndrome

Hemolytic uremic syndrome (HUS) is a rare disease characterized by hemolytic anemia, acute kidney failure, and thrombocytopenia that predominantly affects children. Most cases are preceded by an episode of bloody diarrhea most commonly caused by a *Shigella*-like toxin producing *E. coli* (STEC-HUS).[55] A rare, chronic, and severe form known as atypical hemolytic uremic syndrome (aHUS), is caused by genetic defects resulting in chronic, uncontrolled complement activation and represents 5% to 10% of HUS cases.[56] Reduced serum levels of complement C3 with normal levels of C4 have been reported in patients with atypical HUS, reflecting complement activation and consumption.[57] A variety of mutations in genes of the complement pathway have been described in patients with aHUS (*CFH, MCP, Factor I, Factor B, C3*). These mutations have been found to account for 50% to 60% of cases.[58] Complement factor H (CFH) is a plasma protein that down-regulates the alternative pathway activation. Mutations in the complement factor H gene (*CFH*) are described in 20% to 30% of patients with aHUS.[59] The treatment of aHUS depends partly on the underlying gene/protein defect. CFH for example is a plasma protein, and plasma infusion or exchange provides normal CFH to patients with CFH deficiency, which induces disease remission. Membrane Cofactor Protein (MCP), however, is a cell-associated protein and plasma exchange is unlikely to be effective in patients with *MCP* mutations.[60] Eculizumab is a recombinant humanized monoclonal antibody that blocks the cleavage of C5 to C5a, and is now licensed for the treatment of aHUS[60]

Deficiency of Late Complement Components

Deficiency of C5, although unusual, is more commonly reported in adults and older children.[27] Two adolescents with C5 deficiency had *Neisseria meningitidis* meningitis, but neither had rheumatic complaints. Absence of C6 has been reported in six children younger than 18 years, most of whom had *N. meningitidis* meningitis.[61] Although no child with C6, C7, or C8 deficiency and a rheumatic disease has been reported, adults with these deficiencies have developed discoid lupus erythematosus, Sjögren syndrome, or SLE.[62] Wulffraat et al. reported a 13-year-old boy presenting with a 6-month history of recurrent fever, rash, and arthritis of wrists, knees, and small joints of both hands, who had a deficiency of the β-subunit of C8.[63] Deficiencies of C9 and of components of the alternate complement pathway are very rare.[45,62]

Mannose Binding Lectin

Mannose Binding Lectin (MBL) is a serum protein with a specific role in innate immunity.[64,65] MBL has structural similarities to C1q; it binds to mannose structures on the cell surface of bacteria and yeasts, thus facilitating opsonization by phagocytes. It initiates complement activation through the classical pathway by activation of the mannan-binding lectin–associated serine protease 2 (MASP-2), which then cleaves complement factors C4 and C2, generating the C3 convertase C4bC2b. Activation of C3 initiates the alternative pathway and the formation of the membrane-attack complex. Low MBL serum levels have shown to enhance the risk for infection and high MBL serum levels have been associated with inflammatory autoimmune diseases like SLE.[66] An inherited MASP-2 deficiency has been described in a man with ulcerative colitis from age 13, SLE from age 29, and severe pneumococcal pneumonias.[67] The human MBL2 gene on chromosome 10 has three variant alleles: mutations may cause low serum MBL levels, which are associated with an increased risk of infections, although individuals with MBL deficiency may be asymptomatic.[64,68] Because Kawasaki disease is an acute vasculitis with a possible infectious cause, a possible role of the MBL gene in white patients with Kawasaki disease was investigated.[69,70] In a group of 90 children with Kawasaki disease, there was a higher frequency of mutations in the MBL gene compared to healthy children. Similar studies on MBL gene polymorphisms in SLE, Sjögren syndrome, and sarcoidosis reported contrasting results.[71-76]

RHEUMATIC DISEASES ASSOCIATED WITH OTHER DEFECTS IN THE INNATE IMMUNE SYSTEM

Familial chilblain lupus is inherited in an autosomal dominant fashion and is characterized by cold-induced painful, purple acral lesions.[77] There is a mutation in the DNA exonuclease (TREX1) or the phosphohydrolase (SAMHD1).[78,79] Homozygous TREX1 mutations are the cause of Aicardi–Goutières syndrome, an infancy-onset inflammatory

---

BOX 46-1   Diagnostic Work-up of a Patient with Rheumatic Disease for Potential Primary Immunodeficiency*

Complete blood count: hemoglobin, red cell morphology and indices, WBC, differential count including lymphocyte and eosinophil count, platelet count, platelet volume

Quantitative serum immunoglobulins: IgG, IgA, IgM, IgE, IgG subclasses

Specific serum antibody titers for diphtheria, tetanus, pneumococcus, *Hemophilus influenzae* (if titers abnormal, repeat after immunization), isohemagglutinins, autoantibodies

Complement components (CH_{50}, AP_{50}): Specific assays including complement C3 and C4 in case of abnormal screening tests

Quantitation of B and T cell subsets including naive T cell fraction and switched memory B cell fraction

Histological examination of lymph nodes when suspected for infection or malignancy

Specific studies of phagocytosis (respiratory burst assays), chemotaxis

Genetic testing (gene specific, targeted panel analysis or whole genome sequencing, depending on symptoms)

*Specific tests vary depending on specific presentation of symptoms.

---

encephalopathy mimicking congenital viral infection with chilblain-like cutaneous lesions.[80] It is thought that deficiencies in these enzymes lead to an accumulation of DNA and/or RNA inside cells, causing a danger signal resulting in a release of IFN-α. Overexpression of IFN-α–induced genes in white blood cells, referred as the IFN-α signature, has also been described in patients with SLE and dermatomyositis.[81]

DISORDERS OF ADAPTIVE IMMUNITY ASSOCIATED WITH RHEUMATIC DISEASES

Adaptive immunity is mediated by lymphocytes and their products. Deficiencies are classified according to whether abnormalities predominantly affect T lymphocytes, B lymphocytes, or both cell types.[82] Acquired abnormalities of adaptive immunity are common in children with rheumatic diseases. It is thought that these abnormalities, such as hypergammaglobulinemia, that alter lymphocyte numbers reflect responses to the disease rather than primary abnormalities. Rare but instructive examples of the association of primary immunodeficiencies and rheumatic diseases are discussed below and listed in Table 46-2. The association of immunodeficiency and rheumatic disease has been extensively reviewed.[24,25,83-85] Box 46-1 suggests an immunological diagnostic workup for patients with rheumatic disease and suspected immunodeficiency.

PRIMARY ABNORMALITIES OF T AND B LYMPHOCYTES

Primary immunodeficiencies of T and B lymphocytes are listed in eTable 46-3.[82,84,86-88]

Severe Combined Immunodeficiency

Severe combined immunodeficiency (SCID) is a rare group of disorders (1 in 35,000-75,000 births) characterized by severe congenital defects in both cellular and humoral immunity.[83,84,86,88,90] Because of absent or severely disturbed T cell–mediated immunity, affected children develop upper airway and lung infections (e.g., with *Pneumocystis*

TABLE 46-2   Disorders of Adaptive Immunity Associated With Rheumatic Disease

DISORDERS OF ADAPTIVE IMMUNITY	RHEUMATIC DISEASE ASSOCIATIONS
Severe Combined Immunodeficiencies	AIHA, ITP, vasculitis
Combined Immunodeficiencies	
Wiskott–Aldrich syndrome	AIHA, arthritis, renal disease, vasculitis
STAT1 gain of function mutation	SLE-like symptoms, thyroiditis
Syndromic T Cell Immunodeficiencies	
Di George syndrome	Polyarticular JIA
Cartilage hair hypoplasia	ITP, hypothyroidism, vitiligo, JIA, Crohn disease
Defective Control of Lymphocyte Survival	
ALPS	AIHA, ITP, glomerulonephritis, Guillain–Barré syndrome, urticaria, SLE
Disorders of Regulatory T and NKT Cells	
IPEX syndrome	Autoimmune enteritis, AIHA, DM type I, eczema, hypothyroidism
APECED	Hypothyroidism, DM type I, autoimmune hepatitis, vitiligo, alopecia
CD25 deficiency	Autoimmune enteritis, AIHA, DM type I
STAT5b deficiency	Thrombocytopenia, AIHA, JIA
Il-10RA and IL-10RB deficiency	Early-onset colitis, skin disease, arthritis
Other Well-Defined Immunodeficiencies	
Hyper-IgE syndrome	Vasculitis, erythema nodosum
Humoral Immunodeficiencies	
Selective IgA deficiency	JIA, SLE, RA, and others
Hypogammaglobulinemia	Chronic arthritis, SLE, granulomatous disease
CVID	Arthritis, SLE, dermatomyositis-like syndrome
IgG subclass deficiencies	JIA, SLE, HSP

AIHA, Autoimmune hemolytic anemia; *ALPS,* autoimmune lymphoproliferative syndrome; *APECED,* autoimmune polyendocrinopathy-candidiasis-ectodermal dystrophy; *CVID,* common variable immune deficiency; *DM,* diabetes mellitus; *HSP,* Henoch-Schönlein purpura; *ITP,* idiopathic thrombocytopenic purpura; *JIA,* juvenile idiopathic arthritis; *NKT,* natural killer T-cells; *RA,* rheumatoid arthritis; *SLE,* systemic lupus erythematosus.

jerovecii), chronic candidiasis, persistent diarrhea, and failure to thrive within the first year of life. Lymphopenia is classically noted (although not obligatory), and the thymus is usually undetectable radiographically. Laboratory tests confirm the presence of agammaglobulinemia (although some maternal IgG may be detected in the first months of life) and T cell lymphopenia with absent *in vitro* responses to mitogens. However, in Omenn syndrome (a type of SCID associated with mutations in *RAG1* and *RAG2* [recombination activating genes] as well as Artemis, DNA ligase IV, and IL-2RG, and characterized by erythroderma, eosinophilia, lymphadenopathy and hepatosplenomegaly)

T cell lymphopenia can be absent, which often delays diagnosis. There are different genetic mutations causing SCID. The immunological phenotypes and clinical presentation of these mutations differ, and also depend on the type of genetic defect (i.e., null mutations or hypomorphic mutations with residual activity). X-linked SCID accounts for 50% to 60% of cases: B lymphocytes are present but natural killer (NK) cells are absent. In these patients (with T⁻B⁺ SCID), agammaglobulinemia is a consequence of deficient T cell help. X-linked SCID results from a gene defect located at Xq12–13.1, which encodes the common γ-chain present in the interleukin receptors IL-2R, IL-4R, IL-7R, IL, 9R, and IL-15R.[83,91,92] In the autosomal recessive form of SCID, B cells are lacking and NK cells may be present (T⁻B⁻SCID). In adenosine deaminase (ADA) deficiency, a variety of ADA gene mutations have been described. A lack of ADA in precursor lymphocytes results in a maturation arrest by accumulation of deoxy ATP, which inhibits cell division.[84,86,93,94] The disease is usually fatal within the first 2 years of life if untreated. Genetic causes of autosomal recessive SCID include JAK-3 kinase deficiency caused by a mutation in the JAK-3 kinase gene and ZAP-70 deficiency, a key signal transduction molecule in T cells.[86] The low number of reports of rheumatic diseases in children with SCID[95] may reflect the early mortality in these children, but may also illustrate the essential role of T cells in the initiation of an autoimmune disorder. In general, children with T-B+ type of SCID have less autoimmune symptoms than children with SCID with partly defective T cells. A spontaneous point mutation of the gene encoding an SH2 domain of ZAP-70 caused chronic autoimmune arthritis in mice that resembles human rheumatoid arthritis (RA) in many aspects.[96] However, arthritis has not been described in the human counterpart. Defects in V(D)J recombination, such as caused by RAG mutations, result in a block in B and T cell differentiation because formation of immunoglobulin and T cell receptors is perturbed. Different RAG mutations can result in a broad spectrum of clinical phenotypes; the same mutations can result in different phenotypes from classical SCID to classical Omenn syndrome with erythroderma or even combined immune deficiency (CID) with autoimmune hemolytic anemia.[97] Patients with a skewed V(D)J repertoire seem to be more prone to develop autoimmunity.[98]

In patients with SCID due to purine nucleoside phosphorylase (PNP) deficiency, autoimmune thyroiditis, thrombocytopenia, SLE, and cerebral vasculitis were described before stem cell transplantation was performed.[93] Tokgoz et al. presented two SCID cases with CD3y deficiency presenting with only autoimmunity.[99] Autoimmune hemolytic anemia has been described in patients with graft-versus-host disease (GvHD). Chronic GvHD of the skin leads to skin changes that resemble those that occur in systemic scleroderma. The only curative treatments for SCID are allogeneic hemopoietic stem cell transplantation (HSCT) or gene therapy. HSCT from a human leukocyte antigen (HLA)-matched donor confers significant therapeutic benefit to these patients. However, life-threatening infections and graft-versus-host disease still impose considerable risks to SCID patients who undergo HSCT. In the past decade, substantial progress has been made in treating several primary immunodeficiency disorders (PIDs) with gene therapy. Outcomes from clinical trials targeting different PIDs using lentiviral vectors have been encouraging but not without caveats. As in patients with ADA-SCID, patients with the X-linked IL-2R deficiency, CGD and Wiskott–Aldrich syndrome, may benefit from gene therapy; therapies are still in clinical trial phase.[100-102]

Combined Immunodeficiency

The term "combined immunodeficiency" is applied to a group of disorders of variable clinical severity associated with defects in both cellular and humoral immunity.[83,103]

Signal Transducer and Activator of Transcription-1 (*STAT1*) Mutations

Mutations in *STAT1* are currently defined by four distinct clinical disorders. Loss of function alleles (complete and partial autosomal recessive STAT1 deficiency) confer a predisposition to intracellular bacterial (mostly mycobacteria) and viral illnesses, owing to impaired IFN-γ production and concomitant impairment of IFN-αβ and IFN-λ signaling. The autosomal dominant (AD) form of STAT 1 deficiency selectively predisposes to weakly pathogenic mycobacteria (such as bacille Calmette-Guérin [BCG] vaccine) as IFN-αβ mediated immunity is maintained.[112,113] In contrast, gain-of-function alleles (AD gain of STAT 1 activity) are associated with autoimmunity (typically thyroiditis and, more rarely, other conditions like SLE) and with chronic mucocutaneous candidiasis (CMC). The mechanism underlying CMC involves an impairment of the development of Th17 cells owing to enhanced STAT1 dependent responses to IL-17 inhibitors. The mechanism underlying autoimmunity probably involves enhanced IFN-αβ responses.[114-115]

Syndromic T Cell Immunodeficiencies.

In the syndromic T cell immunodeficiencies, in contrast with SCID, T lymphocytes are present in the peripheral blood, although in reduced numbers. This is a heterogeneous and poorly defined group of disorders. Various functional and genetic defects have been described (eTable 46-3). Clinically, these diseases do not have life-threatening infections in the first months of life but severe and chronic autoimmune manifestations, mostly involving blood cells, develop between 1 and 12 years of age.[103] In addition, vasculitis, autoimmune hepatitis, and thyroiditis have been described. An imbalance between T and B lymphocytes may explain the high incidence of autoimmune disorders, as well as infections, allergies, and malignancies. In younger patients, without severe ongoing infections, stem cell transplantation may be performed.

Wiskott–Aldrich Syndrome

The Wiskott–Aldrich syndrome (WAS) is an X-linked disease characterized by a progressive abnormality in both T and B lymphocyte function. Wiskott–Aldrich syndrome is caused by defects in the gene encoding *WASp*, which leads to defective actin-mediated cytoskeleton reorganization with subsequent defects in lymphocyte polarization and function. The *WAS* gene is located at chromosome Xp11.23.[104] Interestingly, a female WAS patient has been described in whom the gene mutation was discovered to be present on one of the X chromosomes.[104a] The fact that she was nevertheless affected was explained by nonrandom inactivation of the X chromosomes. Discovery of the gene mutation has led to the identification of related male adults with only thrombocytopenia (X-linked thrombocytopenia [XLT]), which is caused by a different set of mutations in the same gene.[105] Patients with Wiskott–Aldrich syndrome usually present with persistent eczema, thrombocytopenia with a low platelet volume, and recurrent ear, nose, and throat infections. They often have reactivations of herpes viruses (e.g., Epstein–Barr virus [EBV] and cytomegalovirus [CMV]). Laboratory abnormalities vary widely. Patients may have normal IgG and elevated IgA and IgE levels, with absent production of antibodies to polysaccharide antigens (such as pneumococcal capsular antigen) and absent blood group isoagglutinins. Without appropriate care and intervention, morbidity and mortality are high. Sullivan et al. found that 36% of patients with WAS experienced non–HSCT-associated deaths at a mean age of 8 years. These deaths were attributed to infection (44%), bleeding (23%), and malignancy (thymomas and sarcomas) (26%).[106] Long-term survival following allogeneic HSCT is

80%.[107,108] About 40% of patients with WAS develop autoimmunity. There is a high incidence of Coombs-positive hemolytic anemia, vasculitis, renal disease and arthritis.[104,106,108,109] Autoimmunity in the setting of WAS may be due to the formation of autoantibodies or the presence of autoreactive T cell clones.[110] For severe manifestations of autoimmunity, immunomodulatory therapy including intravenous immunoglobulin (IVIG) may improve symptoms. Corticosteroids are widely utilized; however, the toxicity associated with the use of these agents is significant. Limited data exist on the use of other immunosuppressive agents and immunomodulatory therapies, such as cyclosporine, azathioprine, cyclophosphamide, and plasma exchange.[111] In a survey on the long-term outcome following hematopoietic stem-cell transplantation in WAS, host autoimmunity (present in 20% of patients) strongly associated with a persistent mixed/split chimerism status.[108]

DiGeorge Syndrome

Patients with 22q11 deletions have a wide spectrum of clinical phenotypes. Thirty-five percent to 90% of patients clinically diagnosed with DiGeorge syndrome (DGS) and 80% to 100% with velocardiofacial syndrome (pharyngeal dysfunction, cardiac anomaly, dysmorphic facies) have the hemizygous deletion. DGS usually presents with cardiac anomalies, hypoparathyroidism, and immunodeficiency. There is a T cell disorder of variable severity caused by mutations in the 22q11 region. Several case reports describe an increased incidence of polyarticular JIA in DGS.[116-119] In a cohort of 80 patients with DGS and a proven chromosome 22q11.2 deletion, 3 patients (3.8%) had polyarticular JIA, a significantly higher prevalence than the general population.[119]

Cartilage-Hair Hypoplasia

Cartilage-hair hypoplasia (CHH) is an autosomal recessive disease and consists of bony dysplasia, short-limbed dwarfism, fine sparse hair, short fingernails, and various immune defects, including neutropenia, and a variable degree of combined immunodeficiency or humoral immunodeficiency.[120] The disease is caused by mutations in the *RMRP* gene (which codes for mitochondrial RNA-processing endoribonuclease) on the short arm of chromosome 9. Affected infants have generalized hypermobility.

Defective Control of Lymphocyte Survival

Apoptosis (programmed cell death) is an essential physiological mechanism to regulate embryonic development, cell differentiation, and tissue turnover. Of the several mechanisms leading to apoptosis, the best studied is the death pathway initiated by the interaction of CD95 (Fas/APO-1) and its Fas ligand (FasL).[121] Recently, the molecular pathways of this process have been unraveled. After binding of Fas ligand to the extracellular part of the Fas molecule, the so-called "death domain" of this molecule associates with Fas-associated death domain (FADD) and procaspase 8 and 10.[122-124] This complex of molecules is called the death-inducing signaling complex (DISC). DISC induces activation of caspase 8/10 and cell death. Activation-induced cell death is important in preventing uncontrolled T cell activation. MRL-lpr/lpr mice have mutations in the Fas-encoding gene leading to faulty Fas (CD95) expression on T cells.[125] This mutation results in a syndrome characterized by lymphoproliferation of CD4⁻CD8⁻ T cells associated with autoimmune manifestations. The severity of disease depends not only on the Fas mutations but also on the genetic background of the mice. Mutations of the *Fas-L* gene (gld mutation in mice) also result in lymphoproliferation.[126] The human counterpart is autoimmune lymphoproliferative syndrome (ALPS). Patients with ALPS

BOX 46-2 Revised Diagnostic Criteria for ALPS*[130]

Required

1. Chronic (>6 months), nonmalignant, noninfectious lymphadenopathy, splenomegaly or both
2. Elevated CD3+TCRαβ+CD4-CD8- DNT cells (≥1.5% of total lymphocytes or 2.5% of CD3+ lymphocytes) in the setting of normal or elevated lymphocyte counts

Accessory

Primary

1. Defective lymphocyte apoptosis (in 2 separate assays)
2. Somatic or Germline pathogenic mutation in *FAS*, *FASLG*, or *CASP10*

Secondary

1. Elevated plasma sFasL levels (>200 pg/mL) OR elevated plasma interleukin-10 levels (>20 pg/mL) OR elevated serum or plasma vitamin B_{12} levels (>1500 ng/L) OR elevated plasma interleukin-18 levels >500 pg/mL
2. Typical immunohistological findings as reviewed by an experienced hematopathologist
3. Autoimmune cytopenias (hemolytic anemia, thrombocytopenia, or neutropenia) AND elevated immunoglobulin G levels (polyclonal hypergammaglobulinemia)
4. Family history of a nonmalignant/noninfectious lymphoproliferation with or without autoimmunity

*A definitive diagnosis is based on the presence of both required criteria plus one primary accessory criterion. A probable diagnosis is based on the presence of both required criteria plus one secondary accessory criterion.

present with chronic nonmalignant lymphoproliferation, autoimmune diseases, and secondary cancers. They have a marked increase in the number of TCRαβ+CD4-CD8- double-negative (DN) T cells. A review including pediatric patients showed that TCRαβ+CD4-CD8- T cells levels between 1% to 1.5% of total lymphocytes may be observed in healthy persons or as a reactive phenomenon in conditions such as SLE.[127-129] As a consequence, the percentage of TCRαβ+CD4-CD8- T cells required for a diagnosis of ALPS has been revised to greater than or equal to 1.5% of total lymphocytes or 2.5% of T lymphocytes (Box 46-2).[130] Elevations of DN T cells above 3% of total lymphocytes are rarely seen in conditions other than ALPS.[127-129,131] There are several known mutations leading to different clinical subtypes of ALPS. Oliveira et al. proposed a classification based on the underlying genetic defect (eTable 46-4).[130] Patients who fulfill the diagnostic criteria but in whom no genetic defect is found are classified as ALPS-U (undetermined). Patients who do not fulfill the diagnostic criteria but have ALPS-like disease are defined as having an ALPS-related disorder (eTable 46-5). Caspase 8 deficiency state (CEDS) is an ALPS-related disease, but these patients also have defective B cell and NK cell activation.[82,122] In homozygous Fas deficiency, lymphoproliferation is already present at birth. Stimulated lymphocytes do not express Fas and are insensitive to *in vitro* treatment by an agonist anti-Fas antibody.[86,132] Heterozygous Fas gene mutations are relatively common in the general population.[132-134] The majority reside in the Fas (TNFRSF6) gene, as well as in genes encoding Fas ligand and caspase 8 and caspase 10, all of which are involved in Fas-mediated signaling.[134] These heterozygotes may have lymphadenopathy at an early age, autoimmune hemolytic anemia, and thrombocytopenia. Less frequently, glomerulonephritis, Guillain–Barré syndrome, and urticaria occur. Variable

heterozygous Fas mutations lead to defective Fas-mediated apoptosis. Parents of affected children have Fas mutations without clinical symptoms. This important observation indicates that for the disease to be expressed, the single allele Fas mutation must be combined with another gene defect (digenic disease).[86] Mutations in the Fas ligand gene can also result in lymphoproliferative diseases associated with autoimmunity.[135] A patient with SLE was shown to have an 84-bp deletion within exon 4 of the Fas ligand gene.[135,125] Both the short- and long-term prognosis of most ALPS-FAS patients appears to be good, with an overall survival of approximately 85% by the age of 50 years in a cohort of 150 ALPS-FAS patients.[136] Many patients do not need any intervention for asymptomatic lymphadenopathy and splenomegaly, which often improve with age. Successful treatments for autoimmune cytopenias are short-term steroids and IVIG; for steroid-sparing alternatives, mycophenolate mofetil and sirolimus have been employed.[137] Interestingly, some ALPS patients have been successfully treated with the antimalarial drug pyrimethamine: however treatment failures are also reported.[138,139] For the more severe cases, allogeneic stem cell transplantation has been performed and can be successful.[86,140,141]

Disorders of Regulatory T Cells and NKT Cells

CD4+CD25+ regulatory T (Treg) cells play a critical role in immune tolerance.[142] The majority of Treg cells are generated in the thymus, express the lineage specific transcription factor Foxp3 and are specific for self-antigens.[143-145] Treg cells exert immune surveillance activity by modifying the function of antigen presenting cells (APCs) and can also induce apoptosis of APCs, T and B cells. These actions of Treg cells are mediated by both soluble factors (IL-10, transforming growth factor-β, perforins, granzymes) and cell-associated molecules such as CTLA4 (cytotoxic T lymphocyte antigen 4). However, in autoimmunity, chronically activated immune cells under the influence of intracellular signaling pathways, such as phosphatidyl inositol 3 kinase, JAK-STAT, MAPK, and nuclear factor-kappa B pathways, can escape surveillance by Treg cells, leading to the activation of T cells that are refractory to suppression by Treg cells. Deficits of Treg cell development, function, numbers, and T cell receptor repertoire are involved in the pathogenesis of autoimmunity in many primary immunodeficiencies, most frequently presenting with autoimmune features.[146] The IPEX syndrome (immunodysregulation, polyendocrinopathy, enteropathy, X-linked syndrome) is a rare disease characterized by absence of Treg cells due to mutations in the *FOXP3* gene, resulting in the defective development of CD4+ CD25+ Treg cells.[147] Disease manifestations include autoimmune enteritis, type 1 diabetes mellitus (often occurring in the first months of life), eczema, hypothyroidism, autoimmune hemolytic anemia (AIHA), membranous nephropathy, and recurrent infections. Patients presenting with IPEX syndrome usually die before the age of 5 years unless allogeneic hematopoietic stem cell transplantation is performed.[148] Autoimmune polyendocrinopathy-candidiasis-ectodermal dystrophy (APECED) syndrome is a recessive autosomal disease that may present with a classical triad of chronic mucocutaneous candidiasis, hypoparathyroidism, and adrenal failure due to Addison disease.[149] Other organ-specific autoimmune manifestations include hypothyroidism, hypogonadism, type 1 diabetes mellitus, autoimmune hepatitis, pernicious anemia, vitiligo, alopecia, primary biliary cirrhosis, and ectodermal dysplasia. APECED syndrome results from a defect in the autoimmune regulator (*AIRE*) gene.[150] In healthy individuals, *AIRE* increases the transcription of these antigens and allows the negative selection of self-reactive T cells, leading to their deletion. Mice deficient in *AIRE* also show evidence of spontaneous organ-specific autoimmunity.

CD25 Deficiency

One of the defining characteristics of Treg cells is the expression of CD25, the IL-2 receptor alpha chain. Deficiencies in CD25 result in a syndrome with features resembling IPEX with inflammatory responses at sites of constant microbial exposure, sites where Treg cells are induced. IL-2 appears critical for the growth of Treg cells, but CD25 deficiency may also result in defective function of Treg cells (failure of producing IL-10 in vitro).[145,151,152]

STAT 5b Deficiency

Signaling through the IL-2 receptor/CD25 requires STAT5. Deficiency in STAT5b leads to a syndrome of immune deficiency with autoimmunity. Patients have growth failure because STAT5 is also involved in growth hormone signaling, and most of these patients develop interstitial lymphocytic pneumonia. These infants can suffer from autoimmune diseases such as thrombocytopenia, hemolytic anemia, eczema, and idiopathic arthritis, which is similar to that seen in CD25 deficiency.[153,154]

IL-10 Receptor and IL-10 Deficiency

IL-10 is a key cytokine for the function of Treg cells. IL-10 deficiency in mice results in inflammatory bowel disease; however, in humans, IL-10 receptor defects result in early onset colitis and folliculitis.[145,155,156] Glocker et al. identified three distinct homozygous mutations in children with early onset severe inflammatory bowel disease in genes encoding the IL10R1 or IL10R2 proteins, which form a hetero-tetramer making up the IL-10 receptor complex.[156] One patient has been cured by HSCT.[156,157]

NKT Cells

Natural killer T (NKT) cells express a highly restricted repertoire of T cell receptors that recognize glycolipid antigens bound with the antigen-presenting molecule CD1d. NKT cells produce high amounts of cytokines upon antigenic stimulation, giving these cells potent immunoregulatory properties and protection against autoimmunity.[158-160] In patients with a variety of autoimmune diseases, numbers and functions of NKT cells are disturbed.[161] In some mouse models of autoimmunity, NKT cell-deficiency exacerbates disease.[158] NK cell deficiencies (NKDs) can be divided into two types, depending on whether NK cells are present or absent in peripheral blood. Classical natural killer cell deficiency (CNKD) is defined as an absence of NK cells and their function among peripheral blood lymphocytes. Functional natural killer cell deficiency (FNKD) is defined as the presence of NK cells with defective NK cell activity. In some forms of SCID ($\gamma\delta$ deficiency/JAK3 deficiency), in XLP1 and STAT5b deficiency, or in patients with mutations in *GATA2* or *MCM4*, NK cells may be absent or defective. NKT cells may also be low in certain primary immunodeficiencies, including XIAP and SHD2D1H deficiency.[82,162] These diseases usually present with lymphoproliferative disorders and/or hemophagocytic lymphohistiocytosis (HLH).

Other Well-Defined Immunodeficiencies
Hyper IgE Syndrome

Hyper IgE syndrome is a primary immunodeficiency with recurrent pneumonia, eczema, elevated immunoglobulin E levels, and eosinophilia. Both autosomal dominant (*STAT3*, also known as Job's syndrome) and autosomal recessive (*DOCK8* deficiency) inheritance have been described.[163,164] Many patients with autosomal dominant hyper-IgE syndrome have delayed shedding of primary teeth, and some patients have formation of pneumatoceles and involvement of central nervous system.[165,166] Autoimmune manifestations that are described

are vasculitis and erythema nodosum.[166,167] It should be differentiated from the Omenn syndrome, which is associated with very high IgE levels and a severe T cell deficiency.

PRIMARY ANTIBODY DEFICIENCIES

These antibody deficiency syndromes result from either impaired intrinsic B cell development or ineffective B cell responses to T cell–derived signals. The association between primary humoral immunodeficiencies and rheumatic disease is a well-known phenomenon.

Selective IgA Deficiency

Selective IgA deficiency (sIgA-D) is the most common primary immunodeficiency in Western countries, with a prevalence ranging between 1 in 330 and 1 in 2200 persons.[168-170] It is defined as serum IgA levels equal to or below 0.07 g/l with normal IgM and IgG levels in individuals of 4 years of age or older.[82] IgA is also absent in secretions, although the secretory component of IgA is normally present in saliva. Patients with sIgA-D identified by routine immunodiffusion assays may have trace amounts of circulating IgA detectable by the more sensitive radioimmunoassay.[168] Although the term sIgA-D denotes an isolated deficiency of IgA, this immunoglobulin is also deficient in 20% of patients with IgG subclass deficiency and in 40% of patients with a defective antipolysaccharide antibody response. Antibodies of the IgM or the IgG class directed against IgA are commonly found in sera from patients with sIgA-D.[171] The etiology of sIgA-D is largely unknown. Anti-IgA autoantibodies may play a role in the induction of IgA deficiency. This is supported by the observation that IgA deficiency is more common in children of affected mothers than in children of affected fathers.[172] Transplacental passage of maternal anti-IgA antibodies might interfere with the developing IgA system. The fact that plasma cells producing anti-IgA could not be detected locally along the mucosal linings has led to the hypothesis that sIgA-D results from systemic exposure to endogenous IgA. sIgA-D with anti-IgA antibodies could thus be regarded as an autoimmune disorder. Moreover, such antibodies are more common in IgA-deficient patients with autoimmune and rheumatic diseases than in asymptomatic IgA-deficient patients. In the majority of patients, B cells expressing IgA on their surface and in the cytoplasm are still present in the blood, albeit in low numbers.[173] Exposure to an oral vaccine induces a normal mucosal immune response by B cells that secrete antigen-specific IgG or IgM. Nevertheless, a B cell maturation defect may be present because, in contrast with B cells of normal persons, B cells from IgA-deficient persons also express surface IgM and IgD. Comparable to common variable immunodeficiency (CVID), T cellular proliferative responses to mitogens are decreased in a small proportion of patients with IgA deficiency.[173] Both defective T-helper cell function and regulatory T cells inhibiting IgA production have been described.[174] sIgA-D can be familial, and in some families an autosomal dominant inheritance pattern is found. The incidence of sIgA-D is increased in families of patients with CVID or hypogammaglobulinemia. sIgA-D may also precede CVID. As in CVID, a putative gene defect resides on chromosome 6 between the HLA-B and the HLA-DQ regions, and an increased incidence in the *TNFSR13B* gene, encoding TACI, (transmembrane activator and calcium-modulator and cyclophilin ligand interactor, a protein central to mediating isotype switching in B cells), have been reported.[175,176] sIgA-D is usually congenital and permanent, although transient cases have been described.[173] In some patients with JIA and sIgA-D, the IgA deficiency developed before antirheumatic drugs were prescribed.[177,178] However, drug-induced IgA deficiency is also well described. In particular, nonsteroidal antiinflammatory drugs such as diclofenac and DMARDS including sulfasalazine, parenteral gold, and

BOX 46-3 Selective IgA Deficiency Disease Associations

- Recurrent sinopulmonary, gastrointestinal, or urogenital bacterial infections
- Rheumatic diseases: chronic arthritis (JRA-like), systemic lupus erythematosus
- Dermatomyositis, scleroderma, ankylosing spondylitis, mixed connective tissue disease
- Chronic active hepatitis, pernicious anemia, autoimmune hemolytic anemia, thrombocytopenia
- Autoimmune disorders: thyroiditis, pulmonary hemosiderosis, sarcoidosis
- Gastrointestinal diseases: nodular lymphoid hyperplasia, celiac disease, inflammatory bowel disease
- Central nervous system disease: ataxia-telangiectasia
- Anticonvulsants (Dilantin), hydroxychloroquine, gold compounds, D-penicillamine, sulfasalazine
- Nonsteroidal antiinflammatory drugs
- Malignancy
- Chromosome 18 deletions
- Other immune deficiencies: chronic mucocutaneous candidiasis
- Chronic granulomatous disease, neutropenia

JRA, Juvenile rheumatoid arthritis.
Data adapted from A.J. Amman, R. Hong, Selective IgA deficiency: presentation of 30 cases and a review of the literature, Medicine (Baltimore) 50 (1971) 223. A. Plebani, V. Monafo, A.G. Ugazio, et al., Clinical heterogeneity and reversibility of selective immunoglobulin A deficiency in 80 children, Lancet 1 (1986) 829. J.T. Cassidy, Selective IgA deficiency antichronic arthritis in children, in: T.D. Moore (Ed.), Arthritis in Childhood. Report of the Eightieth Ross Conference in Pediatric Research, Ross labs, Columbus, 1981, p. 82.

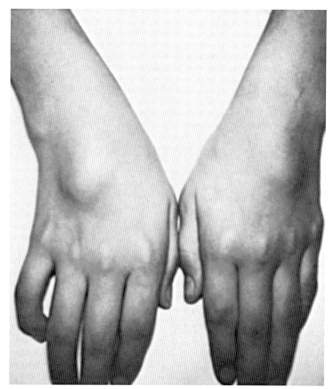

FIGURE 46-1 Hands of an 11-year-old girl with chronic arthritis, tenosynovitis, and selective IgA deficiency. Hand and wrist involvement gradually returned to normal, but a minimally symptomatic effusion of her right knee persisted.

D-penicillamine can be associated with IgA deficiency that is sometimes reversible on discontinuation of the drug.[179,180]

Disease Associations

The clinical spectrum varies from asymptomatic healthy persons to those with recurrent respiratory and gastrointestinal infections. The heterogeneity of this disorder is further illustrated by a variety of associated diseases (Box 46-3). Organ-specific autoimmune diseases are more frequent in patients with sIgA-D, with the exception of those rheumatic diseases listed in the table. The frequency of autoimmune disease as reported in large studies of IgA-deficient individuals ranges between 7% and 36%.[179-181] It has been established that among the rheumatic diseases JIA, SLE, and rheumatoid arthritis are most frequent. Associations of sIgA-D with other rheumatic diseases such as sarcoidosis, scleroderma, dermatomyositis, and Kawasaki disease are more sporadic and may reflect an ascertainment bias. In general, rheumatic diseases in these patients respond to conventional antirheumatic therapy.

Chronic arthritis. The prevalence of sIgA-D in JIA varies from 2% to 4%.[175,181,182] In general, the clinical picture including number of affected joints, sex ratio, and age at onset of arthritis do not differ from those in children with JIA and normal or elevated levels of IgA[173,177] (Figs. 46-1, 46-2, and 46-3). In the majority of patients, the disease course is mild and remains oligoarticular. Erosive arthritis, however, has been described in up to 28%.[183] Patients with sIgA-D associated with oligoarticular JIA may have uveitis and ANA[173,177]

Systemic lupus erythematosus. The prevalence of sIgA-D in patients with SLE is 1% to 4%, which is 20 to 30 times higher than that in the normal population.[169,181,184] In general, the clinical

manifestations of SLE and the response to therapy do not differ between patients with or without sIgA-D, although in a series of 10 children with sIgA-D and SLE, there was more neuropsychiatric disease but nephritis was absent.[185] Resolution of the sIgA-D may follow immunosuppressive therapy, as may be the case in low IgG-associated SLE and sIgA-D–associated JIA.[186]

Other rheumatic diseases. SIgA-D has been described sporadically in other systemic rheumatic diseases such as dermatomyositis, sarcoidosis, scleroderma, and ankylosing spondylitis.[181,187,188] However, these associations may reflect ascertainment bias.

Hypogammaglobulinemia. The term *hypogammaglobulinemia* is applied to a number of disorders characterized by decreased levels of serum IgG and the inability to produce specific antibodies when exposed to an antigen. Unlike SCID and combined immunodeficiency, there are generally no severe T cell abnormalities that would lead to a combined immunodeficiency phenotype, although multiple abnormalities in the laboratory evaluations of T cells have been reported in patients with hypogammaglobulinemia. Among the primary hypogammaglobulinemias are X-linked agammaglobulinemia (Bruton's agammaglobulinemia), CVID (common variable immunodeficiency), and the class switch recombination diseases (also known as the hyper-IgM syndromes) (eTable 46-6). Clinical manifestations of hypogammaglobulinemia include recurrent bacterial infections, often involving the respiratory tract, and an increased incidence of parasitic gastrointestinal infections. Noninfectious complications include autoimmune manifestations, polyclonal lymphoid infiltration, enteropathy, and malignancies. Drug-induced hypogammaglobulinemia has been reported in patients exposed to various anticonvulsants and antirheumatic drugs.

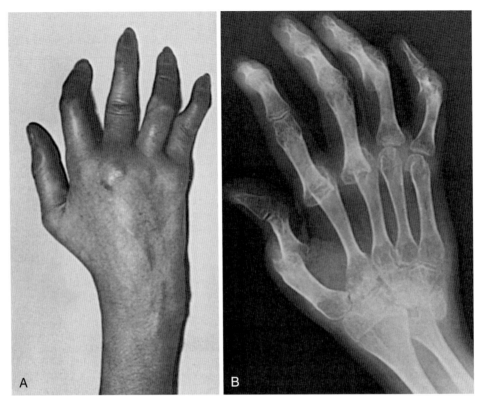

FIGURE 46-2 A, Hand of a 27-year-old patient with sIgA deficiency. A chronic, deforming, erosive arthritis of the wrists and small joints of the hands was slowly progressive from onset. These deformities and subluxation of MCP joints are evident. The second PIP joint had been surgically fused in a functional position. **B,** Hand of an 18-year-old girl with SIgAD and SLE, with onset of arthritis at the age of 7 years. Destruction of joints is already far advanced, with subluxations of ulnar side of wrist, MCP joints 1 to 3, and PIP joints 4 and 5. Erosions, destruction of articulating surfaces, microfractures and bony collapse, and extreme juxta-articular osteoporosis are present. sIgAD: selective IgA deficiency; SLE: systemic lupus erythematodes; MCP: metacarpophalyngeal; PIP: proximal inter phalangeal.

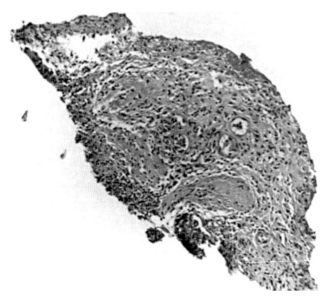

FIGURE 46-3 Needle biopsy of synovium of a patient who developed chronic synovitis of the left knee and was found to have common variable immune deficiency (CVID). There is marked hypertrophy of the subsynovial layers with hyperplasia of vascular endothelium and compaction of collagen. A nonspecific infiltrate of mononuclear cells is seen, but there are no aggregations of round cells. Plasma cells are absent. Fibrin is present on the synovial surface. (From R.E. Petty, J.T. Cassidy, D.G. Tubergen, Association of arthritis with hypogammaglobulinemia, Arthritis Rheum 20 (Suppl) (1977) 441.)

X-linked agammaglobulinemia. X-linked agammaglobulinemia (XLA) is characterized by recurrent severe bacterial infections beginning in males at age 6 to 12 months.[189] The estimated rate of XLA in the United States from 1988 to1997 averaged 1 XLA patient per 379,000 total births per year, or 1 per 190,000 male births per year.[190]

Recurrent otitis media, pneumonia, meningitis, and septic arthritis are caused mainly by extracellular encapsulated organisms such as *Streptococcus pneumoniae* and *Haemophilus influenzae*. The defective *BTK* gene resides at Xq21.3–22 and leads to defective production of the protein Bruton's tyronase kinase, resulting in a block in B cell differentiation at the pre-B cell stage.[191] B cells are therefore absent. Serum IgG is usually less than 2 g/L; IgM, IgA, and IgE are absent. Patients should be treated with life-long immunoglobulin replacement therapy (intravenous or subcutaneous) and should be treated vigorously with antibiotics during breakthrough infections. Gene therapy approaches are likely to be developed in the near future.[192]

Common Variable Immunodeficiency Disorders (CVID)

Common variable immunodeficiency disorders (CVID) comprise a heterogeneous group of primary immunodeficiencies, characterized by hypogammaglobulinemia secondary to defective specific antibody production, and accompanied by recurrent infections, predominantly bacterial. The incidence of CVID is about 5 per 100,000. The age at onset varies from 1 to 71 years,[185-187] with approximately 50% of patients being between 30 and 45 years of age at the onset of their disease. About 25% have onset before the age of 15 years.

Recurrent sinopulmonary infections often cause bronchiectasis, and an increased incidence of parasitic gut infections is observed. Apart from recurrent infections and their sequelae, up to 45% of CVID patients suffer from other disease-related complications: autoimmunity, enteropathy, polyclonal lymphoid infiltration, or malignancies.[193,194] Enteropathy includes different clinical entities; the majority of patients have polyclonal lymphocytic infiltration, but also increased incidences of celiac-like disease, inflammatory bowel disease (IBD), and several other entities have been reported.[195] Patients with CVID have an increased risk (up to 10%) of malignancies of the lymphoid system or gastrointestinal tract.[196,197] The clinical entity of polyclonal lymphocytic infiltration includes granulomatous disease, and may affect the spleen, lungs, gastrointestinal tract, skin, and kidneys. The number of peripheral blood B lymphocytes in patients with CVID may be normal or low. Defects in early and late B cell differentiation, impaired upregulation of CD70 and CD86, impaired somatic hypermutation and impaired antibody affinity maturation are among the defects described. B cells from patients with CVID can synthesize at least some immunoglobulin in the presence of an appropriate *in vitro* stimulus. Although this disease is usually regarded as an intrinsic B cell defect, distinct T cell abnormalities, including a decreased number of CD4+ T cells and decreased *in vitro* T lymphocyte proliferative responses to mitogens have been reported.[196,198] Several genetic defects have been described in CVID patients, including mutations in inducible costimulator (ICOS), CD19, CD21, CD81, transmembrane activator and calcium-modulator and cyclophilin ligand interactor (TACI), and B cell–activating factor of the tumor necrosis factor family receptor (BAFF-R).[199-202] In recent years, mutations in the *CD27* and *LRBA* genes have also been described as leading to a CVID phenotype.[203,204] Except for ICOS, which is expressed on T cells and is involved in costimulation of B cells, defects in these genes affect B cell surface receptors involved in activation and proliferation of B cells. Although defects in *TACI* have clearly been related to CVID, its role in the pathogenesis of CVID is still unclear. Mutations in *TACI* predispose to autoimmunity and other types of immune dysregulation, although this relation is also likely to be influenced by other factors.[176] In more than

85% of patients with CVID the precise B cell defect is still unknown. The hypogammaglobulinemia may also result from a lack of appropriate T cell–derived stimulation necessary for normal B cell maturation, as is the case for ICOS gene mutations.[205] Such a T cell abnormality may account for the observed predisposition of patients with CVID to malignancies and autoimmune disorders. Decreased T cell numbers are observed in up to 30% of CVID patients.[198] In addition, an accelerated decline of thymic output with age has also been described, as shown by a more rapid decline of T cell receptor rearrangement excision circles (TRECS) and reduced numbers of CD31 positive recent thymic emigrants. Specifically, patients' CD4+ cells produce less IL-2, possibly because of a selective defect in the ability to activate the IL-2 gene normally.[206] In addition, some patients with CVID have expanded activated CD8+ populations, a pattern comparable to that in patients infected with cytomegalovirus, Epstein-Barr virus, or human immunodeficiency virus. It was thus speculated that a chronic viral infection in a genetically predisposed person may induce CVID. A similar pathogenesis is thought to apply to the X-linked lymphoproliferative syndrome. Autoimmune disease occurs in 20% to 30% of patients with CVID[195,196] (compared to only a few reports of autoimmune disease in X-linked agammaglobulinemia).[207] Thrombocytopenia and hemolytic anemia are most common.[208] The prevalence of arthritis in hypogammaglobulinemia ranges from 10% to 30 %. It is divided into septic and inflammatory forms. Septic arthritis, both with common and with rare microorganisms, occurs relatively frequently in patients with hypogammaglobulinemia.[206,208] Causative microorganisms are *Staphylococcus aureus*, *Streptococcus pneumoniae*, *Haemophilus influenzae*, *Mycobacteria* species, and *Mycoplasma* species (including *Ureaplasma*). *Mycoplasma* species are difficult to culture. Improved detection techniques (such as specific culture fluids, electron microscopy and PCR) may increase the rate of identification of these microorganisms.[209,210] The association of rheumatic diseases and CVID or X-linked agammaglobulinemia is well established, with reported frequencies between 7% to 42% (eTable 46-6). In a series of 103 patients with CVID, 3 had chronic arthritis similar to JIA.[196] Arthritis is often subtle, characterized by small to moderate effusions, soft tissue thickening, and limitation of motion.[185] In half of the patients, arthritis is the presenting symptom.[211] In the other half, arthritis is preceded by several years of infectious complications. Uluhan described a patient with systemic-onset JIA and CVID who later developed neutropenia, autoimmune hemolytic anemia, and a cellular immune deficiency. Despite immunoglobulin infusions, the patient died at age of 22 from infection.[212]

Whereas the prevalence of sIgA-D in patients with SLE is 20 to 30 times higher than that in the normal population, only 9 cases of SLE with persistent hypogammaglobulinemia have been described.[213-215] After a 24-year disease history of SLE, one of these patients developed fatal extra-pulmonary tuberculosis.[216] Cronin reported 18 patients who developed low IgG levels following the diagnosis of SLE.[186] There was no significant proteinuria that could account for low IgG. These data suggest that the association of SLE and CVID could be coincidental.

IgG Subclass Deficiencies and Rheumatic Diseases

The availability of specific antisera for the IgG subclasses has enabled the detection of subclass deficiencies in a wide variety of normal and abnormal conditions.[217,218] A 10-year-old boy with JIA and Hodgkin disease had low concentrations of IgA and IgG2, whereas another had SLE, undetectable IgA, and an IgG2 concentration of 0.02 g/L. Heiner and colleagues found low IgG4 levels (<30 mg/L) in 12 of 112 patients with "disseminated collagen vascular disease" but provided no further details.[219] Among 450 patients with subclass deficiencies, Aucouturier et al. reported that IgG2 deficiency was associated most frequently with vasculitis and cytopenias.[220] Another study found an increased frequency of Henoch-Schönlein purpura and glomerulonephritis.[221]

CONCLUSIONS

In recent years, knowledge of the genetic basis and the underlying molecular defects of immunodeficiencies has increased extensively. Through understanding of the molecular basis of immunodeficiencies and the consequences for the immune system, we can better understand why autoimmune diseases develop under these circumstances. In this chapter we have provided an overview of primary immune deficiencies that can present with an autoimmune disease or autoimmune symptoms and of the suspected underlying mechanism. In the future, this knowledge may also help us to better understand the molecular basis of other autoimmune diseases like SLE and vasculitis.

REFERENCES

3. C. Meischl, D. Roos, The molecular basis of chronic granulomatous disease, Springer Semin. Immunopathol. 19 (4) (1998) 417–434.

4. D.B. Kuhns, W.G. Alvord, T. Heller, et al., Residual NADPH oxidase and survival in chronic granulomatous disease, N. Engl. J. Med. 363 (27) (2010) 2600–2610.

7. R.A. Seger, T. Gungor, B.H. Belohradsky, et al., Treatment of chronic granulomatous disease with myeloablative conditioning and an unmodified hemopoietic allograft: a survey of the European experience, 1985-2000, Blood 100 (13) (2002) 4344–4350.

8. T. Cole, M.S. Pearce, A.J. Cant, et al., Clinical outcome in children with chronic granulomatous disease managed conservatively or with hematopoietic stem cell transplantation, J. Allergy Clin. Immunol. 132 (5) (2013) 1150–1155.

10. S.S. De Ravin, N. Naumann, E.W. Cowen, et al., Chronic granulomatous disease as a risk factor for autoimmune disease, J. Allergy Clin. Immunol. 122 (6) (2008) 1097–1103.

19. S. Certain, F. Barrat, E. Pastural, et al., Protein truncation test of LYST reveals heterogenous mutations in patients with Chediak-Higashi syndrome, Blood 95 (3) (2000) 979–983.

22. M.A. Karim, K. Suzuki, K. Fukai, et al., Apparent genotype-phenotype correlation in childhood, adolescent, and adult Chediak-Higashi syndrome, Am. J. Med. Genet. 108 (1) (2002) 16–22.

24. G. Bussone, L. Mouthon, Autoimmune manifestations in primary immune deficiencies, Autoimmun. Rev. 8 (4) (2009) 332–336.

28. K.E. Sullivan, Complement deficiency and autoimmunity, Curr. Opin. Pediatr. 10 (6) (1998) 600–606.

29. M.J. Walport, Complement and systemic lupus erythematosus, Arthritis Res. 4 (Suppl. 3) (2002) S279–S293.

36. M.C. Pickering, M. Botto, P.R. Taylor, et al., Systemic lupus erythematosus, complement deficiency, and apoptosis, Adv. Immunol. 76 (2000) 227–324.

49. D. Raum, D. Glass, V. Agnello, et al., Congenital deficiency of C2 and factor B, N. Engl. J. Med. 299 (23) (1978) 1313.

54. B.E. Gilliam, A.E. Wolff, T.L. Moore, Partial C4 deficiency in juvenile idiopathic arthritis patients, J. Clin. Rheumatol. 13 (5) (2007) 256–260.

55. J.J. Corrigan Jr., F.G. Boineau, Hemolytic-uremic syndrome, Pediatr. Rev. 22 (11) (2001) 365–369.

58. J. Caprioli, M. Noris, S. Brioschi, et al., Genetics of HUS: the impact of MCP, CFH, and IF mutations on clinical presentation, response to treatment, and outcome, Blood 108 (4) (2006) 1267–1279.

62. M. Carneiro-Sampaio, B.L. Liphaus, A.A. Jesus, et al., Understanding systemic lupus erythematosus physiopathology in the light of primary immunodeficiencies, J. Clin. Immunol. 28 (2008) S34–S41.

82. R.S. Geha, L.D. Notarangelo, J.L. Casanova, et al., Primary immunodeficiency diseases: an update from the International Union of Immunological Societies Primary Immunodeficiency Diseases Classification Committee, J. Allergy Clin. Immunol. 120 (4) (2007) 776–794.

83. R.H. Buckley, Primary immunodeficiency diseases due to defects in lymphocytes, N. Engl. J. Med. 343 (18) (2000) 1313–1324.

86. A. Fischer, M. Cavazzana-Calvo, B.G. De Saint, et al., Naturally occurring primary deficiencies of the immune system, Annu. Rev. Immunol. 15 (1997) 93–124.

95. J.D. Milner, A. Fasth, A. Etzioni, Autoimmunity in severe combined immunodeficiency (SCID): lessons from patients and experimental models, J. Clin. Immunol. 28 (2008) S29–S33.

97. H. Ijspeert, G.J. Driessen, M.J. Moorhouse, et al., Similar recombination-activating gene (RAG) mutations result in similar immunobiological effects but in different clinical phenotypes, J. Allergy Clin. Immunol. 13 (2014) 10.

100. A. Aiuti, F. Cattaneo, S. Galimberti, et al., Gene therapy for immunodeficiency due to adenosine deaminase deficiency, NEJM 360 (5) (2009) 447–458.

108. H. Ozsahin, M. Cavazzana-Calvo, L.D. Notarangelo, et al., Long-term outcome following hematopoietic stem-cell transplantation in Wiskott-Aldrich syndrome: collaborative study of the European Society for Immunodeficiencies and European Group for Blood and Marrow Transplantation, Blood 111 (1) (2008) 439–445.

116. K. Davies, E.R. Stiehm, P. Woo, K.J. Murray, Juvenile idiopathic polyarticular arthritis and IgA deficiency in the 22q11 deletion syndrome, J. Rheumatol. 28 (10) (2001) 2326–2334.

130. J.B. Oliveira, J.J. Bleesing, U. Dianzani, et al., Revised diagnostic criteria and classification for the autoimmune lymphoproliferative syndrome (ALPS): report from the 2009 NIH International Workshop, Blood 116 (14) (2010) e35–e40.

147. T.R. Torgerson, H.D. Ochs, Immune dysregulation, polyendocrinopathy, enteropathy, X-linked: forkhead box protein 3 mutations and lack of regulatory T cells, J. Allergy Clin. Immunol. 120 (4) (2007) 744–750.

156. E.O. Glocker, D. Kotlarz, K. Boztug, et al., Inflammatory bowel disease and mutations affecting the interleukin-10 receptor, N. Engl. J. Med. 361 (21) (2009) 2033–2045.

163. S.M. Holland, F.R. DeLeo, H.Z. Elloumi, et al., STAT3 mutations in the hyper-IgE syndrome, N. Engl. J. Med. 357 (16) (2007) 1608–1619.

194. C. Wehr, T. Kivioja, C. Schmitt, et al., The EUROclass trial: defining subgroups in common variable immunodeficiency, Blood 111 (1) (2008) 77–85.

Entire reference list is available online at www.expertconsult.com.

CHAPTER 47

Periodic Fever Syndromes and Other Inherited Autoinflammatory Diseases

Karyl S. Barron, Daniel L. Kastner

Fever is one of the most common signs of illness in children. Most episodes are acute, of short duration, and usually caused by upper respiratory infections. When febrile episodes are prolonged beyond 2 to 3 weeks, infection is still the most common etiological factor. However, after acute infectious causes and conditions such as chronic infections have been excluded, rheumatic illnesses and malignancy enter the differential diagnosis.

Repeated febrile episodes lasting for a few days to a few weeks are common in young children attending day care centers and kindergarten. Such episodes are often caused by repeated viral infections, although parents frequently worry about immune system defects. Infections in immunodeficient children are often caused by unusual or opportunistic pathogens. Immunocompromised children often develop failure to thrive and other clinical signs of underlying pathology. Frequent localization of infections to the same organ system should raise the suspicion of anatomical defects.

If repeated infections due to immunodeficiency or organ malformations can be excluded, unexplained bouts of fever with a characteristic frequency and constellation of symptoms fall under the term *recurrent* or *periodic fever syndrome*. Such disorders are defined as three or more episodes of unexplained fever in a 6-month period, occurring at least 7 days apart.[1] These conditions may demonstrate strict periodicity or recur with varying intervals between attacks. Specific genetic mutations have been linked to some syndromes, although the etiology of others remains obscure. With increasing understanding of the genetics and pathophysiology of innate immunity and inflammation, the clinical concepts of periodic fever syndromes may change.

HEREDITARY AUTOINFLAMMATORY SYNDROMES

The term *autoinflammatory* has been used to describe a group of illnesses characterized by attacks of seemingly unprovoked inflammation without significant levels of either autoantibodies or antigen-specific T cells more characteristic of autoimmune disease.[2-5] The hereditary periodic fever syndromes, a group of monogenic disorders manifesting with recurrent fever and inflammation, were the first illnesses to be classified as autoinflammatory, but there are now several other monogenic autoinflammatory diseases. A key insight has been the recognition that the autoinflammatory syndromes represent disorders of the innate immune system. In contrast to adaptive immunity, which is based upon lymphocytes and receptors that rearrange and mutate somatically, the innate immune system is phylogenetically more ancient, based on myeloid cells and hard-wired receptors for pathogen-associated molecular patterns. In general, adaptive immunity plays a

much more prominent role in the more classically recognized autoimmune disorders, such as systemic lupus erythematosus, whereas the monogenic autoinflammatory diseases are primarily inborn errors of innate immunity. Advances in our understanding of the autoinflammatory diseases have sometimes come hand-in-hand with advances in immunomodulatory therapy and have given an added stimulus to research in this area. The identification of the deficiency in interleukin-1 (IL-1) receptor antagonist (DIRA) is a case in point.[6,7]

The range of autoinflammatory diseases has expanded to include several other diseases, such as gout, systemic onset juvenile idiopathic arthritis, and Behçet disease, which are currently not considered simple monogenic hereditary syndromes, but may in fact prove to have a polygenic origin[5] with a contribution of adaptive immunity. Discussed in this chapter are twelve distinct disorders grouped among the hereditary autoinflammatory syndromes, based on clinical findings and patterns of inheritance (Box 47-1). Several of these have been termed *hereditary periodic fevers*, but Table 47-1 reclassifies these syndromes based on the current understanding of innate immunity and the inflammasome, a protein complex containing caspases involved in the proteolytic cleavage of IL-1 precursors to produce active forms of IL-1.[8]

Familial Mediterranean Fever
Genetics and Pathogenesis
Familial Mediterranean fever (FMF) is the most common monogenic autoinflammatory syndrome, resulting from autosomal recessive mutations in the *MEFV* (MEditerranean FeVer) locus on chromosome 16p.[9,10] This disorder occurs most frequently among Sephardi and Ashkenazi Jewish, Arab, Armenian, Italian, and Turkish populations, with carrier frequencies as high as 1:3 to 1:5 in population-based surveys.[11-16] FMF occurs at lower frequencies in other populations and ethnicities.[11,12,17-23]

MEFV comprises 10 exons encoding a 781 amino acid protein called *pyrin* (after the Greek word for fever) or marenostrin (after the Latin word for the Mediterranean Sea), which are expressed primarily in the innate immune system, including granulocytes, cytokine-activated monocytes, dendritic cells, and serosal and synovial fibroblasts.[24] The N-terminal domain of pyrin defines a motif, called the pyrin domain (PYD), which is similar to the structure of the death domain (DD), death effector domains (DEDs), and the caspase recruitment domains (CARDs).[25-29] Through homotypical domain interactions, pyrin binds the apoptosis-associated speck-like protein with a CARD (ASC)[30-34] and participates in at least three important cellular processes: apoptosis; recruitment and activation of procaspase-1 (also known as IL-1β converting enzyme)[31,35-38] with associated processing and secretion of IL-1 and IL-18; and activation of the nuclear factor-κB transcription factor.[30-33,39,40] Recent genetic data on FMF patients with only a single demonstrable mutation,[41,42,43] taken together with data from pyrin knockout mice and mice harboring human FMF mutations,[44] indicate that FMF is likely the result of gain-of-function mutations. A single mutation may result either in subclinical biochemical inflammation or overt FMF, whereas the carriage of two mutations is more likely to be clinically significant. In both knockin mice and human patients, mutations result in increased IL-1β activation and accentuated innate immune activation. There is an emerging body of data supporting the use of IL-1 inhibition in FMF patients who cannot tolerate or do not respond to conventional therapy.[45-48]

Clinical Manifestations

The first clinical episode usually occurs during childhood or adolescence, with 90% of patients having had onset by age 20 years (Table 47-2).[23,49-52] There is often a modest male predominance, perhaps because of underdiagnosis in females.[49,50,53] FMF attacks can last between 12 and 72 hours and consist of inflammation involving the

peritoneum, pleura, joints, or skin; sometimes in combination. Between episodes, patients usually feel completely well and remain so for a few days to a few months. In children, fever may be the only sign of FMF, although other symptoms typically develop progressively with time.[51] The attacks vary not only among patients but also among episodes in a given affected individual.[54] The exact mechanism of triggering periodic attacks in FMF is unclear, with patients often noting menstruation or stress associated with the onset of an attack.

Abdominal symptoms often accompany the fever and range from mild discomfort and distention to severe pain with rigidity.[11,49,52] Constipation is more common than diarrhea, and in extreme cases, peristalsis may cease and result in paralytic ileus. Pain can be generalized or focused in a quadrant, sometimes mimicking acute appendicitis. Pleural pain is generally unilateral, occurring with decreased breath sounds. Less commonly, a small effusion, friction rub, or atelectasis may be present.[55]

Joint manifestations are common and are sometimes the first sign of the disease in children.[56] Arthralgia occurs more frequently than arthritis. Arthritis in adults usually is monoarticular, although children may have involvement of several joints, symmetrically or asymmetrically, with pain and large effusions.[11,52,57] Synovial aspirates from joints are sterile but may demonstrate leukocyte counts as high as 100,000/mm^3. Rarely, in the precolchicine era, arthritis in the knees and hip may have had a protracted course.[58] In these cases, radiographic changes may have included severe juxta-articular osteoporosis, erosions, and osteonecrosis. Muscle pain is a classical manifestation of FMF and occurs in about 20% of patients.[59] Usually the pain is not severe, appears in the lower extremities after physical exertion, mostly in the evenings, lasts from a few hours to 2 to 3 days, and subsides with rest. Treatment with nonsteroidal anti-inflammatory drugs (NSAIDs) may be needed. Protracted febrile myalgia is an uncommon dramatic manifestation of FMF and requires treatment with corticosteroids.[59,60] It is important to differentiate colchicine-induced myopathy, a rare side effect, from an attack of prolonged febrile myalgia, an even rarer disease manifestation. Fever, high erythrocyte sedimentation rate (ESR), normal creatine kinase (CPK) levels, and the evidence of inflammatory myopathy on electromyogram (EMG) should help rule out colchicine as a likely causative factor.[59]

Cutaneous findings are less common than serosal or synovial involvement. Most commonly, there is an erysipeloid erythematous rash on the dorsum of the foot, ankle, or lower leg.[11,52,61,62] The rash

---

BOX 47-1 Inheritance Patterns of the Hereditary Autoinflammatory Syndromes

Autosomal Dominant Pattern

Tumor necrosis factor receptor-associated periodic syndrome (TRAPS)
Familial cold autoinflammatory syndrome (FCAS)
Muckle–Wells syndrome (MWS)
Neonatal-onset multisystem inflammatory disease (NOMID), also called chronic infantile neurological cutaneous and articular syndrome (CINCA)
Cyclic hematopoiesis (CH), also called cyclical neutropenia (CN)
Pyogenic arthritis, pyoderma gangrenosum, and acne syndrome (PAPA)

Autosomal Recessive Pattern

Familial Mediterranean fever (FMF)
Hyperimmunoglobulinemia D with periodic fever syndrome (HIDS)
Deficiency of interleukin-1 receptor antagonist (DIRA)
Deficiency of interleukin-36 receptor antagonist (DITRA)
Autoinflammatory diseases involving the immunoproteasome
Deficiency of adenosine deaminase 2 (DADA2)

TABLE 47-1 Classification of the Hereditary Periodic Fever Syndromes[a]

DISEASE	GENE (CHROMOSOME)	PROTEIN (SYNONYMS)
IL-1β ACTIVATION DISORDERS (INFLAMMASOMOPATHIES)		
Familial Mediterranean fever (FMF)	*MEFV* (16p13.3)	Pyrin (marenostrin)
Hyperimmunoglobulin D with periodic fever syndrome (HIDS)	*MVK* (12q24)	Mevalonate kinase
Familial cold autoinflammatory syndrome (FCAS), Muckle–Wells syndrome (MWS), neonatal-onset multisystem inflammatory disease (NOMID), chronic infantile neurological cutaneous and articular syndrome (CINCA)	*NLRP3/CIAS1* (1q44)	Nucleotide-binding domain, leucine-rich repeat, and pyrin domain containing protein (NALP3, Cryopyrin, PYPAF1)
Pyogenic arthritis, pyoderma gangrenosum, and acne (PAPA)	*PSTPIP1* (15q24-25.1)	Proline serine threonine phosphatase-interacting protein (PSTPIP1); CD2-binding protein (CD2BP1)
Deficiency of the interleukin-1 receptor antagonist (DIRA)	*IL1RN* (2q14.2)	IL-1Ra
PROTEIN FOLDING DISORDERS OF THE INNATE IMMUNE SYSTEM		
TNF receptor–associated periodic syndrome (TRAPS)	*TNFRSF1A* (12p13)	TNF receptor superfamily 1A (TNFRSF1A, TNFR1, p55, CD120a)

[a]Adapted from S.L. Masters, A. Simon, I. Aksentijevich, D.L. Kastner, Horror autoinflammaticus: the molecular pathophysiology of autoinflammatory disease (*), Annu. Rev. Immunol. 27 (2009) 621–668.

TABLE 47-2 Clinical, Demographical, and Genetic Features of Selected Monogenic Autoinflammatory Diseases

	FMF	TRAPS	HIDS	FCAS	MWS	NOMID/CINCA	PAPA	DIRA
Inheritance	Autosomal recessive	Autosomal dominant	Autosomal recessive	Autosomal dominant	Autosomal dominant	Autosomal dominant or *de novo*	Autosomal dominant	Autosomal recessive
Ethnicity	Jewish, Arab, Turkish, Armenian, Italian	Any ethnic group	Dutch, French, other European	Mostly European	Northern European	Any ethnic group	Any ethnic group	Newfoundland, Puerto Rico, Netherlands, Lebanon
Chromosome	16p13	12p13	12q24	1q44	1q44	1q44	15q24	2q14.2
Gene	*MEFV*	*TNFRSF1A*	*MVK*	*NLRP3*	*NLRP3*	*NLRP3*	*PSTPIP1/CD2BP*	*IL1RN*
Protein	Pyrin/marenostrin	TNFRSF1A	Mevalonate kinase	Cryopyrin	Cryopyrin	Cryopyrin	CD2-binding protein 1	Interleukin-1 receptor antagonist
Duration of Episode	1-3 days	Often >7 days	3-7 days	Usually <24 hours	2-3 days	Almost continuous, with exacerbations	Variable	Almost continuous
Cutaneous	Erysipeloid erythema	Migratory rash, underlying myalgia	Nonmigratory maculopapular rash; vasculitis	Cold-induced urticaria-like rash	Urticaria-like rash	Urticaria-like rash	Cystic acne; pyoderma gangrenosum (PG)	Pustulosis, pathergy
Abdominal	Peritonitis, constipation > diarrhea	Peritonitis, diarrhea, or constipation	Severe pain, vomiting, diarrhea > constipation; rarely peritonitis	Nausea	Sometimes abdominal pain	Uncommon	None	Not reported
Serositis	Frequent	Frequent	Rare	Not seen	Rare	Rare	Not seen	Not seen
Joints	Monoarthritis, occasionally protracted in knees or hips	Arthralgia, arthritis in large joints	Arthralgia, polyarthritis	Polyarthralgia	Polyarthralgia, oligoarthritis	Epiphyseal overgrowth, contractures, intermittent or chronic arthritis	Pyogenic, sterile arthritis	Neonatal-onset sterile multifocal osteomyelitis, periostitis
Ocular	Uncommon	Conjunctivitis, periorbital edema	Uncommon	Conjunctivitis	Conjunctivitis, episcleritis	Conjunctivitis, uveitis, optic disc changes, vision loss	Not reported	Conjunctival injection reported
Distinctive Features	Monarthritis, peritonitis, erysipelas-like rash	Migratory myalgia and erythema, periorbital edema	Cervical adenopathy and aphthous ulcers	Cold-induced urticaria-like rash	Sensorineural hearing loss	Aseptic meningitis and arthropathy	Scarring cystic acne, PG, and pyogenic sterile arthritis	Multifocal osteomyelitis, periostitis, pustulosis
Vasculitis	HSP, polyarteritis nodosa	HSP, lymphocytic vasculitis	Cutaneous vasculitis, rarely HSP	Not seen	Not seen	Occasional	Not seen	Uncommon
Amyloidosis	Variable risk depending on *MEFV, SAA* genotypes, family history, gender, residence, compliance	Occurs in 10%	Rare	Uncommon	Occurs in 25%	May develop in portion of patients	Not reported	Not reported

DIRA, Deficiency of the interleukin-1-receptor antagonist; *FCAS*, familial cold autoinflammatory syndrome; *FMF*, familial Mediterranean fever; *HIDS*, hyperimmunoglobulinemia D with periodic fever syndrome; *HSP*, Henoch–Schönlein purpura; *MWS*, Muckle–Wells syndrome; *NOMID/CINCA*, neonatal-onset multisystem inflammatory disease, also called chronic infantile neurologic cutaneous and articular syndrome; *PAPA*, pyogenic arthritis with pyoderma gangrenosum and acne; *TRAPS*, tumor necrosis factor receptor-associated periodic syndrome.

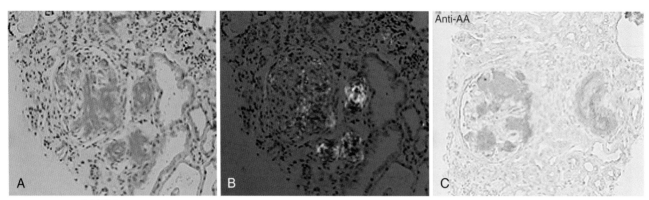

FIGURE 47-1 Amyloidosis in the kidney of an FMF patient. **A,** Stained with Congo red, viewed under non-polarized light. **B,** The same field as in **A,** but viewed under polarizing light. **C,** Stained with a monoclonal antibody to serum amyloid A (Anti-AA). (Courtesy Dr. James E. Balow.)

may occur alone or in conjunction with other manifestations. Biopsies of the rash are characterized by a prominent mixed cellular infiltrate.[62]

Findings less commonly associated with FMF include episodes of unilateral acute scrotal pain in prepubescent boys[52,63,64] and diverse cutaneous manifestations including Henoch–Schönlein purpura.[49,52,65,66] Rarely, pericarditis is observed.[67] Behçet disease,[68-70] polyarteritis nodosa,[71,70] microscopic polyarteritis,[72] and glomerulonephritis[73,74] occur more frequently in FMF patients than in the general population. Although headache and febrile seizures may occur in pediatric patients, other neurological symptoms are rare. There may also be a higher than expected frequency of inflammatory bowel disorders among FMF patients.[75,76]

Laboratory Investigations

During attacks, concentrations of acute phase reactants such as C-reactive protein (CRP), serum amyloid A (SAA), and complement increase. Leukocytosis and an increased ESR are commonly observed.[11] The continuous elevation of these acute phase serum proteins during and even between attacks[77-79] predisposes patients to the development of systemic amyloidosis, the most serious sequela of FMF (Fig. 47-1). SAA deposition occurs in several organs, including the gastrointestinal tract, spleen, kidneys, adrenals, thyroid, and lungs, but usually not the tongue, peripheral nerves, or heart.[49] Before effective treatment was available, renal failure occurred by the age of 40 in many patients. The risk of amyloidosis increases with a positive family history of this complication, male sex, the α/α genotype at the SAA1 locus, and poor compliance with colchicine therapy.[80-83] In most studies, homozygosity for the M694V mutation also predisposes patients to amyloidosis, arthritis, and erysipeloid erythema,[56,81,84-86] although the M694V association with amyloidosis has not been observed universally.[87] For reasons not clear, the country of origin influences the phenotype of FMF and is a key risk factor for amyloidosis in FMF,[88,89] with a decreased incidence of amyloidosis in patients living in the United States. An early indicator of impaired renal function is microalbuminuria, and periodic urinalyses are an important part of continuing care for FMF patients. After proteinuria occurs, amyloidosis can be confirmed by biopsy of the kidney or rectum. Although kidney biopsy is more sensitive, rectal biopsy is preferred because it is safer, less invasive, and still has a sensitivity of 75%.[90]

Diagnosis

The clinical diagnosis of FMF is based on the presence of short (12 to 72 hours), recurrent (three or more) febrile episodes and abdominal,

chest, joint, or skin manifestations with no discernible infectious cause.[91,92] Appropriate ethnicity, positive family history, onset before the age of 20 years, and a favorable response to colchicine also support the diagnosis. Because physicians in the West are not as familiar with FMF as clinicians in regions with a higher prevalence, genetic testing has become a valuable adjunct to clinical diagnosis, particularly in North America and Europe. More than 50 mutations have been described in *MEFV* (http://fmf.igh.cnrs.fr/infevers/),[93] as well as a much larger number of sequence variants that are likely not pathogenic. The majority of FMF-associated mutations are missense changes clustered in exon 10, which encodes the C-terminal B30.2 domain of the pyrin protein. The most common mutations are the substitutions of valine or isoleucine for methionine at position 694 (M694V and M694I, respectively), the substitution of isoleucine for methionine at residue 680 (M680I), and the substitution of alanine for valine at position 726 (V726A). Exon 2 of *MEFV* includes a number of missense substitutions that are variously considered benign polymorphisms or mild mutations, the most notable of which is the substitution of glutamine for glutamic acid at residue 148 (E148Q).

The interpretation of genetic testing for FMF is more complicated than would be expected under a simple recessive model of inheritance, in which FMF patients would be homozygous for a single mutation or compound heterozygous for two different mutations. In some cases patients have complex alleles, most commonly an exon 10 mutation in cis with a polymorphism in exon 2, thus giving the impression of three or even four mutations (counting the exon 2 variants as true mutations). Some rare mutations appear to be inherited in a dominant fashion[94] and, as noted above, approximately 30% of patients with clinical signs of FMF have only one demonstrable mutation[41-43], despite complete sequencing of the coding region of *MEFV*. Moreover, sequencing of the entire MEFV coding sequence fails to identify any abnormalities in a small number of patients who respond well to colchicine and exhibit FMF symptoms, suggesting there may be more than one gene causing FMF.[95,96] A diagnosis of FMF should never be excluded based solely on the results of genetic testing. However, the clinical and ethnic spectra of FMF have definitely expanded with the availability of genetic testing[11], suggesting that a combination of clinical evaluation and genetic testing for selected patients is the most sensible diagnostic approach.

Treatment

Colchicine therapy is highly effective for most patients in preventing febrile episodes and systemic amyloidosis.[52;78-100] Approximately 95% of patients demonstrate a marked improvement in symptoms, whereas almost 75% have a near-complete remission. Daily therapy is generally more effective in controlling the attacks of FMF than intermittent treatment at the time of attacks, and daily therapy has the important added benefit of reducing the subclinical inflammation between episodes that potentially leads to amyloidosis.[77-79,100] Colchicine may have a number of beneficial actions in FMF, including its well-documented effects on the expression of adhesion molecules and on leukocyte migration.

Colchicine is generally safe in children, although colchicine pharmacokinetics may differ in younger patients, and doses adjusted for body weight may be greater in children than those used in adults. Dosage should be started as low as possible (one half of a 0.6 mg tablet once daily in children) and slowly increased, titrating to maximize efficacy and minimize side effects, but usually not exceeding 1.8 mg/day in single or divided doses.[101,102] A gradual increase in dose often prevents or lessens diarrhea, the most common adverse effect. Some patients develop lactose intolerance due to colchicine, and a lactose-free diet may help to control gastrointestinal symptoms. In children with FMF, development of myopathy with progressive proximal muscle weakness and generalized myalgia is rarely observed on regular dosage.[99] Bone marrow alterations (hemolytic or aplastic anemia, pancytopenia, neutropenia, and thrombocytopenia) have been reported in cases of acute intoxication, but are rarely observed in the usual doses given orally. Toxicity is more common with intravenous therapy and when given together with other drugs that are metabolized by CYP3A4 such as erythromycin and cimetidine.[103,104] Based on the role of pyrin, the FMF protein, in IL-1 activation, anakinra and canakinumab have been increasingly used in FMF patients who are unresponsive to or cannot tolerate therapeutic doses of colchicine at doses similar to those used in cryopyrin-associated periodic fever syndromes (CAPS). A recent randomized, placebo-controlled trial suggests that rilonacept, a protein consisting of the extracellular domains of humanized IL-1 receptor and the IL-1 receptor accessory protein fused with the Fc portion of IgG1, may reduce the frequency of FMF attacks and may be a treatment option for patients with colchicine-resistant or colchicine-intolerant FMF.[48] Future larger studies using IL-1 inhibitors in FMF are indicated.

Outcome and Prognosis

Among FMF patients with end-stage renal amyloidosis, the survival rate on hemodialysis is lower than among age-matched dialysis patients, perhaps because of poor vascular access and hemodynamic instability.[105,106,107] Studies have confirmed little difference in patient and graft survival between FMF and control kidney transplant recipients.[108] Transplantation (with oral colchicine administration to prevent amyloidosis in the transplanted kidney) is the preferred treatment for renal failure.

Tumor Necrosis Factor Receptor-Associated Periodic Syndrome

One of the first clinical descriptions of tumor necrosis factor receptor-associated periodic syndrome (TRAPS) was that of a large family of Irish/Scottish ancestry, with an illness denoted as familial Hibernian fever.[109] The current TRAPS nomenclature was proposed as a result of the discovery of mutations in the *TNFRSF1A* gene[2] (located on chromosome 12p13, which encodes the 55-kDa tumor necrosis factor (TNF) receptor) in this family and in several other families of non-Irish ancestry.

Genetics and Pathogenesis

TRAPS is inherited as an autosomal dominant trait, although in some cases, a clear pattern of inheritance cannot be discerned because of

reduced penetrance in mutation-positive relatives or, rarely, because of *de novo* mutation. TRAPS has been reported in patients of many ethnicities. It is the second most common hereditary periodic fever disorder, with more than 90 known mutations in *TNFRSF1A*[2,110-126] (http://fmf.igh.cnrs.fr/infevers/).

The 55 kDa TNF receptor is widely expressed on cell membranes and mediates a number of proinflammatory effects. To date, nearly all TRAPS-associated *TNFRSF1A* mutations lead to single amino acid substitutions in the extracellular domain of the receptor and many involve cysteine residues thereby disrupting highly conserved disulfide bonds. When the first of these mutations was discovered,[2] there were additional data supporting the hypothesis that mutations impair metalloprotease-mediated cleavage of receptors from the cell surface, the most common way of inactivating TNFRSF1A. Impaired receptor shedding might then lead to repeated signaling and prolongation of the immune response. Impaired receptor shedding has been observed by flow cytometry in patients with some but not all mutations.[2,112,118,119,127,128] Impaired cleavage does not seem to correlate with disease severity, suggesting that there must be other mechanisms by which *TNFRSF1A* mutations cause autoinflammatory disease.[129,130] Recent data indicate that mutant TNFR1 accumulates and aggregates within the cytoplasm, activating JNK and p38 signaling.[131] This activation sensitizes cells to the effects of other innate immune stimulation, resulting in enhanced production of proinflammatory cytokines. This process is independent of TNF-TNFR1 interactions and is therefore "ligand independent."

Clinical Manifestations

The clinical manifestations of TRAPS are similar to those of FMF and differ from those of the cryopyrinopathies (Table 47-2). TRAPS causes episodic fever and inflammation with serosal, synovial, and cutaneous manifestations. Distinguishing characteristics of TRAPS include longer attacks (1 to 4 weeks or more) and conspicuous eye and skin symptoms.[132-134] TRAPS attacks may be precipitated by minor trauma or infection or by stress and physical exertion. During attacks, patients exhibit vigorous acute phase responses that sometimes persist into the intercritical period, albeit at lower intensity.[133]

Cutaneous symptoms associated with TRAPS are often distinctive, consisting of macular areas of erythema that occur on the torso or on an extremity (Fig. 47-2).[132,133] These cutaneous lesions are warm and tender, may resemble cellulitis or bruises, and consist of superficial and deep perivascular infiltrates of mononuclear cells. When lesions occur on the limbs, they often migrate distally. There may be associated myalgia caused by inflammation of the underlying fascia.[135] Magnetic resonance imaging (MRI) of affected muscle groups reveals focal areas of edema in discrete muscular compartments and intramuscular septa (Fig. 47-2).[133] Other types of rash may also occur, including annular patches and generalized serpiginous plaques.[132,133]

Clinical attacks may include peritoneal inflammation or pleurisy, or both. Abdominal pain with tenderness is often a major feature resembling an acute abdomen. Recurrent pericarditis has also been reported. Ocular inflammation with periorbital edema or conjunctivitis is common (Fig. 47-2).[133] Arthralgia is more prominent than arthritis, and it generally involves single joints, especially the hip, knees, and ankles. Scrotal inflammation may occur. Amyloidosis, although less common than in untreated FMF, affects about 10% of patients and can lead to renal failure.[17,112-114,133,136]

Laboratory Investigations

Levels of SAA, CRP, and serum complement components are increased during flares, and most patients exhibit leukocytosis and thrombocytosis, with an accelerated ESR. Acute phase reactants may remain

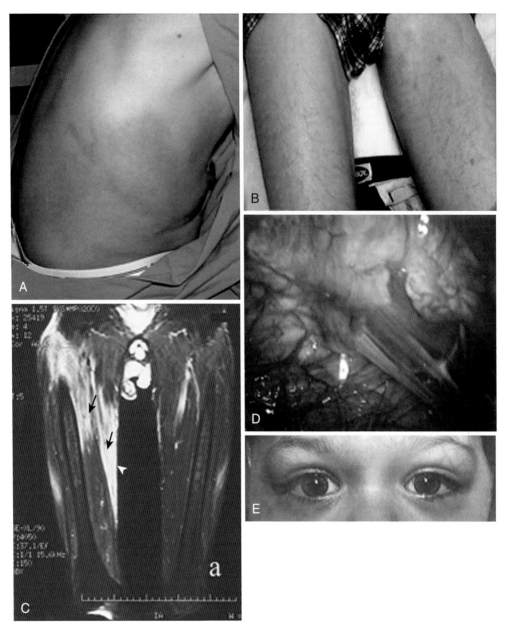

FIGURE 47-2 Cutaneous findings associated with TRAPS may consist of macular areas of erythema on the torso **(A)**[133] or on an extremity **(B)**.[135] **C,** Sagittal views of the proximal thighs of a TRAPS patient demonstrating edematous changes within muscle compartments *(black arrows)*, here and extending to the skin *(white arrows)*[133] **D,** Peritoneal inflammation can lead to adhesions.[133] **E,** Periorbital edema is commonly observed in TRAPS patients during a flare.[133]

elevated between clinical attacks, suggesting an elevated level of baseline inflammatory activity.

Diagnosis

The specific diagnosis is defined by mutations in *TNFRSF1A*. The majority are single nucleotide missense mutations in exons 2-4 encoding the first or second cysteine-rich extracellular domains (CRD1 and CRD2).[2,93] The binding site for TNF is formed by CRD2 and CRD3 of TNFRSF1A, whereas CRD1, also known as the preligand assembly binding domain, is thought to mediate the TNFRSF1A self-assembly. Genotype-phenotype studies have shown that mutations at cysteine residues are associated with a more severe phenotype and a higher incidence of amyloidosis.[112,133] A positive family history of amyloidosis

may increase the risk for other relatives. Although most TRAPS associated mutations are fully penetrant, 2 TNFRSF1A variants, P46L and R92Q, have also been identified in asymptomatic family members and at greater than 1% frequency in healthy populations.[122,129] These variants do not lead to the same signaling abnormalities associated with more severe mutations, raising the question of whether they are mild mutations or functional polymorphisms.

Treatment

Treatment depends on the severity of the underlying disease. For some patients with relatively infrequent episodes, tapering doses of prednisone at the time of attacks may be effective and relatively safe.[133] For patients with more severe disease, etanercept (the recombinant soluble

TNF receptor), given once or twice a week in divided doses, is effective in preventing attacks in some patients.[3,133,137-140] Experience with infliximab (anti-TNF monoclonal antibodies) is limited. Treatment with this agent has led to exacerbation of the disease in some cases,[139-142] possibly a result of the failure to shed infliximab-bound TNF/TNFR1 from the cell surface leading to an increase in cytokine secretion and an increased proinflammatory response.[143] Recent data suggest that IL-1 inhibition may be more effective than inhibiting TNF in TRAPS.[144,145] Both anakinra (IL-1 receptor antagonist) and canakinumab (anti-IL-1 antibody) have been shown to be effective in controlling the clinical and laboratory manifestations in some patients with TRAPS.[144-148] Colchicine usually has no effect on symptoms or the development of amyloidosis.[133,136] In patients with demonstrated amyloidosis, the goal should be to maintain the SAA levels at less than 10 mg/L. The prognosis depends on the development of amyloidosis. More aggressive therapy may be indicated in patients with a positive family history of amyloidosis or mutation at cysteine residues to suppress subclinical inflammation.

Hyperimmunoglobulinemia D with Periodic Fever Syndrome

Hyperimmunoglobulinemia D with periodic fever syndrome (HIDS) is an autosomal recessive disease[149] that was initially described in several patients of Dutch heritage.[150] HIDS is caused by mutations in the *MVK* gene, on chromosome 12, which encodes mevalonate kinase.[151-153] It occurs mainly in patients of northern European ancestry, and approximately 50% of patients are of Dutch ancestry.[134,154-158]

Genetics and Pathogenesis

Mevalonate kinase is the first enzyme to follow 3-hydroxy-3-methyl-glutaryl-CoA reductase (HMG-CoA reductase) in the mevalonate pathway and converts mevalonic acid to 5-phosphomevalonic acid. The mevalonate pathway produces cholesterol, a structural component of cellular membranes and precursor for bile acids and steroid hormones. In addition, the mevalonate pathway produces nonsterol isoprene compounds (Fig. 47-3).[153,159,160] Isoprenes are involved in a variety of cellular functions, including electron transport, protein glycosylation and synthesis, and prenylation of proteins involved in cell proliferation and differentiation. Mutations associated with HIDS lead to markedly reduced mevalonate kinase enzymatic activity,[151,152] whereas the mutations in the clinically more severe mevalonic aciduria result in the absence of enzymatic activity.[161] Although excessive production of proinflammatory cytokines by HIDS mononuclear cells may result from excessive accumulation of mevalonic acid substrate, current data support an alternative hypothesis related to deficiencies in nonsterol isoprenoids synthesized through the mevalonate pathway.[162] Thus, a shortage of geranylgeranylated proteins may be the link between the mevalonate pathway, increased IL-1β production, and the febrile attacks of HIDS.[163]

Clinical Manifestations

HIDS manifests in early childhood, often by the age of 6 months (Table 47-2). Attacks last about 3 to 7 days, usually separated by 1- to 2-month, symptom-free intervals. Episodes are often heralded by chills and headache, a rising fever, abdominal pain, nausea, and vomiting, sometimes precipitated by immunizations, surgery, trauma, and mild infections.[154,164] The mevalonate kinase enzyme in patients with HIDS-associated mutations loses activity at supraphysiological temperatures, perhaps explaining the association of immunizations, upper respiratory infections, and other inflammatory provocations with attacks.[165] Some patients develop a nondestructive arthritis, usually in the large joints, associated with attacks.[154,166,167] This arthritis is often

polyarticular, unlike that associated with FMF. Protracted joint manifestations are rare.

During attacks, widespread erythematous macules that are sometimes painful develop.[157,168] The rash is usually not migratory, differentiating it from the rash associated with TRAPS, and it has no predilection for the lower legs, unlike that of FMF. The HIDS rash may be a diffuse maculopapular eruption (Fig. 47-4) extending to the palms and soles, or it can be nodular, urticarial, or morbilliform. Skin biopsies show perivascular inflammatory cells and deposits of antibody or complement component C3, or both. Oral and vaginal aphthous ulcers may be present. Henoch–Schönlein purpura[169] and erythema elevatum diutinum (a benign type of necrotizing vasculitis)[156] have been reported. Cervical lymphadenopathy is a common manifestation of HIDS, as are severe headache and splenomegaly.[154] Pleurisy is uncommon.

Patients with mevalonic aciduria have complete deficiency of mevalonic kinase and have developmental delays of varying severity, hematological abnormalities, dysmorphic features, and hepatosplenomegaly. These patients have been known to develop periodic crises characterized by fever, rash, and arthralgia. HIDS is one end of the clinical spectrum of deficiency of mevalonate kinase.[161]

Laboratory Investigations

Most patients have elevated serum immunoglobulin (Ig) D levels, but how this observation contributes to the clinical disease is poorly understood. In a recent report, 22% of HIDS patients had normal levels of IgD,[154] suggesting that an elevated IgD concentration may be an epiphenomenon.[152,159,170] Levels of IgA may also be elevated.[171] Patients also exhibit an accelerated ESR, leukocytosis, and elevated levels of CRP[134,154,159,172] during and, less commonly, between attacks. Elevated levels of mevalonic acid may be detected in urine during attacks.[151,152,173,174] Many proinflammatory and inflammatory cytokines, particularly IL-1, IL-6 and TNF-α and their soluble receptors are increased during attacks.[134]

Diagnosis

A diagnosis may involve several lines of inquiry, including clinical observation, genetic testing, serum IgD measurement, and assay of mevalonate in urine. Modest elevations in IgD should be interpreted with caution because this phenomenon is common in several other conditions, including chronic infections, acquired immunodeficiency syndrome, Hodgkin's lymphoma, and other periodic fever syndromes.[164,175-177] Furthermore, the height of the IgD concentration is not related to the severity of disease, nor does IgD concentration necessarily increase further during an inflammatory episode. Many laboratories perform genetic screenings for only the most common V377I and I268T *MVK* mutations.[158,173,178,179] There is general consensus that patients with two mutations in *MVK* and/or elevated levels of mevalonate in the urine during acute attacks have HIDS. However, sizeable minorities of patients with seemingly typical disease have only a single identifiable mutation or are mutation negative.[154] The genetic and biochemical basis of disease, particularly in the latter group, remains to be elucidated.

Treatment

Various treatments have been proposed. Some patients may respond to colchicine. Glucocorticoids, intravenous immune globulin, and cyclosporine have all been tried with varying success rates. Small studies demonstrated improvement with etanercept[154,180] and simvastatin.[181] Consistent with the involvement of IL-1β in this disease, on-demand treatment with anakinra has been shown to effectively treat flares of disease.[182] HIDS is not generally associated with a

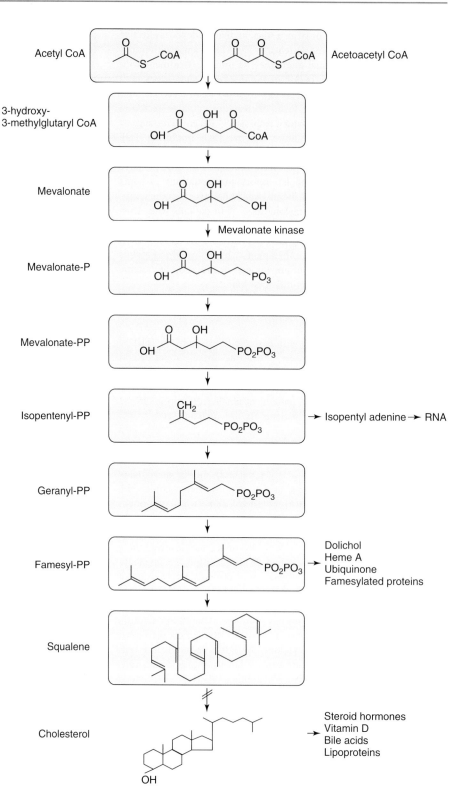

Acetyl CoA

Acetoacetyl CoA

3-hydroxy-
3-methylglutaryl CoA

Mevalonate

Mevalonate kinase

Mevalonate-P

Mevalonate-PP

Isopentenyl-PP → Isopentyl adenine → RNA

Geranyl-PP

Famesyl-PP → Dolichol / Heme A / Ubiquinone / Famesylated proteins

Squalene

Cholesterol → Steroid hormones / Vitamin D / Bile acids / Lipoproteins

FIGURE 47-3 Patients with the hyperimmu-noglobulinemia D with periodic fever syndrome have mutations in mevalonate kinase that result in enzyme activity markedly diminished but not absent. Patients with clinically more severe mevalonic aciduria have mutations leading to an almost total loss of enzyme activity.

shortened life span. Although very rare, HIDS-associated amyloidosis has been reported.[183-186]

CRYOPYRIN-ASSOCIATED PERIODIC FEVER SYNDROMES

Among the episodic or periodic fever syndromes are three clinically distinguishable disorders caused by dominantly inherited abnormalities in cryopyrin (NLRP3), which results from missense mutations in the *NLRP3* gene, formerly denoted *CIAS1* (cold autoinflammatory syndrome 1 gene, discussed later in this chapter). These three disorders include: familial cold autoinflammatory syndrome (FCAS), Muckle–Wells syndrome (MWS), and neonatal-onset multisystem inflammatory disease (NOMID), also called chronic infantile neurological cutaneous and articular syndrome (CINCA). These diseases were originally described as distinct clinical entities, but all phenotypes have

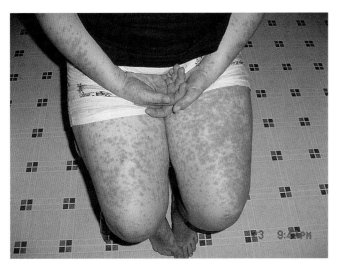

FIGURE 47-4 The rash of HIDS may be a diffuse maculopapular eruption, often extending to the palms and soles.

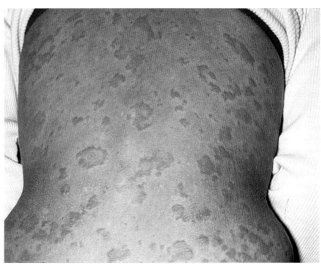

FIGURE 47-5 Urticarial rash is the most common skin manifestation seen in Muckle–Wells syndrome.

some overlapping clinical features; patients often present with fever, neutrophilic urticaria-like skin rash, and joint involvement of varying severity associated with neutrophil-mediated inflammation and an intense acute phase response. In reality, these three syndromes exist on a continuum of severity;[187] however, the clinical description is important regarding disease prognosis. Although patients with FCAS usually have normal life spans, the mortality rate is around 20% in children with NOMID before they reach adulthood.[188,189]

The skin rash—a key feature of all three diseases—is usually the first notable manifestation and develops shortly after birth or in early infancy. This rash exhibits the same clinical and histological characteristics regardless of syndrome: it is migratory, maculopapular, urticaria-like, and usually nonpruritic. Some patients report a burning sensation. The intensity of the skin rash can vary from patient to patient and with disease activity. Microscopic examination of lesional skin reveals a predominant perivascular neutrophilic infiltrate, dermal edema, and dilated blood vessels without the presence of vasculitis, mast cells or mast cell degranulation.[54,190-192] These histological findings are in contrast with the typical lymphocytic and eosinophilic infiltration seen in classical urticaria. For this reason, the rash associated with FCAS, MWS, and NOMID is sometimes called pseudourticaria.[187,192,193]

Familial Cold Autoinflammatory Syndrome

Familial cold autoinflammatory syndrome (FCAS) was first described in 1940.[194] This autosomal-dominant syndrome is characterized by recurrent short and self-limited episodes of fever, rash, and arthralgia precipitated by generalized exposure to cold (Table 47-2).[190,193] The cold sensitivity in FCAS is unlike that in other cold-related disorders such as cryoglobulinemia; it is not only induced by a cool absolute ambient temperature but also by a rapid decrease in temperature. Air conditioning may be very problematic for patients with FCAS in hot climates and provides a clear example of an environmental influence on a genetic disease.[190,195]

Conjunctivitis is frequently observed. Other commonly reported symptoms are muscle pain, profuse sweating, drowsiness, headache, extreme thirst, and nausea. Early onset of the disease, at birth or within the first 6 months of life, is characteristic. Typically, FCAS patients report the development of symptoms beginning 1 to 2 hours after generalized exposure to cold temperatures or to a considerable drop in temperature, and the duration of attacks is usually short (<24

hours). Predictably, attacks are more frequent in winter, on damp and windy days, and following exposure to air conditioning. Most patients describe a correlation between the severity of the crisis and the intensity of cold exposure. Many patients with FCAS also show evidence of chronic inflammation between attacks, particularly a daily pattern of rash developing in the afternoon that can be associated with headache, myalgia, and fatigue by the evening. The typical urticarial rash in FCAS does not necessarily occur on exposed areas of skin, unlike the classic urticarial rash in the more common acquired cold urticaria, in which direct contact with cold objects causes pruritic hives at the site of exposure.[191] The ice cube test is negative, in contrast to what is observed in acquired cold urticaria.[196] Amyloidosis is rarely reported,[196-200] in contradistinction to MWS and NOMID. Leukocytosis and increased acute phase reactants accompany episodes of inflammation.

Hoffman and colleagues[190] proposed a set of diagnostic criteria: (1) recurrent intermittent episodes of fever and rash that primarily follow natural, experimental, or both types of generalized cold exposure; (2) autosomal dominant pattern of disease inheritance; (3) age of onset less than 6 months of age; (4) duration of most attacks less than 24 hours; (5) presence of conjunctivitis associated with attacks; (6) absence of deafness, periorbital edema, lymphadenopathy, and serositis.

Muckle–Wells Syndrome

Muckel–Wells syndrome (MWS) was described in 1962 by Muckle and Wells as a perplexing syndrome of fever, urticarial rash, and limb pain that eventually led to progressive hearing loss and amyloidosis.[201] This disease is usually inherited as an autosomal dominant trait, but apparent sporadic cases also occur.[195,202] MWS is characterized by recurrent episodes of fever and rash associated with joint and eye manifestations, although fever is not always present (see Table 47-2).[187,202,203] Urticarial rash is the most common skin manifestation (Fig. 47-5). In contrast to FCAS, the rash of MWS and its other manifestations are not necessarily triggered by changes in temperature and last longer or can even be continuously present at varying intensity. Precipitating factors cannot usually be identified. The course of the disease varies between individuals from the typical recurrent attacks of inflammation to more persistent symptoms. Joint manifestations can be mild with brief episodes of arthralgia, but recurrent episodes of joint swelling affecting predominantly large joints can be observed.[187,204] Conjunctivitis is

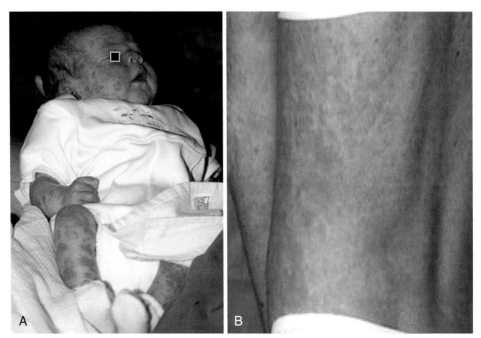

FIGURE 47-6 **A,** An urticaria-like rash is usually present at birth or during the first months of life. **B,** The rash is nonpruritic and papular. (Courtesy Dr. Raphaela Goldbach-Mansky.)

common, and episcleritis and iridocyclitis have been reported.[195] Sensorineural hearing loss is seen in approximately 70% of cases[187,197] and usually begins in late childhood or early adulthood. Abdominal pain and headache may occur in some cases. Amyloid A amyloidosis, due to chronic inflammation, is the primary complication[192,195,205,206] and occurs in approximately one fourth of patients with MWS, reflecting the very intense and prolonged acute-phase response in this particular disorder. It usually manifests as proteinuria, followed by impaired renal function. Amyloid A amyloid fibrils are derived from the circulating acute-phase protein SAA. Other evidence of acute phase response includes elevation of the ESR and leukocytosis,[187,204] and may be observed during episodes of inflammation or nearly constant in severely affected individuals. Clinical manifestations of mild forms of MWS resemble those of FCAS, and more severe phenotypes overlap with NOMID/CINCA.[207,208]

Neonatal-Onset Multisystem Inflammatory Disease

Neonatal-onset multisystem inflammatory disease (NOMID), also known as chronic infantile neurological cutaneous and articular syndrome (CINCA) is associated with the most severe phenotype in the cryopyrin spectrum of diseases, although the clinical manifestations vary in degree (Table 47-2). This syndrome was first described by both Prieur and Goldsmith in the early 1980s[189,209,210] as a chronic inflammatory disease with rash, articular involvement, and chronic aseptic meningitis. Most cases of NOMID appear sporadic, with a few reports of autosomal dominant transmission.[54] With increased quality of life afforded by currently available treatment, more patients with NOMID will reach childbearing potential, and as a result, more patients with autosomal dominant transmission may be recognized.

First symptoms occur at birth or in early infancy. Fever can be intermittent, very mild, or in some cases absent. An urticaria-like, nonpruritic papular rash is usually present at birth or during the first months of life (Fig. 47-6). It varies in intensity from patient to patient, with time, and with disease activity. Bone and joint inflammation also vary in severity: in approximately two thirds of patients, joint manifestations are limited to arthralgia and transient swelling without

effusion, and occur during flare-ups. In one third of patients, joint abnormalities are severe and usually begin within the first year of life. The metaphyses and epiphyses of the long bones are affected, and bony overgrowth can result in gross deformity of the joints, articular and bone pain, and loss of range of motion (Fig. 47-7).[211] Joint involvement is most commonly asymmetrical and chiefly involves the knees; however, the condition can be symmetrical and affect other joints, including the ankles, wrists, and elbows.[211] Radiological manifestations, when present, are distinctive (Fig. 47-7).[211,212] The first recognizable finding is swelling of the periarticular soft tissues, often with visible enlargement of the nonossified portion of the epiphyses. Fraying and cupping of irregular metaphyses follow. The hallmark of this disease is a bizarre enlargement of the ossified portions of the epiphyses of the involved joints. These epiphyses demonstrate erratically ossified, markedly coarsened trabeculae arranged in a random reticular pattern. The borders of the ossified portions of the epiphyses are spiculated and uneven. Eventually, long bones develop bowing of the ends and shortening of the diaphysis. Other radiographic findings include osteoporosis and prominent periosteal new bone formation along the diaphyses and metaphyses of affected long bones. Bone biopsy may show poorly organized cartilaginous columns on hematoxylin-eosin staining, nonhomogeneous spread of chondrocytes with staining for proteoglycans with Alcian blue, and a complementary pattern of calcification seen on von Kossa staining for calcium.[211]

Prematurity and dysmaturity are characteristic of one third of patients. Umbilical cord anomalies were observed in a few children.[189,212,213] Neurological manifestations, including chronic aseptic meningitis, cerebral ventricular dilation, cerebral atrophy, uveitis, optic disc edema, and high-frequency hearing loss are present in various subsets of patients.[187,189,214] High frequency progressive hearing loss is caused by chronic cochlear inflammation that can be seen on gadolinium enhanced images on MRI (Fig. 47-8).[215] Ocular manifestations can progress to blindness, and 25% of patients have a significant ocular disability.[189,203,213,216] Chronic headache, vomiting and papilledema are frequently observed consequences of chronic increased intracranial pressure (Fig. 47-8.). Spastic diplegia and epilepsy may develop.

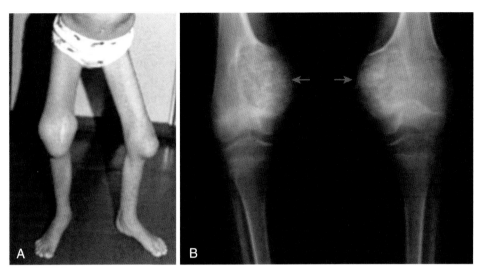

FIGURE 47-7 Joint involvement in NOMID is most commonly asymmetrical and chiefly involves the knees. **A,** The arthropathy can cause gross deformity of the joints with contractures. **B,** A hallmark of NOMID is a bizarre enlargement of the ossified portions of the epiphyses of the involved joints. (Courtesy Dr. Raphaela Goldbach-Mansky.)

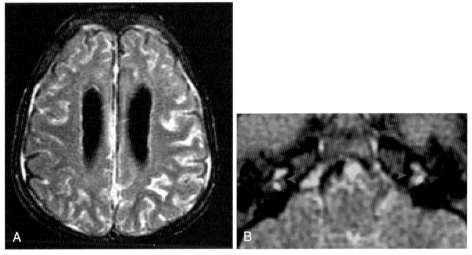

FIGURE 47-8 A, Leptomeningeal enhancement and ventriculomegaly seen on MRI of a patient with NOMID.[215] **B,** Cochlear inflammation seen on gadolinium enhanced MR images. (Courtesy Dr. Raphaela Goldbach-Mansky.)

Progressive cognitive impairment occurs in severely affected patients. Closure of the anterior fontanelle may be delayed, and macrocrania, frontal bossing, and saddle nose appearance are frequently observed due to increased intracranial pressure and the resulting macrocephaly. Cerebral spinal fluid (CSF) examination demonstrates variable hypercellularity with increased polymorphonuclear leukocytes, elevated protein levels, and an increased opening pressure. Computed tomography or MRI can be normal or document mild ventricular dilation and enlarged subdural fluid spaces, suggesting mild cerebral atrophy.[187] Some patients develop progressive calcifications of the falx cerebri and dura mater. Leptomeningeal enhancement can be observed on MRI after gadolinium injection.[215] Amyloid A amyloidosis develops with increasing age in some patients. Severe disabilities are frequent, and premature death is possible in severely affected patients.[189,214]

Findings suggestive of an ongoing inflammatory process include lymphadenopathy, splenomegaly, a prolonged ESR, elevated CRP,

leukocytosis, eosinophilia, and hyperglobulinemia, but autoantibodies are generally not present.[189]

Genetics of Cryopyrin-Associated Periodic Syndromes

Cryopyrin-associated periodic syndromes (CAPS) are associated with missense mutations of the *NLRP3 (CIAS1)* gene and are inherited in an autosomal dominant manner.[195,197,203,214,217,218] Sporadic cases represent *de novo* germline mutations.[214] In approximately half of the patients with typical clinical features of NOMID/CINCA, germline *NLRP3* mutations are not present, but many of these patients have recently been shown to exhibit somatic mosaicism for *NLRP3* mutations.[219-221] This gene encodes the cryopyrin protein, also called NLRP3 or NALP3,[197] which is a member of the nucleotide-binding domain and leucine-rich repeat containing (NLR) family intimately involved in the innate immune system. Cryopyrin contains an N-terminal PYD, a nucleotide binding (NBS/NACHT) domain, and a

C-terminal leucine-rich repeat (LRR) domain.[197,217] More than 100 mutations have been reported (http://fmf.igh.cnrs.fr/infevers/), and almost all are located in the region encoding the NACHT domain and its flanking structures (e.g., exon 3).[187] In the past several years, a small number of mutations have been identified in exons 4 and 6, within the region that encodes the LRR.[187,222-224] While some mutations are specific for a given disorder, particular *NLRP3* mutations may be involved in more than one disease.[54,195,218-225] These findings strongly suggest that additional modifier genes or environmental factors play a role in determining the disease phenotype.[214]

Cryopyrin/NLRP3 is a component of the macromolecular complex, the inflammasome, that senses various microbial products and endogenous "danger signals" and is involved in activation of IL-1β.[5] NLRP3 interacts with apoptosis-associated speck-like protein containing a CARD (ASC) by means of homotypical interaction between its pyrin domain (PYD) and the PYD of ASC.[226] This interaction mediates procaspase-1 activation, and caspase-1 activates pro- IL-1β to its proinflammatory active form, IL-1β. Current evidence suggests that the wild-type NLRP3 is kept in an inactive state either through autoinhibition likely mediated by the interaction between the LRR domains with the NACHT domain of the protein, or through inhibitory interactions with cAMP.[227] Mutations in the NACHT domain or some regions of the LRR domain might disrupt these inhibitory interactions, resulting in increased inflammasome activation and subsequent IL-1β release.[8] *Nlrp3* knockout mice have been described and have established the requirement of NLRP3 for macrophage IL-1β production in response to Toll-like receptor agonists, plus adenosine triphosphate, to Gram-positive bacteria such as *Staphylococcus aureus* or *Listeria monocytogenes*, to bacterial RNA, to dsRNA and viral RNA, and to uric acid crystals.[228-231] Although NLRP3 is required to produce IL-1β in response to these many and varied insults, the disease-causing mutations in this protein do not seem to render CAPS patients clinically overresponsive when faced with these challenges in nature, although some patients anecdotally report increased resistance to common viral infections.[5]

Cryopyrin is expressed on immune cells and chondrocytes.[197,217] Cryopyrin mutations are gain-of-function mutations that lead to constitutive activation of the inflammasome,[8] generating the inappropriate release of IL-1β and leading to the excessive multisystem inflammation responsible for the symptoms associated with CAPS.[232] Consistent with this hypothesis is the finding of oversecretion of IL-1β by peripheral blood leukocytes from patients with CAPS.[8,214,233-236]

Treatment

Elucidation of the pathway involved in IL-1 action has allowed for the development of IL-1 targeted therapies. Targeting the IL-1 pathway has led to new treatment options for patients with CAPS. The use of an IL-1 receptor antagonist (IL-1RA; anakinra), a soluble IL-1 decoy receptor (IL-1 Trap; rilonacept), and an anti-IL-1β monoclonal antibody (canakinumab) have proven to be efficacious in treating CAPS patients.[188,202,215,224,232,234,237-243] In addition to alleviating the fever, rash, conjunctivitis, joint pain, and evidence of systemic inflammation, there are reports of reversal of hearing loss associated with MWS,[234,244,245] and to normalization of the ESR, CRP and SAA levels.[202,246] Treatment with anakinra has also shown to resolve the meningitis, and the ocular and cochlear inflammation of NOMID.[215] Attention must be paid to doses of medications to block the effects of interleukin-1, as studies of CAPS-specific gene expression have suggested incomplete suppression of inflammation at low doses of medications.[247] In some patients, residual central nervous system inflammation and deafness persisted, especially if there had been a delay in diagnosis and treatment.[248] Cochlear enhancement on magnetic resonance imaging correlates with continued hearing loss. Aggressive individual adjustment of IL-1 blockade is

needed to achieve control of inflammation. Unfortunately, treatment with IL-1 blockade does not appear to have an effect on bone lesions. NSAIDs and prednisone may offer temporary clinical relief. Colchicine is ineffective.

Periodic Fever with Aphthous Stomatitis, Pharyngitis, and Adenitis

Periodic fever with aphthous stomatitis, pharyngitis, and adenitis (PFAPA) syndrome (also known as Marshall syndrome) was described in 1987.[249] It is a relatively common condition that has a benign prognosis.[250,251] The precise etiology is unknown; however, it has been suggested that there is a dysregulation of the immune response in patients with PFAPA that may contribute to the etiology.[252] No genetic mutations or ethnic factors have been associated with PFAPA, and although most cases occur sporadically, there have been reports of siblings and parents with similar presentations.[253,254]

Clinical Manifestations

The onset of PFAPA is usually before the age of 5 years. In an American series,[255] febrile episodes occurred approximately every 28 days and lasted for a mean of 5 days. It is the most clock-like of the periodic fevers in children. Children are healthy between episodes and grow normally. Malaise, chills, fatigue, and oral lesions may herald the onset of a cycle. Fever may appear suddenly and reach a maximum of 40° C to 41° C and then resolve over a 24 to 48-hour period. In the largest series reported,[255] 70% of patients had aphthous stomatitis, characterized by shallow ulcers in the buccal mucosa and pharynx that lasted for 3 to 5 days and healed without scarring. Seventy-two percent had pharyngitis,[255] consisting of erythematous, enlarged tonsils.[256] Although cervical adenitis is a major feature of the disease in 88% of patients, generalized lymphadenopathy or noteworthy hepatosplenomegaly suggests a diagnosis other than PFAPA. Arthralgia and abdominal pain may be associated with the fever and are usually mild. Children may also complain of headache with the episodes.

Laboratory Investigations

During episodes, there is an increase in the total white blood cell count and elevation of acute phase reactants. Levels of CRP are substantially increased during the febrile episodes with higher values on days two to four compared to day one of fever.[257] Neutropenia usually is not present, but mild elevations in serum IgG, IgM, and IgA may occur. Elevated levels of IgD were reported in one study[251] but not in another.[255] Increased serum levels of interferon-γ, TNF, IL-1β, and IL-6 have been observed with fevers,[252,258] suggesting that perturbations in the cytokine network contribute to the disease phenotype. Gene expression profiling can distinguish PFAPA flares from asymptomatic intervals, flares due to other hereditary periodic fever syndromes and healthy controls.[259] During PFAPA attacks, complement, IL-1 related and IFN-induced genes were significantly overexpressed. On the protein level, PFAPA flares were accompanied by significantly increased serum levels of chemokines for activated T lymphocytes, G-CSF, and proinflammatory cytokines. One hypothesis is that during a PFAPA flare there is an environmentally triggered activation of complement and IL-1β/-18, with induction of Th1-chemokines and subsequent retention of activated T cells in peripheral tissues.

Diagnosis

PFAPA is diagnosed by exclusion of other probable causes of recurrent fevers in children, such as infectious, autoimmune, and malignant disorders. The differential diagnosis also includes cyclic neutropenia and the hereditary periodic fever syndromes.

- Onset of disease in early childhood, generally prior to the age of 5 years
- Regularly recurring abrupt episodes of fever lasting approximately 5 days, associated with constitutional symptoms, and both of the following:
  - Aphthous stomatitis and/or pharyngitis (with or without cervical adenitis) in the absence of other signs of respiratory tract infection
  - Acute inflammatory markers such as leukocytosis or elevated erythrocyte sedimentation rate
- Completely asymptomatic interval periods (generally lasting less than 10 weeks), benign long-term course, normal growth parameters, and the distinct absence of sequelae
- Exclusion of cyclic neutropenia by serial neutrophil counts, before, during, and after symptomatic episodes
- Exclusion of other episodic syndromes (familial Mediterranean fever, hyper-IgD syndrome, TRAPS, Behçet disease) by family history and the absence of typical clinical features and laboratory markers
- Absence of clinical and laboratory evidence for immunodeficiency, autoimmune disease or chronic infection

From G.S. Marshall, K.M. Edwards, A.R. Lawton, PFAPA syndrome, Pediatr. Infect. Dis. J. 8 (1989) 658–659.

The clinical overlap of PFAPA with these diseases requires their exclusion, but at the same time raises the question of whether PFAPA is a separate entity or whether it represents a collection of other as yet undefined fever syndromes. In order to encourage recognition and facilitate uniform reporting, diagnostic criteria for PFAPA have been established (Box 47-2).[260]

Treatment

Treatment of PFAPA is still a matter of debate. Although NSAIDs may alleviate the fever in some patients, antibiotics and colchicine have generally not been effective in alleviating the spectrum of symptoms observed. The use of prednisone 0.6 mg/kg to 2 mg/kg given orally, as a single dose at the onset of symptoms, on day one and, if necessary, on day two causes a dramatic resolution of febrile episodes, although it does not prevent their recurrence and may actually shorten the interval between episodes.[249,251,255,261] Cimetidine (and, anecdotally, colchicine) may be effective at preventing recurrences.[262-264] Some investigators have reported that tonsillectomy and adenoidectomy may eliminate attacks.[264-270] Two randomized studies on tonsillectomy or adenotonsillectomy have demonstrated that these surgical interventions may induce a remission of fever episodes compared with the control group.[266,269] Although this is certainly promising news to those who care for these children, other nonsurgical interventions should also be considered. Based on the evidence for IL-1β activation, anakinra has been used to treat flares of PFAPA with patients generally demonstrating a prompt clinical and laboratory response.[259]

Outcome and Prognosis

Prognosis seems to be excellent. In long-term follow-up, most patients with PFAPA experienced spontaneous symptom resolution without sequelae in adolescence.[271] Patients with persistent symptoms had episodes of shorter duration and reduced frequency.

BOX 47-3   **Clinical Features of Cyclic Hematopoiesis**

1. Typical cycles recur approximately every 21 days.
2. Absolute neutrophil count is less than 0.2×10^9/L.
3. Absolute neutrophil count is low normal to mildly neutropenic between cycles.

Periodic Fever Due to Cyclic Hematopoiesis

Cyclic hematopoiesis (CH), or cyclic neutropenia, is a rare disorder consisting of febrile episodes due to periodic neutropenia, interspersed between intervals of relatively normal neutrophil counts. CH may occur as a sporadic congenital disorder, an autosomal dominant inherited disease, or an acquired condition.[272-275] Cyclic neutropenia is a more common term for this condition, although cyclic hematopoiesis is more descriptive because other formed elements of blood in addition to neutrophils also demonstrate cyclic variations in numbers.[274] Although the fevers associated with CH are sometimes caused by infectious agents, patients with CH may develop fevers in the absence of apparent infection, perhaps due to the large-scale apoptotic death of bone marrow precursors that underlies the variation in circulating mature forms.[275]

Genetics and Pathogenesis

The clinical features of autosomal dominant familial CH are indistinguishable from those of the sporadic form, suggesting that the sporadic variety may represent unrecognized familial cases or *de novo* mutations in CH genes. Inherited CH is caused by mutations in the neutrophil elastase-2 gene (*ELANE*, formerly *ELA2*),[276-278] which encodes neutrophil elastase (NE), a serine protease of neutrophil and monocyte granules. Mutations in the growth factor independent-1 gene (*GFI1*),[279] which encodes a transcription factor that controls expression of NE, cause severe congenital neutropenia, a noncyclical disorder. In dogs, CH has also been related to mutations in an adaptor protein (AP3B1) bound to NE.[279,280] The equivalent mutation is the cause of the Hermansky-Pudlak syndrome type 2 (HPS2) in humans caused by the absence of AP3B1, and is associated with intermittent neutropenia.[281,282]

There are several hypotheses to account for the periodicity of cyclic neutropenia. One hypothesis is that mutations in *ELANE* lead to altered NE activity, thereby affecting digestion of a number of proteins regulating hematopoiesis, including granulocyte-CSF (G-CSF) and the G-CSF receptor, and most mutations reduce NE activity.[283] Other hypotheses are that CH is a mistrafficking/mislocalization disorder of NE[283] or that CH is caused by low level activation of the unfolded protein response. A more recent hypothesis is that the periodicity of cyclic neutropenia can be explained through a disturbance of a feedback circuit, in which mature neutrophils inhibit cell proliferation, thereby homeostatically regulating progenitor populations.[284]

Clinical Manifestations

Clinical manifestations of CH start in early childhood, with the earliest reported case occurring in the first few weeks of life (Box 47-3).[274] The cycle length is typically 21 days (with a range of 14 to 36 days), and each febrile cycle lasts 3 to 10 days.[274] In older persons, the cycles may not be evident. During attacks, the absolute neutrophil count (ANC) is less than 200/μL and may be 0/μL. Patients who are neutropenic are highly susceptible to infections from normal flora, resulting in recurrent oral ulcers, gingivitis, fever, and lymphadenopathy. Although these infections are usually mild to moderate in severity, severe infections due to *Clostridium* or *Escherichia coli*, with abdominal pain and vomiting rapidly progressing to necrotizing enterocolitis, may occur.[274] *Clostridium septicum* infection has caused enterocolitis, myonecrosis, and death.[285,286] Other symptoms include bone pain, fatigue, malaise, diarrhea, and headache. Symptoms improve rapidly as neutrophils counts recover. Children are well between attacks with ANCs in the low normal to mildly neutropenic range.

Blood monocyte counts cycle in opposite fashion, so that the peak monocyte count coincides with the nadir of the ANC.[287] Reticulocytes, platelets, and eosinophils also may oscillate with neutrophils.[274,276,288] An acute phase response may be observed during the neutropenic episodes. Results of bone marrow examination are characterized by intramedullary destruction of promyelocytes and defects in granulopoiesis[289] due to accelerated apoptosis.[290] Adult-onset CH may be a benign neoplasm with clonal proliferation of large granular lymphocytes.[287,291,292]

Diagnosis

Based on extensive family studies,[274] the diagnosis of autosomal dominant CH can be established with reasonable accuracy based on the following criteria: regular, cyclic fluctuations in peripheral blood neutrophil counts, with a periodicity ranging from 19 to 21 days, and documentation of neutrophil counts less than 200/µL during periods of neutropenia. Complete blood counts should be determined two or three times each week for at least 6 weeks.[274] Genetic testing may play an adjunctive role, especially in families in which formes fruste are suspected or when there is no family history but there is a suspicion of *de novo* mutation.

Treatment

Treatment with granulocyte colony-stimulating factor (G-CSF)[293,294] or granulocyte-macrophage (GM-CSF) may be effective. The recommendation is to administer G-CSF subcutaneously at doses of 1 to 5 µg/kg/day. Symptoms are controlled by this treatment, and the cycles are shortened, with an increase in the nadir ANC.[294]

Infections must be treated promptly and aggressively. *E. coli* and *Clostridium* species precipitate serious and often fatal illness. Appropriate cultures should be obtained, particularly if a child develops abdominal pain with diarrhea and vomiting. Typhlitis (i.e., inflammation of the cecum) and perforating enterocolitis should always be considered.

Outcome and Prognosis

Prognosis appears to be good, except for the increased mortality rate associated with infection.[274] With age, the cycles are less prominent and symptoms improve. Sinusitis and bone pain become more common, whereas fever, lymphadenopathy, and skin infections become rare. Early loss of permanent teeth associated with chronic gingivitis is common to all forms of neutropenia. No association with malignancy has been observed.

Pyogenic Arthritis, Pyoderma Gangrenosum, and Acne Syndrome

Pyogenic arthritis, pyoderma gangrenosum, and acne (PAPA) syndrome is a rare autosomal dominant autoinflammatory syndrome characterized by early onset of recurrent episodes of destructive inflammation of joints and skin (Table 47-2).[295] PAPA syndrome manifests typically with recurrent episodes of sterile, erosive arthritis in early childhood, occurring spontaneously or after minor trauma, occasionally resulting in significant joint destruction.[295-297] Radiographic findings include periosteal proliferation of involved bones and in

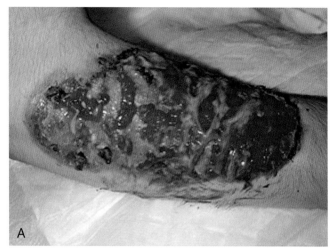

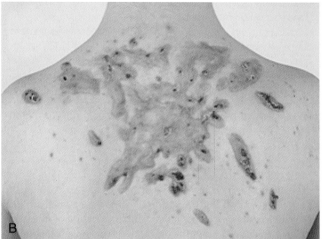

FIGURE 47-9   A, Aggressive ulcerative skin lesions indistinguishable from pyoderma gangrenosum seen in a patient with PAPA. **B,** Cystic acne in PAPA begins in adolescence and persists into adulthood.[302]

some cases ankylosis.[295] The arthritis may respond to corticosteroid therapy; however, the associated adverse effects often limit steroid use. As patients progress to puberty, cutaneous involvement may predominate. Dermatological manifestations are also episodic and recurrent and are characterized by debilitating aggressive ulcerative skin lesions, often of the lower extremities, indistinguishable from pyoderma gangrenosum (Fig. 47-9).[297,298] Although the synovial fluid and skin lesions may have the appearance of an infectious process, culture of skin and joints is sterile. The other component of this triad is cystic acne, which begins in adolescence and persists into adulthood (Fig. 47-9).[296] Other possible manifestations of the PAPA syndrome include pathergy (the formation of sterile abscesses at injection sites), sporadic episodes of irritable bowel syndrome, aphthous stomatitis, and, reported in one family, pancytopenia after administration of sulfa-containing medications.[295,296]

PAPA is caused by mutations in the proline serine threonine phosphatase-interacting protein [PSTPIP1, or CD2 binding protein 1 (CD2BP1)] on chromosome 15[297] that link PEST-type phosphatases to their substrates.[299] The encoded cytoplasmic protein modulates T cell activation,[300] cytoskeletal organization,[301] and IL-1β release.[302] PSTPIP1 interacts with pyrin, and PAPA-associated PSTPIP1 mutations increase the strength of this interaction. Increased PSTPIP1-pyrin interaction, in turn, appears to cause increased IL-1β activation. Increased avidity of PSTPIP1 for pyrin may lead to the formation of macromolecular complexes denoted pyroptosomes, leading to cell death and inflammatory cytokine release.[303]

To date, several missense mutations have been described in an online database of mutations (http://fmf.igh.cnrs.fr/infevers/). Mutations in PSTPIP1 are incompletely penetrant and variably expressed in the PAPA syndrome.[304] Two related syndromes have recently been described: PASH (pyoderma gangrenosum, acne, and suppurative hidradenitis)[305] and PAPASH (pyogenic arthritis, pyoderma gangrenosum, acne, and hidradenitis suppurativa),[306] thus expanding the clinical spectrum associated with mutations in PSTPIP1.

Consistent with the proposed pathogenesis, patient leukocytes produce increased levels of IL-1β in vitro,[302] and increased IL-1β may contribute to TNF production,[307] raising the possibility that treatment with biological agents may be helpful. There are reports of successful treatment with anakinra,[308] etanercept,[307] and infliximab[298] in some patients; however, there is no consistently successful treatment for this syndrome. There is anecdotal evidence that IL-1 inhibition may be more beneficial for joint manifestations and TNF inhibition for pyoderma gangrenosum.

Deficiency of the Interleukin-1 Receptor Antagonist

DIRA is a rare autosomal recessive autoinflammatory disease caused by mutations affecting the gene IL1RN encoding the endogenous IL-1 receptor antagonist.[6,7,309,310] There are founder mutations in Puerto Rico, Newfoundland, the Netherlands, and the Lebanese Israeli border.[6] Children with DIRA present with strikingly similar clinical features, including systemic inflammation in the perinatal period, bone pain, characteristic radiographic findings of multifocal sterile osteolytic bone lesions, widening of multiple anterior ribs, periostitis, pustular skin lesions, skin pathergy, and elevated acute phase reactants (Fig. 47-10). The skin manifestations range from groupings of small pustules to a generalized pustulosis. DIRA-associated IL1RN mutations lead to markedly reduced levels of endogenous IL-1 receptor antagonist, resulting in patient cells being hyperresponsive to IL-1 stimulation, with increased production of proinflammatory cytokines and chemokines. Patients treated with anakinra, a recombinant IL-1 receptor antagonist, exhibit rapid clinical and immunological responses.[6,7,309]

Deficiency of Interleukin Thirty-six Receptor Antagonist

Deficiency of interleukin thirty-six receptor antagonist (DITRA) is a rare life-threatening, multisystem disease involving repeated flare-ups of sudden onset characterized by generalized pustular psoriasis combined with high-grade fever, general malaise, and extracutaneous organ involvement.[311,312] Age of onset is variable. Linkage analysis has identified homozygous mutations in IL36RN, the gene encoding interleukin-36Ra (also known as interleukin-1F5), an antagonist of three cytokines belonging to the interleukin-1 family: interleukin-36α, interleukin-36β, and interleukin-36γ. These cytokines activate several proinflammatory signaling pathways. Mutations of this gene result in a reduction of interleukin-36Ra activity, thus accounting for the name DITRA. Fewer organ systems appear to be affected in DITRA (which primarily involves the skin) then DIRA. Patients with DITRA, in contrast to those with DIRA, have very high-grade fever and general malaise during an attack.

Autoinflammatory Diseases Involving the Immunoproteasome

A common molecular defect involving one component of the immunoproteasome, a protein called PSMB8 (proteasome subunit β type 8)

has been associated with three previously independent clinical syndromes:

- Join contractures, muscle atrophy, microcytic anemia, and panniculitis-induced childhood-onset lipodystrophy (JMP)[313]
- Nakajo-Nishimura syndrome[314]
- Chronic atypical neutrophilic dermatosis with lipodystrophy and elevated temperature (CANDLE)[315]

These conditions are characterized by recurrent fevers, violaceous skin rashes varying from small nodules to annular plaques (also described as pernio-like) covering the trunk and extremities, facial rashes leading to various degrees of edema, violaceous eyelids (mimicking heliotrope rashes), progressive lipodystrophy, arthralgia or arthritis with varying degrees of joint contractures, and increased acute phase reactants (ESR and C-reactive protein). In addition, some patients may have myositis, drumstick widening of the distal fingers, hepatomegaly, lymphadenopathy, a prominent abdomen, low weight and height, and microcytic anemia.

The immunoproteasome is a multi-subunit protease that targets intracellular polyubiquitinated proteins, generating antigenic peptides for class I MHC presentation and maintenance of cell homeostasis. In patients with mutations in PSMB8, the assembly of the inducible proteasome complex is defective and polyubiquitinated proteins accumulate in tissues, leading to an over-activation of a number of proinflammatory intracellular pathways. Microarray analysis suggests a unique interferon signature.

Most clinical symptoms, including cutaneous eruption, joint pain, and fever respond to high doses of steroids (1-2 mg/kg/day), but symptoms often rebound with tapering. Responses to steroid-sparing agents are inconsistent, with variable response observed to anti-TNF, anti-IL1, and anti-IL6 agents, but complete remission has not been achieved with any of these therapies. Additionally, the lipodystrophy tends to progress despite immunosuppressive and cytokine targeted therapy.[315,316] Novel therapies targeting the interferon pathway are investigational.

Deficiency of Adenosine Deaminase 2

Deficiency of adenosine deaminase 2 (DADA2) is a newly recognized recessively inherited disorder caused by loss-of-function mutations in CECR1, encoding adenosine deaminase type 2.[317,318] Patients present usually very early in life with recurrent fevers, a livedoid skin rash, and vascular involvement that can include recurrent lacunar strokes and polyarteritis nodosa. Other possible clinical manifestations are hepatosplenomegaly, portal hypertension, and cutaneous vasculitis. Patients may manifest low-titer antinuclear antibodies, but antineutrophil cytoplasmic antibodies (ANCA) are negative. Hypogammaglobulinemia M is also frequently observed.

The ADA2 protein is a highly glycosylated dimer secreted by myeloid cells, monocytes, T and B lymphocytes, and NK cells, and is considered the prototype for a family of adenosine deaminase growth factors. A total of 14 deleterious mutations have been published to date. Patients have a marked reduction in the levels of ADA2 and ADA2-specific enzyme activity in the blood. Knockdown of a zebrafish ADA2 homologue leads both to intracranial hemorrhage and neutropenia. Immunohistochemical studies of patient skin biopsies demonstrate endothelial damage and perivascular inflammation; cultured monocytes from patients show skewing towards the proinflammatory M1 macrophage subset, and patient monocytes disrupt cocultured monolayers of endothelial cells. Possibly, the deficiency of the ADA2 growth factor leads both to endothelial damage and polarization of monocyte/macrophage subsets toward proinflammatory cells, establishing a vicious circle of vasculopathy and inflammation.

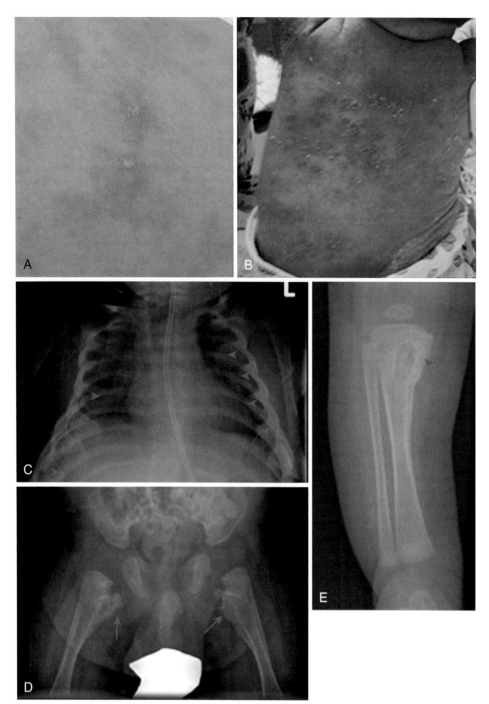

FIGURE 47-10 The skin manifestations range from groupings of small pustules **(A)** to a generalized pustulosis **(B)**. **C,** Typical radiographic manifestations include widening of multiple ribs (with affected ribs indicated with *arrowheads*). **D,** Heterotopic ossification or periosteal cloaking of the proximal femoral metaphysis (*arrows*).[6] **E,** An osteolytic lesion with a sclerotic rim (*arrow*). (Courtesy Dr. Raphaela Goldbach-Mansky.)

Limited observational studies of DADA2 patients with polyarteritis nodosa suggest a possible role for etanercept in the treatment of this disorder. Other potential therapies include replacement either with fresh-frozen plasma or recombinant protein, or bone marrow transplantation.

REFERENCES

1. C.C. John, J.R. Gilsdorf, Recurrent fever in children, Pediatr. Infect. Dis. J. 21 (2002) 1071–1077.

2. M.F. McDermott, I. Aksentijevich, J. Galon, et al., Germline mutations in the extracellular domains of the 55 kDa TNF receptor, TNFR1, define a family of dominantly inherited autoinflammatory syndromes, Cell 97 (1999) 133–144.

3. J. Galon, I. Aksentijevich, M.F. McDermott, et al., TNFRSF1A mutations and autoinflammatory syndromes, Curr. Opin. Immunol. 12 (2000) 479–486.

5. S.L. Masters, A. Simon, I. Aksentijevich, D.L. Kastner, Horror autoinflammaticus: the molecular pathophysiology of autoinflammatory disease (*), Annu. Rev. Immunol. 27 (2009) 621–668.

6. I. Aksentijevich, S.L. Masters, P.J. Ferguson, et al., An autoinflammatory disease with deficiency of the interleukin-1-receptor antagonist, N. Engl. J. Med. 360 (2009) 2426–2437.

7. S. Reddy, S. Jia, R. Geoffrey, et al., An autoinflammatory disease due to homozygous deletion of the IL1RN locus, N. Engl. J. Med. 360 (2009) 2438–2444.

9. International FMF Consortium, Ancient missense mutations in a new member of the RoRet gene family are likely to cause familial Mediterranean fever, Cell 90 (1997) 797–807.

10. French FMF Consortium, A candidate gene for familial Mediterranean fever, Nat. Genet. 17 (1997) 25–31.

12. I. Aksentijevich, Y. Torosyan, J. Samuels, et al., Mutation and haplotype studies of familial Mediterranean fever reveal new ancestral relationships and evidence for a high carrier frequency with reduced penetrance in the Ashkenazi Jewish population, Am. J. Hum. Genet. 64 (1999) 949–962.

41. M.G. Booty, J.J. Chae, S.L. Masters, et al., Familial Mediterranean fever with a single MEFV mutation: where is the second hit?, Arthritis Rheum. 60 (2009) 1851–1861.

44. J.J. Chae, Y.-H. Cho, G.-S. Lee, et al., Gain-of-function pyrin mutations induce NLRP3 protein-independent interleukin 1β activation and severe autoinflammation in mice, Immunity 34 (2011) 755–768.

45. J.J. Chae, G. Wood, S.L. Masters, et al., The B30.2 domain of pyrin, the familial Mediterranean fever protein, interacts directly with caspase-1 to modulate IL-1beta production, Proc. Natl. Acad. Sci. U.S.A. 103 (2006) 9982–9987.

48. P.J. Haskes, S.J. Spalding, E.H. Giannini, et al., Rilonacept for colchicine-resistant or -intolerant familial Mediterranean fever, Ann. Intern. Med. 157 (2012) 533–541.

49. E. Sohar, J. Gafni, M. Pras, H. Heller, Familial Mediterranean fever. A survey of 470 cases and review of the literature, Am. J. Med. 43 (1967) 227–253.

50. A.D. Schwabe, R.S. Peters, Familial Mediterranean fever in Armenians. Analysis of 100 cases, Medicine (Baltimore) 53 (1974) 453–462.

51. H.A. Majeed, M. Rawashdeh, H. el Shanti, et al., Familial Mediterranean fever in children: the expanded clinical profile, QJM 92 (1999) 309–318.

88. I. Touitou, T. Sarkisian, M. Medlej-Hashim, et al., Country as the primary risk factor for renal amyloidosis in familial Mediterranean fever, Arthritis Rheum. 56 (2007) 1706–1712.

93. I. Touitou, S. Lesage, M. McDermott, et al., Infevers: an evolving mutation database for auto-inflammatory syndromes, Hum. Mutat. 24 (2004) 194–198.

109. L.M. Williamson, D. Hull, R. Mehta, et al., Familial Hibernian fever, Q. J. Med. 51 (1982) 469–480.

112. I. Aksentijevich, J. Galon, M. Soares, et al., The tumor-necrosis-factor receptor-associated periodic syndrome: new mutations in TNFRSF1A, ancestral origins, genotype-phenotype studies, and evidence for further genetic heterogeneity of periodic fevers, Am. J. Hum. Genet. 69 (2001) 301–314.

131. A. Simon, H. Park, R. Maddipati, et al., Concerted action of wild-type and mutant TNF receptors enhances inflammation in TNF receptor 1-associated periodic fever syndrome, Proc Nat Acad Sci USA 107 (2010) 9801–9806.

133. K.M. Hull, E. Drewe, I. Aksentijevich, et al., The TNF receptor-associated periodic syndrome (TRAPS): emerging concepts of an autoinflammatory disorder, Medicine (Baltimore) 81 (2002) 349–368.

140. E. Drewe, E.M. McDermott, P.T. Powell, et al., Prospective study of anti-tumour necrosis factor receptor superfamily 1B fusion protein, and case study of anti-tumour necrosis factor receptor superfamily 1A fusion protein, in tumour necrosis factor receptor associated periodic syndrome (TRAPS): clinical and laboratory findings in a series of seven patients, Rheumatology (Oxford) 42 (2003) 235–239.

144. N. ter Haar, H. Lachmann, S. Ozen, et al., Treatment of autoinflammatory diseases: results from the Eurofever Registry and a literature review, Ann. Rheum. Dis. 72 (2013) 678–685.

145. A.C. Bulua, D.B. Mogul, I. Aksentijevich, et al., Efficacy of etanercept in the tumor necrosis factor receptor-associated periodic syndrome: A prospective, open-label, dose-escalation study, Arthritis Rheum. 64 (2012) 908–913.

146. M. Gattorno, M.A. Pelagatti, A. Meini, et al., Persistent efficacy of anakinra in patients with tumor necrosis factor receptor-associated periodic syndrome, Arthritis Rheum. 58 (2008) 1516–1520.

150. J.W. van der Meer, J.M. Vossen, J. Radl, et al., Hyperimmunoglobulinaemia D and periodic fever: a new syndrome, Lancet 1 (1984) 1087–1090.

151. J.P. Drenth, L. Cuisset, G. Grateau, et al., Mutations in the gene encoding mevalonate kinase cause hyper-IgD and periodic fever syndrome. International Hyper-IgD Study Group, Nat. Genet. 22 (1999) 178–181.

152. S.M. Houten, W. Kuis, M. Duran, et al., Mutations in MVK, encoding mevalonate kinase, cause hyperimmunoglobulinaemia D and periodic fever syndrome, Nat. Genet. 22 (1999) 175–177.

154. J.C. van der Hilst, E.J. Bodar, K.S. Barron, et al., Long-term follow-up, clinical features, and quality of life in a series of 103 patients with hyper-immunoglobulinemia D syndrome, Medicine (Baltimore) 87 (2008) 301–310.

182. E.J. Bodar, L.M. Kuijk, J.P.H. Drenth, et al., On demand anakinra is effective in mevalonate kinase deficiency, Ann. Rheum. Dis. 70 (2011) 2155–2158.

189. A.M. Prieur, C. Griscelli, F. Lampert, et al., A chronic, infantile, neurological, cutaneous and articular (CINCA) syndrome. A specific entity analysed in 30 patients, Scand. J. Rheumatol. Suppl. 66 (1987) 57–68.

190. H.M. Hoffman, A.A. Wanderer, D.H. Broide, Familial cold autoinflammatory syndrome: phenotype and genotype of an autosomal dominant periodic fever, J. Allergy Clin. Immunol. 108 (2001) 615–620.

194. R.I.R.H. Kyle, A case of cold urticaria with unusual family history, JAMA 114 (1940) 1067.

197. H.M. Hoffman, J.L. Mueller, D.H. Broide, et al., Mutation of a new gene encoding a putative pyrin-like protein causes familial cold autoinflammatory syndrome and Muckle-Wells syndrome, Nat. Genet. 29 (2001) 301–305.

201. T.J. Muckle, M. Wells, Urticaria, deafness, and amyloidosis: a new heredofamilial syndrome, Q. J. Med. 31 (1962) 235–248.

203. I. Aksentijevich, D.P. C, E.F. Remmers, et al., The clinical continuum of cryopyrinopathies: novel CIAS1 mutations in North American patients and a new cryopyrin model, Arthritis Rheum. 56 (2007) 1273–1285.

207. B. Neven, I. Callebaut, A.M. Prieur, et al., Molecular basis of the spectral expression of CIAS1 mutations associated with phagocytic cell-mediated autoinflammatory disorders CINCA/NOMID, MWS, and FCU, Blood 103 (2004) 2809–2815.

209. A.M. Prieur, C. Griscelli, Arthropathy with rash, chronic meningitis, eye lesions, and mental retardation, J. Pediatr. 99 (1981) 79–83.

210. S.G. Hassink, D.P. Goldsmith, Neonatal onset multisystem inflammatory disease, Arthritis Rheum. 26 (1983) 668–673.

214. I. Aksentijevich, M. Nowak, M. Mallah, et al., De novo CIAS1 mutations, cytokine activation, and evidence for genetic heterogeneity in patients with neonatal-onset multisystem inflammatory disease (NOMID): a new member of the expanding family of pyrin-associated autoinflammatory diseases, Arthritis Rheum. 46 (2002) 3340–3348.

215. R. Goldbach-Mansky, N.J. Dailey, S.W. Canna, et al., Neonatal-onset multisystem inflammatory disease responsive to interleukin-1beta inhibition, N. Engl. J. Med. 355 (2006) 581–592.

217. J. Feldmann, A.M. Prieur, P. Quartier, et al., Chronic infantile neurological cutaneous and articular syndrome is caused by mutations in CIAS1, a gene highly expressed in polymorphonuclear cells and chondrocytes, Am. J. Hum. Genet. 71 (2002) 198–203.

231. F. Martinon, V. Petrilli, A. Mayor, et al., Gout-associated uric acid crystals activate the NALP3 inflammasome, Nature 440 (2006) 237–241.

232. H.M. Hoffman, M.L. Throne, N.J. Amar, et al., Efficacy and safety of rilonacept (interleukin-1 Trap) in patients with cryopyrin-associated periodic syndromes: results from two sequential placebo-controlled studies, Arthritis Rheum. 58 (2008) 2443–2452.

242. H.J. Lachmann, I. Kone-Paut, J.B. Kuemmerle-Deschner, et al., Use of canakinumab in the cryopyrin-associated periodic syndrome, N. Engl. J. Med. 360 (2009) 2416–2425.

243. R. Goldbach-Mansky, Current status of understanding the pathogenesis and management of patients with NOMID/CINCA, Curr. Rheumatol. Rep. 13 (2011) 123–131.

246. P.N. Hawkins, H.J. Lachmann, M.F. McDermott, Interleukin-1-receptor antagonist in the Muckle-Wells syndrome, N. Engl. J. Med. 348 (2003) 2583–2584.

247. J.E. Balow Jt, J.G. Ryan, J.J. Chae, et al., Microarray-based gene expression profiling in patients with cryopyrin-associated periodic syndromes defines a disease-related signature and IL-1 responsive transcripts, Ann. Rheum. Dis. 72 (2013) 1064–1070.

248. B. Neven, I. Marvillet, C. Terrada, et al., Long-term efficacy of the interleukin-1 receptor antagonist anakinra in ten patients with neonatal-onset multisystem inflammatory disease/chronic infantile neurologic, cutaneous, articular syndrome, Arthritis Rheum. 62 (2010) 258–267.

249. G.S. Marshall, K.M. Edwards, J. Butler, A.R. Lawton, Syndrome of periodic fever, pharyngitis, and aphthous stomatitis, J. Pediatr. 110 (1987) 43–46.

255. K.T. Thomas, H.M. Feder Jr., A.R. Lawton, K.M. Edwards, Periodic fever syndrome in children, J. Pediatr. 135 (1999) 15–21.

259. S. Stojanov, S. Lapidus, P. Chitkara, et al., Periodic fever, aphthous stomatitis, pharyngitis, and adenitis (PFAPA) is a disorder of innate immunity and Th1 activation responsive to IL-1 blockade, Proc Natl Acad Sci USA 108 (2011) 7148–7153.

261. H.M. Feder Jr., Periodic fever, aphthous stomatitis, pharyngitis, adenitis: a clinical review of a new syndrome, Curr. Opin. Pediatr. 12 (2000) 253–256.

271. V.M. Wurster, J.G. Carlucci, H.M. Feder, K.M. Edwards, Long-term follow-up of children with periodic fever, aphthous stomatitis, pharyngitis, and cervical adenitis syndrome, J. Pediatr. 159 (2011) 958–964.

273. D.C. Dale, A.A. Bolyard, W.P. Hammond, Cyclic neutropenia: natural history and effects of long-term treatment with recombinant human granulocyte colony-stimulating factor, Cancer Invest. 11 (1993) 219–223.

277. D.C. Dale, R.E. Person, A.A. Bolyard, et al., Mutations in the gene encoding neutrophil elastase in congenital and cyclic neutropenia, Blood 96 (2000) 2317–2322.

302. N.G. Shoham, M. Centola, E. Mansfield, et al., Pyrin binds the PSTPIP1/CD2BP1 protein, defining familial Mediterranean fever and PAPA syndrome as disorders in the same pathway, Proc. Natl. Acad. Sci. U.S.A. 100 (2003) 13501–13506.

305. M. Braun-Falco, O. Kovnerystyy, P. Lohse, T. Ruzicka, Pyoderma gangrenosum, acne, and suppurative hidradenitis (PASH): a new autoinflammatory syndrome distinct from PAPA syndrome, J. Am. Acad. Dermatol. 66 (2012) 409–415.

306. A.V. Marzano, V. Trevisan, M. Gattorno, et al., Pyogenic arthritis, pyoderma gangrenosum, acne, and hidradenitis suppurativa (PAPASH): a new autoinflammatory syndrome associated with a novel mutation of the PSTPIP1 gene, JAMA Dermatol 149 (2013) 762–764.

Entire reference list is available online at www.expertconsult.com.

CHAPTER 48

Autoinflammatory Bone Disorders

Polly J. Ferguson, Ronald M. Laxer

Autoinflammatory disorders (discussed in Chapter 47) result from aberrant activation of the innate immune system.[1,2] They occur in the absence of high titer autoantibodies or autoreactive lymphocytes, thus distinguishing them from the classic autoimmune disorders.[1,3] The concept of autoinflammatory disorders was proposed in 1999, following the identification of the genetic basis of the prototypic periodic fever syndromes, familial Mediterranean fever and TRAPS (TNF receptor-associated periodic syndrome).[1,4-6] There are now more than 30 disorders that are thought to be autoinflammatory, most of which affect children; included are a group of disorders that have bone inflammation as a main phenotypic feature, including chronic recurrent multifocal osteomyelitis (CRMO); synovitis, acne, pustulosis, hyperostosis, osteitis (SAPHO) syndrome; Majeed syndrome; deficiency of interleukin-1 receptor antagonist (DIRA); and cherubism.[1,7,8]

CHRONIC RECURRENT MULTIFOCAL OSTEOMYELITIS

Overview

In 1972, Giedion recognized what is now commonly referred to as chronic recurrent multifocal osteomyelitis (CRMO) as a distinct clinical entity when he described four children with noninfectious multifocal osteomyelitis who presented with subacute and chronic symmetric osteomyelitis.[9] The term *chronic recurrent multifocal osteomyelitis* was coined by Probst, Bjorksten, and Gustavson to describe the recurrent nature of the illness.[10,11] Since that time, the term has been commonly used for this clinical entity despite the fact that the disease is neither always multifocal nor recurrent. The co-occurrence of CRMO with pustulosis palmoplantaris (PPP) was reported in 1967 in a child with bilateral clavicular osteitis, but it was Bjorksten et al. who firmly established the association with CRMO and PPP.[11,12] The association of CRMO with PPP has been confirmed by others and descriptions of additional dermatologic associations with CRMO including psoriasis vulgaris, severe acne, generalized pustulosis and Sweet syndrome followed shortly thereafter.[13-22] Subsequently, reports of the co-occurrence of CRMO and inflammatory bowel disease emerged as well as the observation that CRMO may evolve into spondyloarthropathy over time in some patients, suggesting that CRMO might best fit in the spondyloarthropathy family of disorders.[23-36] Recently, the identification of the genetic basis for a subgroup of early-onset CRMO cases and for murine models of disease has defined CRMO as an autoinflammatory syndrome.[7,37-45]

NOMENCLATURE

It is difficult to review the CRMO literature because many terms have been utilized to describe similar clinical entities. Names that have been used to describe cases of sterile inflammatory bone disorders that occur in the presence or absence of skin or intestinal inflammation are listed in Box 48-1.[35,46-59] The most common terms utilized in the literature are CRMO and SAPHO syndrome. SAPHO is an acronym proposed in 1987 by Chamot et al. as a broad umbrella term to denote a clinical syndrome characterized by inflammation of the bone, joint, and skin.[60,61] The SAPHO syndrome encompasses bone inflammation in the form of sterile osteomyelitis or as hyperostosis; inflammation of the skin, including acne or pustulosis and inflammation of the joint in the form of synovitis. SAPHO syndrome is the term most frequently utilized by adult rheumatologists, whereas the pediatric community has primarily utilized the term CRMO.[33,47,62-65] SAPHO syndrome and CRMO may well be the same disorder presenting in different age groups (CRMO in childhood and SAPHO in adults) or it may be that they are distinct disorders that are part of the same disease spectrum.

Another problem with the term CRMO is that sometimes the disease process is unifocal or is multifocal without recurrence, thus limiting the accuracy of the diagnostic term for many patients' clinical course. For instance, in a German cohort of 89 patients with at least one noninfectious inflammatory bone lesion, approximately 20% had bone inflammation in one location with disease duration longer than 6 months without recurrence (unifocal nonrecurrent), nearly 45% of patients had classic CRMO with multiple bone lesions with recurrent flares with remissions (recurrent multifocal), and the remaining 35% had persistent multifocal bone inflammation for longer than 6 months without remissions (persistent multifocal).[66] In addition, some children present with unifocal disease, yet over time develop classic multifocal recurrent disease.[66] Similarly, in a cohort reported by Girschick et al. of 30 pediatric patients with sterile osteitis, 30% had unifocal nonrecurrent disease, 10% had unifocal recurrent disease, 30% had multifocal nonrecurrent disease and 30% had classic CRMO.[67] Because of this, several authors have proposed other names, including chronic nonbacterial osteomyelitis (CNO) and chronic nonbacterial osteitis (NBO).[66,67] In this chapter, we will utilize the term CRMO.

Incidence, Geographic and Racial Distribution

CRMO is a rare disorder. Several hundred cases have been reported in the literature, but the incidence of the disease is unknown. Early reports of CRMO were predominantly from Scandinavia. However, review of the literature suggests a worldwide distribution of disease affecting multiple ethnicities and races.[12,13,66,68]

Age at Onset and Sex Ratio

CRMO is primarily a disease of young girls, with peak onset between 7 to 12 years of age.[66,69] Females are affected at a rate two to four times more often than males.[34,66,67,69-72] The majority of cases occur in childhood but adults can be affected and are more likely to be reported as SAPHO syndrome.[62,71,73] Onset of CRMO prior to the age of 2 years is unusual and should prompt an evaluation for a syndromic form of CRMO, including DIRA and Majeed syndrome.[37-39,41]

Etiology and Pathogenesis

CRMO best fits into the category of autoinflammatory disorders, a group of innate immune system disorders in which there are "seemingly unprovoked" episodes of inflammation.[1,3,74] In most cases of CRMO (and SAPHO), bone inflammation occurs in the absence of an identifiable trigger. Cultures of the bone are typically sterile, antibiotic therapy is rarely accompanied by clinical improvement, and antiinflammatory medications improve the condition.[66,69-72,75-80] Despite the inability to culture an organism in the vast majority of cases, many have postulated that the osteitis is driven or triggered by exposure to a microbial agent. There are a few reports of bone cultures growing organisms including *Propionibacterium acnes*, *Mycoplasma*, and various *Staphylococcus* species.[26,27,69,76-78,80-87] However, in many cases it is unclear whether it is a contaminated specimen or a true infection.[80] In a cohort of adults with inflammatory osseous anterior chest wall lesions, most of whom also had palmoplantar pustulosis, *Propionibacterium acnes* was cultured in bone biopsy samples from 7 of the 15 patients, suggesting that for this population of adult patients infection may have played a role in pathogenesis.[85] However, in children with CRMO and for most adults with SAPHO syndrome, the vast majority of cultures of pustules and bone are negative.[69,78,79,86]

Girshick et al. looked for evidence of microbial infection in 25 patients with chronic nonbacterial osteomyelitis, all of whom had a bone biopsy performed as part of their diagnostic evaluation.[67] All biopsies were sent for aerobic and anaerobic bacterial, mycobacterial, and fungal organisms. Eubacterial polymerase chain reaction was performed on 12 of the 25 bone biopsy samples, yet no bacterial ribosomal DNA was detected.[67] Serologic testing for evidence of *Borrelia burgdorferi*, *Salmonella*, *Yersinia enterocolitica*, *Campylobacter jejuni* and *Streptococcus pyogenes* showed no evidence of acute or chronic infection with any of these microbes.[67] Supporting the lack of an active infection as an etiology in CRMO or SAPHO syndrome, prolonged antimicrobial therapy rarely results in clinical improvement.[69,70,88,89] Schilling et al. reported that 7 of 13 patients with CRMO treated with azithromycin had rapid clinical and radiologic improvement.[86,90] However, azithromycin has a known antiinflammatory effect, and so a response to azithromycin does not necessarily support an active infection in CRMO.[91,92] Bjorksten et al. and Jurik et al. reported that approximately 25% of CRMO patients reported trauma preceding the development of chronic bone inflammation,[11,73] suggesting tissue damage as another possible trigger, although this has not been found in most series.

The precise immunologic basis of CRMO remains unknown. There is no evidence of immune deficiency in the vast majority of children and the lack of high titer autoantibodies suggests that it does not have an autoimmune basis.[69,77] Although a German cohort was noted to have a positive ANA greater than or equal to 1:120 in approximately one third of cases, this hasn't been found other cohorts.[66] There is no significant association with HLA-B27 positivity.[66,69,77] There are reports of neutrophil dysfunction in CRMO; however, the role of neutrophils in these disorders has not been fully studied.[11,73,93]

There are two murine models of CRMO, which are both due to mutations in proline-serine-threonine phosphatase interacting protein-2 (*Pstpip2*) gene. The chronic multifocal osteomyelitis (cmo) mouse lacks detectable *Pstpip2* and the mice develop multifocal osteomyelitis beginning at 6 to 8 weeks of age.[40,43] Mouse models of CRMO have demonstrated that the adaptive immune system is not needed for disease development[40,42,94] supporting the autoinflammatory nature of the disease. Recently, two groups demonstrated dysregulation of the IL-1 pathway in the pathogenesis of disease in the cmo mouse.[44,45] In this model, both groups demonstrated that the inflammatory phenotype was IL-1 dependent, as the mice were completely protected if the cmo mice lacked a functional IL-1 receptor (IL-1RI).[44,45] Yet, disease occurred in the absence of a functional Nlrp3 inflammasome and occurred in cmo.caspase-1 knockout mice.[44,45] Further, using a genetic approach, they demonstrated that it is IL-1β, not IL-1α, that is needed for disease.[44,45] Cmo neutrophils, but not cmo bone marrow–derived macrophages, secreted increased IL-1β in response to ATP, silica, and *P. aeruginosa* when compared to wild-type neutrophils.[44] The aberrant neutrophil response could be inhibited by serine protease inhibitors.[44] These results demonstrate that bone disease in the cmo mouse is an inflammasome-independent, IL-1β–mediated disease[44,45] and implicates neutrophils and neutrophil serine proteases in disease pathogenesis.[44] In addition, the discovery that infantile-onset noninfectious multifocal osteitis associated with generalized pustulosis (deficiency of the interleukin-1 receptor antagonist [DIRA]) is due to IL-1 pathway dysregulation lends additional support to the notion that CRMO, SAPHO, and related disorders are autoinflammatory.[38,39]

Many authors have noted the tendency for CRMO or SAPHO syndrome to evolve into a picture consistent with spondyloarthropathy over time.[27,47,64,72,95] Rohekar and Inman point out that SAPHO syndrome has many features that fit into the spondyloarthropathy family with features that suggest it lies in the spectrum of disease between ankylosing spondylitis and psoriatic arthritis (Fig. 48-1).[33,36] The connection between CRMO and inflammatory bowel disease also supports the contention that CRMO is part of the spondyloarthropathy spectrum of disease. Crohn disease and ulcerative colitis have both been reported in conjunction with CRMO and SAPHO syndrome.[24-26,28-32,36] When inflammatory bowel disease (IBD) is associated with CRMO, pyoderma gangrenosum may accompany the inflammatory gut and bone disease.[21,32,96] The link between gut inflammation and spondyloarthropathies is well established, with endoscopic gastrointestinal inflammation detectable in greater than 40% of spondyloarthropathy patients.[97,98] In three CRMO cohorts, 13% of affected individuals had a first- or second-degree relative with Crohn disease, further supporting the link between IBD and autoinflammatory bone disease.[7,66,70]

Role of Genetics in CRMO Pathogenesis

There is evidence that genetics plays a prominent role in susceptibility to CRMO. There are reports of affected siblings, concordant monozygotic twins (with unaffected parents), as well as parent/child duos.[15,49,59,66,93,99] There are also reports of first degree relatives with CRMO in one and PPP or psoriasis in at least one other.[7,66,73,99,100] Golla et al. performed an association study in CRMO and found evidence for a susceptibility locus on chromosome 18q21.3-22.[99] More recently, Hofmann et al. detected an association with a promotor polymorphism in the IL-10 gene that has been associated with high IL-10 production.[101] Further support for a genetic basis of CRMO comes from animal models of the disease. Two single gene murine models of disease and a canine model all develop spontaneous sterile multifocal osteomyelitis.[40,42,43,102] And finally, up to half of the first and second degree relatives of individuals with CRMO have another inflammatory disorder, most often some form of psoriasis (palmar plantar pustulosis or psoriasis vulgaris) or inflammatory bowel disease.[7,66,103] Definitive proof that CRMO can be genetically determined came when *LPIN2* was identified as the causative gene for Majeed syndrome, followed by the identification of autosomal recessive mutations in *pstpip2* in two murine models of disease (Fig. 48-2) and by the identification of mutations in *IL1RN* in infants with DIRA.[37-40,42]

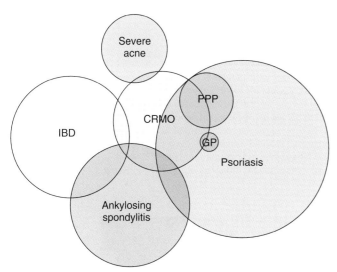

FIGURE 48-1 Overlapping features of the main inflammatory disorders associated with CRMO. *CRMO*, Chronic recurrent multifocal osteomyelitis; *GP*, generalized pustular psoriasis; *IBD*, inflammatory bowel disease; *PPP*, palmoplantar pustulosis.

Clinical Manifestations of CRMO

The typical clinical presentation of CRMO is local bone pain with or without fever.[11,27,69,72] The pain is typically worse at night. Onset is usually insidious, although some patients present with acute pain.[11,27,76] Tenderness, swelling, or warmth are often present overlying the involved bone but may be absent.[11,27,34,69,76-78,104] At any one time, the number of osteomyelitis lesions can vary from one to 18.[69] The symptoms may be intermittent or chronic and persistent, lasting from months to as long as 20 years.[69,70,105] However, many individuals instead have chronic unremitting symptoms that may vary in severity.[70] The disease may affect virtually any bone of the body, but the metaphyseal regions of the long bones, clavicle, vertebral bodies and pelvis are the most commonly affected sites.[27,66,67,69,70,103,106,107] Involvement is symmetric in 25% to 40% of individuals.[66,69]

The local swelling involving the soft tissues adjacent to the inflamed bone may mimic arthritis when the lesions affect the metaphyseal regions of the long bones.[27] Clavicular lesions often present with marked swelling and tenderness, most often involving the medial one third of the bone (Fig. 48-3).[11,72,73,108] When the pelvis or vertebrae are involved, the patient presents with pain (local or referred), limp, or pelvic girdle weakness.[72] Synovitis may accompany the bone lesions and can occur distant from the sites of bone involvement.[66,67,103] In one study 80% of patients had been diagnosed with arthritis in joints adjacent to the lesion; some had synovial biopsies that revealed histologic evidence of synovitis.[67] Fever accompanies the bone pain at presentation in 17% to 33% of patients.[34,69,73,103] Most often the affected individuals appear well, although many complain of malaise and fatigue.[72,73] Twenty-five percent of CRMO patients present with an extra osseous manifestation, most commonly a pustular rash on the palms and soles (Fig. 48-4).[27,67,69]

The majority of affected individuals have modest elevations of the erythrocyte sedimentation rate and C-reactive protein.[66,69,73,80] White blood cell counts are typically normal or only mildly elevated.[27,66,69] High titer autoantibodies are typically absent and there is no strong association with HLA-B27.[34,67,69,76] Tumor necrosis factor alpha (TNF-α)[66,101] and interleukin-6 were elevated in the serum of patients with CNO, suggesting a role for these cytokines in the pathogenesis of the disease.[66,101]

Radiographic Studies

Very early in the disease plain films may be normal or only show osteopenia; however, increased uptake on technetium bone scan or

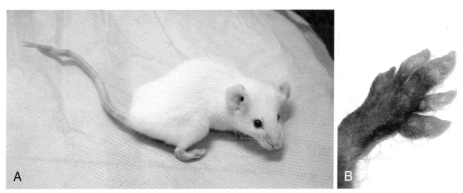

FIGURE 48-2 Tail kinks and hindfoot deformities in the cmo mouse model of CRMO. **A,** A cmo mouse with segmental swelling of the tail, swollen hindfoot, and increased erythema of the left ear. **B,** Swelling and deformity in the hindfoot and digits accompanied by thickening and discoloration of the nails in a cmo mouse. The swelling of the digits resembles dactylitis.

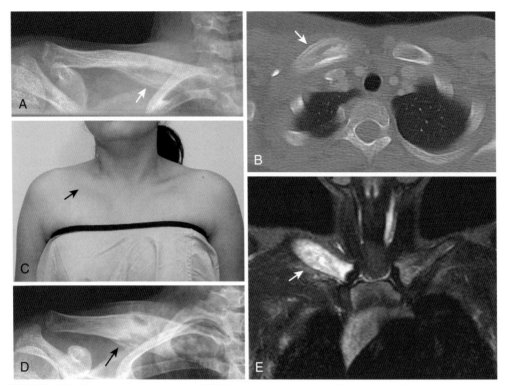

FIGURE 48-3 Clavicular involvement in CRMO. Adolescent female with unilateral clavicular involvement. **A,** Plain radiograph of the right clavicle at presentation reveals widening of the medial two thirds, with associated periosteal reaction. **B,** Corresponding CT scan of the right clavicle demonstrates expansion of the medial right clavicle with areas of increased sclerosis accompanied by a surrounding periosteal reaction (*arrow*). **C,** Flare of disease 18 months later showing further clavicular enlargement (clinical photo). **D,** Plain radiograph of the right clavicle at that time demonstrates marked interval sclerosis and thickening. **E,** MRI at the same time shows increased signal intensity on fat-suppressed contrast-enhanced T1-weighted images of the right medial clavicle consistent with continued inflammation. (Images courtesy Dr. P. Babyn.)

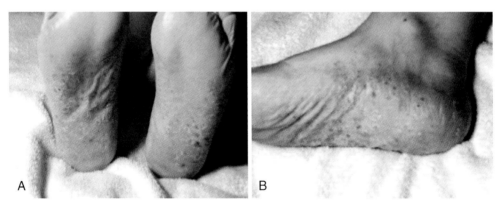

FIGURE 48-4 Palmoplantar pustulosis. Pustules in various phases of healing on the soles of an individual with CRMO **(A)** and PPP **(B)**.

evidence of marrow edema on MRI can be seen at this stage. Mixed osteolytic and sclerotic lesions, with a predilection for the metaphyses of the long bones, are one of the most common radiologic findings (Fig. 48-5).[10,72,105,109,110] Periosteal reaction may be present[10,80]; involvement of the small tubular bones is more likely to be accompanied by a significant periosteal reaction than is typically seen in the long bones.[80,110] Cortical thickening or progressive sclerosis of the lesions occurs later in the course of the disease, followed by gradual normalization of the radiographic appearance over several years.[10,66,70,72,80,105,110]

Epiphyseal involvement is unusual but may occur and when present may lead to premature epiphyseal fusion.[80,110] Likewise, diaphyseal involvement is unusual but is typically adjacent to involved metaphyseal regions.[72]

Clavicular lesions are typically located in the medial clavicle and may have a lytic destructive appearance with periosteal new bone formation when the disease is active.[72,108,111] As the lesions heal, the clavicle becomes increasingly sclerotic in appearance.[72,108] Repeated periods of remission and active disease often results in progressive

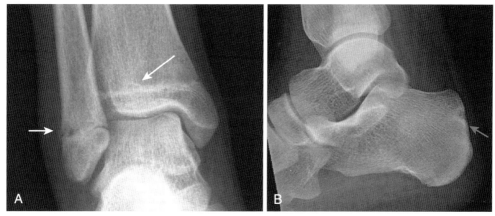

FIGURE 48-5 Typical lesions of CRMO. **A,** Osteolytic lesion with surrounding sclerosis in the metaphyseal area of the distal fibula (*short arrow*) and the distal tibia (*long arrow*). **B,** Osteolytic lesion with surrounding sclerosis in the calcaneus (*arrow*).

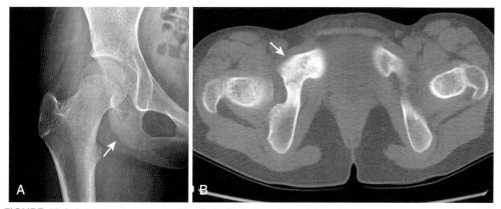

FIGURE 48-6 Pelvic involvement in CRMO. **A,** Plain film of the right pelvis demonstrates expansion of the ischium without visible osteolytic lesions *(arrow)*. **B,** CT of the region demonstrates expansion of the ischium with sclerosis and osteolytic lesions on the right *(arrow)*.

clavicular sclerosis and hyperostosis.[55,72] Vertebral lesions typically display erosion of vertebral plates sometimes accompanied by reduced intervertebral space, which can mimic infectious spondylodiscitis.[10,11,72,112,113] Alternatively, a destructive lytic lesion involving a vertebral body may precede its collapse.[72,114] Vertebra plana may be seen.[36,79,115] Involvement of the bones of the pelvis may occur at joint surfaces or synchondroses and often have a sclerotic appearance (Fig. 48-6).[72] Sacroiliitis may also occur as part of the osseous pelvic lesions (Fig. 48-7).[27,34,70,72,110]

Asymptomatic lesions are common and can be screened for by technetium bone scan.[72,79,80,109] MRI is very useful for gauging activity and extent of the bone lesions and is preferred over bone scan for diagnosis and subsequent management.[72,110,116] In addition, it provides information about the extent of soft tissue involvement.[72,110] Active lesions typically have high signal intensity on T2-weighted images and on short tau inversion recovery (STIR) images accompanied by decreased signal intensity on T1 weighted images.[72] The ability to more clearly discern the extent of soft tissue involvement makes STIR images extremely useful.[72,110] Whole body MRI with STIR images offer an alternative to bone scan for detecting asymptomatic lesions (see Chapter 9.).[106,107,110,117-122] The advantage of MRI over bone scan is that the lesions of CRMO often occur in the metaphyseal regions of the long bones and are often symmetric. In a growing child, symmetric inflammatory lesions in the metaphyses may be read as normal increased uptake due to metabolic activity in the open growth plate. An additional benefit of MRI is that it spares radiation exposure.

A reasonable radiographic approach in a child with suspected CRMO would be to start with plain radiographs of symptomatic regions, perform a whole body MRI with STIR images (or bone scan if whole body MRI is not possible) to detect asymptomatic lesions, obtain plain radiographs of the additional lesions and utilize site specific MRI to further delineate extent of disease as needed.

Histology

Histologic findings in the bone vary depending on the age of the lesion with neutrophils prominent in early lesions while a mixed inflammatory infiltrate consisting primarily of lymphocytes and plasma cells with various degrees of sclerosis and fibrosis are present later.[11,69,71,73,76,77] Abscess formation surrounded by lymphocytes and increased osteoclasts with signs of bone resorption also can be seen early.[71] Later, there is a predominance of lymphocytes, accompanied by plasma cells, histocytes, and a few neutrophils.[69,71,73,77] Noncaseating granulomas have been reported in some biopsies.[11,71] Multinucleated giant cells, necrotic bone, areas of new bone formation, and fibrosis can also be seen in late lesions.[69,71,73,77] The histopathologic picture may vary within the same sample, and it is therefore important to evaluate multiple sections from each biopsy specimen.[77]

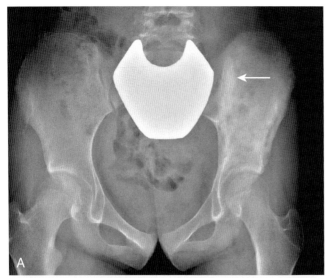

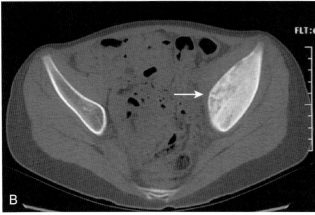

FIGURE 48-7 Involvement of the pelvis with sacroiliitis and osteomyelitis of the ilium. **A,** Unilateral sacroiliitis is present with sclerosis of the SI joint that is most prominent on the iliac side of the joint (*arrow*). There is associated increase sclerosis of the left ilium with multiple moth eaten lesions scattered throughout the left side of the pelvis. **B,** CT scan shows marked expansion of the left ilium with multiple small osteolytic lesions with surrounding sclerosis on the left (*arrow*).

Associated Inflammatory Conditions

There is a firm association of CRMO with inflammatory disorders of the skin and gut. These include palmoplantar pustulosis,[11,12,15,22,23] psoriasis vulgaris,[13,23] generalized pustulosis,[123] Sweet syndrome,[18-21] severe acne[14,17] and pyoderma gangrenosum.[32,70,96] An association also exists with inflammatory bowel disease, most often Crohn disease but also with ulcerative colitis and celiac disease.[24-26,28-32,66,70,124] Peripheral arthritis has been reported with CRMO often adjacent to active bone lesions but can involve joints distant to the osteitis[35,66,67,70]; sacroiliac joint disease has also been reported.[27] Other disorders that have been reported in individuals with CRMO include Takayasu arteritis,[34,125,126] Wegener granulomatosus,[70,75] sclerosing cholangitis,[26,70] Ollier disease,[70] myositis,[103,106,127,128] Still disease,[129] tumoral calcinosis,[130] and parenchymal lung disease.[131,132]

Differential Diagnosis

There are no validated diagnostic criteria and no diagnostic test for CRMO. Jansson et al. developed a clinical score to aid in differentiating nonbacterial osteitis from other bone lesions. They found that a normal complete blood count; symmetric bone lesions; lesions with marginal sclerosis; absence of fever; lesion in a vertebra, clavicle or sternum; the presence of a radiographic-proven lesion, and C-reactive protein level greater than or equal to 1 mg/dl were suggestive of CRMO. A clinical score can then be calculated that ranges from 0 to 63 with a score of greater than or equal to 39 generating a positive predictive value of 97% and a sensitivity of 68% in their cohort.[66] The differential diagnosis includes infectious osteomyelitis; malignant bone tumors, including primary intraosseous lymphoma, osteosarcoma, Ewing sarcoma, leukemia, and neuroblastoma; benign bone lesions, including osteoid osteoma and osteoblastoma; Langerhans cell histiocytosis; Rosai-Dorfman disease; psoriatic arthritis or spondyloarthropathy; hypophosphatasia; and immune deficiency.[10,90,117,133-138] Biopsy is often needed to exclude an infectious etiology and to exclude the possibility of malignancy. It is difficult to definitively rule out malignancy based on the clinical picture and imaging. MRI of the affected region is helpful to guide the site to biopsy.[72] The best site to biopsy is the site that is felt to give the best diagnostic information with the lowest chance for functional or cosmetic consequences.[117] In some cases, a biopsy may not be needed. This occurs when a child has classic radiographic findings of CRMO (particularly if the clavicle is one of the bones involved) and has a comorbid condition such as Crohn disease or psoriasis.

Treatment

Nonsteroidal antiinflammatory drugs (NSAIDs) are used as a first line treatment strategy in CRMO, providing some degree of symptomatic relief in up to 80% of patients.[34,66,67,69,108,139] Indomethacin may be more effective than other NSAIDs.[140] However, many children continue to have symptoms despite NSAIDs.[34,66,67,78,103] In one long-term follow-up study of 22 individuals with CRMO, only 9% had a good response to NSAIDs with 27.2% having no response at all.[78] Beck et al. prospectively followed a group of children with CRMO and gauged their response to antiinflammatory medications (most often naproxen) during the first year of treatment. They found that 43% of individuals treated with naproxen were symptom-free at 6 months after starting treatment.[141] This was accompanied by a statistically significant decrease in pain, functional impairment, and swelling and by more than 50% reduction in radiologically apparent lesions at 12 months.[141] However, 100% of those with arthritis continued to have active synovitis at 3 months; at 6 months that figure was 50%.[141] Two out of 7 patients (28%) in this cohort with spinal involvement developed pathologic fractures during the 12 months of follow-up.[141] This suggests that NSAIDs alone may not be optimal for individuals who present with arthritis or spinal involvement.

The decision to escalate medical therapy must take into consideration the fact that most lesions resolve without significant sequelae, and spontaneous remission can occur (Fig. 48-8).[67,70] Indications for escalation include persistent pain that affects normal activities, frequent recurrences, and functional limitations. Second-line treatment agents that have been utilized include corticosteroids, azathioprine, disease-modifying antirheumatic drugs (DMARDs), bisphosphonates, biologics, and other immune modulators.[66,117,142,143] Most individuals obtain symptomatic relief with corticosteroids, but side effects limit their usefulness in long-term disease management.[34,67] There are reports of improvement in patients with CRMO or SAPHO treated with methotrexate, sulfasalazine, colchicine, hyperbaric oxygen, calcitonin, azithromycin, interferon-α, interferon-γ, TNF-α inhibitors, IL-1 blocking agents, and bisphosphonates; however, there is no randomized trial of any of these agents, and there are also reports of treatment failures.[26,27,34,66,70,80,86,103,139,144-148] Borzutsky et al. performed a retrospective analysis of 70 patients with CRMO/CNO and found that the estimated probability to response was 57% for NSAIDs,

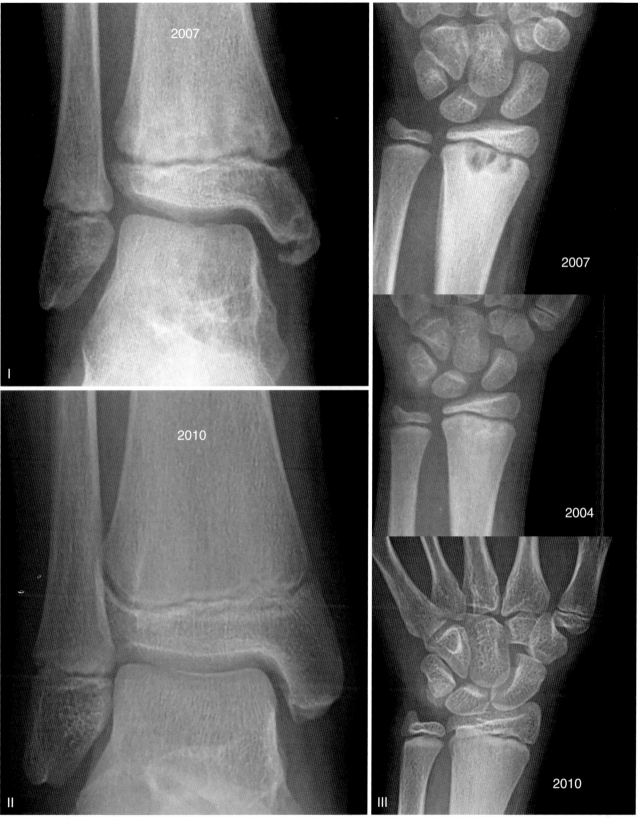

FIGURE 48-8 Spontaneous resolution of lesions in an 8-year-old girl with CRMO over a 3-year time span. Plain radiographs of the ankle *(I and II)* and wrist *(III)* of a female with CRMO whose parents decided to stop treatment after only a couple of days of an NSAID. Over the span of 3 years there is spontaneous healing of all of her bone lesions. (Courtesy Dr. Marilyn Ranson.)

66% for sulfasalazine, 91% for methotrexate, 91% for TNF inhibitors, and 95% for corticosteroids. No individuals were treated with bisphosphonates.[103] The rate of clinical remission (defined as resolution of pain, normalization of inflammatory markers, and radiologic improvement) was highest in the TNF inhibitor group at 46%, followed by corticosteroids at 37%; clinical remission was only achieved in 20% in the methotrexate group, 18% in the sulfasalazine group, and 13% in the NSAID group.[103] For NSAID-resistant disease, there are case reports of marked improvement following treatment with TNF-α blocking agents[29,66,103,149-156] and bisphosphonates.[143,150,152,157-165] The data are strongest regarding the use of bisphosphonates in recalcitrant bone lesions. There is now information in the literature on more than 50 individuals with CRMO, CNO of the jaw, or SAPHO treated with various bisphosphonates with a positive response to initial treatment reported in most of the individuals treated (Fig. 48-9).[66,150,152,157-169] In the series of Miettunen et al., nine patients with CRMO were treated with pamidronate with a mean resolution of

MRI abnormalities of 6 months. Four of the nine subsequently flared but all responded to retreatment.[157] There are also reports in the literature of failure to respond to bisphosphonates as well as failure to respond to TNF inhibitors.[66,159,161,168] Surgical approaches to treatment have included curettage or partial resection of the involved bone; however, surgical intervention is typically limited to obtaining tissue for cultures and histology. The optimal treatment strategy for CRMO remains unknown, and safety questions remain with the long-term use of both TNF inhibitors as well as with bisphosphonates in children. The use of IL-1 inhibitors to treat CRMO remains largely unexplored and needs further investigation given the successful treatment of sterile bone inflammation in both DIRA and Majeed syndrome with these agents.[38,39,170] All children should remain physically active despite ongoing inflammation. Referral to a physical therapist may be needed to regain strength and range of motion lost due to inactivity and guarding the extremity; this is especially true for those with a delay in diagnosis and treatment.

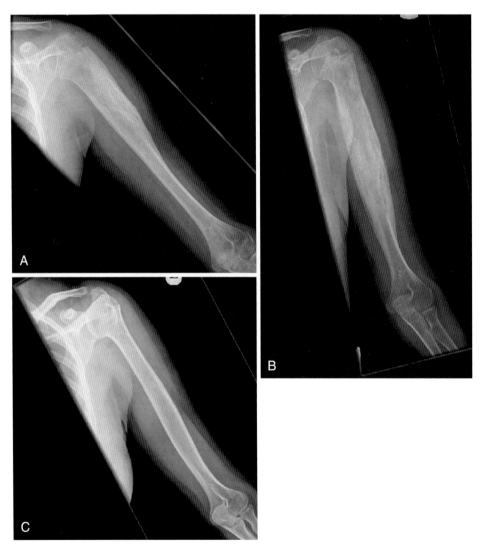

FIGURE 48-9 Plain radiographs of the left humerus. 10-year-old girl with noninfectious osteomyelitis of the left tibia diagnosed 7 months previously presents with a several-month history of left arm pain. **A,** Initial radiograph shows marked proximal expansion with lateral cortical thickening extending down the proximal half of the humerus. She improved clinically on naproxen. **B,** Eighteen months later, she had a recurrence of pain with significant radiologic progression showing areas of lucency and sclerosis with extensive medullary expansion now involving almost the entire humerus. **C,** Plain radiograph taken 1 year after a 1-year course of intravenous pamidronate shows significant healing of the humerus lesion. (Courtesy Dr. Paul Babyn.)

Long-Term Outcome

For most affected individuals, the disease waxes and wanes with periods of exacerbations and remissions, but with resolution of the disease process after several years; reportedly leaving most with no long-term sequelae (Fig. 48-10).[67,69] However, several long-term follow-up (f/u) studies suggest that CRMO might be more persistent, lasting well over a decade in some,[70,71,105] and not as benign as previously reported. For instance, the percentage of individuals with continued disease activity at follow-up ranges from 0% in a German cohort (mean f/u = 5.6 years),[67] 18% in an Australian cohort (mean f/u = 6.2 years),[78] 25% in a Finish cohort (mean f/u = 7.5 years),[75] 26% in an Canadian/Australian cohort (mean f/u = 12.4 years),[70] 57% in a French cohort (mean f/u = 5.3 years),[34] and 100% in a Dutch cohort (mean f/u = 5.5 years).[73] Pathologic fractures, most often of a vertebral body, occurred in 49% of a German cohort.[66] Long-term skeletal deformities, particularly leg length discrepancy, have been reported in up to 58% in one study.[80,105] Other long-term musculoskeletal abnormalities include residual hyperostosis and sclerosis of the bones, difficulty with mastication (following mandibular involvement), valgus deformity of the knee, vertebral collapse, persistent muscle atrophy, thoracic outlet syndrome, persistent arthritis, and evolution into spondyloarthropathy.[66,67,69,70,75,105,171] Disease recurrence may occur as long as 6 years after the last episode of osteitis.[10,105] Difficulty with employment, educational achievement, and participating in recreational sporting activities has been reported in a few cases.[70,105]

DISTINCT GENETIC AUTOINFLAMMATORY BONE SYNDROMES (TABLE 48-1)

Majeed Syndrome

The classic clinical triad in Majeed syndrome (OMIM reference #609628) includes early onset CRMO, congenital dyserythropoietic anemia, and a neutrophilic dermatosis (consistent with Sweet syndrome) (Fig. 48-11).[19] This is a rare syndrome with only three unrelated Arabic families and one Turkish family identified to date.[19,41,68,170] Affected individuals from all four families have homozygous mutations in the gene LPIN2.[37,41,170] Onset of the inflammatory bone disease is typically prior to the second birthday.[41,68,170] Bone pain with or without fever is the typical presenting feature. The histology and radiographic findings are identical to those of CRMO.[19,41,68] Cultures are negative and there is no improvement with antibiotic therapy.[19,68]

Individuals with Majeed syndrome have varying degrees of anemia ranging from mild to transfusion dependent.[19,41,68,170] The red cells are typically microcytic.[19,172] Bone marrow biopsy reveals evidence of dyserythropoiesis with bi- and tri-nucleated normoblasts.[41,68,170] No other cell lines appear to be affected. Other laboratory abnormalities

TABLE 48-1   Autoinflammatory Bone Disorders

	CRMO	MAJEED SYNDROME	DIRA	CHERUBISM	CMO AND LUPO MICE
Ethnicity	Worldwide, but mostly European	Arabic	European, Puerto Rican, Arabic	Worldwide	Occurs in various backgrounds
Fever	Uncommon	Common	Uncommon	No	Not assessed
Sites Of Osseous Involvement	Metaphyses of long bones > vertebrae, clavicle, sternum, pelvis, others	Similar to CRMO	Anterior rib ends, metaphyses of long bones, vertebrae, others	Mandible > maxilla, rarely ribs	Vertebrae, hind feet > forefeet
Extraosseous Manifestations	PPP, psoriasis, IBD, others	Dyserythropoietic anemia, Sweet syndrome, HSM, growth failure	Generalized pustulosis, nail changes, lung disease, vasculitis	Cervical lymphadenopathy	Dermatitis, extramedullary hematopoiesis, splenomegaly
Family History of Inflammatory Disorders	Psoriasis, PPP, arthritis, IBD, others	Psoriasis in some obligate carriers	No known associations	No known associations	Heterozygotes normal
Inheritance	Not clear	Autosomal recessive	Autosomal recessive	Autosomal dominant; incomplete penetrance	Autosomal recessive
Gene Defect	Unknown	LPIN2	IL1RN	SH3BP2 ≫ PTPN11	Pstpip2
Protein Name	Unknown	LIPIN2	IL-1Ra	SH3BP2	PSTPIP2 (MAYP)
Protein Function	Unknown	Fat metabolism: (PAP enzyme activity), ↑ message to oxidative stress, unknown role in mitosis	Antagonist of IL-1 receptor	↑ myeloid cell response to M-CSF and RANKL, ↑ TNF-α expression in macrophages	Macrophage proliferation, macrophage recruitment to sites of inflammation, cytoskeletal function
Cytokine Abnormalities	↑ serum TNF-α	Not tested	↑ IL-1α, IL-1β, MIP-1α, TNF-α, IL-8, IL-6 ex vivo monocyte assay; skin reveals ↑ IL-17 staining	↑ serum TNF-α in mouse model	cmo: ↑serum IL-6, MIP-1α, TNF-α, CSF-1, IP-10Lupo: ↑serum MIP-1α, IL-4, RANTES, TGF-β

CRMO, Chronic recurrent multifocal osteomyelitis; HSM, hepatosplenomegaly; IBD, inflammatory bowel disease; IL, interleukin; MCSF, macrophage colony-stimulating factor; MIP, macrophage inflammatory protein; PPP, palmoplantar pustulosis; RANTES, regulated on activation, normal T cell expressed and secreted; TGF, transforming growth factor; TNF, tumor necrosis factor; ↑, increase.

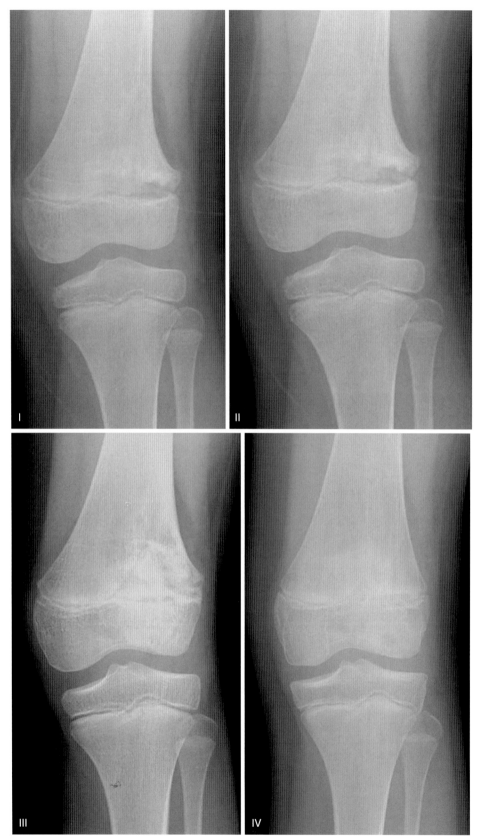

FIGURE 48-10 Radiographic resolution of distal femur lesion in a girl with CRMO over a 5-year time span. In 2002, there is an osteolytic lesion with surrounding sclerosis adjacent to the growth plate in the left distal femoral metaphysis (*I*). Minimal change is seen in the lesion 1 year later (2003; *II*). In 2004, the lesion begins to heal with significant sclerosis (*III*). In 2007, the lesion is nearly completely healed and the bone mineral density is nearly normal (*IV*).

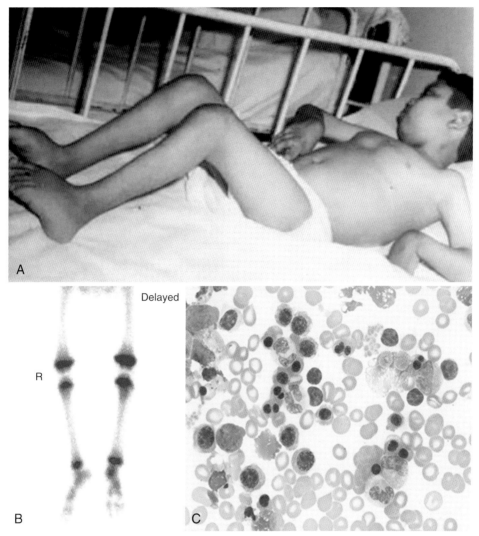

FIGURE 48-11 CRMO and dyserythropoietic anemia in Majeed syndrome. **A,** Affected male with contractures and failure to thrive. **B,** Technetium (Tc-99m) bone scan of a female with Majeed syndrome demonstrating increased radiotracer uptake in the metaphyses of the long bones of the lower extremities consistent with osteomyelitis. **C,** Dyserythropoiesis with multiple bi-nucleated erythrocyte precursors in the bone marrow from a child with Majeed syndrome.

include leukocytosis, thrombocytosis, and a raised erythrocyte sedimentation rate.[19,41,68,170] Despite the evidence that the protein LIPIN2 is involved in fat metabolism, no lipid abnormalities have been reported in children with Majeed syndrome.[41] Cutaneous manifestations include a neutrophilic dermatosis consistent with Sweet syndrome in two affected individuals.[19] Interestingly, several of the carrier parents have psoriasis, which suggests that LIPIN2 may play a role susceptibility to psoriasis.[7]

Treatment with corticosteroids results in only partial clinical improvement in the inflammatory bone and skin disease; anemia is less responsive to treatment. However, undesirable long-term steroid-induced side effects limit their long-term usefulness.[19,41] Nonsteroidal antiinflammatory medications provide some degree of pain relief but do not produce disease control.[68] Colchicine was tried in three individuals without significant clinical improvement.[19] Permanent joint contractures and growth disturbance have been reported after years of chronic inflammation (Fig 48-11).[68] However, Herlin et al. recently reported prompt and sustained improvement in two brothers treated with anakinra who flared upon its discontinuation, followed

by rapid improvement when treated with the IL-1β blocking agent canakinumab.[170] Both boys had previously failed to respond to TNF-α inhibition. This suggests that Majeed syndrome is an IL-1β (not IL-1α) driven disease.

The role of LIPIN 2 in inflammation of the bone and skin remains ill defined. All three members of the *LPIN* gene family act as phosphatidate phosphatases (PAP) and can act as transcription regulators.[173-177] Rue et al. demonstrated *in vitro* that one of the Majeed syndrome–causing mutations, p.Ser734Leu (S734L), abolishes the PAP activity of LIPIN2,[178] suggesting that the inflammatory phenotype may result from the loss of PAP activity. Valdearcos et al. found that in a cell line, under expression of *LPIN2* resulted in increased production of proinflammatory cytokines when exposed to excessive quantities of saturated fatty acid (palmitic acid), and overexpression of *LPIN2* in this setting was associated with lower levels of proinflammatory cytokines.[179] This suggests that *LPIN2* plays a role in the immune response to saturated fatty acids. Yet, how aberrant function in these lipid pathways genes causes autoinflammatory disease of the bone remains unknown.[180] *LPIN2* may play a role in responses to oxidative stress because it is highly upregulated in animal models of tissue damage, including paraquat-induced pulmonary injury and 2,3,7,8-tetrachlorodibenzo-*p*-dioxin induced liver injury.[181,182] *Ned1* is an *LPIN* ortholog that when mutated in yeast *Schizosaccharomyces pombe* results in aberrantly shaped nuclei.[183] This suggests that *LIPIN2* may be involved in mitosis as there are frequent bi- and tri-nucleated pronormoblasts in the bone marrow of children with Majeed syndrome.[184]

Deficiency of the Interleukin-1 Receptor Antagonist

Deficiency of the interleukin-1 receptor antagonist (DIRA) (OMIM reference #612852) is an autosomal recessive autoinflammatory disorder that is cause by mutations in *IL1RN* that encodes the interleukin-1 receptor antagonist [IL-1Ra].[38,39] Affected individuals do not produce functional IL-1Ra, resulting in marked dysregulation of IL-1 pathway signaling.[38,185] DIRA presents in infancy (usually within the first few weeks of life) with pustular rash, sterile osteitis, and periostitis, typically in the absence of fever.[38,39] Half of the infants have been born near-term premature (31 to 36 weeks' gestation).[38,39,186,187] Respiratory problems (respiratory distress, apnea, or aspiration pneumonia) were present in half of the infants shortly after birth.[38,39,185,186,188,189] Hepatomegaly was reported in five of the nine infants in one study.[38] All infants had elevated inflammatory markers including white blood cell counts in the 20,000 to 60,000 cells/mm^3 range, erythrocyte sedimentation rates up to 115 mm/hr, thrombocytosis ranging from 500,000 to 1,000,000 platelets/mm^3 and C-reactive protein levels up to 30 mg/dl.[38,39,185-188,190,191] The majority of affected infants received prolonged courses of antibiotics for presumed sepsis without clinical improvement.[38,39,185,186,188-190] Clinical improvement was noted in most (but not all) when treated with sizeable doses of corticosteroids.[38,39,185,188-190]

Inflammation of the skin has been present in 95% of the affected infants and varies in severity from a few clusters of pustules to severe wide-spread generalized pustulosis to ichthyosiform lesions; pustules were only present transiently in one child.[38,39,185-191] Histologically, involved skin displays a predominantly neutrophilic infiltration of the epidermis and dermis, acanthosis, hyperkeratosis, parakeratosis and subcorneal pustule formation.[38,39,185,187,189] Cultures of the skin lesions are generally negative; however, two infants had positive cultures from pustules, one methicillin-resistant *Staphylococcus aureus* cultured on one occasion[39] and the other coagulase-negative *Staphylococcus.*[188] Other reported mucocutaneous manifestations included pathergy, oral ulcers, and pyoderma gangrenosum.[38,185] Nail abnormalities (nail pits, onychomadesis, nail shedding, and anonychia) have been reported in nearly half of the children.[38,187,190,191]

There may be no objective evidence of osteitis on examination but the infant may appear to be in pain with movement. Only 33% of infants had objective swelling on musculoskeletal examination.[186,188,190] Marked radiologic abnormalities were present in all affected children. Common findings included multifocal osteolytic lesions, marked periostitis, widening of the medial clavicle, and flaring of the anterior rib ends (Fig. 48-12).[38,39] Multifocal osteolytic lesions involving the long bones were present in most affected children.[38,39,185-187,190,191] Involvement of the vertebrae occurred in approximately 25% of children, resulting in vertebral collapse, gibbus deformity, nonunion of the odontoid, C1-C2 instability, and vertebral fusion.[38,185,187] Bone biopsies reveal neutrophilic infiltration with bone destruction, fibrosis, sclerosis, reactive new bone formation, and scattered osteoclasts.[38,39,185] Cultures of the bone were negative for anaerobes, aerobes, fungi, and acid-fast bacilli in all biopsies tested.[38,39,185]

Pulmonary involvement occurs in approximately 50% of infants, most often transient respiratory distress in the perinatal period. However, life-threatening lung disease has been reported in four patients

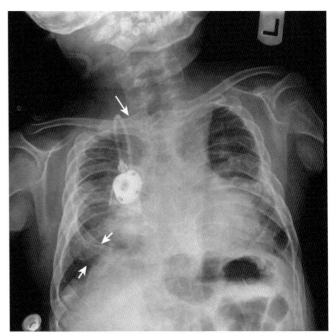

FIGURE 48-12 Chest radiograph in a patient with DIRA. Male infant with multiple bony abnormalities including expansion of the medial clavicles R > L (*long arrow*) and widening of the anterior rib ends (*small arrows*). Patchy opacifications are seen in the lung fields. This child developed interstitial lung disease. (Courtesy Dr. P. Babyn.)

including interstitial lung disease in two infants (pulmonary fibrosis found at autopsy in one and classic computed tomography findings of ground-glass opacities in the other)[38,39] and systemic inflammatory response syndrome (SIRS) requiring mechanical ventilation in two others (one of whom died of respiratory failure).[186,189] Venous thrombosis, either spontaneous or associated with a indwelling catheter, have been reported in four cases.[39,185,188,191] Less common complications include CNS vasculitis, cardiomyopathy, marked abdominal distension with caput medusa, conjunctival injection, hypotonia, and developmental delay.[38,191] Failure to thrive is reported in one third of patients.[38,185,187,190,191]

Antibiotics are ineffective in DIRA and most, but not all, children improved when treated with high doses (2 mg/kg/day) of corticosteroids.[38,39,185,188,191] Prior to the discovery that children with DIRA were deficient in the interleukin-1 receptor antagonist, several steroid-sparing agents were utilized unsuccessfully, including nonsteroidal antiinflammatory drugs, intravenous gamma globulin, methotrexate, cyclosporine, azathioprine, etanercept, thalidomide, and interferon-γ.[38,190] An empiric trial of anakinra in one child led to dramatic and rapid disease improvement, and it was this observation that led investigators to sequence IL-1 pathway genes leading to the discovery of gene defect.[38] Mononuclear cells from DIRA patients produce high levels of inflammatory cytokines (including MIP-1α, TNF-α, IL-8 and IL-6) *in vitro.*[38,39,185] Left untreated, the unopposed action of IL-1 results in life-threatening systemic inflammation that predominately affects skin and bone.[38] Treatment with anakinra results in prompt and dramatic improvement within days of the initiation of treatment.[38,39,187-191]

There is limited information about long-term outcome in this condition given that it was unrecognized as a distinct clinical entity until its description in 2009. The disease is potentially fatal with a 33% mortality rate including the siblings of reported mutation-positive cases(38, 186, 190, 191). Most deaths occurred in the first 2 years of life and were attributed to multisystem failure due to SIRS.[38,186] One child lived until he was 9.5 years of age; he was treated with corticosteroids, methotrexate, and cyclosporin but ultimately died of respiratory failure secondary to chronic interstitial lung disease.[38] Permanent skeletal deformities and failure to thrive occurred in several of the children prior to initiation of anakinra.[38,191] Allergic reaction to anakinra may occur in those who have complete deficiency of the protein and desensitization therapy may allow continued treatment; alternatively, other IL-1 blocking agents may be utilized. Outcomes should improve significantly with early recognition accompanied by prompt initiation of appropriate treatment. Once the diagnosis of DIRA is made, genetic counseling should be offered to each family so that they understand the recurrence risk. When genetic testing for *IL1RN* mutations is commercially available, determination of carrier status and prenatal diagnosis (if desired) would be options for family members of affected individuals.

Cherubism

Cherubism is an autosomal dominant autoinflammatory disorder (OMIM reference #118400) that is almost exclusively confined to the jaw.[192-196] The disorder was described by Jones in 1933. Most children present between 2 and 7 years of age with symmetric, progressive, nontender bony enlargement of the jaw without associated systemic symptoms.[192,194,195,197,198] The expansion of the mandible and maxilla causes a chubby cheeked appearance and an upward gaze; features that Jones felt were thought to be reminiscent of paintings of cherubs in Renaissance art.[198,199] The jaw hypertrophy is disfiguring and associated with significant dental problems, including malocclusion and loss of dentition with secondary difficulty with mastication in severely affected individuals.[198,199] The bony enlargement of the jaw begins to slowly regress after the onset of puberty.[198] Regression may be accompanied by marked sclerosis, which may never fully resolve. Lymphadenopathy may be present during the active phase of the disease.[198] Extra gnathic bone involvement is rare, but there are reports of lesions in the ribs, humerus, femur, and tibia.[198,200,201]

Radiographs reveal large multilocular, cystic appearing lesions predominately affecting the mandible with less severe involvement of the maxilla.[198,199,202-204] The lesions may appear osteolytic or radiopaque with a coarse trabecular pattern associated with thinning of the cortices.[202,203] Computerized tomography reveals osseous expansile lesions, cortical scalloping, dental derangement, and many show secondary maxillary sinus disease.[198,205,206] MRI examination reveals extensive homogeneous isointense (to skeletal muscle) lesions on T1 images and hypointense on fast spin-echo T2-weighted images with fat suppression.[206] Histologically, there are abundant osteoclasts interspersed throughout dense fibrostromal connective tissue without accompanying features of osteomyelitis.[197,207,208] There have been no effective medical or surgical treatments.

A gene defect was identified in 2001, when heterozygous mutations in the SH3 binding protein-2 (SH3BP2) were discovered in affected individuals from 12 affected families.[192] Mutations in SH3BP2 account for the vast majority of gene defects found in individuals with cherubism; however, mutations in *PTPN11* can also result in a cherubism phenotype.[209] To further understand the pathophysiology of cherubism, Ueki et al. created a murine cherubism model by knocking in the most common human *SH3BP2* mutation.[210] One copy of the knockin allele resulted in a surprisingly normal mouse.[210] However, mice homozygous for the knockin allele (double knockin) had widespread bone disease with osteoclast-rich inflammatory jaw lesions, systemic myeloid inflammation, and extensive trabecular bone loss throughout the remainder of the skeleton.[210] The inflammatory phenotype in cherubism mice occurs independent of a functioning

adaptive immune system, is dependent on the presence of TNF-α, and is mediated by hematopoietically derived myeloid cells.[210] Cherubism mutations have been found to abolish the recognition of SH3BP2 by tankyrase, an enzyme that normally targets SH3BP2 for ubiquitylation and subsequent degradation.[211-213] This results in increased stability of mutant SH3BP2 with enhanced activation of SCR, SYK, and VAV pathways, with resultant hyperactivation of osteoclasts.[211,213] These suggest that TNF-α and or SRC inhibition might prove to be an effective therapy for this disfiguring disease.[214] However, a recent report of two children treated with the TNF-α antagonist adalimumab did not prevent lesion expansion in active cherubism.[215]

SUMMARY

Sterile bone inflammation is the cardinal feature of the autoinflammatory bone disorders. Many affected individuals also have a chronic inflammatory condition of the skin or intestinal tract, suggesting common immunologic pathways are involved in CRMO, psoriasis, and inflammatory bowel disease. A genetic defect has been found in two syndromic forms of CRMO and in a mouse model of the disease. The information learned from these single gene disorders implicates the innate immune system in the pathogenesis of CRMO and related disorders.

REFERENCES

2. H. Park, A.B. Bourla, D.L. Kastner, et al., Lighting the fires within: the cell biology of autoinflammatory diseases, Nat. Rev. 12 (8) (2012) 570–580, (eng). [Epub 2012/07/26]; PubMed PMID: 22828911.

7. P.J. Ferguson, H.I. El-Shanti, Autoinflammatory bone disorders, Curr. Opin. Rheumatol. 19 (5) (2007) 492–498. PubMed PMID: 17762617.

8. G.A. Sanchez, A.A. de Jesus, R. Goldbach-Mansky, Monogenic autoinflammatory diseases: disorders of amplified danger sensing and cytokine dysregulation, Rheum. Dis. Clin. North Am. 39 (4) (2013) 701–734. PubMed PMID: 24182851, Pubmed Central PMCID: 3888876.

9. A. Giedion, W. Holthusen, L.F. Masel, D. Vischer, Subacute and chronic "symmetrical" osteomyelitis, Ann. Radiol. (Paris) 15 (3) (1972) 329–342.

33. G. Rohekar, R.D. Inman, Conundrums in nosology: synovitis, acne, pustulosis, hyperostosis, and osteitis syndrome and spondylarthritis, Arthritis Rheum. 55 (4) (2006) 665–669.

37. P.J. Ferguson, S. Chen, M.K. Tayeh, et al., Homozygous mutations in LPIN2 are responsible for the syndrome of chronic recurrent multifocal osteomyelitis and congenital dyserythropoietic anaemia (Majeed syndrome), J. Med. Genet. 42 (7) (2005) 551–557.

38. I. Aksentijevich, S.L. Masters, P.J. Ferguson, et al., An autoinflammatory disease with deficiency of the interleukin-1-receptor antagonist, N. Engl. J. Med. 360 (23) (2009) 2426–2437.

39. S. Reddy, S. Jia, R. Geoffrey, et al., An autoinflammatory disease due to homozygous deletion of the IL1RN locus, N. Engl. J. Med. 360 (23) (2009) 2438–2444.

40. P.J. Ferguson, X. Bing, M.A. Vasef, et al., A missense mutation in pstpip2 is associated with the murine autoinflammatory disorder chronic multifocal osteomyelitis, Bone 38 (1) (2006) 41–47.

42. J. Grosse, V. Chitu, A. Marquardt, et al., Mutation of mouse Mayp/Pstpip2 causes a macrophage autoinflammatory disease, Blood 107 (8) (2006) 3350–3358.

44. S.L. Cassel, J.R. Janczy, X. Bing, et al., Inflammasome-independent IL-1beta mediates autoinflammatory disease in Pstpip2-deficient mice, Proc. Natl. Acad. Sci. U.S.A. 111 (3) (2014) 1072–1077.

45. J.R. Lukens, J.M. Gross, C. Calabrese, et al., Critical role for inflammasome-independent IL-1beta production in osteomyelitis, Proc. Natl. Acad. Sci. U.S.A. 111 (3) (2014) 1066–1071.

62. G. Hayem, A. Bouchaud-Chabot, K. Benali, et al., SAPHO syndrome: a long-term follow-up study of 120 cases, Semin. Arthritis Rheum. 29 (3) (1999) 159–171.

65. M.F. Kahn, A.M. Chamot, SAPHO syndrome, Rheum. Dis. Clin. North Am. 18 (1) (1992) 225–246.

66. A. Jansson, E.D. Renner, J. Ramser, et al., Classification of non-bacterial osteitis: retrospective study of clinical, immunological and genetic aspects in 89 patients, Rheumatology (Oxford) 46 (1) (2007) 154–160.

67. H.J. Girschick, P. Raab, S. Surbaum, et al., Chronic non-bacterial osteomyelitis in children, Ann. Rheum. Dis. 64 (2) (2005) 279–285.

68. H.A. Majeed, M. Al-Tarawna, H. El-Shanti, et al., The syndrome of chronic recurrent multifocal osteomyelitis and congenital dyserythropoietic anaemia. Report of a new family and a review, Eur. J. Pediatr. 160 (12) (2001) 705–710.

69. C. Schultz, P.M. Holterhus, A. Seidel, et al., Chronic recurrent multifocal osteomyelitis in children, Pediatr. Infect. Dis. J. 18 (11) (1999) 1008–1013.

70. A.M. Huber, P.Y. Lam, C.M. Duffy, et al., Chronic recurrent multifocal osteomyelitis: clinical outcomes after more than five years of follow-up, J. Pediatr. 141 (2) (2002) 198–203.

73. A.G. Jurik, O. Helmig, T. Ternowitz, B.N. Moller, Chronic recurrent multifocal osteomyelitis: a follow-up study, J. Pediatr. Orthop. 8 (1) (1988) 49–58.

76. S.M. King, R.M. Laxer, D. Manson, R. Gold, Chronic recurrent multifocal osteomyelitis: a noninfectious inflammatory process, Pediatr. Infect. Dis. J. 6 (10) (1987) 907–911.

87. M. Colina, A. Lo Monaco, M. Khodeir, F. Trotta, Propionibacterium acnes and SAPHO syndrome: a case report and literature review, Clin. Exp. Rheumatol. 25 (3) (2007) 457–460.

93. P.J. Ferguson, M.A. Lokuta, H.I. El-Shanti, et al., Neutrophil dysfunction in a family with a SAPHO syndrome-like phenotype, Arthritis Rheum. 58 (10) (2008) 3264–3269.

94. V. Chitu, P.J. Ferguson, R. de Bruijn, et al., Primed innate immunity leads to autoinflammatory disease in PSTPIP2-deficient cmo mice, Blood 114 (12) (2009) 2497–2505.

99. A. Golla, A. Jansson, J. Ramser, et al., Chronic recurrent multifocal osteomyelitis (CRMO): evidence for a susceptibility gene located on chromosome 18q21.3-18q22, Eur. J. Hum. Genet. 10 (3) (2002) 217–221.

101. S.R. Hofmann, T. Schwarz, J.C. Moller, et al., Chronic non-bacterial osteomyelitis is associated with impaired Sp1 signaling, reduced IL10 promoter phosphorylation, and reduced myeloid IL-10 expression, Clin. Immunol. 141 (3) (2011) 317–327.

102. N. Safra, N.C. Pedersen, Z. Wolf, et al., Expanded dog leukocyte antigen (DLA) single nucleotide polymorphism (SNP) genotyping reveals spurious class II associations, Vet. J. 189 (2) (2011) 220–226.

103. A. Borzutzky, S. Stern, A. Reiff, et al., Pediatric chronic nonbacterial osteomyelitis, Pediatrics 130 (5) (2012) e1190–e1197.

105. C.M. Duffy, P.Y. Lam, M. Ditchfield, et al., Chronic recurrent multifocal osteomyelitis: review of orthopaedic complications at maturity, J. Pediatr. Orthop. 22 (4) (2002) 501–505.

106. S. Guerin-Pfyffer, S. Guillaume-Czitrom, S. Tammam, I. Kone-Paut, Evaluation of chronic recurrent multifocal osteitis in children by whole-body magnetic resonance imaging, Joint Bone Spine 79 (6) (2012) 616–620.

107. T. von Kalle, N. Heim, T. Hospach, et al., Typical patterns of bone involvement in whole-body MRI of patients with chronic recurrent multifocal osteomyelitis (CRMO), Rofo 185 (7) (2013) 655–661.

110. G. Khanna, T.S. Sato, P. Ferguson, Imaging of chronic recurrent multifocal osteomyelitis, Radiographics 29 (4) (2009) 1159–1177.

117. H.J. Girschick, C. Zimmer, G. Klaus, et al., Chronic recurrent multifocal osteomyelitis: what is it and how should it be treated? Nat. Clin. Pract. 3 (12) (2007) 733–738.

118. J. Fritz, N. Tzaribatchev, C.D. Claussen, et al., Chronic recurrent multifocal osteomyelitis: comparison of whole-body MR imaging with radiography and correlation with clinical and laboratory data, Radiology 252 (3) (2009) 842–851.

120. J. Fritz, N. Tzaribatchev, C.D. Claussen, et al., Chronic recurrent multifocal osteomyelitis: comparison of whole-body MR imaging with radiography and correlation with clinical and laboratory data, Radiology 252 (3) (2009) 842–851.

121. C. Falip, M. Alison, N. Boutry, et al., Chronic recurrent multifocal osteomyelitis (CRMO): a longitudinal case series review, Pediatr. Radiol. 43 (3) (2013) 355–375.

122. M.T. Kennedy, T. Murphy, M. Murphy, et al., Whole body MRI in the diagnosis of chronic recurrent multifocal osteomyelitis, Ortho. Traumatol. Surg. Res. 98 (4) (2012) 461–464.

129. J. Rech, B. Manger, B. Lang, et al., Adult-onset Still's disease and chronic recurrent multifocal osteomyelitis: a hitherto undescribed manifestation of autoinflammation, Rheumatol. Int. 32 (6) (2012) 1827–1829.

133. H.J. Girschick, E. Mornet, M. Beer, et al., Chronic multifocal non-bacterial osteomyelitis in hypophosphatasia mimicking malignancy, BMC Pediatr. 7 (2007) 3.

134. T.S. Sato, P.J. Ferguson, G. Khanna, Primary multifocal osseous lymphoma in a child, Pediatr. Radiol. 38 (12) (2008) 1338–1341.

138. A. Reiff, A.G. Bassuk, J.A. Church, et al., Exome sequencing reveals RAG1 mutations in a child with autoimmunity and sterile chronic multifocal osteomyelitis evolving into disseminated granulomatous disease, J. Clin. Immunol. 33 (8) (2013) 1289–1292. Pub Med PMID: 24122031.

141. C. Beck, H. Morbach, M. Beer, et al., Chronic nonbacterial osteomyelitis in childhood: prospective follow-up during the first year of anti-inflammatory treatment, Arthritis Res. Ther. 12 (2) (2010) R74.

142. P.J. Ferguson, M. Sandu, Current understanding of the pathogenesis and management of chronic recurrent multifocal osteomyelitis, Curr. Rheumatol. Rep. 14 (2) (2012) 130–141.

143. M. Twilt, R.M. Laxer, Clinical care of children with sterile bone inflammation, Curr. Opin. Rheumatol. 23 (5) (2011) 424–431.

149. A. Deutschmann, C.J. Mache, K. Bodo, et al., Successful treatment of chronic recurrent multifocal osteomyelitis with tumor necrosis factor-alpha blockage, Pediatrics 116 (5) (2005) 1231–1233.

150. B.E. Tlougan, J.O. Podjasek, J. O'Haver, et al., Chronic recurrent multifocal osteomyelitis (CRMO) and synovitis, acne, pustulosis, hyperostosis, and osteitis (SAPHO) syndrome with associated neutrophilic dermatoses: a report of seven cases and review of the literature, Pediatr. Dermatol. 26 (5) (2009) 497–505.

151. D. Eleftheriou, T. Gerschman, N. Sebire, et al., Biologic therapy in refractory chronic non-bacterial osteomyelitis of childhood, Rheumatology 49 (8) (2010) 1505–1512.

157. P.M. Miettunen, X. Wei, D. Kaura, et al., Dramatic pain relief and resolution of bone inflammation following pamidronate in 9 pediatric patients with persistent chronic recurrent multifocal osteomyelitis (CRMO), Pediatr. Rheumatol. Online J. 7 (2009) 2.

160. S. Compeyrot-Lacassagne, A.M. Rosenberg, P. Babyn, R.M. Laxer, Pamidronate treatment of chronic noninfectious inflammatory lesions of the mandible in children, J. Rheumatol. 34 (7) (2007) 1585–1589.

166. H. Amital, Y.H. Applbaum, S. Aamar, et al., SAPHO syndrome treated with pamidronate: an open-label study of 10 patients, Rheumatology (Oxford) 43 (5) (2004) 658–661.

170. T. Herlin, B. Fiirgaard, M. Bjerre, et al., Efficacy of anti-IL-1 treatment in Majeed syndrome, Ann. Rheum. Dis. 72 (3) (2013) 410–413.

172. H.A. Majeed, H. El-Shanti, H. Al-Rimawi, N. Al-Masri, On mice and men: an autosomal recessive syndrome of chronic recurrent multifocal osteomyelitis and congenital dyserythropoietic anemia, J. Pediatr. 137 (3) (2000) 441–442.

178. J. Donkor, P. Zhang, S. Wong, et al., A conserved serine residue is required for the phosphatidate phosphatase activity but not the transcriptional coactivator functions of lipin-1 and lipin-2, J. Biol. Chem. 284 (43) (2009) 29968–29978.

179. M. Valdearcos, E. Esquinas, C. Meana, et al., Lipin-2 reduces proinflammatory signaling induced by saturated fatty acids in macrophages, J. Biol. Chem. 287 (14) (2012) 10894–10904.

185. A.A. Jesus, M. Osman, C.A. Silva, et al., A novel mutation of IL1RN in the deficiency of interleukin-1 receptor antagonist syndrome: description of two unrelated cases from Brazil, Arthritis Rheum. 63 (12) (2011) 4007–4017.

186. E. Altiok, F. Aksoy, Y. Perk, et al., A novel mutation in the interleukin-1 receptor antagonist associated with intrauterine disease onset, Clin. Immunol. 145 (1) (2012) 77–81.

187. K. Minkis, I. Aksentijevich, R. Goldbach-Mansky, et al., Interleukin 1 receptor antagonist deficiency presenting as infantile pustulosis mimicking infantile pustular psoriasis, Arch. Dermatol. 148 (6) (2012) 747–752.

188. M. Stenerson, K. Dufendach, I. Aksentijevich, et al., The first reported case of compound heterozygous IL1RN mutations causing deficiency of the interleukin-1 receptor antagonist, Arthritis Rheum. 63 (12) (2011) 4018–4022.

189. C. Schnellbacher, G. Ciocca, R. Menendez, et al., Deficiency of interleukin-1 receptor antagonist responsive to anakinra, Pediatr. Dermatol. 30 (6) (2013) 758–760. PubMed PMID: 22471702.

190. W. Sakran, S.A. Shalev, H. El-Shanti, Y. Uziel, Chronic recurrent multifocal osteomyelitis and deficiency of interleukin-1-receptor antagonist, Pediatr. Infect. Dis. J. 32 (1) (2013) 94.

Entire reference list is available online at www.expertconsult.com.

49 | CHAPTER

Macrophage Activation Syndrome

Alexei A. Grom

DEFINITIONS

Macrophage activation syndrome (MAS) is a severe, potentially fatal condition caused by excessive activation and expansion of macrophages and T cells, leading to an overwhelming inflammatory reaction. The main manifestations of MAS include fever, hepatosplenomegaly, lymphadenopathy, severe cytopenias, liver disease, and coagulopathy consistent with disseminated intravascular coagulation.[1-6] Striking hyperferritinemia is another characteristic laboratory finding. Numerous, well-differentiated macrophages phagocytosing hematopoietic elements, the pathognomonic feature of MAS, are often found in bone marrow, liver, spleen, or lymph nodes (Fig. 49-1). These hemophagocytic macrophages can infiltrate almost any organ in the body and may account for many of the systemic features of this syndrome. Although MAS has been reported to occur with many other rheumatic diseases, it is most common in the systemic form of juvenile idiopathic arthritis (JIA). Systemic lupus erythematosus (SLE) and Kawasaki disease are also conditions in which MAS appears to occur more frequently than in other rheumatological diseases.[7-8]

MAS bears a close resemblance to a group of histiocytic disorders known as *hemophagocytic lymphohistiocytosis* (HLH),[9-10] a term that describes a spectrum of disease processes characterized by accumulations of well-differentiated mononuclear cells with a macrophage phenotype.[11-12] Because the macrophages represent a subset of histiocytes distinct from Langerhans cells, this entity should be distinguished from Langerhans cell histiocytosis and other dendritic cell disorders. In the current classification of histiocytic disorders, HLH is further subdivided into primary or familial HLH (FHLH) and secondary or reactive HLH (ReHLH).[11-12] Clinically, however, it may be difficult to distinguish one from the other. Familial HLH is a constellation of rare autosomal recessive immune disorders linked to genetic defects in various genes all affecting the cytolytic pathway. Its clinical symptoms usually become evident within the first two months of life. Reactive HLH tends to occur in older children and is more often associated with an identifiable infectious episode, most notably Epstein–Barr virus (EBV) or cytomegalovirus infection. The group of secondary hemophagocytic disorders also includes malignancy-associated HLH. The distinction between primary and secondary HLH is becoming increasingly blurred as new genetic causes are identified, some of which are associated with less severe and somewhat more distinct clinical presentations.[13] Some of these may present later in life due to heterozygous or compound heterozygous mutations in cytolytic pathway genes that confer a partial dominant negative effect on the cytolytic function.[14]

As with MAS, the clinical course for HLH is characterized by persistent fever and hepatosplenomegaly.[12-13] Neurological symptoms can complicate and sometimes dominate the clinical course. Hemorrhagic rash and lymphadenopathy are observed somewhat less frequently. The laboratory findings—cytopenias (particularly thrombocytopenia), elevated liver enzymes, hypertriglyceridemia, hyperferritinemia, and hypofibrinogenemia—also overlap with MAS. As with MAS, hemophagocytosis in bone marrow is a hallmark of HLH. Despite all these clinical similarities, the exact pathophysiological relationship between MAS and HLH is unclear.

EPIDEMIOLOGY

The epidemiological studies of MAS have been complicated by the lack of well-defined diagnostic criteria. Despite the lack of diagnostic criteria, increasing awareness of MAS has meant that it is recognized more frequently than previously. Approximately 7% to 17% of patients with systemic JIA develop profound disease,[5,15] while mild "subclinical" MAS may be seen in as many as one third of patients with active systemic disease.[16,17] In subclinical MAS, bone marrow examination typically reveals extensive expansion of highly activated macrophages with only few of them exhibiting overt hemophagocytic activity. Based on one report originating from a large tertiary center, MAS can be seen in about 1% of patients with SLE.[18]

MAS occurs with equal frequency in boys and girls. There appears to be no racial predilection, and it may occur at almost any age. The youngest MAS patient reported to date was 12 months old.[1] Although most patients develop this syndrome sometime during the course of their primary rheumatic disease, MAS occurring at the initial presentation is not uncommon.[1,19,20] The vast majority of patients have an active primary rheumatic disease prior to developing MAS. However, in the recent phase III clinical trials of the biologics inhibiting either IL-1 or IL-6, MAS occurred in several patients despite an excellent control of the underlying systemic JIA. Infectious triggers were identified in almost all of these cases.[21,22]

TRIGGERS

A triggering event, such as infection or modification in the drug therapy, can be identified in about half of MAS episodes. It is now evident that development of MAS can be precipitated by virtually any infectious agent: viral, bacterial, fungal, and even parasitic. Viral illnesses, particularly EBV and other members of the herpes family, appear to be the most commonly reported.[3,6] In several reports, the triggering of MAS coincided with the modifications in the drug therapy, most notably administration of gold preparations,[3] methotrexate,[23] and sulfasalazine.[24] These associations, however, should be interpreted cautiously because many of the described patients had very active underlying rheumatic disease and might have been developing MAS as the drugs were started. In many patients, MAS appears to be triggered by a flare of the underlying rheumatic disease.

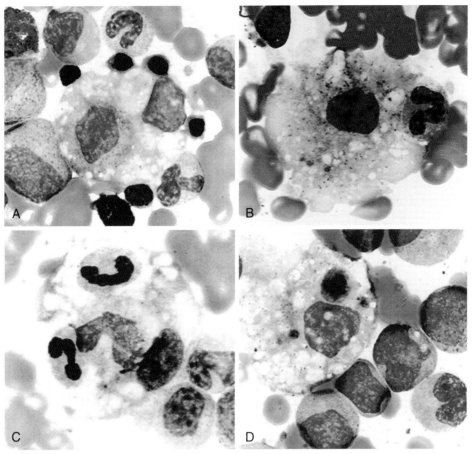

FIGURE 49-1 Activated macrophages phagocytosing hematopoietic elements in the bone marrow of a systemic JIA patient with MAS. Bone marrow aspirate specimen revealing activated macrophages (H&E stain, original magnification ×1000). **A,** Myelocyte within activated macrophage. There are also multiple adherent red blood cell and myeloid precursors. **B,** Activated macrophage engulfing a neutrophilic band form. **C,** Neutrophilic band forms and metamyelocyte within an activated macrophage. Nuclei of band forms appear condensed, a result of destruction. **D,** Activated macrophage with hemosiderin deposits and a degenerating phagocytosed nucleated cell. (Courtesy Prahalad et al., J Rheumatol 28 (2001) 2122.)[77]

GENETIC BACKGROUND

The pathological mechanisms of MAS are not fully understood. In clinically similar FHLH, the uncontrolled proliferation of T cells and macrophages has been linked to decreased natural killer (NK) cell and cytotoxic T cell (CTL) function.[25] In about 30% of FHLH patients, the cytolytic dysfunction is due to mutations in the gene encoding perforin (*PRF1*),[26] a protein which cytolytic cells normally utilize to induce apoptosis of target cells, such as cells infected with viruses. The proteins encoded by several other FHLH-associated genes are generally those involved in the intracellular transport of perforin-containing granules to the cell surface interface with the target cell (*MUNC13-4*, Syntaxin 11 [*STX11*], and syntaxin binding protein 2 [*STXBP2*, also known as *MUNC18-2*]).[27-29] Although the cytolytic cells in these patients with FHLH produce sufficient amounts of perforin, the poor ability to release perforin into the immunologic synapse with the target cell leads to profoundly decreased cytolytic activity. Similar defects have also been implicated in three other genetic diseases associated with the hemophagocytic syndrome. Mutations in the gene-encoding Rab27a, one of the MUNC13-4 effector molecules, have been linked to the development of Griscelli syndrome type 2,[30] mutations in the Lyst gene have been identified as a cause of

Chediak-Higashi syndrome,[31] and mutations in the gene encoding SH2D1A, an adaptor protein critical for lymphocyte activation, including granule-mediated cytotoxicity, have been associated with X-linked lymphoproliferative disease.[32,33] Recent observations suggest that as in HLH, MAS patients have profoundly depressed natural killer cell function, often associated with abnormal perforin expression,[34-37] and these abnormalities are associated with specific *MUNC13-4*[38,39] and *PRF1*[40] gene polymorphisms.

PATHOPHYSIOLOGY

The exact mechanisms to link deficient natural killer cell and cytotoxic T cell function with the expansion of activated macrophages are not clear. One explanation is related to the fact that HLH/MAS patients appear to have a diminished ability to control some infections.[31] More specifically, natural killer cells and cytotoxic T cells fail to kill infected cells and to thus remove the source of antigenic stimulation. Such persistent antigen stimulation leads, in turn, to persistent antigen-driven activation and proliferation of T cells associated with escalating production of cytokines that stimulate macrophages. However, in many cases of MAS, attempts to identify an infectious trigger have not been successful, and some episodes appear to be triggered by a flare of the underlying disease, rather than infection. Because cytolytic cells have also been shown to induce apoptosis of activated immune cells in some experimental systems, it has been hypothesized that in hemophagocytic syndromes, abnormal cytotoxic cells may fail to provide appropriate apoptotic signals for the removal of activated macrophages and T cells during the contraction stage of the immune response.[41,42] One intriguing possibility is that such perforin-dependent apoptotic signals may be delivered by the regulatory T cells.[43] Whatever the exact mechanism might be, the failure to deliver apoptotic signals leads to persistent expansion of T cells and macrophages secreting proinflammatory cytokines. The clinical findings during the acute phase of HLH can largely be explained because of the prolonged production of cytokines and chemokines originating from activated macrophages and T cells.[12,44] In fact, hemophagocytosis, the pathognomonic feature of the syndrome, is a hallmark of cytokine-driven excess activation of macrophages.[12]

One study of liver biopsies in MAS patients demonstrated massive infiltration of the liver by hemophagocytic macrophages producing tumor necrosis factor (TNF) α and IL-6 and CD8+ T lymphocytes producing IFN-γ.[44] Studies in perforin-deficient mice, an animal model of HLH, suggest that these cytotoxic CD8+ cells producing IFN-γ are particularly important in the pathogenesis of excessive macrophage activation.[45] Perforin-deficient mice manifest many features of MAS/HLH after infection with lymphocytic choriomeningitis virus. However, the MAS-like symptoms in these animals can be almost completely prevented by elimination of CD8+ T cells or by neutralization of IFN-γ. Because IFN-γ is a well-known macrophage activator, it has been suggested to be critical to the expansion of macrophages in these animals. Similar results have been obtained in mice deficient in other HLH-associated genes including *Munc13-4* and *Rab27a*.[46,47]

These animals also developed an HLH-like picture upon infection with lymphocytic choriomeningitis virus (LCMV) in an IFNγ dependent manner. Based on these studies, the neutralization of IFNγ has been proposed as a potential alternative treatment of HLH in humans. In all these models, however, the HLH-like clinical features emerge only in response to LCMV infections. Although a viral illness is a very common trigger of hemophagocytic syndromes, many FHLH patients develop the first symptom of the disease spontaneously without an identifiable infection.[13] Similarly, MAS is often associated with a flare of underlying systemic JIA rather than infection. These considerations prompted a search for other animal models that would not be dependent on a viral infection. Recent reports showing the critical need for the TLR signaling adaptor MyD88 in the development of HLH-like disease in LCMV infected *MUNC13-4* deficient mice[48] combined with the evidence of persistently activated TLR/IL1R signaling pathways in SJIA[49,50] provided a rationale for repeated activation of TLR to replicate the environment that would allow MAS to develop in a genetically predisposed host. Indeed, mice given repeated TLR9 stimulation develop some MAS features.[51] Furthermore, this disease also appears to be IFNγ dependent. The exact mechanisms involved in this model and their relevance to the disease in humans still needs to be elucidated. Consistent with the animal data, the increase in serum IFN-γ levels in MAS patients, compared to those in patients with active systemic JIA, is dramatically higher than the increase in the levels of any other cytokine.[52-54] Combined, these observations suggest that, similar to the animal models, massive activation and expansion of cytotoxic CD8+ T cells in MAS patients are associated with the production of IFN-γ and other macrophage-activating cytokines, such as M-CSF (Fig. 49-2). This leads to subsequent activation and expansion of macrophages. The activated macrophages, in turn, exhibit hemophagocytic

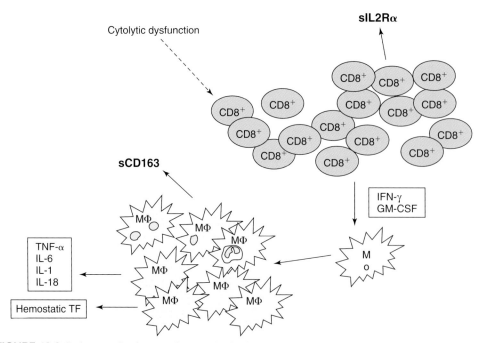

FIGURE 49-2 Pathogenesis of macrophage activation in hemophagocytic syndromes. The underlying cytolytic dysfunction leads to uncontrolled expansion and survival of activated cytotoxic CD8+ T cells. They continue to secrete proinflammatory cytokines, including interferon (INF)-γ and macrophage colony-stimulating factor (M-CSF). Prolonged stimulation of monocytes with cytokines leads to their excessive activation and differentiation into macrophages with hemophagocytic activity. This is also associated with increased production of proinflammatory cytokines, such as tumor necrosis factor (TNF)-α, IL-1, and IL-6. Hemophagocytosis of blood elements in the bone marrow leads to peripheral cytopenias. Production of procoagulant tissue factor (TF) combined with the TNF-α effects on vascular endothelial cells contribute to the development of coagulopathy. *GM-CSF*, Granulocyte-macrophage colony-stimulating factor.

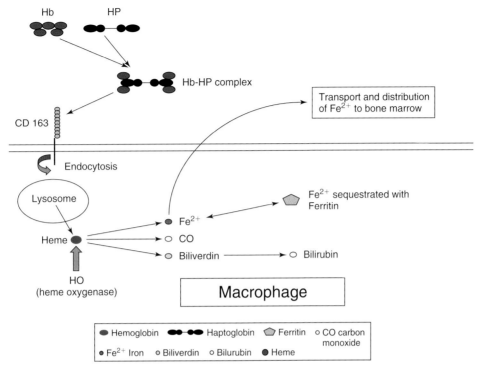

FIGURE 49-3 Role of the hemoglobin-haptoglobin scavenger receptor CD163, heme oxygenase (HO), and ferritin in adaptation to oxidative stress induced by free heme and iron. Free heme is a source of redox-active iron. To prevent cell damage caused by iron-derived reactive oxygen species, haptoglobin forms a complex with free hemoglobin. The haptoglobin-hemoglobin (Hp-Hb) complexes then bind to CD163 and are internalized by the macrophage. Endocytosis of Hp-Hb complexes leads to upregulation of HO enzymatic activity. HO degrades the heme subunit of Hb into biliverdin, which is subsequently converted to bilirubin, carbon monoxide, and free iron. The free iron is either sequestered with ferritin in the cell or transported and distributed to red blood cell precursors in the bone marrow. Increased uptake of Hp-Hb complexes by macrophages leads to increased synthesis of ferritin. Highly elevated levels of serum ferritin are an important diagnostic feature of both MAS and HLH.

activity and secrete proinflammatory cytokines, including interleukin-1 (IL-1), TNF-α, IL-6, and IL-18, which are responsible for many of the clinical manifestations of MAS. Excess of circulating IL-1β, TNF-α, IL-6, IL-18, and IFN-γ is likely to contribute to the early and persistent findings of fevers, hyperlipidemia, and endothelial activation responsible in part for coagulopathy and later sequelae, including hepatic triaditis and central nervous system (CNS) demyelination.[12,52] The activated macrophages also secrete hemostatic tissue factor, which contributes to the development of the coagulopathy reminiscent of the disseminated intravascular coagulation-like syndrome seen in sepsis.

Recently, there has been an increasing interest in the role of IL-18 in systemic JIA and MAS. Strikingly high IL-18 levels have been observed in both primary and secondary hemophagocytic syndromes.[55,56] In these patients, hemophagocytic macrophages and Kupffer cells appear to be the major cellular sources of IL-18,[55] and IL-18 levels strongly correlate with serum ferritin. Although serum levels of IL-18 are strikingly high in MAS, they are also very high in systemic JIA patients in general, particularly in those with pronounced systemic manifestations.[56] Although it may be a useful biomarker, the exact role of IL-18 remains unclear, particularly considering the fact that in many systemic JIA patients, plasma IL-18 levels remain elevated even in remission.

The hemophagocytic macrophages in MAS express the scavenger receptor CD163,[19,57] a feature that provides clues to the understanding of the origin of extreme hyperferritinemia in MAS. The only known function of CD163 is related to its ability to bind hemoglobin-haptoglobin complexes and to initiate pathways important for the adaptation to oxidative stress induced by free heme and iron.[58] Because the sequestration of free iron by ferritin is an important component of these pathways, increased uptake of hemoglobin-haptoglobin complexes by CD163+ macrophages leads to increase synthesis of ferritin (Fig. 49-3). Therefore, increased release of free hemoglobin associated with increased erythrophagocytosis would require more production of ferritin to sequestrate excessive amount of free iron.

Two recent studies have suggested that expansion of CD163+ macrophages in the bone marrow occurs in a substantial proportion of patients with systemic JIA without apparent MAS, and this phenomenon is highly specific to this disease.[16-17] It has been proposed that such expansion may represent early stages of MAS. As shown in Fig. 49-2, the expansion of overly activated T cells and macrophages is associated with shedding off some of their receptors including sIL2Rα and sCD163. The emerging consensus in the HLH literature is that serum levels of sIL2Rα and sCD163 reflect the degree of activation and expansion of T cells and phagocytic macrophages, respectively,[59-60] and thus, serve as useful diagnostic markers. Limited experience in pediatric rheumatology suggests that assessment of serum levels of sIL2Rα and sCD163 may not only help diagnose MAS in patients with systemic JIA at the early stages, but may also provide a new way to monitor response to treatment.[16]

CLINICAL FEATURES

The clinical findings in overt MAS are dramatic.[1-6] Typically, patients with a chronic condition become acutely ill with persistent fever, mental status changes, lymphadenopathy, hepatosplenomegaly, liver dysfunction, easy bruising, and mucosal bleeding. These clinical symptoms are associated with precipitous fall in at least two of three blood cell lines (leukocytes, erythrocytes, and platelets). The fall in platelet count is usually an early finding. Because bone marrow aspiration typically reveals significant hypercellularity and normal megakaryocytes, such cytopenias do not seem to be secondary to inadequate production of cells. Increased destruction of the cells by phagocytosis and consumption at the inflammatory sites are more likely explanations. Precipitous fall in erythrocyte sedimentation rate (ESR) is another characteristic laboratory feature, which probably reflects the degree of hypofibrinogenemia secondary to fibrinogen consumption and liver dysfunction.[2-6] Liver involvement is common in MAS, and significant hepatomegaly is frequently present. Some patients develop mild jaundice. Liver function tests often reveal high serum transaminases activity and mildly elevated levels of serum bilirubin, and moderate hypoalbuminemia has been reported. Serum ammonia levels are typically normal or only mildly elevated.

Encephalopathy is another frequently reported clinical feature of MAS. Mental status changes, seizures, and coma are the most common manifestations of CNS disease.[1-6] Cerebrospinal fluid pleiocytosis with mildly elevated protein has been noted in some studies.[2] Significant deterioration in renal function has also been noted in several series and was associated with particularly high mortality in one report.[5] Pulmonary infiltrates have been mentioned in several reports, and hemophagocytic macrophages can be found in bronchoalveolar lavage.

Additional laboratory findings in MAS include highly elevated serum levels of triglycerides, LDH, and ferritin. The elevation of serum ferritin is particularly marked (often above 10,000 ng/mL)[61] and appears to parallel the degree of macrophage activation. In normal physiological conditions, serum ferritin is usually 60% to 80% glycosylated while intracellular ferritin is not glycosylated. It is not clear what factors determine the balance between the glycosylated versus nonglycosylated forms, but it has been shown that the percentage of glycosylated ferritin in the serum of patients with hemophagocytic syndromes is very low (below 20%).[61] Based on these observations, it has been proposed that the assessment of the glycosylated ferritin may be a useful tool for the diagnosis of hemophagocytic syndromes.

A hemorrhagic syndrome resembling DIC is another striking abnormality in MAS.[1-6,62-63] Hemorrhagic skin rashes from mild petechiae to extensive ecchymotic lesions, epistaxis, hematemesis secondary to upper gastrointestinal bleeding, and rectal bleeding are the most commonly described clinical symptoms caused by coagulation abnormalities observed in MAS. Further laboratory evaluation reveals prolonged prothrombin and partial thromboplastin times, marked hypofibrinogenemia, and moderate deficiency of vitamin K–dependent clotting factors. A decrease in factor V levels is usually mild. Fibrin degradation products are usually present as well.

TISSUE HISTOLOGY

The most common histopathological finding in patients with MAS is tissue infiltration with T lymphocytes and cytologically benign yet actively phagocytic macrophages (see Fig. 49-1). Although the demonstration of macrophages phagocytosing hematopoietic elements in the bone marrow or lymph nodes is virtually diagnostic, negative reports may occur due to sampling difficulties or timing of the procedure. The hemophagocytic macrophages may also be found in tissues other than

bone marrow. Thus, postmortem evaluation of one patient with MAS revealed extensive macrophagic infiltration of the heart, adrenal glands, liver, pancreas, and meninges.[3] In addition to sinusoidal and periportal infiltration with macrophages, histological evaluation of the liver often reveals severe diffuse fatty changes.[62,63] The development of fatty changes in the liver may be related to the metabolic effects of TNF-α. TNF-α has been shown to stimulate hepatic lipogenesis and inhibit synthesis of lipoprotein lipase, an enzyme needed to release fatty acids from circulating lipoprotein so that they can be used by the tissues. The same mechanism also appears to be responsible for high triglyceridemia seen in MAS patients.

The most common cutaneous manifestations of MAS are panniculitis and purpura.[62-64] Most skin biopsy specimens show edema and hemorrhage associated with mononuclear cell infiltration with numerous macrophages occasionally showing hemophagocytosis. Two recent reports described systemic JIA/MAS patients who also had necrotizing histiocytic lymphadenopathy consistent with Kikuchi syndrome.[34,65] Given the rarity of both conditions, this association may not be random.

DIAGNOSIS

There are no validated diagnostic criteria for MAS, and early diagnosis is often difficult. Thus, in a patient with persistently active underlying rheumatological disease, a fall in the ESR and platelet count, particularly in a combination with persistently high C-reactive protein and increasing levels of serum D-dimer and ferritin, should raise a suspicion of impeding MAS. The diagnosis of MAS is usually confirmed by the demonstration of hemophagocytosis in the bone marrow. However, this method may be difficult to use due to sampling errors, particularly at the early stages of the syndrome.[66] In addition, many reports have demonstrated that hemophagocytic macrophages may accumulate in tissues other than bone marrow. In some reports, additional biopsies were performed due to the initial failure to detect hemophagocytosis in the bone marrow, and hemophagocytic macrophages were found in organs, such as the liver, lymph nodes, or the lungs. In these patients, assessment of the levels of sIL2Rα and sCD163 in serum may help with the timely diagnosis of MAS. As discussed earlier, soluble IL2Rα receptors and soluble CD163 are now increasingly recognized as important biomarkers of MAS. Because they shed off the surface of activated T cells and macrophages respectively, their levels are likely to increase in the serum regardless of the tissue localization of the cells. Although mild elevation of sIL2Rα has been reported in many rheumatic diseases, including JIA and SLE,[67] a several-fold increase in these diseases is highly suggestive of MAS.[16,68] One must remember, however, that other clinical entities associated with high levels of sIL2Rα include malignancies and some viral infections, including viral hepatitis, and these conditions should be considered in the differential diagnosis.

In contrast to MAS, the diagnosis of HLH is usually established based on the diagnostic criteria developed by the International Histiocyte Society[69] (Box 49-1). However, the application of the HLH diagnostic criteria to systemic JIA patients with suspected MAS is problematic. Some of the HLH markers, such as lymphadenopathy, splenomegaly, and hyperferritinemia, are common features of active systemic JIA itself and, therefore, do not distinguish MAS from a conventional systemic JIA flare. Other HLH criteria, such as cytopenias and hypofibrinogenemia, become evident only at the late stages. This is because systemic JIA patients often have increased white blood cell and platelet counts and serum levels of fibrinogen as a part of the inflammatory response seen in this disease. Therefore, when patients develop MAS, they reach the degree of cytopenias and hypofibrinogenemia seen in HLH only at the late stages of the syndrome when their management becomes challenging. This is even more problematic for the diagnosis of MAS in patients with SLE in whom autoimmune cytopenias are common and difficult to distinguish from those caused by MAS. In these patients, the presence of extreme hyperferritinemia and LDH elevation should raise suspicion for MAS.[70] Attempts to modify the HLH criteria to increase their sensitivity and specificity for the diagnosis of MAS in rheumatic conditions have been initiated.[71,72]

DIFFERENTIAL DIAGNOSIS

In addition to distinguishing MAS from a flare of an underlying rheumatological disease, one must consider other clinical entities associated with hepatic dysfunction, coagulopathy, cytopenias, or encephalopathy. In some MAS patients, the combination of hepatic dysfunction with encephalopathy may be reminiscent of Reye syndrome. The diagnosis of Reye syndrome, however, is based of viral prodrome, unexplained vomiting, behavioral changes, and a distinctive chemical profile characterized by rapid coordinated increase in serum aminotransferase levels, blood ammonia, and prothrombin time with relatively minimal changes in serum bilirubin. The DIC-like coagulopathy seen in MAS is not a feature of Reye syndrome. Conversely, sharp increase in blood ammonia levels, an important feature of Reye syndrome, is usually very mild in MAS.

The hemorrhagic syndrome seen in MAS may resemble thrombotic thrombocytopenic purpura. However, microangiopathic anemia with the emergence of fragmented red blood cells in peripheral circulation, a central feature of thrombotic thrombocytopenic purpura, is usually not seen in MAS.

It is also important to differentiate MAS from malignancy associated HLH and malignant histiocytic disorders. Some other important differential diagnoses include sepsis, drug reactions, and thorough infectious work up is necessary for the majority of these patients.

TREATMENT

MAS is a life-threatening condition still associated with high mortality rates. Therefore, early recognition of this syndrome and immediate therapeutic intervention to produce a rapid response are critical. Prompt administration of more aggressive treatment in these patients may prevent development of a severe syndrome. To achieve rapid reversal of coagulation abnormalities and cytopenias, most clinicians start with intravenous methylprednisolone pulse therapy (30 mg/kg for three consecutive days) followed by 2 to 3 mg/kg/day divided in four doses. After normalization of hematological abnormalities and resolution of coagulopathy, steroids are tapered slowly to avoid relapses of MAS. However, MAS sometimes appears to be corticosteroid resistant with deaths being reported even among patients treated with massive doses of steroids.

Parenteral administration of cyclosporine A has been shown to be highly effective in patients with corticosteroid-resistant MAS.[73-74] From the primary effect of cyclosporine A, largely, but not entirely confined to T cells, a wide variety of other effects are mediated leading to profound and therapeutically useful immunosuppression. In many patients, parenteral administration of cyclosporine A (2-7 mg/kg/day) not only provides rapid control of the symptoms, but also allows for avoiding of excessive use of steroids.

Patients in whom MAS remains active despite the use of corticosteroids and cyclosporine A present a formidable challenge. In these patients, one might consider using etoposide (or VP16), a podophyllatoxin derivative that inhibits DNA synthesis by forming a complex with topoisomerease II and DNA. The combination of steroids, cyclosporine A, and etoposide is the main component of the HLH-2004 treatment protocol developed by the International Histiocyte Society.[69] This protocol includes a combination of etoposide and CNS-penetrating dexamethasone (with or without methotrexate), followed by a maintenance dose of cyclosporine A and less frequent pulses of etoposide once clinical remission has been established. In accordance with the protocol, patients with familial HLH and patients who experience a relapse after initially responding to HLH 2004 should proceed to definitive therapy with allogeneic hematopoietic stem cell transplantation.

Although successful use etoposide in MAS has been reported,[75] potential toxicity of the drug is a major concern, particularly in patients with hepatic impairment. Etoposide is metabolized by the liver, and then both the unchanged drug and its metabolites are excreted through the kidneys. Because patients who may require the use of etoposide are very likely to have hepatic and renal involvement, caution should be exercised to properly adjust the dosage and thus limit the extent of the potential side effects, such as severe bone marrow suppression, that may be detrimental. Reports describing deaths caused by severe bone marrow suppression and overwhelming infection have been published.[6]

Recently, it has been suggested that antithymocyte globulin (ATG) might be a safer alternative to etoposide in patients unresponsive to the combination of steroids and cyclosporine A, particularly in those with renal and hepatic impairment. ATG depletes both CD4[+] and CD8[+] T cells through complement-dependent cell lysis. Mild depletion of monocytes is noted in some patients as well. Although this treatment was tolerated well by patients in the reported cases,[14,68] one must remember infusion reactions, including anaphylaxis, are frequently reported with the use of ATG, and adequate laboratory and supportive medical resources must be readily available if this treatment is used.

Occasional reports describe successful use of cyclophosphamide to control MAS mainly in patients with SLE.[76]

The effectiveness of biological drugs in MAS treatment remains unclear. Although TNF-inhibiting agents have been reported to be effective in occasional MAS patients,[77-78] numerous recent reports describe patients in whom MAS occurred while they were on the agents.[79-82] Because MAS episodes are often triggered by the disease flare, at least in systemic JIA, biological drugs that neutralize IL-1, a cytokine that plays a pivotal role in systemic JIA pathogenesis, have been tried by some authors. The results, however, have been conflicting. Successful use of anakinra, a recombinant IL1R antagonist, in patients with MAS complicating systemic JIA has been reported,[83-84] but in a larger series that described experience with this treatment in systemic JIA in general, several patients developed MAS while being treated with anakinra.[85-87] Canakinumab, a monoclonal antibody directed against IL-1β, is another IL-1 blocking biological agent.[21] Canakinumab is an effective treatment in systemic JIA; however, based on the recent clinical trials, it does not appear to have a significant effect on MAS rates, even in patients whose underlying systemic JIA is well controlled.[21] Infections appear to be the most prevalent trigger for MAS in this group, and the main clinical features of MAS in patients receiving canakinumab, do not appear to be modified by the treatment.

IL-6 blockade, via the anti-IL-6 receptor monoclonal antibody tocilizumab, has proved to be highly efficacious in treating systemic JIA.[22] IL-6 is produced by activated macrophages in MAS,[44] and one animal model suggests IL-6 may amplify the response of macrophages to proinflammatory stimuli.[88] However, in a Phase III clinical trial of tocilizumab in systemic JIA, several patients developed MAS while being treated with this agent. This corresponded to 1.5 MAS cases per 100 patient years. As with canakinumab, at the time of MAS presentation, underlying systemic JIA in these patients was well controlled.[22] Another recent report from Japan described a patient with severe adult-onset Still disease who showed a very good initial response to tocilizumab, but then rapidly progressed to develop MAS.[89] Furthermore, it has been suggested that treatment with tocilizumab may mask some features of MAS. Thus, Shimizu and colleagues described several systemic JIA patients receiving tocilizumab in whom CRP levels remained normal and the increase in the levels of ferritin was relatively modest, despite the development of MAS.[90]

Based on some success with intravenous immunoglobulin administration in virus-associated reactive HLH,[91] this treatment might be effective in MAS triggered by viral infection. However, if MAS is driven by EBV infection, one might consider rituximab, a monoclonal antibody that depletes B lymphocytes, which are the main type of cells harboring EBV virus.[92,93] This approach has been successfully used in EBV-induced lymphoproliferative disease.[94] The treatment with rituximab may also be effective in MAS presenting as a complication of SLE.[95]

PROGNOSIS

MAS is a life-threatening condition, and reported mortality rates reach 20%. Due to increasing awareness of this syndrome, MAS is now diagnosed relatively early, and the outcome is improving. A substantial proportion of MAS patients experience recurrent episodes, and these patients may require closer monitoring.

REFERENCES

1. E.D. Silverman, J.J. Miller, B. Bernstein, et al., Consumption coagulopathy associated with systemic juvenile rheumatoid arthritis, J. Pediatr. 103 (1983) 872–876.
2. M. Hadchouel, A.M. Prieur, C. Griscelli, Acute hemorrhagic, hepatic, and neurologic manifestations in juvenile rheumatoid arthritis: possible relationship to drugs or infection, J. Pediatr. 106 (1985) 561–566.
3. J.L. Stephan, J. Zeller, P. Hubert, et al., Macrophage activation syndrome and rheumatic disease in childhood: a report of four new cases, Clin. Exp. Rheumatol. 11 (1993) 451–456.
4. A.A. Grom, NK dysfunction: a common pathway in systemic onset juvenile rheumatoid arthritis, macrophage activation syndrome, and hemophagocytic lymphohistiocytosis, Arthritis Rheum. 50 (2004) 689–698.
6. J.L. Stephan, I. Kone-Paut, C. Galambrun, et al., Reactive Haemophagocytic syndrome in children with inflammatory disorders. A retrospective study of 24 patients, Rheumatology (Oxford) 40 (2001) 1285–1292.
7. A. Muise, S.E. Tallett, E.D. Silverman, Are children with Kawasaki disease and prolonged fever at risk for macrophage activation syndrome?, Pediatrics 112 (2003) e495–e497.
8. A. Parodi, S. Davi, A.B. Pringe, et al., Macrophage activation syndrome in juvenile systemic lupus erythematosus: a multinational multicenter study of thirty-eight patients, Arthritis Rheum. 60 (2009) 3388–3399.
9. B.H. Athreya, Is macrophage activation syndrome a new entity?, Clin. Exper. Rheumatol. 20 (2002) 121–123.
11. B.E. Favara, A.C. Feller, M. Pauli, et al., Contemporary classification of histiocytic disorders. The WHO Committee on Histiocytic/Reticulum Cell Proliferations. Reclassification Working Group of the Histiocyte Society, Med. Pediatr. Oncol. 29 (1997) 157–166.
12. H.A. Filipovich, Hemophagocytic lymphohistiocytosis, Immunol. Allergy Clin. N. Am. 22 (2002) 281–300.
13. M.B. Jordan, C.E. Allen, S. Weitzman, et al., How I treat hemophagocytic lymphohistiocytosis, Blood 118 (2011) 4041–4052.
16. J. Bleesing, A. Prada, D.M. Siegel, et al., The diagnostic significance of soluble CD163 and soluble interleukin-2 receptor alpha-chain in macrophage activation syndrome and untreated new-onset systemic juvenile idiopathic arthritis, Arthritis Rheum. 56 (2007) 965–971.
17. E.M. Behrens, T. Beukelman, M. Paessler, R.Q. Cron, Occult macrophage activation syndrome in patients with systemic juvenile idiopathic arthritis, J. Rheumatol. 34 (2007) 1133–1138.
18. O. Lambotte, M. Khellaf, H. Harmouche, et al., Characteristics and long-term outcome of 15 episodes of systemic lupus erythematosus-associated hemophagocytic syndrome, Medicine 85 (2006) 169–182.
19. T. Avcin, S.M.L. Tse, R. Schneider, et al., Macrophage activation syndrome as the presenting manifestation of rheumatic diseases in childhood, J. Pediatr. 148 (2006) 683–686.
25. K.E. Sullivan, C.A. Delaat, S.D. Douglas, et al., Defective natural killer cell function in patients with hemophagocytic lymphohistiocytosis and first degree relatives, Pediatr. Res. 44 (1998) 465–468.
26. S.E. Stepp, R. Dufourcq-Lagelouse, F. Le Deist, et al., Perforin gene defects in familial hemophagocytic lymphohistiocytosis, Science 286 (1999) 1957–1959.
27. J. Feldmann, I. Callebaut, G. Raposo, et al., MUNC13-4 is essential for cytolytic granules fusion and is mutated in a form of familial hemophagocytic lymphohistiocytosis (FHL3), Cell 115 (2003) 461–473.
28. U. zur Stadt, S. Schmidt, A.S. Diler, et al., Linkage of familial hemophagocytic lymphohistiocytosis (FHL) type-4 to chromosome 6q24 and identification of mutations in syntaxin 11, Hum. Mol. Genet. 14 (2005) 827–834.
29. U. zur Stadt, J. Rohr, W. Seifert, et al., Familial hemophagocytic lymphohistiocytosis type 5 (FHL-5) is caused by mutations in munc18-2 and impaired binding to syntaxin 11, Am. J. Hum. Gen. 85 (2009) 482–492.
30. G. Menasche, E. Pastural, J. Feldman, et al., Mutations in Rab27a cause Griscelli syndrome associated with haemophagocytic syndrome, Nat. Genet. 25 (2000) 173–176.
31. M.D. Barbosa, Q.A. Nguyen, V.T. Tchernev, et al., Identification of the homologous beige and Chediak-Higashi syndrome genes (LYST), Nature 382 (1996) 262–265.
33. R.A. Marsh, L. Madden, B.J. Kitchen, et al., XIAP deficiency: a unique primary immunodeficiency best classified as X-linked familial hemophagocytic lymphohistiocytosis and not as X-linked lymphoproliferative disease, Blood 116 (7) (2010) 1079–1082.

34. A.A. Grom, J. Villanueva, S. Lee, et al., Natural killer cell dysfunction in patients with systemic-onset juvenile rheumatoid arthritis and macrophage activation syndrome, J. Pediatr. 142 (2003) 292–296.

37. N.M. Wulffraat, G.T. Rijkers, E. Elst, et al., Reduced perforin expression in systemic onset juvenile idiopathic arthritis is restored by autologous stem cell transplantation, Rheumatology (Oxford) 42 (2003) 375–379.

39. K. Zhang, J. Biroscak, D.N. Glass, et al., Macrophage activation syndrome in systemic juvenile idiopathic arthritis is associated with MUNC13D gene polymorphisms, Arthritis Rheum. 58 (2008) 2892–2896.

40. S.J. Vastert, R. van Wijk, L.E. D'Urbano, et al., Mutations in the perforin gene can be linked to macrophage activation syndrome in patients with systemic onset juvenile idiopathic arthritis, Rheumatology (Oxford) 49 (2010) 441–449.

43. J.W. Verbsky, W.J. Grossman, Hemophagocytic lymphohistiocytosis: diagnosis, pathophysiology, treatment, and future perspectives, Ann. Med. 38 (2006) 20–31.

44. A.D. Billiau, T. Roskams, R. Van Damme-Lombaerts, et al., Macrophage activation syndrome: characteristic findings on liver biopsy illustrating the key role of activated, IFN-γ-producing lymphocytes and IL-6 and TNF-α-producing macrophages, Blood 105 (2005) 1648–1651.

45. M.B. Jordan, D. Hildeman, J. Kappler, et al., An animal model of hemophagocytic lymphohistiocytosis (HLH): CD8+ T cells and interferon gamma are essential for the disorder, Blood 104 (2004) 735–743.

49. V. Pascual, F. Allantaz, E. Arce, et al., Role of interleukin-1 (IL-1) in the pathogenesis of systemic onset juvenile idiopathic arthritis and clinical response to IL-1 blockade, J. Exp. Med. 201 (2005) 1479–1486.

50. N. Fall, M. Barnes, S. Thornton, et al., Gene expression profiling of peripheral blood from patients with untreated new-onset systemic juvenile idiopathic arthritis reveals molecular heterogeneity that may predict macrophage activation syndrome, Arthritis Rheum. 56 (2007) 3793–3804.

51. E.M. Behrens, S.W. Canna, K. Slade, et al., Repeated TLR9 stimulation results in macrophage activation syndrome-like disease in mice, J. Clin. Invest. 121 (2011) 2264–2277.

52. J.I. Henter, G. Elinder, O. Söder, et al., Hypercytokinemia in familial hemophagocytic lymphohistiocytosis, Blood 78 (1991) 2918–2922.

53. T. Imagawa, H. Umebayashi, R. Kurosawa, et al., Differences between systemic-onset juvenile idiopathic arthritis and macrophage activation syndrome from the standpoint of the proinflammatory cytokine profile, Arthritis and Rheum. 50 (Suppl.) (2004) S92.

54. M.F. Ibarra, M. Klein-Gitelman, E. Morgan, et al., Serum neopterin levels as a diagnostic marker of hemophagocytic lymphohistiocytosis syndrome, Clin. Vaccine Immunol. 18 (2011) 609–614.

55. N. Maeno, S. Takei, H. Imanaka, et al., Increased interleukin-18 expression in bone marrow of a patient with systemic juvenile idiopathic arthritis and unrecognized macrophage-activation syndrome, Arthritis Rheum. 50 (2004) 1935–1938.

57. D.J. Schaer, B. Schleiffenbaum, M. Kurrer, et al., Soluble hemoglobin-haptoglobin scavenger receptor CD163 as a lineage-specific marker in the reactive hemophagocytic syndrome, Eur. J. Haemotol. 74 (2005) 6–10.

62. K.J. Smith, H.G. Skeltom, J. Yeager, et al., Cutaneous, histopathologic, immunohistochemical, and clinical manifestations in patients with hemophagocytic syndrome, Arch. Dermatol. 128 (1992) 193–200.

63. A.P. Reiner, J.L. Spivak, Hematophagic Histiocytosis. A report of 23 new patients and a review of the literature, Medicine 67 (1998) 369–388.

68. A. Coca, K.W. Bundy, B. Marston, et al., Macrophage activation syndrome: serological markers and treatment with anti-thymocyte globulin, Clin. Immunol. 132 (2009) 10–18.

69. J.I. Henter, A. Horne, M. Arico, et al., HLH-2004: Diagnostic and therapeutic guidelines for hemopagocytic lymphohistiocytosis, Pediatr. Blood Cancer 48 (2007) 124–131.

70. A. Parodi, S. Davì, A.B. Pringe, et al., Macrophage Activation Syndrome in Juvenile Systemic Lupus Erythematosus. Multinational multicenter study of 38 patients, Arthritis Rheum. 60 (2009) 3388–3399.

71. A. Ravelli, S. Magni-Manzoni, A. Pistorio, et al., Preliminary diagnostic guidelines for macrophage activation syndrome complicating systemic juvenile idiopathic arthritis, J. Pediatr. 146 (2005) 598–604.

72. S. Davi, A. Consolaro, D. Guseinova, et al., An international consensus survey of diagnostic criteria for macrophage activation syndrome in systemic juvenile idiopathic arthritis, J. Rheumatol. 38 (2011) 764–768.

73. R. Mouy, J.L. Stephan, P. Pillet, et al., Efficacy of cyclosporine A in the treatment of macrophage activation syndrome in juvenile arthritis: report of five cases, J. Pediatr. 129 (1996) 750–754.

74. A. Ravelli, F. De Benedetti, S. Viola, et al., Macrophage activation syndrome in systemic juvenile rheumatoid arthritis successfully treated with cyclosporine, J. Pediatr. 128 (1996) 275–278.

75. D. Fishman, M. Rooney, P. Woo, Successful management of reactive haemophagocytic syndrome in systemic-onset juvenile chronic arthritis, Br. J. Rheumatol. 34 (1995) 888.

76. Y. Ueda, H. Yamashita, Y. Takahashi, et al., Refractory hemophagocytic syndrome in systemic lupus erythematosus successfully treated with intermittent intravenous cyclophosphamide: three case reports and literature review, Clin. Rheumatol. (pre-published online).

83. P.M. Miettunen, A. Narendran, A. Jayanthan, et al., Successful treatment of severe paediatric rheumatic disease-associated macrophage activation syndrome with interleukin-1 inhibition following conventional immunosuppressive therapy: case series with 12 patients, Rheumatology (Oxford) 50 (2011) 417–419.

85. P.A. Nigrovic, M. Mannion, F.H. Prince, et al., Anakinra as first-line disease-modifying therapy in systemic juvenile idiopathic arthritis: report of forty-six patients from an international multicenter series, Arthritis Rheum. 63 (2011) 545–555.

86. A. Zeft, R. Hollister, B. LaFleur, et al., Anakinra for systemic juvenile arthritis: the Rocky Mountain experience, J. Clin. Rheumatol. 15 (2009) 161–164.

88. R. Strippoli, F. Carvello, R. Scianaro, et al., Amplification of the response to Toll-like receptor ligands by prolonged exposure to interleukin-6 in mice: implication for the pathogenesis of macrophage activation syndrome, Arthritis Rheum. 64 (2012) 1680–1688.

90. M. Shimizu, Y. Nakagishi, K. Kasai, et al., Tocilizumab masks the clinical symptoms of systemic juvenile idiopathic arthritis-associated macrophage activation syndrome: the diagnostic significance of interleukin-18 and interleukin-6, Cytokine 58 (2012) 287–294.

91. C. Larroche, F. Bruneel, M.H. Andre, et al., Intravenously administered gamma-globulins in reactive hemophagocytic syndrome, Ann. Med. Interne (Paris) 151 (2000) 533–539.

93. D. Chellapandian, R. Das, K. Zelley, et al., Treatment of Epstein Barr virus associated haemophagocytic lymphohistiocytosis with rituximab-containing chemo-immunotherapeutic regimens, Br. J. Haematol. 162 (2013) 376–382.

95. J. Bakshi, S. Hassan, D. D'Cruz, A. Chan, Rituximab therapy in refractory macrophage activation syndrome secondary to systemic lupus erythematosus, Lupus 22 (2013) 1544–1546.

Entire reference list is available online at www.expertconsult.com.

Skeletal Malignancies and Related Disorders

Roger Allen, Karin Tiedemann

INTRODUCTION

One of the challenges of pediatric rheumatology is the broad spectrum of conditions ranging from the benign to the potentially life-limiting childhood malignancies that may present with relatively nonspecific musculoskeletal symptoms and signs. The importance of careful history taking, thorough physical examination, and appropriate use of investigations to arrive at the correct diagnosis, cannot be overemphasized. It is always appropriate in assessing a child with an arthritis or musculoskeletal pain to ask the question: Could this be a neoplastic mimic? Musculoskeletal manifestations of neoplasia in children can be considered under three overall groupings:

1. Primary malignant disease of bone marrow
2. Primary benign or malignant tumors of bone, cartilage, or adjacent tissues (Table 50-1)
3. Malignant diseases metastasizing to bone

In recent decades there have been significant improvements in the overall survival, disease-free survival, and treatment-associated morbidity in most of the childhood malignancies. These improvements have resulted from sequential multi-institutional clinical trials, the progressive refinement of prognostic factors allowing therapy stratification, and the rapidly changing fields of diagnostic tumor cytogenetics and molecular biology in addition to newer techniques in radiologic evaluation and reconstructive surgery.

PRIMARY MALIGNANT DISEASE OF BONE MARROW

Leukemia

Acute lymphoblastic leukemia (ALL) accounts for 80% of leukemia in childhood and is the most common neoplastic mimic of juvenile idiopathic arthritis (JIA). Advances in diagnostic techniques and therapeutic strategies have resulted in a cure rate of approximately 85% in patients with B cell lineage ALL. B-precursor ALL is the most common immunophenotypic subgroup accounting for 75% of childhood ALL, the remainder being of T cell lineage. It is B-precursor ALL that can occasionally present real challenges in diagnosis because marrow replacement occurs slowly and musculoskeletal pain, which is often worse at night, may be present over a protracted period in association with relatively minor, nonspecific symptoms such as lethargy or fever.[1] Pain is usually metaphyseal, but joint swelling can occur. Back pain is relatively common due to leukemic infiltration, which may be associated with diffuse osteopenia with vertebral compression fractures. Conversely, bone pain is unusual in recent onset JIA. Importantly, neither the total number of active joints, the distribution of the arthritis, nor the presence of a positive antinuclear antibody (ANA) can differentiate ALL from JIA. Plain radiographs may be normal or may

show transverse metaphyseal lucencies (Fig. 50-1). MRI shows diffuse marrow changes even when plain radiographs are normal.

Full blood examination may be entirely normal but frequently shows a mild normocytic anemia. The total white blood cell (WBC) count may be normal, elevated, or low and blasts may be absent. A multicenter case control study of children presenting to rheumatology clinics, but ultimately diagnosed with ALL, reported that 75% did not have blasts in the initial peripheral blood film.[2,3] Other features suggestive of ALL include an elevated ESR, particularly if out of keeping with the degree of arthritis, unexplained neutropenia or thrombocytopenia, and elevated levels of lactic dehydrogenase (LDH) and uric acid. Bone marrow evaluation is warranted if there is sufficient uncertainty about the possibility of leukemia.[2,4,5]

In order to afford each child the best chance of cure, it is essential that all appropriate diagnostic investigations be performed before instigation of any therapy. Treatment with corticosteroids or methotrexate for a presumptive diagnosis of JIA may result in amelioration of symptoms in a child with ALL and obscure vital prognostic information because a partial or even complete remission may be induced.[6]

Therapy regimens are "risk adapted"; that is, designed to minimize exposure to drugs with potential long-term effects in the patient groups shown to have the best outcomes and to intensify therapy for patients with poorer prognostic factors. Age and WBC at disease presentation together with the presence or absence of extramedullary disease have prognostic significance and allow initial risk group assignment. "Standard risk" patients must be aged 1 to less than 10 years with a WBC less than $50 \times 10^9/\mu l$ and have no extramedullary disease. Those classified as "high risk" are aged 10 years or greater, have a WBC greater than $50 \times 10^9/\mu l$, and/or central nervous system or testicular involvement at diagnosis. Further refinement of risk groups based on cytogenetic and molecular studies and on the speed of response to induction therapy determines the intensity of postinduction therapy.[7,8]

Given the concerns of delay in correct diagnosis and the potential for inappropriate initiation of therapy, it is perhaps reassuring that the survival rate of children with ALL presenting initially to pediatric rheumatologists is reported to be higher in these children.[9] This probably reflects the fact that the same predictive factors that may heighten a rheumatologists' diagnostic concern (e.g., low WBC) also place the child in the better prognostic group for anticipated treatment response.

TUMORS OF BONE

Benign Tumors of Bone

Osteoid Osteoma/Osteoblastoma

Osteoid osteoma is a common benign bone tumor developing typically in the second decade, although occasionally reported in infants.[10] There is a 3:1 male to female preponderance. Children present with insidious onset of pain, which is classically nocturnal.[11] Other features may include gait disturbance, muscle wasting, or scoliosis. If intraarticular bone is involved there may be joint swelling and reduced range of movement mimicking arthritis.

Osteoid osteomas are small (<15 mm) and typically affect cortical bone, usually of the long bones and less commonly vertebrae or carpal/tarsal bones. Plain radiograph can be diagnostic if demonstrating an area of lysis and surrounding sclerosis. The sclerotic nidus within the area of lysis is more distinct on CT (Fig. 50-2, A). MRI may demonstrate an area of adjacent bone edema around the nidus (Fig. 50-2, B) and technetium radionuclide bone scan reveals a discrete area of increased activity.[12] Osteoblastoma tend to occur in older children with a predilection for medullary bone. They are of larger size (>20mm), but are histologically the same as osteoid osteoma.[13]

The nocturnal pain associated with an osteoid osteoma is reduced by aspirin and nonsteroidal antiinflammatories (NSAIDs). The fact that a thousand-fold increase in prostaglandin concentration has been reported in the nidus material is relevant to this response.[14] A useful diagnostic hint is when parents have used simple analgesia for the nocturnal pain, such as acetaminophen, but note a greater reduction in the degree of pain when aspirin or a nonprescription NSAID, such as ibuprofen, has been used.

Treatment is very successful with CT guided radiofrequency ablation, but CT guided resection is also used to overcome the need for

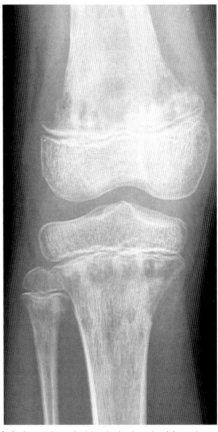

FIGURE 50-1 Acute lymphoblastic leukemia. Metaphyseal lucencies of the right femur, tibia, and fibula in a 5-year-old girl.

TABLE 50-1	Musculoskeletal Tumors and Tumor-like Conditions of Childhood	
HISTOLOGICAL TYPE	**BENIGN**	**MALIGNANT**
Osteogenic	Osteoid osteoma	Osteosarcoma
	Osteoblastoma	
Chondrogenic	Osteochondroma	Chondrosarcoma
	Chondroma	
	Chondroblastoma	
	Chondromyxoid Fibroma	
Fibrogenic	Fibrous cortical defect	Fibrosarcoma
	Juvenile fibromatosis	
	Fibrous dysplasia	
Other	Aneurysmal bone cysts	Rhabdomyosarcoma
	Eosinophilic granuloma	Ewing's sarcoma
	Synovial hemangioma	Synovial sarcoma
	Synovial chondromatosis	
	Pigmented villondoular synovitis	

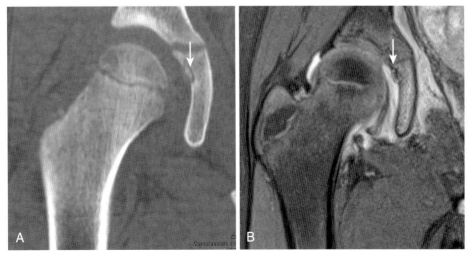

FIGURE 50-2 Osteoid osteoma. Lesion in right acetabulum in a 7-year-old boy. **A,** CT demonstrates nidus of lesion (*arrow*). **B,** MRI of same lesion demonstrates extensive adjacent bone and soft tissue reaction (*arrow*).

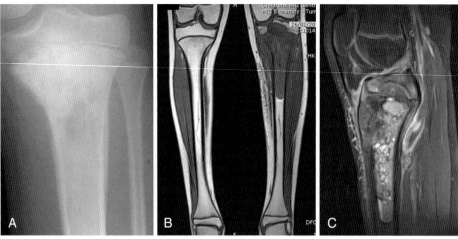

FIGURE 50-3 Osteosarcoma of left proximal tibia in an 11-year-old boy. **A,** plain radiograph shows cortical breach with periosteal reaction. T1 **(B)** and T2 sequences on MRI **(C)**.

open resection.[15,16] Surgical excision is generally required for the larger osteoblastoma lesions. Osteoid osteomas have not been reported to evolve into malignant lesions and typically will resolve spontaneously over some years. As such, long-term medical treatment with NSAIDs is an option,[17] particularly for lesions in sites that may be difficult to access by interventional means, with the reported mean duration of medical therapy required being 1.5 to 2.5 years.[18]

Malignant Tumors of Bone
Osteosarcoma
Osteosarcoma (osteogenic sarcoma) is the most common malignant bone tumor in the pediatric age group. Median peak age at presentation is 16 years, with males more commonly affected (1.6:1). It is very rare in children under 5 years.[19] High cell turnover, as occurs in the metaphyses during puberty, may be a factor in the development of osteosarcomas as presentation is earlier in girls and it appears to occur more commonly in children of taller stature.[20]

A variety of rare genetic conditions with germline mutations in tumor suppressor genes (hereditary bilateral retinoblastoma, Li–Fraumeni syndrome) or in genes associated with maintenance of chromosome stability (Bloom and Rothmund–Thomson syndromes) are associated with an increased risk of developing osteosarcoma.[21] Radiation exposure is the only proven environmental risk factor for the development of osteosarcoma, with a prolonged postexposure latency of 10 to 20 years.[22]

The typical presenting symptom is pain, which may be nocturnal, followed by development of a tender swelling of hard consistency. Systemic symptoms such as fever, weight loss, and fatigue are not common. The metaphysis or metadiaphysis of the long bones are the most common sites: distal femur (40%), proximal tibia (20%), and proximal humerus (10%); the axial skeleton is involved in less than 10% of pediatric cases. Pathological fracture may occur. At diagnosis, classic osteosarcoma is localized to the primary site in 80% of patients, but 20% will already have metastases, typically to the lung or, less frequently, to distant bones. Occasionally, "skip lesions" occur within the same bone as the primary tumor. A lesion typically starts within the medullary cavity, invading through the cortex, elevating the periosteum, creating the classic radiologic appearance of the triangle of immature bone (Codman's sign), and then into surrounding tissue forming a soft tissue mass. The radiologic appearances of lesions vary from osteosclerotic (45%), osteolytic (30%), or mixed (25%). Imaging with technetium bone scan, CT, and MRI will define the site of any metastases and delineate the extent of the primary lesion, enabling a carefully planned biopsy (Fig. 50-3).[21,23]

Preoperative chemotherapy to eradicate micrometastatic disease and to shrink the primary tumor facilitates subsequent resection utilizing limb-sparing techniques rather than amputation.[24] Complete surgical resection remains essential for cure.[24-26] Histological assessment of the degree of tumor necrosis in response to the initial chemotherapy is important in guiding the choice of agents used in postoperative chemotherapy. Osteosarcomas are poorly responsive to radiation therapy, which has a limited role in therapy.

Ten-year survival for patients with nonmetastatic disease at diagnosis is approximately 70% with current treatment approaches; however, 5-year survival is only 20% to 30% in the presence of metastatic disease.[27-29]

Ewing Sarcoma
Ewing sarcoma (EWS) is the second most common primary bone tumor in children and adolescents. The tumor may occur in very young children but more typically occurs in the second decade. It belongs to the spectrum of tumors known as the Ewing Sarcoma family of tumors (ESFT), which includes primary bone tumors (87%), primary extra osseous EWS (8%), and peripheral primitive neuroectodermal tumors (PPNETs) (5%). All are small round cell tumors with differences in their degree of differentiation and expression of neural markers reflecting their neural crest derivation. They share an identical translocation t(11;22) found in up to 95% of ESFT, which has an oncogenic fusion protein. Immunohistochemistry and the identification of translocations within tumor tissue are important aids in differentiating ESFT tumors from other small round cell tumors such as neuroblastoma, lymphoma, or rhabdomyosarcoma.[30]

Ewing sarcoma is more common in males and has a nine times greater incidence in Caucasians than in the African population. That segments of the *EWS* gene are smaller in individuals of African heritage, with fewer polymorphisms, has been postulated as a possible explanation for such marked ethnic variation.[31] Any bone may be affected, with only a slight predominance in the limbs (53%) over bones of the axial skeleton. Metastatic disease is present in about 25% of patients at the time of diagnosis, predominantly to lung (60%), bone (43%), and bone marrow (19%).[32,33]

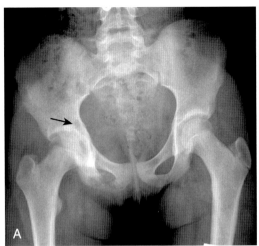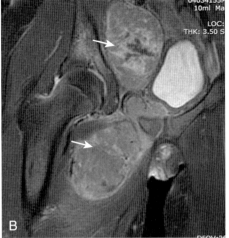

FIGURE 50-4 Ewing sarcoma of right ischium in 12-year-old boy. Plain radiograph demonstrates lytic lesion (*arrow;* **A**), but MRI indicates extent of soft tissue tumor mass (*arrows;* **B**).

The most common presenting symptoms are intermittent pain and a palpable swelling with a median duration of 4 to 6 months between symptom onset and diagnosis. Pathological fracture may be the presenting feature in up to 10% of cases. Systemic features may include fever and weight loss, leading on occasion to misdiagnosis of osteomyelitis, particularly as biopsy specimens may be totally necrotic and mistaken for pus.

Plain radiographs show a destructive lesion of the diaphysis, or within flat bones of the axial skeleton, which may demonstrate the classic "onion-skin" appearance due to areas of tumor lysis accompanied by periosteal reaction, but may also demonstrate a spiculated pattern of new bone formation mimicking an osteogenic sarcoma. The cortex is generally breached and there is typically an associated large soft tissue component. Imaging by MRI, CT, technetium bone scan, and increasingly FDG-PET have become standard modalities for evaluation of the primary tumor and staging and assessment of metastatic disease (Fig. 50-4).[30,34,35]

Treatment involves aggressive preoperative chemotherapy to induce rapid resolution of soft tissue masses enabling resection of the primary bone lesion. Extensive residual tumor within bone or in the associated resected soft tissues requires postoperative radiotherapy in addition to chemotherapy.[30]

Patients with localized disease at diagnosis who receive intensive therapy have a 5-year event-free survival of 73%.[30] Cure rates for those with metastatic disease remain low at approximately 25%, with small pulmonary metastases faring better than for those with bony metastases. Cure rates after disease recurrence are poor.

TUMORS OF CARTILAGINOUS ORIGIN

Benign Cartilage Tumors

Cartilaginous tumors contain foci of chondroid matrix. As many of these entities are asymptomatic, an assessment of the true incidence is difficult but osteochondroma is most common followed by enchondroma, chondroblastoma, and chondromyxoid fibroma. Diagnosis is typically based on radiologic features, such the bone involved, the size, and whether solitary or multiple lesions are present.[35]

Osteochondroma

Osteochondromas are cartilage capped bony projections usually of the metaphyseal region of long bones but also the ileum and scapula. There is an equal sex distribution. Approximately 15% of patients have multiple lesions, of which approximately 62% have a positive family history (e.g., multiple hereditary osteochondromatosis).[36] Although usually asymptomatic, significant growth deformity, symptoms of local impingement, and pain may be presenting features, particularly in those with multiple lesions. Assessment using the Child Health Questionnaire has demonstrated differences in pain and self-esteem in affected individuals compared to normative pediatric data indicating that even these benign lesions can have a negative impact on children and adolescents.[37]

The osteochondroma has three components: perichondrium, cartilage cap, and bony stalk (pedunculated or sessile). Of these, only the cartilage cap is neoplastic (Fig. 50-5). In puberty the cartilage cap thins and undergoes calcification. Although rare, malignant transformation to a secondary peripheral chondrosarcoma can occur in 1% of solitary and 5% of multiple lesions for which the suggestive clinical features include a large cartilage cap (>1.5-2 cm), continued growth post-puberty, and the development of pain. These clinical features appear more predictive of malignant change than many histological features.[38,39]

Mutations of the *EXT1* and *EXT2* genes have shown strong linkage with the development of multiple osteochondromas.[40,41] It has been postulated that the development of osteochondromas following irradiation, including total body irradiation prior to bone marrow transplantation for the treatment of childhood leukemia, results from induction of *EXT* mutations.[42]

Treatment by surgical excision is only warranted if the lesions are causing pain or if significant growth disturbances such as valgus deformities at the ankle or knee, develop. As malignant transformation is rare, prophylactic excision is not recommended.[36]

Enchondroma

Enchondromas are benign hyaline cartilage neoplasms of medullary bone generally affecting adolescents with an equal sex ratio. The hands and feet are affected in 50% of cases (Fig. 50-6) but other sites including the femur and humerus may be affected. The majority are solitary but, if multiple, it is diagnosed as Ollier disease or, if in association with soft tissue hemangiomas, Marfucci syndrome. Calcification around the periphery of the lesions (bone encasement) is characteristic. Malignant transformation into a chondrosarcoma is reported in 15% to 30% of multiple lesions prompting need for appropriate surveillance.[43,44]

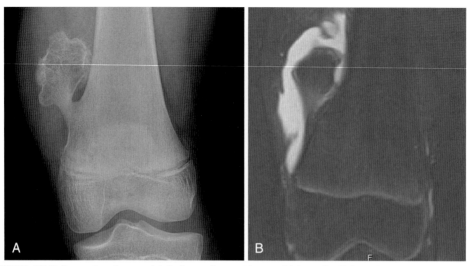

FIGURE 50-5 Osteochondroma of left femur in an 11-year-old boy. **A,** Plain radiograph demonstrates pedunculated lesion. **B,** T2-weighted MRI demonstrates presence of an associated bursa.

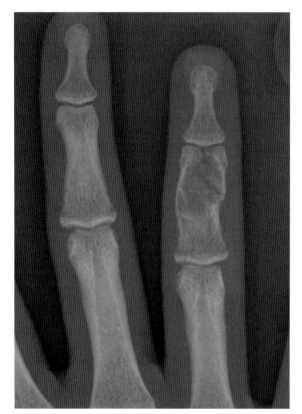

FIGURE 50-6 Enchondroma of middle phalanx in a 15-year-old girl with no involvement of interphalangeal joint.

Chondroblastoma

These rare lesions have a male predilection (2:1) and typically involve the epiphysis of the long bones of prepubertal children, most commonly the humerus, followed by the femur and tibia. Pain is the typical presenting feature and up to one third may involve a secondary aneurysmal bone cyst.[44] On radiograph, the classic appearance is of a well-circumscribed, ovoid lytic lesion with thin sclerotic margins (Fig. 50-7). A variety of genetic rearrangements have been demonstrated but

the relevance to tumor production is unknown. Treatment is by excision and, if relevant, management of the associated bone cyst.

Chondromyxoid Fibroma

These rare tumors have their peak incidence in adolescence with a male predominance. They can be found in any osseous site but the majority occur in the proximal tibia or iliac bone. On plain radiograph they appear as lytic lesions with sclerotic borders. Histology shows abundant myxoid and chondroid matrix. Although differentiation from chondrosarcoma may be necessary, the immunohistochemical appearances are distinct.

Malignant Cartilage Tumors
Chondrosarcoma

Primary chondrosarcoma is primarily a disease of adulthood, however secondary chondrosarcoma due to malignant transformation of benign osteochondromas can develop in multiple hereditary osteochondromatosis or in the syndromes associated with multiple enchondromas. The development of pain, often insidious in nature, is the most consistent feature of malignant transformation. There may be a soft tissue mass and pathological fracture may occur. Radiologic features suggesting chondrosarcoma are endosteal scalloping greater than two thirds of the cortical width on plain radiograph, peritumoral edema, and intense enhancement on T2-weighted MRI and positive uptake on technetium bone scan. Newer modalities such as PET-CT also demonstrate high degrees of sensitivity and specificity.[45]

The preferred treatment is wide surgical excision followed by reconstruction of the affected bone. Most chondrosarcomas are resistant to both chemotherapy and radiotherapy.

TUMORS OF FIBROUS TISSUE

Benign Fibrous Tissue Tumors

Fibrous Cortical Defect (Non Ossifying Fibroma):

These benign fibrous lesions are the most common of all focal bone lesions affecting up to 40% of children between 4 and 8 years. They are generally asymptomatic and resolve spontaneously so that the diagnosis is usually an incidental finding on plain radiograph taken for other reasons. They typically occur near the epiphyseal growth plate at

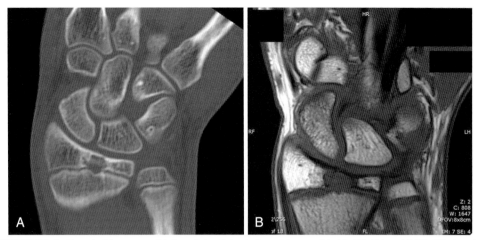

FIGURE 50-7 Chondroblastoma of left radial epiphysis in a 14-year-old girl. CT **(A)** and MRI **(B)** showing lack of any bone edema or inflammatory reaction.

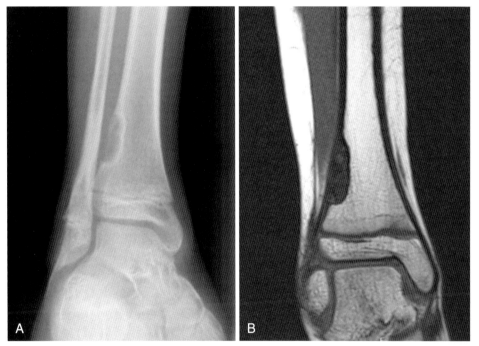

FIGURE 50-8 Fibrous cortical defect in right tibia of an 11-year-old boy. Plain radiograph **(A)** and MRI **(B)**.

sites of tendon or ligament insertions, most commonly at the distal femur or proximal tibia. The characteristic radiographic appearance is of an eccentric, metaphyseal lucency with sclerotic margins (Fig. 50-8). Biopsy is not usually required, and active management is required only for large lesions deemed to be at risk of fracture, in which case curettage and bone grafting may be necessary.[46]

Juvenile Fibromatosis

These uncommon lesions are classified into superficial and deep fibromatoses. They share similar histological appearances but widely divergent growth patterns, genetic changes, and clinical characteristics.[47] The superficial fibromatoses occur predominantly in adults (e.g., Dupuytren contracture); however, superficial plantar fibromatosis does occur during adolescence, with ill-defined thickening in the plantar fascia. Infantile digital fibromas present as discrete nodular lesions over the dorsum of fingers and/or toes in children less than 3 years of age. They can be isolated or multiple and may produce local deformity. Interestingly, spontaneous resolution is not unusual so that decisions regarding timing of potential surgical intervention can be difficult.[48,49]

The deep fibromatoses, also known as aggressive fibromatosis or desmoids tumors, are much rarer, arise from musculoaponeurotic tissues, demonstrate an infiltrative pattern along tissue planes, and may invade adjacent tissues such as bone, but do not have metastatic potential.[50] They occur throughout life but exhibit a relative peak in early childhood and are strongly associated with Gardner syndrome and familial adenomatous polyposis. There is a female predominance.

Lesions typically present as a firm, slow growing and painless swelling attached to underlying soft tissue or bone, with the major sites of

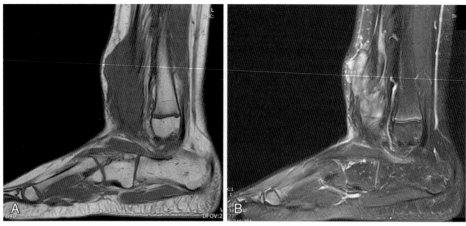

FIGURE 50-9 Juvenile fibromatosis. MRI of an aggressive fibromatosis lesion affecting the right distal tibia. T1-weighted image **(A)** and T2 **(B)** fat-saturated image.

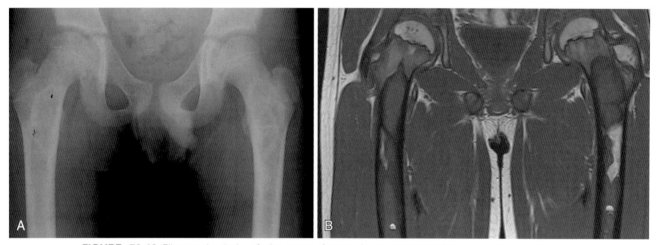

FIGURE 50-10 Fibrous dysplasia of the upper femora in an 11-year-old boy. **A,** Plain radiograph. **B,** T1-weighted MRI image.

involvement being in the head and neck, upper limb, thigh, and trunk (Fig. 50-9).

Biopsy must be undertaken after local tumor staging, most appropriately with MRI. Complete resection with clear histological margins is often not possible to achieve because of the anatomical site and infiltrative behavior of the tumor. Patients with completely resected disease receive no adjuvant therapy. A variety of chemotherapeutic regimens as well as noncytotoxic drug combinations, such as NSAIDs combined with an antiestrogenic agent, predominantly tamoxifen, have shown promise in achieving tumor regression in some children.[51,52] Radiotherapy has a less clear role. Because spontaneous stabilization and regression in tumor extent has been noted to occur, a generally conservative approach is now advocated. Overall survival remains excellent.

Fibrous Dysplasia

Fibrous dysplasia occurs in either a monostotic (75%) or polyostotic (25%) distribution. Common sites include the facial bones and ribs, particularly in the monostotic form, but also the long bones. Initial symptoms are pain, gait disturbance, and growth deformity. On plain radiograph there is a "ground glass" appearance with a lack of trabeculae (Fig. 50-10). Endosteal scalloping may occur but without a periosteal reaction. A classic radiologic feature is the "shepherd's crook" deformity of the femoral head, which may predispose to pathological fracture. Polyostotic forms may be associated with café-au-lait spots and endocrine abnormalities, particularly precocious puberty (McCune–Albright syndrome) or intramuscular myxomas (Mazabraud syndrome).[53,54]

Treatment relies on maintaining maximal bone density by bisphosphonates and parathyroid hormone analogues. Exercise and diet may also play a role. Surgical intervention for bone deformity and pathological fracture with internal fixation and bone grafting may be required. Radiotherapy is no longer used for therapy but has been proposed as an etiologic factor in the rare cases of malignant transformation (1% to 4%).

Malignant Tumors of Fibrous Tissue
Fibrosarcoma

Fibrosarcoma, although rare, is one of the most common soft tissue sarcomas in children and adolescents. There are two age peaks in incidence. More common is the infantile or congenital form, which occurs predominantly in males under 2 years of age, with up to 40% being present at birth. Presentation is usually with a rapidly growing mass in a distal extremity. The tumors are quite vascular so can be confused clinically with hemangiomas,[55] although imaging may demonstrate osseous changes with bowing, cortical thickening, or even bony destruction. On MRI, heterogeneous high-signal T2-weighted changes are important diagnostic features.[56] Histological assessment with immunogenetic analysis is required in differentiating fibrosarcoma from other tumors.[57] Complete surgical excision is curative but often not feasible without significant morbidity. Neoadjuvant chemotherapy may make surgical excision more feasible. Overall prognosis is 90% for 5-year survival, but local relapse requiring retreatment can occur.[58]

Fibrosarcoma in adolescence is more common in males and presents as a mass in the deep soft tissues. Although the histological appearance is similar to that of the infantile form, it lacks the characteristic cytogenetic and molecular abnormalities. Importantly, they behave similar to adult fibrosarcoma being a high-grade sarcoma with a high risk of local recurrences, lymph node and pulmonary metastases, and an overall 5 year-survival of around 55%. Treatment requires a combination of surgery, adjuvant chemotherapy, and radiotherapy.[59]

TUMORS OF MUSCULOSKELETAL SOFT TISSUES

Benign Tumors of Soft Tissues

Pigmented Villonodular Synovitis

Pigmented villonodular synovitis (PVNS) is a locally aggressive synovial proliferative disorder of unknown etiology affecting joints, tendon sheaths, and bursae. When isolated to the tendon sheath it is called a giant cell tumor of the tendon sheath (Fig. 50-11). PVNS can present as a painful, monoarticular effusion predominantly affecting the knee but any joint can be involved. PVNS should be considered, particularly in adolescents, if a joint aspirate suggests hemarthrosis and/or if response to intraarticular corticosteroid injection is poor. Histology demonstrates thickened, reddish-brown synovium due to hemosiderin deposition, with numerous villous projections. Cytogenetic studies have reported monoclonality, leading to the suggestion PVNS is a neoplastic process.[60]

Plain radiographs may be normal, other than nonspecific features of an effusion, or may show erosive disease. MRI demonstrates low signal intensity T1 and T2 sequences within the tissue with evidence of the hemosiderin (Fig. 50-12), which may even exaggerate the true

extent of the synovitis due to the "blooming phenomenon" caused by the magnetic susceptibility effect of the hemosiderin.[61]

Treatment is by local excision, which may require total synovectomy for more extensive involvement. Recurrence is common and consideration of radioactive yttrium synovectomy may be required.[62]

Intraarticular/Periarticular Vascular Anomalies

Vascular anomalies are classified as either vascular tumors, specifically synovial hemangioma, or vascular malformations, which encompass lesions with varying combinations of venous, arterial, and lymphatic components.[63,64]

Synovial hemangiomas usually affect the knee, presenting with recurrent episodes of pain, swelling, and decreased range of movement.[65,66] Marked reduction in adjacent thigh muscle girth may occur. Recurrent episodes of hemarthrosis may result in severe articular cartilage degeneration similar to hemophilic arthropathy. Plain radiographs may be normal, but MRI will usually confirm the diagnosis with low-intensity T1-weighted signal but high T2-weighted images correlating with stagnant blood in vascular spaces.

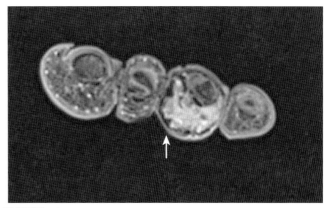

FIGURE 50-11 Giant cell tumor of the left third toe in a 13-year-old boy. T1-weighted MRI contrast study with small hemosiderin deposits within the tendon sheath (*arrow*).

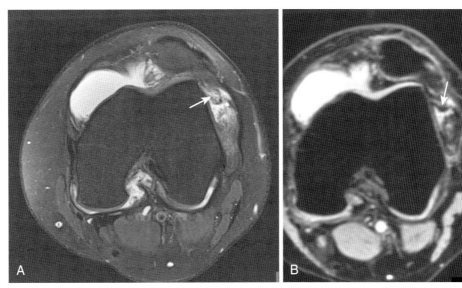

FIGURE 50-12 Pigmented villonodular synovitis in the knee of a 15-year-old girl. **A,** MRI shows synovial thickening (*arrow*) on proton density axial fat-saturation image. **B,** Gradient image demonstrates hemosiderin deposition (*arrow*).

Juxtaarticular vascular malformations can also present with pain and muscle wasting. When associated with cutaneous lesions, they may be part of the Klippel–Trenaunay–Weber syndrome (cutaneous port-wine lesions, varicose veins, and limb hemihypertrophy). If the malformation includes an intraarticular component, hemarthroses can occur. Juxtaarticular low flow lesions may demonstrate phleboliths on plain radiographs, and ultrasound can be useful in diagnosis. A serious complication in both vascular malformations and hemangiomata can be the development of a consumptive coagulopathy with resultant severe thrombocytopenia (Kasabach–Merritt phenomenon).[67]

Treatment depends on the size, location, and predominant aberrant vascular nature of the anomaly. Surgical resection may be curative in localized lesions, but more complex forms of treatment may involve percutaneous embolization (Fig. 50-13) or medical therapy, such as corticosteroids and β-blockers.

Synovial Chondromatosis

Synovial chondromatosis rarely occurs in children. It is usually mono-articular, predominantly involving the knee (50%). The cause is unknown but pathology consists of synovial hyperplasia and the production of small round cartilaginous nodules, which in time undergo ossification. Symptoms and signs are relatively nonspecific with pain, effusions, and mechanical joint symptoms such as locking. Diagnosis is based on imaging findings with plain radiograph being abnormal in 70% of cases demonstrating multiple calcified bodies of uniform size (Fig. 50-14).[68] Periarticular erosions may be present. On MRI the nodules usually are of low signal intensity due to calcification of the nodule. Treatment is by arthroscopic excision, which, unless complete, may allow recurrence. Very rare malignant transformation to a secondary chondrosarcoma is described.

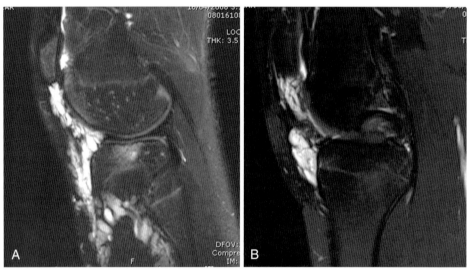

FIGURE 50-13 Vascular (venous) malformation in the left knee of a 17-year-old girl. **A,** Contrast MRI demonstrates extent of vascular anomaly with cartilage loss and an osteochondral defect of the tibial plateau. **B,** Repeat study demonstrates reduction in size after initial sclerotherapy.

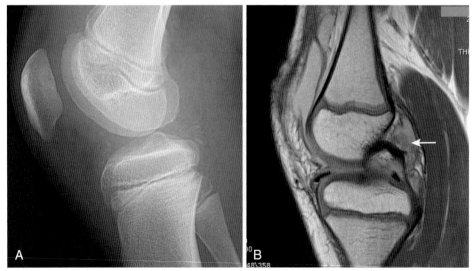

FIGURE 50-14 Synovial chondromatosis in the right knee of an 11-year-old boy. **A,** Plain radiograph demonstrates multiple calcified bodies. **B,** MRI demonstrates multiple lesions with signal characteristics of cartilage (*arrow*) plus large effusion.

Malignant Tumors of Soft Tissue

Rhabdomyosarcoma

Rhabdomyosarcoma is the most common soft tissue sarcoma in children, representing approximately 5% of all childhood malignancies. It is one of the most challenging pediatric tumors to treat because of the complex sites of origin and young age at presentation of many patients.[69,70]

The tumor can arise in striated or smooth muscle at any site, particularly affecting the head and neck and genitourinary tract; 20% occur in the limbs. Histologically, tumors are broadly divided into embryonal (60% to 70%) and alveolar subtypes (25% to 30%). Specific cytogenetic translocations are described, which vary between the subtypes and clinical aspects, including prognosis, of these tumors.[71]

The median age at presentation is 5 years with two thirds of all patients diagnosed being under 10 years of age. Embryonal histology is more common in younger children with predominantly head and neck and genitourinary primaries. Extremity and truncal lesions are less common, affect predominantly adolescents, and are usually of the alveolar subtype. They typically present as a painless mass. There is a high incidence of regional lymph node involvement, which, together with the unfavorable alveolar histology, impacts negatively on prognosis.

Radiologic evaluation of the primary tumor is required prior to any biopsy (Fig. 50-15) to determine the potential for complete primary excision prior to initiation of chemotherapy. Complete pretreatment resection may have considerable impact on treatment intensity, potentially reduce the irradiation dose required, or obviate the need for radiotherapy altogether.

Risk group assignment and therapy is based on the site and extent of the primary tumor, histology and cytogenetics, presence or absence of nodal involvement, degree of resectability, and the presence or absence of metastatic disease.[72] Low risk indicates the tumor is less than 5 cm and completely resected resulting in an overall survival of 90% at 5 years. The majority of limb and truncal tumors fall into the intermediate-risk group, whereas metastatic disease at diagnosis indicates high risk. The reported 3-year survival is 55% to 75% and 30% for the intermediate and high-risk groups, respectively.[71]

Radiotherapy for primary tumor control is used if initial resection is incomplete.

Synovial Sarcoma

Although uncommon in the pediatric age group, synovial sarcoma is the most common nonrhabdomyosarcoma soft tissue sarcoma of childhood. Despite the name, the characteristic epithelial appearance is not consistent with synovium, and tumors are rarely intraarticular.[73] The tumor occurs slightly more frequently in males and is rare under the age of 10 years. Synovial sarcoma can occur anywhere in the body but the most common presenting sign is of a slowly growing painless mass, usually in a lower limb, in periarticular proximity to tendon sheaths and bursae.[74,75] The tumor spreads to regional lymph nodes and metastasizes predominantly to the lungs. Plain radiographs demonstrate calcification in 30% of cases. MRI most accurately differentiates tumor from normal tissue and elucidates evidence of neurovascular and lymph node involvement (Fig. 50-16).[76,77]

Tumor size and resectability correlate strongly with outcome. Complete surgical resection of tumors less than 5 cm leads to a cure rate of up to 90% without adjuvant chemotherapy or irradiation. Larger tumors, those with local extension, lymph node involvement, or metastases (predominantly pulmonary) at diagnosis have a poorer prognosis.[78,79] Radiotherapy may be used as adjunctive therapy for primary tumor control if complete resection is not achieved.

Malignant Diseases Metastasizing to Bone

The pediatric malignancy with the highest incidence of metastases to bone is neuroblastoma. Ewing sarcoma, osteosarcoma, rhabdomyosarcoma, clear cell sarcoma of the kidney, and retinoblastoma also metastasize to bone but at a much lower frequency.

Neuroblastoma

Neuroblastoma is the most common extra cranial solid tumor occurring in children under the age of 5 years, and is metastatic at presentation in approximately two thirds of patients. The tumor derives from

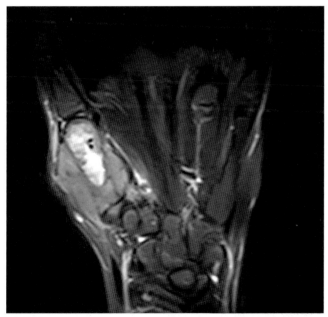

FIGURE 50-15 Rhabdomyosarcoma. MRI of localized tumor mass of the thenar muscles with first metacarpal involvement.

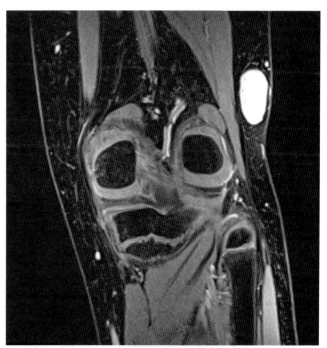

FIGURE 50-16 Synovial sarcoma of the left thigh in a 12-year-old boy demonstrates no direct connection with the adjacent knee joint.

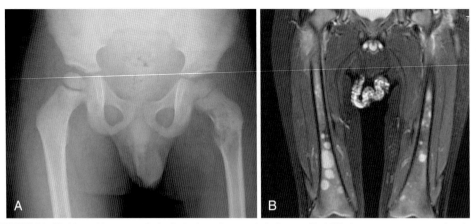

FIGURE 50-17 Neuroblastoma. **A,** Lytic lesion of upper left femur. **B,** MRI demonstrates extensive bone marrow involvement.

the primitive neural crest, arising within tissues of the sympathetic nervous system. Marrow involvement usually accompanies bony metastases, and both are more common in children with abdominal primaries as compared with those with thoracic or cervical primaries (Fig. 50-17). Pulmonary metastases rarely occur in neuroblastoma.[80,81]

Children present most often with weight loss, pallor, and limb and abdominal pain. They are typically miserable, irritable, and often reluctant or unable to walk. Some will have orbital metastases with proptosis and the pathognomonic periorbital bruising ("racoon eyes"). Abdominal ultrasound or CT will usually demonstrate an often large, extrarenal mass.

The majority of neuroblastomas are metabolically active and adrenergic metabolites, such as homovanillic acid, dopamine, adrenaline, and noradrenaline are usually elevated in the urine. Tumor metabolic activity, as measured by a metaiodobenzylguanidine (MIBG) scan, enables more accurate initial staging and also serial assessment of the response to chemotherapy.[82]

Bone marrow aspirate will frequently confirm the diagnosis, but a primary tumor sample allows better definition of important biological factors that impact prognosis. Serum ferritin is frequently elevated. Initial treatment involves intensive myelosuppressive chemotherapy. For patients achieving at least a good partial response, resection of the primary tumor is undertaken where feasible, followed by radiotherapy to the tumor bed. Myeloablative chemotherapy with autologous peripheral blood stem cell support is usually given as consolidation therapy.[82] Current trials are achieving overall survival of around 80% at 2 years in patients for whom, until relatively recently, the prognosis was dismal.[83,84] Unfortunately, late recurrences continue to occur.

Hypertrophic Pulmonary Osteoarthropathy

Secondary hypertrophic osteoarthropathy (HPOA) is a rare musculoskeletal complication of malignancy in children.[85] This condition is more common in cyanotic congenital heart disease or in chronic suppurative lung disease. Clubbing and joint swelling occurs with painful long bones, which on imaging demonstrate extensive periosteal reaction. In the largest reported series of HPOA complicating childhood malignancy carcinoma of the nasopharynx, osteosarcoma, and Hodgkin's lymphoma were the predominant causes.[86,87] A minority had no radiologic evidence of pulmonary disease when the HPOA was diagnosed. Treatment for secondary HPOA involves treatment of the primary malignancy, which may include metastasectomy of pulmonary lesions and symptomatic treatment with bisphosphonates and NSAIDs.[88,89]

BENIGN TUMORS OF MISCELLANEOUS ORIGIN

Unicameral Bone Cysts

These lesions of unknown etiology usually present in later childhood, typically occurring in the metaphysis of the proximal humerus or femur. Presentation is usually due to pain or pathological fracture, but the lesion may be an incidental radiologic finding. They are well-defined, expansile lesions, but with minimal sclerosis on plain radiograph. The cysts contain yellowish tissue fluid and are lined by a fibrous capsule. Although cystic, there are often irregular internal septa. Management is by corticosteroid injection, curettage with bone grafting and/or intramedullary rod fixation determined by the size, site, and likelihood of fracture. Recurrence is relatively common, necessitating retreatment.

Aneurysmal Bone Cysts

These lesions are more common in adolescent girls. Presenting symptoms are pain and swelling. Plain radiograph demonstrates an expansile lesion, the aggressiveness of which is suggested by the presence or lack of distinct margins. Although more commonly found in the long bones, involvement of spine/pelvis accounts for 10 to 30% of cases. MRI may demonstrate fluid levels within the cysts (Fig. 50-18). Management may require surgical excision, saucerization and/or curettage with grafting. Nonsurgical approaches for pelvic lesions include selective embolization and bisphosphonate therapy.[90] Recurrence occurs in up to 60% of cases, particularly in children under 10 years of age.

Giant Cell Tumors

These are painful tumors, which occur mainly in adolescent females. They are typically metaphyseal or epiphyseal in location with an eccentric expansile lytic appearance on radiograph with no associated sclerosis or periosteal reaction. Treatment requires curettage and grafting or thermoablation. Although benign, they can be quite aggressive demonstrating local invasion and/or recurrence in up to 25% of cases.

Langerhans Cell Histiocytosis

Langerhans cell histiocytosis (LCH) varies in its clinical presentation throughout childhood. LCH is staged into single system and multisystem disease, encompassing the previously named eosinophilic granuloma, Hand–Schüller–Christian disease, and Letterer–Siwe disease.[91,92] Single system bony lesions occur mainly in children below 10 years of age, with a peak incidence from 3 to 5 years. Posterior pituitary involvement with resultant diabetes insipidus and potential growth hormone

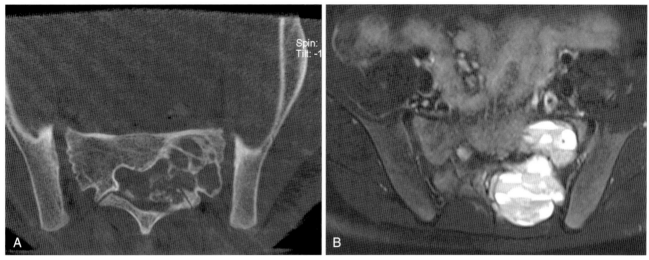

FIGURE 50-18 Aneurysmal bone cyst involving the left sacral alar in a 15-year-old girl. **A,** CT shows lytic cystic lesion. **B,** T2 MRI study demonstrating fluid levels within cysts.

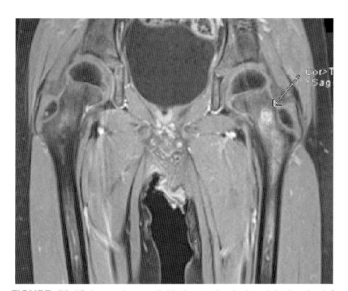

FIGURE 50-19 Langerhan cell histiocytosis. Isolated lesion in left femoral neck in an 8-year-old boy (*arrow*).

resolution of soft tissue masses, but bony healing may occur slowly and in some instances residual lytic areas remain. Large lesions, particularly in weight-bearing bones and lesions potentially compromising function, are treated with systemic corticosteroids and/or chemotherapy for 6 to 12 months. Lesions presenting a fracture risk or risk of spinal instability may require immobilization during the healing phase. Although new lesions, which may require retreatment, develop in up to 30% of children, the prognosis for LCH remains excellent.

SUMMARY

In pediatric rheumatology clinics a wide variety of potential diagnoses and pathological processes warrant consideration for what might appear to be a relatively limited number of symptoms and/or signs (e.g., joint pain, joint effusion, gait disturbance). Neoplastic disorders, both malignant and benign, must be considered when the clinician approaches any child with such features. The ability to treat children with the spectrum of malignancies that have musculoskeletal aspects now falls in to the realm of allowing a realistic expectation of cure in what previously were invariably fatal conditions.

deficiency may accompany bony lesions of the base of the skull in young children. The disorder is postulated to be one of immune dysregulation rather than a true malignancy. While clonal changes have been reported, lesions do not metastasize; some will undergo spontaneous resolution and, despite recurrences, lesions remain sensitive to therapy. The prognosis is generally excellent for patients without systemic involvement.

The most common site of involvement is the skull, but any long bone or vertebrae may be involved (Fig. 50-19). Lesions in weight-bearing bones or in the spine usually present with pain in the involved area, including signs of nerve root or cord compression with spinal lesions.

Radiographs classically demonstrate well-defined lytic areas, but some may show periosteal reaction. Involvement of individual vertebrae may cause collapse of the vertebral body producing vertebra plana on plain radiograph. Initial diagnostic biopsy should be undertaken, but resection of the whole lesion is not required. Simple curettage or injection of intralesional corticosteroids frequently results in rapid

REFERENCES

2. O.Y. Jones, C.H. Spencer, S.L. Bowyer, et al., A multicenter case-control study on predictive factors distinguishing childhood leukemia from juvenile rheumatoid arthritis, Pediatrics 117 (2006) e840–e844.

4. R.K. Marwaha, K.P. Kulkarni, D. Bansal, et al., Acute lymphoblastic leukemia masquerading as juvenile rheumatoid arthritis: diagnostic pitfall and association with survival, Ann. Hematol. 89 (2010) 249–254.

5. D. McKay, L. Adams, G. Ostring, et al., In a child presenting with features consistent with a diagnosis of juvenile idiopathic arthritis, what clinical features or laboratory findings (at presentation) predict a diagnosis of acute lymphoblastic leukaemia? J. Paed. Child Health. 10 (2010) 442–445.

6. L. Zomboni, G. Kovacs, M. Csoka, et al., Rheumatic symptoms in childhood leukaemia and lymphoma—a ten year retrospective study, Pediatr. Rheumatol. Online J. 11 (2013) 20.

7. K.R. Schultz, J. Pullen, H.N. Sather, et al., Risk and response based classification of childhood B-precursor acute lymphoblastic leukemia: a combined analysis of prognostic markers from the Pediatric Oncology Group (POG) and Children's Cancer Group (CCG), Blood 109 (2007) 926–935.

9. P.J. Hashkes, B.M. Wright, M.S. Lauer, et al., Survival rates of children with acute lymphoblastic leukemia presenting to a pediatric rheumatologist in the United States, J. Pediatr. Hematol. Oncol. 33 (2011) 424–428.

12. E.H. Lee, M. Shafi, J.H. Hui, Osteoid osteoma: a current review, J. Ped. Orthop. 26 (2006) 695–700.

14. G. Ciabattoni, F. Tamburrelli, F. Greco, Increased prostacyclin biosynthesis in patients with osteoid osteoma, Eicosanoids 4 (1991) 165–167.

15. D. Neumann, H. Berka, U. Dorn, et al., Follow-up of thirty-three computed-tomography guided percutaneous radiofrequency thermoablations of osteoid osteoma, Int. Orthop. 36 (2012) 811–815.

17. T. Goto, Y. Shinoda, T. Okuma, et al., Administration of nonsteroidal anti-inflammatory drugs accelerates spontaneous healing of osteoid osteoma, Arch. Orthop. Trauma Surg. 131 (2011) 619–625.

18. I. Ilyas, D.A. Younge, Medical management of osteoid osteoma, Can. J. Surg. 45 (2002) 435–437.

19. M. Horner, L.A.G. Ries, M. Krapcho, et al., SEER Cancer Statistics Review, National Cancer Institute, Bethesda, MD, 2009, pp. 1975–2006.

20. S.J. Cotterill, C.M. Wright, M.S. Pearce, et al., Stature of young people with malignant bone tumors, Pediatr. Blood Cancer 42 (2004) 59–63.

23. P. Picci, Osteosarcoma (Osteogenic sarcoma), Orphanet J. Rare Dis. 2 (2007) 1–4.

24. H.T. Ta, C.R. Dass, P.F.M. Choong, et al., Osteosarcoma treatment: state of the art, Cancer Metastasis Rev. 28 (2009) 247–263.

25. H.J. Kim, P.N. Chalmers, C.D. Morris, Pediatric osteogenic sarcoma, Curr. Opin. Pediatr. 22 (2010) 61–66.

26. R. Abed, R.J. Grimer, Surgical modalities in the treatment of bone sarcoma in childen, Cancer Treat. Rev. 36 (2010) 342–347.

28. A. Longhi, C. Errani, M. De Paolis, et al., Primary bone osteosarcoma in the pediatric age: state of the art, Cancer Treat. Rev. 32 (2006) 423–436.

30. J. Potratz, U. Dirksen, H. Jürgens, et al., Ewing Sarcoma: clinical state of the art, Pediatr. Hematol. Oncol. 29 (2012) 1–11.

31. J. Potratz, H. Jurgens, A. Craft, et al., Ewing Sarcoma: biology based therapeutic perspectives, Pediatr. Hematol. Oncol. 29 (2012) 12–27.

33. R. Gorlick, K. Janeway, S. Lessnick, et al., Children's Oncology Group's 2013 blueprint for research: bone tumors, Pediatr. Blood Cancer 60 (2013) 1009–1015.

34. J.M. Bestic, J.J. Peterson, L.W. Bancroft, Use of FDG PET in staging, restaging and assessment of therapy response in Ewing Sarcoma, Radiographics 29 (2009) 1487–1501.

35. S.L. Miller, F.A. Hoffer, Malignant and benign bone tumors, Radiol. Clin. North Am. 39 (2001) 673–699.

36. J.V.M.G. Bovee, Multiple osteochondromas, Orphanet J. Rare Dis. 3 (2008) 3.

37. H. Chhina, J.C. Davis, C.M. Alvarez, Health related quality of life in people with hereditary multiple exostoses, J. Pediatr. Orthop. 32 (2012) 210–214.

38. C.E. De Andrea, H.M. Kroon, R. Wolterbeek, et al., Interobserver reliability in the histopathological diagnosis of cartilaginous tumors in patients with multiple osteochondromas, Mod. Path. 25 (2012) 1275–1283.

40. G. Duncan, C. McCormick, F. Tufaro, The link between heparin sulphate and hereditary bone disease: finding a function for the EXT family of putative tumor suppressor proteins, J. Clin. Invest. 108 (2001) 511–516.

43. D.R. Lucas, J.A. Bridge, Chondromas: enchondroma, periosteal chondroma and enchondromatosis, in: C.D.M. Fletcher, K.K. Unni, F. Mertens (Eds.), World Health Organization Classification of Tumours, *Pathology and Genetics of Tumours of Soft Tissue and Bone*, IARC Press, Lyon, 2002, pp. 237–240.

44. S. Romeo, P.C.W. Hogendoorn, A.P. Dei Tos, Benign cartilaginous tumors of bone: from morphology to somatic and Germ-line genetics, Adv. Anat. Pathol. 16 (2009) 307–315.

45. S.M. Mosier, T. Patel, K. Strenge, et al., Chondrosarcoma in childhood: the radiologic and clinical conundrum, J. Radiol. Case Rep. 6 (2012) 32–42.

46. J.S. Biermann, Common benign lesions of bone in children and adolescents, J. Pediatr. Orthop. 22 (2002) 268–273.

49. M.S. Ruparelia, D.K. Dhariwal, Infantile fibromatosis: a case report and review of the literature, Br. J. Oral Maxillofac. Surg. 49 (2011) e30–e32.

50. C. Maezza, G. Bisogno, A. Gronchi, et al., Aggressive fibromatosis in children and adolescents, Cancer 116 (2010) 233–240.

51. H. Lackner, C. Urban, R. Kerbl, et al., Noncytotoxic drug therapy in children with unresectable desmoid tumors, Cancer 80 (1997) 334–340.

52. J. Janinis, M. Patriki, L. Vini, et al., The pharmacological treatment of aggressive fibromatosis: a systemic review, Ann. Oncol. 14 (2003) 181–190.

55. K. Kerl, M. Nowacki, I. Leuschner, et al., Infantile fibrosarcoma—an important differential diagnosis of congenital vascular tumors, Pediatr. Hematol. Oncol. 29 (2012) 545–548.

56. E.A. Abdel-Gawad, H. Bonatti, P.T. Norton, et al., Infantile fibrosarcoma: surgical treatment and MRI/MRA findings, Eur. J. Pediatr. Surg. 20 (2010) 276–278.

58. D. Orbach, A. Rey, G. Cecchetto, et al., Infantile fibrosarcoma: management based on the European experience, J. Clin. Oncol. 28 (2010) 318–323.

59. A. Bahrami, A.L. Folpe, Adult-type fibrosarcoma: a re-evaluation of 163 putative cases diagnosed at a single institution over a 48-year period, Am. J. Surg. Pathol. 34 (2010) 1504–1513.

61. N.A. Al-Nakshabandi, A.G. Ryan, H. Choudur, et al., Pigmented villonodular synovitis, Clin. Radiol. 59 (2004) 414–420.

62. H. Sharma, M.J. Jane, R. Reid, Pigmented villonodular synovitis: diagnostic pitfalls and management strategy, Curr. Orthop. 19 (2005) 215–222.

63. J.T. Huang, M.G. Liang, Vascular malformations, Pediatr. Clin. North Am. 57 (2010) 1091–1110.

67. L.H. Lowe, T.C. Marchant, D.C. Rivard, et al., Vascular malformations: classification and terminology the radiologist needs to know, Semin. Roentgenol. 47 (2012) 106–117.

68. G. McKenzie, N. Raby, D. Ritchie, A pictorial review of primary synovial osteochondromatosis, Eur. Radiol. 18 (2008) 2662–2669.

70. R. Dasgupta, D.A. Rodeberg, Update on Rhabdomyosarcoma, Semin. Pediatr. Surg. 21 (2012) 68–78.

71. A. Hayes-Jordan, R. Andrassy, Rhabdomyosarcoma in children, Curr. Opin. Pediatr. 21 (2009) 373–378.

74. R.L. Randall, K.S. Schabel, Y. Hitchcock, et al., Diagnosis and management of synovial sarcoma, Curr. Treat. Options Oncol. 6 (2005) 449–459.

75. B. Brennan, M. Stevens, A. Kelsey, et al., Synovial sarcoma in childhood and adolescence: a retrospective series of 77 patients registered by the Children's Cancer and Leukaemia Group between 1991 and 2006, Pediatr. Blood Cancer 55 (2010) 85–90.

78. A. Ferrari, G.L. De Salvo, O. Oberlin, et al., Synovial sarcoma in children and adolescents: a critical reappraisal of staging investigations in relation to the rate of metastatic involvement at diagnosis, Eur. J. Cancer 48 (2012) 1370–1375.

80. T. Ara, Y.A. DeClerck, Mechanisms of invasion and metastasis in human neuroblastoma, Cancer Metastasis Rev. 25 (2006) 645–657.

82. K.A. Cole, J.M. Maris, New Strategies in refractory and recurrent neuroblastoma: translational opportunities to impact patient outcome, Clin. Cancer Res. 18 (2012) 2423–2428.

86. E.G. Utine, B. Yalcin, I. Karnak, et al., Childhood intrathoracic Hodgkin lymphoma with hypertrophic pulmonary osteoarthropathy: a case report and review of the literature, Eur. J. Pediatr. 167 (2008) 419–423.

89. S. Nguyen, M. Hojjati, Review of current therapies for secondary hypertrophic pulmonary osteoarthropathy, Clin. Rheumatol. 30 (2011) 7–13.

90. P.J. Simm, M. O'Sullivan, M.R. Zacharin, Successful treatment of a sacral aneurysmal bone cyst with zoledronic acid, J. Pediatr. Orthop. 33 (2013) e61–e64.

91. K. Windebank, V. Nanduri, Langerhans cell histiocytosis, Arch. Dis. Child. 94 (2009) 904–908.

92. O. Abla, R.M. Egeler, S. Weitzman, Langerhans cell histiocytosis, Cancer Treat. Rev. 36 (2010) 354–359.

Entire reference list is available online at www.expertconsult.com.

CHAPTER 51

Noninflammatory Musculoskeletal Pain

Claire LeBlanc, Kristin Houghton

Musculoskeletal pain of noninflammatory origin is common in childhood and is a frequent cause of referral to pediatric rheumatologists, orthopedic surgeons, sports medicine specialists, and primary care physicians. Noninflammatory causes of pain are more common than inflammatory ones, and early identification and differentiation from other causes of musculoskeletal pain, such as infection or malignancy, are essential to institution of appropriate therapy and avoidance of inappropriate investigations. Children and adolescents with inflammatory arthritis may develop mechanical pain secondary to muscle tendon imbalances exaggerated by anatomical alignment, neuromuscular or proprioceptive deficits, rapid growth, or change in activity level.

PAIN ASSOCIATED WITH HYPERMOBILITY

Generalized Hypermobility

The term *joint hypermobility syndrome* (JHS) was first described in 1967 as musculoskeletal symptoms associated with generalized hypermobility without any associated congenital syndrome or connective tissue abnormality.[1] The criteria for hypermobility have evolved over the years, and currently most authors use either the nine-point Beighton scale or the modified criteria of Carter and Wilkinson (Box 51-1).[2,3] Prevalence estimates vary from 7% to 36% depending on tests and criteria cutoff points.[4] Hypermobility is more common in girls and decreases with age.[5] Asian and African children are more hypermobile than Caucasians.[5] A family history of hypermobility is common.

Some children with generalized joint hypermobility develop pain.[4] Hypermobile adolescents from the United Kingdom were shown in a prospective study to have a higher risk of chronic widespread pain and a 2-fold greater risk of localized pain in specific joints (e.g., shoulder, knee, ankle/foot) but not the lower back.[6] A significantly higher odds ratio of knee pain was seen in obese youth.[6] Children with benign hypermobility may also have fibromyalgia.[7] The cause of pain in hypermobile children is not known but may be related to joint instability, impaired proprioception and related microtrauma, or a central sensitization and disturbance in the autonomic nervous system.[8,9] Premature osteoarthritis has been suggested to be a result of hypermobility, but longitudinal studies have not confirmed an association.[4,10]

Other musculoskeletal conditions reported to be associated with hypermobility include temporomandibular joint dysfunction with disc

displacement, patellofemoral pain syndrome (PFP), and frequent ankle sprains.[11-13] Reduced muscle strength, balance, and head and trunk stability are more prevalent in hypermobile children, suggesting delayed locomotor development.[4,14] Children with developmental coordination disorder (motor coordination below expected for chronological age and intelligence) are also frequently hypermobile.[15]

The revised Beighton criteria for benign joint hypermobility syndrome (BJHS) in Box 51-2 incorporate the Beighton score plus musculoskeletal and extraskeletal symptoms.[16] These criteria suggest that BJHS is a multisystem disorder, which includes symptoms of chronic pain, autonomic dysfunction (orthostatic intolerance, poor concentration, fatigue), and gastrointestinal dysmotility.[9] While these associations are reported, there is no universal agreement on the causal relationship with BJHS.[4]

It is important that heritable disorders of connective tissue (HDCT) are considered in patients presenting with hypermobility. Several such syndromes are listed in Box 51-3; in most, characteristic phenotypes suggest an underlying HDCT, but conditions such as Ehlers Danlos III (hypermobility syndrome), Stickler and Marfan syndromes can be overlooked if they are not specifically considered. The latter should be evaluated using the revised Ghent criteria.[17]

Treatment

Reassurance is the initial treatment of hypermobility. Although hypermobility may enable a child to be a good gymnast or ballet dancer, injuries may be more frequent.[18] Supportive footwear is helpful for many. Some children benefit from a post-activity or evening dose of acetaminophen or a nonsteroidal antiinflammatory drug (NSAID). Older, more severely affected children may be helped by formal physical therapy that focuses on reestablishment of normal muscle power and overall reconditioning.[4,9] Taping or bracing of troublesome joints and the use of orthotics may be advantageous.[19] Those with more widespread pain may benefit from cognitive behavioral techniques.[9] Children who "crack their knuckles" are frequently hypermobile. Parents are often concerned that this activity might lead to joint damage, but it is probably not a cause of later osteoarthritis.[20]

Pes Planus

The flexible flat foot is common in infants; development of an arch with age is part of normal growth.[21] It is defined by a normal arch when

Children with flexible flat feet are often asymptomatic, but affected preschoolers seen in follow-up at 16 years of age had occasional pains in the neck back knee, leg, or foot.[24] Anterior knee pain was more common in 17-year-old military recruits with flexible flat feet.[25] The Framingham foot study found that men with pes planus had more arch pain and those with pronated feet had more generalized foot and heel pain.[26] Interestingly, pes planus does not appear to be associated with significant lower extremity injuries in young adult athletes or impair athletic performance in children and youth.[27,28]

Most children do not require treatment unless they develop symptoms or do not acquire an arch by 9 years of age.[22] Those who are symptomatic may benefit from supportive footwear as well as stretching and strengthening exercises. Corrective orthotics may improve symptoms or have no impact.[24,29] Surgery to lengthen the heel cord is indicated only in the extreme cases in skeletally mature adolescents.[30]

In contrast to the mobile flat foot, a rigid flat foot is always pathological. This is defined by reduced range of motion of the tarsal and subtalar joints and a longitudinal arch that does not increase with standing on the toes. It may result from a tarsal coalition in which a fibrous or bony connection between two or more tarsal bones is present at birth (Fig. 51-2). It occurs in 1% of the population, affects boys twice as often as girls, and is bilateral in up to 80% of patients.[31] There is often a family history of this condition. Ninety percent of cases are calcaneonavicular and talocalcaneal coalitions. Symptom onset usually occurs at the time of ossification: 8 to 12 years of age for calcaneonavicular and 12 to 16 years of age for talocalcaneal coalitions.[31] Children may report ankle pain that is aggravated by activity or frequent "ankle sprains." On examination, valgus rearfoot and equinus ankle deformities are noted along with restricted and possibly painful subtalar range of motion. The peroneal muscles may spasm from adaptive shortening in response to heel valgus. Radiographs (oblique and axial views) may show calcaneonavicular coalitions, but computerized tomography (CT) or magnetic resonance imaging (MRI) is needed for fibrous or cartilaginous union and other tarsal coalitions (see Fig.

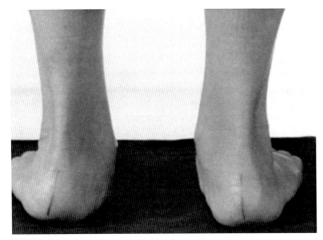

FIGURE 51-1 Pes Planus with hindfoot valgus.

toe standing or lying down and flattening on weight bearing. The reported prevalence is higher in young children (up to 60% of 2 to 6 year olds) but reduces to less than 19% by 8 to 13 years of age.[22] Other factors associated with flatfoot include male gender, family history, generalized ligamentous laxity, shoe wearing before 6 years of age, obesity and developmental coordination disorder.[22,23] A patient with flat feet and hindfoot valgus is shown in Fig. 51-1.

BOX 51-3 Selected Conditions Associated With Hypermobility

Marfan Syndrome
- Tall and thin
- Arm span greater than height
- Lower ratio of upper-body segment to lower-body segment (long legs); normal ratio is 0.85 in whites and 0.92 in blacks
- Arachnodactyly
- Pectus excavatum or carinatum
- Kyphoscoliosis
- Dislocation of the lens of the eye
- Aortic root dilatation
- Heart murmurs, midsystolic click
- Hernias
- Autosomal dominant disorder due to mutations of fibrillin gene on chromosome 15

Homocystinuria
- Marfanoid habitus
- Major risk of thrombotic events
- Autosomal recessive disorder usually associated with cystathionine β-synthase deficiency due to mutations of gene on long arm of chromosome 21

Stickler Syndrome
- Marfanoid habitus
- Typical facial appearance: malar hypoplasia, depressed nasal bridge, epicanthal folds, micrognathia
- Cleft palate (Pierre Robin sequence)
- Severe myopia (may lead to retinal detachment)
- Sensorineural hearing loss
- Mitral valve prolapse
- Autosomal dominant disorder due to mutations of type II collagen gene on chromosome 12

Ehlers-Danlos Syndromes
- Skin abnormalities: thin, hyperelastic, cigarette paper scars, easy bruising
- Dislocation of joints
- Rarely, artery aneurysms; hollow organ rupture
- Heterogeneous conditions; at least nine types with different inheritance patterns

Osteogenesis Imperfecta
- Blue sclerae
- Fragile bones with multiple fractures and deformities
- Short stature
- Spinal deformity
- Different types; usually autosomal dominant inheritance
- Involves abnormalities of type I collagen

Williams Syndrome
- Short stature
- Characteristic elfin facial appearance
- Hoarse voice
- Friendly and loquacious
- Developmental delay
- Supravalvular stenosis
- Occasionally hypercalcemia
- Initially hypermobile but later become hypomobile without pain
- Sporadic and inherited cases due to deletion of elastin allele on chromosome 7

Down Syndrome (Trisomy 21)
- Hypotonia
- Developmental delay
- Characteristic facial appearance; epicanthal folds
- Short stature
- Endocardial cushion defects
- Broad hands with simian creases
- Brushfield (depigmented) spots of the iris
- Usually occurs in a sporadic fashion

For further details about these conditions, the reader is referred to K.L. Jones, Smith's recognizable patterns of human malformation, fifth ed., Saunders, Philadelphia, 1997; and P. Beighton, McKusick's heritable disorders of connective tissue, fifth ed., Mosby, St. Louis, 1993.

51-2).[32] Children with symptomatic coalitions require orthopedic assessment for casting and/or orthoses, physiotherapy, and possible surgical excision of the bony bar.[31]

Genu Recurvatum

Genu recurvatum, like pes planus, may be part of a generalized hypermobility syndrome or may occur as an isolated phenomenon. Symptoms are worse with standing or walking and are relieved by rest. Athletes may have particular difficulty.[33] Symptomatic genu recurvatum occurs most commonly in adolescent girls and is associated with popliteal pain and an increased incidence of anterior cruciate ligament injury.[33-35] Obese children are also more likely to be affected and suffer lower extremity pain.[36] Treatment includes orthotic correction of biomechanical faults, improving knee proprioception, muscle control (especially quadriceps strength) and gait, and maintaining good knee alignment during functional activities.[34,35]

PAIN ASSOCIATED WITH HYPOMOBILITY

Symptomatic generalized hypomobility (JHypoS) is an entity in which decreased ranges of joint motion and pain in periarticular tissue are probably caused by an increased stiffness in joint ligaments.[37] Physical activity-induced lower extremity pain and habitual toe walking are typically associated with JHypoS, and boys appear to be more frequently affected. Reduced exercise tolerance is associated, which is likely related to a pain-related deconditioned state.[38] Although familial hypomobility has been described, prevalence data are not yet available. This condition may be caused by changes in collagen metabolism, perhaps because of greater hydroxylation of lysine residues in collagen telopeptides due to an upregulation of telopeptide lysyl hydroxylase.[37] There are other relatively uncommon disorders, including hyalinosis and familial fibrosing serositis,[39,40] in which pain may relate to very stiff joints (Box 51-4). Most children with marked stiffness/contractures

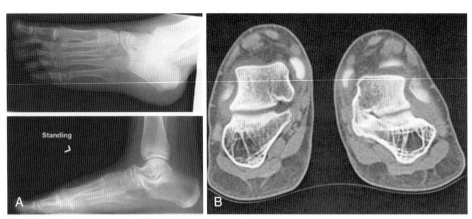

FIGURE 51-2 A, Standing lateral images of the left foot together with oblique images in this 10-year-old patient with left flat foot clinically. Alignment of midfoot and hindfoot looks normal. There is, however, evidence of calcaneal-navicular coalition with both talar and calcaneal beaking. **B,** Computed tomography illustrates the bony bridge between the calcaneus and talus on the right side. The left hindfoot is normal. This feature may not be detectable on plain radiographs. (Courtesy Dr. R. Cairns.)

BOX 51-4   Selected Conditions Associated With Hypomobility and Joint Contractures

Diabetes mellitus (diabetic cheiroarthropathy)
- Tightening of skin and soft tissues of fingers
- Short stature

Scleroderma and scleroderma-like conditions

Mucopolysaccharidoses and mucolipidoses with dysostosis multiplex
- Autosomal recessive inheritance (except in Hunter syndrome, which is X-linked)

Hyalinosis

Familial fibrosing serositis
- Progressive contractures of fingers and toes
- Fibrosing pleuritis and constrictive pericarditis
- Probably autosomal recessive inheritance

Camptodactyly syndromes (several familial conditions including Blau syndrome)
- Flexion contractures of fingers

Beals contractural arachnodactyly syndrome
- Marfanoid features
- Crumpled ears
- Cardiac abnormalities unusual
- Linked to fibrillin-l-like gene on chromosome 5 (autosomal dominant inheritance)

Winchester syndrome
- Multicentric osteolysis particularly of fingers, starting in infancy
- Autosomal recessive inheritance

For further details about the inherited conditions listed here, the reader is referred to K.L. Jones, Smith's recognizable patterns of human malformation, fifth ed., Saunders, Philadelphia, 1997; and P. Beighton, McKusick's heritable disorders of connective tissue, fifth ed., Mosby, St. Louis, 1993.

TABLE 51-1   Patellofemoral Pain Syndromes

Age At Onset	Adolescence to young adulthood
Sex Ratio	Girls > boys
Symptoms	Insidious onset of activity related knee pain, difficulty descending stairs and squatting, need to sit with legs straight ("theatre sign")
Signs	Vastus medialis atrophy, patellar facet tenderness, positive quadriceps setting/grind and patellar compression tests, lateral tracking of patella. Weakness of the quadriceps, hip external rotators and abductors, and trunk muscles.

COMMON OVERUSE INJURIES

Lower Extremity

Patellofemoral Pain Syndrome

Patellofemoral pain (PFP) is one of the most common knee conditions among children, with a prevalence of approximately 7%.[42] PFP affects active and inactive children, is more common in girls, and is most common during the adolescent growth spurt (Table 51-1). Symptoms usually affect both knees with one side more affected. The etiology of PFP is unknown and believed to be due to biomechanical factors, malalignment of the patella relative to the femoral trochlea, and excessive mechanical loading.[43,44] The most common presenting complaint is dull, achy peripatellar or retropatellar pain and stiffness during and after activity, and after prolonged sitting with the knee in flexion ("theatre sign"). Pain is worse with weight-bearing sport, stair use, and squatting. True instability does not occur, but patients often report "giving way" due to pain-related reflex inhibition of the quadriceps muscle or deconditioning. On examination, children may have lower extremity malalignment (genu valgum, varum, or recurvatum, leg length discrepancy, femoral anteversion, external tibial torsion, laterally displaced tibial tubercle, pronated subtalar joint), vastus medialis wasting, increased Q-angle (angle formed between the line joining anterior superior iliac spine and center of the patella and the patella and tibial tuberosity), patellar facet tenderness, tightness (hamstrings,

due to conditions such as arthrogryposis, Williams syndrome, and cerebral palsy, do not seem to have arthralgias, so careful evaluation for other explanations for pain needs to be undertaken. Treatment of these conditions requires an effective stretching exercise program to allow plastic deformation of collagen tissue.[41]

BOX 51-5 Safe Return-to-Play Guidelines

Pain free

No swelling

Full range of motion (compare the injured part with the uninjured opposite side)

Full or close to full (90%) strength (compare with the uninjured side)

For lower body injuries—able to perform full weight bearing without limping

For upper body injuries—able to perform athletic movements (throwing, swimming, etc.) with proper form and no pain

Always start with aerobic exercise, followed by functional and sport specific skills (jumping, pivoting, etc.), and practice before competitive play.

quadriceps, iliotibial band, gastrocnemius), and weakness (quadriceps, hip external rotators, abductors, trunk muscles) of the lower extremity muscles. A painful quadriceps setting/grind test (suprapatellar resistance while the patient performs isometric quadriceps contraction with knee in full extension), and patellar compression test (direct compression of the patella into the trochlea) aid diagnosis.[45]

The aim of treatment is to correct unbalanced tracking of the patella. Longer pain duration before initiation of treatment is associated with poorer long-term prognosis.[46] Treatment includes activity modification, cryotherapy, short-term NSAID therapy, and physiotherapy. Physiotherapy focuses on patellar tracking exercises, flexibility, and strengthening around the hip and knee.[47] Patellofemoral orthoses, patellar taping, and shoe orthoses (to improve alignment and patellar tracking) may reduce symptoms but have no benefit unless combined with exercise therapy.[48-50] Box 51-5 shows guidelines for safe return to sport.

Patellofemoral Instability

Patellofemoral instability is more common in children with hypermobility and anatomic variants (ligamentous laxity, patella alta, trochlear dysplasia, external tibial torsion, genu valgum). Children complain of anterior knee pain, episodic giving way and locking, and recurrent swelling. On examination, findings are similar to PFP and the patellar apprehension test (contraction of the quadriceps muscle when the examiner attempts to displace the patella laterally), or frank lateral dislocation may be elicited. Radiographs are recommended to rule out osteochondral fracture associated with patellar dislocation. Treatment is the same as for PFP. Patellofemoral orthoses (stabilization braces) may prevent recurrent episodes of instability. Orthopedic referral is recommended for acute patellar dislocation and recurrent instability. A Cochrane review failed to find evidence to support surgical management over conservative management for acute patellar dislocation.[51] A systematic review found better outcomes for surgical stabilization in patients with recurrent instability.[52]

Synovial Plica

The knee has normal synovial folds that are residual embryonic remnants persisting from when the knee cavity was a septated structure.[52] Plicas around the knee are common and generally asymptomatic. Occasionally, plica becomes symptomatic due to inflammation from acute trauma or repetitive microtrauma. The mediopatellar plica syndrome is most common; presenting with medial knee pain, patellar snapping, and catching during flexion. The plica may be palpable as a tender thickened band when pressed against the edge of the condyle and there may be localized tenderness at the medial and inferior patellar border. Dynamic ultrasonography has good sensitivity and

specificity to detect abnormalities of medial plicae.[53] MRI may show thickening of the plica and any associated synovitis or reactive changes in subchondral bone. Management includes patellar mobilization and massage, physiotherapy, and NSAIDs. Surgical removal of the plica is reserved for recalcitrant symptoms.

Fat Pad Irritation/Impingement ("Hoffa Syndrome")

The infrapatellar fat pad is richly innervated, and injury may cause anterior knee pain. Impingement of the infrapatellar fat pad between the patella and the femoral condyle may be secondary to direct trauma or acute hyperextension injury. Chronic irritation may be associated with patellar tendinopathy, PFP, or recurrent synovitis. Pain is often present with knee extension, prolonged standing, and kneeling. On examination, there is localized tenderness and swelling in the fat pad with posterior displacement of the inferior pole of the patella. Squatting, active extension of the knee, or passive pressure into extension may reproduce pain. Associated predisposing biomechanical factors include genu recurvatum and anterior tilting of the pelvis. Treatment includes local cryotherapy, taping the patella to reduce the amount of tilt and impingement, physiotherapy, and correcting lower limb biomechanics as in PFP. Surgery is usually not necessary.[54]

Patellar Tendinopathy

"Jumper's knee," or patellar tendinopathy, is a common cause of infrapatellar pain in skeletally mature individuals. Maximum discomfort is usually at the inferior patellar pole at the site of the proximal patellar tendon attachment, and is aggravated by jumping. On examination, there is tenderness over the proximal patellar tendon; thickening or nodules may be palpable. There may be secondary PFP. Treatment requires load reduction (activity modification, biomechanical correction), cryotherapy, transfriction massage (massage transverse to the direction of muscle fibers), and progressive eccentric strengthening.[55,56] In skeletally immature children and adolescents the osteochondroses/traction apophysitis Osgood–Schlatter (OSD) and Sinding–Larsen–Johansson (SLJD) disease present similarly, but tenderness is at the tibial tuberosity and inferior patellar pole, respectively. (See discussion of osteochondroses.)

Iliotibial Band Syndrome

The ITB emanates from the tensor fasciae latae and gluteus medius and maximus muscles, and extends laterally down the leg as a tight band of fascial tissue. It has multiple attachments at the lateral knee before inserting at Gerdy tubercle just lateral to the tibial tubercle. ITB syndrome is associated with repeated knee flexion to or through a 30-degree angle and is common in runners and cyclists. Risk factors include anatomical factors (genu varum, subtalar pronation, internal tibial torsion, leg length discrepancy), weak hip abductors, tight calf muscles, and increased activity.[57,58]

Adolescents present with activity-related lateral knee pain and tenderness. Occasionally, pain is localized proximally at the greater trochanter due to an associated trochanteric bursitis. On examination, pain and snapping can often be reproduced by palpating over the lateral femoral condyle with passive movement of the knee through a 60-degree arc of flexion; pain is typically maximal at 30 degrees of knee flexion. ITB is often tight with a positive Ober test (patient lying on their side with their affected leg uppermost. Abduct the leg and flex the knee to 90 degrees while keeping the hip joint in neutral position. On release of the leg, the thigh should drop into an adducted position; the thigh will remain abducted in a positive test) for contraction of iliotibial band.

Imaging is not usually necessary; ultrasound and MRI can confirm the diagnosis in difficult cases.[59] Management in the acute phase includes rest, cryotherapy, and analgesics. Physiotherapy is important to correct deficits in muscle strength and mobility and promote a gradual return to activity. In refractory cases, surgical release of the ITB may be required.[60]

Apophysitis and Apophyseal Avulsion Injuries

Apophyseal injuries are common in young athletes, affect boys more often than girls, and are usually secondary to forceful or repetitive traction of the attached muscle. The apophyses of the pelvis appear and fuse later than physes in long bones. The physes are the weakest structures of the immature skeleton, placing adolescents at increased risk of apophyseal injury, especially during a growth spurt. Adolescents have tight soft tissues during rapid growth, placing additional stress on the apophyses. Apophysitis refers to an overuse stress injury at the insertion site of major abdominal and hip muscles around the pelvis. Adolescents usually present with dull, activity-related pain. Radiographs are generally normal or show widening of the affected apophyses. Management includes rest, ice, modified activity, and physiotherapy. Most adolescents return to sport within 4 to 8 weeks.

Apophyseal avulsion fractures occur with sudden forceful muscle-tendon contraction. Common sites of avulsions are at the iliac crest (abdominal muscles), anterior superior iliac spine (sartorius), anterior inferior iliac spine (rectus femoris), ischial tuberosity (hamstrings), and lesser trochanter (iliopsoas) (Fig. 51-3). Adolescents usually present with localized pain, swelling, and reduced range of motion. Pain on resisted contractions of involved muscles, where hip joint motion is restricted, confirms pain is extrinsic to the hip joint. Radiographs demonstrate displacement of the apophyseal center, callus formation, and bony reaction. MRI is useful in suspected avulsion injuries with normal radiographs.[61,62] Management is usually nonoperative and includes rest, ice, modified activity, and physiotherapy. Most adolescents return to sport within 4 to 8 weeks.

Osteochondritis Dissecans

Osteochondritis dissecans (OCD) is an idiopathic lesion of bone and cartilage, resulting in bone necrosis and loss of continuity with subchondral bone. There may be partial or complete separation of articular cartilage with or without involvement of subchondral bone. Proposed etiologies include acute trauma, repetitive microtrauma, genetic factors, vascular insufficiency, ossification variants, inflammation, or normal growth variant.[63] The knee is most commonly affected (75% of cases).[64] Classically, the lateral aspect of the medial femoral condyle is affected, but the lateral femoral condyle, patella, ankle (talus), and elbow (capitellum) are also affected.[65,66] OCD may be asymptomatic and present as an incidental finding on radiographs, or adolescents may present with activity-related pain and swelling. Locking may be present if there is instability of the fragment. On examination, there may be focal bony tenderness, joint effusion, and evidence of a loose fragment with extension block or palpable loose body. Radiographs may show a radiolucent lesion, subchondral fracture, and a loose body.[63] OCD lesions of the knee can be missed on routine nonweight-bearing anteroposterior and lateral radiographs; tunnel (notch) and axial (skyline patellar profile) views are required to view the articular surfaces of the distal femoral condyles and patella (Fig. 51-4).[67] MRI may show cartilage changes earlier with contrast enhancement of intact cartilage lesions.[68] Staging of lesions has been done based on radiographic,[69] MRI, and arthroscopic[70] appearance. The Berndt and Harty classification characterizes OCD lesions based on radiographical appearance.[69] Stage I reflects small areas of compression, stage II lesions are separate fragments, stage III includes detached hinged fragments, and stage IV lesions are loose bodies.[69] Treatment depends on the site and stage of the lesion and the skeletal maturity

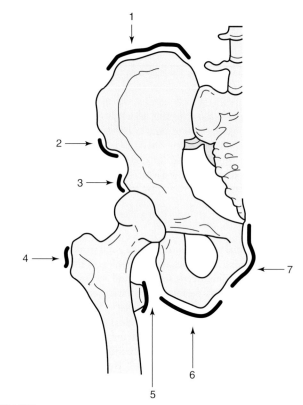

FIGURE 51-3 Hip and pelvis anatomy. **1,** Iliac crest (abdominal muscle attachment); **2,** Anterior superior iliac spine (sartorius attachment); **3,** Anterior inferior iliac spine (rectus femoris attachment); **4,** Greater trochanter (gluteal attachment); **5,** Lesser trochanter (psoas attachment); **6,** Ischial tuberosity (hamstring attachment); **7,** Pubic symphysis and inferior pubis ramus (gracilis and adductor attachments)

of the patient with early lesions in skeletally immature patients having the best prognosis.[68] Conservative treatment (protected weight bearing, immobilization, cryotherapy, NSAIDs, and up to 6 to 18 months of rehabilitation (range of motion, proprioceptive, strength, and endurance exercises)[71] is recommended for stable, nondetached, smaller lesions in children with open physes.[71] Children with symptomatic lesions, salvageable unstable, or displaced OCD lesions require surgery.[72] Approximately one third of all lesions progress to surgery.[73] Surgical treatment is effective in most cases. Treatments include "microfracture" (subchondral drilling), debridement, fragment excision, fragment fixation, osteochondral autograft, osteochondral allograft, and autologous chondrocyte implantation.[74]

Shin Splints (Posteromedial Tibial Stress Syndrome)

Activity-related pain and tenderness along the posteromedial border of the tibia is often referred to as "shin splints" or periostitis. Posteromedial tibial stress syndrome describes the periostitis and fasciitis caused by repetitive traction at the origins of the muscle fascial attachments along the middle and distal posterior medial tibia. Adolescents usually complain of shin pain at onset and toward the end of weight-bearing activity that resolves with rest. Alignment (hindfoot pronation), relative inflexibility (tight gastrosoleus complex, hip abduction), recent increase in activity levels, and change in footwear may be contributing factors.[75,76] Physical examination demonstrates generalized tibial boney tenderness. Radiographs are normal and radionuclide bone scans show diffuse increased uptake classically at the junction of

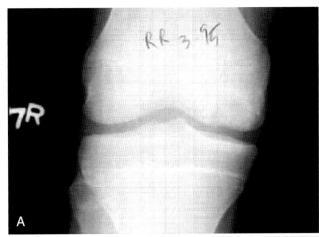

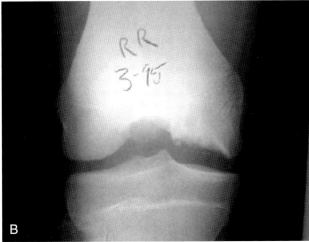

FIGURE 51-4 **A,** Anteroposterior radiograph shows minimal cystic changes affecting the lateral condyle. **B,** Tunnel or notch views show the cystic changes more clearly. (From E. Wall, D. Von Stein, Juvenile osteochondritis dissecans, Orthop. Clin. North. Am. 34 (2003) 341–353.)

the middle and distal one third of the posteromedial tibia. The differential diagnoses include stress fracture and posterior compartment syndrome. Management includes rest, ice, modified activity, improving gastrosoleus and posterior tibialis strength and flexibility, change in footwear or orthotic, and correction of any training errors. There is emerging evidence that extracorporeal shockwave therapy (ESWT) may be effective treatment.[77,78]

Stress Fractures

Stress fracture occurs when repetitive and excessive stress is applied to normal bone and represents a disturbance between bone resorption and bone regeneration. Stress fractures are believed to be a fatigue fracture or overuse injury and are more common in athletic children who report a recent increase in activity. Low levels of 25-hydroxyvitamin D and the female athlete triad (eating disorders, amenorrhea, osteoporosis) are also risk factors.[79,80] A study of a prospective cohort of 6712 preadolescent and adolescent girls found that Vitamin D intake was predictive of a lower risk of developing a stress fracture, especially among girls participating in physical activity.[81] The distal to middle third of the tibia is the most common site of stress fracture. The second and third metatarsals are commonly injured in older adolescents and adults and represent the classic "March fracture" seen in the military.[82] Several site-specific stress fractures are high risk for nonunion, complete fracture, or avascular necrosis (AVN), including the proximal fifth metatarsal, tarsal navicular, scaphoid, anterior tibial diaphysis, and femoral neck.[79] Children with stress fractures usually present with progressively worsening pain, aggravated by weight-bearing activity and relieved with rest. Pain may be present at rest or even at night. On examination, the fracture site is tender to palpation and there may be swelling. Early radiographs may be normal and late radiographs detect callus formation (Fig. 51-5), physeal widening, or apophyseal fragmentation. Early lesions are best detected by MRI, which is more specific than radionucleotide bone scan.[83] CT is useful for evaluation of tarsal navicular stress fractures. Management depends on symptoms and the site of injury. Treatment includes activity modification and, if required, a short period of nonweight bearing and immobilization. A pneumatic brace and early mobilization are recommended for tibial stress

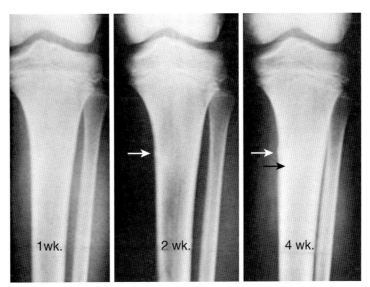

FIGURE 51-5 Serial radiographs document the evolution of a stress fracture in a 10-year-old girl. Two weeks after the onset of leg pain, the fracture line is evident. After four weeks, the fracture callus is seen. (Courtesy Dr. R. N. Hensinger.)

fractures.[84] High-risk stress fractures often require nonweight bearing and immobilization for 6 to 8 weeks, or surgical intervention.[85]

Upper Extremity

Little League Shoulder

Overuse injuries of the shoulder are common in young athletes involved in throwing sports, tennis, and swimming. Little league shoulder occurs when excessive traction and rotational torque forces cause microfractures across the proximal humeral physis. It typically affects males between 11 and 16 years of age, and is likely due to the properties of collagen and cartilage in this age group as well as excessive pitching and poor throwing techniques.[86] These athletes usually present with progressive shoulder pain during the throwing motion. Tenderness of the proximal lateral upper arm is common. Many have at least 25 degrees less internal rotation of the dominant shoulder compared to the other side.[87] Radiographs (AP, scapular Y, and axillary views) demonstrate irregularity and widening of the proximal humeral physis. Because similar findings can be seen in asymptomatic pitchers, T2 MRI confirms the diagnosis, demonstrating high intensity signal changes in the adjacent metaphysis. Treatment is almost exclusively nonsurgical, consisting of education, prolonged relative rest from shoulder activity, and rehabilitation to maximize range of motion and strength. Prior to return to play, modification in throwing technique, intensity, and frequency needs to be addressed. Prevention is the key, and, for young baseball pitchers, Little League Baseball Inc. recommends an age-appropriate restriction in number of pitches per day and mandatory rest periods between pitching appearances.[88]

Tennis Elbow

Overuse of the arm related to excessive wrist extension can cause lateral elbow pain, which is commonly called tennis elbow or lateral epicondylitis. One percent to 3% of the general population is affected; both genders equally. The peak prevalence is in the fourth and fifth decades of life.[89] The pathological process consists of tendinosis of the extensor carpi radialis brevis tendon origin. Patients present with lateral elbow pain and maximal tenderness 1 to 2 cm distal to the lateral epicondyle. Resisted middle finger or wrist extension, especially with the forearm pronated and radially deviated reproduces the discomfort. Although generally not required to confirm diagnosis, MRI demonstrates a thickened common extensor tendon with increased signal intensity.[89] Most cases are asymptomatic at 1 year, regardless of treatment. Relative rest, a short course of NSAIDS, and nitric oxide patching followed by rehabilitative therapy (elbow manipulation, strengthening exercises) may provide benefit. Refractory cases treated with a steroid injection at the site of pain derive short-term benefits (under 6 weeks), but high recurrence is reported. Autologous blood injection, platelet-rich plasma, and dry needle injection therapy may be helpful in refractory cases.[90,91] Surgery is rarely required. Prior to returning to sport, correction of inappropriate sport technique and equipment and the use of a counterforce brace are recommended.[92]

Children are more likely to suffer a valgus compressive injury to the lateral elbow. Repetitive valgus forces during a vulnerable period of growth damages the end-arterial blood supply to the capitellum and can lead to Panner osteochondrosis. Children between the ages 5 and 11 years present with vague lateral elbow pain and stiffness. Radiographs demonstrate flattening and fragmentation of the ossific nucleus, but the condition resolves with no long-term sequelae.[93] OCD of the capitellum is another possible sequela; it may present with lateral elbow pain, swelling, and inadequate extension in older youth. MR imaging best confirms the diagnosis. Rest and immobilization can allow adequate healing, but surgery may be necessary. Prevention of

such injuries in all sports is essential. In baseball, Little League Inc. preventive guidelines are recommended.[88]

Golfer Elbow

Overuse of the arm may also result in medial elbow pain or "golfer elbow." This condition is 7 to 10 times less common than "tennis elbow" but affects a similar age group.[94] In the skeletally mature, this represents a tendinosis at the origin of the flexor/pronator muscles. Localized tenderness at or below the medial epicondyle and pain on resisted wrist flexion and forearm pronation in elbow flexion are characteristic. As with lateral epicondylitis, MRI demonstrates increased signal intensity. Treatment is similar to tennis elbow with recalcitrant cases deriving benefit from ultrasound-guided steroid or autologous blood injection.[94]

Medial elbow pain is more common than lateral pain in skeletally immature throwing athletes. Repeated valgus stress to the medial epicondyle typically presents with local swelling and tenderness. Radiographs may be normal or show fragmentation and sometimes avulsion of the medial epicondyle.[93] MRI may detect stress injury of the medial epicondyle apophysis before plain radiograph changes occur. Treatment consists of rest until symptoms abate, followed by gradual stretching and strengthening to regain full range of motion and power. Surgery is rarely necessary but may be considered for avulsions displaced greater than 5 mm. Prevention of this injury is key.[88]

Wrist Overuse Injuries

Overuse tendon injury may occur in children participating in sports requiring repetitive wrist motion such as throwing, rowing, and racquet sports. DeQuervain's tenosynovitis, extensor carpi ulnaris tendonitis, and intersection syndrome present with insidious onset of localized pain coincident with increased activity.

Stress injury to the distal radius physis occurs in skeletally immature children participating in hand weight-bearing activity such as gymnastics. Children present with dorsal wrist pain during weight-loading activities (handsprings) and focal tenderness over the distal radial physis. Bone marrow edema may be apparent on MRI before early radiographic changes of widening and irregularity of the physis are apparent. Late radiographic changes may include distal radial deformity or distal ulna overgrowth.[95] Treatment of overuse injuries of the wrist includes ice, NSAIDs, bracing, relative rest, and physiotherapy.

DISORDERS OF THE TRUNK

Chest Pain

Chest pain is not a frequent complaint in the pediatric population. Rowe and colleagues reported that six of 1000 children's emergency department visits were for chest pain, and boys and girls were equally affected.[96] Twenty-eight percent were diagnosed with chest wall pain; however, only 1% had cardiac causes.[96] One of the most common reasons for chest wall pain is precordial catch syndrome or Texidor twinge, which is a benign and self-limited condition. Affected children have a history of recurrent, well-localized, sharp chest wall pain of sudden onset lasting a few seconds to minutes, with negative findings on examination or laboratory testing.[97]

Costochondritis

Costochondritis is a poorly understood condition affecting up to 14% of pediatric patients presenting with chest pain. It is often associated with a history of prolonged cough or chest wall strain. Brief, acute, and stabbing pain affecting one side of the anterior chest that is worse with deep breathing is typical.[98] Tenderness of one or more of the second to fourth costal cartilages is noted without associated swelling, heat, or erythema. Routine laboratory testing is not usually necessary unless the diagnosis is uncertain. The syndrome can be self-limited or chronic and intermittent, but most resolve by 1 year. Treatment is generally directed at pain control with analgesics and NSAIDS, but physical therapy and taping may also help.[99] Refractory cases are occasionally injected with a local anesthetic/corticosteroid into the costochondral region.

Tietze Syndrome

This is a localized form of costochondritis that affects one costochondral, costosternal, or sternoclavicular joint. There is associated swelling, warmth, and tenderness of the second or third costochondral junction.[98] Etiology is unknown, but it may be triggered by an upper respiratory tract infection with cough. Plain films are usually normal, but MRI may reveal enlarged and edematous cartilage and contrast enhancement of subchondral bone.[100] Treatment is similar to costochondritis. Injury, septic arthritis, spondyloarthritis, and lymphoma may present similarly and should be excluded.

Slipping Rib Syndrome

This condition is believed to be due to hypermobility of the eighth to twelfth ribs causing the cartilage of one rib to slip superiorly and impinge on the adjacent intercostal nerve. It may be a result of direct trauma or repetitive trunk motion during certain sports.[98,101] Patients have severe, sharp chest or upper abdominal pain, which may fade over a few hours or persist as a dull ache. Exacerbations can occur with periodic resubluxations precipitated by vigorous physical activity, trauma, or coughing. Physical findings include tenderness of the affected ribs, worsening pain on direct pressure over these ribs, and asymmetry of rib position. Reproduction of the pain, often with a click, occurs when the examiner hooks their fingers under the inferior margins of the affected ribs and pulls anteriorly and superiorly. This "positive hooking maneuver" is usually performed with an intercostal nerve block.[102] Radiological imaging does not confirm the diagnosis but helps to exclude other conditions. Treatment consists of reassurance, avoidance of exacerbating movements, taping, manipulation, and injection of local anesthetic nerve blocks. In severe cases, excision of the anterior rib end and costal cartilage may be curative.[102]

Back Pain

Nonspecific back pain in the general pediatric population is common. A recent meta-analysis of 59 studies found a 40% mean lifetime point prevalence, a 33.6% 1-year period prevalence and a point prevalence of 12%.[103] It may be more common in girls and rates rise with increasing age. Recurrent back pain mirrors that of recurrent abdominal pain with a 6-month point prevalence of 21% to 31%.[104] Most children have mild and self-limited symptoms, but they frequently report avoidance of heavy work at home or at school and greater relaxation time. The etiology of back pain in children is believed to be multifactorial relating to genetic and environmental factors, but body mass index and heavy backpacks do not appear to be associated.[105] Children who have more problems with peers experienced a higher risk of persistent low back pain.[106] Treatment for idiopathic back pain in children has not been well studied. A meta-analysis of physical treatment options suggests the combination of therapeutic physical conditioning and manual therapy is best but education and exercise are also important.[107] Other causes of back pain such as spondylolysis, lordotic pain, disk prolapse, and Scheuermann disease should be considered, especially in young athletes.[108]

Spondylolysis and Spondylolisthesis

Spondylolysis is the most common (47%) cause of back pain in young athletes, especially those participating in activities such as football, rugby, ballet, diving, and gymnastics.[108] Both acute and overuse injuries can occur, although the latter are more common. Repetitive hyperextension causes a stress fracture of the pars interarticularis, most commonly of the fifth (85% to 95%) and fourth (5% to 15%) lumbar vertebrae.[109] Spondylolysis is rare before the age of 5 years and uncommon (6%) in adults. Factors that increase lumbar lordosis (weak abdominal muscles, tight hip flexors, tight thoracolumbar fascia) may increase stress on these posterior spine elements. Other risk factors include European ancestry, family history, and a preexisting developmental spine defect.

Isthmic spondylolisthesis occurs with bilateral pars defects and is defined by forward translation of one vertebra on the next caudal segment, most commonly at L5-S1.[108] This condition is graded based on the percentage of slip of one vertebral body on the vertebra below (grade 1 slip [0% to 25% slip], grade 2 [25% to 50%], grade 3 [50% to 75%] and grade 4 [>75%]).[110] Spondylolisthesis is more common in females, and typically occurs during the adolescent growth spurt. It is less common than spondylolysis, and progression of a slip is rare after skeletal maturity.[111]

The usual presentation of spondylolysis and spondylolisthesis is the insidious onset of extension-related low back pain. Symptoms generally increase over months, and pain may radiate to the buttocks and posterior thigh. If there are radicular symptoms of numbness and weakness, spondylolisthesis and disk herniation need to be considered. On examination, lumbar hyperlordosis, ipsilateral paraspinal muscle spasm, and tight hamstrings with posterior thigh pain on forward flexion are often found. Discomfort is worsened by hyperextension of the spine and this may localize to the affected side on single-leg back extension. There is usually focal tenderness to palpation over the site of the pars lesion and there may be a palpable step-off at the lumbosacral junction with spondylolisthesis. Strength, sensation, and lower extremity reflexes are normal unless a slip causes nerve root irritation.[108]

Radiographs (standing lateral, coned lateral of the lumbosacral junction, AP) are the first line of investigation (Fig. 51-6). Additional oblique views may demonstrate a break in the pars interarticularis (Scottie dog neck), but a low (32%) sensitivity has been demonstrated especially early in the course of this condition. A single-photon emission computerized tomography (SPECT) bone scan is more sensitive and identifies lesions with active bone turnover. CT shows better bony detail and is useful in assessing the healing process; however, the risk of radiation exposure to pelvic organs should be considered.[112] Bone marrow edema on MRI may be useful in detecting early lesions and can also be helpful when neurological symptoms accompany spondylolisthesis.

The goals of management are to achieve bony or fibrous union, relieve pain, optimize and restore function, and prevent or minimize the degree of spondylolisthesis. Initial management includes avoidance of activities that cause pain with a restriction of sport for 3 to 6 months. Physiotherapy is important to reduce lumbar lordosis, strengthen core muscles, and stretch tight hamstring muscles. The use of thoracolumbar orthoses to limit extension and rotation is variable and largely physician and center specific. A meta-analysis comparing bracing to conservative nonbracing treatments suggests both provide a successful outcome 1 year later in 84% of patients.[113] Adolescents can return to sport when they are pain-free with or without a brace, usually within a few months. Standing lateral

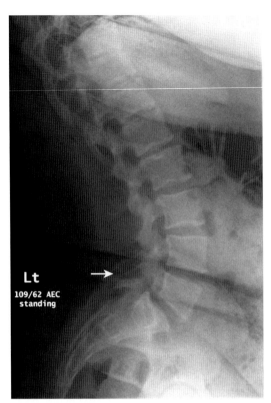

FIGURE 51-6 Spondylolysis of L5 is visible on this lateral radiograph. There is also Grade 1 spondylolisthesis with anterior slip of L5 on S1 *(arrow).* Endplate changes are seen throughout the lumbar spine. (Courtesy Dr. R. Cairns.)

radiographs are recommended at 4- to 6-month intervals until skeletal maturity. Progressive spondylolisthesis with greater than 50% slip (grade 3 or 4), youth with neurological deficit, or painful nonunion with persistent back pain warrant orthopedic referral.[108]

Lordotic Low Back Pain/Posterior Element Overuse Syndrome

This condition occurs in young athletes during their growth spurt, and is associated with tightening of the interspinous ligaments, thoracolumbar fascia and tendinous attachments on the spine. It is a diagnosis of exclusion. Athletes typically complain of low back pain with activity, especially in sports that require repetitive hyperextension of the lower back. As a result, traction apophysitis, impingement of the spinous processes, and even pseudoarthrosis of the developing vertebrae may occur.[108] Physical examination demonstrates tight hamstrings and pain on back hyperextension. Radiographs can be used to rule out other etiologies. Physical therapy strategies used for spondylolysis are usually effective.

Lumbar Disk Herniation

Discogenic pain has been estimated to occur in about 11% of pediatric athletes, especially those over 12 years of age. Ninety-two percent of affected adolescents experience herniation at the L4-5 or L5-S1 regions.[108] Trauma from collision sports or strength training is often associated with disc protrusion in young athletes, especially those with preexisting spinal deformity (scoliosis, lumbarization/sacralization, canal narrowing) or those with lumbar Schmorl nodes and Scheuermann disease.

Low back pain with or without sciatica is often noted, but overt neurological deficits are uncommon in this age group. Coughing, sneezing, and bending may aggravate the pain. Examination reveals limitation of forward flexion, and over 60% have an abnormal straight-leg test with either localized pain or radicular features.[114] Adolescents may assume a scoliotic posture as a compensatory attempt to relieve nerve root irritation. MRI confirms the diagnosis, with herniated disc material often larger than in adults at the L4-L5 or L5-S1 region. Careful inspection for apophyseal fracture is recommended, especially in youth with large or central herniations.[114]

Conservative treatment with education, rest, analgesics, and physical therapy is successful in most cases.[108] Operative therapy is indicated for those with persistent or progressive neurological deficits.[114] Over 90% of surgically treated adolescents achieve symptom relief; however, reoperation is required in 20% at 10 years and 26% at 20 years postoperatively.[108]

Diskitis

Diskitis is a rare but well-recognized entity affecting toddlers and young children typically between the third and fourth lumbar vertebrae. The pathogenesis is unclear but may reflect self-limited infectious or inflammatory causes.[115] Children may present with back pain, limp, neck stiffness, irritability, and gastrointestinal upset. Toddlers often refuse to stand or sit. Tenderness on palpation of the spinous processes is infrequently found, but the child may refuse to bend down to pick up an object. These poorly localized symptoms and the normal or mildly elevated complete blood count and inflammatory markers contribute to delays in diagnosis. Plain radiographs demonstrate disk space narrowing and irregular endplates of adjacent vertebrae by 10 days; bone scan and MRI have excellent sensitivity, but MRI can also exclude abscesses and spinal tumors.[115] Treatment consists of antiinflammatory agents, antibiotics, and immobilization. The natural course of the disease is benign with the majority being asymptomatic by three weeks. Chronic spinal restriction may develop and persistent intervertebral narrowing on radiographs is common, hence ongoing follow-up is suggested.

Calcific diskitis is a relatively uncommon childhood condition that presents with acute onset of neck pain, torticollis, and calcification of the cervical or thoracic intervertebral disks. The etiology is unclear, but interruption of a tenuous blood supply is suggested. Plain radiographs and MRI are usually diagnostic.[116]

Scheuermann Disease

Scheuermann disease is the most common cause of a structural kyphotic deformity in adolescence with an incidence of 0.4% to 10%. It is most frequently diagnosed between the ages of 12 and 17 years, and is more common in boys.[108,117,118] The pathogenesis is unclear, but disorders in endochondral vertebral ossification or collagen aggregation, and biomechanical abnormalities may play a role.[110] Eighty percent of patients are asymptomatic and concerned about cosmetic appearance, but pain may be noted with activity, especially in athletes with high demands on their back. The most common "thoracic" type consists of over 40 degrees of kyphosis usually between T7 and T9. It is not reducible with back hyperextension or by lying supine, which is in contrast to postural kyphosis. It may be associated with nonstructural hyperlordosis of the cervical or lumbar spine with greater rates of back pain and risk of spondylolysis. Tightness of the thoracolumbar fascia and hamstring muscles has been noted.[108] Neurological deficits are rare, and cardiopulmonary insufficiency occurs only with severe curves measuring greater than 100 degrees.[119] Classic standing lateral radiological features include anterior wedging of at least three adjacent vertebral bodies each by 5 degrees or more, end plate irregularities, loss

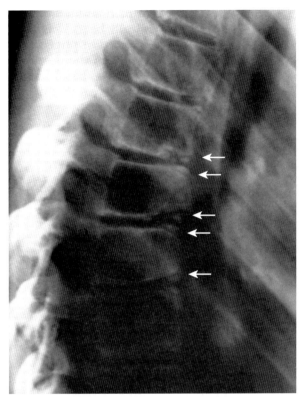

FIGURE 51-7 Lateral radiograph of the spine illustrating the abnormalities of the anterior margins of the vertebral bodies *(arrows)* that are characteristic of Scheuermann disease and result in anterior wedging. (Courtesy Dr. R. Cairns.)

TABLE 51-2	The Osteochondroses	
TYPE	**CONDITION/ EPONYM**	**SITE**
Articular Upper Extremity	Kienböck	Lunate
	Thiemann	Basal phalanges
	Mauclaire	Second metacarpal head
	Preiser	Carpal navicular
	Burns	Distal ulna
	Brailsford	Radial head
	Panner	Capitellum
	Osteochondritis dissecans (OCD)	Capitellum
	Hass	Head of humerus
	Friedrich	Sternal end clavicle:
Articular Lower Extremity	Legg-Calvé-Perthes	Femoral head
	Meyer dysplasia	Femoral epiphysis
	Diaz	Talus
	Kohler	Tarsal navicular
	Frieberg	Metatarsal head (2nd, 3rd)
	Köhler	Primary patellar center
	Buschke	Medial cuneiform
	Osteochondritis dissecans (OCD)	Femoral condyles, talar dome
Nonarticular Upper Extremity	Adams	Medial epicondylitis
Nonarticular Lower Extremity	Osgood–Schlatter disease (OSD)	Tibial tuberosity
	Sinding–Larsen– Johansson (SLJD)	Inferior pole of patella
	Sever	Calcareous
	Iselin	Fifth metatarsal tuberosity
	Milch	Ischial apophysis
	Buchman	Iliac crest
	Oldberg	Ischiopubic region
	Van Neck	Pubic symphysis
	Mandl	Greater trochanter
	Liffert–Arkin	Distal tibia
Spine	Schmorl	Disk
	Calve	Vertebral body
Physeal	Scheuermann	Thoracic spine epiphysis
	Blount	Proximal tibia
Normal Variation		

Adapted from A.C. Brower, The osteochondroses, Orthop. Clin. North Am. 14 (1983) 99; R.S. Siffert, Classification of the osteochondroses, Clin. Orthop. Rel. Res. (1981) 158; and other sources.

of disk space height, and Schmorl nodes (Fig. 51-7).[108] The infrequent thoracolumbar subtype is associated with greater pain and restriction in exercise. It is more likely to progress into adulthood.

Treatment recommendations for youth with nonrigid Scheuermann disease, from the SOSORT panel of experts, consist of simple analgesia, exercise, and the use of a back brace to prevent flexion. Physical therapy to teach postural self-control and 20 minutes of home exercises daily to auto-elongate the spine with isometric stabilization is advised prior to bracing.[110] The use of a day and night custom back orthotic at the onset of puberty is preferred to restore the alignment of muscle forces and decrease mechanical stress on the anterior wall of the vertebral body. Bracing should continue for 2 years and stop once growth is completed but before bony maturity is reached. Overall, nonsurgical outcome is very good. Surgical intervention is rarely indicated in patients with persistent pain and curves over 75 degrees.

Osteochondroses

Osteochondroses are unique to the growing skeleton and are believed to be due to AVN caused by repetitive stress and disruption of the vascular supply to bone. Articular sites are most common, but nonarticular and physeal osteochondroses also occur.[120,121] There are over 70 osteochondroses, and they have been named after individuals who first described them (Table 51-2).[122] The etiology is unclear and probably includes normal variants of development, stress injury, and vascular insufficiency.[123] The typical presentation is localized pain aggravated by exercise and/or swelling. With the exception of Freiberg disease (2nd and 3rd metatarsal), they are more common in boys than in girls. Onset of symptoms is related to skeletal maturity with girls usually presenting earlier than boys do. Kienböck disease (lunate) is the only

osteochondroses to occur after skeletal maturity. Symptoms of osteochondroses last from several months up to 2 years, generally resolving with skeletal maturity. Some sites are associated with long-term problems secondary to bony incongruity and subsequent positional deformity or early degenerative osteoarthritis. Some of the more common osteochondroses are discussed.

Osgood–Schlatter and Sinding–Larsen–Johansson. Osgood–Schlatter (OSD) and Sinding–Larsen–Johansson (SLJD) disease are microavulsion fractures due to the patellar tendon traction forces on the apophyses. OSD involves the growth plate of the tibial tuberosity at the inferior attachment of the patellar tendon, is bilateral in 30% of cases, and is more common than SLJD, which occurs at the inferior pole of the patella at the proximal attachment of the patellar tendon.

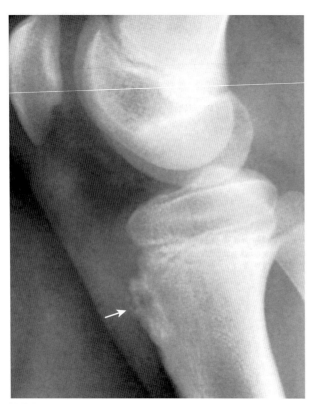

FIGURE 51-8 Radiograph of the knee of a boy with Osgood Schlatter disease. In addition to fragmentation of the apophysis, the soft tissues overlying the tibial tubercle are thickened *(arrow)*. (Courtesy Dr. R. Cairns.)

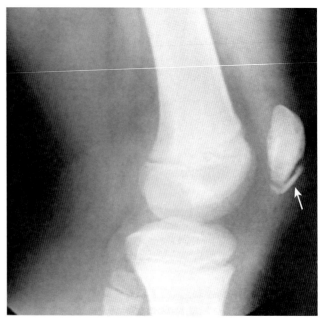

FIGURE 51-9 Radiograph of the knee of a boy with Sinding–Larsen–Johansson disease. The lower pole of the patella has been separated from the patella *(arrow)*. (Courtesy Dr. R. Cairns.)

TABLE 51-3	Osgood–Schlatter Disease
Age At Onset	Adolescence
Sex Ratio	Boys > girls
Symptoms	Pain localized to tibial tuberosity worsened by running and jumping, pain with kneeling
Signs	Tenderness and swelling over tibial tuberosity at site of inferior patellar tendon attachment, tightness of surrounding muscles
Radiographs	Soft tissue swelling, enlarged and sometimes fragmented tubercle

Both conditions are more common in active children and occur during the adolescent growth spurt. Children present with localized pain during activity (especially running and jumping), focal tenderness, and soft tissue swelling (Table 51-3). Tightness of surrounding muscles (quadriceps, hamstrings, gastrocnemius) is common. Radiographs are not usually required, but if presenting symptoms and signs are atypical, radiographs can exclude bony tumor, fracture, or infection. Typical radiographs of OSD show enlargement and fragmentation of the tubercle (Fig. 51-8). Radiographs of SLJD may show ossification and calcification of the inferior patellar pole (Fig. 51-9). Ultrasound allows visualization of changes to the tibial tuberosity and depiction of deep and superficial infrapatellar bursitis and fibrosis.[124] Recent studies report that positive Doppler ultrasound correlate with patient-reported pain and ultrasound may help guide management plans.[125] Laboratory evaluation shows no evidence of chronic inflammation and no association with human leukocyte antigen-B27, so it is not a forme fruste of enthesitis-related arthritis (JIA).[126]

Management is conservative; these are self-limited conditions that resolve with skeletal maturity, but symptoms may persist for up to 24 months. Treatment includes activity modification, cryotherapy, local muscle stretching and strengthening (quadriceps, hamstrings, gastrocnemius), and correction of any predisposing biomechanical factors (e.g., subtalar pronation) with physical therapy, bracing, and/or orthotics. Occasionally in OSD, symptoms may persist after skeletal maturity due to nonunion of the tibial tuberosity. Excision of a symptomatic ossicle often relieves symptoms.[127]

Sever disease. Sever disease (calcaneal apophysitis), a traction apophysitis of the os calcis at the insertion of the Achilles tendon, affects children aged 7 to 14 years, is more common in active boys, and is bilateral in 60%.[128] Children present with heel pain during running and jumping activities, tenderness and variable swelling over the posterior heel at the insertion of the Achilles tendon, pain with medial and lateral squeeze of the calcaneal apophysis, and weakness of dorsiflexion and Achilles tendon contracture.[129] Radiographs demonstrate a normally irregular apophysis, and are not required unless there are atypical presenting features.[130] A recent systematic review found little evidence to support traditional management of ice, NSAIDS, activity modification, and physiotherapy. There is some evidence that taping, heel lift, and heel cups decrease pain during sport.[131] Children who do not respond to usual therapies require further imaging with MRI. Ogden and colleagues showed that children with persistent pain had calcaneal metaphyseal trabecular stress fracture, not traction apophysitis, and required immobilization.[132]

Iselin disease. Iselin disease refers to traction apophysitis of the tuberosity of the fifth metatarsal. The apophysis is within the peroneus brevis tendon insertion site. The secondary ossification center usually fuses by age 11 years in girls and 14 years in boys.[133] Pain with weight-bearing activity, tenderness over the base of the fifth metatarsal, and pain with resisted eversion are common. Radiographs differentiate Iselin disease from avulsion fracture: the apophysis is parallel to the long axis of the fifth metatarsal, and fractures are usually transverse. Technetium bone scan may help confirm apophysitis. Management includes cryotherapy, modified activity, immobilization, and physiotherapy. In rare instances of persistent pain due to nonunion of the apophysis, surgery is required.[134]

Köhler disease. Köhler disease is an osteochondroses of the tarsal navicular that affects children between 5 and 9 years of age and may be bilateral in up to 25% of cases.[135] It can be an incidental finding on radiographs, or children may complain of midfoot pain with weight-bearing activity. On examination, there is localized swelling, erythema, and tenderness over the navicular. Children characteristically walk on the lateral aspect of the foot.[136] Radiographs show increased sclerosis of the navicular. Management includes cryotherapy, NSAIDs, activity modification, and immobilization in a walking boot for severe cases. Mild pain persists in some, but complete resolution of symptoms is the rule.[137]

Freiberg disease. Freiberg disease is an osteonecrosis of the metatarsal heads.[138] The second and third metatarsals are the most commonly affected, and it is more common in athletic adolescent females.[139] The pathophysiology is unknown; studies suggest a multifactorial etiology, including trauma, vascular, genetic, and altered biomechanics.[140] Adolescents present with forefoot pain and focal tenderness over the affected metatarsal head. Radiographs show initial widening of the MTP joint space, followed by collapse and sclerosis of the articular surface of the metatarsal head, which eventually reossifies. Radiographic healing is complete over 2 to 3 years. MRI and bone scan can detect disease earlier than radiographs. Management is aimed at decreasing foot pressures and unloading the affected metatarsal. Nonoperative treatment includes activity modification, NSAIDs, stiff-soled shoes, casting, and orthotics. Surgical management is reserved for those failing conservative strategies.[140,141]

Thiemann disease. Thiemann disease is a rare osteochondrosis of the phalangeal epiphyses, which has an unknown etiology but appears to be genetic with autosomal dominant transmission.[142] It is also considered to be a form of epiphyseal dysplasia and typically affects the PIP joints of the fingers and toes in adolescence.[143,144] Distal interphalangeal joints of the hands and the interphalangeal joints of the first toes may also be affected.[145] There is fusiform swelling and tenderness of the affected joints. Radiographs aid diagnosis; the affected epiphyses demonstrate sclerosis, flattening, cup-shaped widening, and eventual fragmentation. Thiemann disease often follows a benign course with normalization of the phalangeal dimensions after growth plate closure. Trauma may worsen the prognosis.[145-150]

DEVELOPMENTAL CONDITIONS

Legg–Calvé–Perthes Disease

Legg–Calvé–Perthes (LCP) disease was independently and simultaneously described by Legg,[151] Calvé,[151] and Perthes[152] in 1909. It is an idiopathic AVN/osteonecrosis of the femoral epiphysis that usually affects children between 4 and 10 years of age, peaking between 5 and 7 years. It is four to five times more common in boys, and it is more common in Caucasians and in children with low socioeconomic status. It is bilateral in 10% to 15%.[153,154] Bilateral Perthes disease is usually asynchronous; synchronous bilateral Perthes should raise the suspicion of an alternative diagnosis, such as epiphyseal dysplasia.

LCP has been associated with delayed skeletal maturation and growth hormone deficiency.[155,156] Disruption of the blood supply to the femoral head is the inciting pathogenic event. When hip joint loading overcomes the weakened mechanical strength of the necrotic femoral head, the femoral head deforms. The etiology is not known; however, the current leading theory is that mechanical overloading causes disruption of the blood supply to the femoral head in a genetically susceptible individual. Proposed etiologies include type II collagen

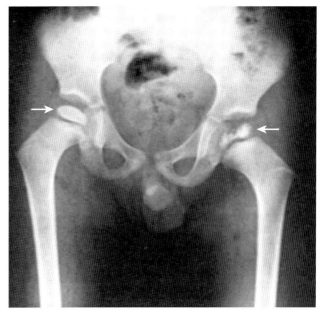

FIGURE 51-10 Legg–Calvé–Perthes disease. On the right side, the capital femoral epiphysis is flattened and sclerotic *(arrow)*; on the left, it is fragmented *(arrow)*. The femoral metaphyses are widened, especially on the left side. (Courtesy Dr. R. Cairns.)

mutation, insulin-like growth factor-1 pathway abnormality, inflammatory process, coagulopathy/thrombophilia, vasculopathy, venous congestion, arterial occlusion, and maternal or passive smoking.[157-169] Osteonecrosis of the proximal femoral epiphyses may also be associated with systemic disease (leukemia, lymphoma, systemic lupus erythematosus), hemoglobinopathies, coagulopathies, and as a complication of corticosteroid treatment or trauma.

Children usually present with a limp or pain in the hip, thigh, or knee. Examination reveals limited and painful internal rotation and abduction of the affected hip. The Trendelenburg sign may be positive. Four radiographical stages are described (1) avascular necrosis stage (decreased size or increased density of the proximal femoral epiphyses on an AP view, widening of the joint space and crescent sign (subchondral fracture that correlates with the extent of necrosis) on the lateral view); (2) fragmentation stage (patchy areas of increased radiolucency and radiodensity); (3) reossification, or healing, stage (radiodensities develop in previously radiolucent areas and abnormalities of the shape of the femoral head and neck appear); and (4) residual, or healed, stage (bone density is normal and the femoral head is healed but deformed) (Fig. 51-10).[170] These changes may take several years to develop, and MRI has greater sensitivity to detect early changes.[171] Treatment consists of rest from aggravating activities and exercises to preserve hip range of motion; femoral and/or pelvic surgery may be required. Current literature does not support the use of bracing, with the exception of short-term treatment with a Petrie cast in patients with deformed femoral heads before complete reossification.[172] Experimental studies suggest bisphosphonates may decrease femoral head deformity, but the few clinical studies to date have not demonstrated definitive benefit.[173] A recent consensus statement on the management of LCP emphasizes the aim of all treatments is to maintain the femoral head well covered within the acetabulum and to minimize the deformity of the head.[174] The main long-term concern is early osteoarthritis. Femoral acetabular impingement is another complication that may result in pain and poor function.[175]

Femoral head involvement, lateral pillar classification, and age strongly correlate with outcome. A Norwegian prospective study with

5-year follow-up on 358 children reported that having more than 50% of femoral head involvement was the strongest predictor of poor outcome.[176] A prospective multicenter study with follow-up at skeletal maturity on 345 affected hips in 337 children found that children with loss of less than 50% of the femoral head lateral height (Group A and B lateral pillar hips) under age 8 years (with 6-year-old skeletal age) had a good outcome regardless of treatment, whereas those with more than 50% loss of lateral height (Group C hips) had poor outcome, regardless of age. Children aged 8 years (with 6-year-old skeletal age) or older at onset and loss of 50% or less of the original height of the lateral pillar (Group B, B/C) had better outcome with surgical treatment than with nonoperative treatment.[177,178] A meta-analysis of 1232 patients and 1266 hips found that among patients younger than 6 years, nonoperative and operative procedures had the same likelihood of a good radiologic outcome, whereas operative treatment was almost twice as likely to result in a good outcome as nonoperative treatment in patients aged 6 years and older.[175] Timely operative treatment may improve outcome in older and more severely affected children. A recent study reported that only 26% of children with LCP treated nonoperatively had a spherical femoral head at a mean follow-up of 20 years.[179] Better outcomes are reported if surgery is done during the AVN process or early part of fragmentation.[180]

Slipped Capital Femoral Epiphyses

Slipped Capital Femoral Epiphyses (SCFE), displacement of the proximal femoral epiphysis on the femoral neck, is more common in obese children, boys, African Americans, Hispanics, Polynesians, and Native Americans.[181,182] It is bilateral in 20% to 40%; the second SCFE usually occurs within 1 year of the initial slip.[183,184] There has been an increase in the incidence of SCFE over the last few decades and a younger age of onset for boys (12.7 to 13.5 years) and girls (11.2 to 12 years).[181,185] These trends of increased rates of SCFE in younger children reflect the increasing obesity rates.[186] The pathogenesis of SCFE is not known and growth plate failure is felt to be due to mechanical, endocrine, and metabolic changes at puberty.

Children usually present with a limp and may have hip, groin, thigh, or knee pain. An acute slip may develop after a moderate injury, resulting in more severe pain and inability to bear weight. The affected hip is often preferentially held in abduction and external rotation with decreased active and passive internal rotation and adduction. The Trendelenburg test may be positive, reflecting gluteus medius weakness. SCFE is classified as stable or unstable based on a child's ability to weight bear on the affected leg.[187] Radiographs (AP and frog leg lateral) of the hip may show widening and irregularity of the physis with posterior inferior displacement of femoral head. On the AP view, a line drawn from the superior femoral neck (Klein line) should intersect some portion of the femoral head (Fig. 51-11). Standard radiographs may underestimate the severity of SCFE and MRI can be helpful in diagnosing a "pre-slip" and may show physeal widening, synovitis, periphyseal edema, and joint effusion.

SCFE may compromise the vascular supply to the femoral head and lead to AVN; all cases warrant urgent orthopedic referral. A systematic review reported that patients with unstable slips have a 9.4-fold greater risk of developing AVN.[188] Pretreatment bone scan and MRI are sensitive predictors for the development of AVN.[189] Treatment includes nonweight-bearing, traction, and surgery with epiphyseal fixation and osteotomy. Most patients do well after surgical fixation. Complications include AVN and chondrolysis, which may occur in both treated and untreated children.[190] Femoral acetabular impingement may be associated with SCFE-related deformity and dysfunction in both the short- and long-term outlooks.[191,192] Patients require long-term follow-up because SCFE may develop within 12 to 18 months in the contralateral

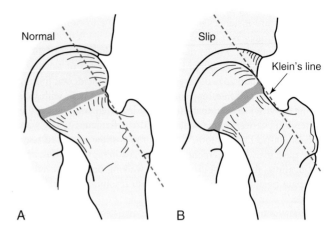

FIGURE 51-11 The Klein line in normal situation versus in slipped capital femoral epiphysis. Klein line is drawn along the radiographic border of the neck of the femur. This line should intersect the epiphysis. **A,** Klein line in normal situation. **B,** Alignment of Klein line with slip: the epiphysis is out of alignment. (Redrawn from R.A. Reynolds, Diagnosis and treatment of slipped capital femoral epiphysis, Curr. Opin. Pediatr. 11 (1999) 76–79.)

hip if prophylactic pinning is not performed.[193] Children under the age of 10 years or over the age 16 years who are thin and do not fit the typical profile for SCFE should undergo evaluation for endocrinopathies (thyroid disease, growth hormone abnormalities) associated with SCFE.[194]

Bipartite Patella

The patella ossifies between the ages of 3 and 5 years of age with gradual coalescence of multiple ossification centers. Accessory ossification centers occur in 2% of the population, are more common in boys, and usually involve the superolateral patella. A bipartite patella is usually an asymptomatic, incidental radiographical finding. Tripartite patella may also occur but is less common. Radiographs show regular smooth fragment margins with no evidence of soft tissue swelling, differentiating the lesion from acute fracture. Occasionally, bipartite patella may cause anterior knee pain, with a peak incidence in early adolescence.[195] Clinically there is soft tissue tenderness at the superolateral patellar pole. MRI may show bone marrow edema in symptomatic cases.[196] Initial treatment is conservative with modified activity and local flexibility and strengthening exercises. Surgical options include excision or fixation of the bipartite patella or release of the vastus lateralis insertion.[197,198]

Sesamoid Pathology

The medial and lateral sesamoid bones are intratendinous in the flexor hallucis brevis muscle and act as pulleys to help stabilize the first MTP joint. The sesamoids ossify by 8 years in girls and 12 years in boys.[199] Bipartite or multipartite sesamoids are present in 10% to 33% of feet.[135] More than half of body weight is transmitted through the first MTP joint during gait, and the sesamoids are susceptible to inflammation, avascular necrosis, fracture, or sprain of bipartite sesamoid. Injury is usually seen in young athletes or dancers who repetitively push off the ball of their feet during jumping or ballet.[135] Presenting symptoms include pain with forefoot weight bearing and compensatory weight bearing on the lateral foot border. On examination there may be localized tenderness and swelling. Treatment includes rest, cryotherapy, NSAIDS, modified activity, modified footwear (wide toe box, stiff sole, low heel), orthoses (metatarsal bar, donut pad), and physiotherapy. Surgical excision of a sesamoid bone should be avoided unless significant osteonecrosis occurs.

Accessory Bones of the Foot

Accessory ossification centers in the foot and ankle are normal growth variants, and approximately 22% of children have at least one accessory bone.[200] They are commonly asymptomatic, but may become painful with activity.

Accessory navicular occurs in 2% to 21% of the general population, and is bilateral in 50% of cases.[201] When symptomatic, adolescents present with medial foot pain due to synchondrosis disruption and/or posterior tibialis tendinopathy and dysfunction. On examination, tenderness is localized over the prominent navicular and resisted strength testing of the posterior tibialis reproduces pain. Radiographs confirm the presence of an accessory navicular and MRI may show abnormal bony signal and bone marrow edema as well as changes in the synchondrosis, posterior tibialis tendon, and adjacent soft tissues.[201] Conservative treatment with physiotherapy and/or boot and rigid orthotics is usually successful. Surgical excision is considered for recalcitrant cases.

Failure of the secondary ossification center at the posterior aspect of the talus to fuse creates an os trigonum. It is usually unilateral and occurs in 7% to 25% of the population.[201] It can be congenital (persistent separation of secondary ossification center) or acquired (fracture nonunion). Most are asymptomatic, but children participating in sport involving repetitive ankle plantar flexion or inversion may complain of pain in the posterolateral ankle. On examination, tenderness is localized over the posterior talus and calcaneus, and there is pain with forced plantar flexion. Radiographs of the ankle, including a lateral view in plantar flexion show os trigonum and may show soft tissue swelling. CT is useful to delineate fractures or fragmentation and synchondrosis disruption. MRI is the best imaging modality to characterize posterior impingement of the talus that may involve soft tissue structures, including synovitis, capsular hypertrophy, and tenosynovitis.[202] Management of posterior impingement syndrome includes rest, NSAIDS, physiotherapy, taping, and orthopedic referral for possible resection.

MISCELLANEOUS

Traumatic Arthritis

Joint swelling associated with trauma usually occurs in older school-aged children and adolescents. Acute injury may result in hemorrhage from an intraarticular fracture, joint dislocation, or tear of a large intraarticular ligament. Chronic injury from overuse and/or structurally abnormal joints may cause transient joint swelling. JIA is far more common than traumatic arthritis in the very young.

Chondrolysis

Chondrolysis of the hip is characterized by pain and limp due to progressive loss of articular cartilage space by an undefined but presumed inflammatory process. It may be idiopathic or secondary to other hip pathology, particularly SCFE or LCP disease. Chondrolysis has also been associated with prolonged immobilization, severe trauma, septic arthritis, inflammatory arthritis, Marfan syndrome, and Stickler syndrome.[203] An association with spondyloarthropathy has been postulated but not confirmed; some authors consider this condition an independent subform of juvenile arthritis.[204]

Chondrolysis usually occurs in the second decade of life, girls are affected more than boys, and African Americans may be more severely affected.[203] Children present with unilateral hip pain, stiffness, limp,

and reduced hip range of motion in all planes. There are no systemic features and investigations (hematological, microbiological, immunological, and acute phase reactants) are normal. Early radiographs may be normal, and late radiographs show regional osteoporosis, premature closure of the femoral capital physis, narrowing of the joint space, and lateral overgrowth of the femoral head. Early MRI findings include a geometric region of abnormal signal intensity centered in the proximal femoral epiphysis, acetabular bone marrow edema, mild synovial hypertrophy, and minimal or no joint fluid.[205]

The natural history of chondrolysis is described in two distinct phases: an acute inflammatory phase (up to 18 months) characterized by joint inflammation, pain, and decreased range of motion; and a chronic phase (3 to 5 years). The chronic phase results in three different outcomes: restoration of joint space with clinical improvement; ankyloses of the hip with pain-free but limited function; and malpositioned ankyloses associated with pain and limited function.[203] Approximately 50% to 60% of patients recover with acceptable hip function, but many go on to develop painful and disabling osteoarthritis of the hip.[203] Management includes protective weight bearing, NSAIDs, physiotherapy, and orthopedic intervention, as necessary.[206] The role of intraarticular steroid injections is unclear, and there is no current treatment regimen with proven benefit.

Femoral Acetabular Impingement

Femoral acetabular impingement (FAI) is increasingly recognized as a cause of hip pain, dysfunction, and early degenerative hip disease. FAI describes abnormal dynamic contact between the femoral head and acetabular labrum due to a misalignment of the femoral and acetabular sides of the joint.[207] In FAI, osteophytes develop around the femoral head and/or along the acetabulum (Fig. 51-12). There are three types of FAI: CAM impingement due to a nonspherical femoral head; pincer impingement due to excessive acetabular covering; and a combination of both.[207,208] The prevalence of FAI is 10% to 15%, and it is more common in males.[207] It may be idiopathic or develop secondary to

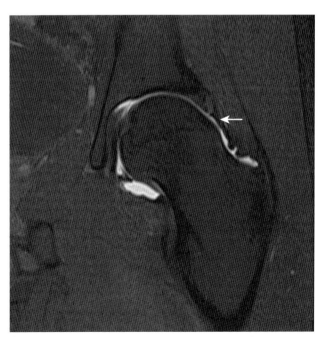

FIGURE 51-12 Femoral acetabular impingement. Coronal T1 fat-saturation sequence shows an abnormal bump at the femoral head/neck junction *(arrow)*, consistent with cam type femoroacetabular impingement. (Courtesy Dr. R. Cairns.)

primary hip disease, including LCP, SCFE, developmental dysplasia, prior infection, trauma, or JIA.

FAI usually presents in young adults with activity related groin pain, stiffness and limp. On examination there is reduced range of hip motion and positive impingement tests (hip flexion with adduction). If there is labral pathology, catching, locking or clicking may be present.

FAI is important in pediatrics because early radiographic changes may be apparent in adolescence. Management includes activity restriction, NSAIDS and physiotherapy. Surgery can correct FAI in some cases.

Growing Pains

Growing pains are the most common cause of episodic childhood musculoskeletal pain, affecting 3% to 37% of school-aged children.[209,210] The term *growing pains* is actually a misnomer, as the peak incidence of pain is in children between the ages of 3 to 12 years and not coincident with the peak adolescent growth period.[211-213] The term *benign idiopathic nocturnal pains of childhood* has been suggested; however, no generally accepted alternative term exists.[214-216] The cause of growing pains is not known but probably represents a pain amplification syndrome.[210] Children with growing pains are more likely to have abdominal pain and migraine.[217,218] A recent twin study of growing pains found familial occurrence and possible shared genetic determinants with restless leg syndrome.[219]

Children classically present with episodic nonarticular leg pain in the thigh, calf, or shin at night (Table 51-4). Pain is often bilateral and usually responds to massage and over-the-counter analgesics. Children are pain-free during the day and are normally active. Increased daily activity may be associated with episodes of growing pains.[220] The physical examination is normal during and between episodes and motor milestones are normal. There are no diagnostic tests and laboratory and radiography are normal. Growing pains are not associated with any organic disease but may have a significant impact on a family due to daytime fatigue, school and work absences, and chronic analgesia use.

As growing pains are a diagnosis of exclusion, it is important to rule out other causes. Investigations should be considered if there are atypical symptoms, including articular or unilateral pain, pain in the back or upper extremities, pain that is present during the day, daily pains (not episodic), systemic symptoms, or abnormalities on physical examination. Treatment includes education and reassurance that the pains are self-limited and benign. Over-the-counter analgesics, passive stretching and orthotics for children with hypermobility and pes planus may be helpful for symptom management.[221]

Restless Legs Syndrome

Restless legs syndrome (RLS), also known as Willis–Ekbom disease, is a sensorimotor disorder characterized by a strong irresistible urge to move the lower extremities. The prevalence of RLS in the pediatric population is 2% to 4%, with boys and girls equally affected in childhood and girls more commonly affected in late adolescence and young adulthood.[222,223] The cause is unknown, but a genetic mechanism is suggested by the high familial prevalence (40% to 92%) among individuals with RLS with onset before age 40.[224,225] In a pediatric population-based study, 71% of affected children aged 8 to 11 years and 80% of those aged 12 to 17 years reported a family history of RLS.[223]

Genome-wide studies report an association of RLS with genetic variants of BTBD9, MEIS1, and *MAP2K5/LBXCOR,* as well as a possible association with PTPRD and A2BP1.[226,227]

Brain dopamine dysfunction and low brain iron stores are hypothesized to play a role in RLS.[228] Increased prevalence of small intestinal bacterial overgrowth in controlled studies and case reports of postinfectious RLS have led some researchers to hypothesize an inflammatory/immune-mediated mechanism of disease.[229]

Revised criteria for pediatric RLS have been developed to include a description of characteristic leg discomfort in a child's own words.[230] Key diagnostic criteria include: the urge to move legs (usually accompanied by an uncomfortable sensation), symptoms begin or worsen during rest, symptoms are relieved with movement, symptoms occur in the evening or at night, symptoms are not accounted for by another medical or behavioral condition, and symptoms cause significant distress or functional impairment.[230]

Attention deficit hyperactivity disorder, depression, and anxiety are more common in children with RLS.[223,231] A recent twin study of growing pains found possible shared genetic determinants with restless leg syndrome, although the majority of children with growing pains are unlikely to have RLS.[219]

Management includes identification and discontinuation of possible triggering factors (seratonergic antidepressants, dopamine blockers, nonsedating antihistamines, nicotine, caffeine, alcohol, sleep deprivation), physical activity, and better sleep hygiene. In adults, there is good evidence to support the use of dopamine agonists and gabapentin.[232] In pediatrics, experts recommend a trial of iron therapy.[233] Of interest, a Cochrane Review did not find sufficient evidence for iron therapy in adult[234] but a smaller pediatric study (n = 97) reported iron supplementation is effective in treating RLS, with improvement or resolution of symptoms in approximately 4 months.[235]

Carpal Tunnel Syndrome

Carpal tunnel syndrome is a rare condition in children. A review of 163 cases found most were secondary to lysosomal storage diseases (58% mucopolysaccharidosis; 13% mucolipidosis) and the rest were secondary to a variety of syndromes, as well as posttraumatic and familial etiologies. Only one was rheumatologic; a patient with scleroderma.[236] Fabry's disease has been recently implicated with increased extracellular matrix material and inclusions of globotriaosylceramide (GL3) in retinacular fibroblasts causing compressive carpal tunnel symptoms despite enzyme replacement.[237]

Children with carpal tunnel syndrome often have atypical presentations with clumsiness or weakness, and wrist or hand pain. By the time of diagnosis, weakness and thenar wasting are often marked, suggesting longstanding compression. Physical examination should include provocative median nerve testing. A controlled study in adults with electrophysiologically confirmed carpal tunnel syndrome found that the wrist-flexion test (Phalen maneuver) was more sensitive, whereas the nerve-percussion test (Tinel sign) was least sensitive but more specific.[238] In children, these clinical tests are often normal, hence electrophysiological testing is essential. Operative release is often the only effective treatment in children, and some suggest that early surgery should be performed to minimize damage.[239]

TABLE 51-4	Growing Pains (Benign Nocturnal Pains of Childhood)
Age At Onset	4 to 12 years
Sex Ratio	Probably equal, slightly more girls in some series
Symptoms	Deep aching, cramping pain in thigh or calf, usually in the evening or during the night; never present in the morning; bilateral; responds to massage; and analgesia
Signs	Physical examination results are normal
Investigations	Laboratory and radiographical studies (if done) have normal results

Cervical Neurapraxia

Athletes participating in contact sports may experience brachial plexus or cervical nerve root injuries or a cervical cord neurapraxia. Athletes with the former ("stinger") present with transient burning pain or paresthesia in a unilateral shoulder and arm following a multidermatomal (usually C5-C6) distribution, often associated with weakness of the proximal arm muscles.[240] "Stingers" represent a stretching injury of the brachial plexus by contralateral neck flexion or a direct blow to this neural tissue. Alternatively, cervical nerve root compression at the neural foramen occurs from ipsilateral C-spine side flexion or neck extension with contralateral rotation. These are diagnosed clinically and imaging is not required unless symptoms persist, there are neurological deficits, or the athlete has two or more episodes. MRI is helpful to identify foraminal narrowing or disk herniation and can distinguish compression on the brachial plexus or enlargement of the "stretched" neural structures with increased T2 signal intensity.[241] Electrodiagnostic studies may be useful in differentiating cervical radiculopathy from brachial plexopathy for those with persistent weakness. Most athletes are able to continue contact sport after a single "stinger" that resolves quickly. For those with more complex episodes or persistence of symptoms, the extent and recovery of any associated neurological deficit, recurrence pattern, and anatomical factors determine return to play.[242]

Cervical cord neurapraxia is described as a spinal cord contusion resulting in transient bilateral upper extremity paresthesias with variable motor weakness. The mechanism of injury is neck hyperextension and/or axial load. Although affected children may have hypermobile ligaments, central canal spinal stenosis must be ruled out through MRI or CT myelography.[240] Athletes with transient symptoms and no evidence of cervical spinal stenosis can return to full sporting activity.

Neuralgic Amyotrophy

Neuralgic amyotrophy (brachial plexus neuritis) is a rare peripheral nerve disorder with an incidence of 2 to 3 per 100,000 individuals in the general population.[243] Age of onset is usually the second or third decade, but it can occur in children. Over 96% of cases present with acute episodes of extreme pain in the upper extremities, neck, and/or trunk, usually lasting 4 weeks followed by shooting pains to the arms or trunk that dissipate over a period of weeks to months.[243] Typically there is also multifocal paresis and atrophy of the upper extremity muscles. One third of cases demonstrate asymmetric bilateral motor, sensory, and autonomic symptoms.

The pathogenesis is unknown but seems to involve an interaction between genetic predisposition, an autoimmune trigger, and mechanical vulnerability. Idiopathic forms may be preceded by infection, vaccination, pregnancy, and immunotherapy, suggesting an inflammatory process. Peripheral sensory nerve biopsies support this theory, showing T-cell infiltrates in the epineural perivascular tissue, elevated terminal complement components, and low levels of C3 and CD8 T suppressor cells. Biomechanical triggers have included physical exercise and overuse of the upper extremity in the work setting. The hereditary type, with mutations in the SEPT9 gene on chromosome 17q25, is found in over 50% of patients. This type is thought to be 10 times less common than the idiopathic forms and may be associated with dysmorphic features and short stature.

Investigations to support the diagnosis include electromyography, nerve conduction studies, and MRI.[244] Thickening and patches of brachial plexus hyperintensity have been seen on MRI performed early in the course of this disease and are thought to represent plexitis. Administration of oral prednisolone within the first month of an attack can shorten the duration of pain and accelerate recovery. A physical therapist and physiatrist can provide the necessary rehabilitation to minimize risk of permanent joint contractures and any associated musculoskeletal pain. This process may respond to NSAIDs. Patients with neuralgic amyotrophy recover up to 90% of their prior health after 2 to 3 years but more than 70% are left with residual paresis and exercise intolerance.[243] Almost half experience persistent pain, about one third of patients have severe fatigue and one quarter develop recurrent episodes within two years of onset.

REFERENCES

1. J.A. Kirk, B.M. Ansell, E.G. Bywaters, The hypermobility syndrome. Musculoskeletal complaints associated with generalized joint hypermobility, Ann. Rheum. Dis. 26 (1967) 419–425.
2. P. Beighton, L. Solomon, C.L. Soskolne, Articular mobility in an African population, Ann. Rheum. Dis. 32 (1973) 413–418.
4. M.C. Scheper, R. Engelbert, E.A. Rameckers, et al., Children with generalised joint hypermobility and musculoskeletal complaints: state of the art on diagnostics, clinical characteristics, and treatment, Biomed. Res. Int. 2013 (2013) 121054.
5. G. McCluskey, E. O'Kane, D. Hann, et al., Hypermobility and musculoskeletal pain in children: a systematic review, Scand. J. Rheumatol. 41 (2012) 329–338.
8. M. Castori, S. Morlino, C. Celletti, et al., Re-writing the natural history of pain and related symptoms in the joint hypermobility syndrome/Ehlers-Danlos syndrome, hypermobility type, Am. J. Med. Genet. A 161 (2013) 2989–3004.
9. A. Fikree, Q. Aziz, R. Grahame, Joint hypermobility syndrome, Rheum. Dis. Clin. North Am. 39 (2013) 419–430.
11. L. Westling, A. Mattiasson, General joint hypermobility and temporomandibular joint derangement in adolescents, Ann. Rheum. Dis. 51 (1992) 87–90.
14. S. Falkerslev, C. Baagø, T. Alkjær, et al., Dynamic balance during gait in children and adults with Generalized Joint Hypermobility, Clin. Biomech. 28 (2013) 318–324.
15. L.D. Jelsma, R.H. Geuze, M.H. Klerks, et al., The relationship between joint mobility and motor performance in children with and without the diagnosis of developmental coordination disorder, BMC Pediatr. 13 (2013) 35.
16. R. Grahame, H. Bird, A. Child, The revised (Brighton 1998) criteria for the diagnosis of benign joint hypermobility syndrome (BJHS), J. Rheumatol. 27 (2000) 1777.
19. L.M. Barton, H.A. Bird, Improving pain by the stabilization of hyperlax joints, J. Orthop. Rheumatol. 9 (1996) 46–51.
21. L.T. Staheli, D.E. Chew, M. Corbett, The longitudinal arch. A survey of eight hundred and eighty-two feet in normal children and adults, J. Bone Joint Surg. Am. 69 (1987) 426–428.
26. H.B. Menz, A.B. Dufour, J.L. Riskowski, et al., Association of Planus Foot Posture and Pronated Foot Function With Foot Pain: The Framingham Foot Study, Arthritis Care Res. 65 (2013) 1991–1999.
29. D.R. Wenger, D. Mauldin, G. Speck, et al., Corrective shoes and inserts as treatment for flexible flatfoot in infants and children.[see comment], J. Bone Joint Surg. Am. 71 (1989) 800–810.
31. A.D. Cass, C.A. Camasta, A review of tarsal coalition and pes planovalgus: clinical examination, diagnostic imaging, and surgical planning, J. Foot Ankle Surg. 49 (2010) 274–293.
34. J.K. Loudon, H.L. Goist, K.L. Loudon, Genu recurvatum syndrome, J. Orthop. Sports Phys. Ther. 27 (1998) 361–367.
37. R.H. Engelbert, C.S. Uiterwaal, E. van de Putte, et al., Pediatric generalized joint hypomobility and musculoskeletal complaints: a new entity? Clinical, biochemical, and osseal characteristics, Pediatrics 113 (2004) 714–719.
42. M. Rathleff, S. Skuldbol, M. Rasch, et al., Care-seeking behaviour of adolescents with knee pain: a population-based study among 504 adolescents, BMC Musculoskelet. Disord. 14 (2013) 225.

44. N. Lankhorst, S. Bierma-Zeinstra, M. van Middelkoop, Factors associated with patellofemoral pain syndrome: a systematic review, Br. J. Sports Med. 47 (2013) 193–206.

47. R.A. van der Heijden, N.E. Lankhorst, R. van Linschoten, et al., Exercise for treating patellofemoral pain syndrome [Protocol], Cochrane Database Syst. Rev. 2 (2013)

50. N. Swart, R. van Linschoten, S. Bierma-Zeinstra, M. van Middelkoop, The additional effect of orthotic devices on exercise therapy for patients with patellofemoral pain syndrome: a systematic review, Br. J. Sports Med. 46 (2012) 570–577.

51. C.B. Hing, T.O. Smith, S. Donell, F. Song, Surgical versus non-surgical interventions for treating patellar dislocation, Cochrane Database Syst. Rev. 11 (2011)

56. M.E.H. Larsson, I. Käll, K. Nilsson-Helander, Treatment of patellar tendinopathy: a systematic review of randomized controlled trials, Knee Surg. Sports Traumatol. Arthrosc. 20 (2012) 1632–1646.

57. W. Strash, R. Perez, Extracorporeal shockwave therapy for chronic proximal plantar fasciitis, Clin. Podi. Med. Surg. 19 (2002) 467–476.

61. T.G. Sanders, M.B. Zlatkin, Avulsion injuries of the pelvis, Semin. Musculoskelet. Radiol. 12 (2008) 42–53.

65. J.I. Kessler, H. Nikizad, K.G. Shea, et al., The demographics and epidemiology of osteochondritis dissecans of the knee in children and adolescents, Am. J. Sports Med. 2013 (2013)

67. J.W. Milgram, Radiological and pathological manifestations of osteochondritis dissecans of the distal femur. A study of 50 cases, Radiology 126 (1978) 305–311.

69. A.L. Berndt, M. Harty, Transchondral fractures (osteochondritis dissecans) of the talus, J. Bone Joint Surg. Am. 41 (1959) 988–1020.

72. H.G. Chambers, K.G. Shea, A.F. Anderson, et al., American Academy of Orthopaedic Surgeons Clinical Practice Guideline on the diagnosis and treatment of osteochondritis dissecans, J. Am. Acad. Orthop. Surg. 94 (2012) 1322–1324.

73. J.I. Kessler, H. Nikizad, K.G. Shea, et al., The demographics, epidemiology, and incidence of progression to surgery of osteochondritis dissecans of the knee in children and adolescents, Orthop. J. Sports Med. 1 (2013)

77. M. Winters, M. Eskes, A. Weir, et al., Treatment of medial tibial stress syndrome: a systematic review, Sports Med. 43 (2013) 1315–1333.

79. D.S. Patel, M. Roth, N. Kapil, Stress fractures: diagnosis, treatment, and prevention, Am. Fam. Physician 83 (2011) 39–46.

83. R.H. Daffner, B.N. Weissman, M. Appel, et al., ACR appropriateness criteria; stress (fatigue/insufficiency) fracture, including sacrum, excluding other vertebrae, Agency for Healthcare Research and Quality (AHRQ), American College of Radiology, 1/10/2014. Available at: <http://www.guideline.gov/content.aspx?id=32618&search=stress+fracture>. Accessed January 10, 2014, 2014.

84. K. Rome, H.H. Handoll, R. Ashford, Interventions for preventing and treating stress fractures and stress reactions of bone of the lower limbs in young adults, Cochrane Database Syst. Rev. (2005) CD000450

86. D.C. Osbahr, H.J. Kim, J.R. Dugas, Little league shoulder, Curr. Opin. Pediatr. 22 (2010) 35–40.

89. N.A. Kotnis, M.M. Chiavaras, S. Harish, Lateral epicondylitis and beyond: imaging of lateral elbow pain with clinical-radiologic correlation, Skeletal Radiol. 41 (2012) 369–386.

93. R.M. Greiwe, C. Saifi, C.S. Ahmad, Pediatric sports elbow injuries, Clin. Sports Med. 29 (2010) 677–703.

98. M.B.F. Son, R.P. Sundel, Musculoskeletal causes of pediatric chest pain, Pediatr. Clin. North Am. 57 (2010) 1385–1395.

103. I. Calvo-Muñoz, A. Gómez-Conesa, J. Sánchez-Meca, Prevalence of low back pain in children and adolescents: a meta-analysis, BMC Pediatr. 13 (2013) 14.

108. B.M. Haus, L.J. Micheli, pain in the pediatric and adolescent athlete, Clin. Sports Med. 31 (2012) 423–440.

110. J. De Mauroy, H. Weiss, A. Aulisa, et al., 7th SOSORT consensus paper: conservative treatment of idiopathic & Scheuermann's kyphosis, Scoliosis 5 (2010) 9.

115. S.J. Spencer, N.I. Wilson, Childhood discitis in a regional children's hospital, J. Pediatr. Orthop. B 21 (2012) 264–268.

122. R.S. Siffert, Classification of the osteochondroses, Clin. Orthop. Relat. Res. 158 (1981) 10–18.

131. A.M. James, C.M. Williams, T.P. Haines, Effectiveness of interventions in reducing pain and maintaining physical activity in children and adolescents with calcaneal apophysitis (Sever's disease): a systematic review, J. Foot Ankle Res. 6 (2013) 16.

135. E.G. Manusov, W.A. Lillegard, R.F. Raspa, T.D. Epperly, Evaluation of pediatric foot problems: Part I. The forefoot and the midfoot, Am. Fam. Physician 54 (1996) 592–606.

151. J. Calve, On a particular form of pseudo-coxalgia associated with a characteristic deformity of the upper end of the femur, Clin. Orthop. Relat. Res. 451 (1910) 14–16.

177. J.A. Herring, H.T. Kim, R. Browne, Legg-Calvé-Perthes disease. Part I: Classification of radiographs with use of the modified lateral pillar and Stulberg classifications, J. Bone Joint Surg. Am. 86 (2004) 2103–2120.

178. J.A. Herring, H.T. Kim, R. Browne, Legg-Calvé-Perthes disease. Part II: Prospective multicenter study of the effect of treatment on outcome.[see comment], J. Bone Joint Surg. Am. 86 (2004) 2121–2134.

179. A.N. Larson, D.J. Sucato, J.A. Herring, et al., A prospective multicenter study of legg-calvé-perthes disease functional and radiographic outcomes of nonoperative treatment at a mean follow-up of twenty years, J. Am. Acad. Orthop. Surg. 94 (2012) 584–592.

181. C.L. Lehmann, R.R. Arons, R.T. Loder, M.G. Vitale, The epidemiology of slipped capital femoral epiphysis: an update, J. Pediatr. Orthop. 26 (2006) 286–290.

183. R.A. Reynolds, Diagnosis and treatment of slipped capital femoral epiphysis.[see comment], Curr. Opin. Pediatr. 11 (1999) 80–83.

192. C.R. Fraitzl, W. Käfer, M. Nelitz, H. Reichel, Radiological evidence of femoroacetabular impingement in mild slipped capital femoral epiphysis a mean follow-up of 14.4 years after pinning in situ, J. Bone Joint Surg. Br. 89 (2007) 1592–1596.

196. D. Biko, A. Miller, V. Ho-Fung, D. Jaramillo, MRI of congenital and developmental abnormalities of the knee, Clin. Radiol. 67 (2012) 1198–1206.

205. T. Laor, A.H. Crawford, Idiopathic chondrolysis of the hip in children: early MRI findings, AJR Am. J. Roentgenol. 192 (2009) 526–531.

207. C.N. Anderson, G.M. Riley, G.E. Gold, M.R. Safran, Hip-femoral acetabular impingement, Clin. Sports Med. 32 (2013) 409–425.

208. D. Hendry, E. England, K. Kenter, R.D. Wissman, Femoral acetabular impingement, Semin. Roentgenol. 48 (2013) 158–166.

209. A.M. Evans, S.D. Scutter, Prevalence of "growing pains" in young children. [Review] [22 refs], J. Pediatr. 145 (2004) 255–258.

211. J.M. Naish, J. Apley, "Growing pains": a clinical study of non-arthritic limb pains in children, Arch. Dis. Child. 26 (1951) 134–140.

233. E. Frenette, Restless legs syndrome in children: a review and update on pharmacological options, Curr. Pharm. Des. 17 (2011) 1436–1442.

236. N. Van Meir, L. De Smet, Carpal tunnel syndrome in children.[see comment], J. Pediatr. Orthop. B 14 (2005) 42–45.

243. N. van Alfen, Clinical and pathophysiological concepts of neuralgic amyotrophy, Nat. Rev. Neurol. 7 (2011) 315–322.

Entire reference list is available online at www.expertconsult.com.

CHAPTER 52

Pain Amplification Syndromes

David D. Sherry

Pediatric rheumatologists encounter children with acute and chronic pain for which an overt primary cause for the pain cannot be found. In these disorders the pain seems disproportional or amplified. In this chapter, the approach and evaluation of pain in children will be addressed, followed by a review of the presentation and treatment of children with amplified musculoskeletal pain syndromes.

HISTORICAL REVIEW

Chronic musculoskeletal pain in children received scant attention until the latter half of the twentieth century. In 1951, Naish and Apley published their landmark study on pediatric limb pains due to nonarthritic causes,[1] in which they considered emotional factors to play a causative role. Since then, it has been increasingly recognized that a significant number of children suffer from both chronic and amplified musculoskeletal pain.[2,3] Reflex sympathetic dystrophy (complex regional pain syndrome [CRPS]) was first described in a child in 1971.[4] This 12-year-old girl had resolution of all signs and symptoms of CRPS on the day she was to see the psychiatrist, an indicator of the psychological aspects of this condition. The first description of childhood fibromyalgia was published in 1985.[5] CRPS and fibromyalgia are the subject of most studies, whereas other, less clearly classified amplified musculoskeletal pain conditions are less frequently reported.[6-8]

DEFINITION AND CLASSIFICATION

In this chapter, the term *amplified musculoskeletal pain* is used because it is descriptive, does not presume an etiology, and differentiates children from adults with chronic pain. The word *amplified* refers to the idea that the body amplifies the pain and does not imply that the child is willfully exaggerating the symptoms.

Current terms used to describe these conditions are inadequate and confusing because many children have features that are shared among different subsets.[6,8] Children are categorized depending on the presence of physical features (e.g., the presence of overt autonomic signs, number of painful points with a variety of systemic symptoms) or location (localized [one or two body regions] or diffuse [three or more body regions]).[6,7,9,10] At times, the different terms used to describe these conditions can be helpful in defining a specific subset of children with amplified pain for studies; however, there is a great deal of similarity between the subsets of amplified pain regarding the presentation, evaluation, and treatment.[7,10]

When evaluating any particular study of pain amplification, it is important to know which classification criteria were used (Box 52-1). Discrete subsets exist in each of the groups. Specifically, criteria for diffuse idiopathic musculoskeletal pain include those with fibromyalgia, and localized idiopathic musculoskeletal pain includes those with

CRPS. Children with intermittent amplified musculoskeletal pain in whom the criterion for duration is not satisfied are nevertheless included in some reports due to the severity of their pain and marked dysfunction that may reoccur over years.[11] Because CRPS and fibromyalgia are very distinctive and each has its own literature, these terms are used in this chapter when discussing these specific subsets.

There are two kinds of CRPS: type I and type II.[9] Type II CRPS is similar to the older term causalgia and implies the presence of nerve damage. It is exceedingly rare in children and all subsequent discussion refers to CRPS Type I. Many children present with more than one form of amplified pain such as CRPS of a limb and localized pain to the back or abdomen or even total body pain. Some children meet the definition for both fibromyalgia and CRPS but actually there is only one underlying condition (e.g., amplified pain); however, both have overlapping clinical characteristics, demographics, and response to therapy.[6,15]

EPIDEMIOLOGY

Incidence and Prevalence

Population surveys of school children confirm that musculoskeletal pain is common; back pain occurs in as many as 20%, and limb pain has been reported in 16%.[2,16,17] A systematic review noted the prevalence of chronic and recurrent musculoskeletal pain in up to 40% of children.[18] Fibromyalgia, and widespread pain, has been reported to have a frequency in children and adolescents of 2% to 6%.[19-23] The incidence of complex regional pain syndrome in adults is estimated to be 5 to 26 per 100,000.[24,25] There are no data regarding the incidence of childhood CRPS or specific data regarding the other amplified musculoskeletal pain syndromes, but 5% to 8% of new patients presenting to North American pediatric rheumatology centers most likely have a form of amplified musculoskeletal pain.[26-28] Many pediatric rheumatologists believe they are seeing increasing numbers of children with amplified musculoskeletal pain in the past two decades, although this may represent a recall bias.

Age at Onset

Amplified musculoskeletal pain has been described in patients as young as 2 years of age, but the majority of reports involve children in late childhood and adolescence.[5,6,8,29-33] Older adolescents may be underrepresented in pediatric series, presumably because they are referred to adult specialists.

Sex Ratio

Girls are more commonly affected than boys in a ratio of approximately 4:1,[5,6,8,29,31-33] and the difference increases with age.[18,34,35] Because women seek medical advice more often than men, there may be a

---

BOX 52-1   Sets of Criteria for Different Subsets of Amplified Musculoskeletal Pain

Budapest Clinical Diagnostic Criteria for Complex Regional Pain[12]

All of the Following Four Criteria Must Be Met:

1. The patient has continuing pain, which is disproportionate to any inciting event.
2. The patient has at least one sign in two or more of the categories below.
   - Sensory: hyperalgesia or allodynia
   - Vasomotor: asymmetric temperature or skin color
   - Sudomotor/edema: edema or asymmetric sweating
   - Motor/trophic: decreased range of motion, motor dysfunction, or trophic changes (hair, skin, nail)
3. The patient reports at least one symptom in three or more of the categories below.
   - Sensory: reports hyperesthesia or allodynia
   - Vasomotor: reports asymmetric temperature or skin color
   - Motor/trophic: reports decreased range of motion, motor dysfunction, or trophic changes
4. No other diagnosis can better explain the signs and symptoms.

1990 American College of Rheumatology Criteria for Fibromyalgia[13]

Both Criteria Must Be Satisfied

1. Widespread pain (bilateral, and above and below the waist and axial pain) present for at least 3 months
2. Pain (not tenderness) upon digital palpation with 4 kg of pressure on 11 of the following 18 sites:
   - Occiput: at insertion of suboccipital muscle
   - Low cervical: at anterior aspect of the intertransverse spaces of C5-C7
   - Trapezius: at the midpoint of the upper border
   - Second rib: just lateral to the second costochondral junction at the upper rib border
   - Scapula: the medial border just above the spine of the scapula
   - Lateral epicondyle: 2 cm distal to the epicondyle
   - Gluteal: in the upper outer quadrant of the buttocks

- Greater Trochanter: 1 cm posterior to the trochanteric prominence
- Knees: at the medial fat pad 1 cm proximal to the joint mortise

2010 American College of Rheumatology Criteria for Fibromyalgia[14]

All Three Conditions Must Be Satisfied:

1. Absence of a disorder to explain the pain
2. Symptoms present for 3 months
3. At least one of the following
   - Widespread pain* index ≥7 and symptom severity score ≥5
   - Widespread pain* index 3-6 and symptom severity score ≥9

Yunus & Masi Criteria for Childhood Fibromyalgia[5]

All Four Major and Three Minor or the First Three Major and Four Painful Sites and Five Minor Need to Satisfied

Major:

1. Generalized musculoskeletal aching at three or more sites for three or more months
2. Absence of underlying condition or cause
3. Normal laboratory tests
4. Five or more typical tender points (see sites under 1990 ACR criteria above)

Minor:

1. Chronic anxiety or tension
2. Fatigue
3. Poor Sleep
4. Chronic headaches
5. Irritable bowel syndrome
6. Subjective soft tissue swelling
7. Numbness
8. Pain modulation by physical activities
9. Pain modulation by weather factors
10. Pain modulation by anxiety or stress

*Widespread pain equals the number of areas of pain in the last week (scale: 0-19). Areas include: shoulder girdle, upper arm, lower arm, buttocks/trochanter, upper leg, lower leg, jaw, upper back, lower back (2 points if bilateral) and 1 point each for chest, abdomen, neck. Symptom severity score (0-12).
Fatigue, waking unrefreshed, cognitive symptoms scored 0 to 3 each.
(0 = no problem, 1 = mild or intermittent, 2 equals moderate or considerable, 3 = severe, continuous).
Plus considering a host of somatic symptoms rated as 0 = no symptoms, 1 = few symptoms, 2 = moderate number of symptoms, 3 = great deal of symptoms (somatic symptoms include muscle pain, irritable bowel syndrome, tiredness, thinking problems, muscle weakness, headache, abdominal pain, numbness and tingling, dizziness, insomnia, depression, constipation, upper abdominal pain, nausea, nervousness, chest pain, blurred vision, fever, diarrhea, dry mouth, itching, wheezing, Raynaud phenomenon, hives, tenderness, vomiting, heartburn, oral ulcers, dysgeusia, seizures, xerophthalmia, shortness of breath, loss of appetite, rash, sensitivity, hearing difficulties, easy bruising, hair loss, urinary frequency, dysuria, bladder spasms).

---

selection bias; however, given the disability involved, this is most likely not a major factor in children. In Finland, predictors of widespread pain in children were older age, being female, reporting more depressive symptoms, and having back pain.[18,23]

Geographic and Racial Distribution

There have been no formal investigations regarding the relationship of amplified pain syndromes to ethnicity; however, a series from Philadelphia reported a disproportionate number of white patients (15 of 15).[36] All reports are from developed countries and comparisons with developing nations are not possible.[37]

ETIOLOGY AND PATHOGENESIS

The cause, or causes, of amplified musculoskeletal pain syndromes are unknown. Childhood pain syndromes seem to differ from those occurring in adults. For example, compared to adults, children with CRPS more frequently have lower rather than upper extremity involvement, the technetium bone scintigraphy shows decreased rather than increased uptake, and in both complex regional pain syndrome and fibromyalgia, children have different outcomes.[38,39] Children respond more readily to physical and occupational therapy.[8,11,29,31,36,38] Nevertheless, in many children, as in adults, these syndromes seem to be causally related to injury, illness, or psychological distress, either singly or in combination.

Physical Trauma

Injury, including surgery, frequently precedes complex regional pain syndrome in adults, and minor injury is commonly reported in children. Rarely, overt trauma may be the inciting event.[40-43] Minor trauma may play a role in localizing the site of amplified musculoskeletal pain. CRPS has been reported following vaccinations.[44-46] An adult developed CRPS following a corticosteroid injection for tenosynovitis.[47] Children who are hypermobile may be at increased risk of developing the fibromyalgia form of amplified musculoskeletal pain, perhaps due to chronic microtrauma; however, Mikkelsson et al. found no relationship between hypermobility and musculoskeletal pain in 1637 grade 3 and grade 5 Finnish children.[44,48-50]

The role of ischemia in the production of pain in CRPS and fibromyalgia has been a recurring theme. Ischemic injury has been noted on biopsy, and decreased blood flow to the painful region has been demonstrated by contrast-enhanced ultrasound.[45,46,51,52]

Comorbidities

Amplified musculoskeletal pain has been observed in children with a variety of illnesses,[17,53] including arthritis, cerebral palsy, muscular dystrophy, new-onset diabetes, systemic lupus erythematosus, and leukemia. These associations may or may not be coincidental. A series of eight children with mitochondrial disease had CRPS in the setting of multiple other, generally neurologic, symptoms.[54] There are abnormalities in the mitochondria in the muscles of adults with end-stage CRPS who underwent amputation, but their significance is not clear because none had other symptoms to suggest mitochondrial dysfunction.[55]

Sleep Disorders

Fibromyalgia was thought to be a manifestation of a sleep disorder, and many adults and children with fibromyalgia have abnormal polysomnography, specifically, increased α-δ sleep.[5,53,56] However,[57] children who resolved their fibromyalgia with an intense exercise program had normal sleep but no change in the abnormal amount of α-δ sleep.[58] Likewise, sleep abnormalities are not always present, and treating the sleep disorder does not correlate with improvement in symptoms.[57] Only three of 108 (3%) consecutive adult patients presenting to a disorder sleep clinic had fibromyalgia, which is similar to the normal population.[59] Therefore, sleep does not seem to play a role in the etiology of amplified pain.

Psychological Factors

Psychological distress is a recurring theme in most reports of children with amplified musculoskeletal pain, although controlled studies are lacking.[1,8,29,32,44,60-68] School is more stressful in children with amplified pain than in those with chronic arthritis.[32,60,69] Missing school is a frequent problem and can be the nidus for school avoidance.[70] Children with amplified pain may have inappropriate roles within the school (taking classes that are too advanced) or family (caretakers, peacemakers, or being overly busy).[8,32,71] Clearly, there are children and families who are overtly psychologically dysfunctional or distressed, but whether this is the cause of, the effect of, or unrelated to the development of an amplified musculoskeletal pain syndrome is not known. Two Finnish population studies indicate that children who are depressed subsequently develop chronic pain or fibromyalgia.[23,72] Geertzen et al. found 79% of patients with CRPS to have recent stressful life events compared to 21% of controls.[73] Stress directly relates to the endocrine and immune system and may play a pivotal role in some of the mechanisms discussed below.[74] However, it is important to note that not all families with a child with amplified pain are inappropriately distressed.

Gender Differences

The reason girls are more frequently affected is not clear. Contraceptive or hormonal replacement therapy is not associated with fibromyalgia, nor are there differences in estrogen, progesterone, luteal hormone, follicular-stimulating hormone, or testosterone during the menstrual cycle between women with fibromyalgia and controls.[75,76] However, stress hormones may be at play in fibromyalgia because patients have lower baseline cortisol levels and lower expression of corticosteroid receptors.[77] Women with fibromyalgia reporting childhood abuse have higher diurnal cortisol.[78] Girls have lower pain thresholds as well as differences in coping and cultural expectations, especially in Western countries.[19,79-81] Girls are also more frequently hypermobile but hypermobility may or may not be associated with amplified pain.[48-50,82-85]

Neurologic Abnormalities

Amplified pain is related to increased sympathetic nervous system activity and α-adrenoceptor responsiveness.[86-90] Deconditioning increases sympathetic tone, which leads to ischemia, which can be ameliorated by exercise.[91] Ackerman and Ahmad studied the sympathetic activity with laser Doppler imaging in adults who had CRPS following carpal tunnel surgery who required repeat surgery.[92] Of those with increased sympathetic activity, eight of 11 had recurrent CRPS, whereas only three of 23 with normal sympathetic activity had recurrent CRPS. It is postulated that this may be modulated at the level of the spinal cord.[93]

Functional magnetic resonance imaging (fMRI) has shown abnormal activation in the basal ganglia and parietal lobe in children with CRPS and that these abnormalities persist when the children are symptom-free, possibly partially explaining the risk for recurrent CRPS.[94,95] Adults with fibromyalgia showed enhanced brain activity as measured by magnetoencephalography when presented with a painful stimulus.[96] Many patients complain of inability to concentrate and Maihofner et al. showed decreased tactile learning in adults with CRPS.[97] LeBel suggests there are significant brain circuitry changes in the "CRPS brain."[94] This may be another factor in creating central sensitization in which neurons regulating the pain pathway are hyperexcitable.[98] Quantitative sensory testing in children suggests central sensitization may play a significant role.[99] Browning et al. surmise that neuroimaging may eventually help classify somatoform disorders such as the amplified pain syndromes.[100]

There is recent evidence of small fiber dysfunction in fibromyalgia and CRPS manifested by decreased intraepidural nerve fiber density.[101,102] Oaklander et al. has also reported this phenomenon in children with a host of somatic, neurologic, and immunologic abnormalities and in erythromelalgia.[102,103] It is unknown if this is a primary process or an epiphenomenon.

Inflammation and Immune Response

There has been recent interest in the role of inflammation in the amplified pain syndromes.[104] There is localized, but not systemic, cytokine imbalance with high levels of TNFα and IL-6 in experimentally obtained blister fluid from the involved limb compared to the uninvolved limb and in skin biopsies, but not serum, in adults with CRPS; however, the degree of TNFα and IL-6 did not correlate with clinical characteristics or the duration of CRPS.[105-107] Autoantibodies directed against sympathetic and myenteric plexus neurons have been found in 13 of 30 (43%) adult patients with CRPS but none of 30 controls and in only one of 20 patients with noninflammatory neuropathy, such as in diabetes, and in one of 20 patients with peripheral nerve lesions.[108] Involvement of the innate immune system is suggested by the presence of elevated L-selectin on monocytes and elevated spontaneous hydrogen peroxide production by neutrophils in adults with fibromyalgia.[109,110]

Genetic Background

Amplified musculoskeletal pain syndromes have been described in siblings, parent–child pairs, spouses, and multiple family members.[61,111-117] Buskila et al. noted fibromyalgia in 28% of 58 offspring of 20 mothers with fibromyalgia. Pellegrino and colleagues reported that 52% of 50 parents or siblings of 17 patients with primary fibromyalgia also had fibromyalgia, and a set of identical twins developed fibromyalgia within 6 months of each other.[112,115] Others have noted that not only fibromyalgia but other chronic pain conditions are more common in family members of children with fibromyalgia.[118] In the Netherlands, 31 families were identified with up to five family members with CPRS, but a clear mode of inheritance was not observed.[119] No particular gene has been implicated, although one small study of CRPS suggested that women with HLA-DR2(15) may be more resistant to treatment.[120] There is interest in the role of catechol-O-methyltransferase (COMT) because it controls the metabolism of catecholamines. COMT polymorphisms found in fibromyalgia may influence the degree of central sensitization, psychological distress, and outcome.[121-124] If genetic factors are important in amplified pain conditions, it is probable that multiple genetic polymorphisms are involved that predispose the individual to develop amplified pain when inciting environmental and cultural factors are present.

EVALUATION OF MUSCULOSKELETAL PAIN

Pain is the subjective expression of an unpleasant sensation or emotional experience associated with actual or perceived tissue damage.[9] It is difficult, if not impossible, for an observer to know with any certainty to what extent another person is in pain. Although parents and children tend to make a similar assessment of the degree of pain, parents may over- or underestimate their child's pain in relation to the child's own self-report. An important premise in the evaluation and management of a child in pain is that the child's report of pain and its severity must be accepted at face value. "Pain is what the patient says it is, and exists when he says it does."[125] Prolonged malingering in childhood is exceedingly rare. Effective management requires that the child knows that he or she is believed. Many interacting issues determine whether a child's pain disturbs the child's and the family's functioning, and when, if ever, medical help is sought (Fig. 52-1).

Many children with pain amplification have been seen by multiple healthcare providers, have undergone multiple investigations, and have failed multiple therapeutic trials before the correct diagnosis is made. Unfortunately, attempts to identify an increasingly rare and unlikely cause for the pain or escalating empiric treatment aimed at organic pain can result in perpetuating the amplified pain.

History and Physical Examination

It is imperative to obtain a complete history of pain-related symptoms (Box 52-2), as well as a complete past history and review of systems, and to perform a directed physical examination to ascertain the child's overall health status. This is especially important in children with amplified pain because it is the initial step in establishing a trusting relationship with the child and family, who often feel that their concerns have not been considered seriously. A few key observations to be made during the physical examination are listed in Box 52-3.

Amplified pain is a clinical diagnosis with the presence and absence of salient features (Box 52-4). Although there are differences between

---

> **BOX 52-2 History of Musculoskeletal Pain**
>
> **What Is the Character of the Pain?**
> Which body parts are painful?
> How long has it been present?
> Is the pain getting better, worse, or staying the same?
> What makes the pain better?
> What makes the pain worse?
> Is there diurnal variation in the severity of the pain?
> Is the pain present at night and if so, does it waken him or her?
> Does the pain interfere with function, and if so, what specifically?
> What descriptive terms are used to describe the pain?
> Does the pain radiate, migrate, or spread?
> Is the painful area tender to touch or to clothing?
> Is the painful area either cool or warm to the touch?
> Does the painful part look abnormal or swollen?
> What is the child's or parent's assessment of the pain severity?
>
> **Are There Other Symptoms?**
> Fever?
> Rash?
> Change in gastrointestinal function?
> Weight loss?
> Upper or lower respiratory tract symptoms?
> Muscle weakness?
> Sleep disturbance?
> Depression?
> Anxiety?
>
> **Family and Social History**
> Ankylosing spondylitis, reactive arthritis, or inflammatory bowel disease?
> Back pain, heel pain, or acute iritis?
> Psoriasis?
> Fibromyalgia, complex regional pain syndrome or other chronic pain condition?
> Is there an identifiable stressor in the family, school, or peer group?
> Are there significant or recent life changes?
> Where is the child sleeping?
> What activities does the child participate in and how busy are they during the week?
> How does the child perform in school?
> How do the parents describe the child's personality?
> If there was inciting injury, is there a lawsuit in place or contemplated?

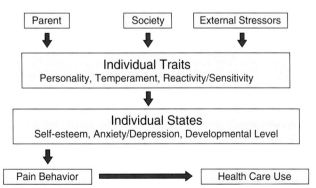

FIGURE 52-1 Factors influencing pain nexpression and seeking health care.

BOX 52-3 The Clinical Examination: Several Key Observations

Does the child look well or ill?

Is the child's affect consistent with the reported level of pain?

Does the child exhibit *la belle indifference*?

Is there any joint swelling?

Is there any muscle weakness or atrophy?

Is there any tenderness to palpation and if so, is it over joints, entheses, or muscles?

Is there any area of allodynia, and if so, is the area constant or does it vary over time?

Is there any color, temperature or perspiration change?

Does function vary when observed or when an activity is being focused on and when the child does do not realize he or she is being observed or is distracted?

Are there any inconsistencies on repeat examination?

If asked to perform an activity that has been reported as being unable to do can the child do it?

Is there any neurologic dysfunction?

Does the pain occur in an area defined by a dermatome or peripheral nerve distribution?

Are there abnormal child-parent interactions such as enmeshment, hostility, berating?

Is there evidence of concurrent conversion symptoms?

In children with back pain, are signs of nonorganic back pain present?

BOX 52-4 Common Patterns Observed in Amplified Pain

- Insufficient inciting event to cause such pain and disability (minor trauma or illness)
- Increasing pain over time
- Increasing dysfunction over time
- Disproportionate pain
- Disproportionate dysfunction
- Lack of response to medicinal and physical treatments
- Incongruent affect
- *La belle indifference*
- Typical personality (mature, perfectionistic, pleaser, driven)
- Multiple life changes or psychological stressors present
- Allodynia with a variable border
- Able to do things that they previously were not able to do when asked

localized and diffuse amplified musculoskeletal pain syndromes, the medical history and physical examination are surprisingly similar.

Even when reporting severe pain or other somatic symptoms, the child often has a markedly incongruent affect, smiling even when reporting severe pain (up to 10 out of 10), and display *la belle indifference* about the pain and dysfunction it causes. A few children, usually but not exclusively those with localized amplified musculoskeletal pain, demonstrate marked pain behaviors such as crying or screaming. Children with amplified musculoskeletal pain often seem mature for their age, are accomplished in school and extracurricular activities, and are described by their parents as perfectionistic, empathetic, and pleasers.[8,32,126]

In all forms of amplified musculoskeletal pain, conversion symptoms are not uncommon.[7,8,127] Numbness is frequently reported, but children can manifest paralysis, pseudoseizures, or conversion spells,

shaking or rigidity, blindness, or a bizarre (histrionic) gait. Eating disorders may be present.[128,129]

Additionally, patients may have symptoms of an altered autonomic system, including lightheadedness when standing, orthostatic tachycardia, functional abdominal pain, or headaches. They frequently complain of not being able to think clearly; however, most children maintain their usual grades in school.[130]

Assessment of Pain and Its Effects in Children with Amplified Musculoskeletal Pain

There are two major independent variables to consider when assessing pain: the quality and quantity of the pain complaint itself, and the amount of dysfunction as a consequence of the pain. The report of pain is always valid because, by definition, pain is subjective.[9] Therefore, the most useful measurement of pain is the self-report on a verbal or visual analog scale. The quality of pain can be assessed using various instruments, such as the McGill Pain Questionnaire or Pediatric Pain Questionnaire.[131,132]

The amount of reported pain does not directly correlate with the degree of incapacity, which can vary from almost none to being bedridden. An important observation is that with treatment function usually returns before the pain diminishes. Functional measurements vary depending on the location of the pain and the presence of coexisting conditions, such as arthritis or, more commonly, conversion symptoms. Children with both amplified musculoskeletal pain and conversion paralysis can be extremely dysfunctional.

Children with amplified musculoskeletal pain appear to suffer more than children with other musculoskeletal conditions, which may indicate the degree of psychological distress present. In one comparison of the degree of well-being, children with CRPS ranked themselves as significantly more disabled as measured by a visual analog scale than did those with juvenile rheumatoid arthritis.[32]

Psychological dysfunction is almost universally present by the time the diagnosis is made.[8,29,32,44,133,134] The psychological toll on the child and family is often severe although these syndromes are not necessarily psychological in cause. The degree of psychosocial pathology is highly variable and may range from mild anxiety or poor coping to borderline personality disturbance, or may involve siblings and other family members. Not only are such symptoms frequent, but the author has observed an increase in self-cutting (Sherry D.D., unpublished observation).

CRPS

In children with CRPS, minor trauma that might not be clearly recalled is common ("someone must have stepped on my foot"). The pain and consequent disability increase over time in spite of medication. A cast or splint may increase the pain or, at best, minimize the pain while it is worn. Immobilization is an important factor in perpetuating the pain, and once the cast is removed the limb should not be further immobilized. In adults with wrist fractures, the presence of pain of 5/10 or greater after one week in a cast was very predictive of the development CRPS.[135] Autonomic signs (edema, cyanosis, coolness, increased perspiration) may be persistent or transient, or may not occur. In a study of 70 children with CRPS, all had pain; 86% had allodynia (pain caused by normally nonpainful stimuli), 77% edema, 77% coolness to the limb, 73% cyanosis, and only 31% had hyperhidrosis.[33] Allodynia can be marked ("the breeze of someone walking by hurts") and can lead to significant impairment. This phenomenon, too, can be transient. Any body part can be involved, and the child may have several areas of pain. The lower extremity is more commonly involved than the upper extremity, and peripheral body parts are more commonly involved than central areas. Occasionally, only one small area is involved, such as a finger, the nose, or a tooth.[136] Localized pain is usually continuous.

Notable points on physical examination include the absence of findings suggesting an underlying disease, a normal neurologic examination, and frequently the presence of allodynia. Careful sensory testing, with special attention to dermatomal and peripheral nerve innervation, is required. Allodynia is present if pain is reported when lightly touching the skin or gently pinching a fold of skin. The border of the allodynia can vary dramatically and may occur in a glove-and-stocking distribution. Signs of autonomic dysfunction, especially coolness and cyanosis, may only be present after exercising the limb, or may become apparent if the limb is held in a dependent position for a few minutes. Many children have near total body allodynia but the face, genitalia, and breasts are frequently spared.

Diffuse Amplified Musculoskeletal Pain

In diffuse amplified musculoskeletal pain, the onset is usually more gradual and may be vague in location and character. Autonomic nervous system signs are absent, but affected children complain of poor sleep and depression more often than do those with localized pain.[137] However, some children with diffuse amplified musculoskeletal pain initially have very localized pain, which may spread to involve the entire body. Children with diffuse amplified musculoskeletal pain frequently report a multiplicity of symptoms. The pain is often centrally located involving the back, chest, abdomen, and head, as well as the extremities.

Older criteria for fibromyalgia include counting painful points (although frequently called *tender* points, the patient needs to identify them as causing *pain* not just *tenderness* when 4 kg of pressure is applied) as outlined in Box 52-3. Pressure should also be applied at control points such as the forehead, shin, and thumbnail to define the extent of the amplified pain.[138] A number of children with diffuse amplified pain do not have the painful points of fibromyalgia, although they are otherwise indistinguishable.

Prolonged back pain in childhood may be due to a serious illness and should be carefully investigated.[139] However, some children have nonorganic back pain, usually in conjunction with diffuse amplified musculoskeletal pain. Distinguishing signs include the axial loading test, distracted straight leg raising, passive rotation test, overreaction, and allodynia (Table 52-1).[140]

Laboratory Examination

After taking a history and performing an examination, the diagnosis of an amplified pain syndrome is often certain and no further investigations are required. It is unwise to make a diagnosis of a noninflammatory condition in a child with an abnormal blood count, or increased acute-phase reactants, unless the abnormalities can be clearly ascribed to an intercurrent illness. The most common "abnormal" test is a low-titer positive antinuclear antibody (1:40 to 1:160), which should be discounted if the clinical presentation is typical.[141] There may be normal or slightly slowed nerve conduction velocity in patients with CRPS.[142,143] Any laboratory testing should be done with caution because the more tests that are performed, the more likely is the occurrence of false positive results leading to unjustified doubt about the diagnosis, anxiety concerning more serious illnesses, and delay in initiating treatment.

Radiographic Examination

Imaging studies should be directed to rule in or out a specific diagnosis (e.g., plain radiographs or bone scintigraphy to exclude trauma or tumor and magnetic resonance imaging to exclude spinal cord lesions).[144,145]

TABLE 52-1	**Signs of Nonorganic Back Pain**
TEST	**DESCRIPTION**
Axial loading test	A positive test occurs when back pain is reported while the examiner exerts downward pressure on the top of a standing patient's head. Neck pain may be elicited and is not a positive test.
Distracted straight leg raising	In a positive test, flexion of the hip causes back pain when the patient is supine but not when sitting.
Passive rotation test	A positive test occurs when the patient reports back pain with passive rotation at the ankles and knees, keeping the pelvis, back, and shoulders in the same plane.
Overreaction	Overreaction is defined as excessive wincing, muscle tremors, screaming, or collapsing with pain. "Excessive" is quite subjective and may vary based on age, mental status, cultural influences, or fear.
Allodynia	Report of pain to light touch or a gentle pinch of the skin, usually with a border that varies on repeat testing.

Data from G. Waddell, J.A. McCulloch, E. Kummel, et al., Nonorganic physical signs in low-back pain, Spine 5 (1980) 117–125.

Radiographic findings are normal or demonstrate disuse osteoporosis depending on the duration and degree of disability; rarely children have the spotty osteoporosis that occurs in adults with CRPS.[29] Technetium radionuclide bone scans are probably the most useful study if the diagnosis is in doubt.[36,38,146] The most frequent abnormality is decreased radionuclide uptake in the affected limb. A normal study is evidence against an underlying bone disease such as osteomyelitis, osteoid osteoma, or a stress fracture, but abnormal scans are subject to differing interpretations, especially if the finding are subtle, because interobserver variation in reading mildly abnormal scans is common.[145-147] Bone scintigraphy in adults with CRPS had a sensitivity of only 0.80 and a specificity of 0.73.[144] Magnetic resonance images in children with localized amplified pain document regional bone marrow edema with T1-weighted images of low signal intensity and T2-weighted images with high signal intensity; it has been reported that MRI is more sensitive than scintigraphy; however, early in the disease course, there may be difficulty distinguishing between the edema of amplified musculoskeletal pain and the edema of trauma, including subtle fractures.[145,148,149]

Pathology

There is a dearth of information concerning the histopathology of connective or nerve tissues from children with amplified musculoskeletal pain syndromes. Three children with CRPS had findings on biopsies of skin, muscle, and nerve consistent with ischemic injury.[51] Endothelial swelling, basement membrane thickening and reduplication, and patchy fiber atrophy of muscle were observed. The author had one patient with CRPS with ischemic changes present in the synovium of her knee. Various abnormalities have been demonstrated in the muscles of adults with fibromyalgia although it is not clear that these are related to the etiology or are an effect of another process such as ischemia.[46,52] Skin biopsies have shown decreased intra-epidural nerve fiber density interpreted as a small fiber neuropathy.[101-103]

TABLE 52-2 Differential Diagnoses in Children Presenting with Marked Pain

DIAGNOSIS	TYPICAL AGE	DISTINGUISHING CHARACTERISTICS
Fabry disease	Adolescents	Episodic, excruciating, burning pain in the distal extremities; blue maculopapular, hyperkeratotic lesions clustered on the lower trunk and perineum; erythrocyte sedimentation rate is usually elevated
Neoplasia	Any	Episodic or migratory pain or arthritis, generalized malaise, anorexia, and bone pain
Spinal cord tumors	Any	Abnormal neurological examination, altered gait, or spinal curvature
Erythromelalgia	Adolescents	Pain with erythematous, warm, swollen hands or feet that is eased by cold to the point that patients refuse to remove ice or cold water from their affected limbs
Pernio (chilblains)	Any	Burning pain with associated red to purple, swollen papules on exposed fingers or toes after cold injury
Raynaud disease	Adolescents	Tricolor change (white, blue, red), associated with tingling; usually not very painful
Hypermobility	Children	Intermittent nocturnal pains that may occur after certain activities
Restless legs syndrome	Adolescents	Nocturnal discomfort in, and an inability to keep from moving, the legs; paresthesias, not pain per se, are common and rarely cause awakening
Myofascial pain	Adolescents	Sustained contraction of part of a muscle, especially those about the head, jaw, and upper back; pain well localized and reproduced when that part of the muscle is palpated
Chronic recurrent multifocal osteomyelitis	Any	Specific point tenderness
Chronic compartment syndrome	Adolescents	Severe muscle pain (usually calf) after exercising
Progressive diaphyseal dysplasia	Adolescents	Severe leg pain, fatigue, headaches, weight loss, weakness, and an abnormal, waddling gait; radiographs show cortical thickening and sclerosis of the diaphysis of the long bones
Peripheral mononeuropathy	Adults	Posttraumatic mononeuropathy
Transient migratory osteoporosis	Adolescents	Rapidly developing, painful osteoporosis
Vitamin D deficiency	Adults	Hyperesthetic pain in debilitated patients with multiple reasons to be deficient in vitamin D
Thyroid disease	Any	Widespread musculoskeletal pain with either hypothyroidism or hyperthyroidism with associated symptoms of thyroid dysfunction

DIFFERENTIAL DIAGNOSES

A number of other painful conditions should be considered in the evaluation of a child who may have an amplified musculoskeletal pain syndrome. Table 52-2 lists disorders that may be confused with amplified pain syndromes. In children with back pain, enthesitis-related arthritis is a consideration.[139,150,151] The most common misdiagnoses for children who actually have an amplified pain syndrome are trauma, especially Salter-Harris I fractures, mechanical pain, or arthritis.

TREATMENT

The plethora of widely disparate treatments attests to the fact that there are no proven therapies demonstrated by well-controlled therapeutic trials in children with amplified musculoskeletal pain.[7,68] Therefore, treatment is based largely on clinical experience and a very few larger patient series. Extrapolation of results from studies in adults to children is of limited value because children with CRPS or fibromyalgia significantly differ from adults with these disorders.[33,38,94,152-155] Furthermore, a recent Cochrane review concluded that there was no high quality evidence for most therapies for adults with CRPS.[156] When considering therapy for children with amplified pain syndromes, it is best to exercise great circumspection and consider the risks involved compared to more standard, conservative therapy.[157]

Treatment has two goals: restoration of function and relief of pain. Although less than ideal, restoration to full function without total pain relief occasionally has to be accepted. Helping the child to develop skills to cope with the pain is often effective in relieving distress and dysfunction even if the pain persists.[158]

Psychological Therapy and Support

Chronic pain significantly affects individual and family dynamics.[32,60,61,64,69,72,155,159-165] All children and their families should have a psychological assessment to explore the individual and family psychodynamics and to address psychological issues that may exist. School issues, both social and academic, need to be explored.[32,60,69,70] Therapy needs to address the family or marital dynamics.[8,32,71,162] Cognitive-behavioral therapy (CBT) can help the child develop coping strategies to deal with pain and dysfunction.[166-169]

Using progressive muscle relaxation and guided imagery, Walco and Ilowite treated five girls with fibromyalgia for four to nine sessions and four reported no pain an average of 10 months later.[169] Gedalia et al. reported that only two of five children with fibromyalgia found CBT to be helpful.[49] In a randomized controlled trial of CBT involving 114 children (half in an education group) Kashikar-Zuck et al. showed that both groups resolved depressive symptoms but there was no significant difference in sleep quality, physical activity, pain severity, or meaningful reduction in pain.[167,170] Those treated with CBT, however, had a greater reduction in their Functional Disability Inventory (FDI) score, although final scores were in the moderately disabled range.[171] fMRI data in adults suggests that CBT may alter pain pathways, however this was not shown by lower pain scores or pain sensitivity.[172] It is the author's experience that children benefit from CBT primarily as an adjunct to intense physical and occupational therapy and further psychotherapy and family therapy.[31,32,58] More attention to family issues has been advocated (Sherry D.D., unpublished observation).[173,174] Some children, especially those who have difficulty with verbal expression, may benefit from creative arts therapy such as music therapy or art therapy. A Cochrane review concluded that psychological treatments are effective for long-term pain control in children with headache and may improve pain control in children with musculoskeletal and recurrent abdominal pain, but there was little evidence available to estimate effects on disability or mood.[175] Guite et al. found parental worry about their child's physical health but not their emotional health fostered more functional disability and suggested education and support of the parents to reduce protective behaviors.[162] Formal psychotherapy based on an initial psychological evaluation has been advocated by some.[10,118,176] Children with fibromyalgia are less prone to depression than adults but have a higher incidence of anxiety that may interfere with function and may warrant psychiatric evaluation for medication.[155]

Physical and Occupational Therapy

Physical and occupational therapy aimed at increasing function are recommended for all children[29,31,58,116,126,142,168,177-182]; however, patient response to various intensities of physiotherapy varies widely. Understanding that it is not physiologically damaging to use the affected limb enables some children to work through the pain, restore function, and resolve the pain without formal therapy.[31] Others respond with home exercises or local physical therapy, whereas some others require a very intense program.

Bernstein et al.[29] and others[31,126,179] reported outstanding results in a large number of children with CRPS treated exclusively with physical and occupational therapy, without medication. In children who do not respond to limited treatment with physical and occupational therapy, a very rigorous program of 5 to 6 hours of daily therapy has been successful in children with CRPS and fibromyalgia.[31,58,126] Using such a regimen, Sherry et al. reported a 92% success rate in 103 consecutive children with CRPS and over 5 years later, 88% were symptom free.[31] Similar programs in Pittsburgh and Portland reported 32 children with CRPS in whom 89% became pain-free.[126] Children with CRPS treated with physical and occupational therapy only had a relatively low relapse rate, and many were able to treat themselves if they relapsed, without needing subsequent formal treatment.[31,126] Using a less rigorous therapy program together with pain medications Logan et al. reported significant improvement in Functional Disability Inventory (FDI) and decreased pain in 56 children with CRPS.[179] A systematic review of adults with CRPS found strong evidence for the use of rehabilitation physical therapy interventions to reduce pain and improve function.[183] However, there still remains a paucity of controlled trials of physical and occupational therapy in children with amplified musculoskeletal pain.[182]

There are fewer reports of children with fibromyalgia being treated with intense physical and occupational therapy. A randomized control pilot study of weekly aerobic training (n = 14) versus anaerobic (Qigong) training (n = 18) demonstrated a significant drop in pain rating in the aerobic training group compared to the anaerobic group.[185] There were no exacerbations of fibromyalgia symptoms despite aerobic training. Nine children with fibromyalgia treated with 5 hours of physical and occupational therapy daily along with psychotherapy improved from severely debilitated (FDI 31) to normal (FDI 4), and their pain level dropped from 65 (with 100 being the highest) to 17.[58]

Vierck and Thompson make a compelling argument that physical therapy in adults with fibromyalgia be first-line therapy based on its salubrious effects on muscle vasoconstriction, stress, depression, fatigue, concentration, and sleep.[186,187] A meta-analysis by Kelley and Kelley confirms improved well-being in adults with fibromyalgia who exercise.[188] A recent review of three evidence-based guidelines for management of fibromyalgia in adults emphasizes individualization of therapy, especially self-management strategies, including exercise and cognitive-behavioral techniques.[189]

There are reports of the use of transcutaneous nerve stimulation (TENS) in small numbers of children with CRPS,[33,42,142,178,190] but no controlled trials. In experimentally induced ischemic pain in normal volunteers, there was no difference between actual TENS and placebo.[191]

There are no efficacy trials of acupuncture in children with amplified pain. Sham acupuncture was as effective and needle placement was not critical when treating 114 adults with fibromyalgia.[192,193] Leo documented the successful use of electrical stimulation at several acupuncture sites together with physical therapy in a 10-year-old girl;[194] However, the author has had several children report significantly increased pain after acupuncture (Sherry D.D., unpublished observation).

Medical Treatment

No drugs are approved for the treatment of amplified pain syndromes in children and most reports in pediatrics are single case studies or small series.

Tricyclic Antidepressants

Tricyclic antidepressants block the reuptake of serotonin and norepinephrine. Amitriptyline, and to a lesser extent, nortriptyline, have been used extensively in adults with fibromyalgia with mixed results. A recent systematic Cochrane review noted that there is no supportive unbiased evidence to substantiate its use.[195] Initially, amitriptyline was proposed to restore normal sleep pattern because sleep studies in patients with fibromyalgia showed excessive α-δ sleep non–rapid eye movement (NREM). However, a placebo-controlled trial showed it had no effect on the NREM abnormalities.[57] In an open label study of 175 adults with fibromyalgia, amitriptyline was equally effective as routine physical therapy over 6 months.[196] Frequently, amitriptyline has been used in conjunction with other medications and procedures making it hard to discern its effect.[197-201,202] It is important to note that a significant number of children will have electrocardiographic findings that contraindicate the use of amitriptyline.[203] Side effects of amitriptyline include gastrointestinal upset, drowsiness, dizziness, weakness, insomnia, weight gain, and headaches as well as blurred vision, photosensitivity, and dry mouth. Young people taking tricyclic antidepressants need to be warned of the increased risk of suicide, especially initially, and monitored for this.

Other Antidepressants

Selective serotonin reuptake inhibitors, dual serotonin and noradrenalin reuptake inhibitors, and monoamine oxidase inhibitors have been tested in adults with fibromyalgia in randomized controlled trials. Uceyler et al. systematically reviewed these trials and found all the studies were limited by short durations (6-12 weeks) and that there was little evidence of superiority of one class of antidepressant over another.[204] The mean improvement in pain was 26% and improvement in quality of life was 30%; generally these findings were independent of an effect on depression. They concluded that antidepressant medication can be recommended for the short term in adults, but there are no data regarding their long-term use. Side effects were common and may have interfered with the blinding and, in children and young adults, these medications are associated with increased risk of suicide.

Antiepileptics

The antiepileptics most commonly used for CRPS and fibromyalgia are gabapentin and pregabalin, although pregabalin is not presently approved for pediatric use. The mechanism of action is unknown, although pregabalin binds to calcium channels in the central nervous system and may act by reducing insular glutamatergic activity as evidenced by neuroimaging.[205,206] A meta-analysis of both agents in fibromyalgia in adults concluded that pregabalin reduced pain by 30%, but that its use was limited by side effects, including dizziness, drowsiness, dry mouth, weight gain, and edema leading to one quarter of patients stopping therapy.[207] Reports of gabapentin use in children are limited to a few case studies.[208-213] A meta-analysis concluded that moderate to higher doses of pregabalin were effective in a minority of patients with fibromyalgia, and side effects were frequent.[214] Roskell et al. systematically reviewed nine drugs (duloxetine, fluoxetine, gabapentin, milnacipran, pramipexole, pregabalin, amitriptyline, cyclobenzaprine, and tramadol plus acetaminophen) in adults with fibromyalgia and concluded that all were equally effective, but that milnacipran and pregabalin were more likely to be discontinued due to side effects.[215] Topiramate, another anti-epileptic drug, was not shown to be effective in adult fibromyalgia.[216]

Bisphosphonates

Kubalek et al. reported the use of pamidronate in 29 adults with CRPS related to trauma, diabetes, drugs or cancer.[217] The pain resolved in 86% in the short term. Resolution of pain in an 11-year-old patient treated with pamidronate and physical therapy has been reported.[218] Neridronate was studied in a double blind placebo, controlled trial in 40 adults within 4 months of onset of CRPS and showed marked benefit at 40 days, but there was a surprisingly good initial response to placebo.[219] A systematic review found strong evidence for the use of bisphosphonates used early in the disease course, but long-term studies are needed.[183] There are concerns of serious side effects, including osteonecrosis of the jaw and optic neuritis.[220,221]

Corticosteroids

Oral corticosteroids were reported by Ruggeri et al. to be without benefit in six children, although a small, randomized study in adults showed short term benefit in 13 adults with CRPS.[222,223] A study of intrathecal methylprednisolone in CRPS was stopped early due to lack of effect.[224] Many authors use corticosteroids in combination with other treatments, so it is difficult to discern any specific effect. Systemic and injected corticosteroids have too many side effects to recommend their use.

Cyclobenzaprine

Cyclobenzaprine acts in the central nervous system to reduce tonic muscle activity probably due to actions on both the α and γ motor neurons. It is structurally related to the tricyclics. Eleven of 15 children (73%) with fibromyalgia judged cyclobenzaprine to be helpful but the durability of benefit was not reported.[225] Another study reported that only three of 33 children with fibromyalgia indicated that they would recommend cyclobenzaprine to other individuals with similar pain.[226] There has been an absence of reports studying the efficacy of cyclobenzaprine in children since the 1990s, and it is one among many poorly studied agents in adults.[225]

Opioids

Opioids should not be used in children with amplified pain. A recent Cochrane review concluded there is, at best, only equivocal evidence of the efficacy of opioids in adults with neuropathic pain.[227] The author knows of two children who died following opioid use for the treatment of pain amplification, and several others who have required drug rehabilitation (Sherry D.D., personal observation).

Ketamine

Ketamine is an anesthetic agent that is an antagonist of the NMDA receptor, which may be activated and upregulated in the spinal cord in patients with chronic pain. However, it is associated with psychomimetic side effects; that is, it can produce hallucinations or paranoid delusions identical to psychotic symptoms. In a 12-week study of 60 patients with CRPS there was a significant decrease in pain at week 1 but by week 12 there was no difference between those receiving ketamine and those receiving placebo.[228] Niesters et al. showed no difference between ketamine, morphine, and placebo in conditioned pain modulation using a cold water bath model in patients with neuropathic pain.[229] Even when there is an initial response to ketamine, the duration of effect is brief (3-4 weeks).[230,231] There is an increasing recognition of untoward effects, including hepatotoxicity and prolonged mania.[232-235] Ketamine coma is not approved in the United States, is very controversial, and is unproven to have any lasting benefit.[236] Side effects are significant, including paralysis, pneumonia, and pulmonary embolus.

Sympathetic Blocks and Sympathectomy

Sympathetic blockade, by a variety of agents and techniques, was frequently used in adults because it was thought that blocking the sympathetic overactivity would be curative. Sympathetic blocks have included guanethidine or reserpine blockades, lumbar, axillary, or stellate ganglion blocks, or sympathectomy (surgical, chemical, and radioablation).[33,120,212,237-246] However, it was recognized not to have lasting effects and, in one report, results were felt to be good or lasting in only 7% of 273 patients treated with sympathetic blockade.[247] In 55 adults, guanethidine blocks gave less than 10% significant long-term relief and 34% had significant side effects.[248] There have been no specific studies of sympathetic blockade in children, but a Cochrane review found little evidence to support sympathetic blocks as standard of care in CRPS.[249] Wilder emphasizes that sympathetic blocks should not be used to treat CRPS in children but, if used, should be in conjunction with physical therapy.[182] Sympathetic blocks have been done for fibromyalgia and as there are individual cases of success, there are also cases of failure, such as a 14-year-old girl resistant to corticosteroids, surgical ganglionic blockade, and sympathectomy.[242]

Peripheral Nerve Blocks

Daudure et al. report 13 children treated with a peripheral block followed by a Bier block (intravenous regional anesthesia) and all did well at 2 months.[250] Three patients (two children) had continuous peripheral blockade to allow for physical therapy with good results at 2 and 5 months in two patients, but one child continued receiving multiple medications.[251,252] Side effects include seizures.[253]

Epidural infusions

A variety of agents have been infused in the epidural space for treatment of amplified pain (usually CRPS), including baclofen, clonidine, morphine, ketamine, and bupivacaine.[254-256] Patients in these case reports generally had unsatisfactory outcomes with minimal to moderate functional or pain benefit over repeated or prolonged (months) treatment. Untoward effects included sepsis in one child and epidural abscess in two children.[257,258]

Spinal Cord Stimulators

Spinal cord stimulators are surgically implanted with leads in the epidural space at the level of the spinal cord determined by a trial procedure to decrease pain in the area of amplified pain. They are reported to transiently decrease pain but do not prevent the spread of CRPS.[259] Wilder reported mild improvement or worsening of pain in 6 children.[182] There is a high rate of migration of the leads[260] as well as other complications.[261-278] Olsson reported the use of spinal cord stimulators in seven children; two failed to have any benefit, one became infected, and the rest had prolonged relief and the stimulator was eventually removed.[279] There have been no systematic reviews of spinal cord stimulators in the amplified pain syndromes; however, a Cochrane review of cancer-related pain concluded there was insufficient evidence to establish a role of spinal cord stimulators in treating refractory cancer-related pain.[280]

Amputation

Amputation has been performed in adults for intractable CRPS and although few get pain relief, the outcome is better in those with a high level of resilience.[55,255,281,282] Amputation is extremely rarely indicated in children, perhaps in those with intractable infection as a complication of CRPS.[283] The author has seen two children with CRPS with amputations; one was associated with Munchausen by proxy (Sherry D.D., personal observation).

Miscellaneous

A host of allopathic and nonallopathic therapies have been used to treat the various forms of amplified pain. There is no evidence of benefit, and none is recommended. Rodrigo found a large percentage of adults with fibromyalgia and irritable bowel syndrome to have celiac disease and reported that they improved on a gluten-free diet.[284,285] Only one of 50 children with fibromyalgia was found to have celiac disease and she did not improve when on a gluten free diet.[286] It is unlikely that amplified pain is due to a food sensitivity or dietary deficiency.

Sleep

Sleep disturbance is frequently mentioned as an important aspect of childhood fibromyalgia, and good sleep hygiene (Box 52-5) is always advocated; however, its value is uncertain. Low dose tricyclic antidepressant medication has been recommended to facilitate sleep initiation, but it is not helpful or needed in most children with fibromyalgia or other amplified musculoskeletal pain syndromes.[58,226,287] It is well documented that children with fibromyalgia have altered α-δ sleep, which does not change with medication or even when they have no pain and sleep well.[56-58] Increased periodic limb movements during sleep have been reported in one small series.[53] It is the author's experience that no specific treatment is necessary or indicated for the sleep disturbance. Even if children report not sleeping at all at night, it is rare that they fall asleep during school or during the daytime.

A Philosophy of Therapy for Amplified Musculoskeletal Pain

A team approach is indicated for children with either localized or diffuse amplified musculoskeletal pain directed to the restoration of full function.[8,10,31,288,289] The intensity of physical and occupational therapy varies, but if routine outpatient therapy fails, the time is escalated to 5 to 6 hours a day on weekdays for a mean of 3 to 4 weeks.

BOX 52-5   Elements of Good Sleep Hygiene

- No caffeine
- No television or radio in the bedroom
- Do not exercise within 2 hours before bedtime
- Have a set bedtime and awake time 7 days a week
- Have the bedroom completely dark
- Sleep in your own bed
- Do not lie in bed except when trying to sleep at night (not for homework or naps)
- If not asleep in 30 minutes, get up and do a quiet, boring activity
- Do not disturb parents or other family members

The children are treated one-on-one, with the therapist encouraging both speed and quality of movement. Exercises are focused on normal function and aerobic training such as walking times, rope jumping, climbing stairs, dressing, and other activities of daily living.[7,10,31,126,158] Allodynia is treated with desensitization using towel and lotion rubs, vibration, wearing normal clothing, and footwear. Most children are treated as day patients and are expected to engage in normal family activities at night and on weekends while doing a home exercise program. Children who are very dysfunctional, or have severe postexercise pain behaviors, require inpatient treatment. Others have used a more prolonged inpatient treatment program (3 months) with graded physical exercises, graded activities, and counseling with good outcomes.[290]

There is no consistent evidence of benefit from any medication, most of which are not approved for use in children, and many of which have significant risk of side effects. In adult women who sustained a wrist fracture, the prevalence of complex regional pain syndrome was reduced from 10% to 2% by giving vitamin C for 50 days postinjury.[291] The ingestion of 500 to 1000 mg of vitamin C daily in children who have had an amplified musculoskeletal pain syndrome may minimize the risk of relapse if they suffer an injury or undergo surgery.

COURSE AND PROGNOSIS

There are no long-term studies of the natural history of amplified pain syndromes in children. Many children have spontaneous remission of illness; 11 of 15 children incidentally diagnosed with fibromyalgia were asymptomatic after 30 months.[153] In a population survey of children with widespread pain, 30% still had widespread pain at either 1 or 4 years after baseline.[23] However, 92% of children with fibromyalgia who sought care at one pediatric rheumatology center still had significant pain 15 to 60 months (mean, 33 months) later.[291] A much better short- and long-term outcome is reported with intense physical and occupational therapy and psychotherapy.[10,31,58,126,179] In general, children fulfilling criteria for CRPS have a better outcome than children with regional pain without signs of autonomic dysfunction, who, in turn, have a better outcome than those with diffuse amplified musculoskeletal pain or fibromyalgia. After a mean of 5 years, 88% of children with CRPS were free of pain and fully functional.[31] On follow-up after a mean of 5 years, 30% had had a recurrence, but half of those had treated themselves without needing formal therapy. Brooke and Janselewitz treated 32 children with CRPS with an intense inpatient rehabilitation program and eventually 89% resolved all pain.[126] Recurrences were seen in seven patients, but five treated themselves without needing formal retreatment. Logan et al. treated 56 children with CRPS with a day hospital approach and, of those with complete data, 100% were functionally better and they reported a significant improvement in anxiety as well.[179] Most (90%) of the children without autonomic signs, with either localized or diffuse amplified pain, were functional, but only 78% were without pain.[8] Initially, 90% of the group with fibromyalgia was pain-free, but this declined to 50% over 5 years. However, 90% still remained fully active in school or employment. No difference in outcome between girls and boys or between younger children and older adolescents was observed.

Relapses may occur in all forms of amplified musculoskeletal pain. The clinical manifestation of the second episode may be different from the first, even changing between localized and diffuse disease.[6,8] In one study, children with relapses were more likely to have significant underlying psychopathology, specifically a prior suicide attempt.[31] The age, sex, and duration of symptoms did not predict relapses.

In addition to recurrent episodes of amplified musculoskeletal pain, children may develop chronic pain involving other organ systems, especially headaches or abdominal pains, and other psychological problems, including conversion disorders (blindness, paralysis), suicide attempts, self-cutting, panic attacks, incapacitating dizziness or fatigue, gastroparesis, or eating disorders. It is unclear whether these problems occur at a greater frequency than in the general population but recognizing these as possibly part of the spectrum of an aberrant sympathetic nervous system or a manifestation of psychological stress is prudent.

CONCLUSION

Musculoskeletal pain is common in childhood and an accurate diagnosis and a logical and consistent approach to its management is important. A careful history and examination combined with judicious laboratory or radiographic investigations usually allow a correct diagnosis to be made in a timely fashion. Once the diagnosis of amplified musculoskeletal pain is made, reassurance about the nature of condition and treatment with appropriate physiotherapy should be promptly instituted. The effect of the pain and dysfunction on the child and family needs to be appreciated and addressed. Many children with amplified musculoskeletal pain need complex medical and psychological management involving a multidisciplinary team. It is challenging to care for these children, but the outcome is usually very rewarding. The treating team can help these children with their immediate problem by helping them resolve the pain and dysfunction, but also help many with long-term and, possibly, more important issues by improving the psychological functioning of the child and family.

REFERENCES

4. A.I. Matles, Reflex sympathetic dystrophy in a child. A case report, Bull. Hosp. Joint Dis. 32 (1971) 193–197.
5. M.B. Yunus, A.T. Masi, Juvenile primary fibromyalgia syndrome. A clinical study of thirty-three patients and matched normal controls, Arthritis Rheum. 28 (1985) 138–145.
6. P.N. Malleson, M. al-Matar, R.E. Petty, Idiopathic musculoskeletal pain syndromes in children, J. Rheumatol. 19 (1992) 1786–1789.
8. D.D. Sherry, T. McGuire, E. Mellins, et al., Psychosomatic musculoskeletal pain in childhood: clinical and psychological analyses of 100 children, Pediatrics 88 (1991) 1093–1099.
9. H. Merskey, N. Bogduk, Classification of chronic pain: descriptions of chronic pain syndromes and definitions of pain terms, second ed., IASP press, Seattle, 1994.
10. D.D. Sherry, Pain syndromes, in: J.I. Miller (Ed.), Adolescent Rheumatology, Martin Duntz, London, 1998, pp. 197–227.
12. R.N. Harden, S. Bruehl, R.S. Perez, et al., Validation of proposed diagnostic criteria (the "Budapest Criteria") for complex regional pain syndrome, Pain 150 (2010) 268–274.
13. F. Wolfe, H.A. Smythe, M.B. Yunus, et al., The American College of Rheumatology 1990 criteria for the classification of fibromyalgia. Report of the Multicenter Criteria Committee, Arthritis Rheum. 33 (1990) 160–172.
14. F. Wolfe, D.J. Clauw, M.A. Fitzcharles, et al., The American College of Rheumatology preliminary diagnostic criteria for fibromyalgia and measurement of symptom severity, Arthritis Care Res. (Hoboken) 62 (2010) 600–610.
23. M. Mikkelsson, A. El-Metwally, H. Kautiainen, et al., Onset, prognosis and risk factors for widespread pain in schoolchildren: a prospective 4-year follow-up study, Pain 138 (2008) 681–687.
29. B.H. Bernstein, B.H. Singsen, J.T. Kent, et al., Reflex neurovascular dystrophy in childhood, J. Pediatr. 93 (1978) 211–215.
31. D.D. Sherry, C.A. Wallace, C. Kelley, et al., Short- and long-term outcomes of children with complex regional pain syndrome type I treated with exercise therapy, Clin. J. Pain 15 (1999) 218–223.
32. D.D. Sherry, R. Weisman, Psychologic aspects of childhood reflex neurovascular dystrophy, Pediatrics 81 (1988) 572–578.
33. R.T. Wilder, C.B. Berde, M. Wolohan, et al., Reflex sympathetic dystrophy in children. Clinical characteristics and follow-up of seventy patients, J. Bone Joint Surg. Am. 74 (1992) 910–919.
38. R.M. Laxer, R.C. Allen, P.N. Malleson, et al., Technetium 99m-methylene diphosphonate bone scans in children with reflex neurovascular dystrophy, J. Pediatr. 106 (1985) 437–440.
44. G.J. Reid, B.A. Lang, P.J. McGrath, Primary juvenile fibromyalgia: psychological adjustment, family functioning, coping, and functional disability, Arthritis Rheum. 40 (1997) 752–760.
48. A. Gedalia, C.O. Garcia, J.F. Molina, et al., Fibromyalgia syndrome: experience in a pediatric rheumatology clinic, Clin. Exp. Rheumatol. 18 (2000) 415–419.
50. M. Mikkelsson, J.J. Salminen, H. Kautiainen, Joint hypermobility is not a contributing factor to musculoskeletal pain in pre-adolescents, J. Rheumatol. 23 (1996) 1963–1967.
58. M.N. Olsen, D.D. Sherry, K. Boyne, et al., Relationship between sleep and pain in adolescents with juvenile primary fibromyalgia syndrome, Sleep 36 (2013) 509–516.
70. D.E. Logan, L.E. Simons, M.J. Stein, et al., School impairment in adolescents with chronic pain, J. Pain 9 (2008) 407–416.
92. W.E. Ackerman 3rd, M. Ahmad, Recurrent postoperative CRPS I in patients with abnormal preoperative sympathetic function, J. Hand Surg. [Am] 33 (2008) 217–222.
94. A. Lebel, L. Becerra, D. Wallin, et al., fMRI reveals distinct CNS processing during symptomatic and recovered complex regional pain syndrome in children, Brain 131 (2008) 1854–1879.
99. N.F. Sethna, P.M. Meier, D. Zurakowski, C.B. Berde, Cutaneous sensory abnormalities in children and adolescents with complex regional pain syndromes, Pain 131 (2007) 153–161.
103. A.L. Oaklander, M.M. Klein, Evidence of small-fiber polyneuropathy in unexplained, juvenile-onset, widespread pain syndromes, Pediatrics 131 (2013) e1091–e1100.
106. H.H. Krämer, T. Eberle, N. Üçeyler, et al., TNF-alpha in CRPS and "normal" trauma—Significant differences between tissue and serum, Pain 152 (2011) 285–290.
118. L.E. Schanberg, F.J. Keefe, J.C. Lefebvre, et al., Social context of pain in children with Juvenile Primary Fibromyalgia Syndrome: parental pain history and family environment, Clin. J. Pain 14 (1998) 107–115.
121. J. Desmeules, J. Chabert, M. Rebsamen, et al., Central Pain Sensitization, COMT Val158Met polymorphism, and emotional factors in fibromyalgia, J. Pain 15 (2014) 129–135.
126. V. Brooke, S. Janselewitz, Outcomes of children with complex regional pain syndrome after intensive inpatient rehabilitation, PM & R 4 (2012) 349–354.
129. T.J. Silber, Eating disorders and reflex sympathetic dystrophy syndrome: is there a common pathway?, Med. Hypotheses 48 (1997) 197–200.
138. A. Okifuji, D.C. Turk, J.D. Sinclair, et al., A standardized manual tender point survey. I. Development and determination of a threshold point for the identification of positive tender points in fibromyalgia syndrome, J. Rheumatol. 24 (1997) 377–383.
140. G. Waddell, J.A. McCulloch, E. Kummel, R.M. Venner, Nonorganic physical signs in low-back pain, Spine 5 (1980) 117–125.
153. D. Buskila, L. Neumann, E. Hershman, et al., Fibromyalgia syndrome in children—an outcome study, J. Rheumatol. 22 (1995) 525–528.
157. B. Zernikow, M. Dobe, G. Hirschfeld, et al., Please don't hurt me!: a plea against invasive procedures in children and adolescents with complex regional pain syndrome (CRPS), Der Schmerz 26 (2012) 389–395.
162. J.W. Guite, D.E. Logan, R. McCue, et al., Parental beliefs and worries regarding adolescent chronic pain, Clin. J. Pain 25 (2009) 223–232.
167. S. Kashikar-Zuck, T.V. Ting, L.M. Arnold, et al., Cognitive behavioral therapy for the treatment of juvenile fibromyalgia: a multisite, single-blind, randomized, controlled clinical trial, Arthritis Rheum. 64 (2012) 297–305.

168. B.H. Lee, L. Scharff, N.F. Sethna, et al., Physical therapy and cognitive-behavioral treatment for complex regional pain syndromes, J. Pediatr. 141 (2002) 135–140.

179. D.E. Logan, E.A. Carpino, G. Chiang, et al., A day-hospital approach to treatment of pediatric complex regional pain syndrome: initial functional outcomes, Clin. J. Pain 28 (2012) 766–774.

181. T.J. Silber, M. Majd, Reflex sympathetic dystrophy syndrome in children and adolescents. Report of 18 cases and review of the literature, Am. J. Dis. Child. 142 (1988) 1325–1330.

182. R.T. Wilder, Management of pediatric patients with complex regional pain syndrome, Clin. J. Pain 22 (2006) 443–448.

183. L. Cossins, R.W. Okell, H. Cameron, et al., Treatment of complex regional pain syndrome in adults: a systematic review of randomized controlled trials published from June 2000 to February 2012, Eur. J. Pain 17 (2013) 158–173.

186. C.J. Vierck, A mechanism-based approach to prevention of and therapy for fibromyalgia, Pain Res. Treat. 2012 (2012) 951354.

189. J. Ablin, M.A. Fitzcharles, D. Buskila, et al., Treatment of fibromyalgia syndrome: recommendations of recent evidence-based interdisciplinary guidelines with special emphasis on complementary and alternative therapies, Evid. Based Complement. Alternat. Med. 2013 (2013) 485272.

195. R.A. Moore, S. Derry, D. Aldington, et al., Amitriptyline for neuropathic pain and fibromyalgia in adults, Cochrane Database Syst. Rev. (12) (2012) CD008242.

202. M. Saps, N. Youssef, A. Miranda, et al., Multicenter, randomized, placebo-controlled trial of amitriptyline in children with functional gastrointestinal disorders, Gastroenterology 137 (2009) 1261–1269.

203. K.P. Patra, S. Sankararaman, R. Jackson, S.Z. Hussain, Significance of screening electrocardiogram before the initiation of amitriptyline therapy in children with functional abdominal pain, Clin. Pediatr. (Phila) 51 (2012) 848–851.

204. N. Uceyler, W. Hauser, C. Sommer, A systematic review on the effectiveness of treatment with antidepressants in fibromyalgia syndrome, Arthritis Rheum. 59 (2008) 1279–1298.

207. T.G. Tzellos, K.A. Toulis, D.G. Goulis, et al., Gabapentin and pregabalin in the treatment of fibromyalgia: a systematic review and a meta-analysis, J. Clin. Pharm. Ther. 35 (2010) 639–656.

215. N.S. Roskell, S.M. Beard, Y. Zhao, T.K. Le, A meta-analysis of pain response in the treatment of fibromyalgia, Pain Pract. 11 (2011) 516–527.

219. M. Varenna, S. Adami, M. Rossini, et al., Treatment of complex regional pain syndrome type I with neridronate: a randomized, double-blind, placebo-controlled study, Rheumatology 52 (2013) 534–542.

222. K. Christensen, E.M. Jensen, I. Noer, The reflex dystrophy syndrome response to treatment with systemic corticosteroids, Acta Chir. Scand. 148 (1982) 653–655.

223. S.B. Ruggeri, B.H. Athreya, R. Doughty, et al., Reflex sympathetic dystrophy in children, Clin. Orthop. Relat. Res. (1982) 225–230.

226. D.M. Siegel, D. Janeway, J. Baum, Fibromyalgia syndrome in children and adolescents: clinical features at presentation and status at follow-up, Pediatrics 101 (1998) 377–382.

227. E.D. McNicol, A. Midbari, E. Eisenberg, Opioids for neuropathic pain, Cochrane Database Syst. Rev. (8) (2013) CD006146.

228. M.J. Sigtermans, J.J. van Hilten, M.C. Bauer, et al., Ketamine produces effective and long-term pain relief in patients with Complex Regional Pain Syndrome Type 1, Pain 145 (2009) 304–311.

236. P. Henson, S. Bruehl, Complex regional pain syndrome: state of the art update, Curr. Treat. Options Cardiovasc. Med. 12 (2010) 156–167.

247. P.H. Veldman, H.M. Reynen, I.E. Arntz, R.J. Goris, Signs and symptoms of reflex sympathetic dystrophy: prospective study of 829 patients, Lancet 342 (1993) 1012–1016.

249. M.S. Cepeda, D.B. Carr, J. Lau, Local anesthetic sympathetic blockade for complex regional pain syndrome, Cochrane Database Syst. Rev. (2005) CD004598.

280. P. Lihua, M. Su, Z. Zejun, et al., Spinal cord stimulation for cancer-related pain in adults, Cochrane Database Syst. Rev. 2 (2013) CD009389.

289. D.D. Sherry, C.A. Wallace, Resolution of fibromyalgia with an intensive exercise program, Clin. Exp. Rheumatol. 10 (1992) 196.

290. A.C. de Blecourt, H.R. Schiphorst Preuper, C.P. Van Der Schans, et al., Preliminary evaluation of a multidisciplinary pain management program for children and adolescents with chronic musculoskeletal pain, Disabil. Rehabil. 30 (2008) 13–20.

291. P.E. Zollinger, W.E. Tuinebreijer, R.S. Breederveld, R.W. Kreis, Can vitamin C prevent complex regional pain syndrome in patients with wrist fractures? A randomized, controlled, multicenter dose-response study, J. Bone Joint Surg. Am. 89 (2007) 1424–1431.

Entire reference list is available online at www.expertconsult.com.

CHAPTER 53

The Impact of Rheumatic Diseases and Their Treatment on Bone Strength Development in Childhood

Rolando Cimaz, Leanne Ward

NORMAL SKELETAL MATURATION

The complex structure and composition of bone is directly related to the two primary functions of the skeleton: to support the tissues of the body in order to permit locomotion and to provide a reservoir of ions critical to metabolic functions.[1-4] Bone is composed of 70% mineral and 30% organic constituents. Hydroxyapatite, consisting primarily of calcium and phosphorus, accounts for 95% of the mineral content. Magnesium, present in smaller amounts, is also important in homeostasis. The organic component consists of 98% matrix, which is predominantly type I collagen. Noncollagenous proteins, such as osteocalcin, fibronectin, osteonectin, and osteopontin, make up 5% of the matrix. Cells occupying the remaining 2% of the organic component of bone are responsible for formation, resorption, and maintenance of the remodeling cycle. Osteoclasts are derived from mononuclear cells and resorb bone. Osteoblasts form osteoid and osteoid matrix. Osteocytes differentiate from osteoblasts and maintain the integrity of bone through a network of canaliculi.

PHYSIOLOGY OF THE DEVELOPING SKELETON

Genetic Determinants of Bone Mass

It is estimated that heredity determines 75% to 85% of the skeletal mass.[5-9] Environmental variables, including those related to endocrine and nutritional influences, mechanical forces, and other risk factors, account for the remainder. The genetic basis at the molecular level by which bone mass and strength are determined have yet to be fully elucidated. Many genes may be involved, and several polymorphisms have been implicated, including those for interleukin-6 (IL-6), vitamin D receptors, calcitonin receptor, transforming growth factor-β, estrogen receptor-α, osteocalcin, apolipoprotein E, osteoprotegerin (OPG), androgen receptor, osteopontin, osteonectin, and type I collagen.[9,10] Data suggest that genetic variations at multiple genetic loci are important in bone accrual, and that the combination of genotypes at several loci may have a major role in determining bone mineral density (BMD) and bone mineral content (BMC).[10] Among extrinsic factors, an adequate intake of calcium and vitamin D is a relatively important factor in achievement of peak bone mass.[11-14]

Bone Modeling, Remodeling, and Biochemical Markers of Bone Formation and Resorption

Bone remodeling is the process by which the skeleton refreshes itself by working on the same bone surfaces, engaging first in resorption to remove old, damaged bone, and then formation to replace the old, damaged bone with new, healthy tissue. On the contrary, modeling is the process by which the skeleton changes in size and shape, working on different bone surfaces. For example, as the tibia grows there is bone formation-driven periosteal apposition on the external cortical surfaces causing growth in width, and at the same time, there is resorption taking place on the endocortical surface making the bone marrow cavity bigger. Both children and adults can undergo bone modeling and thereby repair damaged bone, whereas bone modeling is largely unique to the pediatric skeleton and as such, has important clinical implications. For example, because of bone modeling children have a much greater capacity to restitute bone density spontaneously or in response to bone-targeted therapy (such as bisphosphonates). Similarly, children have the unique potential to reshape vertebral bodies following spine fractures, a clinical phenomenon described later in this chapter.

Bone turnover in a growing skeleton is a linked phenomenon of facilitating bone formation and limiting bone resorption in order for skeletal growth to occur. Studies of bone mineral metabolism generally assay a specific set of markers of bone formation and resorption in blood or urine.[15-17] Table 53-1 summarizes the principal characteristics of commonly used biochemical markers of bone remodeling. However, there are many confounding factors in using these measures (e.g., urinary acidity, medications, magnesium concentration, and renal function). Moreover, additional difficulties are intrinsic in the interpretation of pediatric measurements, mainly because these markers reflect growth and remodeling. Therefore, geographical reference data for age, sex, and ethnicity are essential. Although these markers cannot be used for the *diagnosis* of osteoporosis, they are important in the study of bone turnover in pathological conditions, and they can be useful in the follow-up of patients during anti-osteoporotic treatment, for evaluation of compliance, and are a consideration in prognosis.

Measures of bone formation include the activity of bone-specific alkaline phosphatase, which is released during osteoblastic activity. Osteocalcin (also called bone-gla protein) is a vitamin K-dependent, γ-carboxylated protein derived from osteoblasts. Its serum concentration reflects the portion of newly synthesized protein that does not bind to the mineral phase of bone and is released into the circulation. Serum carboxylterminal propeptide of type I procollagen (PICP) is also a marker of bone formation.[18] PICP is a globular protein cleaved by a specific peptidase at the C-terminal end of the procollagen triple helix. Its concentration in blood directly reflects the number of collagen fibrils formed.

TABLE 53-1 Biochemical Markers of Bone Remodeling

MARKERS OF BONE FORMATION

Alkaline phosphatase (ALP)	Enzyme secreted by osteoblasts, but also by other cells (e.g., liver, gut, kidneys). In children, about 80% of ALP is derived from bone. Bone-specific ALP is a constituent of osteoblast membrane and can be assayed in serum (no circadian variations).
Osteocalcin	Small noncollagenous protein synthesized by osteoblasts and chondrocytes and deposited in the extracellular bone matrix. A small amount enters the circulation and can be measured in serum. It is a sensitive and specific marker of bone formation.
Procollagen type I propeptides	N-terminal and C-terminal extension peptides are cleaved during the extracellular processing of type I collagen, prior to fibril formation, and can be measured in serum.

MARKERS OF BONE RESORPTION

Tartrate-resistant acid phosphatase (TRAP)	Enzyme present in the osteoclast and released during osteoclastic activity. Serum TRAP is not bone-specific.
Hydroxyproline	Amino acid found in collagenous proteins of bones and other soft connective tissue. A product of post-translational hydroxylation of proline in the procollagen chain. Can be measured in urine, but not specific (can be released by noncollagenous proteins and dietary proteins).
Collagen crosslinks (pyridinoline, deoxypyridinoline)	Pyridinoline and deoxypyridinoline are generated from lysine and hydroxylysine during post-translational modification of collagen. They are released during matrix resorption and excreted in urine, but new assays are available for serum determination. Of the two, deoxypyridinoline is more specific for bone.
Collagen type I N- terminal (Ntx) and C-terminal (ICTP or Ctx) telopeptides	Derived from degradation of type I collagen. Ntx is more sensitive. Both can be measured in serum and Ntx also in urine.

Plasma tartrate-resistant acid phosphatase is a marker of bone resorption.[19,20] This labile enzyme is released during osteoclastic activity. The urinary concentration of the deoxypyridinoline crosslinked telopeptide of type I collagen represents hydroxylysyl and lysyl post-translational components of the crosslinkage of type I collagen that stabilize the molecule. It is measured in the urine in relation to the concentration of creatinine. These crosslinks are reflective of mature collagen breakdown and are also a marker of bone resorption.[21] Deoxypyridinoline is found in large amounts only in type I collagen; therefore, its urinary excretion reflects the metabolic breakdown of that molecule. Urinary hydroxyproline has been used similarly. The urinary calcium/creatinine ratio is also a marker of bone resorption.

Calcium-Regulating Hormones

Assessment of bone mineral metabolism includes assays for calcium-regulating hormones such as parathyroid hormone (PTH), 25-hydroxyvitamin D_3 [25-$(OH)D_3$], and 1,25-dihydroxyvitamin D_3 [1,25-$(OH)_2D_3$].[22] The primary function of PTH is to maintain the ionized calcium concentration of the blood within a narrow physiological range. Hypocalcemia stimulates PTH secretion, whereas hypercalcemia suppresses its secretion. PTH regulates calcium homeostasis by acting on the major calcium reservoir of the body, the skeleton. It stimulates osteoclastic activity and thereby bone resorption. It also stimulates the conversion of 25-$(OH)D_3$ to 1,25-$(OH)_2D_3$. The principal source of 25-$(OH)D_3$ is dietary vitamin D_2. Ultraviolet light also endogenously stimulates the production of vitamin D_3 from 7-dehydrocholesterol in the skin. 25-$(OH)D_3$ is biologically inactive and is hydroxylated in the kidneys to the 1,25-$(OH)_2D_3$ hormone. This hormone, calcitriol, stimulates intestinal absorption of calcium, thereby elevating the serum calcium concentration. Receptors for 1,25-$(OH)_2D_3$ are present on intestinal cells. Care must be taken in interpreting the results of measurement of the vitamin D hormones, because diet, malnutrition, the presence of diseases leading to malabsorption or a catabolic state, and geographical location and season of the year (sun exposure) influence the results.

The Receptor Activator of Nuclear Factor-κB (RANK), RANK ligand (RANKL), OPG System

Discovery of the RANK signaling pathway in the osteoclast provided insight into the mechanisms of osteoclastogenesis and activation of bone resorption.[23-30] Osteoprotegerin (OPG), RANK, and the RANKL are parts of a family of biologically related tumor necrosis factor receptor (TNFR)/TNF-like proteins that regulate osteoclast function. RANK, a transmembrane signaling receptor, is mainly expressed by monocytes and macrophages; it is essential for osteoclast differentiation and activation and therefore for bone resorption. Its activation depends on binding with RANKL. OPG is a soluble protein that acts as a decoy receptor of RANKL, inhibiting osteoclast differentiation and activation, and thereby reducing bone resorption. To maintain bone homeostasis, balance in the RANKL, RANK, OPG system is required. The mature osteoclast, in response to activation of RANK by RANKL, undergoes internal structural changes that enable it to resorb bone.

The Mechanostat Model of Bone Strength Development in Childhood

According to mechanostat theory, the development of bone strength in childhood is driven by mechanical loads. These loads induce bone tissue strain, which is monitored by the osteocyte system. When bone tissue strain exceeds a given threshold, osteocytes initiate an effector cascade that induces osteoblasts and osteoclasts to reinforce bone at the site of strain,[31,32] thus effectively adapting to mechanical stimuli. The key mechanical loads in childhood that stimulate bone strength development are increases in muscle forces and increases in bone length, both of which are maximal around the time of puberty.[33] In children with rheumatic disorders, there are two potent risk factors that interfere with the mechanostat model of bone strength development: glucocorticoid (GC) therapy and loss of muscle strength.

The skeletal toxicity of GC therapy is highlighted by data showing that 15% to 20% of adult chronic GC users have a new vertebral fracture each year.[34,35] Similarly, a recent pediatric study reported that 6% of children with GC-treated rheumatic disorders developed vertebral fractures in the first 12 months of therapy alone[36]; a number of other studies have also linked GC exposure to increases in vertebral and/or nonvertebral fractures in this setting.[37-40] GC therapy exerts its osteotoxicity in childhood via a number of mechanisms. First, GC treatment attenuates linear growth, removing a critical mechanical impetus that normally fosters bone strength. GC therapy also has a more direct, adverse effect on bone cells, by blunting bone formation and inducing excessive bone resorption through promotion of osteoblast/osteocyte apoptosis and prolonged osteoclast survival.[41,42] The effect is not only to reduce BMD[40] but also to alter bone microarchitecture with a predilection for the trabecular-rich spine.[43] This explains why children with GC-treated illnesses are at particular risk for vertebral fractures compared to those who have not had GC exposure.

The fact that muscle strength is essential for bone development is clear from animal[44] and human[45,46] studies, and is underscored by the fact that children with congenital neuromuscular disorders consistently manifest low bone mass and bone fragility.[47] Burnham et al.[48] showed significant reductions in tibial muscle cross-sectional area in children with polyarticular juvenile idiopathic arthritis (JIA) and spondyloarthritis compared to healthy controls with corresponding deficits in volumetric BMD and section modulus (an index of bone strength). Overall, severe and long-standing disease was most strongly associated with musculoskeletal deficits in this study. Rodd et al.[36] showed a 6% incidence of vertebral fractures after 12 months of GC therapy in a longitudinal cohort of children with GC-treated rheumatic disorders; among the children in this study with incident fractures, 40% held a diagnosis of juvenile dermatomyositis compared to 20% with systemic lupus erythematosus (SLE), 20% with systemic vasculitis, 20% with systemic arthritis, and 10% with nonsystemic JIA. These observations support the hypothesis that the myopathy of juvenile dermatomyositis may pose an additional threat to bone health beyond the osteotoxicity of GC therapy.

OSTEOPOROSIS IN PEDIATRIC RHEUMATIC DISORDERS: CLINICAL MANIFESTATIONS AND RISK FACTORS

Mechanisms of Bone Strength Loss in Pediatric Rheumatic Disorders

The Impact of Inflammation on Bone Metabolism

Increasing evidence suggests that inflammation exerts a direct and detrimental effect on bone, as highlighted by the common finding of generalized bone loss in children with rheumatic diseases independently from GC exposure. The cell populations of the innate and adaptive immune system are activated during the inflammatory response and produce pro-inflammatory cytokines that are currently considered to be the main mediators of inflammation-associated osteoporosis. Cytokines such as tumor necrosis factor alpha (TNF-α), interleukin-1 (IL-1) and IL-6 profoundly affect the differentiation and function of osteoblasts and osteoclasts and uncouple the tightly regulated bone remodeling cycle, resulting in a negative bone balance. These proinflammatory cytokines promote osteoclastogenesis[49] either directly, by acting on cells of the osteoclast-lineage,[50] or indirectly, by modulating expression in target cells of key molecules such as RANKL.[51] Moreover they can upregulate RANK on osteoclast precursors thus increasing their sensitivity to prevailing RANKL concentrations.[52] In this regard, a reduced OPG/RANKL ratio in vivo was observed in patients affected by dermatomyositis[53] and juvenile idiopathic arthritis.[54-57] In another study,[58] however, Masi and colleagues observed significantly higher levels of serum OPG and a higher OPG/RANK-L ratio in a cohort of patients with JIA; in this study OPG levels were higher in patients affected by polyarticular and extended oligoarticular disease, and the authors explained these apparently paradoxical results as a compensatory response for preventing bone loss.

In the course of inflammatory diseases the function of osteoblasts has also been found to be impaired, and in vitro studies have shown that the pro-inflammatory cytokines can inhibit osteoblast differentiation and enhance their apoptosis.[59] Moreover, it has been shown that cytokines such as TNF-α are capable of inducing inhibitors of the Wnt protein-signaling pathway (i.e., sclerostin and Dickkopf 1 [DKK-1])[60-63] and inhibiting the osteoblast differentiation factor RUNX2.[64-66]

The impaired proliferation and function of osteoblasts in JIA has been demonstrated by Caparbo and colleagues.[67] Human osteoblasts exposed to sera obtained from children with polyarticular JIA showed reduced activity (indicated by low levels of alkaline phosphatase, calcium production, and osteocalcin) and higher rate of apoptosis when compared to osteoblasts cultured with sera obtained from healthy controls. In this study, serum IL-6 levels appeared to be the main determinant of the effects on bone cells, a finding that has been confirmed by others.[68-70]

The hypothesis that IL-6 might have detrimental effects on bone has been confirmed in studies by De Benedetti and colleagues.[71,72] They showed that a transgenic murine model with high circulating levels of IL-6 since birth had growth defects and a bone morphology comparable to those of children with chronic inflammatory disease. The same group also recently demonstrated in the same mouse model the efficacy of sequential anabolic treatments with osteoprotegerin and PTH in preventing bone defects and restoring normal osteoblast and osteoclast activity.[73]

Although cytokines are considered to be the final executors of chronic inflammation on bone, T and B lymphocytes have emerged as novel crucial regulators of bone health.[74] According to in vitro experiments, an important role can be attributed to the T helper 17 (Th17) population.[75] This cell type shows high expression of RANKL, which allows a direct activation of osteoclasts. Compared with Th1 and Th2 lymphocytes, these cells secrete a particular array of cytokines (mainly IL-17), whereas the secretion of IFNγ e IL-4, with an inhibitory effect on osteoclastogenesis, is reduced.[76] IL-17 activates osteoclast differentiation by increasing the expression of RANK/RANKL in target cells and suppresses the expression of OPG in osteoblasts.[77]

Effects of Glucocorticoids on Bone Metabolism

Glucocorticoids (GC) continue to represent an important adjunct in the treatment of many rheumatic diseases, even if, with the availability of new immunosuppressants and biological therapies, their role is now less prominent than in the past. Even though a physiological amount of endogenous GCs is necessary for efficient osteoblast differentiation,[78-80] systemic treatment with GC in childhood and adolescence is associated with detrimental effects on bone mass and growth[81] by means of multiple pathogenic mechanisms. GC-induced osteoporosis is characterized by a decreased bone turnover with a disproportionate reduction in bone formation over bone resorption.[82] Trabecular bone, a major constituent of vertebral bodies, is more vulnerable to GC than cortical bone[83]; therefore a progressive thinning and a reduction in the number of trabecular plates and consequently of bone strength occurs during such treatment.[84] This process is the result of a direct effect of GC on bone cells, through impairment of the replication and differentiation of osteoblasts.[85] Moreover, in the presence of GC, bone marrow stromal cells differentiation is redirected toward an adipocyte cell lineage mainly by the transactivation of CCAAT/enhancer-binding protein δ, which increases the expression of the pivotal adipogenic transcription factor peroxisome proliferator-activated receptor γ2 (PPAR γ2).[86,87] In addition to osteoblast differentiation, GC also impair bone matrix composition by reducing the synthesis of type I collagen and osteocalcin,[88] hence decreasing the bone matrix available for mineralization. The function of the mature osteoblasts and osteocytes is also impaired because the supraphysiological concentration of GC activate Caspase 3[41] and induce apoptosis. This progressive depletion of bone-forming cells disrupts the osteocyte-canalicular network, impairing the capacity of the bone to repair microdamage and determining a poor bone quality.[89] Although reduction of bone formation persists throughout the duration of GC therapy, bone resorption is an early and transient phenomenon[43] that follows an increased osteoclastogenesis[90] and prolongation of osteoclast lifespan.[42] GC promote osteoclast activity by increasing the RANKL/OPG ratio and enhancing the production of macrophage colony stimulating factor.[91-94]

Several extraskeletal effects of GC can also contribute to bone mass loss because they decrease gastrointestinal calcium absorption, increase its urinary excretion, and decrease the synthesis of IGF-1 and gonadotropins.[95]

The clinical effects of GC on bone health in children have been known for a long time; a large epidemiological study on more than 37,000 children treated with GC for a variety of underlying conditions[37] showed that patients with a history of frequent use of oral GCs or those taking greater than or equal to 30 mg prednisolone/day were at increased risk of fracture. Similarly, a recent study reported that 6% of children with GC-treated rheumatic disorders developed vertebral fracture in the first 12 months of therapy[36] and that a significant bone loss occurs soon after the initial exposure to GC[96]; children with more severe inflammation and more systemic involvement, such as those with systemic-onset JIA or connective tissue diseases, appear to be at higher risk. The effects of inflammation (i.e., disease activity) add to the burden of GC treatment, and the two factors are so tightly linked that it is difficult to extrapolate their relative weight in inducing bone loss.[97]

Disease-Specific Clinical Manifestations
Low Bone Mass in Children with JIA

Failure to develop adequate bone mineralization is common in children with chronic arthritis. Juxtaarticular osteopenia can be evident in plain radiographs even in early disease, whereas diffuse osteopenia or osteoporosis can develop later and lead to the risk of vertebral collapse and long bone fractures after minimal trauma.

Multiple risk factors are known to be associated with decreased bone mass (Box 53-1).[98-120]

Pepmueller and colleagues[112] measured BMC and BMD in 41 children with juvenile rheumatoid arthritis (JRA) and 62 healthy geographical controls, and analyzed serum markers of bone metabolism. Decreased BMD was found at all sites in the patient group with a negative correlation between measures of disease severity and bone mass. These researchers hypothesized that decreased mineralization, rather

than increased resorption, was the primary pathophysiological mechanism. However, the balance between bone formation and resorption is controlled by a variety of factors, and further studies on this subject have yielded conflicting results.[110,121] Although BMD may be decreased at all sites in children with arthritis, the appendicular skeleton is predominantly affected.[122]

Henderson and coworkers[116] evaluated predictors of BMD in prepubertal patients with JRA who had not been treated with GC. Almost 30% of mild to moderately ill patients had low total body BMD. Parameters of disease severity (number of swollen joints, articular severity score, erythrocyte sedimentation rate) exerted a negative effect on bone mineralization. In another study of postpubertal females who had never received systemic GC, approximately 30% of the subjects with mild to moderate disease demonstrated low bone mass.[117] A stepwise logistic regression model was used to identify contributing factors, and the only variable that significantly contributed to BMC was lean body mass, which accounted for the majority of the variance in total body BMC. This decreased lean body mass could be the result of altered body composition, which often occurs in chronic inflammatory arthritis.

In a 2-year controlled study,[123] Lien and colleagues evaluated bone mass and bone turnover in 108 children with JIA and 108 healthy controls matched for age, sex, race, and county of residence. Bone mass and changes in total body, spine, femur, and forearm BMD and BMC, body composition, growth, and biochemical parameters of bone turnover were examined at baseline and at follow-up a mean of 24 months later. Low or very low total body BMC was observed in 24% of the patients and 12% of the healthy children. Bone formation, bone resorption, and weight-bearing activities were reduced in patients when compared to controls. Total body BMC was lower in patients with polyarticular onset than in those with oligoarticular disease onset. Patients with JIA have moderate reductions in bone mass gains, bone turnover, and total body lean mass early in the disease course.

Stagi and colleagues demonstrated that BMD correlated with the JIA subtypes.[124] Dual-energy x-ray absorptiometry (DXA) examination was performed on 219 subjects with JIA (104 oligoarticular, 61 polyarticular, 34 enthesitis-related arthritis, 20 systemic disease) and on 80 age-matched and sex-matched healthy controls. Children with JIA showed a reduction in bone mineral apparent density when compared with controls. Bone mineral apparent density (BMAD, a technique used to correct for bone size) was -0.41 ± 0.7 for subjects with oligoarticular disease, -0.63 ± 0.8 for polyarticular disease, and -1.41 ± 0.7 for systemic disease. On the contrary, patients with enthesitis-related arthritis did not show a significant difference in BMAD than controls (-0.09 vs. 0.02). Children with systemic arthritis had a higher bone loss and a higher cumulative GC dose than those with polyarticular or oligoarticular disease. A subgroup of 89 patients was enrolled in a longitudinal study and underwent a second and a third DXA examination; most subjects with a reduced bone mass did not improve over time. BMAD significantly improved only in subjects with systemic-onset JIA, from -1.41 at baseline to -1.11 at the third DXA examination.

An abnormal body composition with low muscle mass and increased fat are well known features of children with JIA, as demonstrated by several studies conducted using peripheral quantitative computerized tomography (pQCT).[125-127]

A significant role has been therefore ascribed to the deficit of muscle mass in the bone loss and altered bone geometry seen in JIA.[128] According to the theory of the "functional muscle-bone unit" as described in the description of the mechanostat model of bone development, muscles are strongly related to bone and essentially drive bone

---

BOX 53-1   Risk Factors for Osteoporosis in Children With Chronic Arthritis

Active inflammatory disease
Glucocorticoid treatment
Decreased mobility
Protein/caloric malnutrition
Inadequate calcium/vitamin D intake
Decreased sun exposure
Decreased height and weight
Pubertal delay

strength development through application of a dynamic stimulus to the cortical bone via the tendons.[129] Consequently, the reduction in muscle force acting on bones may contribute to the pathological alterations in bone structure and strength, resulting in an increased risk of fractures.[130]

To assess the status of the functional muscle-bone unit, Burnham and colleagues[48] used pQCT at the tibia in a cohort of 101 patients with JIA (79% female; median age 10.5 years; median disease duration 40 months). Diagnosis was oligoarticular JIA in 24, polyarticular JIA in 40, systemic JIA in 18, and enthesitis-related arthritis in 19. Active disease was present in 29%. A significant reduction of tibial muscle cross-sectional area (mCSA) was observed in children with polyarticular JIA and spondyloarthritis compared to healthy controls, with corresponding deficits in volumetric BMD and section modulus (an index of bone strength). Trabecular volumetric BMD was significantly low in all subtypes apart from oligoarticular disease. Overall, severe and long-standing disease was most strongly associated with musculoskeletal deficits in this study. Therefore, the impaired muscular function likely contributes to, but does not fully account for, the bone deficits seen in children with JIA: bone loss can be viewed as a mixed disorder of altered bone development and lower muscular forces.

In addition to efficient disease control, mechanical load through physical activity appeared to increase muscle strength and bone density in children with JIA.[127,131] A study conducted on 48 subjects with JIA, randomized in an exercise group (n = 28) and a control group (n = 20), recently demonstrated that a short-term exercise program (three times a week for 12 weeks) resulted in a significant BMD increase in the exercise group.[132]

Effects of Childhood Arthritis on Bone Health in Adulthood

Chronic inflammatory diseases occurring during childhood and adolescence that are associated with a loss of bone mass may predispose patients to premature osteoporosis and fractures during adulthood.

Zak and colleagues[133] assessed BMD of the hip and spine in 65 young adults (mean age, 32.2 years) with a history of juvenile chronic arthritis. They found that BMD was significantly lower in these patients than in age-, sex-, height-, and weight-matched healthy controls. Moreover, significantly more patients than expected had osteopenia and osteoporosis. Factors associated with a lower BMD included active disease at the time of the study, baseline erosions, higher Steinbrocker functional class, polyarticular course, and chronic steroid treatment. The presence of juvenile chronic arthritis by itself explained about 20% of BMD variation.

French and colleagues[134] also determined the extent of osteopenia in a population-based cohort of adults with a history of JRA. Forty-one percent of the patients had a T score of 1 or lower at either the lumbar spine or the femoral neck. In another study,[135] the impact of disease activity on peak bone mass was assessed in 229 young adults in their mid-20s with juvenile arthritis at a mean of 15 years after disease onset. Patients with persistent disease had a significantly lower BMD than did healthy subjects, whereas patients whose disease was in remission had, overall, a normal bone mass. However, even in women with only a history of arthritis in childhood, total body BMD was significantly lower, although this was not true for the lumbar spine or radius. In a later report,[136] a large proportion (41%) of adolescents with early-onset disease were found to have a low bone mass more than 10 years after onset, and their low BMC was related to the duration of active disease, disease severity, measures of bone resorption, and anthropometric parameters such as height and weight.

In another study,[137] Thornton and colleagues retrospectively evaluated bone status in 87 young adults with a history of JIA (mean disease duration 21.2 years). In half of them a previous exposure to systemic GC was reported. At DXA examination the mean Z-score was lower in women compared to men at both lumbar spine (−0.328 vs. −0.251) and hip (−0.542 vs. −0.176); risk factors for a low BMD were a higher BMI, a more severe disease, a higher Health Assessment Questionnaire (HAQ) score, history of large-joint arthroplasty, and a previous exposure to GC.

Other Connective Tissue Diseases

Children and adolescents with SLE, juvenile dermatomyositis (JDM), and the vasculitides are also at risk for the development of osteopenia and osteoporosis, both from the disease itself and from its medical treatment. GC therapy, often in high doses and for prolonged periods, is the basis of treatment for most of these disorders. Avoidance of sun exposure and limited mobility in these patients can also contribute to decreased mineralization.

In SLE, despite evidence that in adults osteopenia is common,[138] scant pediatric data exist.[39] Reports in childhood-onset SLE provide evidence of a high frequency of osteopenia and a higher risk of osteoporosis later in life when the disease develops before achieving peak bone mass. In these studies the lumbar spine was the most seriously affected skeletal site, followed by the femoral neck, and higher cumulative steroid doses were associated with lower bone mass.[139,140] In another study, Compeyrot and colleagues studied 64 consecutive patients with juvenile SLE (JSLE) in whom routine DXA scanning was performed in order to determine the prevalence of low BMD and to identify associated risk factors. Lumbar spine osteopenia was defined as a BMD Z-score between −1 and −2.5, and osteoporosis as a BMD Z-score of less than 2.5. Their results indicated that osteopenia and osteoporosis are common in JSLE and are associated more closely with increased disease duration than with cumulative steroid dose.[141] More recently, Lim and colleagues[142] conducted a study on 80 newly diagnosed patients with JSLE in order to determine the prevalence of low BMD in the first 3 months after diagnosis. In this series of patients with active disease (mean Systemic Lupus Erythematosus Disease Activity Index (SLEDAI) score at diagnosis of 11), low BMD prevalence, defined as a lumbar spine (LS) Z-score less than −2, was 15%, whereas an additional third of the cohort had a LS BMD Z-score between −1 and −2. The result of this study suggests that disease activity affects bone metabolism from the early phase of disease. The same group also showed that a long disease duration can significantly impair long-term bone health in patients with JSLE, impairing peak bone mass achievement.[143] In this longitudinal study, 68 consecutive newly diagnosed JSLE patients aged 11 to 14 years were enrolled; the authors showed that LS BMD followed a deteriorating trend over time despite optimal vitamin D and calcium supplementation. DXA scans were performed within 6 months of diagnosis and annually thereafter. At the baseline only 9% of patients showed a low BMD (Z-score <−2); however, this proportion increased to 19% after 3 years. Overall, 35% of all patients' DXA Z-scores declined and only 6% improved. The rate of Z-score decrease was higher for patients who had entered into puberty at the time of the diagnosis, and for those with a higher cumulative prednisone dose. Another recent study[144] on 56 subjects with JSLE aged 13 to 24 years confirmed that peak bone mass is reduced compared with age-matched healthy controls. Bone status was assessed with lumbar DXA, radius pQCT, and phalangeal quantitative ultrasound (QUS); most of the patients were also revaluated after 3 years. Compared with age- and sex-matched healthy controls, at baseline JSLE subjects showed a reduced bone mass, altered bone architecture, and an increased value of fat cross-sectional area.

The progressive decline in bone mass can predispose JSLE patients to a high risk of osteoporosis later in the life. A recent study conducted on 395 adult patients with SLE by Mok and colleagues[145] demonstrated that patients who had disease onset in childhood had a lower BMD at any sites compared with patients who had adult-onset SLE.

The main role of GC in bone loss in JSLE has been analyzed by Baker-LePain and colleagues in a study conducted on 90 JSLE patients.[146] The association between bone turnover markers and disease activity was evaluated by measuring physical parameters, bone turnover markers (osteocalcin, serum tartrate-resistant acid phosphatase, urinary N-terminal telopeptide/creatinine ratio), disease activity indexes (SLEDAI, erythrocyte sedimentation rate (ESR), complement levels), serum level of interferon beta, and bone density by DXA. Their results indicated a decreased bone formation as result of GC use as indicated by the negative association between GC dose and serum osteocalcin; unexpectedly, an increased disease activity was associated with a reduced bone resorption. This finding may suggest that GC may be a more important determinant of bone loss than the disease itself; however, the two factors are so tightly linked that it is difficult to draw firm conclusions.

Vitamin D deficiency is also frequent in patients with JSLE, and is linked to multiple factors (e.g., avoidance of sun exposure, chronic renal insufficiency, long-term GC therapy, and insufficient dietary intake). Recent studies report an inverse relationship between serum levels of 25OHD and SLE activity.[147,148] Vitamin D deficiency can affect bone health in children with JSLE. In a cohort of 57 JSLE patients, Casella et al.[149] found that hypovitaminosis D was an independent risk factor for low BMD and vertebral fracture. Furthermore, a persistent state of 25-OHD deficiency was reported despite supplementation at currently recommended levels. Recently, lean mass has been identified as a major determinant of bone density, suggesting that muscle rehabilitation may be an additional target for bone therapeutic intervention in reducing the risk of fractures in JSLE.[150]

Another disease that can be associated with low bone mass is JDM: a report from 15 patients with JDM showed low BMD values in the majority and persistent or worsening osteopenia in patients with ongoing active disease.[151] Another recent study on 10 girls aged 7 to 16 years with JDM reported that lumbar BMD was significantly lower than age-matched healthy controls.[152] A correlation was observed between BMD and weight, suggesting that reduced bone mass in JDM may be related to other intrinsic mechanisms in addition to steroid treatment, and that some aspects of the disease itself (e.g., muscle involvement) may contribute to this condition.

Moreover, Omori and colleagues suggested a beneficial role of physical exercise on bone health in JDM[153]; after a short-term supervised exercise program (12 weeks) bone mineral apparent density (BMAD) was significantly increased at both the lumbar spine (+2.85%) and the whole body (+1.44%) in 10 children with mild JDM.

Finally, juvenile-onset systemic sclerosis has also been shown to be associated with low bone mass.[154] Ten young adults (mean age 20.9 years) with this disorder had a BMD significantly lower than healthy controls in femoral neck (0.2946 ± 0.060 vs. 0.395 ± 0.048, respectively) and total femur (0.134 ± 0.021 vs. 0.171 ± 0.022, respectively). However, all patients showed vitamin D insufficiency with lower serum levels when compared with controls (18.1 ± 6.4 vs. 25.1 ± 6.6, respectively), despite values of calcium, phosphorus, alkaline phosphatase, and PTH within normal range and comparable in both groups.

Fractures as a Key Manifestation of Osteoporosis in Pediatric Rheumatic Diseases

The most important clinical outcome arising from lack of bone strength development in childhood rheumatic disorders is fragility fractures, with loss of bone mass and density being one of the factors on the causal pathway to bone fragility. Fragility fractures have also been referred to as low trauma, atraumatic, pathological, or osteoporotic fractures. A commonly used guideline to define low trauma fractures is that they arise from falls, which occur from a standing height or less. Fragility fractures are typically further classified according to their skeletal site as nonvertebral or vertebral fractures. Nonvertebral fractures refer to those occurring at the hip and pelvis (both rare in childhood), long bones of the upper and lower extremities, hands, feet, nose, fingers, and toes. Vertebral fractures occur within the vertebral bodies of the spine, and are usually quantified from T4 to L4 on a lateral spine radiograph. In adults, both hip and vertebral fractures are associated with increased mortality (an observation that has not been assessed in the pediatric population), and, overall, fractures of the long bones, spine, hips, and pelvis are considered the most clinically significant.

A large study recently showed that children with a diagnosis of arthritis are indeed at increased risk for nonvertebral fractures. Using the United Kingdom General Practice Research Database, Burnham et al[155] reported (in a longitudinal, population-based study comparing over 1,900 children with various forms of arthritis to more than 200,000 healthy controls) that incident fracture rates at the forearm, wrist, lower leg, and ankle were increased threefold around the time of puberty. In this series, the most common fracture sites were the forearm and wrist. However, vertebral fractures presenting to medical attention (e.g., symptomatic fractures) did not occur more frequently in children with arthritis compared to healthy controls. Furthermore, GC therapy was not significantly associated with fractures in this study, an observation that may have been related to the fact that only a small percentage of children had received GC therapy in this study (4.9%).

Vertebral fractures are increasingly recognized as an important, but underrecognized, manifestation of osteoporosis in children with GC-treated rheumatic disorders. A number of studies assessed the prevalence of vertebral fractures after years of GC therapy and showed that spine fractures were evident in 10% to 34% of children with GC-treated rheumatic disorders.[38,150,156] Vertebral fractures can also be detected before or soon after GC exposure, as demonstrated by Huber et al,[157] who reported that 7% of children with a variety of rheumatic disorders showed signs of vertebral collapse before or within 30 days following GC initiation. When this cohort was studied 12 months later,[36] 6% of children had incident (i.e., new) vertebral fractures, and one patient in this follow-up cohort presented urgently to medical attention with painful vertebral fractures after only 4 months of GC therapy. Interestingly, those with incident vertebral fractures manifested discrete clinical features in this study compared to those without[36]; within the first 6 months of GC therapy, children with GC-treated rheumatic disorders and incident vertebral fractures had greater increases in weight and body mass index Z-scores, as well as greater declines in spine BMD Z-scores. The observed changes in body habitus are reminiscent of cushingoid features, suggesting that patients with cushingoid features (and declines in spine BMD Z-scores) within the first 6 months of GC therapy may be at increased risk for incident vertebral fractures. In both the Huber[157] and Rodd[36] studies, children with vertebral fractures were frequently asymptomatic, which adds credence to the concern that vertebral fractures as an overt sign of bone fragility in children with rheumatic disorders is clinically underrecognized. This is an important clinical observation, because even mild and/or asymptomatic vertebral fractures have been shown to predict incident vertebral fractures in children with GC-treated illnesses.[158]

Of the techniques available to assess vertebral fractures in children, the Genant semiquantitative method[159] has been studied on the largest number of pediatric patients to date,[38,157,158,160-162] and has shown clear biological relevance to children because Genant-defined fractures are

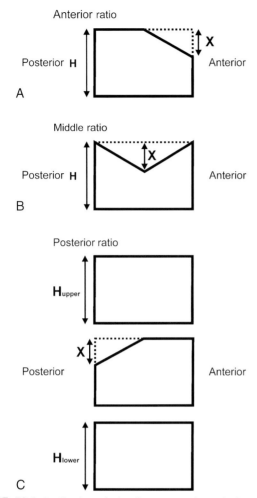

Anterior ratio

Posterior **H**   Anterior

A

Middle ratio

Posterior **H**   Anterior

B

Posterior ratio

Hupper

X

Posterior   Anterior

Hlower

C

FIGURE 53-1 Application of the Genant semiquantitative method. Loss of vertebral body height is visually estimated as a ratio of a reference vertebral height for each of three locations on a vertebral body: anterior, middle, and posterior. The loss of anterior vertebral body height **(A)**, designated X, is assessed in relation to the posterior height of the same vertebral body, designated H. Loss of middle vertebral body height **(B)** is similarly evaluated in comparison the posterior vertebral height of the same vertebral body. Loss of posterior vertebral body height **(C)** is assessed by comparison to the posterior vertebral body of the vertebrae above (H$_{upper}$) and below (H$_{lower}$). In the case of T4 and L4, only one adjacent vertebra is available, as the complete assessment is from T4 to L4. (Adapted from K. Siminoski, B. Lentle, M.A. Matzinger et al., Observer agreement in pediatric semiquantitative vertebral fracture diagnosis. Pediatr Radiol 44 (2014) 457–466.)

associated with clinically relevant outcomes including low BMD Z-scores, back pain, GC exposure, and an increased risk of future vertebral fractures.[38,158,160] In the Genant method (Fig. 53-1), vertebral bodies are graded according to the extent of the reduction in height ratios when the anterior vertebral height is compared with the posterior height (anterior wedge fracture), the middle height to the posterior height (biconcave fracture), and the posterior height to the posterior height of adjacent vertebral bodies (crush fracture). The scores correspond to the following reductions in height ratios: grade 0, 20% or less (normal); grade 1 fracture (mild), more than 20% to 25%; grade 2 fracture (moderate), more than 25% to 40%; grade 3 fracture (severe), more than 40%. Therefore, the critical loss of vertebral height ratio to define a Genant fracture is 20%, a threshold cutoff, which appears biologically relevant for the reasons stated above.

Vertebral Body Reshaping

A clinical phenomenon unique to children, compared with adults, is that children have the potential to reshape vertebral bodies following fracture, whereas adults do not. This is because vertebral body reshaping (that is, restoration of normal vertebral dimensions) is a growth-dependent phenomenon that comes about as a result of endochondral bone formation (growth of the vertebral body in height) and periosteal apposition (growth of the vertebral body in width). It is extremely important to recognize the child with potential for vertebral body reshaping because it obviates the need for bone-specific osteoporosis rescue therapy. Vertebral body reshaping has been consistently described in children with osteogenesis imperfecta undergoing bisphosphonate therapy[163]; however, bisphosphonate-independent reshaping in children with transient threats to bone health and vertebral collapse (e.g., GC-treated rheumatic disorders), is not well-recognized. Fig. 53-2 provides an example of this phenomenon in a girl with juvenile dermatomyositis who developed vertebral fractures while on GC therapy. She was subsequently treated with intravenous cyclical pamidronate therapy and demonstrated vertebral body reshaping on antiresorptive as well as GC therapy. GC therapy was ultimately withdrawn, at which time antiresorptive therapy was also discontinued as she was well clinically from both skeletal and underlying disease perspectives. Following bisphosphonate withdrawal, she had ongoing vertebral body reshaping through endochondral bone formation and periosteal apposition, and near-complete restoration of normal vertebral dimensions at the time of the last evaluation. As such, the presentation and subsequent evolution of this patient are important for three reasons: (1) clinically significant vertebral collapse can be present in patients with rheumatic disorders (and may not be symptomatic, so a surveillance program in at-risk children is necessary); (2) children have the potential to reshape vertebral bodies while on bisphosphonate therapy, provided they have adequate linear growth; and (3) with transient bone health threats, children have the potential to undergo vertebral body reshaping in the absence of bisphosphonate therapy (again, provided they are growing). Because bone-targeted therapies such as bisphosphonates are not without side effects, their judicious use is paramount and should typically be reserved for patients who are unlikely to spontaneously reshape vertebral bodies and restitute BMD, and they should be discontinued when risk factors abate, including vertebral body morphology as a clinical outcome in pediatric bone health; assessment is therefore recommended.

Diagnosis and Monitoring of Osteoporosis in Pediatric Rheumatic Disorders
Definition and Diagnosis of Osteoporosis in Childhood

Due to concerns about the misdiagnosis of children with osteoporosis based on BMD or bone mineral content testing alone, the International Society for Clinical Densitometry created a Task Force that went on to publish guidelines in 2008 to reasonably define osteoporosis in the pediatric population.[164] In this position statement, the diagnosis of osteoporosis was proposed to be based on two requirements: (1) the presence of a clinically significant fracture history (defined as a two or more fractures of the upper extremity, one or more fractures of the lower extremity, or a vertebral fracture), and (2) a low bone mineral content or BMD (further defined as a Z-score for either that is less than or equal to −2 SD, adjusted for age, gender, and body size, as appropriate). This definition encourages practitioners to reserve the term *osteoporosis* for children who have significant bone morbidity, a view that came about after significant concerns were raised that children were being diagnosed with osteoporosis in the absence of clinical evidence for bone fragility.

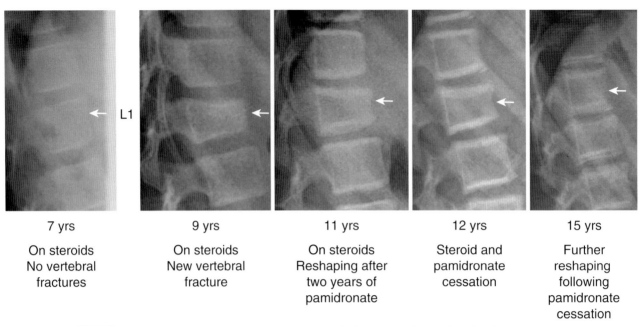

7 yrs	9 yrs	11 yrs	12 yrs	15 yrs
On steroids No vertebral fractures	On steroids New vertebral fracture	On steroids Reshaping after two years of pamidronate	Steroid and pamidronate cessation	Further reshaping following pamidronate cessation

FIGURE 53-2 Vertebral body reshaping *during* and *after* bisphosphonate therapy in a girl with dermatomyositis and a prior history of vertebral fractures associated with glucocorticoid therapy.

While this definition was embraced by the pediatric bone health community to the extent that it would prevent unnecessary intervention in children without a history of fractures, it did not recognize that some children, particularly those with risk factors for bone strength loss (i.e., prolonged GC therapy, underlying inflammatory states, and loss of ambulation) demonstrate clinically significant bone fragility with spine BMD Z-scores that are better than −2 SD.[158,165] One potential explanation for this observation is that the standard posterior-anterior areal BMD measurement by DXA is not sensitive in detecting GC-induced changes at the spine. Along this line of thinking, Dubner et al.[166] proposed the use of width-adjusted BMD to capture vertebral body BMD deficits, which represents the bone mineral content from the lateral projection of the spine, excluding the dense cortical spinous processes, divided by the estimated vertebral body volume based on paired posterior-anterior-lateral bone dimensions. The rationale for this approach was that width-adjusted BMD may be more sensitive to JIA effects on the predominantly trabecular vertebral body. Indeed, this group found that children with JIA had significantly lower width-adjusted BMD Z-scores compared to healthy controls and further, that width-adjusted BMD Z-scores were significantly lower than areal BMD Z-scores. Furthermore, these investigators found that the magnitude of the difference between width-adjusted BMD Z-scores and areal BMD Z-scores was greater in younger children.

A second issue in the use of a specific BMD Z-score cutoff as part of the definition of osteoporosis in children is that different pediatric reference databases generate different Z-scores.[167] Kocks et al. showed that the magnitude of the disparity in spine BMD Z-scores generated by different Hologic reference data were as much as 0.5 SD, and that the percentage of patients assigned a spine BMD Z-score worse than −2 varied from 15% to almost 30% depending on the reference database that was implemented.[168]

Given the widespread view that the definition of osteoporosis in a child should include a clinically significant fracture history, this continues to form the basis for the diagnosis in children. However, the observations that different pediatric reference data generated very different BMD Z-scores and that at-risk children can manifest overt bone fragility at spine BMD Z-scores better than −2 SD both call into question the −2 cutoff for BMD or bone mineral content Z-score as part of the definition. As such, the fracture history remains the cornerstone of the definition, with additional consideration for the magnitude and duration of the risk factors, and the overall BMD Z-score trajectory.

Diagnostic Techniques

Evaluation of mineralized bone mass using simple radiography is insensitive. Bone mass may have already diminished by 30% to 40% by the time osteoporosis is detectable on conventional x-ray films. Several additional noninvasive methods for measuring bone mass and mineral content have been developed. Table 53-2 includes the characteristics of the most commonly used methods of measuring bone density.

Dual-energy x-ray absorptiometry (DXA) is the technique most appropriate for children because of low radiation (3 mrem), speed, and accuracy. DXA employs two beams of 70 and 140 KeV to distinguish soft tissue from bone. The ratio of cortical to trabecular bone differs in various parts of the skeleton; therefore, DXA measures a composite of trabecular and cortical bone mass. Sites often measured clinically by absorptiometry include the one-third distal radius (95% cortical and 5% trabecular), the one-tenth distal radius (25% cortical and 75% trabecular), the lumbar vertebral bodies (5% cortical and 95% trabecular), the femoral neck (75% cortical and 25% trabecular), and the greater trochanteric area of the femur (50% cortical and 50% trabecular).

Quantitative computerized tomography (QCT) is applicable to measurement with the axial skeleton with a radiation exposure comparable to that of plain radiography. Peripheral quantitative computed tomography (pQCT) has lower radiation exposure and permits analysis of volumetric bone density of appendicular cortical and trabecular sites.

pQCT has become very important in recent years. Measurements can be done at the radius or the tibia. Radiation exposure is very low, less than 0.03 mrem. It is currently the only technique in clinical use that differentiates between trabecular and cortical bone and

TABLE 53-2   Comparison of Different Methods for Bone Density Measurement

METHOD	SITE	DOSE (mrem)	AVERAGE TIME FOR SCANNING (min)	COMMENTS
DXA	Lumbar spine, hip, radius, total body	1-3 (0.1 if peripheral, i.e., distal radius)	<5 for lumbar spine	Gold standard (best method available today)
QCT/pQCT	Lumbar spine radius, tibia	6/<1	10	True volumetric density can be measured. Allows for selective measurements of cortical and trabecular density, bone area, cortical area, cortical thickness, periosteal and endosteal circumferences, muscle cross-sectional area, and biomechanical strain strength indices. Not available yet for clinical routine use.
US	Phalanges, heel, tibia	0	1-2	Ease of scan, fast, no radiation, inexpensive, portable. Downsides: operator-dependent, needs standardization and more reference data.

DPA, Dual-photon absorptiometry; *DXA*, dual-energy x-ray absorptiometry; *pQCT*, peripheral quantitative computed tomography; *QCT*, quantitative computerized tomography; *SPA*, single-photon absorptiometry; *US*, ultrasound.

determines bone density, bone geometry, and muscle cross-sectional area. Variables of bone geometry like cortical thickness, marrow area, and bone area are particularly suitable as indicators of bone strength, which is the most important outcome variable in the assessment of pediatric bone.

In younger children, the precision of pQCT measurements might be compromised by the partial volume effect. This term reflects the fact that partially filled voxels (volumetric pixel) will not be included in the data analysis. As the voxel size is fixed, the cortical bone mass may be underestimated in a young child with a relatively thinner cortical thickness. Another point of concern is whether pQCT measurements at the appendicular skeleton adequately reflect the situation of the whole skeleton, including axial sites.[169] However, this technique is promising, and clinical studies for JIA have already been performed.[48,125-128]

Quantitative high-frequency sonography (ultrasonography) is a new and noninvasive method of estimating bone quality. This radiation-free procedure measures the transmission of ultrasound waves through bones and has been proposed for the assessment of bone density. Two parameters can be simultaneously determined from the measured signal: speed of sound and broadband ultrasound attenuation (BUA). BUA measures the loss of sound caused by bone as a function of frequency; in normal adults and children, it may be the parameter that demonstrates the highest correlation with BMD determined by DXA. In addition, sonographic measurements of bone may provide additional information about bone quality, such as stiffness and elasticity. Normative values for healthy children have been published.[170,171] Also, pilot studies in children with rheumatic diseases have provided relatively good correlations between ultrasonographic bone density measured in the calcaneum[172] or at the midtibia[173] and BMD determined by DXA, supporting the clinical use of ultrasound densitometry. This technique is a promising tool to assess bone mass and quality in children in view of the absence of radiation exposure, low cost, and portability of the equipment.[174-178]

Asymptomatic spine abnormalities in JIA determined by magnetic resonance imaging (MRI) are common in patients treated with GC as recently shown by Toiviainen-Salo et al.[179] This group conducted a study on 50 patients (41 females; median age 14.8 years; mean disease duration 10.2 years) with treatment-resistant JIA (27 patients affected by RF-negative polyarthritis; 14 patients with extended oligoarticular arthritis; 6 patients with systemic disease; 2 patients with psoriatic arthritis; 1 patient with RF-positive polyarthritis). Almost all of them were receiving biological drugs, and for 90% of the patients a previous exposure to systemic GC was reported. The median total duration of GC treatment was 7.1 years (range 0 to 15.5 years) and the median weight-adjusted cumulative GC dose for the preceding 3 years was 72 mg/kg. At the MRI examination, 14 (28%) patients had evidence of at least one wedged or compressed vertebra and 31 patients (61%) showed one or more imaging abnormality. The vertebral deformity was scored as severe in 27% of cases; the thoracic spine was more affected than lumbar spine. The main risk factor for fracture was a higher cumulative dose of GC in the previous 3 years; of note, none of the patients was symptomatic. The same group also assessed this same cohort with conventional x-rays[180]: the prevalence of vertebral fractures using traditional spinal radiographs was 22%, which is lower than the prevalence estimated using MRI.

Considerations in Monitoring Bone Health Among Children at Risk for Osteoporosis

Bone health monitoring is increasingly part of the overall care of children with rheumatic disorders, particularly those with risk factors for bone fragility such as prolonged GC therapy, refractory inflammation, compromised nutrition, and muscle disuse. Given the main predictors of osteoporosis outlined previously in this chapter, it is reasonable to consider a bone health monitoring program for children with any one of the following clinical features: (1) history of low trauma nonvertebral fractures; (2) history of vertebral fractures; (3) back pain; (4) systemic GC therapy for 3 months or more; (5) poorly controlled inflammation; (6) significant increases in weight and BMI Z-scores in the first 6 months of GC therapy; and (7) significant decreases in spine BMD Z-scores, particularly in the first 6 months of GC therapy. In the baseline bone health monitoring assessment of at-risk children with these features, it is reasonable to include an evaluation of the child's fracture history, a lateral thoracolumbar spine radiograph for detection of vertebral fractures, a spine BMD (the most reliable skeletal site for monitoring BMD in children), a 25-hydroxyvitamin D level (preferably at the end of winter to capture the value's nadir), a dietary assessment of calcium intake and a urinary calcium/creatinine to determine the child's total body calcium status, an evaluation of the child's growth and pubertal development (i.e., Tanner staging), and a musculoskeletal examination to assess back pain and ambulatory status. This approach provides concrete information about the child's *functional* bone health status, and serves as a baseline for any future comparative evaluations that may be needed depending upon the child's overall clinical evolution and persistence of risk factors. The tempo of future evaluations depends upon the magnitude of the child's risk factors and current functional status, with reassessments in at-risk children typically ranging from 6 months to 2 years (on average, annually).

IMPACT OF MEDICAL THERAPIES ON SKELETAL HEALTH IN CHILDHOOD

The Prevention and Treatment Effect of Medical Therapies Used for JIA

The osteopenic effect of methotrexate (MTX) has been described in children with malignancies treated with high-dose protocols and confirmed by in vitro studies.[181-185] However, lower-dose MTX is not associated with this osteopenic effect.[186-188] Most likely, the significant beneficial effect on arthritis counterbalances in vivo the demonstrated inhibitory effect on osteoblasts.

Biological drugs exert a potent antiinflammatory effect by selectively blocking specific targets in the inflammatory cascade, such as cytokines, T cell function, or B cell function. TNF-α inhibitors such as infliximab, etanercept, adalimumab, certolizumab, and golimumab are biological therapies commonly used in adults with RA or spondyloarthropathies; the beneficial effects of these agents on bone health seems to be related mainly to their efficacy in controlling inflammation.[189] In JIA, studies on this subject are lacking; a recent paper on adults with a history of JIA[190] showed that anti-TNF-α use avoided the deleterious effect of GC on bone formation and allowed a fast restoration of new bone formation. In 19 adult patients (mean age 25.6 ± 5.8 y) with active JIA, BMD was measured using DXA at baseline and after 1 year of anti-TNF treatments (infliximab, etanercept, or adalimumab). In all the subjects, calcium metabolism and bone turnover markers were assessed and concurrent medications were reported. After 1 year, a significant reduction in disease activity and C-reactive protein (CRP) and a significant increase in lumbar spine BMD and total BMD were found. The beneficial effect of therapy on bone was thought to be a consequence of increased bone formation rather than a reduction in bone resorption because levels of circulating N-terminal propeptide of type I procollagen (PINP) (a marker of bone formation) were observed, whereas levels of the bone resorption marker beta C-terminal telopeptide of type I collagen (βCTX) did not show significant changes. In the pediatric population, a positive effect of anti-TNF-α treatment on bone loss reduction has been documented in two studies: initially, Simonini et al. showed that 1 year of etanercept therapy conferred a sustained benefit on bone loss, again by controlling the underlying disease activity[191]; subsequently, the efficacy of etanercept in improving bone mineralization has been confirmed by Billiau et al.[192] In this latter study, 16 patients with polyarticular JIA who were previously nonresponders to methotrexate showed a sustained reduction in disease activity, a prompt catch-up growth and a significant improvement of bone mineralization after etanercept was added to the treatment regimen. The lumbar Z-score improved from −1.4 at baseline to −1 at 12 months after etanercept commencement; at the same time serum levels of IL-6 rapidly abated while OPG levels significantly increased. However, BMD improved similarly in a group of patients treated with MTX only. A significant increase of bone mineral content and lean to fat mass ratio was seen in the etanercept plus MTX group, but not in the MTX only group. These data confirm the hypothesis that improved bone health seen in children with JIA after treatments is related to antiinflammatory action rather than drug-specific mechanisms.

An abnormal body composition with low muscle mass and increased fat is a well-known feature of children with rheumatic

diseases and might contribute to the abnormal bone changes seen in these patients.[193] Growth hormone (GH) has been used in children with JIA[194] and has shown to exert a positive effect on BMD, bone geometry and body composition.[195-197] In a longitudinal study conducted on 12 children with systemic and polyarticular JIA, the long-term consequences of GH treatment on height, muscle cross sectional area (CSA), fat CSA and BMD were evaluated.[198] All patients underwent pQCT examination at yearly intervals until final height; data were compared with a control group (n = 13) matched for age, height, weight, JIA subtype, and disease duration. GH administration (mean treatment duration 5.3 years) resulted in a significant increase in muscle CSA and in a reduction of fat CSA when compared with the baseline values and with the control group. GH treatment resulted in an increase in total and cortical CSA and in cortical BMD, whereas trabecular BMD and total bone mineral content increased only slightly and remained persistently low.

The Prevention and Treatment Effect of Bone-Targeted Therapies

Knowledge about the main risk factors for osteoporosis in pediatric rheumatic disorders serves to guide clinicians in the prevention and treatment of osteoporosis. Because risk factors include GC exposure, reduced mobility, delayed growth and puberty, compromised nutrition, and inflammatory cytokines, these are the foci to target in prevention strategies. Many,[36,38,81,199] but not all,[155] studies have shown a relationship between GC therapy and an increased risk for bone fragility in this setting; therefore, the benefits of reducing inflammatory cytokines may outweigh the adverse effects of GC on bone. Correction of nutritional deficits is an important component of treatment that is often neglected. Given the potential for vitamin D to reduce inflammation as well as enhance skeletal health,[200] it is prudent to screen for and correct vitamin D deficiency in patients with rheumatologic diseases,[201] with optimal levels considered above 75 nmol/L.[202] Calcium is necessary for adequate skeletal mineralization, and may require supplementation in a select population of children with inadequate dietary intake to meet current daily requirements.[203] However, there is no convincing evidence that calcium supplementation in children with adequate intakes will sustain additional health benefits, and moreover excessive calcium supplementation in children may cause harm. As such, routine calcium supplementation without regard for the child's regular dietary calcium intake is not advised.

Physical activity has been shown to be of benefit to skeletal strength development in children, particularly at the proximal femur (hip). The hip enhances bone strength in response to increased exercise in children by redistributing bone to optimize geometry more than by increasing bone mass, as summarized in a recent review.[204] Therefore, attention has turned in recent years to measurement of a more functional outcome of bone strength. Bone strength can be readily estimated by applying a validated algorithm (Hip Structure Analysis [HSA])[205] to standard, DXA-based hip scans. With HSA, from the DXA-based anterior-posterior proximal femur (hip) scan, the proximal femur narrow neck section modulus is calculated as the cross-sectional moment of inertia (cm^4) divided by half of the subperiosteal width (cm) at the narrow neck in cm^3. This methodology provides a more functional index of bone health (i.e., bone strength) and has been shown to increase in response to loaded exercise in the pediatric population.[206,207] The proximal femur is the skeletal site of most consistent benefit among healthy children undergoing exercise intervention, as summarized in a recent review.[208] Recently, Omori et al.[153] showed that a 12-week supervised exercise training program was safe and led to significant improvements in muscle strength and function, aerobic conditioning, bone mass, disease activity, and health-related quality of

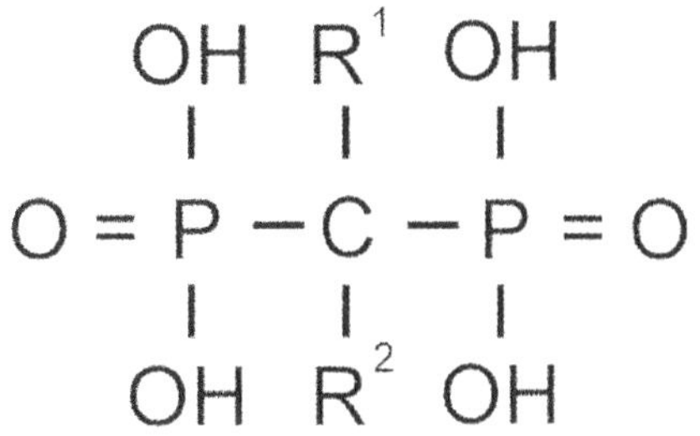

$$O = \underset{\underset{OH}{|}}{\overset{\overset{OH}{|}}{P}} - \underset{\underset{R^2}{|}}{\overset{\overset{R^1}{|}}{C}} - \underset{\underset{OH}{|}}{\overset{\overset{OH}{|}}{P}} = O$$

FIGURE 53-3 Chemical structure of bisphosphonates. R^1 and R^2, side chains.

BOX 53-2   Adverse Effects of Bisphosphonates

Observed

Increase in body temperature following intravenous infusion, flulike symptoms

Nausea, dyspepsia, esophagitis, abdominal pain, diarrhea, constipation

Hypocalcemia, hypophosphatemia, hypomagnesemia

Transient lymphopenia

Iritis, uveitis, scleritis, conjunctivitis

Mineralization defects (with etidronate), transient skeletal pain, epiphyseal and metaphyseal radiological sclerosis in growing bones

Delayed osteotomy-related fracture healing following rodding surgery in osteogenesis imperfecta

Feared but not Observed in Children

Irreversible and permanent effect on bone remodeling

Impaired healing and nonunion of spontaneous fractures

Osteonecrosis of the jaw

Damage to growth plates and impairment in linear growth

Fetal abnormalities

OI, osteogenesis imperfecta.

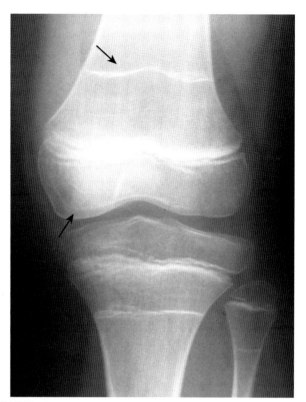

FIGURE 53-4 Metaphyseal dense lines following treatment with bisphosphonates in a prepubertal child (*arrows*).

life in patients with active and nonactive, mild and chronic juvenile DM. These encouraging results suggest a physical activity prescription is beneficial even beyond muscle and bone health. Bisphosphonates are the most frequently recommended therapy for children with overt bone fragility and chronic childhood illnesses.[209] Bisphosphonates, which are analogues of pyrophosphate characterized by P-C-P bonds, were first studied in humans about 30 years ago. Several chemical features contribute to their biological action: the P-C-P moiety facilitates the ability of these compounds to adsorb to hydroxyapatite, and therefore target the bone, while variations in their side chains determine the potency and spectrum of action of each individual compound (Fig. 53-3). Bisphosphonates are selectively concentrated in bone and inhibit bone resorption by interfering with the action of osteoclasts.[210]

Adverse effects of these drugs[209,211-214] are summarized in Box 53-2, and an example of radiological alterations described in a prepubertal patient following treatment with alendronate is shown in Fig. 53-4.

While treatment of low BMD in the absence of fractures is not advised given the lack of prevention studies in this setting, careful monitoring of at-risk children for the early signs of osteoporosis (including vertebral fractures) will identify those who may be candidates for bone-targeted therapy. At the same time, given the potential for children to spontaneously reshape previously fractured vertebral bodies and restitute BMD following transient threats to bone health, bone-targeted therapy should be reserved for children with either

significant impact of fractures on quality of life necessitating prompt treatment to relieve back pain and/or interrupt the extremity fracture-refracture cycle, or less symptomatic children who, because of a persistence of risk factors, are at risk for either further deterioration (i.e., further vertebral collapse, declines in BMD parameters, recurrent extremity fractures) or an inability to spontaneously reshape vertebral bodies. The goal of close monitoring and early intervention in at-risk children is ultimately to avoid permanent vertebral deformity due to spine fractures, to prevent recurrent extremity fractures, and at the same time optimize BMD parameters.

The effects of bisphosphonate therapy for rheumatologic disorders have been assessed in few controlled studies.[215-218] A 1-year randomized trial of weekly oral alendronate versus placebo found significantly greater gains in spine BMC and areal BMD (aBMD) with the active drug; however, neither group had significant changes in spine aBMD Z-score.[215] In a 1-year open-label study, children with diffuse connective tissue disorders given daily alendronate had significant gains in spine aBMD, decreased urinary N-telopeptides, and no new fractures or bone pain. An untreated group of patients with less severe disease not requiring GC therapy served as controls; they had no significant gains in aBMD in the same period.[216] A third study found that 1 to 2 years of intravenous pamidronate given to children with renal or rheumatologic disorders produced significant increases in spine aBMD, reshaping of vertebral bodies and resolution of bone pain.[217] Finally, patients with JIA given daily oral clodronote for a year had an 8% increase in spine volumetric BMD (by QCT) as compared with a 7% decrease in untreated controls.[218] The heterogeneity in diagnoses, outcome measures and drug regimens in these studies preclude pooling of the results. Only one study was randomized and blinded, all had fewer than 40 subjects, and none were powered to examine fracture prevention. For these reasons, the evidence is insufficient to justify routine use of oral or IV bisphosphonates for children with rheumatologic disorders as osteoporosis prevention agents; compassionate use for those with early signs of osteoporosis identified through monitoring of at-risk individuals is in line with current recommendations.[209,211]

FUTURE DIRECTIONS

In recent years there have been significant advances in our understanding of the pathophysiological basis, the clinical manifestations, and the predictors of osteoporosis in pediatric rheumatic disorders. The effect of bone-targeted therapy such as bisphosphonates on the developing skeleton has also been explored in pediatric rheumatology-specific studies and in numerous other osteoporotic conditions of childhood. The main goal facing clinicians and scientists in the future is to develop strategies for effective prevention of osteoporosis in this population. This is best achieved through efforts that target large number of patients and include measures that evaluate overt bone strength loss and functional impairment such as fragility fractures, pain, quality of life, and motor function in response to bone-targeted therapy. Given the clear relationship between muscle and bone strength development in children with rheumatic disorders, interventions that target muscle strength as sole or adjuvant therapy are also meritorious in this setting.

REFERENCES

30. W.J. Boyle, W. Scott Simonet, D.L. Lacey, Osteoclast differentiation and activation, Nature 423 (2003) 337–342.

32. H.M. Frost, E. Schonau, The "muscle-bone unit" in children and adolescents: a 2000 overview, J. Pediatr. Endocrinol. Metab. 13 (2000) 571–590.

36. C. Rodd, B. Lang, T. Ramsay, et al., Incident vertebral fractures among children with rheumatic disorders 12 months after glucocorticoid initiation: a national observational study, Arthritis Care Res. 64 (2012) 122–131.

37. T.P. Van Staa, H.G.M. Leufkens, L. Abenhaim, et al., Use of oral corticosteroids and risk of fractures, J. Bone Miner. Res. 15 (2000) 993–1000.

38. M. Nakhla, R. Scuccimarri, K.N. Duffy, et al., Prevalence of Vertebral Fractures in Children with Chronic Rheumatic Diseases at Risk for Osteopenia, J. Pediatr. 154 (2009) 438–443.

45. F. Rauch, D.A. Bailey, A. Baxter-Jones, et al., The "muscle-bone unit" during the pubertal growth spurt, Bone 34 (2004) 771–775.

46. L.M. Ward, F. Rauch, M.A. Matzinger, et al., Iliac bone histomorphometry in children with newly diagnosed inflammatory bowel disease, Osteoporos. Int. 21 (2010) 331–337.

48. J.M. Burnham, J. Shults, S.E. Dubner, et al., Bone density, structure, and strength in juvenile idiopathic arthritis: importance of disease severity and muscle deficits, Arthritis Rheum. 58 (2008) 2518–2527.

59. H. Wang, S.R. Young, R. Gerard-O'Riley, et al., Blockade of TNFR1 signaling: a role of oscillatory fluid shear stress in osteoblasts, J. Cell. Physiol. 226 (2011) 1044–1051.

60. M. Almeida, L. Han, E. Ambrogini, et al., Glucocorticoids and tumor necrosis factor alpha increased oxidative stress and suppress Wnt protein signaling in osteoblasts, J. Biol. Chem. 286 (2011) 44326–44335.

71. F. De Benedetti, N. Rucci, A. Del Fattore, et al., Impaired skeletal development in interleukin-6 transgenic mice. A model for the impact of chronic inflammation in growing skeletal system, Arthritis Rheum. 54 (2006) 3551–3563.

73. A. Del Fattore, A. Cappariello, M. Capulli, et al., An experimental therapy to improve skeletal growth and prevent bone loss in a mouse model overexpressing IL-6, Osteoporos. Int. 25 (2) (2014) 681–692.

74. K. Okamoto, H. Takayanagi, Regulation of bone by the adaptive immune system in arthritis, Arthritis Res. Ther. 13 (2011) 219.

77. M. Wang, T. Tian, S. Yu, et al., Th17 and Treg Cells in Bone Related Diseases, Clin. Dev. Immunol. (2013) 203705.

97. M.B. Leonard, Glucocorticoid-induced osteoporosis in children: impact of the underlying disease, Pediatrics 119 (2007) S166–S174.

98. R. Cimaz, M. Biggioggero, Osteoporosis, Curr. Rheumatol. Rep. 3 (2001) 365–370.

104. L. Hillman, J.T. Cassidy, L. Johnson, et al., Vitamin D metabolism and bone mineralization in children with juvenile rheumatoid arthritis, J. Pediatr. 121 (1994) 910–916.

112. P.H. Pepmueller, J.T. Cassidy, S.H. Allen, et al., Bone mineralization and bone mineral metabolism in children with juvenile rheumatoid arthritis, Arthritis Rheum. 39 (1996) 746–757.

116. C.J. Henderson, G.D. Cawkwell, B.L. Specker, et al., Predictors of total body bone mineral density in non-corticosteroid-treated prepubertal children with juvenile rheumatoid arthritis, Arthritis Rheum. 40 (1997) 1967–1975.

117. C.J. Henderson, B.L. Specker, R.I. Sierra, et al., Total-body bone mineral content in non-corticosteroid-treated postpubertal females with juvenile rheumatoid arthritis: frequency of osteopenia and contributing factors, Arthritis Rheum. 43 (2000) 531–540.

123. G. Lien, A.M. Selvaag, B. Flatø, et al., A two-year prospective controlled study of bone mass and bone turnover in children with early juvenile idiopathic arthritis, Arthritis Rheum. 52 (2005) 833–840.

124. S. Stagi, L. Masi, S. Capannini, et al., Cross-sectional and longitudinal evaluation of bone mass in children and young adults with juvenile idiopathic arthritis: the role of bone mass determinants in a large cohort of patients, J. Rheumatol. 37 (2010) 1935–1943.

127. J. Roth, M. Linge, N. Tzaribachev, et al., Musculoskeletal abnormalities in juvenile idiopathic arthritis: a four year longitudinal study, Rheumatology 46 (2007) 1180–1184.

128. J.M. Burnham, Inflammatory diseases and bone health in children, Curr. Opin. Rheumatol. 24 (2012) 548–553.

130. J. Roth, C. Palm, I. Scheunemann, et al., Musculoskeletal abnormalities of the forearm in patients with juvenile idiopathic arthritis relate mainly to bone geometry, Arthritis Rheum. 50 (2004) 1277–1285.

137. J. Thornton, S.R. Pye, T.W. O'Neill, et al., Bone health in adult men and women with a history of juvenile idiopathic arthritis, J. Rheumatol. 38 (2011) 1689–1693.

142. S.H.L. Lim, S.M. Benseler, P.N. Tyrell, et al., Low bone mineral density is present in newly diagnosed paediatric systemic lupus erythematosus patients, Ann. Rheum. Dis. 70 (2011) 1991–1994.

143. L.S.H. Lim, S.M. Benseler, P.N. Tyrell, et al., Predicting longitudinal trajectory of bone mineral density in paediatric systemic lupus erythematosus patients, Ann. Rheum. Dis. 71 (2012) 1686–1691.

146. J.C. Baker-LePain, M.C. Nakamura, J. Shepherd, et al., Assessment of bone remodelling in childhood-onset systemic lupus erythematosus, Rheumatology 50 (2011) 611–619.

149. C.B. Casella, L.P.C. Seguro, L. Takayama, et al., Juvenile onset systemic lupus erythematosus: a possible role for vitamin D in disease status and bone health, Lupus 21 (2012) 1335–1342.

153. C.H. Omori, C.A.A. Silva, A.M.E. Sallum, et al., Exercise training in juvenile dermatomyositis, Arthritis Care Res. 64 (2012) 1186–1194.

154. S.K. Shinjo, E. Bonfá, V. de Falco Caparbo, R.M.R. Pereira, Low bone mass in juvenile onset sclerosis systemic: the possible role for 25-hydroxyvitamin D insufficiency, Rheumatol. Int. 31 (2011) 1075–1080.

155. J.M. Burnham, J. Shults, R. Weinstein, et al., Childhood onset arthritis is associated with an increased risk of fracture: a population based study using the General Practice Research Database, Ann. Rheum. Dis. 65 (2006) 1074–1079.

156. H. Valta, P. Lahdenne, H. Jalanko, et al., Bone health and growth in glucocorticoid-treated patients with juvenile idiopathic arthritis, J. Rheumatol. 34 (2007) 831–836.

157. A.M. Huber, I. Gaboury, D.A. Cabral, et al., Prevalent vertebral fractures among children initiating glucocorticoid therapy for the treatment of rheumatic disorders, Arthritis Care Res. 62 (2010) 516–526.

159. H.K. Genant, C.Y. Wu, C. van Kuijk, M.C. Nevitt, Vertebral fracture assessment using a semiquantitative technique, J. Bone Miner. Res. 8 (1993) 1137–1148.

160. J. Halton, I. Gaboury, R. Grant, et al., Advanced vertebral fracture among newly diagnosed children with acute lymphoblastic leukemia: results of

the Canadian Steroid-Associated Osteoporosis in the Pediatric Population (STOPP) research program, J. Bone Miner. Res. 24 (2009) 1326–1334.

161. J. Feber, I. Gaboury, A. Ni, et al., Skeletal findings in children recently initiating glucocorticoids for the treatment of nephrotic syndrome, Osteoporos. Int. 23 (2012) 751–760.

164. F. Rauch, H. Ploktin, L. Di Meglio, et al., Fracture prediction and definition of Osteoporosis in children and adolescents: The ISCD 2007 Pediatric Official Position, J. Clin. Densitom. 11 (2007) 22–28.

165. A.M. Sbrocchi, F. Rauch, M. Matzinger, et al., Vertebral fractures despite normal spine bone mineral density in a boy with nephrotic syndrome, Pediatr. Nephrol. 26 (2011) 139–142.

166. S.E. Dubner, J. Shults, M.B. Leonard, et al., Assessment of spine bone mineral density in juvenile idiopathic arthritis: impact of scan projection, J. Clin. Densitom. 11 (2008) 302–308.

167. J. Kocks, K. Ward, Z. Mughal, et al., Z-score comparability of bone mineral density reference databases for children, J. Clin. Endocrinol. Metab. 95 (2010) 4652–4659.

168. L.M. Ward, F. Rauch, N. Shenouda, D.R. Mack Vertebral Fractures, Tibial Muscle-Bone Structural Changes and Muscle Hypofunction in Children with Crohn's Disease. Annual Meeting of the American Society of Bone and Mineral Research, Toronto, Ontario, 2010, p SU0023.

169. B. Zemel, S. Bass, T. Binkley, et al., Peripheral quantitative computed tomography in children and adolescents: the 2007 ISCD Pediatric official position, J. Clin. Densitometry 11 (2008) 59–74.

170. G.I. Baroncelli, G. Federico, S. Bertelloni, et al., Bone quality assessment by quantitative ultrasound of proximal phalanxes of the hand in healthy subjects aged 3-21 years, Pediatr. Res. 49 (2001) 713–718.

172. F. Falcini, G. Bindi, M. Ermini, et al., Comparison of quantitative calcaneal ultrasound and dual energy x-ray absorptiometry in the evaluation of osteoporotic risk in children with chronic rheumatic diseases, Calcif. Tissue Int. 67 (2000) 19–23.

173. C.F. Njeh, N. Shaw, J.M. Gardner-Medwin, et al., Use of quantitative ultrasound to assess bone status in children with juvenile idiopathic arthritis: a pilot study, J. Clin. Densitom. 3 (2000) 251–260.

174. F. Falcini, G. Bindi, G. Simonini, et al., Bone status evaluation with calcaneal ultrasound in children with chronic rheumatic diseases. A one year followup study, J. Rheumatol. 30 (2003) 179–184.

178. C. Wuster, C. Albanese, D. De Aloysio, et al., Phalangeal osteosonogrammetry: age-related changes, diagnostic sensitivity, and discrimination power. The Phalangeal Osteosonogrammetry Study Group, J. Bone Miner. Res. 15 (2000) 1603–1614.

179. S. Toiviainen-Salo, K. Markula-Patjas, L. Kerttula, et al., The thoracic and lumbar spine in severe juvenile idiopathic arthritis: magnetic resonance imaging analysis in 50 children, J. Pediatr. 160 (2012) 140–146.

180. K. Markula-Patjas, H.L. Valta, L. Kerttula, et al., Prevalence of vertebral compression fractures and associated factors in children and adolescents with severe juvenile idiopathic arthritis, J. Rheumatol. 39 (2012) 365–373.

186. M.L. Bianchi, R. Cimaz, E. Galbiati, et al., Bone mass change during methotrexate treatment in patients with juvenile rheumatoid arthritis, Osteoporos. Int. 10 (1999) 20–25.

189. V.K. Kawai, C.M. Stein, D.S. Perrien, et al., Effects of anti-tumor necrosis factor α on bone, Curr. Opin. Rheumatol. 24 (2012) 576–585.

190. K. Brabnikova Maresova, K. Jarosova, K. Pavelka, et al., Bone status in adults with early-onset juvenile idiopathic arthritis following 1-year anti-TNFα therapy and discontinuation of glucocorticoids, Rheumatol. Int. 33 (2013) 2001–2007.

192. A.D. Billiau, M. Loop, P.Q. Le, et al., Etanercept improves linear growth and bone mass acquisition in MTX-resistant polyarticular-course juvenile idiopathic arthritis, Rheumatology 49 (2010) 1550–1558.

198. S. Bechtold, P. Ripperger, R. Dalla Pozza, et al., Dynamics of body composition and bone in patients with juvenile idiopathic arthritis treated with growth hormone, J. Clin. Endocrinol. Metab. 95 (2010) 178–185.

201. E. von Scheven, J.M. Burnham, Vitamin D supplementation in the pediatric rheumatology clinic, Curr. Rheumatol. Rep. 13 (2011) 110–116.

209. L.K. Bachrach, L.M. Ward, Clinical review 1: Bisphosphonate use in childhood osteoporosis, J. Clin. Endocrinol. Metab. 94 (2009) 400–409.

211. L. Ward, A.C. Tricco, P. Phuong, et al., Bisphosphonate therapy for children and adolescents with secondary osteoporosis, Cochrane Database Syst. Rev. (2007) CD005324

216. M.L. Bianchi, R. Cimaz, M. Bardare, et al., Efficacy and safety of alendronate for the treatment of osteoporosis in diffuse connective tissue diseases in children, Arthritis Rheum. 43 (2000) 1960–1966.

Entire reference list is available online at www.expertconsult.com.

Primary Disorders of Connective Tissue

William G. Cole, Outi Mäkitie

INTRODUCTION

Primary disorders of connective tissue encompass a diverse range of single gene disorders that alter the function of connective tissue cells and their extracellular matrices.[1,2] The mutations have major gene effect sizes with autosomal dominant, autosomal recessive, or X-linked patterns of inheritance. The resultant connective tissue phenotypes can manifest during fetal life but usually do so for the first time during childhood, adolescence, and early adulthood. Many of the phenotypes involve the musculoskeletal system and thus patients are often referred to a pediatric rheumatologist. The reasons for referral are usually joint pain and/or swelling or restricted movement. Some are associated with significant impairment during growth and increased susceptibility to premature osteoarthritis in early adulthood.[2]

Many studies have shown that different mutations of a given gene expressed by connective tissue cells may have different effect sizes with severe, moderate, and mild phenotypes.[1,2] In general, the severity of the phenotypes correlates with the ages of clinical onset of the disorders with severe phenotypes manifesting earlier and milder phenotypes later. Severe phenotypes associated with particular mutations are usually of similar severity in other individuals with the same mutations. However, phenotypes of moderate and mild severity are often more variable in other individuals bearing the same mutations. It is likely that the latter variability is due to interactions with other gene variants and the environment that modify the phenotype to a greater extent than is usually observed in individuals bearing mutations with larger effect sizes. This makes the clinical diagnosis especially challenging in the absence of genetic testing.

Recent advances in mutational analyses have resulted in the identification of causative genes and their variants in an increasing number of primary connective tissue disorders.[1,2] These and previous studies over the past few decades have identified genes that are important for normal musculoskeletal health—a musculoskeletal gene set. These findings are of great value in the diagnosis and care of children with primary connective tissue disorders. In addition, these findings have contributed to the identification of gene variants associated with common adult musculoskeletal phenotypes, such as primary osteoarthritis and postmenopausal osteoporosis. In the latter disorders, genetic variants contribute to about 60% to 80% of the phenotypes, but each of the numerous identified genetic variants accounts for only a small percentage of the total genetic contribution.[3]

For many decades, the rare primary disorders of connective tissue and the common adult disorders of primary osteoarthritis and postmenopausal osteoporosis have been considered separately. However, it is likely that these common disorders of adulthood have their origins at conception and during the subsequent years leading up to their clinical manifestations in adulthood. As a result, an alternative approach is to consider the rare and common primary connective tissue disorders as part of a spectrum. For example, a genetic arthritis spectrum may comprise rare fetal and childhood disorders at one end and common forms of primary osteoarthritis at the other end. Such an integrated approach to these disorders is likely to enhance the identification of potential new therapies for children and adults with genetic disorders of the musculoskeletal (MSK) system.[4] This chapter focuses on the primary disorders of connective tissue that manifest during childhood–the childhood part of such spectra.

Classifications of primary connective tissue disorders were started in the 1950s and have undergone regular revisions since then. In 1956, McKusick reported a structured approach to the classification of heritable disorders of connective tissue.[5] A large number of these disorders alter the radiographic appearance of the skeleton and are referred to as skeletal dysplasias. The nosology and classification of genetic skeletal disorders was revised in 2010 by the International Skeletal Dysplasia Society.[2] A smaller number of disorders produce connective tissue laxity syndromes, such as the Ehlers–Danlos syndrome, in which the major impact is on the structure and function of soft tissues such as ligaments, tendons, vessels, and skin.[6] A revised nosology was produced by the Ehlers–Danlos National Foundation (United States) and the Ehlers–Danlos Support Group (United Kingdom) in 1997.[7] A consortium, which arose out of the first international meeting on Ehlers–Danlos syndrome convened in Ghent in 2012, plans to update the current classification.

This chapter will describe some of the more important disorders of connective tissue that may present initially to a pediatric rheumatologist, with specific focus on skeletal dysplasias and Ehlers–Danlos syndrome.

SKELETAL DYSPLASIAS

Classification

The classification of skeletal dysplasias has undergone revisions as new clinical and molecular information has become available. The International Skeletal Dysplasia Society is responsible for the current revision, which was prepared in 2010 by an expert group with clinical, radiological, and molecular expertise.[2] Four hundred fifty-six different conditions were included and placed into 40 groups defined by molecular, biochemical, and radiographic criteria—a hybrid system (Table 54-1).

The large number of skeletal dysplasias was grouped in accordance with their phenotypic or molecular characteristics. Groups 1 to 8 are defined by their molecular characteristics. They include disorders with heterogeneous, although often overlapping, clinical phenotypes due to molecular anomalies of fibroblast growth factor receptor 3 (*FGFR3*), type 2 collagen, type 11 collagen, sulfation, perlecan, aggrecan, filamin,

TABLE 54-1 Outline of Classification of Skeletal Dysplasias[2]

GROUP NUMBER AND NAME OF DISORDER

1.	Fibroblast growth factor receptor 3 (FGFR3) chondrodysplasia group	2.	Type 2 collagen group and similar disorders
3.	Type 11 collagen group	4.	Sulfation disorders group
5.	Perlecan group	6.	Aggrecan group
7.	Filamin group and related disorders	8.	Transient receptor potential cation channel, subfamily V, member 4 (TRPV4) group
9.	Short-ribs dysplasias (with or without polydactyly) group	10.	Multiple epiphyseal dysplasia (MED) and pseudoachondroplasia (PSACH) group
11.	Metaphyseal dysplasias	12.	Spondylometaphyseal dysplasias (SMD)
13.	Spondyloepi(meta)physeal dysplasias (SE[M]D)	14.	Severe spondylodysplastic dysplasias
15.	Acromelic dysplasias	16.	Acromesomelic dysplasias
17.	Mesomelic and rhizomesomelic dysplasias	18.	Bent bones dysplasias
19.	Slender bone dysplasia group	20.	Dysplasias with multiple joint dislocations
21.	Chondrodysplasia punctata (CDP) group	22.	Neonatal osteosclerotic dysplasias
23.	Increased bone density group (without modification of bone shape)	24.	Increased bone density group with metaphyseal and/or diaphyseal involvement
25.	Osteogenesis imperfecta and decreased bone density group	26.	Abnormal mineralization group
27.	Lysosomal storage diseases with skeletal involvement (dysostosis multiplex group)	28.	Osteolysis group
29.	Disorganized development of skeletal components group	30.	Overgrowth syndromes with skeletal development
31.	Genetic inflammatory/rheumatoid-like osteoarthropathies	32.	Cleidocranial dysplasia and isolated cranial ossification defects group
33.	Craniosynostosis syndromes	34.	Dysostoses with predominant craniofacial involvement
35.	Dysostoses with predominant vertebral with or without costal involvement	36.	Patellar dysostoses
37.	Brachydactylies (with or without extraskeletal manifestations)	38.	Limb hypoplasia—reduction defects group
39.	Polydactyly-syndactyly-triphalangism group	40.	Defects in joint formation and synostoses

and transient receptor potential cation channel, subfamily V, and member 4 (*TRPV4*). Each of the remaining groups is defined by its clinical and radiological phenotypes. Ambiguities in the current hybrid classification are likely to be resolved as disease-genes are identified in the dysplasias without currently assigned genotypes. Three classifications of skeletal dysplasias may emerge: one using the clinical phenotypes, a second using the molecular characteristics, and a third using both. Each of the classifications may have their strengths and weaknesses depending on whether they are being used for clinical or research purposes.

Diagnosis

There are many comprehensive resources available that can help with the approach to the diagnosis of skeletal dysplasias. For example, many relevant databases are available online from the National Center for Biotechnology Information (NCBI), USA. Included within its many options is the "Online Mendelian Inheritance in Man" (OMIM) database (available at www.ncbi.nlm.nih.gov/omim), which provides up-to-date summaries of each skeletal dysplasia and their associated gene variants. Links are embedded within the summaries to many related databases. Other useful diagnostic resources include: Pictures of Standard Syndromes and Undiagnosed Malformations (POSSUM), available from the Murdoch Research Institute, Melbourne (www.possum.net.au/), and the Winter-Baraitser Dysmorphology Database from London Medical Databases Ltd (available at www.lmdatabases.com/).[8] Key phenotypic features are entered and a list of possible diagnoses is presented in sorted order. Both systems can display clinical photographs and radiographs for each of the listed potential diagnoses thus allowing the user to rapidly include and exclude potential diagnoses.

Thorough assessment of a patient with a suspected skeletal dysplasia involves detailed prenatal, perinatal, postnatal, and family histories as well as detailed general and musculoskeletal examinations. A review of growth charts and head circumference is extremely helpful and important in considering a diagnosis.

Many skeletal dysplasias produce typical dysmorphic clinical features that are instantly recognizable to expert clinicians. Achondroplasia with its rhizomelic short stature and characteristic craniofacial and hand features is an example of a relatively common skeletal dysplasia that is easily diagnosed clinically. However, dysplasias that produce mild short stature without dysmorphic features cannot be diagnosed clinically. Genetic testing is extremely important to confirm the clinical impression and to provide genetic counseling and management.

Diagnostic imaging is an essential requirement in the evaluation of children with a suspected skeletal dysplasia. A complete skeletal survey is recommended and should include plain radiographs of the lateral skull; lateral thoracic and lumbar spines; thorax; pelvis, including the hips; long bones; and hands. Detailed evaluations of the size, shape, and structure of each bone and joint are undertaken. The findings are often summarized in accordance with the predominant pattern of changes in the skeleton, such as spondylo, epiphyseal, metaphyseal, and diaphyseal abnormalities. These terms may be grouped together to reflect the diversity of skeletal phenotypes. Examples include multiple epiphyseal dysplasia, spondyloepiphyseal dysplasia, and spondyloepimetaphyseal dysplasia. Other patterns may involve changes in the density and shape of bones of the appendicular and axial skeletons.

The clinical plus radiographic features are usually sufficient to enable a diagnosis or differential diagnosis to be made. It is important to note that the radiographic features often change with growth. Many of the typical radiographic features may not be manifested early, while many other features may be lost following skeletal maturity. Consequently, it is advisable to assess all radiographs because they may provide valuable diagnostic information concerning epiphyseal, physeal, and metaphyseal growth abnormalities. Similarly, serial radiographs of selected bones are often useful in establishing a diagnosis in a child when their initial clinical and radiographic evaluations are inconclusive.

Magnetic resonance imaging (MRI) and computerized tomography (CT) are rarely used to establish the diagnosis of a skeletal dysplasia. However, they are often used to evaluate specific complications that can usually be predicted when the underlying diagnosis is known. For example, MRI is often used to evaluate cervical spinal cord compression in patients with achondroplasia or various forms of spondyloepiphyseal dysplasia as a result of stenosis of the foramen magnum or instability of the atlantoaxial joints.

Biochemical investigations should be performed in children with suspected rickets, mucopolysaccharidoses, mucolipidoses, or chondrodysplasia punctata. These investigations, coupled with molecular diagnosis, should be undertaken as soon as these dysplasias are suspected so that appropriate treatments can also be commenced early, when they are most effective.

Most of the diagnoses can be made without pathological confirmation. However, histology of autopsy material, usually skeletal tissues from lethal skeletal dysplasias, can confirm clinical and radiographic diagnoses.[9] Postnatal iliac crest cartilage biopsy has limited value in the diagnosis of chondrodysplasias, but quantitative histomorphometry of iliac crest bone is routinely undertaken in many centers to monitor bisphosphonate therapy of patients with osteopenia due to osteogenesis imperfecta and related conditions.[10] Histological studies of excised tissue from dysplasias that predispose to malignancy, for example multiple hereditary exostosis, is routine.[11] Bone marrow histology is also undertaken in skeletal dysplasias that are associated with bone marrow anomalies including predisposition to malignancies such as the leukemias and lymphomas. Examples include patients with cartilage-hair hypoplasia or Schwachman–Bodian–Diamond syndrome.[12,13]

Molecular diagnosis is an important tool for the confirmation of the clinical and radiological diagnosis of a skeletal dysplasia. It is valuable in confirming inheritance patterns and risks of recurrence as well as for genetic counseling. Molecular diagnosis has also rapidly expanded the amount of genetic information concerning skeletal dysplasias and the wide spectrum of genes involved in normal skeletal development.

Treatment

Few of the molecular advances in the skeletal dysplasias have been translated into specific therapies directed to the disease genes, the disease gene products, or to physiological or biochemical pathways that are impaired by the mutations. In mucopolysaccharidoses, enzyme replacement therapy by administration of exogenous enzyme or by endogenous production from transplanted allogeneic bone marrow hematopoietic stem cells, may normalize hepatic and splenic abnormalities but is less effective in normalizing the skeletal phenotypes.[14] In contrast, the bone phenotype and bone marrow function improves in some children with severe forms of osteopetrosis treated by allogeneic bone marrow hematopoietic stem cell transplantation.[15]

Therapies for some of the other skeletal dysplasias involve pharmacological modulation of physiological processes that are impaired because of the mutations, and include the administration of phosphate and vitamin D to patients with various forms of genetic rickets and the administration of bisphosphonates to decrease the abnormally high levels of bone turnover in many forms of osteogenesis imperfecta.[10,16] Recent studies in a mouse model of osteogenesis imperfecta

---

BOX 54-1   Features Suggesting a Skeletal or Connective Tissue Disorder Versus JIA

More than one family member affected
Family history of joint replacement at an early age (<40 years old)
Absence of evidence of systemic or synovial inflammation
Absence of ANA and rheumatoid factor
Absence of joint erosions despite chronic disease
Congenital camptodactyly
Generalized hypermobility
Presence of two or more dysmorphic features

(Adapted from Ref 18.)

---

provided evidence that a neutralizing antibody to the osteocyte secreted protein, sclerostin, increased bone formation and, as a result, it may be suitable for clinical trials as a much needed bone anabolic agent for this disorder.[17]

For the majority of patients with skeletal dysplasias there are currently no specific treatments. Rehabilitation services are frequently required because of the musculoskeletal impairments. Surgical treatments may be needed to correct progressive skeletal deformity, stenosis, or instability. Surgery often has high complication and recurrence rates. Total joint replacements may be needed for premature osteoarthritis in patients with epiphyseal dysplasias. Other specialists, such as ophthalmologists, otolaryngologists, and endocrinologists, may need to be involved depending on the extraskeletal manifestations. Some dysplasias are associated with bone marrow dysfunction and the risk of malignancies. Careful surveillance of such patients enables preventative care and early treatments to be provided.

Some of the skeletal dysplasias that may present to the pediatric rheumatologist because of musculoskeletal pain or restricted joint range of motion are discussed below. Some features that can lead to suspicion of a suspected skeletal disorder versus juvenile idiopathic arthritis (JIA) are shown in Box 54-1.

Multiple Epiphyseal Dysplasia

The multiple epiphyseal dysplasias (MED) have been selected for review as a typical example of a group of skeletal dysplasias. The anomalies of epiphyseal and physeal development are shared with large numbers of other skeletal dysplasias such as the heterogeneous spondyloepiphyseal and spondyloepimetaphyseal dysplasias.

The MEDs (see Tables 54-1 and 54-2) are a relatively common group of conditions that are included within groups 4, 6, and 10 of the current classification of genetic skeletal disorders.[2] They are characterized by abnormal development of the epiphyses of the appendicular skeleton (Figs. 54-1 & 54-2) with mild or no visible changes in the axial skeleton.

The autosomal dominant forms are more common than the autosomal recessive forms. Children with the autosomal dominant forms appear to be normal at birth, although families with affected members are often able to identify affected babies because of their short and broad hands and feet. In early childhood, parents often note slowing of longitudinal growth, painful hips and knees, altered gait, and genu valgum (see Fig. 54-2).[19] At initial presentation, these changes may be quite mild. Nonetheless, a skeletal survey may reveal delayed and abnormal development of multiple small and misshapen upper and lower limb epiphyses. The femoral heads may show similar changes but may also show multiple small centers of ossification that coalesce in late childhood and adolescence. Many such children are referred with a diagnosis of Perthes disease, a form of avascular necrosis of the

TABLE 54-2 Multiple Epiphyseal Dysplasias[2],*

NAME OF DISORDER	INHERITANCE	GENE	PROTEIN
Multiple epiphyseal dysplasia type 1 [EDM 1]	AD	COMP	Cartilage oligomeric matrix protein [COMP]
Multiple epiphyseal dysplasia type 2 [EDM 2]	AD	COL9A2	Collagen 9, α2 chain
Multiple epiphyseal dysplasia type 3 [EDM 3]	AD	COL9A3	Collagen 9, α3 chain
Multiple epiphyseal dysplasia type 4 [EDM 4]	AR	DTDST	SLC26A2 sulfate transporter
Multiple epiphyseal dysplasia type 5 [EDM 5]	AD	MATN3	Matrilin 3
Multiple epiphyseal dysplasia type 6 [EDM 6]	AD	COL9A1	Collagen 9, α1 chain
Multiple epiphyseal dysplasia, other types	AD		
Familial osteochondritis dissecans	AD	AGC1	Aggrecan
Stickler syndrome, recessive type	AR	COL9A1	Collagen 9, α1 chain
Familial hip dysplasia (Beukes)	AD		
Multiple epiphyseal dysplasia with microcephaly and nystagmus (Lowry-Wood)	AR		

*EDM (epiphyseal dysplasia multiple) and MED (multiple epiphyseal dysplasia) are alternative abbreviations for the same group of dysplasias. *AD*, Autosomal dominant; *AR*, autosomal recessive.

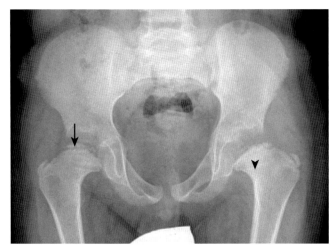

FIGURE 54-1 Pelvic radiograph of a 9-year-old child with type V multiple epiphyseal dysplasia due to autosomal dominant inheritance of a *MATN3* mutation. The femoral necks are short and broad *(arrowhead)* and the secondary ossification centers of the femoral head are small and malformed *(arrow)*.

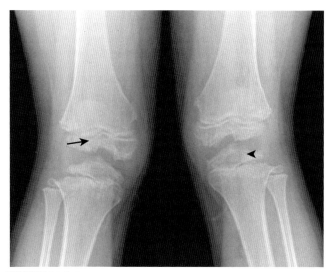

FIGURE 54-2 Radiograph of the knees of the same child shown in Fig. 54-1. There is bilateral genu valgum associated with markedly abnormal formation of the secondary ossification centers of the distal femur *(arrow)* and proximal tibia *(arrowhead)*.

hip. A skeletal survey is essential because of the difficulty in distinguishing Perthes disease from multiple epiphyseal dysplasia if radiological studies are limited to the pelvis and hips. This distinction is also important because some patients with multiple epiphyseal dysplasia may develop typical changes of Perthes disease in one or both hips during childhood. The vertebrae are often normal but may be ovoid with mild irregularity of the vertebral endplates.

Table 54-2 lists the known genes associated with autosomal dominant forms of multiple epiphyseal dysplasia. They include the genes encoding cartilage oligomeric matrix protein (COMP), matrilin 3, and the three α-chains of collagen 9.[20-24] Although their clinical and radiological features are similar, there are also some differences. For example, joint laxity and a mild myopathy are found in those with *COMP* mutations, MED1, because of the expression of COMP protein in ligaments, tendons and muscles as well as in hyaline cartilage and bone. Patients with MED1 also have ovoid vertebral bodies and mild irregularity of the vertebral end plates. Their clinical and radiological features indicate that MED1 is a mild form of pseudoachondroplasia (PSACH) which is a form of spondyloepimetaphyseal dysplasia also caused by

mutations of *COMP* (Fig. 54-3). Muscular weakness, usually without the joint laxity of MED1, is also observed in some patients with mutations of *COL9A2* and *COL9A3*.[24,25] In the latter patients, the muscle weakness involves the proximal muscles of the limbs.

The radiographic features of familial osteochondritis dissecans caused by an autosomal dominant mutation of *AGC1*, that encodes aggrecan, overlap with those of MED2 due to mutations of *COL9A2* in that some epiphyses show features typical of multiple epiphyseal dysplasia while others show features typical of osteochondritis dissecans.[25,26]

All forms of autosomal dominant multiple epiphyseal dysplasia are associated with progressive skeletal impairments.[27] Some patients develop progressive genu valgum, which may require surgical correction, usually lateral hemiepiphyseodesis of the distal femoral physes (see Fig. 54-2). Progressive osteoarthritis, particularly of the hips and knees, is common. Total joint replacements of hips or knees or both are often needed in the fourth decade but may be needed earlier, particularly in those with severe deformities of the femoral heads at skeletal maturity.[28]

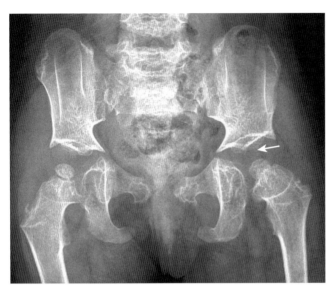

FIGURE 54-3 Pelvic radiograph of an 8-year-old child with the clinical and radiographic features of pseudoachondroplasia due to an autosomal dominant mutation of *COMP*. The pelvic bone and hip joint architectures *(arrow)* are abnormal. There were also severe abnormalities in spinal development and in other appendicular joints in keeping with pseudoachondroplasia, which is a form of spondyloepimetaphyseal dysplasia.

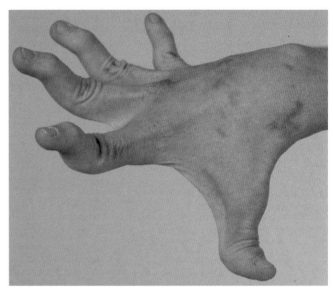

FIGURE 54-4 Clinical photograph of the hand of an adult with classical Ehlers–Danlos syndrome. The joints are hypermobile and the skin is thin, hyperextensible, and has multiple poorly healed scars.

It is often difficult to diagnose the particular type of autosomal dominant multiple epiphyseal dysplasia based on clinical and radiological findings alone. Specific clinical features such as ligament laxity, muscle weakness, and the pattern of skeletal findings may be helpful in suggesting the specific type of MED that the patient has. However, clinical and radiographic typing is often inaccurate because of overlap in phenotypes between the types and because of phenotypic variability within each type.[19] Consequently, each of the genes associated with autosomal dominant multiple epiphyseal dysplasia and familial osteochondritis dissecans need to be included in the genetic analyses. Despite this, molecular studies of a large cohort of patients with autosomal dominant multiple epiphyseal dysplasia did not identify mutations in the known genes in over one half of a series of 29 patients with MED.[29] The latter finding suggests that many autosomal dominant mutations may reside beyond the sequenced regions of the known MED genes or reside in other genes. The latter patients are classified as multiple epiphyseal dysplasia—other types (Table 54-2).

Multiple epiphyseal dysplasia type 4 (MED4) is the most common autosomal recessive variant. Patients with MED4 are born with club feet and later develop clinical and radiological features of multiple epiphyseal dysplasia.[30] Some patients also have recurrent subluxation and dislocation of the patellae.[31] Homozygous or double heterozygous mutations of the *DTDST* (*SLC26A2*) gene, which encodes a sulfate transporter, have been identified in patients with MED4.[32] The femoral heads are often severely affected and progressive osteoarthritis requiring total hip joint replacements in the second decade may develop.[31] A double-layered patella is common in patients with MED. It is noted on lateral radiographs of the knee as a result of separate anterior and posterior centers of ossification. However, the patella findings are not confined to patients with MED because similar radiographic findings have been observed in patients with pseudoachondroplasia due to autosomal dominant mutations of *COMP* and in MED2 due to autosomal dominant mutations of *COL9A2*.[33,34]

SELECTED SYNDROMES

Examples of Syndromes Associated with Joint Hypermobility

Joint mobility changes with increasing age. When the joints are excessively mobile children may develop joint pain with or without swelling. The Beighton criteria (see Chapter 51) are used to define patients with the hypermobile joint syndrome. A number of well-defined syndromes are associated with hypermobile joints and must be recognized by the pediatric rheumatologist.

Ehlers–Danlos Syndrome

Classification. The Ehlers–Danlos syndrome is heterogeneous with severe, moderate, and mild soft tissue laxity phenotypes, particularly affecting the dermis and joints.[7] The current numerical classification is shown in Table 54-3 and is based on clinical phenotypic patterns and gene mutations that resulted in abnormal fibrillogenesis of the collagen fibrils found in affected soft tissues. However, the classification needs to be upgraded because some of the previously included types were poorly characterized or were reclassified. In addition, many newly recognized types of Ehlers–Danlos syndrome, often associated with a more diverse range of molecular anomalies, need to be incorporated into the classification or reclassified elsewhere. The new types are included within the group labeled "other" in Table 54-3.

In the 1960s, major abnormalities of collagen fibril structure were observed by transmission electron microscopy of dermal samples from the severely lax and fragile skin of patients with classical Ehlers–Danlos syndrome (Figs. 54-4 and 54-5).[35] These early findings focused subsequent investigations into the composition of the extracellular matrix of the dermis, which shares many components with other affected tissues, such as ligaments, joint capsules, tendons, vessels, heart valves, cornea, sclera, adventitial layers of viscera, as well as septa, and fascia. Of particular interest in the early studies, was the synthesis and assembly of the heterotypic collagen fibrils, which contain predominately type I collagen, moderate amounts of type III collagen, and minor amounts of type V collagen. Vascular tissues and cornea can contain up to 30% of type III or type V collagen, respectively.[36] Recent advances indicate that the underlying molecular anomalies also involve

TABLE 54-3   Classification of Ehlers–Danlos Syndrome[1,7]

NUMBER	NAME	GENES	INHERITANCE	MAIN CLINICAL FEATURES
I	Classical (gravis)	COL5A1	AD	Severe joint and skin laxity; bruising; poor skin healing
II	Classical (mitis)	COL5A2	AD	Milder form of classical (gravis) EDS
III	Hypermobility	TNXB Mostly unknown	AD	Marked joint laxity with minor skin anomalies
IV	Vascular	COL3A1	AD	Easy bruising; vascular and bowel ruptures; thin skin
VIA	Kyphoscoliosis	PLOD1	AR	Joint hypermobility, severe kyphoscoliosis with fragility of skin and eyes
VIB	Musculocontractural	CHST14	AR	Digit contractures; hypermobility; scoliosis; thin, lax skin; and ocular anomalies
VIIA	Arthrochalasia multiplex congenita	COL1A1	AD	Severe joint hypermobility and hip dislocations
VIIB	Arthrochalasia multiplex congenita	COL1A2	AD	Severe joint hypermobility and hip dislocations
VIIC	Dermatosparaxis	ADAMTS2	AR	Severe skin fragility, joint hypermobility, and blue sclerae
VIII	Periodontitis	Unknown but one locus at 12p13	AD	Periodontal loss, soft skin, and joint hypermobility
Other				
	Progeroid	B4GALT7	AR	Dysmorphic with thin elastic skin
	B3GALT6 related	B3GALT6	AR	Skin fragility, joint laxity, contractures, and spondyloepimetaphyseal dysplasia
	Cardiac valvular	COL1A2	AR	Cardiac valve incompetence with skin and joint laxity
	Classical EDS with vascular ruptures	COL1A1	AD	Features of type I/II EDS and vascular ruptures
	FKBP14 related	FKBP14	AR	Scoliosis, joint hypermobility, hearing loss, and myopathy
	Spondylocheiro dysplasia	SLC39A13	AR	Lax skin, easy bruising, spondyloepiphyseal dysplasia
	Tenascin-X deficient	TNXB	AR	Joint laxity, skin laxity, easy bruising with normal skin healing
	Periventricular heterotopia	FLNA	XL	Joint laxity with periventricular heterotopia

AD, Autosomal dominant; AR, autosomal recessive; EDS, Ehlers–Danlos syndrome; XL, X-linked.

proteoglycans and other proteins that bridge between the various components of the extracellular matrix as outlined below.

Type I collagen defects. The first biochemical anomaly detected in humans and an animal model with Ehlers–Danlos syndrome was a deficiency in lysyl hydroxylase (*PLOD1*).[37,38] This enzyme is required for the hydroxylation of lysyl residues of collagens, including those residues that are involved in the formation of glycosylated hydroxylysyl residues and hydroxylysyl-derived collagen cross-links. This form of Ehlers–Danlos syndrome is now called type VIA (the kyphoscoliosis type) with severe kyphoscoliosis, joint hypermobility, and fragility of vessels and the eye.

A bovine model with severe skin fragility (dermatosparaxis) provided further evidence of the importance of collagen fibrillogenesis in the pathogenesis of Ehlers–Danlos syndrome.[39] The dermatosparactic cattle had an autosomal recessive deficiency of ADAMTS2, which is the enzyme that normally excises the amino-terminal propeptides of the type I procollagen chains as part of the posttranslational processing of procollagen to collagen. Persistence of the amino-terminal propeptides impaired the formation of the collagen fibrils and the structural properties of the dermis and other type I collagen-containing tissues. Investigation of humans showed that patients with arthrochalasia multiplex congenita had autosomal dominant mutations involving the ADAMTS enzyme cleavage sites of the amino-terminal propeptides of either the pro-α1(I) or pro-α2(I) chains of type I procollagen. Mutations of this region of the pro-α1(I) chain were classified as EDS-VIIA while those of the pro-α2(I) chains were classified as EDS-type VIIB.[40–42] Babies with arthrochalasia multiplex congenita had extreme hypotonia and joint laxity, usually with bilateral dislocations of the hip, as well as soft skin. In 1992, a human form of dermatosparaxis, type VIIC, was identified with autosomal recessive inheritance of *ADAMTS2* mutations

with severe skin fragility, joint hypermobility and blue sclerae.[43,44] Severe phenotypes were associated with complete loss of enzyme activity in those with nonsense mutations and milder phenotypes were associated with some residual enzyme activity in those with missense mutations of *ADAMTS2*.[45]

Joint laxity is a common feature of children with osteogenesis imperfecta due to nonsense and missense mutations of the type I collagen. However, joint and skin laxity can be more severe in those with amino acid substitutions near the amino-terminal end of the helical domains of the type I collagen chains. The combined osteogenesis imperfecta and Ehlers–Danlos syndrome phenotypes of such children appear to be due to conformational changes in the procollagen molecules that impair the ADAMTS2 cleavage of their amino-terminal propeptides.[46]

Type I collagen mutations have also been recorded in two other forms of Ehlers–Danlos syndrome. Homozygosity or compound heterozygosity for null mutations of *COL1A2* were detected in individuals with polyvalvular cardiac involvement and laxity of the skin and joints.[47] A small number of individuals with features of classical type I/II Ehlers–Danlos syndrome and vascular ruptures had substitutions of arginine by cysteine within the triple helical domain of pro-α1(I) chains.[48] Recently, an autosomal recessive form of Ehlers–Danlos syndrome with scoliosis, joint hypermobility, and myopathy was shown to be due to mutations of *FKBP14*, which encodes a member of the prolyl cis-trans isomerase family.[49] It is likely that the deficiency in this enzyme impaired cis-trans isomerization of peptidyl-prolyl bonds, which is an essential process in the normal folding of fibrillar collagens.

Type III collagen defects. Mutations of type III collagen are found in type IV Ehlers–Danlos syndrome (the vascular form). Affected

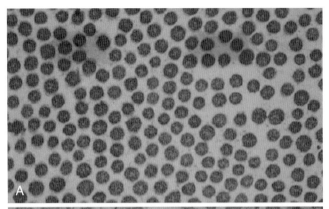

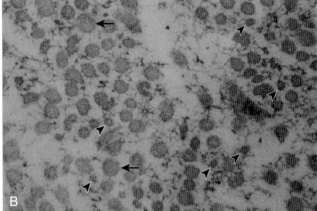

FIGURE 54-5 Transmission electron microscopy of the dermis of the volar aspect of the forearm of the same patient with classical Ehlers–Danlos syndrome shown in Fig. 54-4. **A,** Normal appearance of regular and uniform diameter collagen fibrils in an aged-matched control. **B,** Reduced number of collagen fibrils with abnormal shapes and sizes of the fibrils in the patient (abnormally small fibrils, *arrowheads;* abnormally large fibrils, *arrows*).

individuals have thin translucent skin, wide scars, with prominent subcutaneous veins, easy bruising, vascular fragility, and bowel ruptures. Mild joint hypermobility is usually limited to the hands. Affected individuals have a significant risk of acute vascular ruptures and death.

In the 1970s, analyses of collagens produced by cultured dermal fibroblasts showed reduced amounts and abnormal electrophoretic migration of type III collagen.[50] Subsequent studies showed that autosomal dominant mutations of *COL3A1* were the cause of the vascular type of Ehlers–Danlos syndrome.[51] *Col3a1*-deficient mice had severe vascular abnormalities and abnormally small collagen fibrils. These studies confirmed that type III collagen is an essential component of the heterotypic type I collagen fibrils that normally contain types I, III, and V collagens. The phenotypic impact of *COL3A1* mutations on the vascular system likely reflects the normally much higher proportion of type III collagen in the heterotypic type I collagen fibrils of the vascular system when compared to other connective tissues. To date, there is only a single report of an autosomal recessive inheritance of bi-allelic *COL3A1* mutations in type IV Ehlers–Danlos syndrome.[52]

Type V collagen defects. Type V collagen is present in only minor amounts within heterotypic type I collagen fibrils. However, it appears to play an important role in the nucleation of collagen fibrillogenesis and in limiting the size of the heterotypic type I collagen fibrils. It is found in greatest concentration in the cornea, where it is proposed to strictly control collagen fibril sizes in order to maximize transmission of light.

Most individuals with classical type I/II Ehlers–Danlos syndrome have autosomal dominant mutations of the *COL5A1* or *COL5A2* genes that encode the pro-α1(V) and pro-α2(V) chains of type V procollagen, respectively.[53] Most mutations result in *COL5A1* haploinsufficiency. Mutations of *COL5A2* are less frequently found and are usually missense mutations. *Col5a1* knockout mice do not survive embryogenesis and their tissues lack large collagen fibrils.[54]

Proteoglycan defects. Proteoglycans, such as decorin and biglycan, are important extracellular matrix components of the dermis and other connective tissues. A progeroid type of Ehlers–Danlos syndrome results from impaired addition of glycosaminoglycans to several proteoglycan core proteins due to autosomal recessive mutations of *B4GALT7*.[55] This gene encodes galactosyltransferase I which transfers galactose to the O-linked xylose of the core proteins. Autosomal recessive mutations of *B3GALT6*, a related gene involved in the synthesis of galactosyltransferase II, is associated with joint laxity and contractures, skin fragility, and spondyloepimetaphyseal dysplasia.[56]

The musculocontractural type of Ehlers–Danlos syndrome has been classified as type VIB because the clinical features are similar to those of type VIA. It results from autosomal recessive mutations in *CHST14*, which encodes dermatan 4-O-sulfotransferase I.[57] This enzyme normally sulfates some of the N-acetylgalactosamine residues in dermatan sulfate side chains.

Other protein defects. Several types of Ehlers–Danlos syndrome occur with mutations of *TNXB*, which encodes tenascin X protein within the extracellular matrix of connective tissues. Tenascin X deficient Ehlers–Danlos syndrome is an autosomal recessive disorder that resembles classical Ehlers–Danlos syndrome except that skin healing is normal.[58] Heterozygous carriers of null mutations have a joint hypermobility phenotype similar to type III Ehlers–Danlos syndrome.[59] However, mutations in *TNXB* were detected in only 2.5% of a cohort of patients with type III Ehlers–Danlos syndrome. Studies in *TNXB*-null mice suggest that tenascin X plays a role in collagen deposition and in bridging interactions with fibrillar collagens, fibril-associated collagens, decorin, and other matrix proteins.[60]

A phenotype of lax skin, easy bruising, and spondylocheiro (spine and hand) dysplasia due to autosomal recessive mutations of *SLC39A13* has been added to the "other" category of Ehlers–Danlos syndrome.[61] The gene normally encodes ZIP13, a zinc transporter within punctate vesicles. It appears that deficient availability of zinc may have pleiotropic effects as shown by the combined Ehlers–Danlos syndrome and skeletal dysplasia phenotypes.

An X-linked type of Ehlers–Danlos syndrome associated with periventricular heterotopia of the brain was shown to be due to mutations of *FLNA*.[62] The gene normally encodes filamin A, which is a widely expressed actin-binding protein that regulates the organization of the actin cytoskeleton of cells. Mutations of this gene have been associated with a wide variety of phenotypes that reflect the importance of filamin A in the normal structure and function of most cells.

Protein defects to be discovered. Review of the classification of Ehlers–Danlos syndrome shows that considerable progress has been made in identifying causative genes and their mutations in many forms of Ehlers–Danlos syndrome. Studies of well-characterized cohorts of patients have shown that the genes associated with types I/II, IV, and VII Ehlers–Danlos syndrome are found in most patients. However, little progress has been made in identifying the genes associated with type III Ehlers–Danlos syndrome. Mutations of *TNXB* were only identified in 2.5% of patients. However, type III Ehlers–Danlos syndrome is likely to be clinically and genetically heterogeneous. The genes associated with type VIII Ehlers–Danlos syndrome (the periodontitis type) have also not been identified as yet.

Diagnosis and treatment. The clinical features of classical types I/II Ehlers–Danlos syndrome are characteristic, even from an early age. Severe skin and joint hyperextensibility are evident at birth. Easy bruising and fragility of the skin become more noticeable as the child starts to stand and walk. Lacerations are difficult to suture and heal poorly. Complications due to laxity and fragility of the type I/III/V collagen containing tissues are frequent and often life threatening. Stabilization of subluxing and dislocating joints by arthroscopic or open surgery is often unsuccessful and is associated with high complication rates. Similarly, surgical corrections of progressive spinal deformities have high complication rates. Nonoperative orthotic stabilization of unstable joints and spinal deformities is difficult because of the skin fragility. The clinical diagnosis can be confirmed by sequencing of *COL5A1* and *COL5A2*.

Type III Ehlers–Danlos syndrome (the hypermobility type) is difficult to diagnose and to treat. There is a need to standardize the criteria for diagnosis.[63] Molecular diagnosis is not feasible at present because the disease loci have not be identified in the majority of cases. Ultrastructural studies of the skin can reveal abnormal collagen fibrils but care is needed to avoid skin with sun damage, which can alter the collagen structure of the dermis. Common symptoms include painful joints that sublux or dislocate. In many instances, the pain is more widespread and chronic.[64] The skin may be soft, but it is not hyperextensible or fragile as it is in classical Ehlers–Danlos syndrome. Surgical procedures to stabilize joints have high failure rates.

The clinical features of type IV Ehlers–Danlos syndrome are usually characteristic. The thin, translucent skin with prominent subcutaneous veins, acrogeric hands, and the pinched facial features are commonly observed. Joint hypermobility is mild and often limited to the hands. Many patients present with acute problems, such as vascular rupture, intestinal rupture, or volvulus. Once the diagnosis has been made and confirmed by mutational analysis of *COL3A1*, a vascular surveillance program is usually recommended. Open surgical repairs of vascular ruptures and fistulae have high complication rates because of vascular fragility. Endovascular procedures appear to be more effective.

The clinical features of type VI Ehlers–Danlos syndrome are well characterized and usually enable clinical diagnoses to be made and then confirmed by genetic analyses. Patients with type VI Ehlers–Danlos syndrome need ongoing care with ophthalmologists, spinal surgeons, and rehabilitations services. Corrections of spinal deformities are associated with high complication rates. Affected individuals are also prone to vascular ruptures.

Types VIIA and VIIB have indistinguishable clinical features but differ genetically. Patients with type VIIC Ehlers–Danlos syndrome have a more severe phenotype, which includes skin fragility. Babies with type VIIA and VIIB Ehlers–Danlos syndrome are often born with bilateral hip dislocations that are usually difficult to reduce and hold reduced using standard orthotic methods. Surgical reductions are often unsuccessful and premature osteoarthritis is common.[65] Rehabilitation services with physical therapy and orthotic support of unstable joints are often useful to assist children to stand and walk.

Marfan Syndrome

Dominant mutation of fibrillin 1 leads to Marfan syndrome (OMIM #154700), which is highly variable in severity and is characterized by tall stature, with the arm span exceeding height, and arachnodactyly. Many MSK findings form part of the revised diagnostic criteria and include the wrist and thumb signs, pectus carinatum, hindfoot deformity with pes planus, protrusio acetabuli, kyphoscoliosis, and reduced elbow extension. Other features include high arched palate, hypotonia and joint pain, and effusion, which may bring the patient to the attention of the pediatric rheumatologist.[66] Fibrillin 1 is ubiquitously expressed in the connective tissue of the skin, heart, muscle, cornea, tendon, vasculature, lungs, kidney, and bone. Clinical difficulties involve the skeleton, the eyes (upward dislocation of the lens and iridodonesis), the skin (striae distensae and elastosis perforans serpiginosa), and, in 30% of patients, the cardiovascular system (aortic root dilation and aneurysm formation, mitral valve prolapse, and conduction defects). Affected patients can die unexpectedly from cardiac complications. Recognition is critical in leading to a diagnosis, which may ultimately prevent catastrophic dissection of the aorta. Overviews of the management of Marfan syndrome are provided by Keane and Pyeritz[67] and Dean.[68]

Stickler Syndrome

Stickler syndrome, initially also known as hereditary arthro-ophthalmopathy, includes progressive osteoarthritis as an important manifestation, with an estimated 15% prevalence by age 20.[69] Stickler syndrome includes both autosomal dominant and recessive forms; one of which, Stickler syndrome type 4 (STL4), is a form of multiple epiphyseal dysplasia. The distinguishing features of Stickler syndrome includes moderate to severe sensorineural hearing loss and moderate to high myopia with vitreoretinopathy. Neither of these phenotypes is present in patients with MED1 to MED6. Homozygous mutations of *COL9A1*, which is expressed in the tectorial membrane of the inner ear, the vitreous humor, and hyaline cartilage, have been identified in patients with STL4.[70] In childhood MSK, features of Stickler syndrome include joint hypermobility with pronated feet, kyphoscoliosis, pectus carinatum, joint stiffness (develops later), genu valgum, long limbs with slender extremities and moderate arachnodactyly, and some degree of hypotonia. There are characteristic craniofacial features that include a flattened appearance of the face with mid-facial hypoplasia, cleft palate, micrognathia, and shortening of the nose with anteverted nares. About 25% of patients with Stickler syndrome are born with the Pierre Robin sequence of facial abnormalities. Severe myopia is common and patients are at high risk for retinal detachment. Congenital sensorineural hearing loss may also occur.

Examples of Syndromes Associated With Joint Hypomobility

Hypomobility may reflect the effects of inflammatory joint or muscle disease, or result from misshapen ends of long bones (e.g., from skeletal dysplasias, rickets, or previous fracture), which can lead to an often symmetrically restricted range of motion. Bowing deformities can mimic flexion contractures (e.g., anterior femoral bowing, appearing to be a flexion contracture of the knee).

Kniest Syndrome and Spondyloepiphyseal Dysplasia Congenita

Kniest syndrome and spondyloepiphyseal dysplasia (SED) congenita are autosomal dominant disorders resulting from mutations of *COL2A1*, the same gene associated with type I STL. Kniest syndrome, or Swiss-cheese cartilage syndrome (OMIM #156550) is characterized by congenitally short limbs and trunk, macrocephaly with a round face and a depressed nasal bridge,[71] progressive stiffness of the fingers, dislocation of the hips, and kyphoscoliosis. Other features include cleft palate, myopia, retinal detachment, deafness, and enlargement of the joints. Significant contractures interfere with mobility and are associated with pain. In SED congenita (OMIM #183900), diminished joint mobility, short stature, platyspondyly, and equinovarus deformities of the feet are common. Radiographs show dysplastic and late-developing femoral heads. An associated immunodeficiency has been reported in some patients.

Congenital Contractural Arachnodactyly

Type 2 fibrillin (*FBN2*) plays a large role in prenatal life. Autosomal dominant mutation of *FBN2* leads to congenital contractural arachnodactyly (OMIM #121050), a condition that may be confused with Marfan syndrome.[72-74] Congenital contractures of the knees, elbows, and proximal interphalangeal joints tend to improve during childhood. Long hands and feet and accelerated linear growth occur in both syndromes. There is an associated ear helix abnormality, an early progressive kyphoscoliosis, and an elongated head. Aortic root dilation has also been reported.

Homocystinuria

Recessively inherited homocystinuria caused by cystathionine β-synthase (CBS) deficiency (OMIM #236200) mimics Marfan syndrome in body habitus and the presence of osteoporosis. Downward dislocation of the lens occurs in homocystinuria by the age of 8 years. Hypotonia is present, but the joints are usually stiff rather than hyperextensible. Early identification is crucial in CBS- deficient patients since the thrombosis and mental retardation that accompanies the disorder can be ameliorated in some individuals through targeted dietary restriction (methionine) and/or medicinal intervention (pyridoxine).[75]

Melorheostosis

Tight, bound-down skin occurs in sporadic melorheostosis (OMIM #155950), a rare, idiopathic, sclerosing bone disease (Fig. 54-6) typically affecting one or only a few neighboring long bones. Although sometimes asymptomatic, melorheostosis can be associated with intermittent swelling and pain around joints, asymmetrical growth, unilateral Raynaud-like symptoms, soft tissue fibrosis, vascular anomalies, and contractures.[76] Buschke-Ollendorff syndrome (osteopoikilosis with dermatofibrosis lenticularis disseminata—orange papular skin

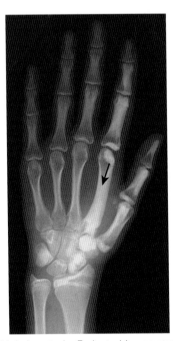

FIGURE 54-6 Melorheostosis. Endosteal hyperostosis *(arrow)* occurring in one or a few neighboring bones in a sclerotomal distribution is characteristic for melorheostosis in childhood. This patient had shortened first and second digits, smaller thenar eminence, overlying bound-down skin, and Raynaud-like phenomena affecting one hand. Later radiographs typically show a "melted candle wax" appearance when the hyperostosis becomes periosteal.

lesions of increased elastin fibers) (OMIM #166700) results from an autosomal dominant mutation in *LEDM3*, and can be associated with areas of dermal fibrosis, foreshortened limbs and contractures, and rarely with melorheostotic lesions.[76,77]

Examples of Mimics of Arthritis

Primary disorders of connective tissue (including some of those discussed previously) may present with arthritis or what can be mistaken for arthritis[77,78] (Table 54-4); often with pain worsening with activity. Some mimics of arthritis, however, have elevated erythrocyte sedimentation rates[78] and/or morning stiffness, gelling, and may appear to respond to nonsteroidal antiinflammatory drugs.[77,78] A congenital or hereditary arthropathy is suggested if there are multiple affected family members, parental consanguinity, and absence of autoantibodies (rheumatoid factor or antinuclear antibody),[18] symmetry of abnormalities, or multiple organ involvement. Osteoarthritis can occur in children who have abnormal cartilage.[79] Irregular joint surfaces, ligamentous laxity, or poor alignment can lead to osteoarthritis in early adulthood, especially in the weight-bearing joints.

Dysostosis Multiplex

Although classified as osteochondrodysplasias, the dysostosis multiplex group of disorders differs from other osteochondrodysplasias in that they are storage disorders.[80-82] They include mucopolysaccharidoses, mucolipidoses, mannosidosis, fucosidosis, gangliosidosis, sialidosis, sialic storage disease, galactosialidosis, and mucosulfatidosis. The manifestations of these progressive diseases result from an accumulation of substrate within the lysosomes of the cells that normally express the missing enzyme. They variably include the development of corneal clouding, dwarfism, mental retardation, joint effusions, face coarsening, stiffness or hypermobility, skeletal dysplasia of skull, thorax, vertebrae, pelvis, hands, and feet; and, in the case of Morquio disease, odontoid hypoplasia. Early intervention with bone marrow transplantation and enzyme replacement, available for some of these disorders, may interrupt some aspects of the otherwise unrelenting, devastating progressive mental and multisystem degeneration.[83]

Mucopolysaccharidoses

The mucopolysaccharidoses are genetically determined deficiencies of enzymes involved in the metabolism of glycosaminoglycans (Table 54-5).[81] Progressive skeletal dysplasia particularly affects the vertebrae, hips, and hands.[84] In the more severe types, such as Hurler syndrome (i.e., mucopolysaccharidosis [MPS] type IH), dwarfism, and marked coarsening of the facial features develops. Deposition of mucopolysaccharide leads to mental retardation and corneal clouding. A claw-hand deformity is often the first clue to the diagnosis.

Two of these storage diseases (Morquio and Scheie syndromes) mimic inflammatory arthritis. The comparatively mild dysostosis but severe dwarfing of the autosomal recessive Morquio syndrome (MPS Type IVA OMIM #253000; MPS Type IVB OMIM #253010; Morquio syndrome Type C OMIM #252300) may suggest juvenile idiopathic arthritis (JIA). Children with this syndrome, who have normal intelligence, may present with an effusion of a large joint (particularly the knee) or with progressive musculoskeletal stiffness, usually by the age of 3 or 4 years. The small joints of the hands become enlarged and stiff, a valgus deformity of the knees develops, and the gait becomes stiff and waddling. The joints are not always hypomobile, however, and some joints (such as the wrists), although enlarged, may be hypermobile. A pectus deformity and barrel chest are usual features. Characteristic radiographical findings include platyspondyly and odontoid hypoplasia, and should help differentiate this disorder from the various forms of SED.[85]

TABLE 54-4 Examples of Heritable Disorders with Skeletal Disturbances That May Manifest as Arthritis

DISORDER	OMIM #	JOINT AND BONE ABNORMALITIES SEEN IN CHILDHOOD	OTHER FEATURES (SOMETIMES)	GENE(S)
CACP (camptodactyly, arthropathy, coxa vara, pericarditis) syndrome	#208250	Polyarthritis with contractures, camptodactyly at birth	Pericarditis, coxa vara	Proteoglycan-4 gene AR
Carpal-tarsal osteolyses	Including #259600 and #166300	"Arthritis" in wrists, ankles, and elbows; knees with pain; swelling; AM stiffness; limitation of motion; rapid destruction of carpals, tarsals; "sucked candy" appearance of metacarpals; and metatarsals	With or without hirsutism, short stature, osteoporosis, nephropathy, dysmorphic appearance	*MMP2, MAFB* or other genes, AR and AD
Mucopolysaccharidoses, mucolipidoses, mannosidosis, fucosidosis, gangliosidosis, sialidosis, sialic storage disease, galactosialidosis, and mucosulfatidosis	Multiple	Dysostosis multiplex (odonto hypoplasia, J-shaped sella, broad oar-shaped ribs, oval vertebrae with gibbus, pelvic and femoral head abnormalities); joint effusions, stiffness, and/or hypermobility	With or without: progressive face coarsening, corneal clouding, mental retardation, hernias, and hepatosplenomegaly	
Stickler syndrome	#108300, #604841, #184840	Spondyloepiphyseal dysplasia, scoliosis, osteoarthritis, "Legg-Perthes disease"	Marfanoid habitus, hearing loss, visual loss, mitral valve prolapse, flat face, small mandible, cleft palate	*COL2A1; COL11A1; COL11A2; COL9A1* (AD and AR)
Progressive pseudorheumatoid arthritis of childhood	#208230	Arthritis, periarticular osteoporosis, coxa vara, platyspondyly, flattened enlarged epiphyses, wide metaphyses	Disease onset: age 3 to 8 years old, progressive disorder; muscle weakness with waddling gait	WNT-1-inducible signaling pathways protein 3 (AR)
Metaphyseal and epiphyseal dysplasias	Multiple	Osteoarthritis	Variable with and without spine involvement	Multiple
Trichorhinophalangeal syndrome	#190350, #150230, and #190351	Enlarged proximal interphalangeal joints, coned epiphyses, short fourth and fifth metacarpals, progressive hip arthritis, scoliosis	Bulbous nose, thin hair, large ears, micrognathia, short stature, "Legg-Calvé-Perthes" and in type II: exostoses +/- mental retardation	Putative transcription factor (TRPS1) (type 1 and 3) or TRPS1 and EXT1 (type 2) (AD)

AD, Autosomal dominant; *AR,* autosomal recessive; *MMP2* and other gene abbreviations are expanded in OMIM; *OMIM,* Online Mendelian Inheritance in Man.

In an autosomal recessive, mild form of Hurler disease, Scheie syndrome (MPS type IS) (OMIM #607016), intelligence is normal, the face is without coarsening, and stature is preserved. However, without intervention, there is a progressive restriction of range of motion the joints of the hands, elbows, and knees without swelling or pain. Corneal clouding and cardiac valvular disease develop generally in adulthood. Enzyme replacement or hematopoietic stem cell transplantation may mitigate the skeletal and cardiovascular abnormalities. All acute phase reactants are normal and urinary excretion of dermatan sulfate is increased, but a demonstration of decreased enzymatic activity of α-L-iduronidase activity is a more reliable screening test, and genetic testing is available.

Mucolipidoses

The term *mucolipidosis* (ML) is applied to a group of four disorders characterized by the intracellular accumulation of glycosaminoglycans and sphingolipids but without excess urinary glycosaminoglycan excretion. Progressive neurological and ocular abnormalities occur in all of these autosomal recessive disorders (Table 54-6).[86]

ML type I (OMIM #256550), an isolated neuraminidase (sialidase) deficiency, causes a Hurler-like syndrome with joint contractures,

short trunk and stature, and dysostosis multiplex (see discussion of dysostosis multiplex). Urinary excretion of sialated urinary oligosaccharides (bound sialic acid) is markedly elevated.

I-cell disease (ML type II α/β) (OMIM #252500) also causes a Hurler-like syndrome with progressive limitation of joint range of motion. The name is derived from the presence of prominent intracytoplasmic inclusions in cultured fibroblasts. I-cell disease[87] and pseudo-Hurler polydystrophy (ML type III α/β) (OMIM #252600)[88] are caused by mutations in the GNPTAB (the α/β subunit of the UDP-N-acetylglucosamine lysosomal-enzyme N-acetylglucosamine-1-phosphotransferase) gene. In pseudo-Hurler polydystrophy, restriction of joint mobility becomes apparent by the age of 2 years, but there is no inflammatory arthritis. Radiological findings are those of dysostosis multiplex. By the age of 6 years, features of Hurler syndrome dominate the clinical picture. A number of other primary disorders of the skeleton are characterized by the presence of stiff or enlarged joints and may be confused with inflammatory arthritis.

Diastrophic Dysplasias

Diastrophic dysplasia (OMIM #222600, #600972) and its variants, achondrogenesis type IB (#600972), multiple epiphyseal dysplasia 4

TABLE 54-5   Mucopolysaccharidoses

TYPE	NAME	INHERITANCE	MPS	ENZYME DEFECT	CLINICAL FEATURES
IH	Hurler	AR	DS, HS	α-L-iduronidase	Corneal clouding, dysostosis multiplex, heart disease, severe mental retardation, death in childhood
IS	Scheie*	AR	DS, HS	α-L-iduronidase	Milder skeletal disease, normal intelligence, normal life span (?)
II	Hunter	XR	DS, HS	Iduronate sulfatase	Milder than type I; no corneal clouding
IIIA	Sanfilippo	AR	HS	Heparan-N-sulfatase	Mild skeletal, severe CNS abnormalities
IIIB				N-acetyl-α-D-glucosaminidase	
IIIC				Acetyl-CoA-glucosaminidase acetyltransferase	
IIID				N-acetyl-glucosamine-6-sulfatase	
IVA	Morquio	AR	KS	N-acetylgalactosoamine-6-sulfatase	Severe skeletal changes; corneal clouding; normal intelligence
IVB				β-Galactosidase	
VI	Maroteaux-Lamy	AR	DS	N-acetylgalactosoamine-4-sulfatase	Severe skeletal changes, corneal clouding, heart disease, normal intelligence
VII	Sly	AR	DS, HS	β-Glucuronidase	Dysostosis multiplex, variable intelligence, hepatosplenomegaly, white blood cell inclusions

*Formerly classified as Type V.
DS, Dermatan sulfate; *HS,* heparan sulfate; *KS,* keratan sulfate; *MPS,* mucopolysaccharide found in urine.
Modified from P. Beighton, McKusick's Heritable Disorders of Connective Tissue, fifth ed., St. Louis, Mosby-Year Book, 1993.

TABLE 54-6   Mucolipidoses

TYPE	NAME	ENZYME DEFECT	MUSCULOSKELETAL FEATURES
I	Sialidase deficiency	Sialidase deficiency	Contractures, short stature, dysostosis multiplex
II	I-cell disease	Phosphotransferase deficiency	Progressive limitation of range of motion
III	Pseudo-Hurler polydystrophy	Phosphotransferase deficiency	Progressive limitation of range of motion; dysostosis multiplex
IV	Sialolipidosis	Uncertain	No characteristic skeletal changes

(OMIM #226900), and atelosteogenesis type II (OMIM #256050), are caused by autosomal recessive mutation in the sulfate transporter gene.[32,89-91] These are characterized by short limbs, small chest, radial dislocation, enlarged joints (particularly the knees), hitchhiker thumb, gap between first and second toes, clubfoot, and limitation of finger movement. Features include progressive fragmentation and calcification of the cartilage with swelling and eventual fusion of the joints, particularly the small joints of the phalanges. Calcification of the cartilage occurs in the ears, trachea, and costochondral junctions.

Dyggve–Melchior–Clausen dysplasia (OMIM #223800) and Smith-McCort dysplasia (OMIM #607326) are rare autosomal recessive disorders caused by deactivating mutation of the ubiquitously expressed dymeclin gene. Affected newborns present with some limitation of movement. Patients are often short, have an exaggerated lumbar lordosis and sternal prominence, and have progressive mental retardation. They develop claw-hand deformities. Radiographs show platyspondyly, epiphyseal dysplasia, irregular metaphyses, and a lacy appearance of the iliac crests. Biopsy shows widened cisternae of rough endoplasmic reticulum in chondrocytes.[92]

Progressive Pseudorheumatoid Arthropathy

This autosomal recessive disorder (OMIM #208230) presents between the ages of 3 and 8 years in healthy appearing children, and is caused by mutation in *WISP3* (WNT1 inducible signaling pathway protein 3, felt to play a role in BMP and WNT signaling).[93] It is a progressive disorder manifesting with stiffness, swelling, weakness with waddling gait, joint space narrowing, and periarticular osteopenia, and progresses to metaphyseal enlargement, contractures, and kyphoscoliosis with platyspondyly (Fig. 54-7). This disorder is sometimes labeled "rheumatoid arthritis with Scheuermann disease" but has none of the laboratory abnormalities of JIA.

Camptodactyly-Arthropathy-Coxa Vara-Pericarditis (CACP) Syndrome

Camptodactyly-arthropathy-coxa vara-pericarditis (CACP) syndrome (OMIM #208250) is an autosomal recessive disorder resulting from a mutations in the proteoglycan-4 gene encoding for the protein lubricin.[94] Affected children are frequently born with camptodactyly ("trigger fingers") and may have undergone surgical correction before presenting with large and small joint noninflammatory arthropathy marked by synovial hypertrophy. Pericarditis and pleuritis develop in some patients and may require aspiration for relief. Bony deformities develop, including coxa vara and large synovial cysts. No effective treatment has been found to date other than rehabilitation.[95]

Trichorhinophalangeal Syndrome

Trichorhinophalangeal syndrome type 1 and the more severe type 3 are autosomal dominant disorders (OMIM #190350 and #190351), arising from mutation of a putative transcription factor (TRPS1). Both disorders are characterized by craniofacial and skeletal abnormalities, including a bulbous nose, short stature, sparse hair, enlarged interphalangeal joints, cone-shaped epiphyses, short metacarpals and metatarsals, and small, flat, fragmented capital femoral epiphyses suggestive of Legg–Calvé–Perthes disease.[96,97] Trichorhinophalangeal syndrome type II, the Langer–Giedion syndrome (OMIM #150230), is a contiguous gene syndrome deriving from the deletion of TRPS1 as well as its neighboring gene, *EXT1*. It is additionally associated with multiple exostoses, causing pain when occurring around joints and variably associated with mental retardation.

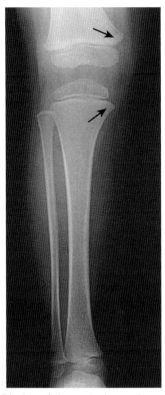

FIGURE 54-7 Widening of the metaphyses *(arrows)* in a child with platyspondyly and progressive pseudorheumatoid arthropathy.

Disorders Characterized by Lytic Bone Lesions

True lytic bone diseases appear radiographically as hypodense areas within the skeleton and occur in metastatic cancer and a number of inherited syndromes, often with a distinctive distribution and sometimes with other organ system involvement.

The *idiopathic osteolyses* are grouped according to the area predominantly affected. Cherubism (OMIM #118400) manifests at the ages of 3 or 4 years with jaw osteolysis; other osteolyses involve phalangeal[98] or carpal-tarsal bones,[99,100] or are multicentric.[101] Acro-osteolysis (progressive loss of tips of distal phalanges) occurs as a feature of a number of different disorders.[102] Carpal-tarsal osteolysis syndromes (Fig. 54-8) begin before the age of 1 year with restricted joint mobility, swelling and pain of the proximal interphalangeal joints, and enlargement of the wrists.[80,103,104] Torg-Winchester and nodulosis-arthropathy-osteolysis syndromes (OMIM #259600) are two types of osteolysis syndromes that result from mutations in type IV collagenase (MMP2). These disorders are also complicated by the development of corneal clouding, coarsening of the face, joint contractures, osteoporosis, bone erosion, and atlantoaxial subluxation. Carpal-tarsal osteolysis associated with nephropathy (OMIM #166300) is an autosomal dominant disease associated with mutations in the *MAFB* gene resulting in abnormalities in the RANK ligand pathway.[105] Patients are often misdiagnosed as having JIA before the radiographic changes have progressed.[106,99,102,106,107] Early radiographs of the wrists in carpal-tarsal osteolyses are often misinterpreted as showing a delayed bone age.[70]

Phantom bone disease (i.e., Gorham disease) occurs between the ages of 5 and 10 years and is not hereditary.[101] A carpal-tarsal osteolysis is usual. Osteolysis can also occur from overactivation of osteoclasts. Other disorders, such as neurofibromatosis Type I (OMIM #162200), can be misinterpreted as showing osteolysis. Metaphyseal enchondromas (at risk for malignant transformation) occurs in multiple enchondromatosis (OMIM #166000), including Ollier and Maffucci syndromes, cystic angiomatosis of bone (OMIM 123880), and disorders of metaphyseal undermineralization.

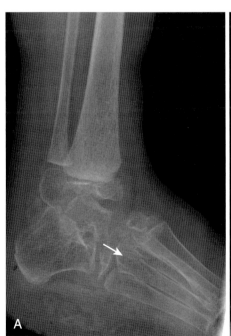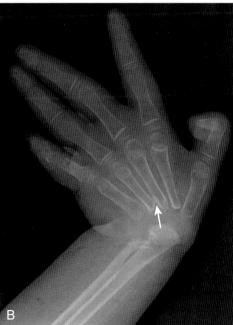

FIGURE 54-8 Idiopathic multicentric osteolysis (IMO), the progressive loss of tarsal (**A;** *arrow*) and carpal bones (**B;** *arrow*), occurs during childhood with eventual destruction of the metacarpals, metatarsals, distal tibia, radius, and ulna, as can be seen in this 4-year-old child with IMO and nephropathy. Early in the course of the disease, hand films can be misread as showing "delayed bone age."

SUMMARY

There are many hundreds of genetically determined primary connective tissue disorders. Impressive advances have been made in identifying new disease genes in known disorders as well as identifying and characterizing new disorders. The information gained from these studies can be expected to have a major impact on the provision of diagnostic and treatment services for affected individuals and their families. In addition, the information expands knowledge about the biology of connective tissues that can also be applied to advancing the investigation of common disorders in the community such as osteoarthritis and osteoporosis.

REFERENCES

1. P.H. Byers, M.L. Murray, Ehlers-Danlos syndrome: a showcase of conditions that lead to understanding matrix biology, Matrix Biol. 33 (2014) 10–15.
2. M.L. Warman, V. Cormier-Daire, C. Hall, et al., Nosology and classification of genetic skeletal disorders: 2010 revision, Am. J. Med. Genet. A 155A (5) (2011) 943–968.
3. B.D. Mitchell, L.M. Yerges-Armstrong, The genetics of bone loss: challenges and prospects, J. Clin. Endocrinol. Metab. 96 (5) (2011) 1258–1268.
5. V.A. McKusick, Heritable disorders of connective tissue. VIII. Concluding comments. Introduction; fibrodysplasia ossificans progressiva; osteopoikilosis; Leri's pleonosteosis; Paget's disease of bone; other possible hereditary and generalized disorders of connective tissue; the future in the study of heritable disorders of connective tissue; general summary and conclusions, J. Chronic Dis. 3 (5) (1956) 521–556.
6. P. Beighton, A. Price, J. Lord, E. Dickson, Variants of the Ehlers-Danlos syndrome. Clinical, biochemical, haematological, and chromosomal features of 100 patients, Ann. Rheum. Dis. 28 (3) (1969) 228–245.
7. P. Beighton, A. De Paepe, B. Steinmann, et al., Ehlers-Danlos syndromes: revised nosology, Villefranche, 1997. Ehlers-Danlos National Foundation (USA) and Ehlers-Danlos Support Group (UK), Am. J. Med. Genet. 77 (1) (1998) 31–37.
8. R.M. Winter, M. Baraitser, The London Dysmorphology Database, J. Med. Genet. 24 (8) (1987) 509–510.
9. P. Smits, A.D. Bolton, V. Funari, et al., Lethal skeletal dysplasia in mice and humans lacking the golgin GMAP-210, N. Engl. J. Med. 362 (3) (2010) 206–216.
12. O. Makitie, I. Kaitila, Cartilage-hair hypoplasia–clinical manifestations in 108 Finnish patients, Eur. J. Pediatr. 152 (3) (1993) 211–217.
14. A.D. Dornelles, L.L. de Camargo Pinto, A.C. de Paula, et al., Enzyme replacement therapy for Mucopolysaccharidosis Type I among patients followed within the MPS Brazil Network, Genet. Mol. Biol. 37 (1) (2014) 23–29.
18. E.C. Chalom, J. Ross, B.H. Athreya, Syndromes and arthritis, Rheum. Dis. Clin. North Am. 23 (3) (1997) 709–727.
19. O. Makitie, G.R. Mortier, M. Czarny-Ratajczak, et al., Clinical and radiographic findings in multiple epiphyseal dysplasia caused by MATN3 mutations: description of 12 patients, Am. J. Med. Genet. A 125A (3) (2004) 278–284.
20. M.D. Briggs, S.M. Hoffman, L.M. King, et al., Pseudoachondroplasia and multiple epiphyseal dysplasia due to mutations in the cartilage oligomeric matrix protein gene, Nat. Genet. 10 (3) (1995) 330–336.
21. K.L. Chapman, G.R. Mortier, K. Chapman, et al., Mutations in the region encoding the von Willebrand factor A domain of matrilin-3 are associated with multiple epiphyseal dysplasia, Nat. Genet. 28 (4) (2001) 393–396.
22. M. Czarny-Ratajczak, J. Lohiniva, P. Rogala, et al., A mutation in COL9A1 causes multiple epiphyseal dysplasia: further evidence for locus heterogeneity, Am. J. Hum. Genet. 69 (5) (2001) 969–980.
23. Y. Muragaki, E.C. Mariman, S.E. van Beersum, et al., A mutation in COL9A2 causes multiple epiphyseal dysplasia (EDM2), Ann. N. Y. Acad. Sci. 785 (1996) 303–306.
24. P. Paassilta, J. Lohiniva, S. Annunen, et al., COL9A3: a third locus for multiple epiphyseal dysplasia, Am. J. Hum. Genet. 64 (4) (1999) 1036–1044.
27. R. Damignani, N.L. Young, W.G. Cole, et al., Impairment and activity limitation associated with epiphyseal dysplasia in children, Arch. Phys. Med. Rehabil. 85 (10) (2004) 1647–1652.
28. N.J. Treble, F.O. Jensen, A. Bankier, et al., Development of the hip in multiple epiphyseal dysplasia. Natural history and susceptibility to premature osteoarthritis, J. Bone Joint Surg. Br. 72 (6) (1990) 1061–1064.
29. E. Jakkula, O. Mäkitie, M. Czarny-Ratajczak, et al., Mutations in the known genes are not the major cause of MED; distinctive phenotypic entities among patients with no identified mutations, Eur. J. Hum. Genet. 13 (3) (2005) 292–301.
30. D. Ballhausen, L. Bonafé, P. Terhal, et al., Recessive multiple epiphyseal dysplasia (rMED): phenotype delineation in eighteen homozygotes for DTDST mutation R279W, J. Med. Genet. 40 (1) (2003) 65–71.
31. O. Makitie, R. Savarirayan, L. Bonafé, et al., Autosomal recessive multiple epiphyseal dysplasia with homozygosity for C653S in the DTDST gene: double-layer patella as a reliable sign, Am. J. Med. Genet. A 122A (3) (2003) 187–192.
32. A. Superti-Furga, L. Neumann, T. Riebel, et al., Recessively inherited multiple epiphyseal dysplasia with normal stature, club foot, and double layered patella caused by a DTDST mutation, J. Med. Genet. 36 (8) (1999) 621–624.
35. H.L. Wechsler, E.R. Fisher, Ehlers-Danlos syndrome. pathologic, histochemical and electron microscopic observations, Arch. Pathol. 77 (1964) 613–619.
47. U. Schwarze, R. Hata, V.A. McKusick, et al., Rare autosomal recessive cardiac valvular form of Ehlers-Danlos syndrome results from mutations in the COL1A2 gene that activate the nonsense-mediated RNA decay pathway, Am. J. Hum. Genet. 74 (5) (2004) 917–930.
49. M. Baumann, C. Giunta, B. Krabichler, et al., Mutations in FKBP14 cause a variant of Ehlers-Danlos syndrome with progressive kyphoscoliosis, myopathy, and hearing loss, Am. J. Hum. Genet. 90 (2) (2012) 201–216.
50. F.M. Pope, G.R. Martin, J.R. Lichtenstein, et al., Patients with Ehlers-Danlos syndrome type IV lack type III collagen, Proc. Natl. Acad. Sci. U.S.A. 72 (4) (1975) 1314–1316.
53. S. Symoens, D. Syx, F. Malfait, et al., Comprehensive molecular analysis demonstrates type V collagen mutations in over 90% of patients with classic EDS and allows to refine diagnostic criteria, Hum. Mutat. 33 (10) (2012) 1485–1493.
57. F. Malfait, D. Syx, P. Vlummens, et al., Musculocontractural Ehlers-Danlos Syndrome (former EDS type VIB) and adducted thumb clubfoot syndrome (ATCS) represent a single clinical entity caused by mutations in the dermatan-4-sulfotransferase 1 encoding CHST14 gene, Hum. Mutat. 31 (11) (2010) 1233–1239.
58. J. Schalkwijk, M.C. Zweers, P.M. Steijlen, et al., A recessive form of the Ehlers-Danlos syndrome caused by tenascin-X deficiency, N. Engl. J. Med. 345 (16) (2001) 1167–1175.
59. M.C. Zweers, J. Bristow, P.M. Steijlen, et al., Haploinsufficiency of TNXB is associated with hypermobility type of Ehlers-Danlos syndrome, Am. J. Hum. Genet. 73 (1) (2003) 214–217.
63. L. Remvig, L. Flycht, K.B. Christensen, B. Juul-Kristensen, Lack of consensus on tests and criteria for generalized joint hypermobility, Ehlers-Danlos syndrome: hypermobile type and joint hypermobility syndrome, Am. J. Med. Genet. A 164A (3) (2014) 591–596.
64. L. Rombaut, M. Scheper, I. De Wandele, et al., Chronic pain in patients with the hypermobility type of Ehlers-Danlos syndrome: evidence for generalized hyperalgesia, Clin. Rheumatol. (2014).
65. C. Giunta, A. Superti-Furga, S. Spranger, et al., Ehlers-Danlos syndrome type VII: clinical features and molecular defects, J. Bone Joint Surg. Am. 81 (2) (1999) 225–238.
66. R.P. Morse, S. Rockenmacher, R.E. Pyeritz, et al., Diagnosis and management of infantile marfan syndrome, Pediatrics 86 (6) (1990) 888–895.
67. M.G. Keane, R.E. Pyeritz, Medical management of Marfan syndrome, Circulation 117 (21) (2008) 2802–2813.

69. T. Couchouron, C. Masson, Early-onset progressive osteoarthritis with hereditary progressive ophtalmopathy or Stickler syndrome, Joint Bone Spine 78 (1) (2011) 45–49.

70. G. Van Camp, R.L. Snoeckx, N. Hilgert, et al., A new autosomal recessive form of Stickler syndrome is caused by a mutation in the COL9A1 gene, Am. J. Hum. Genet. 79 (3) (2006) 449–457.

71. E. Gilbert-Barnes, L.O. Langer Jr., J.M. Opitz, et al., Kniest dysplasia: radiologic, histopathological, and scanning electronmicroscopic findings, Am. J. Med. Genet. 63 (1) (1996) 34–45.

73. B.L. Callewaert, B.L. Loeys, A. Ficcadenti, et al., Comprehensive clinical and molecular assessment of 32 probands with congenital contractural arachnodactyly: report of 14 novel mutations and review of the literature, Hum. Mutat. 30 (3) (2009) 334–341.

74. E. Tuncbilek, Y. Alanay, Congenital contractural arachnodactyly (Beals syndrome), Orphanet J. Rare Dis. 1 (2006) 20.

75. G.H. Boers, A.G. Smals, F.J. Trijbels, et al., Heterozygosity for homocystinuria in premature peripheral and cerebral occlusive arterial disease, N. Engl. J. Med. 313 (12) (1985) 709–715.

78. A.C. Offiah, P. Woo, A.M. Prieur, et al., Camptodactyly-arthropathy-coxa vara-pericarditis syndrome versus juvenile idiopathic arthropathy, AJR Am. J. Roentgenol. 185 (2) (2005) 522–529.

79. G.B. Stickler, P.G. Belau, F.J. Farrell, et al., Hereditary progressive arthroophthalmopathy, Mayo Clin. Proc. 40 (1965) 433–455.

81. J.E. Wraith, The mucopolysaccharidoses: a clinical review and guide to management, Arch. Dis. Child. 72 (3) (1995) 263–267.

82. D.A. Stevenson, R.D. Steiner, Skeletal abnormalities in lysosomal storage diseases, Pediatr. Endocrinol. Rev. 10 (Suppl. 2) (2013) 406–416.

83. J. Muenzer, J.E. Wraith, L.A. Clarke, International Consensus Panel on Management and Treatment of Mucopolysaccharidosis I, Mucopolysaccharidosis I: management and treatment guidelines, Pediatrics 123 (1) (2009) 19–29.

84. R. Cimaz, F. La Torre, Mucopolysaccharidoses, Curr. Rheumatol. Rep. 16 (1) (2014) 389.

85. M. Mikles, R.P. Stanton, A review of Morquio syndrome, Am. J. Orthop. (Belle Mead NJ) 26 (8) (1997) 533–540.

86. E.F. Gilbert-Barness, L.A. Barness, The mucolipidoses, Perspect. Pediatr. Pathol. 17 (1993) 148–184.

89. J. Hastbacka, A. de la Chapelle, M.M. Mahtani, et al., The diastrophic dysplasia gene encodes a novel sulfate transporter: positional cloning by fine-structure linkage disequilibrium mapping, Cell 78 (6) (1994) 1073–1087.

90. A. Superti-Furga, J. Hästbacka, W.R. Wilcox, et al., Achondrogenesis type IB is caused by mutations in the diastrophic dysplasia sulphate transporter gene, Nat. Genet. 12 (1) (1996) 100–102.

93. N. Garcia Segarra, L. Mittaz, A.B. Campos-Xavier, et al., The diagnostic challenge of progressive pseudorheumatoid dysplasia (PPRD): a review of clinical features, radiographic features, and WISP3 mutations in 63 affected individuals, Am. J. Med. Genet. C Semin. Med. Genet. 160C (3) (2012) 217–229.

94. J. Marcelino, J.D. Carpten, W.M. Suwairi, et al., CACP, encoding a secreted proteoglycan, is mutated in camptodactyly-arthropathy-coxa vara-pericarditis syndrome, Nat. Genet. 23 (3) (1999) 319–322.

95. I. Albuhairan, S.M. Al-Mayouf, Camptodactyly-arthropathy-coxavara-pericarditis syndrome in Saudi Arabia: clinical and molecular genetic findings in 22 patients, Semin. Arthritis Rheum. 43 (2) (2013) 292–296.

97. P.R. Carrington, H. Chen, J.A. Altick, Trichorhinophalangeal syndrome, type I, J. Am. Acad. Dermatol. 31 (2 Pt 2) (1994) 331–336.

101. L.W. Gorham, A.P. Stout, Massive osteolysis (acute spontaneous absorption of bone, phantom bone, disappearing bone); its relation to hemangiomatosis, J. Bone Joint Surg. Am. 37-A (5) (1955) 985–1004.

103. D.W. Hollister, D.L. Rimoin, R.S. Lachman, et al., The Winchester syndrome: a nonlysosomal connective tissue disease, J. Pediatr. 84 (5) (1974) 701–709.

105. A. Zankl, E.L. Duncan, P.J. Leo, et al., Multicentric carpotarsal osteolysis is caused by mutations clustering in the amino-terminal transcriptional activation domain of MAFB, Am. J. Hum. Genet. 90 (3) (2012) 494–501.

106. S. Mumm, M. Huskey, S. Duan, et al., Multicentric carpotarsal osteolysis syndrome is caused by only a few domain-specific mutations in MAFB, a negative regulator of RANKL-induced osteoclastogenesis, Am. J. Med. Genet. A (2014).

Entire reference list is available online at www.expertconsult.com.

INDEX

Page numbers followed by "*f*" indicate figures, "*t*" indicate tables, and "*b*" indicate boxes.

Diffuse cutaneous systemic sclerosis *(Continued)*
   Sjögren syndrome, 393
   skin disease, 389-390
   telangiectasias, 389-390, 389f, 400f
  collagen, abnormalities in, 388
  course of, 400-401
  differential diagnosis of
   chemically induced scleroderma-like disease, 403
   chronic graft-*versus*-host disease, 402
   diabetic cheiroarthropathy, 404
   localized idiopathic fibroses, 403-404
   nephrogenic systemic fibrosis, 402-403
   phenylketonuria, 403
   pseudoscleroderma, 403-404
   scleredema, 404
  endothelial cell factors, 387-388
  epidemiology of, 385
  etiology of, 385-388
  fibrosis in, 387
  gender ratios in, 385
  genetic background of, 388
  growth factors in, 386t, 387
  immunological factors of, 386-387, 386t
  laboratory examination of, 395-396
  mononuclear cell infiltrates, 386-387
  musculoskeletal involvement, 400
  organ system involvement, 398t
  pathogenesis of, 385-388, 386f
  pathology of, 393-395, 393f
  prognosis for, 400-401, 400f
  pulmonary function in, 395
  radiological examination of, 391f, 396-397, 396f-397f
  renal function in, 395
  signs and symptoms of, 388, 388t
  skin involvement in, 400
  skin scoring in, 395-396
  treatment of, 398-400
   digital vasculopathy, 398-400
   disease process and complications, 398-400
   mycophenolate mofetil, 399
   rituximab, 399
   supportive measures in, 398
  vascular factors in, 387
Diffusion-weighted imaging, 102
DiGeorge syndrome (DGS), 602
Digital ischemia, Raynaud phenomenon
  management of, 445
  treatment algorithm for, 443f
Digital scores, 84
Digits, polyarteritis nodosa lesions of, 463f
Dihydrofolate reductase, 144-145, 145f
1,25-Dihydroxyvitamin D_3 [1,25-$(OH)_2D_3$], 694
Dipstick analysis, 125-126
Direct enzyme-linked immunosorbent assay, 117, 117.e1f
Direct immunofluorescence, 117
Discriminant instrument, 78.e1t
Disease. *see also* specific disease
  diagnosis of, 57
  etiology of, 56-57
  frequency and prognosis of, 55-56
  risk of, 56-57, 56t
Disease-modifying antirheumatic drugs, 144-150
  antimalarials, 149
  for autoimmune arthritis, 39
  juvenile psoriatic arthritis treated with, 265
  leflunomide, 150
  methotrexate. *see* Methotrexate

Disease-modifying antirheumatic drugs *(Continued)*
  for rheumatoid factor-positive polyarticular JIA, 226
  sulfasalazine. *see* Sulfasalazine
  for systemic juvenile idiopathic arthritis, 212
Diskitis, 544, 544f-545f, 672
Distracted straight leg raising test, 686t
DNA methylation, 46
Domain/dimension, 78.e1t
Doppler sonography, 100, 101f
Double-blind designs, 62-63
Double-dummy design, 63
Down syndrome, 194, 665b
Drug(s)
  absorption of, 140
  bioavailability of, 140
  biotransformation of, 141
  clearance of, 140-141
  elimination of, 140-141
  half-life of, 140-141
  volume of distribution of, 140
Drug safety, 60-61
Drug tolerability, 61
Drug-associated vasculitis, 511-512
Dual-energy X-ray absorptiometry, 102, 700, 701t
Duchenne muscular dystrophy, 367
Duloxetine, 159
Dupuytren contracture, 404
Dyslipoproteinemia, 153-154, 198
Dysostosis multiplex, 714
Dystrophic calcification, forms of, 361b

E
Early onset sarcoidosis, 517
Effect size, 72
Efficacy sample, 66
E-health formats, 92
Ehlers-Danlos syndrome, 665b, 710-713
  classification of, 710-711, 710f, 711t, 712f
  diagnosis and treatment of, 713
  other protein defects and, 712
  proteoglycan defects, 712
  type I collagen defects, 711
  type III collagen defects, 711-712
  type V collagen defects, 712
Ehlers-Danlos type IV, vasculitis and, 515t
Eicosanoids, 30
Eigenvalue, 76
Elastic ligaments, 10
Elastin, 10
Electromyography, 372-373, 372b
Elimination half-life, 60
Emotions, pain and, 89
En coup de sabre linear scleroderma, 406-408, 408f
Enchondroma, 653, 654f
ENCODE project, 45
Endarteropathy, 364
Endocarditis, 306
  in acute rheumatic fever, 576
  prophylaxis for, 581
  in systemic juvenile idiopathic arthritis, 208
Endochondral ossification, 5
Endocrine disorders, 592-594
Endocrinopathies, 367
Endomysium, 11
Endopeptidases, 8
Endotenon, 10

Endothelial cells
  in antiphospholipid syndrome, 321-322, 323f
  in diffuse cutaneous systemic sclerosis, 387-388
  in Raynaud phenomenon, 438
Endothelial-selectin, 25
Endothelin inhibitors, for Raynaud phenomenon, 444
Endothelin-1, 399-400
End-point driven protocol, 64
End-stage disease, 185-186
Enthesis, 10-11, 109, 112f
Enthesitis, 242, 242f-243f
Enthesitis-related arthritis, 108-115, 238-255
  age at onset, 240
  of appendicular skeleton, 108-109
   magnetic resonance imaging in, 111
   radiography in, 108-109, 111b, 112f
   sonography in, 109-111, 112f-113f
  arthritis in, 242-243
  of axial skeleton, 111, 244-245, 244f
   computed tomography in, 115, 115f
   magnetic resonance imaging in, 111-112, 114f
   radiography in, 111
   scintigraphy in, 115
  biologic agents for, 250-252
  cardiopulmonary disease in, 245-246
  classification of, 238-239, 239b
  clinical manifestations of, 241-243
  course of, 252-254, 253t
  definition of, 238-239
  description of, 190
  differential diagnosis of, 246-247
  disease modifying antirheumatic drugs for, 250
  in entheses, 249-250
  enthesitis and, 242, 242f-243f
  epidemiology of, 239-240
  etanercept for, 250-251
  etiology of, 240-241
  gastrointestinal disease in, 245
  genetic background of, 241, 241t
  geographic distribution of, 240
  glucocorticoids for, 250
  incidence of, 239-240
  International League of Associations for Rheumatology classification of, 238, 239b
  intertarsal joint inflammation in, 243-244
  juvenile psoriatic arthritis and, 261-262
  laboratory examination of, 247
  methotrexate for, 250
  nonsteroidal antiinflammatory drugs for, 250
  oligoarticular juvenile idiopathic arthritis and, 246
  pathogenesis of, 240-241
  pathology of, 246
  peripheral joint arthritis and, 243-246, 244f
  physical and occupational therapy for, 252
  prevalence of, 239-240
  prognosis for, 252-254, 253t
  racial distribution of, 240
  radiological characteristics of, 247b
  renal disease in, 246
  rheumatoid factor-negative polyarticular JIA and, 220
  in sacroiliac joint, 247-248, 248f
  sex ratio of, 240
  in spine, 248-249, 249f
  surgery for, 252
  TNF inhibitors for, 250
  treatment of, 250-252, 251f-252f
  uveitis in, 245

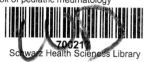
		DATE DUE	